Complex and Revision Problems in Shoulder Surgery

Second Edition

Complex and Revision Problems in Shoulder Surgery

Second Edition

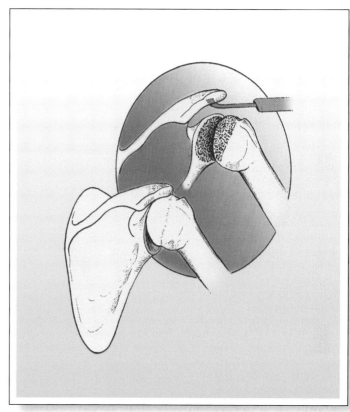

EDITORS

JON J. P. WARNER, M.D.

Chief, The Harvard Shoulder Service
Professor of Orthopaedic Surgery
Harvard Medical School
Massachusetts General and Brigham and Women's Hospitals
Boston, Massachusetts

JOSEPH P. IANNOTTI, M.D.

Chairman, Department of Orthopaedic Surgery
The Cleveland Clinic
Cleveland, Ohio

EVAN L. FLATOW, M.D.

Lasker Professor of Orthopaedic Surgery
Chief of Shoulder Surgery
Mount Sinai Medical Center
New York, New York

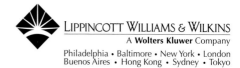

LIPPINCOTT WILLIAMS & WILKINS
A **Wolters Kluwer** Company

Philadelphia • Baltimore • New York • London
Buenos Aires • Hong Kong • Sydney • Tokyo

Acquisitions Editor: Robert Hurley
Developmental Editors: Joanne Bersin and Eileen Wolfberg
Marketing Director: Sharon Zinner
Project Manager: Fran Gunning
Manufacturing Manager: Ben Rivera
Production Services: Maryland Composition
Printer: Quebecor-Kingsport

First Edition reprinted by Lippincott Williams & Wilkins
530 Walnut Street
Philadelphia, PA 19106 USA
LWW.com

Library of Congress Cataloging-in-Publication Data

Complex and revision problems in shoulder surgery / [edited by] Jon J.P. Warner, Joseph P.
Iannotti, Evan L. Flatow.— 2nd ed.
      p. ; cm.
   Includes bibliographical references.
   ISBN 0-7817-4658-2
   1. Shoulder—Surgery. 2. Shoulder—Surgery—Complications. 3. Shoulder—Reoperation.
I. Warner, Jon J. P. II. Iannotti, Joseph P. III. Flatow, Evan L.
   [DNLM: 1. Shoulder—surgery. 2. Intraoperative Complications. 3. Surgical Procedures,
Operative—methods. WE 810 C736 2005]
RD557.5.C64 2005
617.5'72059—dc22

                                                    2004029976

Printed in the United States of America
ICP
10 9 8 7 6 5 4 3

Dedications

To James H. Herndon, M.D., MBA, my mentor and friend. Who always said what he meant, meant what he said, and led by example.
—JJPW

To my son Matthew, whose inner strength through a very difficult time in his life will always be my strength.
—JPI

To my wife and family, for their love and support.
—ELF

Introduction

Three highly recognized and respected American editors have revised their indispensable text with the latest methods on treating complex and revision problems of the shoulder. Their effort is timely: the interest in shoulder surgery has grown considerably and, hence, the number of interventions has increased. Problems of increasing complexity are being handled, and revisions have become more frequent and more difficult. In addition, the methods of treatment have changed dramatically, resulting in enormous progress made in surgical outcomes brought about by the modern inverse prostheses, among many other new developments.

The subject is a difficult one by nature of its specialization: complex and revision problems are not commonplace operations, and, thus, are difficult to subject to evidence-based criteria. Rather than referring to large series in the literature, the authors must base their approaches on personal experience and judgment; their texts, therefore, become by definition more worthwhile but also more controversial the more complex the subject of the individual chapter is. The senior authors of all chapters are in the prime of their professional careers and are undoubtedly the leading international experts, representing a wide variety of approaches. So, even if a reader should disagree with any methodologies in this text, it would be wise to remember that there are "many streets that lead to Rome." The shoulder surgeon should review the respective chapters in detail and incorporate the knowledge offered in this text into his or her judgment. In the field of complex shoulder problems, it would be an error not to have consulted this essential reference book, for which the editors should be congratulated.

Christian Gerber, MD
Professor and Chairman
Department of Orthopedics
University of Zurich
Zurich, Switzerland

Editors' Introduction and Overview

We are pleased to present the second edition of our book, *Complex and Revision Problems in Shoulder Surgery*. Since publication of the first edition, there has been an explosion of articles concerning management of problems affecting the shoulder, and numerous other books have been published as well. This intense interest has developed partly due to the aging baby boomer population and its desire to remain active, performing overhead sports such as tennis, swimming, and golf. Shoulder injuries that may affect the members of this demographic can occur through trauma or repetitive overuse, and threaten their quality of life. More and more shoulder surgery is being performed and, unfortunately, complications and the need for revision surgery have grown exponentially.

The use of shoulder arthroplasty, for instance, has increased at a rate of more than 15% per annum; currently, there is a global market in shoulder arthroplasty that approaches $200,000,000 annually.

Many other textbooks on shoulder surgery have been written as extensive overviews of the problems that affect the shoulder. Our book is intended to be a different type of publication. We have purposefully kept the book succinct and focused on specific problems, and have attempted to organize these problems into logical sections. Each chapter is contributed by author(s) who we believe are experts based on their demonstrated surgical skill. We qualify this statement by further saying that these individuals have been selected based on our opinion that we would permit them to perform the surgery they describe on us or our family members. This is the highest compliment one can pay another surgeon, namely that he or she is a surgeon's surgeon.

The three of us routinely encounter patients with failed prior treatments and complex problems. We felt that the book should be organized into clear, succinct, case-based presentations so that surgeons can cut to the chase, not have to wade through extraneous information, and find examples that may help them with similar cases. This, after all, is the way we continue to learn from each other. Thus experience becomes a shared benefit.

Section I deals with Shoulder Instability. In this edition of the book, we have included two chapters on Traumatic Anterior Instability and two on Multidirectional and Posterior Instability. In each case, experts in arthroscopic management explain their approaches and their success with their chosen technique. In the two chapters on open approaches,

an important emphasis is on decision making for selection criteria for open surgery. For example, in the chapter by Clavert, Millett, and Warner there is a clear description of the degree of bone loss on the glenoid that requires an open approach. Historically, this has been either ignored or trivialized in the literature. There is also consideration given to management of capsular and tendon insufficiency in the setting of failed anterior repairs.

The chapter by Miller and Flatow on Posterior and Multidirectional Instability: Open Solutions nicely summarizes all prior experience with these techniques and clearly illustrates the surgical approach to these problems.

Gerber's consideration of Chronic, Locked Anterior and Posterior Dislocations is one of the only detailed accounts of salvage and replacement of a severely damaged humeral head in the setting of this rare condition. The chapter uses a number of clinical cases to illustrate the methods for optimal treatment.

Section II considers Rotator Cuff Tears. The chapter on Anterior Superior Rotator Cuff Tears: Repairable and Irreparable Tears, by Edwards, Walch, Nove-Josserand, and Gerber, considers problems that affect the subscapularis in combination with the supraspinatus tendon. The biceps tendon is also commonly involved and often overlooked, and is considered in detail in this chapter as well. Clinical examination and radiographic imaging are documented extensively. Surgical treatment steps and outcomes are clearly presented, as are alternatives in the case of an irreparable tendon tear.

The chapter on Massive Tears of the Posterosuperior Rotator Cuff, by Higgins and Warner, presents a step-by-step approach to open surgical repair of these injuries and illustrates details of latissimus tendon transfer in the case of an irreparable rotator cuff tear. Management of the unstable os acromiale is also described.

Two chapters on Arthroscopic Rotator Cuff Repair are presented. The reason for this is to illustrate two experts' approaches and their individual techniques. LaFosse, in his chapter, beautifully illustrates his surgical steps for arthroscopic rotator cuff repair and reports his extensive experience. Esch and Tucker's chapter is somewhat different in its approach but no less elegant. The reader will be able to pick and choose the methods that seem best for his or her skill and experience.

Section III considers Shoulder Stiffness. The chapter on Idiopathic and Diabetic Stiff Shoulder by Cuomo, Flatow,

Schneider and Bishop describes the classification, pathology, and epidemiology of frozen shoulder. These are very important concepts to embrace as they are the basis for understanding the natural history of these conditions, which is essential for selecting the most appropriate treatment options. The chapter on Acquired Shoulder Stiffness: Posttraumatic and Postsurgical, by Holovacs and Warner, describes the variable pathology and the biomechanical consequences for shoulder function in patients with a stiff shoulder after trauma or surgery. Arthroscopic and open treatments are illustrated with particular attention to proper patient selection.

Section IV deals with Fractures of the Shoulder. This is the largest section of the book because we believe it represents one of the most difficult set of shoulder problems to manage.

Two-Part Proximal Humerus Fractures are considered by Bishop and Flatow; surgical techniques such as closed reduction and percutaneous pinning and open plate fixation are illustrated in their contribution. Of special importance is the consideration of greater tuberosity fractures, which may be missed with dire functional consequences.

Three-Part Fractures: Open Reduction and Internal Fixation, or Arthroplasty, by Park, Stanwood and Bigliani, describes the advantages and methods of open reduction and internal fixation, and also provides practical rules for deciding between open reduction and internal fixation and hemiarthroplasty for these difficult fracture configurations.

Aschauer and Resch write about Four-Part Proximal Humerus Fractures; ORIF. While they clearly describe their thinking about why fixation is better than replacement in some cases of four-part fractures, the description of closed reduction and minimally invasive osteosynthesis is very informative. Indeed, Resch has been a pioneer in this revolutionary approach to management of these complex fractures, and he has shown that, with skill, the articular segment and its relationship to the tuberosities can be recreated anatomically while preserving vascularity and avoiding avascular necrosis in many cases.

The chapter on Four-Part Fractures: Arthroplasty, Preoperative Planning and Surgical Management, by Warner and Gerber, describes the authors' approach to humeral head replacement when salvage articular and tuberosity reconstruction is not possible. The clearest and most helpful part of this chapter is their description about preoperative planning, which includes practical guidelines for the surgeon, such as how to place the prosthesis at the correct height with proper humeral offset and version.

Bishop and Flatow describe their approach to Nonunion of Proximal Humerus Fractures in the next chapter. A variety of cases are used to illustrate the authors' best methods for fixation and for humeral head replacement when reconstructing these fractures.

The chapter on Malunions of the Proximal Humerus, by Ritzman and Iannotti, illustrates their best methods for

treatment of these very challenging fractures and provides an instructive summarizing algorithm for treatment.

Scapular and Glenoid Fractures are considered in the chapter by Getz, Deutsch, and Williams. This extensive contribution describes the epidemiology, anatomy and biomechanics of these problems as a basis for selection of the best methods for treatment. Extensive drawings and case illustrations provide guidelines for surgeons who must manage this kind of fracture.

Acute Fractures, Malunions, and Nonunions of the Clavicle are described in the chapter by Ring and Jupiter. The authors' extensive experience with these problems is illustrated through numerous case examples that consider plate and intramedullary fixation.

Kwon and Iannotti in their chapter write about Acromioclavicular Joint: Difficult Problems and Revision Surgery. The issue of superior-inferior instability is considered, but particular attention is given to the clinical relevance of anterior-posterior instability and management of excessive distal clavicle resection.

Finally, Wirth and Rockwood describe how they manage Sternoclavicular Joint: Primary and Revision Reconstruction. A clear illustration of sternoclavicular reconstruction is provided through drawings and cases.

Section V considers Shoulder Arthritis. Cameron and Iannotti describe Alternatives to Total Shoulder Arthroplasty in their chapter, which leads off this section. The natural history of the different forms of shoulder arthritis is presented and options for arthroscopic debridement, osteotomy, and interpositional arthroplasty are illustrated, with results presented as well.

Shoulder Arthroplasty in the Young, Active Patient, by Lee, Flatow, and Warner, provide case presentations in which no other alternative but arthroplasty exists. The concept of anatomic reconstruction and modern surgical techniques are emphasized as a basis for reconstructive techniques likely to yield a durable result in these "young" individuals. The controversy of hemiarthroplasty versus total shoulder replacement is reconsidered in the context of new available clinical and basic science data, and novel new techniques that offer promise, such as meniscal allograft resurfacing of the glenoid and humeral resurfacing, are also illustrated.

Ian Kelley provides the benefit of a lifetime of experience dealing with Special Issues in Inflammatory Arthritis in his contribution. Rheumatoid arthritis and rotator cuff insufficiency are illustrated in detail.

Rotator Cuff Arthropathy: The Unconstrained Arthroplasty is described in the chapter by Safran and Iannotti. Experience with hemiarthroplasty is illustrated clearly.

The Reverse Prosthesis chapter contributed by Sirveaux, Molé, and Boileau is a detailed presentation of a new technique now available to North American surgeons for the treatment of difficult reconstructive problems where the rotator cuff is no longer functional. This includes rotator cuff tear arthropathy, failed prior rotator cuff surgery, fracture malunions, and failed prosthesis. They describe more than a decade of experience using this type of prosthesis, with many case examples of dramatic functional improvement in their patients.

Bishop and Flatow in their chapter on Management of Bony Insufficiency of the Glenoid and Humerus with Arthroplasty illustrate management techniques for reconstructing a shoulder with glenoid and humeral deficiency, which often occurs in the setting of failed prior surgery.

The Failed Arthroplasty: Options for Revision, by Bishop and Flatow, present many examples to illustrate the list of reasons why an arthroplasty fails. Their solutions to each scenario are also clearly documented.

The final chapter in this section is on Arthrodesis and Other Salvage: When Arthroplasty is not Indicated, contributed by Richards. The especially challenging problem of bone and soft-tissue loss after failed arthroplasty is considered, with options for vascularized and intercalated bone grafts to achieve a solid fusion.

*Section VI, t*he final section of this book, *considers a variety of Miscellaneous Conditions: Nerve Injuries and Soft-Tissue Problems.* The chapter on The Painful, Snapping Scapula by Millett, Clavert, and Warner describes their experience with the particularly difficult patient who has chronic pain in a periscapular region. Their surgical technique of arthroscopic bursectomy and superior scapulectomy has been reliable in these patients; it is clearly illustrated in drawings and intraoperative photographs.

Scapular winging is considered in two chapters. In the first chapter, which describes Scapular Winging Caused by Serratus Anterior Dysfunction: Recognition and Treatment, Clavert and Warner illustrate their method of pectoralis

major transfer with small incisions and use of autogenous hamstring graft. Their method of scapulothoracic fusion is also clearly shown. In the companion contribution, Bishop and Flatow write about Scapular Winging: Trapezius Dysfunction and distinguish this form of winging from the pattern seen with a serratus anterior dysfunction. Their approach to tendon transfer is shown in drawings and intraoperative photographs.

Kozin contributes a chapter on Nerve Lesions: Suprascapular, Axillary, Thoracic Outlet and Brachial Plexus. He provides a unique description of conditions that are frequently missed on first glance and that unfortunately contribute greatly to patient morbidity and medicolegal problems.

Deltoid Injuries are considered in the chapter by Sher and Iannotti. Deltoidplasty technique is illustrated and a case of latissimus reconstruction of the deltoid is also shown.

We have aspired to make this book a unique and useful reference for all shoulder surgeons faced with complex and revision problems. It is constructed so that it can be used as *the* go-to reference when specific problems are encountered. In most cases, the surgeon will find a similar case illustrated in this book, in the chapter on that specific problem. This should help as a template for how to best manage their particular patient.

We wish you great results in your care of patients with complex and revision shoulder problems, and hope that this text will be a part of improving their quality of life.

Jon J.P. Warner, M.D.
Joseph P. Iannotti, M.D.
Evan L. Flatow, M.D.

Contents

Contributors

ROBERT A. ARCIERO, MD
Professor
Department of Orthopaedic Surgery
University of Connecticut
Farmington, Connecticut
Fellowship Director, Sports Medicine
Department of Orthopaedics
John Dempsey Hospital
Farmington, Connecticut

ERWIN ASCHAUER, MD
Landesklinik für Unfallchirurgie
Salzburg, Austria

LOUIS U. BIGLIANI, MD
Frank E. Stinchfield Professor
Department of Orthopaedic Surgery
Columbia University
New York, New York
Chairman
Department of Orthopaedic Surgery
New York–Presbyterian Hospital
New York, New York

JULIE Y. BISHOP, MD
Clinical Shoulder Fellow
Department of Orthopaedic Surgery
Mount Sinai Medical Center
New York, New York

PASCAL BOILEAU, MD
Professor
Faculté de Médecine
University of Nice
Nice, France
Chairman
Orthopaedic Surgery and Sports
    Traumatology
Hôpital de L'Archet
Nice, France

BRIAN D. CAMERON, MD
Stevens Orthopaedic Group
Edmonds, Washington

PHILIPPE CLAVERT, MD
Associate Professor
Service d'Orthopédie
CHRU Hautepierre
Strasbourg Cedex, France

BRIAN J. COLE, MD
Associate Professor
Department of Orthopaedic Surgery
Rush Presbyterian Medical Center
Chicago, Illinois

FRANCES CUOMO, MD
Insall Scott Kelly Institute
Beth Israel Medical Center
New York, New York

ALLEN DEUTSCH, MD
Department of Orthopaedic Surgery
Kelsey-Seybold Clinic
Houston, Texas

T. BRADLEY EDWARDS, MD
Clinical Assistant Professor
Department of Orthopaedic Surgery
Fondren Orthopaedic Group
Houston, Texas

JAMES C. ESCH, MD
Assistant Clinical Professor
Department of Orthopaedics
University of California, San Diego,
    School of Medicine
San Diego, California
San Diego Arthroscopy and Sports
    Medicine Fellowship
Department of Orthopaedics
Tri-City Orthopaedics
Oceanside, California

LARRY D. FIELD, MD
Clinical Instructor
Orthopaedic Surgery
University of Mississippi School of
    Medicine
Jackson, Mississippi
Co-Director
Upper Extremity
Mississippi Sports Medicine &
    Orthopaedic Center
Jackson, Mississippi

EVAN L. FLATOW, MD
Lasker Professor of Orthopaedic Surgery
Chief of Shoulder Surgery
Mount Sinai Medical Center
New York, New York

ARIANE GERBER, MD
Associate Professor
Clinic for Trauma and Surgery
Chief, Hand, Elbow, and Shoulder
    Division
Humboldt University
Clinic for Trauma and Reconstructive
    Surgery
Berlin, Germany

CHRISTIAN GERBER, MD, FRCS(ED)
Professor and Chairman
Department of Orthopaedics
University of Zürich
Balgrist Hospital
Zürich, Switzerland

CHARLES GETZ, MD
Fellow, Shoulder and Elbow Service
Department of Orthopaedic Surgery
University of Pennsylvania Medical
    Center
Philadelphia, Pennsylvania

LAURENCE D. HIGGINS, MD
Director
Sports Medicine and Shoulder
    Fellowship
Assistant Professor of Orthopaedic
    Surgery
Duke University
Durham, North Carolina

THOMAS F. HOLOVACS, MD
The Harvard Shoulder Service
Massachusetts General Hospital
Boston, Massachusetts

JOSEPH P. IANNOTTI, MD, PHD
Chairman
Department of Orthopaedic Surgery
The Cleveland Clinic
Cleveland, Ohio

JESSE B. JUPITER, MD
Hansjorg Wyss Professor of
    Orthopaedic Surgery
Department of Orthopaedic Surgery
Harvard Medical School
Boston, Massachusetts
Chief, Hand and Upper Extremity
    Service
Department of Orthopaedic Surgery
Massachusetts General Hospital
Boston, Massachussetts

IAN G. KELLY, BSC, MB, CHB, MD,
FRCS (EDIN), FRCPS (GLAS)*
Consultant Orthopaedic Surgeon
Glasgow Royal Infirmary
Glasgow, Scotland
Honorary Clinical Senior Lecturer
University of Glasgow
Glasgow, Scotland

SCOTT H. KOZIN, MD
Associate Professor
Orthopaedic Surgery
Temple University
Philadelphia, Pennsylvania
Chief
Hand and Upper Extremity
Shriner's Hospital for Children
Philadelphia, Pennsylvania

YOUNG W. KWON, MD, PHD
Assistant Professor
Department of Orthopaedic Surgery
NYU School of Medicine
New York, New York
Attending Surgeon
Department of Orthopaedic Surgery
NYU–Hospital for Joint Disease
New York, New York

LAURENT LAFOSSE, MD
Clinique Générale
Annecy, France

EDWARD W. LEE, MD
Clinical Instructor of Orthopaedic
    Surgery
Albert Einstein College of Medicine
Montefiore Medical Center
Bronx, New York

AUGUSTUS D. MAZZOCCA, MD
Assistant Professor
Department of Orthopaedic Surgery
University of Connecticut
Farmington, Connecticut
Shoulder and Elbow Surgeon
Department of Orthopaedic Surgery
John Dempsey Hospital
Farmington, Connecticut

*deceased

ROBERT E. MCLAUGHLIN, MD
Coastal Orthopaedics
Beverly, Massachusetts

SUZANNE MILLER, MD
Sports Medicine Fellow
UPMC Center for Sports Medicine
Pittsburgh, Pennsylvania

PETER J. MILLET, MD
Assistant Professor
Associate Director, Harvard Shoulder
    Service
Department of Orthopaedic Surgery
Brigham and Women's Hospital
Boston, Massachusetts

DANIEL MOLÉ, MD
Professor
Orthopaedic Surgery
University of Nancy
Nancy, France
Medical Director
Clinique de Traumatologie et
    d'Orthopédie
Nancy, France

LAURENT NOVÉ-JOSSERAND, MD
Orthopaedic Surgeon
Clinique Ste Anne Lumière
Lyon, France

MAXWELL C. PARK, MD
Fellow
Sports Medicine
Kerlan-Jobe Orthopaedic Clinic
Los Angeles, California

HERBERT RESCH, MD
Professor and Chairman
Landesklinik für Unfallchirurgie und
    Sporttraumatologie
Salzburg, Austria

ROBIN R. RICHARDS, MD, FRCSC
Professor of Orthopaedic Surgery
Sunnybrook and Women's College
    Health Sciences Centre
Toronto, Ontario, Canada

DAVID RING, MD
Instructor
Department of Orthopaedic Surgery
Harvard Medical School
Boston, Massachusetts
Orthopaedic Hand and Upper
    Extremity Service
Massachusetts General Hospital
Boston, Massachusetts

TODD F. RITZMAN, MD
Resident
Department of Orthopaedic Surgery
The Cleveland Clinic Foundation
Cleveland, Ohio

CHARLES A. ROCKWOOD, MD
Chair
Department of Orthopaedics
University of Texas Health Science
    Center at San Antonio
San Antonio, Texas

ORI SAFRAN, MD
Fellow
Orthopaedic Department
The Cleveland Clinic
Cleveland, Ohio

FELIX H. SAVOIE III, MD
Clinical Associate Professor
Orthopaedic Surgery
University of Mississippi School of
    Medicine
Jackson, Mississippi
Co-Director, Upper Extremity
Mississippi Sports Medicine and
    Orthopaedic Center
Jackson, Mississippi

JASON A. SCHNEIDER, MD
Clinical Shoulder Fellow
Beth Israel Medical Center
Insall Scott Kelly Institute for
    Orthopaedics
New York, New York

JERRY S. SHER, MD
Clinical Assistant Professor
Department of Orthopaedics and
    Rehabilitation
University of Miami School of Medicine
Miami, Florida
Orthopaedic Specialists of Miami Beach
Miami Beach, Florida

FRANÇOIS SIRVEAUX, MD, PHD
Assistant Professor
Faculté de Médecine
Université de Nancy
Nancy, France
Orthopaedic Surgeon
Clinique de Traumatologie et
    d'Orthopédie
Nancy, France

WALTER G. STANWOOD, MD
Partner
Orthopaedic Surgery
Plymouth Bay Orthopaedics
Duxbury, Massachusetts

BRADFORD S. TUCKER, MD
Active Surgeon
Department of Surgery
Division of Orthopaedic Surgery
Atlantic City Medical Center
Atlantic City, New Jersey

GILLES WALCH, MD
Clinical Associate Professor
Department of Orthopaedic Surgery
University of Lyon
Clinique Ste Ann Lumière
Lyon, France

JON J. P. WARNER, MD
Chief
The Harvard Shoulder Service
Professor of Orthopaedic Surgery
Harvard Medical School
Massachusetts General and Brigham
   and Women's Hospitals
Boston, Massachusetts

GERALD R. WILLIAMS, JR., MD
Professor and Chief
Shoulder and Elbow Service
Orthopaedic Surgery
University of Pennsylvania Medical
   Center
Philadelphia, Pennsylvania
Chief
Orthopaedic Surgery
Presbyterian Medical Center
Philadelphia, Pennsylvania

MICHAEL A. WIRTH, MD
Professor of Orthopaedics
University of Texas Health Science
   Center
San Antonio, Texas

Instability

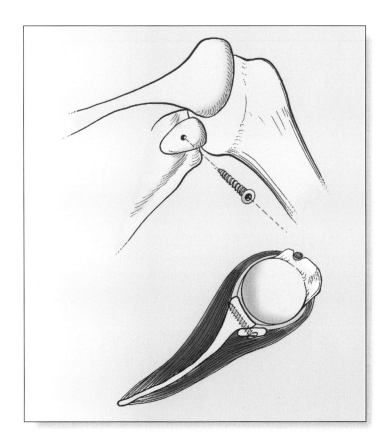

Traumatic Anterior Instability: Arthroscopic Solutions

1

Augustus D. Mazzocca   *Robert A. Arciero*   *Brian J. Cole*

INTRODUCTION

Instability of the shoulder is a common and complex problem. Classifying traumatic unidirectional instability from those patients with a traumatic multidirectional instability is important in the successful treatment of these patients.[34] One of the most common mechanisms of an acute dislocation involves a collision or fall when the arm is in an abducted and externally rotated position. Although open Bankart repair has been the gold standard for treatment of this problem, arthroscopic techniques have improved and now provide results approaching the open method. The main tenet of the arthroscopic technique is to perform the same procedure that is done in the open technique, using arthroscopic methods. This entails the use of suture anchors, permanent sutures, and a method to address capsular redundancy. This will allow the surgeon to have all of the advantages of the arthroscopic technique while also assimilating all of the advantages of the open technique.

This chapter will review the pathology and biomechanics of specific lesions encountered in patients with traumatic anterior instability. It will review various imaging techniques for assistance in preoperative planning. The chapter will describe various arthroscopic techniques for capsular plication, anterior labrum repair, and rotator interval closure. Rehabilitation, postoperative care, results of surgery, and complications will also be detailed.

PATHOLOGY OF ANTERIOR INSTABILITY

This section will describe the specific pathoanatomy associated with various diagnoses. Understanding the anatomy and biomechanics of lesions observed in patients with traumatic anterior instability will facilitate repair of these lesions, essential in a successful outcome. The arthroscope is a tool that will allow the surgeon to evaluate tissue both visually and tactilely.

The overall stability of the glenohumeral joint involves passive and active mechanisms. Static or passive factors include joint conformity, adhesion/cohesion, finite joint volume, and ligamentous restraints, including the labrum.[35] The ligaments and capsule are aided by receptors that provide proprioceptive feedback. When capsuloligamentous structures are damaged, alterations in proprioception occur that is partially restored with operative repair.[29] The active mechanisms are primarily provided by the rotator cuff muscles. The static stabilizers are affected by congenital factors, which include glenoid hypoplasia, and disorders of

A. D. Mazzocca: Department of Orthopaedic Surgery, University of Connecticut, Connecticut.
R. A. Arciero: Department of Orthopaedic Surgery, University of Connecticut, Connecticut.
B. J. Cole: Department of Orthopaedic Surgery, Rush Presbyterian-St. Luke's Medical Center, Chicago, Illinois.

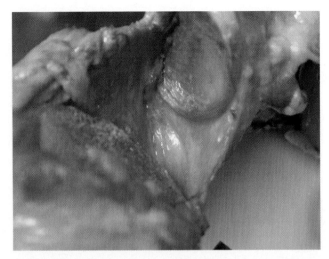

Figure 1-1   Cadaveric image of the inferior glenoid humeral ligament (IGHL) and anterior inferior labral complex.

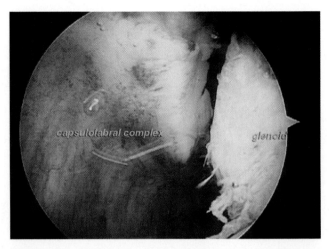

Figure 1-2   Arthroscopic view of a Bankart lesion, left shoulder, sitting position viewed from posterior (70-degree arthroscope).

collagen structure that result in excessive joint laxity. The severity of the instability pattern may be influenced by patient age, seizure disorders, and psychological or secondary gain factors.

The Bankart Lesion

The inferior glenohumeral ligament (IGHL) complex is the primary ligamentous restraint to anterior glenohumeral translation, specifically with the arm in an abducted and externally rotated position[60] (Fig. 1-1). The specific anatomy of the IGHL has been described as having anterior and posterior bands with an intervening axillary pouch.[41] In a classic description of the pathology associated with a traumatic anterior dislocation, detachment of the anterior-inferior labrum and capsule (comprising the anterior band of the IGHL as a capsulolabral complex) is considered one of the major pathoanatomical features. This has subsequently been named the Perthes-Bankart lesion[5,43] (Fig. 1-2).

The mechanism of how the Bankart lesion leads to instability has been studied extensively. A study was conducted that demonstrated that detachment of the anterior inferior labrum and capsule from the glenoid resulted in a nearly doubling of anterior translation. A Bankart repair was then performed, repairing the anterior IGHL and labrum back to the glenoid, which restored glenohumeral stability.[21] In a follow-up study, the strain before failure for all bone-ligament-bone preparations was 27% in a cadaver study, and the authors concluded that plastic deformation of the capsule was a fundamental component of anterior instability.[6] This is an important concept in capsular plication. It is important to mention that, in contradiction to Harryman's study, Speer et al. reported that, after creating a Bankart lesion, there were only small increases in anterior translation when the specimens were loaded. These data have not been duplicated.

There was also some evidence that suggests that age plays a role in the type of pathology seen with anterior dislocations.[21,52] Age has been determined to have an impact on instability. In a 1969 study of young and old primates, Reeves observed that IGHL detachment occurred in young shoulders and that the capsular ligaments tended to tear in the older ones.[44] In a similar study of computed tomography (CT) arthrograms in humans, Ribbans found avulsion of the anterior glenoid labrum in 100% of the young patients and 75% of the older ones (greater than 50 years old).[45] Associated fractures, tears of the rotator cuff, and capsular injuries were more common in those patients over 50 years of age.

Neviaser in 1993 added a differentiation between the Bankart lesion and what he termed the *anterior labral ligamentous periosteal sleeve avulsion* (ALPSA) lesion (Fig. 1-3).

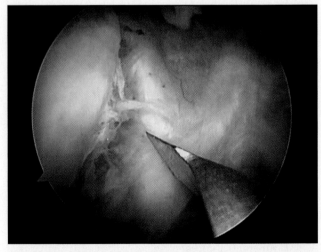

Figure 1-3   Arthroscopic anterior labrum periosteal sleeve avulsion lesion (ALPSA). Anterior view of left shoulder. Lesion being mobilized.

In his description of both acute and chronic anterior dislocations, the anterior scapular periosteum does not rupture as in a Bankart lesion, and the anterior IGHL, labrum, and the anterior scapular periosteum are stripped and displaced in a sleeve-type fashion medially on the glenoid neck. This is an important diagnostic variant to recognize, because, in a chronic situation, a cursory inspection of the anterior inferior quadrant of the glenoid may not reveal evidence of trauma. However, closer inspection more medially will elicit a large, scarred labrum on the anterior portion of the glenoid neck[38] in a medial location.

Superior Labrum Extension

The advantage of an arthroscopic examination of the shoulder joint frequently leads to observations of additional lesions associated with anterior instability. Occasionally, the injury may extend inferiorly into the capsule or the axillary pouch. Taylor and Arciero reported one capsular tear in a series of 63 primary shoulder dislocations.[56] These same authors described injuries that may also extend superiorly into attachment of the biceps tendon, producing a concomitant superior labrum anterior posterior (SLAP) lesion (Fig. 1-4, A and B). This lesion is generally observed when the dislocation involves an extreme type of trauma.[14]

In a variation of the anterior superior labrum lesion, the anterior supraspinatus can have partial or complete tears resulting in various amounts of instability. This has been called the SLAC (superior labrum, anterior cuff) lesion. This can be caused by both acute and chronic trauma and is addressed with suture anchor fixation.[51]

Humeral Avulsion of Glenohumeral Ligament Lesions

A third type of lesion can be observed, which is a lateral detachment of the IGHL from the humeral neck.[39] This has been subsequently described as a humeral avulsion of glenohumeral ligament (HAGL)[3,32] lesion (Fig. 1-5, A and B). Nicola described this entity and its proposed mechanism in 1942.[39] A force applied in continued abduction tears the capsule from the neck of the humerus. A force started in abduction of 90 to 105 degrees, supplemented by impaction, tears the capsule from the neck of the humerus. Bach, in 1988, reported two cases fixed by open repair.[3] Wolf et al., in 1995, found an incidence of 9.3% in a series of anterior instability patients. They also described an arthroscopic technique for repair. In this repair, a standard anterior inferior portal is made, and the bone is burred through this portal. An anterior lateral portal is created 2 cm lateral and 2 cm inferior to the coracoid process. A suture hook places monofilament absorbable suture through the capsule, and these are tied through the anterolateral portal over the subscapularis tendon.[63] Both Field and Warner, in 1997, cited case reports of anterior instability

treated with open techniques. Bokor et al., in 1999, reported 41 cases of a HAGL lesion in 547 shoulders, an incidence of 7.5%. Bui-Mansfield, in 2002, in a retrospective review of 307 patients with anterior instability, identified six cases, an incidence of 2%. Although relatively rare, this lesion must be examined for any anterior instability arthroscopic case. Taylor and Arciero described HAGL lesions after an acute anterior dislocation.[56]

Traumatic Bone Deficiency

Fractures or various bone deficiencies can exist, involving both glenoid and humeral surfaces (Fig. 1-6). The anatomy of the glenoid and proximal humerus is consistent. The articular surface of the proximal humerus is similar to that of a sphere. It is composed of cartilage, subchondral and trabecular bone and is relatively soft even in young athletes. The glenoid has a consistent morphology

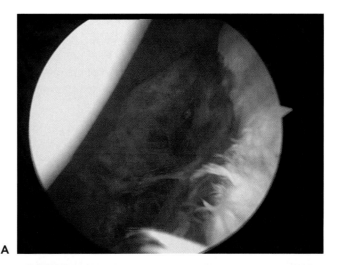

A

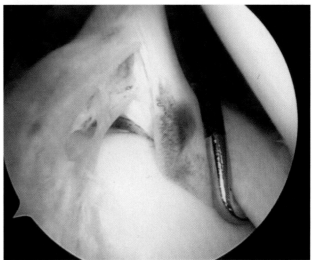

B

Figure 1-4 (A) Arthroscopic capsular tear. Sitting position, left shoulder viewed from posterior. (B) Arthroscopic superior labrum anterior to posterior lesion (SLAP), type IV.

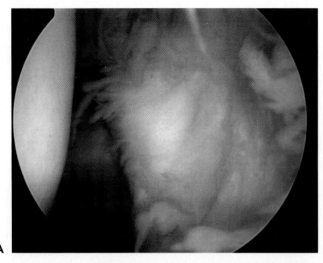
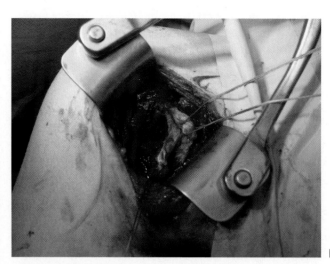

A   B

Figure 1-5 (*A*) Arthroscopic view of a humeral avulsion glenohumeral ligament lesion (HAGL), sitting posterior, left shoulder, scapularis muscle seen as shadowed area in background. (*B*) Open example of HAGL lesion-right shoulder, subscapularis tagged with suture to the right. HAGL lesion tagged with sutures inferiorly.

as well. It is pear-shaped with the inferior portion approximating that of a true circle enface.[55] Bone lesions of the glenoid or humeral head place greater demand of soft tissue repairs and have been shown to cause recurrent anterior instability of the shoulder.[6,23,50]

Humeral Bone Deficiency

The Hill-Sachs lesion is found on the humerus and is an impression fracture caused by the humeral head being dislocated anterior and impacting on the anterior glenoid. This is generally located on the posterior superior part of the humeral head. Burkhart and De Beer reported and defined what they describe as an engaging Hill-Sachs lesion, defined as a lesion in a functional position of abduction and external rotation. The long axis of the Hill-Sachs lesion

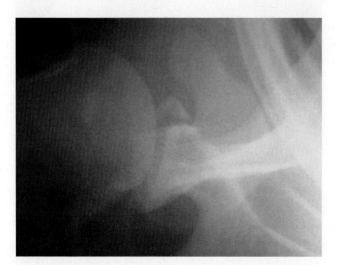

Figure 1-6 Radiograph of a bony Bankart lesion.

is parallel to the glenoid and engages its anterior corner. A nonengaging Hill-Sachs lesion is where the impression fracture occurs when the arm is in a nonfunctional position of shoulder extension or shoulder abduction is less than 70 degrees. The nonengaging Hill-Sachs lesion passes diagonally across the anterior glenoid with external rotation, so there is continual contact with the articular surfaces. These shoulders are reasonable candidates for arthroscopic Bankart repair.[9] It is important to understand that the Hill-Sachs lesion is created by the position of the arm when the dislocation occurs. The Hill-Sachs lesion that develops when the arm is at one's side but with some extension of the shoulder will be located more vertically and superiorly than the lesion that occurs with the shoulder abducted and externally rotated. The Hill-Sachs lesion that develops with the arm at the side is generally a nonengaging lesion.

Burkhart and De Beer report three ways to address the engaging Hill-Sachs lesion. The first is with an open capsular shift procedure that restricts external rotation, not allowing the lesion to engage. The second approach fixes the impression fracture with a size-matched humeral osteoarticular allograft, which is reserved for large defects. The third is a rotational proximal humeral osteotomy that internally rotates the articular surface of the humerus.

Glenoid Bone Deficiency

Two types of lesions can occur involving the anterior inferior glenoid: the impression fracture and the avulsion fracture. The compression Bankart lesion is secondary to compression of the anterior inferior bony articulation of the glenoid or the humeral head. Repeated episodes of instability create the "inverted pair" lesion as well as a typical bony Bankart. Investigators in the past have recommended cora-

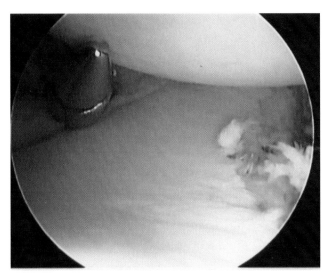

Figure 1-7 Arthroscopic example of an inverted pear-shaped glenoid. Left shoulder, anterior–superior viewing portal, lateral posterior. Note the bony deficiencies of the anteroinferior glenoid to the right.

coid transfer when the glenoid rim fracture comprised 25% of the anterior/posterior diameter of the glenoid.[7] Burkhart et al. comment on the containment of the humeral head by the glenoid as a result of two geometric variables.[10] The first is the deepening effect of a wire glenoid due to the longer arc of its concave surface; the second is the arc length of the glenoid itself. They caution in their article that if the bony fragment is excised or if there is an "inverted pair"-shaped glenoid, and if there is no bone augmentation, arthroscopic techniques may fail (Fig. 1-7). To diagnose this arthroscopically, the arthroscope is placed in the anterior superior portal, looking inferiorly on the glenoid. The bare spot of the glenoid is roughly in the center of the glenoid, and, with a calibrated probe, the distance from the anterior rim of the glenoid to the bare spot is measured, as well as the distance from the bare spot to the posterior glenoid rim. If there is a 25% reduction in the length from the anterior glenoid to the bare spot compared to the bare spot to the posterior glenoid, a bone procedure is indicated.[10]

Version and Hypoplasia Lesions

Increased glenoid retroversion and glenoid hypoplasia have been implicated in posterior or multidirectional instability.

IMAGING

Radiographs

Radiographic evaluation is required in assessment of shoulder instability. Fractures as well as assessment of anatomy are critical to evaluate prior to treatment. A standard anterior-posterior view of the arm in slight internal rotation is used to identify a fracture of the greater tuberosity. A true scapular anterior-posterior radiograph permits evaluation of a glenoid fossa fracture, if present. The West Point axillary view is used to assess bony avulsions of the attachment of the IGHL or bony Bankart lesions,[47] or anterior-inferior glenoid deficiency. The Hill-Sachs lesion can be quantified and evaluated by examining the Stryker Notch view.

Computed Tomography Scan

The CT scan can be a very accurate means of determining glenoid version and overall glenoid morphology. The ability to reconstruct the anatomy of the glenoid in three dimensions by subtracting the humerus is an excellent technique. Knowing the character and shape of the articular surface can aide the surgeon in preoperative planning. Substantial bone loss may be a contraindication to arthroscopic stabilization.

Magnetic Resonance Imaging

Magnetic resonance imaging (MRI) is used for assessment of associated pathology. Stoller, in 1997, reviewed contrast enhancement with intra-articular gadolinium diethylene-triamine pentaacetic acid (Gd/dtpa), which improved diagnostic ability for assessment of labral tears (both superior and anterior inferior), rotator cuff tears (both partial thickness and full), and articular lesions. When identifying a humeral avulsion of the glenoid labrum, MRIs identifying the humeral detachment of the inferior glenoid labrum (IGL) show that, as the IGL drops inferiorly, a midsagittal coronal oblique arthrographic image located toward the axillary pouch is converted from a full, distended U-shaped structure to a J-shaped structure[53] (Fig. 1-8, *A* and *B*). This has been further defined by a follow-up study that describes the MRI appearance of a HAGL as an avulsion fracture from the neocortex in the humeral neck. A thin radiolucency was observed inferior to the anatomical neck of the humerus, and once again as the fluid-filled distended U-shaped axillary pouch transforms into a J-shaped structure by the extravasation of contrast material.[8] The pressure of this lesion may also be a relative contraindication to arthroscopic stabilization.

SURGICAL OPTIONS: DECISION MAKING

The controversy surrounding open versus arthroscopic techniques for anterior labral stabilization has been ongoing since Johnson published his technique of arthroscopic staple fixation in *Techniques of Anterior Glenohumeral Ligament Repair*.[26] Both open and arthroscopic procedures have involved using bone tunnels, staples, transglenoid sutures, rivets, bioabsorbable tacks, and suture anchors. Initial

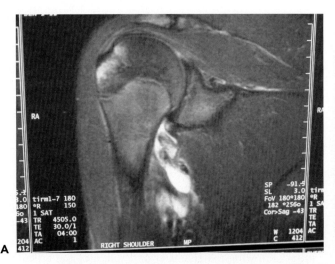
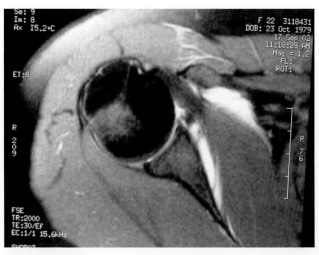

Figure 1-8   (*A*) Magnetic resonance imaging (MRI) example of a HAGL lesion. (*B*) MRI example of a Bankart lesion.

studies reported recurrence rates of arthroscopic techniques from 0% to 44%. The earlier arthroscopic techniques were applied to many types of instability patterns and featured techniques that did not resemble principles of established open methods. The major advantage of arthroscopic repair for instability is the ability to accurately identify and treat the specific pathoanatomy, less iatrogenic damage to normal tissues (subscapularis), lower postoperative pain, and improved cosmesis. Some authors also report an easier functional recovery and improved motion than with the open repair method.[11] Greater than five dislocations/subluxations has been thought of as a relative contraindication for arthroscopic repair.[28,62] Indications for open technique would be bone abnormality, such as an "inverted pair" glenoid or a Hill-Sachs lesion involving greater than 20% to 30% of the articular surface. Some surgeons still advocate the open procedure in high-demand athletes; however, as arthroscopic techniques continue to improve and closely mimic what is done in an open procedure, recurrence rates are similar compared to open.

SURGICAL TECHNIQUES

A surgical technique, based on the idea of a 180-degree repair (Fig. 1-9), that is currently used with various modifications. This technique involves an inferior capsular plication, an anterior shift, a Bankart lesion repair with suture anchors, and a rotator interval closure. In operative treatment of an acute anterior dislocation within three weeks, only the Bankart lesion or the anterior inferior glenoid labrum tear is repaired with suture anchors. Generally, the inferior capsular plication and rotator interval closure are deferred for the late repair of the recurrent dislocator. When the repair is later than 3 weeks after the acute

dislocation, capsular imbrication and rotator interval closure will be required because it is thought that there is capsular elongation that is commonly associated with repetitive microtrauma. Bigliani et al., in 1992, reported that there was a significant amount of elongation with any type of capsular failure, suggesting a plastic deformation of the capsule occurred.[6] Some type of shortening is then required to return the capsule to its anatomical length.

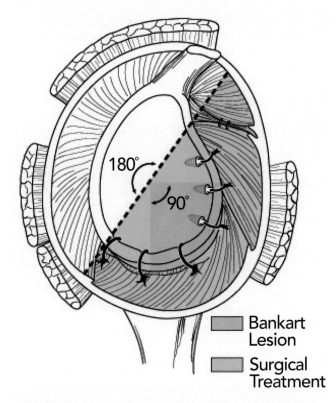

Figure 1-9   180-degree arthroscopic repair. Diagrammatic representation of surgical reconstruction.

Patient Position

The lateral decubitus, or beach-chair, position can be employed for instability surgery. The beach-chair position offers the advantage of being able to convert to an open procedure easily. When the beach-chair position is used, a sterile arm holder (Tennet Medical Engineering, McConnell, TX) is helpful for both holding a desired arm position and for applying a distraction force to the arm. For the lateral decubitus, a three-point distraction device that allows both longitudinal and vertical traction, enabling the humeral head to be lifted reproducibly from the glenoid, is used (Arthrex Inc., Naples, FL) (Fig. 1-10, *A* and *B*). A beanbag is used to stabilize the patient, and a hip-holder is used to stabilize the beanbag in case air is liberated. The patient is positioned in a 30-degree backward tilt to account and place the glenoid in a parallel orientation to the floor. In most cases, general endotracheal intubation is used for anesthesia, with an interscalene block for pain control. Due to the uncomfortable nature of the position, we advocate general anesthesia with or without the block. Preoperative antibiotics are administered intravenously prior to skin incision for portal placement.

Exam Under Anesthesia

An examination of both shoulders, with the patient under anesthesia and in the supine position, is performed, documenting forward elevation, external and internal rotation with the arm at the side, and external and internal rotation with the arm abducted to 90 degrees. An anterior load shift, a posterior "jerk" test, and sulcus tests are performed to assess dominance in instability. This exam under anesthesia is used to confirm and add further information, such as crepitus and/or other pathology that may be present, *not* to make the diagnosis. When performing the load and shift testing, care should be taken to compare both shoulders for the degree of humeral head translation. In addition, the amount of translation should be noted for each arm position with respect to the degree of humeral rotation and the position of the arm in relation to the plane of the scapula. Arm rotation and position will influence the degree of translation because of the changes that they have on ligament length.

Portal Placement

A standard posterior portal should be placed slightly more lateral than the joint line. If the portal is placed medial to the joint line, then it will require the surgeon to lever the arthroscope against the glenoid, making the stabilization procedure quite difficult.

An 8- to 10-mm incision is made, and then the blunt scope sheath and trocar is inserted atraumatically into the space between the glenoid rim and humeral head.

The anterior series of portals are then made using spinal needles for localization. The first anterior portal is made su-

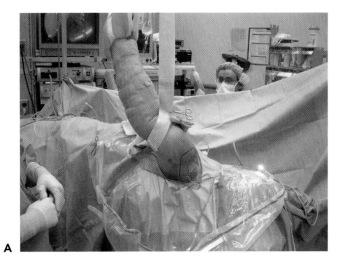

A

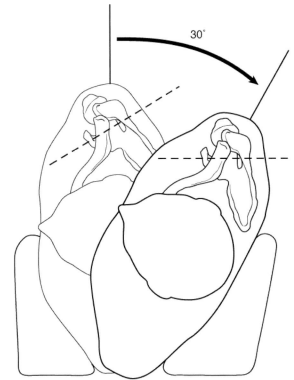

B

Figure 1-10 (*A*) Lateral position traction device (Arthrex Inc., Naples, FL). (*B*) 30-degree tilt positioning.

perior and lateral in the rotator interval, which should be made as high in the anterior superior quadrant as possible, still allowing the cannula to be placed anterior to the biceps tendon. Medial placement of the cannula will compromise access to the glenoid. Care should be taken not to allow the cannula to be posterior to the biceps tendon to avoid entrapment of the tendon with sutures. In general, a 7-mm by 7-cm cannula, either smooth or ridged, is placed for suture shuttling.

The second portal is the anterior inferior portal. This portal can be created in two different manners. The first creates a 5 o'clock portal, which, by needle localization, is through the subscapularis tendon. This allows accurate and easy inferior anchor placement. The difficulty is in placing an 8.25-mm by 7-cm cannula through the subscapularis tendon. This is accomplished after accurate placement by needle localization with a pointed switching stick and then a dilator system. The second is the standard anterior inferior portal that is made at the superior rolled edge of the subscapularis, angled inferiorly. Once again, this is also made with spinal needle localization and avoids the trauma of going through the subscapularis tendon. Potential difficulties involve inferior anchor placement because the angle is more oblique. If this does happen, a stab incision can be made, and the anchor can be placed through the subscapularis tendon with the standard anterior inferior portal maintained and sutures shuttled through that cannula after insertion.

The final portal that is made is the 7 o'clock portal. This is a posterior inferior portal, allowing inferior capsular plication. This portal is made roughly 2 cm lateral and 1 cm inferior to the standard posterior portal. An 18-gauge spinal needle is used under direct visualization to assess the position, and an 8.25-cm by 9-cm cannula is then placed. This allows very accurate inferior capsular plication under direct visualization, as the arthroscope is kept in the posterior portal, and suture shuttling devices are used and placed through the large 7 o'clock cannula (Fig. 1-11).

Care should be exercised in creating portals and in evaluating pumps and pump pressure. Shoulder distention is a problem and is compounded by improper portal development and a lengthy procedure. It is important to always establish accurate and small portals eliminating fluid extravasation, to use cannulas at all times to create a seal in the glenohumeral joint, and to monitor the amount of fluid pressure at all times. An ideal pressure to perform

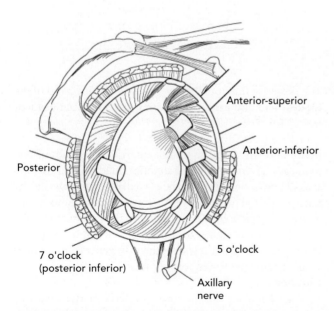

Figure 1-11 Portals that can be utilized for "180-degree" repair technique.

arthroscopic stabilization has not been reported. However, analysis and evaluation of pressure and shoulder distention as the procedure progresses are critical.

Diagnostic Arthroscopy

In an attempt to accurately diagnose the amount of synovitis and other abnormalities found, the initial part of the arthroscopic examination is performed dry. This allows assessment of synovitis, specifically in the anterior superior quadrant of the shoulder, as well as evaluation of the biceps tendon and articular defects. Once the dry exam is completed, fluid is then allowed to flow into the joint.

A systematic evaluation and recoding of the anatomical findings in each region of the glenohumeral joint is one of the major advantages to arthroscopy. These regions include the superior, superoanterior, anterior, inferior, posterior, and rotator cuff insertion.

Superior Region

The superior region includes the triangle formed by the biceps tendon superiorly, the humeral head laterally, and the subscapularis inferiorly. The biceps tendon and the glenoid labrum surrounding the entire glenoid have the appearance of an inverted comma or Q.[15] The biceps tendon attaches to the supraglenoid tubercle at the posterior superior aspect of the glenoid rim. The biceps origin is either attached to the superior labrum or sends fibers to the anterosuperior and posterosuperior labrum. The first portion of this exam can be done prior to distention of the capsule with fluid. This allows visualization and quantification of the amount of erythema on the biceps tendon. Once the fluid has been introduced, the pressure tamponades the microinflammation and "washes it out." This can be a helpful adjunct to diagnosis of biceps tendinosis (Yamaguchi K. Personal Communication, AAOS Advanced Shoulder Course, July 2002).

The superior labrum should be evaluated for tears, detachment, or other abnormalities representing the clinical entity known as the SLAP lesion. A probe can be used from the anterior portal to look under the labrum to evaluate whether it is detached. Rao et al., in 2003, have quantified the four types of anatomical variants of the anterosuperior aspect of the labrum that evaluate the size of the sublabral foramen and type of middle glenohumeral ligament (MGHL). They found a 13.4% incidence of anatomical variability in their group of 546 patients.

Anterosuperior Region

The coracohumeral ligament (CHL) should be evaluated because it encircles the biceps tendon. This ligament originates at the base of the coracoid and then spans out, sending fibers that encircle the biceps tendon, intertwine with the supraspinatus tendon, and insert in front of the sub-scapularis tendon insertion. The superior glenohumeral ligament (SGHL) also attaches to the superior portion of the glenoid, but is in a different plane than the CHL. The SGHL runs from the anterior superior aspect of the glenoid to the upper part of the lesser tuberosity and is considered by some to be the medial wall and floor of the bicipital groove. The SGHL works with the CHL in preventing anterior translation of the humeral head with the arm adducted and externally rotated. The SGHL also prevents inferior subluxation of the humeral head (sulcus sign) with the arm at the side. It becomes taught with external rotation of the arm, further decreasing the inferior translation of the humeral head. The biceps can be followed distally into the bicipital groove. Forward elevation with the elbow flexed, combined with internal rotation of the arm, may assist in viewing the biceps as it passes underneath the transverse humeral ligament. The probe can also be placed superior to the tendon and the tendon "pulled" down into the joint, allowing visualization of the biceps tendon that is located in the intertubercular groove.

The bicipital groove is further bordered by the sub-scapularis tendon medially and the supraspinatus tendon laterally. The supraspinatus tendon can be seen adjacent to the biceps with abduction and external rotation. The SGHL and CHL form the medial sling of the biceps. Damage to these structures can result in biceps instability and/or pain.

Finally, the anterosuperior labrum can be evaluated. The labrum has been described as being triangular in cross section with its free edge directed at the glenoid center. It is made up of dense fibrous connective tissue and anchored to the osseous rim of the glenoid. The hyaline cartilage of the glenoid articular surface frequently extends under and beyond this free edge. Significant normal variability exists in the appearance of the anterosuperior labrum that can include physiologic detachment and confluence with the MGHL (Buford Complex), simple detachment (sublabral hole), or complete absence. A probe can be inserted through the anterior portal, as previously described, and used to examine all labral and ligamentous structures. Noting labral atrophy, fraying, and/or amount of movement should always be done because this information may aid in establishing or confirming the diagnosis and aid in treatment.

Anterior Region

With the arthroscope in the posterior portal and the 30-degree objective facing laterally, the rolled upper edge of the subscapularis is examined. The MGHL is variable in thickness and intersects the subscapularis at a 60-degree angle.[39] The MGHL arises from the anterior humeral neck just medial to the lesser tuberosity and inserts on the medial and superior glenoid rim and scapular neck. Its function is to resist anterior translation of the humeral head at 45 de-

grees of abduction.[24] In a diagnostic glenohumeral arthroscopy, it is also important to examine the subscapularis recess. Loose bodies can be lodged here and will not be discovered unless this area is actually visualized. Inferiorly, the anterior and anterior inferior labrum can be inspected. Any detachment of the labrum below the glenoid equator, however (at the level of the rolled-edge insertion of the subscapularis), is generally considered pathologic.

The articular surface of the glenoid and humerus must be examined in detail. The articular cartilage of the glenoid thins at the center. The surrounding cartilage should be examined for full-thickness lesions, fibrillation, and softening. The treatment of these lesions is still controversial, but they must be noted. Large articular lesions can manifest in a patient as a feeling of instability because the humeral head articulates with the lesion and "clunks" in various positions of rotation and abduction.

Inferior Region

The inferior region is examined for evidence of synovitis and presence of loose bodies. Inferiorly, with the assistant holding traction in 20 to 30 degrees of abduction on the arm in a beach-chair position, the anterior band of the IGHL can be inspected. The IGHL runs from the glenoid to the anatomical neck of the humerus. The anterior band of the IGHL prevents anterior translation of the humeral head when the arm is abducted 90 degrees and externally rotated. It also restricts inferior translation when the arm is abducted and internally rotated. The humeral attachment of the anterior band is best visualized from the anterior portal. It is from this view that a HAGL lesion can be seen. The axillary pouch is then inspected. The capsule of the axillary pouch is thin, and beneath it lays the axillary nerve. This relationship should always be considered when doing suture capsular plication or thermal capsulorrhaphy.

Posterior Region

The posterior inferior labrum and the posterior band of the inferior glenohumeral ligament can be inspected sequentially. The posterior band of the IGHL prevents inferior translation of the humeral head when the arm is abducted 90 degrees and externally rotated. It also prevents posterior translation when the arm is abducted and internally rotated.[25] From this position, the posterior insertion of the rotator cuff can be evaluated for fraying associated with internal impingement. The arm should be abducted to 90 to 110 degrees and maximally externally rotated. Fraying and contact of the posterior labrum and the rotator cuff tendon in a patient with pain can be indicative of internal impingement.

Evaluating the supraspinatus tendon insertion beginning just posterior to the biceps tendon is performed with slight forward elevation, abduction, and external rotation of the humerus. Placing an 18-gauge spinal needle percutaneously and passing a monofilament suture into the joint assists in identifying partial thickness tears by viewing the suture from within the subacromial space following intra-articular arthroscopy. By observing the posterior and inferior humerus, the bare area can be visualized. This is an area of bare bone with remnants of old vascular channels. This bare area also correlates to the attachment of the infraspinatus tendon. It can be used as a landmark in rotator cuff surgery to align the infraspinatus to its footprint. Once the glenohumeral exam is complete, preparation of the tissue can begin.

Preparation

Preparation of the capsule prior to plication has been advocated to "excite the synoviocytes." This has not been scientifically proven, but makes logical sense and can be accomplished with either a shaver or a handheld burr from either the anterior or 7 o'clock portal. Preparation of the glenoid bed for the labrum is also critical. With the viewing arthroscope in the posterior portal, the soft tissue and cortical surface can be removed. This is completed after the periosteal-labral-IGHL complex has been dissected free from the subscapularis tendon. A sharp elevator combined with an arthroscopic shaver or tissue ablation device are used to dissect and liberate the entire labrum, IGHL, and periosteum of the glenoid neck until the subscapularis muscle is seen. The anterior inferior labrum should be released so that it "floats" to the glenoid rim. A small burr is then used to create a bleeding surface on the anterior glenoid neck (Fig. 1-12). To evaluate this preparation of the bed the arthroscope is placed in the anterosuperior or inferior portal. This allows excellent visualization of the labral complex and bone preparation.[6]

Inferior Plication

Inferior plication is accomplished by imbricating the axillary pouch. The importance of capsular plication (capsulorrhaphy) has been shown by the irreversible plastic deformation of the capsule that occurs during an anterior dislocation.[6] Arthroscopically, this can be completed with suture, suture anchors, or thermal energy. Tibone et al., in 2000, reported that thermal treatment to the IGHL produced a 41% decrease in anterior translation and a 36% decrease in posterior translation of the humeral head to the glenoid with a 15N load.[57] Arthroscopic plication with suture or suture anchor has recently been evaluated. Alberta et al., in 2003, reported a 61% decrease in anterior and a 11% decrease in posterior translation with a 1-cm imbrication of the capsule.[2]

There are multiple methods to plicate or decrease capsular redundancy. One such method, the pinch-tuck method, involves penetrating the tissue approximately 1 cm away

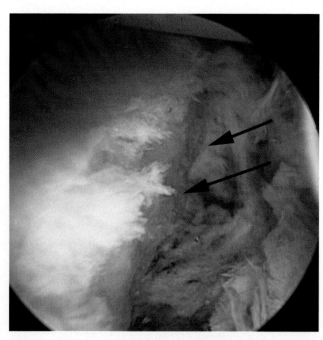

Figure 1-12 Arthroscopic example of anterior glenoid preparation. Left shoulder, lateral position viewed from anterosuperior portal.

from the labrum, then penetrating the labrum itself, with a suture-passing device in a "corkscrew configuration" (Fig. 1-13, A–C). When this knot is tied, it creates a blind pouch that then scars in. If the labrum is friable, or an adequate bite cannot be secured, a suture anchor can be placed into the labrum. The suture can then be shuttled through the inferior capsule and then tied. Two to three of these inferior capsular plication sutures are then placed from posterior inferior to anterior inferior positions (Positions 8, 7, 6 on a right shoulder). An accessory posterior portal can be used (7 o'clock portal), or the camera can be changed to the anterior superior portal and a cannula placed in the posterior portal. Suture management at this stage is important. The surgeon can tie individual sutures, which makes suture management more straightforward but can run the risk of "closing yourself out." The second method involves shuttling the suture out the anterior cannula, then removing the cannula and replacing it, thus removing the suture pair from within. All pairs can then be shuttled back at the end for tying. Once two or three inferior capsular plication sutures are made, attention is turned to the anterior inferior Bankart lesion.

Bankart Repair with Suture Anchors

Repair of the Bankart lesion is the critical step in this procedure. The suture anchor repair is the most similar to the open repair technique and is extremely versatile and reproducible. Two variations of execution are the suture-first or

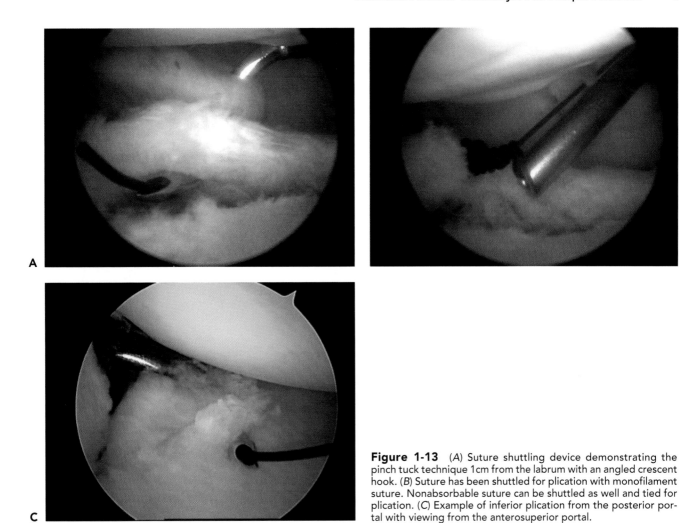

Figure 1-13 (*A*) Suture shuttling device demonstrating the pinch tuck technique 1cm from the labrum with an angled crescent hook. (*B*) Suture has been shuttled for plication with monofilament suture. Nonabsorbable suture can be shuttled as well and tied for plication. (*C*) Example of inferior plication from the posterior portal with viewing from the anterosuperior portal.

the anchor-first techniques. A third, highly successful technique is that of the Knotless Suture Anchor (Mitek Inc., Norwood, MA). Clinically, there is no reported difference between any of these techniques, and use is based on surgeon preference. The anchors themselves can be either metal or bioabsorbable. We recommend bioabsorbable anchors because most instability patients are young and we attempt to avoid the theoretical possibility of migration. There are no differences reported clinically based on the material of the anchor. Proper anchor placement is the most critical, and no material can help an improperly placed anchor.

Anchor-First Technique

The anchor-first technique involves placing an anchor first through the anterior inferior cannula and then shuttling the suture limb (Fig. 1-14, *A* and *B*). It is important to note at this time the position of the anterior inferior cannula and the position in which the anchor should be placed into the glenoid. There are times when the position of the cannula is appropriate for suture shuttling but not

for placement of the anchor. In this case, a percutaneous approach can be followed to insert an anchor into the glenoid at the 5:30 position. The advantage of this technique is that it allows a more appropriate perpendicular placement of the anchor into the glenoid face at approximately 2 to 3 mm over the articular service without "bubbling" or causing any articular damage. After the anchor has been successfully inserted, one of the suture limbs is passed out of the anterior superior cannula. This limb, if using a metal anchor or an anchor with fixed eyelet, is the limb on the tissue side of the suture. The eyelet should be perpendicular to the labrum. A tissue penetrator or suture shuttling device is used to place a passing suture into the tissue inferior to the anchor. The end of the suture will then be grasped and pulled out of the anterior superior cannula. A small square knot will be tied in the line, and then the monofilament suture line will be tied to the nonabsorbable braided suture and pulled through the anterior inferior cannula, hence shuttling the suture through labrum, inferior-glenoid ligament, and scapular periosteal complex. Upon tightening this suture, a shift of tissue from inferior to superior should be observed. If the tissue

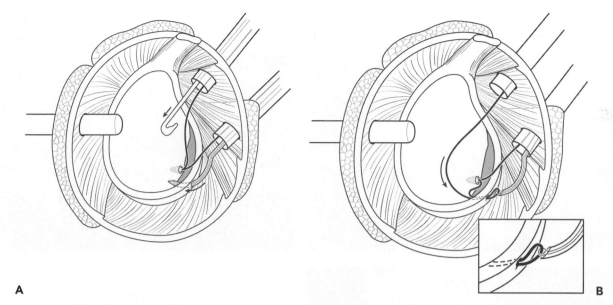

Figure 1-14 (*A*) Example of an anchor first shuttling technique with tissue penetrator inferior to anchor. (*B*) Nonabsorbable suture shuttled through inferior labrum and inferior glenohumeral ligament complex.

bite is not inferior enough to the anchor, then this should be redone at the point. The knot pusher should then be placed on the suture limb to make sure that the post is identified and is on the tissue side. A sliding knot (Duncan Loop, SMC knot, Tennessee slider, etc.) can be tied, or a nonslider knot (multiple half hitches) can be tied at this time. It has been determined that, after placing a sliding knot or multiple half hitches, three alternating half hitches, while switching the post, is the most secure final fixation.[33] The knot should be on the tissue side so that the labrum can create a bumper effect. The next two or three anchors are then placed approximately 5 to 7 mm apart from each other in the same fashion as has been previously described. Upon completing this portion of the procedure, a "bumper" should be observed at the anterior inferior glenoid between the 3 and 6 o'clock positions.

Suture-First Technique

The suture-first technique involves placing a suture to ensure adequate soft tissue shift and then placement of the anchor (Fig. 1-15, *A–D*). A suture-passing device is placed thru the anterior inferior cannula. The tissue is clasped inferior to what would be the 5 o'clock anchor position, thus enabling the tissue from anterior inferior or inferior glenohumeral ligament to be shifted superiorly. The suture is passed through the tissue and shuttled through the anterior superior portal. The suture-passing device is then removed, and the suture limb that is in the anterior inferior portal is switched to the anterior superior portal. Tension is placed on this suture to observe the amount of shift that can be ac-

complished by placement of the anchor in the appropriate position. If it is determined that this suture was not inferior enough, a second suture can be placed. When an appropriate amount of tissue tension is established by direct visualization, the anchor can be placed through the anterior inferior portal in the exact location. As was described before, once the anchor is placed the two limbs of the suture are separated one through the anterior superior cannula, and the other limb is then shuttled through the tissue. This is repeated two or three times depending on repair quality and injury (Fig. 1-16).

Extension of Anterior Inferior Labrum Tear into the Superior Labrum

If the labral tear extends from the anterior inferior up into the superior labrum, the same cannula can be used to continue placing anchors. We recommend two to three anchors for superior labrum tears, one being placed in front of the biceps tendon anchor with one or two behind, depending on the instability being placed behind the biceps tendon anchor. The anchor that is placed in front of the biceps tendon anchor can be placed through the anterior superior portal. The one to two anchors placed posterior to the biceps anchor can be placed percutaneously in a spot that is 1 cm lateral and 1 cm anterior to the posterior lateral corner of the acromion. This portal or area of entrance is known as the "Port of Wilmington."[37] This allows placement of the anchor through the musculotendinous junction of the rotator cuff to the appropriate position on the superior glenoid rim poste-

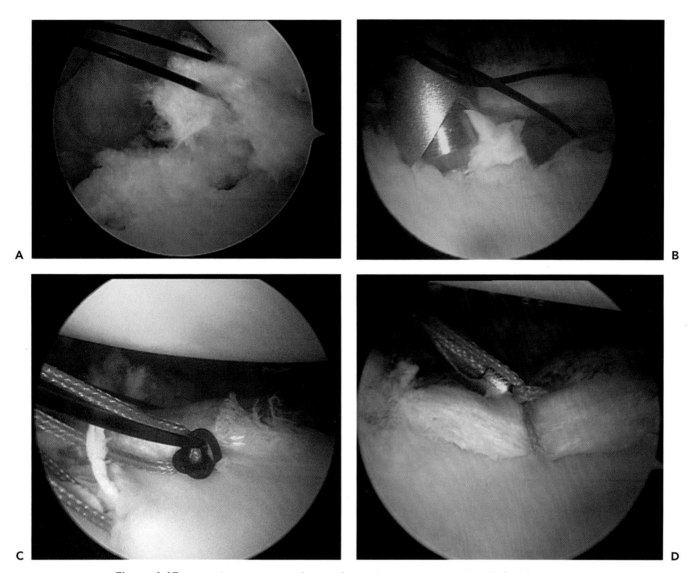

Figure 1-15 (A) Arthroscopic view of suture first technique. "O" PDS placed inferiorly and traction applied. (B) Anchor placement more cephalad to suture so that with eventual knot tying labrum and capsule shifted superiorly. (C) Nonabsorbable suture being shuttled with "O" PDS. (D) Knot tying.

rior to the biceps anchor. Generally, the anchor anterior to the biceps can be placed, using the anterior superior portal.

The Rotator Interval

The rotator interval is an important anatomical region with respect to anterior inferior shoulder stability. The anatomical region is defined as the articular capsule bounded superiorly by the anterior portion of the supraspinatus tendon, inferiorly by the superior portion of the subscapularis tendon, medially by the base of the coracoid process, and laterally by the long head of the biceps tendon. The capsular tissue is reinforced by the coracohumeral ligament and the superior glenohumeral ligament.

The rotator interval is of variable size and is present in the fetus as well as in the adult.[12] Harryman et al. found that sectioning the rotator interval in cadaveric specimens resulted in increased glenohumeral translation in all planes tested.[22] Imbrication of rotator interval lesions resulted in a decreased posterior and inferior glenohumeral translation when compared to the intact state. Gartsman found that repair of the rotator interval was a critical factor in 14 of 53 shoulders treated arthroscopically for anterior inferior glenohumeral instability and contributed to the improved clinical outcomes observed in the study.[18] Field et al. reported good or excellent results in 15 patients who underwent surgical repair of isolated rotator interval defects.[17]

Many authors have reported techniques enclosing the rotator interval.[13,19,27,40,59] There are various techniques

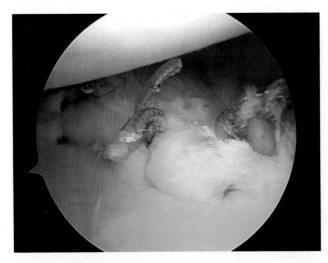

Figure 1-16   Complete Bankart repair.

that have been published. There is no literature evaluating the type of suture material that ensures success. One technique involves removing the anterior inferior cannula and placing all instrumentation through the anterior superior cannula. The MGHL and/or a small portion of the sub-

scapularis is pierced with either a spinal needle or suture shuttling device, and a monofilament suture is deployed (Fig. 1-17A). The SGHL/CHL complex is pierced with a penetrator and grasps the monofilament suture (Fig. 1-17B). This tissue can then be tied through a cannula internally or externally with a guillotine knot cutter (Fig. 1-17C). The final repair involves capsular plication, anterior inferior labral repair, and rotator interval closure (Fig. 1-18).

Thermal Energy Applied to the Anterior Inferior Instability

The concept of using heat to alter the structure of collagen and affect changes in tissue length in treating anterior inferior instability has been around since the time of Hippocrates. Thermal treatment of collagen molecules affects the heat-labile bonds, and, as these re-form, the overall tissue length decreases.[16] There are two types of radiofrequency circuitry for the use in orthopaedic application. The monopolar radiofrequency system uses a current between the treatment probe and the grounding pad or plate. This current passes through the tissue, releasing energy into it so

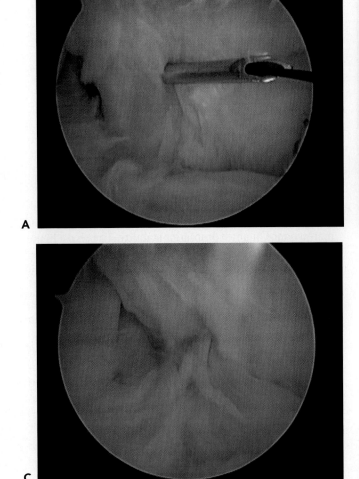

A

C

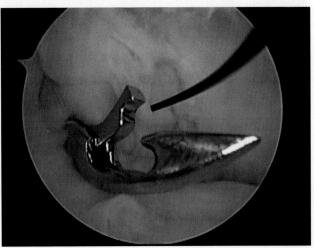

B

Figure 1-17 (A) Suture shuttling device through the middle glenohumeral placing a monofilament suture into joint. (B) Tissue penetrator through superior glenohumeral ligament and coracohumeral ligament retrieving monofilament suture. (C) Tying rotator interval closed extra-articularly.

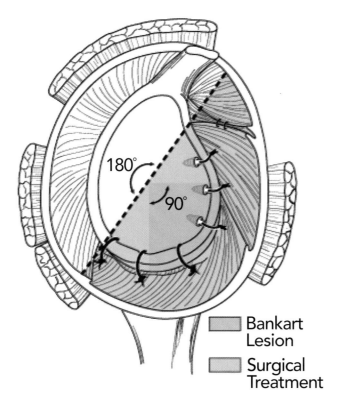

Bankart Lesion

Surgical Treatment

Figure 1-18 Example of 180-degree repair with three inferior plication sutures, three anchors repairing the labrum, and rotator interval closure.

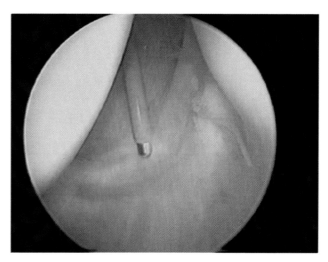

Figure 1-19 Arthroscopic view of thermal capsulorrhaphy.

neously resolving. Stiffness is also a complication of this procedure.[64] Shoulder proprioception is not influenced by the application of thermal energy.[30]

The use of thermal alteration in the aid of elite athletes with traumatic anterior instability has yet to be determined. The indications for thermal energy are for augmentation after the anatomy has been repaired.

that the tissue becomes hot, not the probe. Lintner and Speer have shown that the thermal effect gradient seen up to a depth of 4.5 mm is adequate for capsular response.[32] The bipolar radiofrequency device applies energy by having a current flow from the tip of the probe through the irrigating solution and back to the probe. This causes very high temperatures at the probe. This applies a very high tissue temperature with the very little or low depth of penetration, which is 1 mm or less.

The proposed technique offering the greatest benefit with the least amount of potential complication is the "striping" pattern technique, which leaves a 1- to 2-mm space between each row (Fig. 1-19). This is done to the anterior band, posterior band, and axillary pouch of the shoulder. This has been shown to significantly reduce the anterior translation of the humeral head.[58] Clinically, success has been found with this technique in high-level throwing athletes who have been treated with thermal augmentation for internal impingement.[31]

There have also been cases of dramatic failures to go along with this success. Cases of complete capsular necrosis and ablation following thermal treatment have been reported.[49] There has also been injury to the axillary nerve that lies close to the inferior capsule at the 6 o'clock position.[16] The overall axillary nerve injury incidence has been reported at 1.4% (196 out of 236,015), with most cases involving the sensory portion of the nerve and then sponta-

POSTOPERATIVE CARE

The biological healing response of the inferior capsule after plication, the inferior glenohumeral ligament and the anterior inferior labral complex to bone, and the rotator interval must be respected. One observation that may have led to some of the earlier anterior inferior arthroscopic failures has been the concept that due to significant reduction in pain postoperatively, these patients move their arms more with stress to the repair and eventually failure of it. The first concern when addressing postoperative success is maintenance of anterior inferior stability. The second concern is the restoration of adequate motion, specifically external rotation. The third concern is a successful return to sports or the physical activities of daily living in a reasonable amount of time.

The University of Connecticut postoperative protocol for anterior inferior instability treated by arthroscopy involves immobilization in an abduction arthrosis. This allows the arm to be fixed in a slight amount of external rotation. Codman exercises combined with pendulum exercises are started immediately. Active assisted range-of-motion exercises, external rotation (0–30 degrees), and forward elevation (0–90 degrees) are started at this time. This regime is maintained for the first 6 weeks. From 6 weeks to 12 weeks, active assisted as well as active range-of-motion exercises are started, with the goal as establishing full range of motion. No strengthening exercises or any type of repetitive exercises are started until after full range of motion has been established. This protocol is based on tendon-to-bone healing in a dog model.[46,54] Early resistance exercises and aggressive postoperative rehabilitation do not appear to offer substantial advantages and could compromise the repair. Strengthening is begun once there is full, painless, active range of motion. Strengthening is begun at 12 weeks to 16 weeks. Sports-specific exercises are then started at 16 weeks to 20 weeks, and between 20 and 24 weeks contact athletics are initiated. The use of cold therapy devices has been successful in reducing postoperative pain.

Pagnani and Dome reported on open stabilization in American football players.[42] Their postoperative program is quite similar to ours as mentioned here for further reference. At 0 to 4 weeks, the arm is immobilized with a sling and internal rotation, double range-of-motion, and pendulum exercises are begun. From 4 to 8 weeks, passive- and active-assisted shoulder range-of-motion exercises with external rotation limited to 45 degrees is done. When 140 degrees of active forward elevation is obtained, rotator cuff strengthening is begun, with internal and external rotation strengthening completed with the arm at a low abduction. From 8 to 12 weeks, they start deltoid isometric exercises with the arm in low abduction angles, as well as body blade exercises. They then slowly increase abduction during rotator cuff and deltoid strengthening. Scapular rotator strengthening and horizontal abduction exercises are also begun. From 12 to 18 weeks, restoration of terminal external rotation is achieved. Proprioceptive neuromuscular feedback patterns are employed, and plyometric exercises as well as sports-specific motion using pulley, wand, or manual resistance are begun. After 18 weeks or later, conventional weight training is begun and rehabilitation is orientated toward return to sports, progressing from field drills to contact drills. They report using an abduction harness for selected football positions (linemen). They return to full contact when abduction and external rotation strength are symmetrical on manual muscle testing.[42]

TECHNICAL ERRORS

For successful treatment of arthroscopic anterior inferior instability adequate visualization is imperative. The lateral decubitus position with a traction device has been able to provide both vertical distraction, enabling the humeral head to float superiorly, and horizontal distraction, pulling the humeral head inferiorly. Traction allows the surgical team to work unencumbered by not having to hold the arm. If adequate visualization of the anterior inferior glenoid and pathology cannot be established, an open procedure is recommended.

Mobilization of the Glenoid Labrum and Inferior Glenohumeral Ligament

The labral capsular complex must be elevated so that it floats to the level of the glenoid. Adequate mobilization both anteriorly off the neck of the glenoid as well as inferiorly down to the 6 o'clock position is essential. The adequate release and mobilization of the tissue can be checked in two ways. First, while looking through the posterior portal, the scope can be advanced over the anterior labral rim; if subscapularis fibers are seen, an adequate release has been accomplished. The second way to check is by moving the arthroscope to the anterior superior portal and visualizing inferiorly. If mobilization is not complete capsulorrhaphy, labral repair and tissue shift will be incomplete and may lead to failure.

Glenoid Preparation

The anterior inferior glenoid neck must be debrided with a shaver or burr to a bleeding bed. To ensure that this has been adequately performed, viewing through the anterior superior portal or viewing with a 70-degree scope can be accomplished. A rasp or shaver blade can be used to prepare the inferior capsule. Failure to prepare the bed for soft tissue placement may lead to incomplete healing.

Incorrect Portal Placement

Portal placement is critical to the adequate visualization as well as execution of an arthroscopic anterior inferior stabilization using capsular plication and suture anchors. In establishing the first portal, generally the posterior portal, in the lateral position, it is important to make this slightly more lateral than normal. Obviously, a direct entrance from the posterior skin through the infraspinatus muscle through the capsule is ideal. However, if an error is going to be made, or if the patient is a large person, the portal should be placed more laterally. Medial portal placement in the lateral position will force the arthroscope to be placed at an angle where it has to look over the posterior glenoid. This will make many of the following procedures more difficult. If the surgeon needs to look over the top of the glenoid, a new posterior inferior portal should be established immediately. If the surgeon is worried about extravasation of fluid into the posterior compartment, or fluid dynamics are altered by making a second portal posteriorly, a cannula can be placed in this portal and just not used. This will seal off all potential extravasation of fluid.

When establishing the anterior portals, two important concepts must be maintained. The first is the concept that the two cannulas should be separated as far from each other as possible both internally and externally. This allows for easier passage when shuttling sutures. The second concept is to make sure that the anterior superior portal is not placed into the posterior aspect of the biceps. If it does, care must be taken not to shuttle sutures around, thus locking the proximal biceps tendon in the suture loop.

Suture Anchors

Suture anchor placement should be 2 to 3 mm on the articular margin. Visualization should be maintained as the anchor is inserted. An improper anchor insertion angle can cause articular surface damage or inadequate bone placement, allowing anchor migration and possible articular cartilage damage.

Two types of anchors are available on the market, metal and bioabsorbable. Each has its advantages and disadvantages. Metal anchors can generally be inserted after drilling or punching, thus eliminating a potential step in the process of insertion. Also, these are mechanically stronger, so physical anchor breakage is not as common. The problem sometimes encountered is that in long-term follow-ups, the anchor or cartilage will subside and there may be erosion of the metal anchor on the articular surface.

Bioabsorbable anchors have the advantage of being incorporated into the body over time but have the disadvantage of having various amounts of reactions to this process. They generally require an additional step, which would be a drill or punch, tap, then anchor placement. This can lead to anchor-hole mismatch, which may cause anchor fracture. The advantage of the bioabsorbable anchor at this point is that a second anchor can be placed right on top of the first anchor by either retapping or drilling the original hole. The bioabsorbable anchors also have the advantage of having a suture loop placed inside of them (Arthrex, Bio-FastTac, and BioSutureTac, Naples, FL), in which a suture is embedded into the bioabsorbable anchor. This will allow for consistent sliding of variable sutures.

Suture Shuttling and Knot Tying

A significant amount of frustration can surround passing the suture through the tissue. It is important to make sure that the suture shuttled through the tissue is inferior to the anchor, allowing a superior shift of tissue. This can be done either directly, with a sharp penetrator, by penetrating the tissue, grabbing the sutures, and then pulling the sutures out, or indirectly, with a shuttle system, by using a suture-passing device that passes a monofilament suture into the tissue. This is then retrieved through a cannula, and the suture to be shuttled through is then tied to this and is brought back through the tissue. Tangling and confusion of the sutures can occur at this time, and it is important to be very methodical. Also, anchor unloading can occur at this point. To prevent this, the arthroscope should visualize the anchor directly. If both limbs of the suture are seen moving, then the anchor is being unloaded. This is fine for the initial portion because the loop is pulled out of the cannula.

However, once the loop is out of the cannula, special attention should be paid that no further suture is removed from the anchor. It may be difficult to determine which one this is, so, while looking at the anchor, pull on one limb and, if there is no further movement of the suture through the anchor, then this is the free limb and it can be removed without further concern. For further safety, a hemostat can be placed on the limb that is not sutured, not allowing it to be pulled through the cannula. Although sometimes time-consuming and cumbersome, these small checks can prevent the unfortunate complication of an unloading anchor. If sutures do become tangled intra-articularly (Fig. 1-20), the suture needs to be withdrawn from the joint, pulled out of the cannula, the suture untied, before the process can proceed. If there is not enough room or remaining suture length, a second suture can be tied to the end of the tangled suture, and this can be pulled through, allowing more length of the suture to be untied outside of the cannula and then easily brought back in through the anchor.

There are two classifications of knots that can be tied. The first is the sliding knot; the second, the nonsliding knot. It is not the purpose of this chapter to describe all of the different knots that are available. However, it is important to realize that this is a potential area of difficulty, if the knot prematurely locks or if there is not either knot security or loop security. It is important to observe in the tissue after tying the initial throw that all the excess suture has been taken out of the system and that the knots and loops are indenting the tissue. If this has not been achieved, then the knots should not be locked until this is observed. To avoid twisting of the sutures and loose knots, the knot pusher can be placed on one of the limbs. This is then slid down, and, if there is a twist, it can be untwisted at this time; also, any other abnormalities in the suture can be observed. If a knot prematurely locks or if it is tied and it is not securing the tissue adequately, a second anchor and suture must be placed

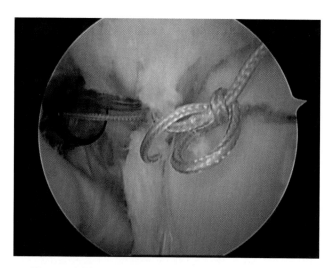

Figure 1-20 Example of suture tangled in the shoulder.

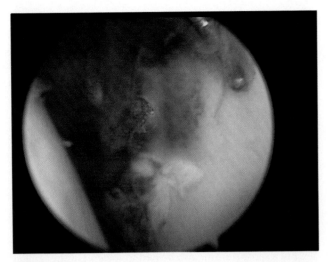

Figure 1-21   Example of labral repair three weeks after arthroscopic repair.

those techniques used in the past. This discussion will attempt to focus on techniques that are similar to what have been described previously. Abrams et al. reported on 662 patients with traumatic anterior instability treated by suture anchor reconstruction techniques with a minimum of a 2-year follow-up. They reported 35 recurrences for a stabilization rate of 95%.[1] Romeo et al. reported on 45 patients with a follow-up of 2 years, with no reports of recurrent dislocation and 96% experiencing good-to-excellent results.[48] In patients at the highest risk, which were high-school contact athletes, specifically football players, Mazzocca et al. reported on 18 collision athletes in high school.[36] They had an average return to contact competition after 6 months and had two subluxation events for a recurrence rate of 15%. It is important to note when evaluating the literature whether recurrences are subluxations that prevent the athletes from returning to their sport versus redislocation. A recurrence is any subluxation event that causes the athlete to lose a day of practice. It is then noted whether they require further stabilization or whether they can return to play unencumbered. The 15% arthroscopic recurrence rate is quite similar to that noted by Uhorchak.[61] Bacilla et al. reported a 10% failure rate with recurrent subluxation in a study population that included 21 American football players.[4] Pagnani et al. reported 52 out of 58 patients returned to full participation in American football for at least one year. They had two patients, with subluxation events, who did not require further treatment.[42]

Current arthroscopic stabilization techniques utilize suture anchors, permanent suture, and address capsular redundancy with plication techniques. The arthroscopic technique now mirrors more closely the open method and, consequently, more recent reports demonstrate results that are comparable. The rates of recurrence (dislocation and

as close to the original knot as possible. A loose knot will never get stronger over time.

Postoperative Glenohumeral Noise

This is an inconsistent physical exam finding that occasionally plagues the postoperative course. Normally, there is a synovialization of the sutures (Fig. 1-21). If this does not happen, a squeak can be detected that may necessitate the removal of the knot after healing has been established.

Overall Operative Failure/Redislocation

Arthroscopic stabilization for anterior inferior instability has evolved over the past 25 years. It is quite difficult to compare redislocation rates and subluxation rates with

TABLE 1-1
ARTHROSCOPIC RECONSTRUCTION USING SUTURE ANCHORS

Author	# of Pt	Mean F/U(mon)	Recurrence (%)	Comments
Wolf (1993)	50	"short"	0	
Belzer (1995)	37	22	11	13%→"Apprehension"
Hoffman (1995)	30	24	11	
Guanche (1996)	25	27	33	Comparative series
Bacilla (1997)	40	30	7	High-demand patients
Sisto (1998)	27	47	13	Refined indications
Field (1999)	50	33	8	Comparative series
Romeo(2000)	32	26	0	3–4 anchors/shoulder
Gartsman (2000)	53	33	8	"Rx all pathology"
Mishra (2001)	42	28	7	RF augmentation
Kim (2002)	58	39	10	Comparative series
Abrams (2002)	61	35	6.6	

SUMMARY: Current techniques can lead to "success" rate greater than 90%.

TABLE 1-2
COMPARISON OF SAME SURGEON ARTHROSCOPIC VS. OPEN STABILIZATION (VARIED TECHNIQUES)

Author	# of Pt Scope/Open	Mean F/U(mo) Scope/Open	Recurrence (%) Scope/Open
Geiger (1993)	16/8	23/24	43/8
Guanche (1996)	25/12	27/25	33/8
Steinbeck (1998)	30/32	36/40	17/6
Field (1999)	50/50	33/30	8/0
Cole (2000)	37/22	52/55	24/18
Karlsson (2001)	66/53	32	15/10
Sperber (2001)	30/26	13/10	23/12
Kim (2002)	30/58	39	10/10

subluxation) results in at-risk collision athletes, and outcomes have been similar with both methods. Table 1-1 and Table 1-2 are a compilation of studies addressing the open-versus-arthroscopic issue.

In cases of recurrent subluxation or recurrent dislocation, either open stabilization for recurrence or arthroscopic stabilization can be performed. In either case, we recommend arthroscopic examination of the glenohumeral joint to assess any or all pathology. If, upon assessment of the intra-articular pathology, there is a recurrent Bankart lesion, or if, in the original surgery, inferior plication and rotator interval closure were not accomplished, there does not seem to be a contraindication to revising with arthroscopic techniques. If in fact this is not the case, and the surgeon along with the patient feel that an open procedure would be more reliable, then this is absolutely indicated at this time as well.

ACKNOWLEDGMENTS

The authors would like to specifically acknowledge the following people for their efforts in preparation of this manuscript. These efforts all go beyond their job description: Anita M. Fowler, Sue Ellen Pelletier, Nancy Ortiz, Sandy Tolisano, Steve Santangelo, Carl W. Nissen, MD, and Joanne D'Aprile. We would also like to acknowledge the residents and fellows at both the University of Connecticut Health Center and Rush-Presbyterian St. Luke's Medical Center for their inspiration.

REFERENCES

1. Abrams JF, Savoie FH, Tauro JC, et al. Recent advances in the evaluation and treatment of shoulder instability: anterior, posterior, and multidirectional. Arthroscopy 2002;18(9):1.
2. Alberta FG, Teruhisa Mihata, McGarry MH, et al. Arthroscopic anteroinferior suture plication results in decreased glenohumeral translation and external rotation in an anterior instability model. Submitted for presentation at the AAOS 2004 Specialty Day, San Francisco, CA, March 13, 2004.
3. Bach BR Jr, Warren RF, Fronek J. Disruption of the lateral capsule of the shoulder: a cause of recurrent dislocation. J Bone Joint Surg Br 1988;70(2):274.
4. Bacilla P, Field LD, Savoie FH. Arthroscopic Bankart repair in a high demand patient population. Arthroscopy 1997;13(1):51.
5. Bankart ASB. The pathology and treatment of recurrent dislocation of the shoulder joint. Br J Surg 1938;26:23.
6. Bigliani LU, Pollack RG, Soslowsky LG. Tensile properties of the inferior glenohumeral ligament. J Orthop Res 1992;10:187.
7. Bigliani LU, Newton PM, Steinmann SP, et al. Glenoid rim fractures associated with a current anterior dislocation of the shoulder. Am J Sports Med 1998;26:41.
8. Bui-Mansfield LT, Taylor DC, Uhorchak JM, et al. Humeral avulsion to the glenohumeral ligament: imaging features in a review of the literature. Am J Roentgenol 2002;179(3):649.
9. Burkhart SS, De Beer JF. Traumatic glenohumeral bone defects and their relationship to failure of arthroscopic Bankart repairs: significance of the inverted pear glenoid and the humeral engaging Hill-Sachs lesion. Arthroscopy 2000;16(7):677.
10. Burkhart SS, DeBeer JF, Tehrany AM, et al. Quantifying glenoid bone loss arthroscopically in shoulder instability. Arthroscopy 2002;18(5):488.
11. Cole BJ, Romeo AA. Arthroscopic shoulder stabilization with suture anchor: technique, technology, and pitfalls. Clin Orthop 2001;390:17.
12. Cole BJ, Rodeo SA, O'Brien SJ, et al. The anatomy and histology of the interval capsule of the shoulder. Clin Orthop 2001;390:129.
13. Cole BJ, Mazzocca AD, Meneghini RM. Indirect arthroscopic rotator interval repair. Arthroscopy 2003;19(6):E28–31.
14. DeBerardino TM, Tenuta JJ, Arciero RA. Combined Bankart and unstable superior labral lesions associated with acute initial anterior shoulder dislocations: evaluation, treatment, and early results. Presented at the 66th annual meeting of the American Academy of Orthopedic Surgeons, Anaheim, CA, February 7, 1999.
15. Ellman H, Gartsman GM. Arthroscopic shoulder surgery and related procedures. Philadelphia, Lea & Febiger, 1993.
16. Fanton GS. Monopolar electrothermal arthroscopy for treatment of shoulder instability in the athlete. In: Drez D, DeLee JC, eds. Operative techniques in sports medicine. vol 8. Philadelphia, WB Saunders, 2000:242.
17. Field LD, Warren RF, O'Brien SJ, et al. Isolated closure of rotator interval defects for shoulder instability. Am J Sports Med 1995;23(5):557.
18. Gartsman GM, Roddey TS, Hammerman SM. Arthroscopic treatment of anterior inferior glenohumeral instability: two- to five-year follow-up. J Bone Joint Surg 2000;82A:991.

19. Gartsman GM, Taverna E, Hammerman SM. Arthroscopic rotator interval repair in glenohumeral instability: description of an operative technique. Arthroscopy 1999;15(3):330.

20. Gohlke F, Essigkrug B, Schmitz F. The pattern of the collagen fiber bundles of the capsule of the glenohumeral joint. J Shoulder Elbow Surg 1994;3:111.

21. Harryman DT, Ballmer FP, Harris SL, et al. Arthroscopic labrum repair to the glenoid rim. Arthroscopy 1994;10:20.

22. Harryman DT, Sidles JA, Harris SL, et al. The role of the rotator interval capsule in passive motion and stability of the shoulder. J Bone Joint Surg 1992;74A:53.

23. Itoi S, Newman SR, Kuechle DK, et al. Dynamic anterior stabilizers of the shoulder with the arm in abduction. J Bone Joint Surg Br 1994;76B:834.

24. Jobe CM. Posterior superior glenoid impingement: expanded spectrum. Arthroscopy 1995;11:530.

25. Jobe FW, Giangarra CE, Kvitne RS, et al. Anterior capsulolabral reconstruction of the shoulder in athletes in overhand sports. Am J Sports Med 1991;19:428.

26. Johnson L. Techniques of anterior glenohumeral ligament repair. In: Johnson L, ed. Arthroscopic surgery: principles and practice. 3rd ed, vol 2. St. Louis, CV Mosby, 1986:1405.

27. Karas SG. Arthroscopic rotator interval repair and anterior portal closure: an alternative technique. Arthroscopy 2002;18:436.

28. Koss S, Richmond JC, Woodward JS. Two- to five-year follow-up of arthroscopic Bankart reconstruction using suture anchor technique. Am Orthop Soc Sports Med 1997;25(6):809.

29. Lephart SM, Warner JP, Borsa PA, et al. Proprioception of the shoulder joint in healthy, unstable, and surgically repaired shoulder. JSES 1994;3(6):371.

30. Lephart SM, Myers JB, Bradley JP, et al. Shoulder proprioception and function following thermal capsulorrhaphy. Arthroscopy 2002;18(7):770.

31. Levitz CL, Dugas J, Andrews JR. The use of arthroscopic thermal capsulorrhaphy to treat internal impingement in baseball players. Arthroscopy 2001;17(6):573.

32. Lintner SA, Speer KE. Traumatic anterior glenohumeral instability: the role of arthroscopy. J Am Acad Orthop Surg 1997;5:233.

33. Lo IK, Burkhart SS. Biomechanical principles of arthroscopic repair of the rotator cuff. In: Romeo AA, Mazzocca AD, eds. Oper Tech Orthop 2002;12(3):152.

34. Matsen FA, Thomas FC, Rockwood CA Jr. Anterior glenohumeral instability. In: Rockwood CA Jr., Matsen FA, eds. The shoulder. 1st ed, vol 1. Philadelphia, JB Lippincott, 1990:526.

35. Matsen FA, Thomas FC, Rockwood CA, et al. Glenohumeral instability. In: Rockwood CA Jr., Matsen FA, eds. The shoulder. 2nd ed, vol 2. Philadelphia, WB Saunders, 1990:633.

36. Mazzocca AD, Brown FM, Carriera DS, et al. Arthroscopic anterior stabilization of collision and contact athletes. Am J Sports Med 2005;33:52–60.

37. Morgan CD, Burkhart SS, Palmeri M, et al. Type II SLAP lesions: three subtypes and their relationships to superior instability and rotator cuff tears. Arthroscopy 1998;14(6):553.

38. Neviaser TJ. The anterior labral ligamentous periosteal sleeve avulsion lesion: a cause of anterior instability of the shoulder. Arthroscopy 1993;9(1):17.

39. Nicola T. Anterior dislocation of the shoulder: the role of the articular capsule. J Bone Joint Surg 1942;25:614.

40. Nobuhara K, Ikeda H. Rotator interval lesion. Clin Orthop 1987;223:44.

41. O'Brien SJ, Neves MC, Arnoczky SP. The anatomy and histology of the inferior glenohumeral ligament complex to the shoulder. Am J Sports Med 1990;18:579.

42. Pagnani MJ, Dome DC. Surgical treatment of traumatic anterior shoulder instability in American football players. J Bone Joint Surg 2002;84A(5):711.

43. Perthes G. Über operationen bei: habitueller schulterlusation. Dtsch Ztschr Chir 1906;85:199.

44. Reeves B. Acute anterior dislocation of the shoulder: clinical and experimental studies. Ann R Coll Surg Engl 1969;44:65.

45. Ribbans WJ, Mitchel R, Taylor JG. Computerized arthrotrography of primary anterior dislocation of the shoulder. J Bone Joint Surg 1990;72B:181.

46. Rodeo SA, Arroczhy SP, Tobilli PA, et al. Tendon healing in a bone tunnel: a biomechanical and histological study in the dog. J Bone Joint Surg 1993;75A(12):1795.

47. Rokous JR, Feagin JA, Abbott HG. Modified axillary roentgenogram. A useful adjunct in the diagnosis of recurrent instability of the shoulder. Clin Orthop 1972;82:84.

48. Romeo AA, Cohen BS, Carreira DF. Traumatic anterior shoulder instability. In: Drez D, DeLee JC, eds. Operative techniques in sports medicine. vol 8. Philadelphia, WB Saunders, 2000:188.

49. Romeo AA, Cole BJ, Mazzocca AD, et al. Autologous chondrocyte repair of an articular defect in the humeral head. Arthroscopy 2002;18(8):925.

50. Rowe CR, Zarins B. Recurrent transient subluxation of the shoulder. J Bone Joint Surg 1981;63:863.

51. Savoie FH, Field LD, Atchinson S. Anterior superior instability with rotator cuff tearing: SLAC lesion. Oper Tech Sports Med 2000;8(3):221.

52. Spear KP, Deng X, Borero S. Biomechanical evaluation of a simulated Bankart lesion. J Bone Joint Surg 1994;76A:1819.

53. Stoller DW. MR arthrography of the glenohumeral joint. Radiol Clin N Am 1997;35(1):97.

54. St Pierre P, Olsen E, Elliott JJ, et al. Tendon healing to cortical bone compared with healing to a cancellous trough. J Bone Joint Surg 1995;77A(12):1858.

55. Sugaya H, Moriishij J, Dohi M, et al. Glenoid rim morphology in recurrent anterior glenohumeral instability. J Bone Joint Surg 2003;85A(5):878.

56. Taylor BC, Arciero RA. Pathologic changes associated with shoulder dislocations. Arthroscopic and physical examination findings in first-time traumatic anterior dislocations. Am J Sports Med 1997;253:306.

57. Tibone JE, Lee TQ, Black Ad, et al. Glenohumeral translation after arthroscopic thermal capsuloplasty. J Shoulder Elbow Surg 2000;9(6):514.

58. Tibone JE, McMahon RJ, Shrader TA, et al. Glenohumeral translation after arthroscopic, nonablative, thermal capsuloplasty with a laser. Am J Sports Med 1998;26:495.

59. Treacy SH, Field LD, Savoie FH. Rotator interval capsule closure: an arthroscopic technique. Arthroscopy 1997;13(1):103.

60. Turkel SJ, Panio MW, Marshall JL. Stabilizing mechanism preventing anterior dislocation of the glenohumeral joint. J Bone Joint Surg 1981;638:1208.

61. Uhorchak JM, Arciero RA, Huggard D, et al. Recurrent shoulder instability after open reconstruction in athletes involved in collision and contact sports. Am J Sports Med 2000;28:794.

62. Uribe JW, Heckman KS, Vijac JE. Arthroscopic Bankart suture repair for recurrent anterior shoulder instability: 51 cases with a minimum two-year follow-up. Arthroscopy 1994;10(3):349.

63. Wolf EM, Cheng JC, Dickson K. Humeral avulsion of glenohumeral ligaments as a cause of anterior shoulder instability. Arthroscopy 1995;11(5):600.

64. Wong KL, Williams GR. Complications of thermal capsulorrhaphy of the shoulder. J Bone Joint Surg 2001;83A(suppl 2):151.

Traumatic Anterior Instability: Open Solutions

2

Philippe H. Clavert   *Peter Millett*   *Jon J. P. Warner*

THE "GOLD STANDARD"

Arthroscopic treatment of instability has evolved into an accepted method used by many surgeons to treat shoulder instability. This treatment method is now the preference for some surgeons because many recent studies have clearly demonstrated that this type of surgical stabilization procedure is the equal of open capsulolabral repair, as long as the patient selection is appropriate and the surgical procedure is performed with skill.[32,78,79,124] Nevertheless, some surgeons choose to treat primary instability with open repair techniques, and, historically, because the success rate with these methods is so proven, it has been called the "Gold Standard."[49,97,134,138]

In the case of primary repair for traumatic anterior shoulder instability, whether performed arthroscopically or openly, careful preoperative determination of relevant pathology is critical to surgical success. In open repair, there are two basic concepts of surgical stabilization: "anatomical" and "nonanatomical." In the former group, the surgical philosophy is to repair the capsulolabral injury with a variant of the Bankart and capsular shift procedures.

Most surgeons are familiar with these methods, some of whom have revised and modified these methods.[4,7,10,49,93,134,138,150,170,178]

In the latter group, the surgeon attempts to compensate for capsulolabral injury and bony injury by using procedures, which include the Bristow,[62] Latarjet,[81] Magnuson-Stack,[96] and Putti-Platt procedures[121], that substitute for these injured structures. A sequela of these procedures has been loss of motion, higher recurrence rate, and, in some cases, acceleration of arthritis.[41,66,74,95,96,101,138] For these reasons, many surgeons in North America tend to avoid them.[49,138,184,186] Nevertheless, many series[2,8,35,92,159] have reported excellent outcome with some of these procedures, and they may be of value in certain revision situations.

This chapter will present the authors' preferred indications for open repair in the treatment of primary recurrent anterior instability as well as in the setting of failed prior surgery.

ANATOMY AND BIOMECHANICS

Mechanisms of Stability: What the Surgeon Should Know

It is important to distinguish "laxity" from "instability." Laxity is an inherent passive quality of the joint required for the large, full range of motion, which permits overhead use of the shoulder in work, recreation, and sports. Instability

P. H. Clavert: Department of Orthopaedic Surgery, Massachusetts General and Brigham and Women's Hospitals, Boston, Massachusetts.
P. Millett: Department of Orthopaedic Surgery, Massachusetts General and Brigham and Women's Hospitals, Boston, Massachusetts.
J. J. P. Warner: Department of Orthopaedic Surgery, Massachusetts General and Brigham and Women's Hospitals, Boston, Massachusetts.

is a dynamic event, which represents the inability of the patient to maintain the humeral head in the glenoid during active shoulder motion.[1,17,19,98,104]

Since the larger humeral head is articulated with a smaller glenoid fossa, the surface contact of the glenohumeral articulation represents only a small portion of the humeral head. Indeed, less than one-third of the humeral head articulates with the glenoid; thus the joint is inherently unstable. Factors that control stability are both dynamic and static and function in combination during all aspects of daily living and sport.[14,33,56,166,167,171]

Many other articles and chapters[31,106,164] have elegantly presented these factors, but they will be briefly listed here from their standpoint of surgical relevance in treatment of recurrent anterior shoulder instability.

Static Stability

Static stability is provided by the bony anatomy of the humeral head and glenoid,[63,76,91,144,145] as well as the cartilage and labrum, which enhance glenoid depth and breadth.[67,91] The glenohumeral joint capsule and its ligaments function as limits to excessive translations and rotations at the end-ranges of joint motion.[1,19,116,155,168]

There is also a joint vacuum effect because a negative pressure is present in the sealed compartment of the shoulder.[53,166] This helps maintain the humeral head on the glenoid when the arm is dependent and adducted at the patient's side.

Dynamic Stability

Dynamic stability is conferred by the rotator cuff and biceps actively contracting during joint motion. An added level of dynamic stability is also provided by coordinated scapulothoracic motion during glenohumeral motion. This positions the glenoid underneath the humeral head and is important in limiting forces, which might otherwise add to shoulder instability.[33,77,85,171] This concept is presented further in the chapter on scapular winging due to serratus anterior palsy.

It is very important to understand that static and dynamic factors work together to maintain stability. One example of this is the concept of "Concavity-Compression," described by Lippitt et al.[91] Contraction of the rotator cuff and biceps provide a force that compresses a convex humeral head into a glenoid-labrum articulation with a matched concavity. This may be one of the most important mechanisms of stability during forceful overhead use of the arm.[166] As noted previously, proper scapular rotation is imperative to position the glenoid underneath the humeral head to provide a platform on which the humeral head may rotate (Fig. 2-1).

Another mechanism in which static and dynamic factors work together is afferent feedback provided by proprioceptive nerve endings in the joint capsule and tendons, which

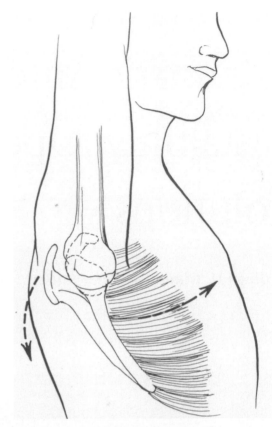

Figure 2-1 Proper scapular rotation while the arm is forward flexed. (Drawing from Kuhn JE, Hawkins RJ. Evaluation and treatment of scapular disorder. In: Warner JJP, Iannotti JP, Gerber C, eds. Complex and revision problems in shoulder surgery. 1st ed. Philadelphia, Lippincott-Raven, 1997.)

modulate muscular contraction so that the joint is actively splinted against excessive translation during overhead shoulder motions.[86,87]

Mechanisms of Instability: What the Surgeon Should Know

Just as normal shoulder stability is an interplay between multiple factors, dynamic and static, instability occurs when the stabilizing structures fail; and this may often involve more than one anatomical structure. Indeed, many studies have observed that instability cannot occur without a combination of dynamic and static failure.[5,9,12,146] When traumatic anterior instability occurs, this is usually a sudden explosive event that exceeds the strength of the capsulolabral structures and dynamic stabilizing effect of the intrinsic muscles around the joint. This may be due to a sudden force applied when the ligamentous structures are taught and the muscles are momentarily at a mechanical disadvantage or unable to contract fast enough to splint the joint.[17] The result is usually a Bankart lesion; however, many surgeons believe that there is also a significant plastic deformation or stretch of the anterior and inferior joint capsule.[3,9,125,146,163,164,169] Clinically, the degree of plastic deformation is hard to assess. Lippitt et al.,[90] in an in vitro study, found no difference in laxity between patients with or without glenohumeral instability.

In the majority of cases, a capsulolabral repair can be performed by either arthroscopic or open methods, and many surgeons have accepted the concept of not only repairing the Bankart lesion but also performing some kind of controlled capsular shift as well to deal with capsular stretch.

The rotator interval is the region between the cranial border of the subscapularis tendon and the anterior edge of the supraspinatus.[29,30,55,73] The capsular components of this region include the superior and *middle glenohumeral* ligaments as well as the coracohumeral ligament.[14,119] The chapter on multidirectional instability will consider management of capsular lesions and laxity of this portion of the capsule; however, capsular deficiency here has been recognized in the setting of anterior instability.[4,10,108,136,170] It is likely that capsular deficiency in this region may be due to a combination of constitutional development (dysplasia of capsular structures) and recurrent trauma with stretching. In any case, when present as a defect, this portion of the capsule should be closed.

Less commonly, pathology may be present in addition to capsulolabral injury, which is significant in recurrence of instability. The relevance of this other pathology is that it may mandate an open treatment approach because anatomical repair using arthroscopic methods cannot restore adequate biomechanical stability. These lesions include glenoid rim fracture,[11,128,149,169] glenoid erosion from recurrent instability,[11,20,37,72,149,177] capsular rupture and capsular insufficiency after multiple failed surgeries,[69,105,126,174] huge Hill-Sachs lesions[20,182] (usually in combination with anterior glenoid erosion), and the so-called humeral avulsion of the glenohumeral ligament (HAGL) lesion.[16,141,163,180] Management of each case scenario is discussed in the following text; however, the biomechanical relevance of each is briefly presented here.

Bony Lesions of the Anterior Glenoid

Either an acute traumatic anterior dislocation or recurrent anterior dislocations can cause an associated fracture or erosion of the glenoid rim. The consequence of such an injury is disruption of the normal Concavity-Compression mechanism of joint stability, discussed previously. In effect, the socket of the glenoid looses both its breadth and its depth. Howell and Galinat[67] demonstrated that the glenoid socket is enhanced by the labrum and cartilage height, and Lippitt et al.[91] demonstrated that this is important for glenohumeral stability (Fig. 2-2). Although Burkhart and DeBeer[20] have provided clinical evidence for the consequence of missing this pathology, it seems that most literature has not considered this important factor for

glenohumeral stability. Burkhart and DeBeer described the "inverted pear"[20] appearance of the glenoid at time of arthroscopy (Fig. 2-3) and found that the recurrence rate of arthroscopic Bankart repair was greater than 80% in contact athletes. They recommended a Latarjet procedure to treat these kinds of patients.

Several other authors[20,71] have noted the incidence of anterior glenoid rim erosion being significant in cases of recurrent anterior instability; however, the exact threshold of bone loss, which requires bony restoration of the joint, was not clarified. More recently, Gerber et al.[48] provided a quantitative method for determining biomechanically relevant anterior glenoid rim defects (Fig. 2-4). In cases where we suspect glenoid erosion or fracture, we image the shoulder to determine whether such pathology is present and relevant to treatment. This approach is described in the following text.

Large Hill-Sachs lesions, which contribute to shoulder instability, are rare. These are usually associated with chronic locked dislocations and accompany an associated anterior glenoid erosion (Fig. 2-5). This pathology requires open stabilization and is considered in the chapter on chronic locked dislocations.

Associated Rotator Cuff Tears

An associated rotator cuff tear can occur with traumatic anterior dislocation and usually occurs in individuals more than 40 years old.[140] In the case where this is a tear of the supraspinatus, many surgeons will treat these arthroscopically at the same time that they repair the capsuloligamentous injury arthroscopically; however, complete tears of the subscapularis tendon may be difficult to repair arthroscopically for most surgeons.[22] Furthermore, subscapularis insufficiency must be carefully assessed in individuals who have recurrent instability after a failed open anterior repair. In such cases, open surgical repair of the disrupted tendon is appropriate, in addition to capsulolabral repair.

HAGL Lesions

This injury was first recognized and reported as a case report by Bach et al.[6] Subsequently, Wolf[180] described the arthroscopic identification of this capsular lesion. Bigliani et al.[13] studied the pattern of capsular failure with instability and found that a small percentage of experimental traumatic instability is associated with avulsion of the humeral insertion of the inferior glenohumeral ligament and middle glenohumeral ligament. Warner[163] and Savoie[39] have also recognized the combination of a humeral avulsion of the insertion of the inferior glenohumeral ligament in combination with a concomitant Bankart lesion (Fig. 2-6). Although some surgeons may attempt to repair this HAGL lesion arthroscopically, most prefer open reinsertion of the capsule on the neck of the humerus.

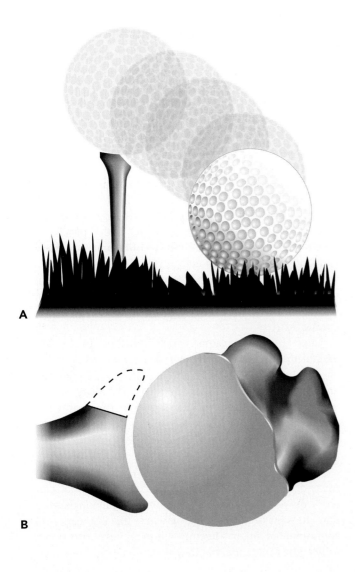

A

B

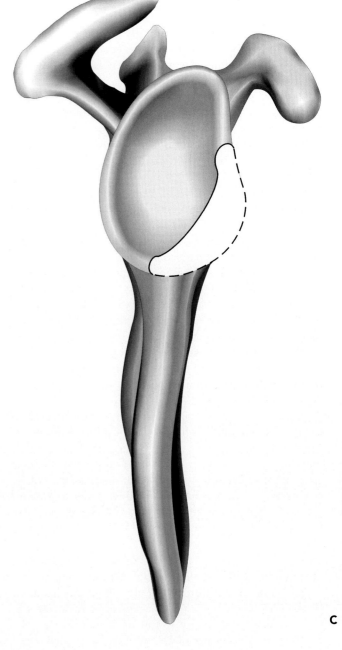

C

Figure 2-2 (*A*) A glenoid erosion is like a broken golf tee, which allows the golf ball (humeral head) to fall off of it. (*B*) A typical severe glenoid erosion results in loss of the anteroinferior glenoid (*dotted line*) and gives the appearance of an inverted pear on the oblique sagittal orientation of the glenoid. (*C*) A significant anterior glenoid erosion is shown in the axial plane (*dotted line*).

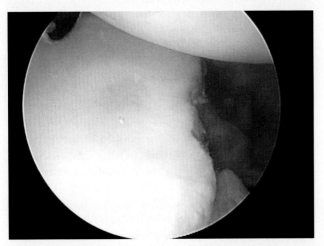

Figure 2-3 An arthroscopic view from the anterior-superior portal-shows the anterior-inferior glenoid rim erosion corresponding to Figures 2-2, *A* and *B*.

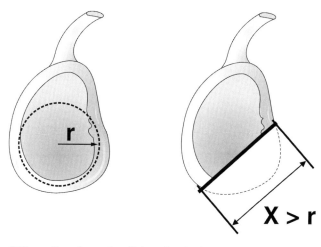

If X > r, then force for dislocation is decreased by 70%

Figure 2-4 Drawing showing the biomechanical consequences of an anterior-inferior glenoid erosion. If X > r, then the force necessary for an anterior dislocation to occur is decreased from 70% over the normal intact glenohumeral joint. (Adapted from Gerber C, Nyffeler RW: Classification of glenohumeral joint instability. Clin Orthop 2002;400:65.)

Capsular Rupture

Acute capsular rupture can occasionally occur with traumatic anterior dislocations, but it is quite rare. Bigliani et al.,[13] in their experimental instability study, noted this occurrence in only a few cases of anterior dislocation. Occasionally, arthroscopic inspection may demonstrate capsular rupture in some cases of traumatic instability (Fig. 2-7). However, this rare pathology is mostly encountered in the setting of instability after many prior failed repairs, and sometimes after failed thermal capsular shift (Fig. 2-7). In this latter case, it is believed that the capsule is severely damaged by thermal necrosis and then fails with recurrent anterior instability.[181] Open surgical repair is required in these cases, which is discussed in the following text.

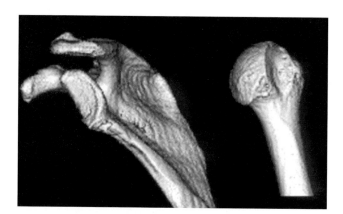

Figure 2-5 A three-dimensional computed tomography (CT) scan reconstruction demonstrating a severe anterior glenoid erosion (*left*) and a corresponding large Hill-Sachs lesion (*right*).

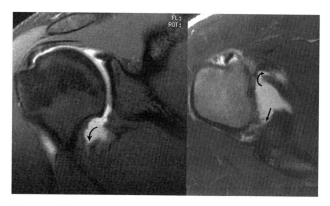

Figure 2-6 A magnetic imaging resonance (MRI) arthrogram demonstrating a BHAGL lesion (Bankart humeral avulsion of the glenohumeral ligament). The coronal view (*right*) shows the humeral avulsion (*curved arrow*) and the axial view shows the humeral avulsion (*curved arrow*) as well as the Bankart lesion (*open arrow*).

PATIENT SELECTION FOR OPEN REPAIR

As described previously, careful preoperative determination of pathology is critical in selecting the best method of treatment.[20,153,163] Burkhart and DeBeer's[20] observation of such a high rate of recurrent anterior instability, when a glenoid erosion was missed, is evidence supporting this statement.

History

The history given by the patient can often give clues as to the pathology, which may be present. For example, a patient who described a traumatic event as the initial cause of instability and then multiple recurrences with lesser degrees of trauma or no trauma, should be suspected of having severe capsular laxity or loss of anterior glenoid through either fracture or erosion.

The complaint of instability developing by simply placing the arm in a position of abduction should suggest the possibility of constitutional laxity. This concept is discussed further in the chapter on multidirectional instability. Complaint of instability with the arm at the side may be consistent with a rotator interval lesion and multidirectional instability as well.

In some instances, the patient may report a fall with loss of memory but without documented seizure activity. In such cases, a neurological cause should be suspected, and proper consultation with a neurologist is appropriate.

Physical Examination

A detailed discussion of the shoulder examination for instability is beyond the scope and purpose of this chapter. Many other chapters[3,99,100] in other textbooks have dealt with this topic, and there are many videos[173] available on the subject. Several important findings should be highlighted, however.

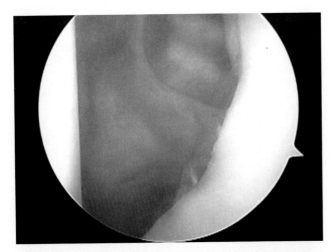

Figure 2-7 Arthroscopic view of an anterior capsular rupture viewed with an arthroscope through the posterior portal. The subscapularis muscle is clearly seen through the area where the anterior capsule has torn.

The first step of any physical examination should be an adequate neuromuscular assessment because axillary nerve injury is not uncommon with traumatic anterior instability. Moreover, loss of axillary nerve sensation may not be an accurate representation of nerve injury, so it is important to assess motor strength carefully. External rotation strength may be weak due to either an associated rotator cuff tear or a rare suprascapular nerve injury. Visual inspection may also detect atrophy from either rotator cuff tear or nerve injury. In some patients this can be quite subtle.

In the case of documented anterior dislocation, the physical exam should focus on determining other lesions, such as rotator cuff and superior labrum lesions, but it is not necessary to forcefully externally rotate the abducted arm to elicit apprehension. Indeed, dislocation can be caused by such an examination. Assessing active and passive motion, mechanical symptoms, such as catching, and patterns of pain are important. For example, marked weakness of active forward flexion may indicate a rotator cuff tear, and the classic findings of a subscapularis tendon disruption include painful passive external rotation, increased passive external rotation of the adducted shoulder, weak internal rotation, a positive lift-off and belly press sign.[46,47] O'Brien[117] has described a sign felt to be sensitive for an associated superior labrum injury, pain felt with resisted flexion of the pronated hand but not of the supinated hand. We and others[64,148] have found this to be sensitive but not specific for superior labrum tears.

In cases where subtle anterior instability is suspected, when there has not been a documented episode of dislocation, the apprehension and relocation tests are valuable.[147] Most surgeons understand how to perform these tests. We perform this test with the patient supine and the arm slowly brought into abduction, external rotation, and extension. Posterior pressure is then applied to the humerus when the patient becomes apprehensive. Speer[147] has

shown that true apprehension, not simply pain, is required for this test to be specific as well as sensitive.

Inferior laxity is always assessed as well; however, we have found that in an office setting, patients often guard against pain by contracting their muscles, making it difficult to truly assess symptomatic instability. Nevertheless, an observable inferior translation of the humeral head, when the adducted arm is pulled inferiorly, suggests inferior instability, which is the hallmark of multidirectional instability.[108,109] If such inferior laxity and symptoms are observed when the arm is in external rotation as well, this suggests pathologic laxity of the rotator interval capsular region.[27,38,61,150,156,175]

Imaging

Plain Radiographs

Orthogonal views of the shoulder are very important to document the direction of instability and to look for relevant osseous lesions. A standard trauma series, which we employ, consists of a true anterior-posterior view of the glenohumeral joint with the shoulder in internal and external rotation, an axillary view (standard or West Point), and a Stryker-Notch view.[123,129,130] The combination of these views has been shown to be very accurate for detecting glenoid fractures and Hill-Sachs lesions[123] (Fig. 2-5). The appearance of static anterior subluxation of the

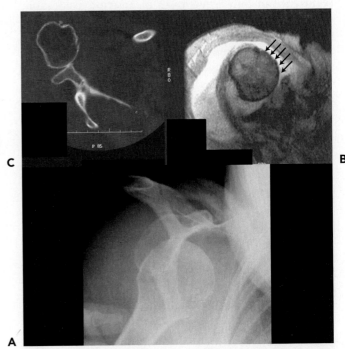

Figure 2-8 Subscapularis rupture in association with an anterior glenohumeral dislocation. (*A*) The plain x-ray demonstrates an anterior, subcoracoid dislocation. (*B*) The MRI shows a fixed anterior subluxation of the humeral head on the glenoid and absence of any subscapularis tendon (*arrows*). (*C*) The CT scan shows a fixed anterior subluxation of the humeral head on the glenoid.

humeral head on the axillary radiograph should suggest severe disruption of the glenoid concavity or a subscapularis rupture (Fig. 2-8). In some cases, an associated anatomic neck fracture or greater tuberosity fracture, which is not displaced, may be identified as well (Fig. 2-9). Furthermore, inferior dislocation of the adducted humerus, the so-called subglenoid dislocation, has a high association with rotator cuff tears (Fig. 2-10).

Three-Dimensional Imaging

If the surgeon considers the range of pathology described previously, it will be impossible to detect all lesions simply using two-dimensional plain radiographs. In all cases, we perform additional imaging to better visualize the three-dimensional nature of the injury. This is either by magnetic resonance imaging (MRI) or by computed tomography (CT).

Magnetic resonance imaging is ordered with intra-articular gadolinium in cases where a capsulolabral injury is suspected. Bankart lesions and superior labrum anterior posterior lesions (SLAP) may be accurately identified, but, occasionally, HAGL lesions and capsular ruptures are also identified (Fig. 2-6). Furthermore, anterior glenoid fractures and erosions may also be seen (Fig. 2-11); however, we do not feel that quantitative assessment of the degree of bone loss is always accurate with this method. Moreover, in the case of failed prior surgery where metal or absorbable anchors have been placed in the anterior glenoid, artifact signal may obscure the degree of glenoid injury (Fig. 2-12). In cases where an anterior glenoid lesion and/or a large Hill-Sachs lesion are suspected, we obtain a CT-arthrogram.[51,70,80,143]

A CT-arthrogram will accurately define the glenoid articular surfaces because the dye will outline cartilaginous erosion (Fig. 2-13). In some circumstances, a three-dimensional reconstruction can give more accurate representation of the degree of osseous injury.

Method for Assessing Anterior Glenoid Erosion

Gerber et al.[48] have demonstrated a method of measuring either oblique sagittal images of the glenoid surface or three-dimensional reconstructions of the glenoid surface (Fig. 2-4). In this method, if the length of the glenoid defect exceeds the maximum radius of the glenoid, then the force required for anterior dislocation is reduced by 70% from an intact glenoid. In such cases, a standard Bankart repair is likely to fail, and some kind of bony augmentation is recommended.

Radiographic evaluation should include plain radiographs. Magnetic resonance imaging or CT with contrast can demonstrate labral tears, capsular injuries, or bony deficiencies. Patients with concomitant glenoid fractures, large Hill-Sachs lesions, or bony erosions will benefit from three-dimensional reconstruction of the glenoid for preoperative planning. These imaging studies are also needed to

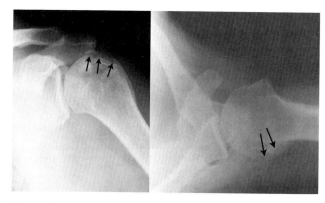

Figure 2-9 A greater tuberosity fracture is observed (*arrows*) after an anterior shoulder dislocation that has been reduced.

identify coexisting pathology (i.e., rotator cuff tears), the degree of capsular laxity, and the extent of labral pathology preoperatively so that the appropriate surgical procedure can be selected and planned.[51,70] Computed tomography is preferred if osseous pathology is suspected.

INDICATIONS AND CONTRAINDICATIONS FOR OPEN ANTERIOR STABILIZATION—AUTHORS' PREFERENCE

In most cases, traumatic anterior instability is associated with a Bankart lesion with some degree of associated capsular stretch. In these cases, we prefer to perform arthroscopic capsulolabral repair. This surgical technique is discussed in another chapter. In some cases where there is constitutional laxity and prior arthroscopic surgery has failed, we then perform an open capsular shift. In cases

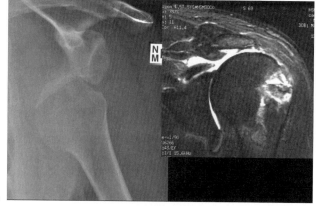

A   B

Figure 2-10 (*A*) A subglenoid dislocation is often associated with a massive rotator cuff tear. (*B*) The MRI demonstrates after reduction of the dislocation that there is a massive rotator cuff tear (superior displacement of the humeral head), which in this case is due to an anterosuperior tear involving the subscapularis and supraspinatus tendons.

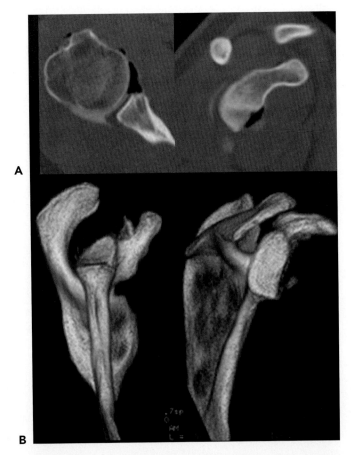

A

B

Figure 2-11   (*A*) A severe anterior glenoid rim erosion is demonstrated on standard axial CT and oblique-sagittal reconstruction as well (*B*) as on a three-dimensional reconstruction.

where there is significant anterior glenoid erosion, according to the criteria described previously, we perform an osseous reconstruction. In rare cases, when we feel a huge Hill-Sachs lesion is playing a role in instability recurrence, open surgery is performed as well. When there is a signifi-

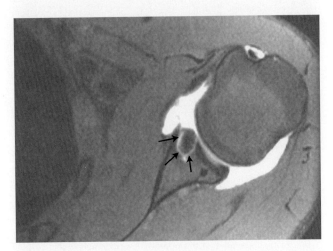

Figure 2-12   An artifact due to an anterior anchor in the glenoid (*arrows*) obscures articular anatomy on this MRI arthrogram.

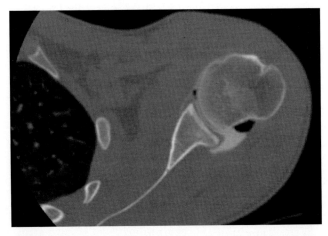

Figure 2-13   A CT-arthrogram of a normal joint demonstrates congruity of the articular surfaces with a normal concavity-convexity match.

cant disruption of the subscapularis, usually in the setting of prior surgery, an open repair is performed.

In cases of concomitant severe arthritis, open instability repair may not be effective. Depending on the status of the osseous glenoid and surrounding rotator cuff, arthroplasty or arthrodesis may be more appropriate. Paralysis may also be associated with chronic instability and, in such cases, arthrodesis may be more successful in eliminating pain.[26,36,50,132]

Other absolute contraindications for open repair of anterior instability are voluntary instability[57,89,135] and the presence of active infection.

OPERATING ROOM SETUP AND PATIENT POSITIONING

Once surgery has been elected, it is prerequisite for success to have the appropriate retractors, implants, and assistants to accomplish the task. It should not be taken for granted that some revision cases and surgical procedures on large individuals may require an additional assistant. We prefer to place the patient in a semi-sitting position, the so-called beach-chair position, with the head of the bed at about 30 degrees of elevation. This can be accomplished by using either a special beach-chair device (Fig. 2-14) or a long bean-bag, which can be contoured to effectively position the patient. The shoulder should be completely free for full rotation, with the anterior and posterior shoulder girdle exposed. If a bone graft is required from the anterior iliac crest, this region is elevated by placing a towel roll underneath the hip. We also prefer to use an articulated arm holder because we have found this to be invaluable for consistent positioning (Fig. 2-15); it also eliminates the need for an additional assistant.

The retractors we find useful are a self-retaining deltopectoral retractor (Innovasive-Mitek, Marlborough, MA), a deltoid retractor (Browne Retractor, Innomed, Savannah, GA), a humeral head retractor (Fukuda Retractor, Innomed, Savannah, GA), modified Cobra retractors (Synthes, Paoli, PA), Hawkins and Bell retractors (Black Handle retractors) (DePuy Inc., Warsaw, IN), and an assortment of osteotomes (Fig. 2-16).

EXAM UNDER ANESTHESIA

Prior to beginning surgery, it is imperative to document passive motion and patterns of laxity, because this can define associated adhesions from prior surgery as well as the extent of capsular laxity. Furthermore, degree and direction of instability may be confirmed. Several authors have emphasized the value of such testing.[27,38,61,150,175] Laxity is graded using a scale of 0−3+, where 0 = no translation; 1+ = translation to the edge of the glenoid; 2+ = translation over the glenoid rim but spontaneous reduction when force is released from the arm; and 3+ = frank dislocation with locking of the humeral head over the glenoid rim.[4] Although side-to-side comparisons are considered helpful for determining the degree of instability, the reliability of such testing has been drawn into question by some surgeons.[54,176] Nevertheless, several important findings should be noted.

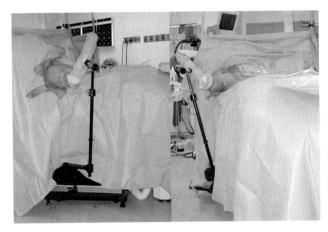

Figure 2-15 One type of mechanical arm holder (McConnell Arm Holder, McConnell Co., Greenville, TX).

Marked inferior laxity with the arm adducted and externally rotated will correlate to either dysplasia (marked underdevelopment) or aplasia (no capsule) of the rotator interval capsular region (Fig. 2-17). A shoulder that rests out of the glenoid and requires a force to reduce it, but won't remain reduced, suggests either interposed soft-tissue or loss of the anterior bony glenoid.

ANATOMIC CAPSULOLABRAL REPAIR: OPEN BANKART AND CAPSULAR SHIFT REVISITED

Open Bankart and capsular shift procedures have been modified by many surgeons, with excellent results reported by most.[28,49,134,170] In most cases, the success rate in the treatment of traumatic recurrent anterior instability exceeds 92%. Indeed, this is the basis for the "Gold Standard" as-

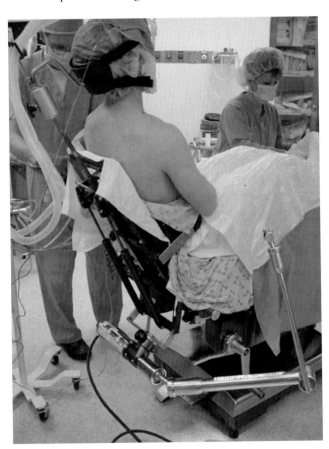

Figure 2-14 Beach Chair positioning device (Tenet Medical T-Max and Spider Arm Holder, Tenet Medical Engineering, Calgary, Canada).

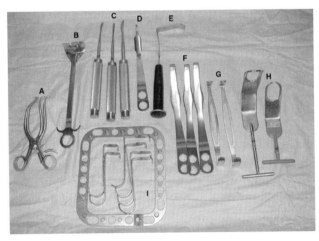

Figure 2-16 Retractors used for open instability surgery (*A:* gelpi; *B:* deltoid retractor; *C:* Cobb elevators; *D:* Spiky Homan; *E:* Hawkins and Bell retractors; *F:* modified Cobra retractors; *G:* Army navy retractor; *H:* humeral head retractor; *I:* self-retaining deltopectoral retractor).

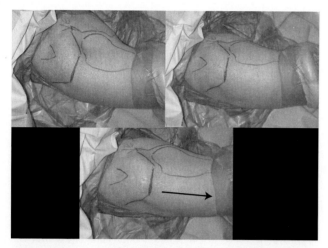

Figure 2-17 Examination under anesthesia is performed for anterior instability (*top two figures*). With an anterior drawer the humeral head is displaced out of the glenoid (*upper right figure*). A sulcus sign is demonstrated in the lower figure as a space between the acromion and humeral head with a downward pull (*arrow*) on the adducted arm.

sertion applied to these open repair techniques, All of these procedures have the common goal of restorating normal anatomy. The labrum is reattached to its anatomic position at the anterior articular margin of the joint, and the capsule is shifted to reestablish adequate tension while preserving sufficient laxity for joint rotation.[7,133]

Authors' Preferred Method of Capsulolabral Repair: The Selective Capsular Shift

The concept of a "Selective Capsular Shift" is based on the observation that the capsuloligamentous static stabilizers function at extreme positions of rotation as checkreins to excessive rotation and translation.[170] The Bankart lesion is anatomically repaired and the capsule is shifted in a manner that preserves physiological laxity so that overconstraint of the joint is avoided.

The patient is positioned as described previously, and an incision is made in the anterior axillary line. We have found it helpful to use an articulated arm holder and maintain the arm slightly abducted and forward flexed anterior to the plane of the body because this allows the deltoid and deeper soft-tissues to be sufficiently lax for easier dissection (Fig. 2-15). If the patient is very thin, the incision can be kept quite inferior in a skin crease in the axilla to provide best cosmesis. In more muscular or obese patients, the incision is carried up to the coracoid process to ensure adequate exposure. Dissection then proceeds in a layer-by-layer fashion with meticulous hemostasis. Subcutaneous undermining of the skin allows enlargement of the incision, which can be very helpful in revision situations. The deltopectoral interval is identified and the cephalic vein retracted laterally with the deltoid. Care is taken to open this interval proximally above the coracoid process because it will allow broader exposure for the deeper portion of the dissection and also take tension off the deltoid during retraction (Fig. 2-18). A self-retaining retractor is placed at this point to retract the deltoid from the pectoralis (Fig. 18). The clavipectoral fascia is identified, and the interval between the conjoined tendon and the subscapularis is sharply defined. A long thin retractor (Hawkins-Bell Black Handle) is then placed underneath the conjoined tendon, and a narrow Hohman retractor is placed over the coracoacromial ligament (Fig. 2-19). The circumflex vessels are identified and ligated with suture ligatures. The subscapularis is then removed from the underlying capsule. It is helpful to place a cobra retractor over the upper border of the subscapularis tendon. The tendon usually comes over the cranial portion of the humeral head and pushes the humeral head inferiorly. There is usually a thin region above the tendon corresponding to the rotator interval capsular area, and, in some cases, this capsular region is deficient. The subscapularis is removed using a needle-tip electrocautery, being careful to start about 2 cm medial to the lesser tuberosity (Fig. 2-20). The capsule is normally inti-

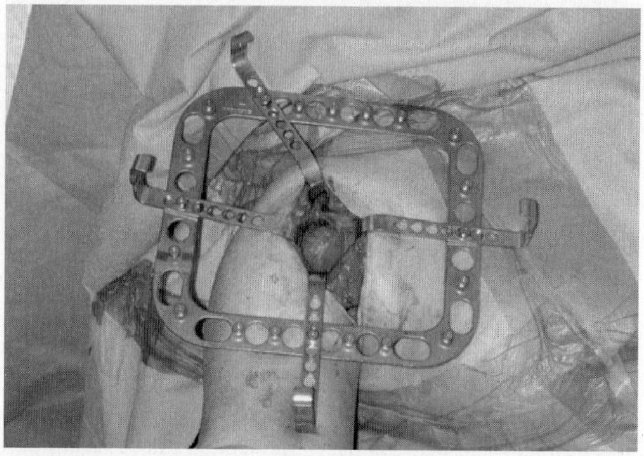

Figure 2-18 Opening of the deltopectoral interval. Deltoid and pectoralis major muscle are retracted with a self-retaining retractor.

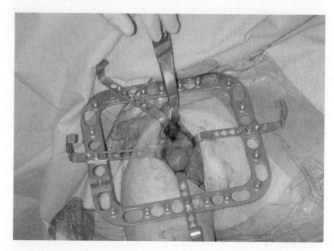

Figure 2-19 Homan retractor over the coracoacromial ligament.

mately conjoined with the subscapularis tendon superiorly and laterally for only a centimeter or so, so that this dissection becomes more defined as one moves medially. In cases of revision surgery, however, the dissection may be more difficult due to adhesions. It is often easier to elevate the subscapularis from the capsule inferiorly, where there is mainly a muscular attachment of the subscapularis. We use a sharp Cobb elevator, Metzenbaum scissors, and a needle-tip electrocautery. The subscapularis is then tagged with No. 2 braided, nonabsorbable sutures.

In revision cases where there may be significant scarring, and in such cases where the subscapularis tendon is also torn, it is imperative to define the axillary nerve. We do so by placing a long thin retractor (Hawkins-Bell Black Handle retractor) inferiorly and maintaining tension on the subscapularis laterally. It may also be easier to define the axillary nerve once the capsulotomy has been performed and the humeral head can be retracted posteriorly. The axillary nerve will be found medial to the anterior humeral circumflex vessels, which may actually form a leash over it. The nerve is elevated on a right angle clamp, and a vessel loupe is placed around it. It can then be protected during the remainder of the procedure (Fig. 2-20).

The capsulotomy can be performed in a variety of ways. It is our preference to do so by opening the rotator interval region. This area is often deficient. The capsule is then removed along the neck of the humerus, leaving a 5- to 10-mm cuff of tissue intact on the humeral neck for repair later. Thus, an inverted-L capsulotomy is performed (Figs. 2-21, 2-22). The capsule is removed inferiorly off the neck of the humerus to the 6 o'clock position. The subscapularis muscle is cleared off inferiorly with an elevator, and a cobra may help expose the humeral head inferiorly.

Bankart Lesion Repair

The anterior glenoid rim is exposed by placing a Fukuda humeral head retractor into the joint to retract the humeral head posteriorly. A cobra retractor is placed over the glenoid rim and inside the capsule. In doing so, the capsule can be folded back, exposing the labrum attachment. If there is a Bankart lesion, the capsuloperiosteal sleeve is elevated using a curved quarter-inch osteotome. Stripping the periosteum medially enlarges the Bankart lesion, allowing for better exposure of the glenoid rim. The Bankart lesion is also often partially healed so such stripping of periosteum may be necessary. The glenoid rim is exposed from just below the coracoid process to the 6 o'clock position. The glenoid rim is then abraded with an osteotome or a burr. Usually, three anchors are placed along the glenoid rim. These are positioned at the 6, 4, and 2 o'clock positions for a right glenoid, carefully positioned so that they are just over the articular margin (Fig. 2-21). This ensures that the capsule and labrum will be attached directly at its anatomic site on the articular margin. We prefer to use push in anchors, which are absorbable and have at least two No. 2 braided, nonabsorbable sutures on them. Thus, a total of three anchors and six sutures are used for the Bankart repair. Shea et al.[142] have shown that two sutures per anchor result in an overall capsulolabral repair, which has greater ultimate failure strength than simply one suture per anchor.

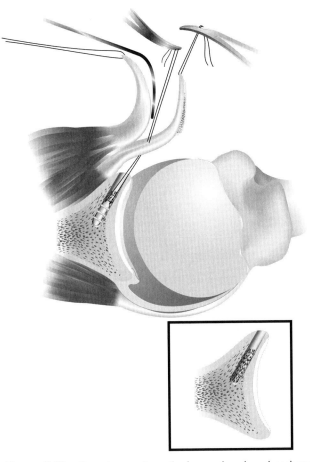

Figure 2-21 Capsulotomy from the humeral neck and anchors placement on the anterior glenoid rim. (Drawing from Ticker JB, Warner JJP. The selective capsular shift for anterior glenohumeral instability. In: Fu FH, Ticker JB, Imhoff AB. An atlas of shoulder surgery. London, Martin Duniz, 1998:8.)

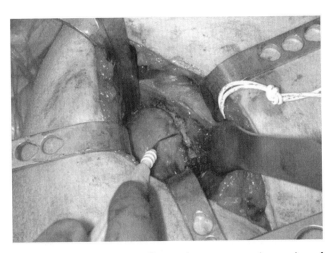

Figure 2-20 Using a needle tip electrocautery, the tendon of the subscapularis muscle is cut.

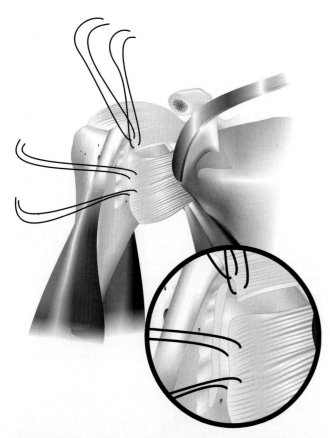

Figure 2-22 T-shape capsulotomy. (Drawing from Ticker JB, Warner JJP. The selective capsular shift for anterior glenohumeral instability. In: Fu FH, Ticker JB, Imhoff AB. An atlas of shoulder surgery. London, Martin Duniz, 1998:8.)

A cobra retractor is then placed over the anterior scapula in the interval between the capsule and the subscapularis so that the latter is retracted medially. Each suture is then brought through the capsule and labrum in a horizontal mattress fashion so that an inside-out anatomic reattachment of the Bankart lesion is performed (Fig. 2-21). The selective capsular shift is then performed.

Selective Capsular Shift

The selective capsular shift is based on the anatomic observation that the inferior glenohumeral ligament is closest to its maximum length when the shoulder is abducted and externally rotated, while the superior capsular region is maximally lengthened when the shoulder is externally rotated and adducted (Fig. 2-23).[167,170]

The inferior capsular flap is first shifted superiorly and laterally. Once the Fukuda humeral head retractor has been removed, the arm is positioned with the mechanical arm holder in 20 degrees of forward flexion and approximately 45 degrees of abduction, with 45 degress of external rotation (Fig. 2-23). In this position, the humeral head will sit reduced on the glenoid. This position can be changed according to concern for maintaining motion. For example, in an overhead athlete, such as a baseball pitcher, external rotation would be increased to close to 90 degrees. The

neck of the humerus is abraded with an osteotome or burr. An absorbable anchor appropriate for humeral bone with two No. 2 braided, nonabsorbable sutures is then placed along the inferior neck of the humerus because there is usually little tissue here for reattachment of the capsule. The capsule is then repaired along the humeral neck using this anchor as well as the cuff of tissue remaining superiorly.

The superior capsular shift is then performed. The rotator interval closure is performed with the arm held in adduction and external rotation. The degree of external rotation should be similar to what is normal for the patient on the contralateral side, typically 20 to 60 degrees. The inferior capsular flap is then closed over the superior capsule, thus reinforcing the rotator interval region (Fig. 2-23).

The subscapularis is then closed anatomically to its insertion using a Mason-Allen stitch and anchors where

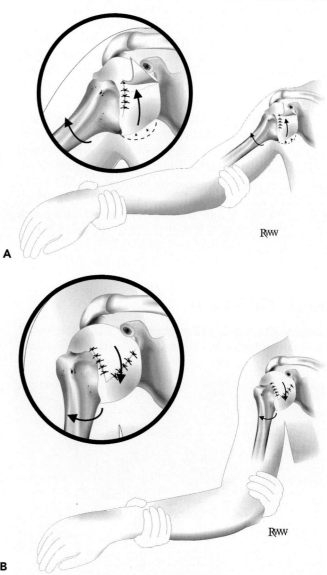

Figure 2-23 Selective capsular shift. (*A*) Interior shift. (*B*) Superior shift. (Drawing from Ticker JB, Warner JJP. The selective capsular shift for anterior glenohumeral instability. In: Fu FH, Ticker JB, Imhoff AB. An atlas of shoulder surgery. London, Martin Duniz, 1998:8.)

needed. The remainder of the incision is closed in layers, and the skin is closed using a subcuticular running stitch of absorbable suture and then steristrips. The shoulder is dressed sterilely; we prefer to use Tegaderm (3M Health Care, St. Paul, MN) for a water occlusive dressing.

In most patients, prior to incision closure, a pain catheter that administers 0.25% bupivacaine 2 cc/hour for 48 hours is inserted through a separate point through the deltoid and into the wound (Painbuster, Donjoy, Vista, CA). We have found this treatment useful for postoperative pain control. In addition to a padded shoulder immobilizer (Ultrasling, Donjoy, Vista, CA), we also prefer to use a cold compressive device (Cryocuff, Aircast, Boca Raton, FL).

Postoperative Program

The shoulder immobilizer is worn for 4 weeks, though the patient is permitted to remove it to go in the shower each day. Until the sutures are removed at 10 days, an occlusive dressing is maintained over the incision. Afterward, the patient is encouraged to go in the shower and perform pendulum exercises each day. Elbow motion is permitted as long as the arm remains against the side, allowing the patient to eat and type on a computer with the repaired arm. After 4 weeks, the immobilizer is removed and active-assisted exercises are begun under a physical therapist's supervision. Physical therapy is directed at recovering glenohumeral motion and scapulothoracic motion. Aquatherapy, if available, is commenced, and the patient is encouraged to actively stretch in the zero gravity environment. After 4 weeks, the patient is permitted to use the arm for all daily living activities. At 6 weeks, light isometric ex-

ternal rotation strengthening is permitted. At 2 months, gentle strengthening with elastic bands is begun. Strengthening progresses after 3 months, and, at the 4th month mark, the patient is permitted to return to noncontact and noncollision skill sports, such as swimming, tennis, and golf. Contact and collision sports are delayed for at least 6 months after surgery.

REVISION AND COMPLEX PROBLEMS

These challenging scenarios include revision surgery with associated scarring, but good tissues; capsular insufficiency after multiple prior surgeries or thermal capsulorrhaphy[103,181]; bony deficiency of the anterior glenoid rim; and associated subscapularis deficiency.

Capsular Deficiency

The dilemma of the "absent capsule" is a rare condition, which most surgeons may never face. This is why there are few published guidelines for surgical reconstruction of soft-tissue deficiency in relation to shoulder instability.[69,105,126,174] Nevertheless, this deficiency may be a reality in some revision situations, so a method for treating instability in such cases is presented here.

Several options exist when the capsule is deficient. In some revision situations, the soft-tissue deficiency may also include the subscapularis as well as the capsule. Lazarus et al.[83] presented a method using hamstrings to repair such deficiencies (Fig. 2-24) with good success. Iannotti

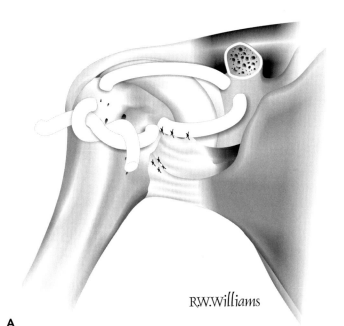
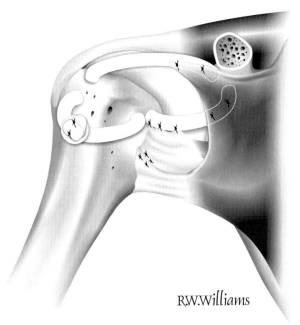

A   B

Figure 2-24 (*A,B*) Anterior capsule reconstruction with hamstrings tendons. (Drawing from Lazarus MD, Harryman DT. Open repairs for instability. In: Warner JJP, Iannotti JP, Gerber C, eds. Complex and revision problems in shoulder surgery. 1st ed. Philadelphia, Lippincott-Raven, 1997.)

and Williams described the use of a variety of capsular substitutes, advocated the use of the iliotibial band, and presented a series of seven patients in which this tissue was used[69] (Fig. 2-25). Also, Moeckel et al.[105] described using an Achilles allograft to manage recurrent anterior instability in the setting of subscapularis and capsular deficiency following shoulder arthroplasty. Some authors have described using the iliotibial band for capsular reconstruction to treat glenohumeral instability associated with an irreparable capsule.[44,69] Others have described using the long head of the biceps tendon.[174]

Autografts and Allografts

Authors' Preferred Method Using Autograft Hamstrings

The patient is positioned so that the ipsilateral leg and thigh are freely mobile and both the arm and shoulder as well as the leg are sterilely prepared and draped. A sterile tourniquet is used for harvesting of the hamstring tendons.

In most cases, this problem is the sequela of multiple failed prior surgeries. Thus, there is significant scarring and distortion of the soft tissues, which may obscure a layer-by-layer dissection. It is extremely important to clearly define each layer and to identify and protect the neurovascular structures. We usually dissect and protect the axillary nerve as described previously. The subscapularis is then carefully dissected from the capsule to the degree possible. The capsule may either be completely absent or be a thin, friable remnant (Fig. 2-26). It is important not to compromise integrity of the subscapularis by creating a capsular flap at the expense of the subscapularis tendon. A Fukuda retractor is then used to retract the humeral head, and the medial remnant of the capsule is exposed with a Cobra retractor over the anterior scapular neck. Braided No. 2 nonabsorbable sutures are then placed into the medial remnant of the capsule, and, if needed, anchors are placed along the glenoid rim as described previously. The semitendinosis and gracilis tendons are then harvested.

The technique of hamstring harvesting has been described in detail elsewhere.[122,172] Both the gracilis and semitendinosis are harvested through a small incision lateral and inferior to the tibial tubercle (Fig. 2-27). These tendons are then sewn side to side (Fig. 2-28).

The shoulder is positioned in about 20 degrees of forward flexion and 45 degrees of abduction and external rotation so that the humeral head is centered in the glenoid and the shoulder is in a midrange position of rotation. The graft is then fixed inferiorly on the glenoid, using a suture anchor, and sewn into any remnant of the capsule medially and inferiorly. The tendon graft is then brought to the humeral neck and fixed here with an anchor as well. The graft is woven back and forth from the glenoid anterior rim to the humeral neck fixing it with anchors (Fig. 2-28). Because the

graft length is usually around 22 cm, it is possible to weave it back and forth between the glenoid rim and humerus three to four times. Remnants of the capsule are then sewn into the tendon graft. The subscapularis is repaired anatomically as described previously, and the incision is closed in layers.

Postoperative care consists of a more conservative approach to regaining motion so as not to place any loads on the autograft tendon graft during healing. Active range of motion is avoided for 6 weeks, during which time the shoulder remains in an immobilizer. The standard protocol is then followed.

Clinical Experience

This procedure has been performed on a small number of patients with good outcomes in all cases[174] (Fig. 2-29).

Achilles Allograft (Authors' Preferred Method)

In place of autogenous hamstring tendons, allograft tendons can be used. This avoids host-site morbidity and, if the Achilles allograft is used, a flat, broad, strong tendon replaces the absent capsule. The method of repair is similar to that described previously, with the arm positioned as described. Moekel et al.[105] described an experience using this allograft in the setting of anterior instability after shoulder arthroplasty. The results were generally fair to good, with loss of motion but restoration of stability. Our experience has been similar.

Concomitant Subscapularis Tear

Primary Repair

Rupture of the subscapularis in association with primary anterior shoulder instability is a rare condition, though it may be commonly missed because the diagnosis can be subtle. More recently, it has been described after failed instability repair,[82] and failure to treat this condition properly can result in a very poor outcome for the patient.

In all cases of failed instability, we perform a careful physical examination to assess function of the subscapularis, as described previously in this chapter. A CT-arthrogram or MRI-arthrogram can be very helpful to identify partial and complete tears of the tendon (Fig. 2-8).

In most cases, a direct repair of the tendon is possible, if there has not been an extensive delay in diagnosis; however, in the case of chronic tear of the subscapularis, the tendon may retract and the muscle can involute, become fat, and scar. This will result in a stiffer muscle tendon, which may not be repairable. In such circumstances, a pectoralis major tendon transfer is employed, in addition to treatment of underlying instability.

There is limited published information on rupture of the subscapularis tendon associated with instability.[34,45,58,114,126,151,162,178] Hauser[58] was the first author to

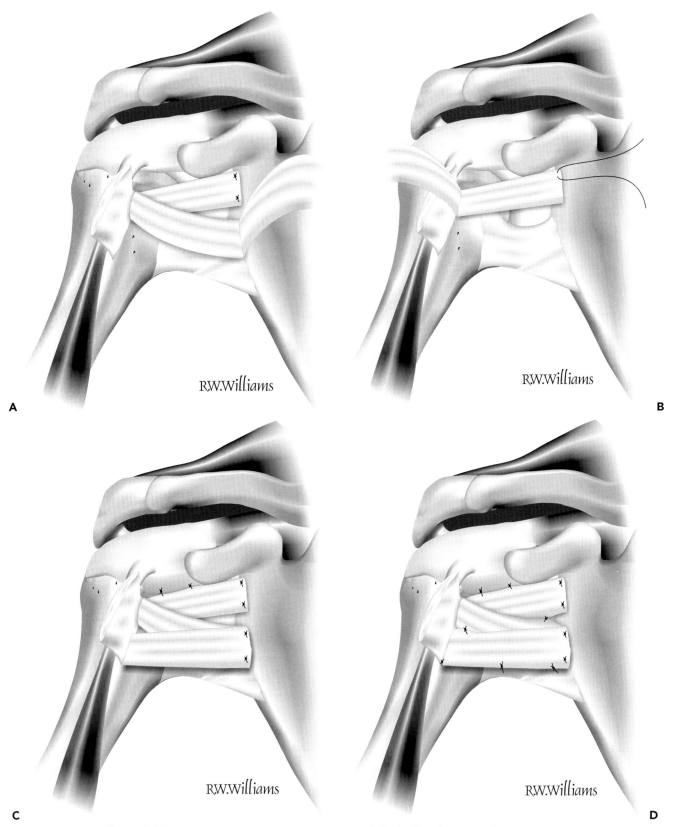

A

B

C

D

Figure 2-25 *(A–D)* Anterior capsule reconstruction with iliotibial band. (Drawing from Iannotti JP, Antoniou J, Williams GR, et al. Iliotibial band reconstruction for treatment of glenohumeral instability associated with irreparable capsular deficiency. J Shoulder Elbow Surg 2002;11(6):618.)

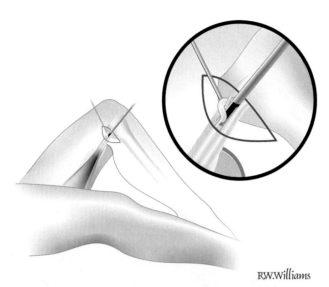

Figure 2-26 Deficient anterior capsule. (Drawing from Warner JJP, Venegas AA, Lehtinen JT, et al. Management of capsular deficiency of the shoulder. J Bone Joint Surg 2002;84(A):1668.)

describe an isolated tear of the subscapularis tendon in two patients associated with instability. Neviaser et al.[110] have emphasized that a rupture of the subscapularis tendon should be suspected in all cases of recurrent instability and in older patients after an initial anterior dislocation of their shoulder. Results of surgical treatment for subscapularis tendon tears are less successful than those

Supraspinatus muscle

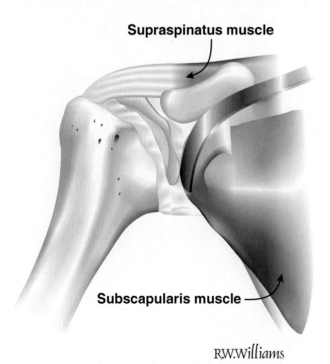

Subscapularis muscle

Figure 2-27 Technique of hamstring tendons harvesting. (Drawing from Warner JJ, Navarro RA. Serratus anterior dysfunction. Recognition and treatment. Clin Orthop 1998;(349):139.)

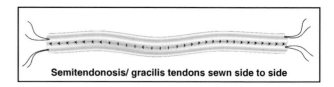

Semitendonosis/ gracilis tendons sewn side to side

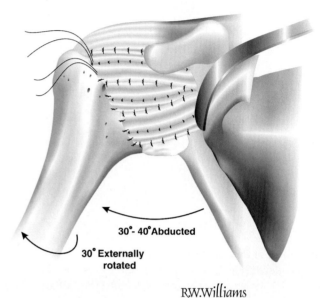

30°- 40° Abducted

30° Externally rotated

Figure 2-28 Hamstrings tendons sewn side to side. Capsule reconstruction. (Drawing from Warner JJP, Venegas AA, Lehtinen JT, et al. Management of capsular deficiency of the shoulder. J Bone Joint Surg 2002;84(A):1668.)

reported for supraspinatus tears. Gerber and Krushell[47] have emphasized the importance of timely diagnosis and early surgical management; results are significantly better if the duration between the traumatic event and the repair is short. Delay leads to retraction and atrophy of the ten-

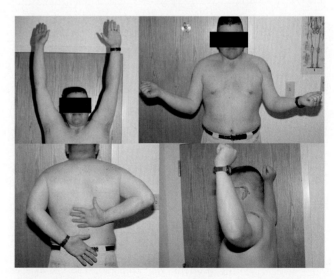

Figure 2-29 Clinical result after an anterior capsule reconstruction, using hamstring tendons.

don, making tendon mobilization impossible. Results of surgical repair are usually good for pain and instability, but patients continue to have mild-to-moderate internal rotation weakness.[47,162]

Surgical Procedure

The patient is positioned as previously described, and dissection is also similar to the method described previously. One important distinction is that there may be extensive adhesions between the conjoined tendon and the underlying subscapularis, depending on prior surgery. In such cases, dissecting and isolating the axillary nerve is required.[18] The biceps tendon, if present, may be subluxated medially because the subscapularis is one of the major medial stabilizing structures against such subluxation. In most cases, this tendon is tenodesed inferiorly in the bicipital groove. A thin layer of bursal scar may still be connected to the lesser tuberosity because the tendon may be in continuity with this but dissinserted and retracted medial to the glenoid rim. This layer is released from the neck of the humerus and dissected inferiorly until a few remaining fibers of the muscular portion of the subscapularis are encountered (Fig. 2-30). The subscapularis is then dissected medially with a retractor placed deep to the axillary nerve to protect it and the rest of the brachial plexus. Sutures are placed in the edge of the tendon, and then the tendon is released from the labrum on its deep surface, and sharp mobilization is performed into the subscapularis fossa. Adhesions to the conjoined tendon are released, as are any adhesions between the tendon and the base of the coracoid process. Thus, a circumferencial tendon release is performed. The capsule is then repaired by the method described previously, and the subscapularis is reinserted into the neck of the humerus and lesser tuberosity, using either anchors or transosseous suture technique with, at least, No. 2 gauge braided, nonabsorbable sutures. We believe the latter method provides a more secure repair because it distributes force over a broader surface of bone and also enhances surface area contact of tendon onto the bone. Furthermore, cortical augmentation can be performed, if the bone is osteopenic.

Postoperative care is very conservative with active motion not permitted for 6 weeks. The program then progresses as described previously.

Management of Irreparable Subscapularis Tear: Pectoralis Major Muscle Transfer (Authors' Preferred Method)

When the subscapularis tendon is deficient or irreparable, a pectoralis major muscle transfer may be used to augment or subsitute for the subscapularis. Gerber et al.[47] originally described the surgical technique for the mobilization and repair of the subscapularis tendon and recommended that

the inferior portion of the subscapularis tendon be repaired so that the pectoralis major transfer can be used simply to augment the function of the deficient upper part of the tendon. There are several reports of transfer of the pectoralis major tendon for anterior shoulder instability in the literature.[43,47,126,161,179] Decreased pain and restored stability are the main benefits of this surgery. Usually, functional gains in terms of mobility are variable and, unfortunately, more limited. Even when motion is improved in flexion and abduction, patients remain limited in overhead activities. In the majority of instances, the lift-off test and the belly-press test remain positive postoperatively.

There are several techniques for pectoralis major transfer. The authors prefer a split pectoralis major transfer, transferring the sternal head beneath the clavicular head to create the appropriate vector to substitute for the deficient subscapularis. We prefer not to pass the tendon beneath the conjoined tendon so as to avoid injuring the musculocutaneous nerve and to avoid the acute angle around the tendon.[161]

Surgical Procedure

Position and dissection are as described previously; however, the inferior border of the pectoralis major is dissected

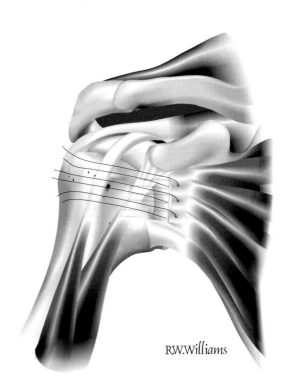

Figure 2-30 Dissection of the bursal scar connected to the lesser tuberosity until the inferior fibers of the muscular portion of the subscapularis are encountered.

laterally to medially. The interval between the clavicular and sternal portion of the tendon is then identified, and the sternal portion of the tendon is harvested (Figs. 2-31 and 2-32). This portion is then brought underneath the clavicular portion of the tendon and sewn into the upper portion of the lesser tuberosity as well as into the subscapularis inferior remnant (Fig. 2-33). Finally, the edge of the tendon is sewn into the supraspinatus tendon insertion. It is important to perform this transfer with the arm in neutral rotation so as to tension the tendon so it can have adequate strength to be effective.

The shoulder is immobilized in a sling for 4 weeks. During this time, passive range-of-motion exercises are allowed for abduction and flexion below the horizontal under a physical therapist's supervision. External rotation is limited to about 30 degrees, depending on the intraoperative repair security. After 4 weeks, active assisted motion is started. Strengthening exercises and full loading are delayed for 4 months.

GLENOID BONY DEFICIENCIES

Osteoarticular pathology is rarely a cause of recurrent anterior instability, but, when present, is often missed, and,

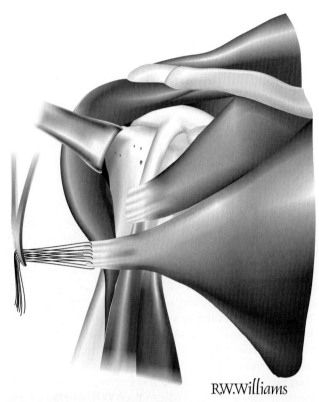

Figure 2-32   Pectoralis major tendon harvesting. (Drawing from Warner JJP. Management of massive irreparable rotator cuff tears: the role of tendon transfer. Instr Course Lect 2001;50:63.)

thus, more likely to be a relevant pathology in patients who present for revision surgery. Both glenoid version and shape are well defined in prior literature.[31,115,139,158,168] There is a range of normal glenoid version, and the glenoid concavity closely matches the humeral convexity, forming a ball-in-socket articulation, which permits nearly pure rotation without translation when the shoulder joint moves.[31,75,76] In a small percentage of patients, there may be a developmental anomaly of glenoid dysplasia where the glenoid shape is flatter than normal or the glenoid rim may be underdeveloped. This is analogous to congenital hip dysplasia. Morrey and Janes[107] believed that this accounted for less than 2% of all patients who required surgical repair of instability. Our experience is that this is more of a relevant pathology, though still rare, in patients with posterior and multidirectional instability than in those presenting with instability after a trauma.

Significant loss of the glenoid articular surface through fracture or erosion is a more likely articular sequela after a single traumatic dislocation or after recurrent episodes of instability. The anterior glenoid rim can actually become rounded and flattened from recurrent dislocations[149] (Figs. 2-2, 2-11). Experience has shown that when such defects are present, there is an increased risk of failure after soft-tissue Bankart repair performed either openly or arthroscopi-

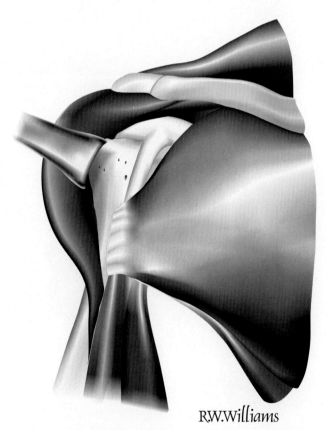

Figure 2-31   Pectoralis major tendon landmarks. (Drawing from Warner JJP. Management of massive irreparable rotator cuff tears: the role of tendon transfer. Instr Course Lect 2001;50:63.)

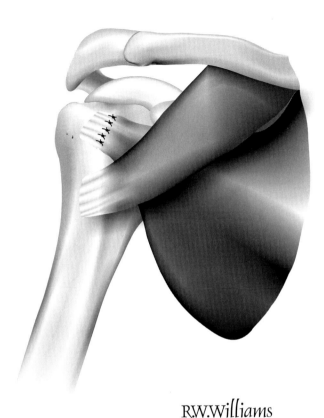

R.W.Williams

Figure 2-33 Fixation of the pectoralis major tendon to the lesser tuberosity. (Drawing from Warner JJP. Management of massive irreparable rotator cuff tears: the role of tendon transfer. Instr Course Lect 2001;50:63.)

cally.[48,72,84,91] Indeed, Burkhart and DeBeer[21] observed that, in patients who were identified at arthroscopy to have a significant glenoid erosion, which they described as an "inverted pear" (Fig. 2-3), the failure rate of arthroscopic capsulolabral repair was over 80% in contact and collision sport athletes. They studied 194 patients who had undergone arthroscopic Bankart repair of the shoulder: in those subjects without bone defects (173 patients), they found a recurrence rate of 4%; in those with significant bone defects, they found a recurrence rate of 67%. In the subset of patients who were contact athletes and had significant bone defects, the recurrence rate was 87%, whereas contact athletes without bone defects had a recurrence rate of only 6.5%.

This is consistent with experimental work performed by Howell and Galinat[67] and Lippitt et al.,[91] which has demonstrated that glenoid labrum and peripheral articular cartilage add height to the glenoid rim and thus enhance the socket effect of stability. Lippitt et al. termed this the concavity-compression effect for stability.

Until recently, there was little recognition of this potentially important risk factor for failure, and bone loss assessment was usually anecdotal at the time of open or arthroscopic surgery, with descriptions being mild, moderate, or severe. Rowe[136] described that up to 30% of the glenoid may be absent without concern for increased risk of failure with an open Bankart repair; however, it may be very difficult to determine the exact degree of glenoid loss even with direct inspection because one does not have the denominator of the whole glenoid as a point of comparison (because a portion of the glenoid is absent). More recent experimental observations have provided quantitative methods of assessing glenoid bone loss prior to surgery.[48,72,149] We prefer the method of Gerber et al.[48] He created experimental anterior glenoid defects and assessed the biomechanical consequences to joint stability. He found that, when the length of the glenoid defect exceeded the maximum radius of the glenoid, the force required to dislocate the humeral head out of the glenoid was reduced by 70% compared to an intact normal glenoid (Fig. 2-4). Furthermore, if a soft-tissue Bankart repair is experimentally performed in this situation, the force required for dislocation is not increased; thus, it is likely that such a soft-tissue repair will fail in a patient with this lesion.[28,46] This is further evidence for the importance of a matched ball-in-socket congruity and the so-called concavity-compression effect of Lippitt.[91]

We suspect significant glenoid erosion in all cases of recurrent traumatic anterior instability, especially if there have been a large number of recurrences or if the force required for dislocation has become significantly less than the original injury force. In these cases, a CT scan is ordered, usually with gadolinium intra-articular enhancement. A three-dimensional CT may also be helpful in demonstrating the extent of erosion and allowing preoperative measurements by the Gerber's method[48] (Fig. 2-4).

Many surgeons now recognize the need for an open surgical stabilization, which attempts to either reconstruct or compensate for anterior glenoid bone loss.[21,48,72,118] The method for such reconstruction basically includes two options: articular reconstruction with bone graft and boney buttress substitution, as with the Bristow or Latarjet procedures. The authors' preference is the former and will be described in the following text.

Iliac Crest Bone Graft—Authors' Preferred Method

Few have reported the results of this procedure. Bodey et al., in 1983, were the first to report this technique for recurrent anterior dislocation in 16 shoulders.[15] Results were good. All patients returned to their level of work and sporting activities. Results of this technique were then reported for sporting activities, military duty, and patients suffering anterior shoulder dislocation from epilepsy.[52,68] Patients were satisfied. No dislocations occurred and less than 10 degrees of range-of-motion loss were noted.

Surgical Procedure

The patient is positioned as previously described, although the head of the bed is kept at 30 degrees so that the ipsilateral anterior iliac crest is exposed. The arm and hemithorax, as well as the anterior iliac crest region, are then prepared and draped sterilely, and the patient receives preoperative intravenous antibiotics for infection prophylaxis. An articulated arm holder is also used, as described previously.

As already described, an incision is made in the anterior axillary line, and a layer-by-layer dissection is performed. The humeral head is retracted posteriorly with a Fukuda humeral retractor, and the glenoid rim is exposed (see previous discussion). We take special care to use a curved Lambotte osteotome to strip the periosteal sleeve as far medial as possible off of the anterior juxta-articular scapular neck, because this region of the anterior scapula will form the bone bed for the contoured graft. The extent of the glenoid defect is then confirmed, and a direct measurement may be made with a malleable or paper ruler just as was performed on the preoperative CT scan oblique sagittal or three-dimensional image.

A tricortical iliac crest bone graft is then harvested just posterior to the anterior-superior iliac spine. The graft is usually 3-cm long by 2-cm deep. This will allow for graft contouring to fit the defect (Fig. 2-34). The graft is then cut with a small oscillating saw so that the inner table of the iliac crest becomes the articular surface when positioned on the anterior scapula. The graft is cut at an angle so that it recreates the glenoid concavity (Fig. 2-35). Once properly positioned, the graft is fixed with K-wires and then definitively fixed to the scapula using cannulated 4.0 cancellous screws. Prior to tightening the screws down, a No. 2 braided nonabsorbable suture is looped around each screw so that, when tightened down against the bone, the suture is fixed in place (Fig. 2-35). The capsule-periosteal sleeve is then sewn over the graft using the sutures from these screws in a horizontal mattress fashion. The articulation is then checked for congruity by removing the Fukuda retractor and rotating the arm. A burr may be used to smooth off the interface between the graft and the glenoid. The capsule may often be shortened, due to scarring and added volume of the anterior bone graft, so direct reinsertion into the humeral neck may not be possible without loss of external rotation. Therefore, the subscapularis tendon can be used as an autogenous graft extension of the capsule. This is accomplished by sewing the capsule into the undersurface of the subscapularis with horizontal mattress sutures and then reattaching the subscapularis to the neck of the humerus and lesser tuberosity (Fig. 2-36). Thus, with external rotation the capsule will be tensioned along with the subscapularis. Postoperative care is similar to that used for capsulolabral reconstruction as described previously.

Authors' Clinical Experience

Osseous reconstruction of the glenoid is relatively rare, and, in the authors' experience over a 3-year period, this accounted for only 11 of 262 surgeries (4%) performed for recurrent anterior instability. In all 11 cases, stability was reestablished even in those patients who had over 20 episodes of dislocation and large Hill-Sachs lesions. Rarely is the Hill-Sachs lesion relevant for the repair, because restoration of the width of the glenoid socket avoids engagement of the Hill-Sachs lesion with the anterior glenoid rim. Of these 11 patients, there had been an average of 2 failed prior instability surgeries. The average Rowe score at a minimum 24-month follow-up was 94, and 3 of these patients were professional Hockey players who resumed their competitive careers. Range of motion is usually preserved with this anatomic procedure (Fig. 2-37).

Bristow-Latarjet Procedure

Latarjet first described a technique of coracoid abutment in 1958[81] that was later popularized by Helfet,[62] a fellow of Bristow. The aim of these procedures is to stabilize the shoulder with the static action of the transferred bone block and the attached coracobrachial tendon. Although, in the Latarjet procedure, the coracoid process is os-

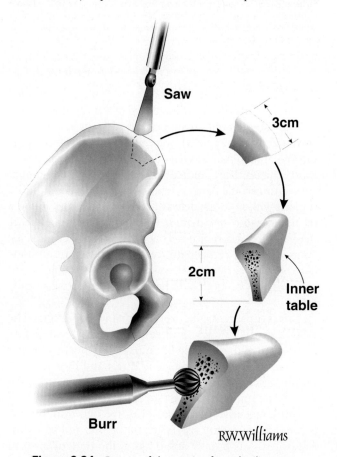

Figure 2-34 Bone graft harvesting from the iliac crest.

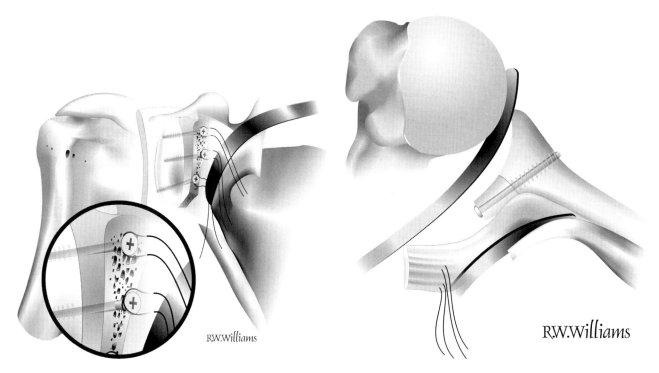

Figure 2-35 Contouring the bone graft and fixing it to the scapular neck.

teotomized at the junction's horizontal–vertical part and then transferred, in the Bristow procedure, only the tip of the coracoid process is transferred and then sutured to the capsuloperiosteal tissue through a short horizontal incision made in the subscapularis. The Latarjet procedure reconstructs the glenoid depth and width with the bone block and creates a dynamic reinforcement of the inferior capsule through the coracobrachial muscle, particularly while the arm is abducted and externally rotated. These techniques are nonanatomic reconstructions; they do not correct the initial lesion, the Bankart lesion. Furthermore, the capsular reinsertion is only partial.

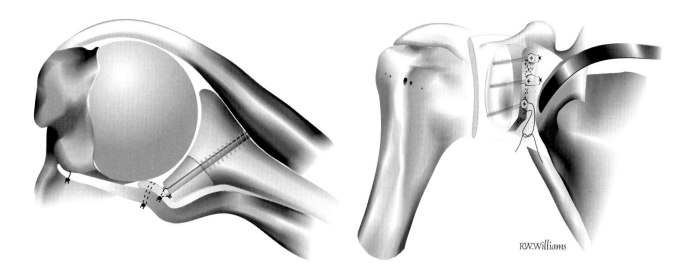

Figure 2-36 The subscapularis is repaired and reattached to the lesser tuberosity.

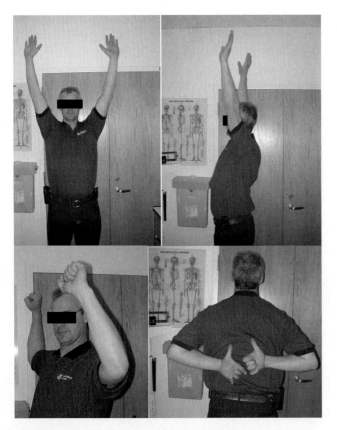

Figure 2-37 Clinical result after an anterior glenoid rim reconstruction with an iliac crest bone graft.

The Latarjet Surgical Procedure

The incision is similar to the basic approach described previously, except that the coracoid process is more extensively exposed. The arm is first abducted and externally rotated. The coracoacromial ligament is then exposed and harvested 1 cm from the coracoid process. The arm is then adducted and internally rotated. The insertion of the pectoralis minor is released from the coracoid process. The entire coracoid is exposed, and, with a saw, an osteotomy is performed at the level of the knee of the coracoid process (junction of the horizontal and the vertical part of the coracoid) (Fig. 2-38).

With a Kocher clamp (Theiman Co., Philadelphia, PA), the bone block is grasped; adhesions and attachments are released from the coracoid, and the first 2 cm of the lateral and posterior aspect of the conjoined tendon, avoiding injuries to the musculocutaneous nerve.[40] The deep surface of the coracoid is abraded with a burr. Two 3.2-mm drill holes are made through the bone block from its superficial to its deep surface.

The arm is then brought in maximal external rotation. The upper and lower part of the subscapularis tendon are identified. The muscle is split horizontally at its junction between the inferior one-third junction and the superior two-third. The capsule is exposed. The plane between the muscle and the capsule is then developed laterally to the lesser tuberosity and medially in the glenoid fossa. The arm is put in neutral rotation. The capsule is exposed and opened vertically at the level of the anteroinferior margin of the glenoid, under the level of the equator (Fig. 2-39). The upper and lower parts of the subscapularis are retracted with 2 Hohmann retractors inserted superiorly and inferiorly; a Fukuda retractor is inserted in the joint. The medial capsule is retracted, and the anteroinferior margin of the glenoid is abraded with a burr.

The bone block is inserted through the soft tissues and positioned on the edge of the anteroinferior margin of the glenoid. Lateral overhang of the bone block must be avoided. Using the two holes of the coracoid, drill holes are made in the glenoid neck, parallel to the articular surface of the glenoid. Two bicortical AO-malleolar screws are driven through the bone block and the scapula (Figs. 2-40, 2-41).

The Fukuda retractor is released. The arm is brought in external rotation. The harvested coracoacromial ligament is then sewn to the lateral flap of the capsule. The remnant pectoralis minor is sewn to the surrounding soft tissues.

Clinical Results

Transferring the coracoid process provides reliable and durable shoulder stabilization.[2,8,35,92,159] Recurrence rates

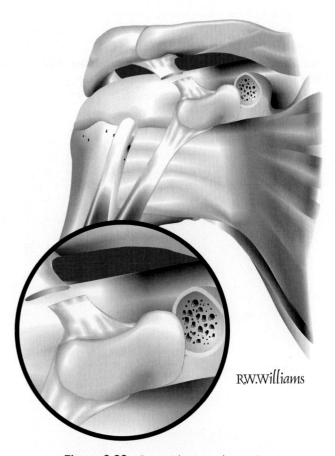

Figure 2-38 Coracoid process harvesting.

vary from 0% to 6%.[2,8,65,88] The average external rotation loss varies from 6 degrees to 23 degrees,[2,88,152] which is greater than after an open Bankart procedure (usually around 10 degrees).[28,49,134] More recently, some surgeons have advocated the addition of a coracoid bone block transfer to a standard Bankart repair for collision athletes.[183]

RECURRENT, "END STAGE" INSTABILITY

In rare cases, patients will continue to complain of instability, despite attempted surgical reconstructions. In certain salvage settings, glenohumeral arthrodesis may remain the only option available.[36,127] Results are variable. A sobering observation was presented by Richards,[127] in his series of fusion cases; he found that many patients who had a subjective sense of instability did not lose this sensation even after radiographic evidence of a solid fusion. Moreover, some of these patients may also have problems with their scapulothoracic joint due to severe posturing, secondary scapular winging, pseudowinging, and snapping scapula. These symptoms may occur after the arthrodesis or may be aggravated by the fusion.[127] Despite these concerns, there may be no other reasonable solution for these difficult patients, and a fusion may be the only acceptable option.

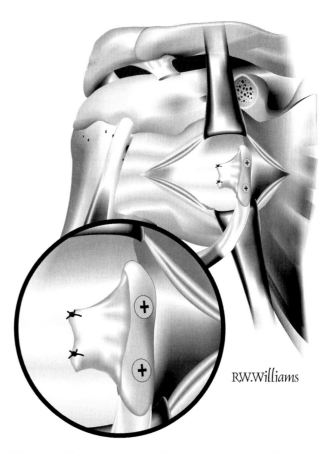

Figure 2-40 Subscapularis split and coracoid bone block fixation; the coracoacromial ligament is sewn to the capsule.

AVOIDING COMPLICATIONS AND PITFALLS

Recurrence

Recurrence is the most frequently reported complication after open surgery for anterior instability.[23,60,66,83,101,111–113,138,160,187] Recurrences may be secondary to new trauma or to atraumatic events.[23,59,185] Patients with traumatic recurrence of their instability usually have better postoperative results after revision surgery than patients with atraumatic recurrence of their instability.[89] The recurrence rate also relates to the number of prior surgeries. For Levine et al.[89] the recurrence rate in subjects who have had one prior surgery is 17%, which rises to 44% in those with multiple failed prior surgeries. The damage to the subscapularis and the capsule after each injury and each surgery undoubtedly compromises further surgery and the outcome. A variety of factors can contribute to failure after an anterior instability surgery, the most common of which are incorrect diagnosis, incorrect or technically inaccurate surgical procedure, bone defect with loss of glenoid concavity, and anterior capsular deficiency.

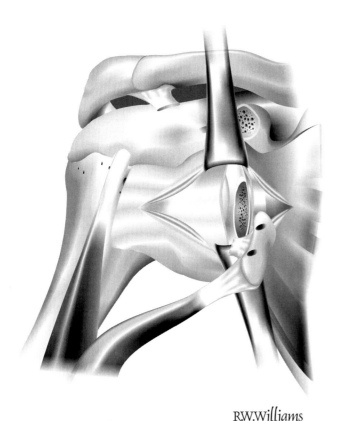

Figure 2-39 Anteroinferior capsulotomy.

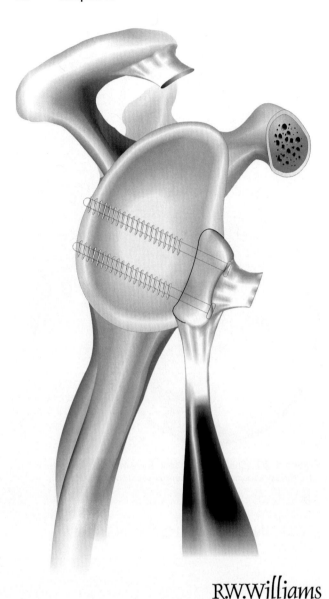

R.W.Williams

Figure 2-41 Coracoid positioning.

Incorrect Diagnosis

Examples of misdiagnosis are failure to recognize posterior or multidirectional instability[23,48,60,98,101] or voluntary instability.[42,135]

Inaccurate Surgical Procedure

An anatomic repair of the injured anterior structures is the goal of surgery. Numerous studies have determined that factors leading to recurrence include residual Bankart lesions,[137] undercorrected excessive anterior capsular redundancy, and unrecognized laxity of the rotator interval.[89,109,111,137,138,186] Furthermore, nonanatomic repairs (i.e., untreated or underrepaired Bankart lesions) lead to high rates of recurrences.[66,89,101,137,138,186]

Loss of Glenoid Concavity

Defects in the glenoid concavity due to an osseous Bankart lesion or an anterior glenoid fracture lead to an increased recurrence rate of instability after reconstruction.[48,72,84,91] Appropriate preoperative imaging and planning should avoid this. In the setting of failed prior surgery or numerous preoperative dislocations, a CT scan with three-dimensional reconstructions should be performed to evaluate the osseous anatomy. In this way, the cartilage of the glenoid and the anterior glenoid rim are assessed, and the appropriate procedure can be selected. When significant bone loss is noted, an anterior glenoid reconstruction with iliac crest bone graft or a coracoid bone block transfer, such as a Latarjet procedure, should be performed. In our institution, we prefer to reconstruct the anterior glenoid rim with an iliac crest bone graft.

Stiffness

Stiffness after surgery for anterior instability is infrequently reported in literature, and the incidence of this complication is probably underrepresented.[59,84,94] In certain settings (e.g., capsular reconstruction), some limitation of external rotation may be expected and should be conveyed to the patients preoperatively.

Although loss of 10 degrees or less of external rotation may have no functional consequences, it may be devastating for an overhead athlete, who must have sufficient external rotation to generate forceful torque when throwing a fastball pitch or serving a tennis ball at high speed. Furthermore, severe reduction of external rotation can have major consequences for joint kinematics and joint reactive forces. Harryman et al.[56] have shown that certain passive motions of the glenohumeral joint are reproducibly accompanied by translation of the head of the humerus on the glenoid. When the anterior capsule is tight, the humeral head translates excessively posteriorly because the arm is externally rotated. The posteriorly translated humeral head creates shearing forces on the posterior glenoid rim, which may result in cartilage erosion and early osteoarthrosis,[59,98,157] also called "capsulorrhaphy arthropathy." There is no accepted threshold for external rotation loss for such biomechanical consequences to become a real concern; however, we believe that a reduction of external rotation greater than 30% of the contralateral shoulder places the patient at risk for capsulorrhaphy arthropathy.

Such motion loss can be avoided by physiologically tensioning the capsule to avoid overconstraint, by the method described previously. Furthermore, proper therapy is also necessary postoperatively. When refractory motion loss persists formal capsular release is recommended, and this is discussed in detail in the chapter considering acquired shoulder stiffness.

Subscapularis Failure

Rupture of the subscapularis after an anterior open instability repair causes significant functional disability, which may or may not be associated with recurrence of instability. Often such a tear is unrecognized when the patient presents postoperatively with weakness and pain but not any clear evidence of recurrence of instability. An index of suspicion in such cases and careful physical examination is necessary to detect this problem.

When this occurs, repair of the subscapularis poses significant surgical challenge and risk for the surrounding neurovascular structures.[18,40,102] The subscapularis muscle and tendon are often retracted and adherent to the surrounding structures. This problem is better avoided, but when it occurs, revision repair is often possible through direct reinsertion of the tendon. In chronic cases tendon transfer of the pectoralis is necessary, as previously described.

Osteoarthrosis

Glenohumeral osteoarthrosis has been well described as a complication of surgical procedures to correct shoulder instability.[2,25,59,107,120,131,154,159,188]

As described previously, overtightening the anterior structures leads to stiffness and can drive the humeral head posteriorly, creating shear on the cartilage and early osteoarthrosis, or capsulorrhaphy arthropathy. In these patients the treatment may be difficult. Some patients paradoxically may have instability and stiffness. They feel unstable because of excessive laxity in the axillary pouch and an untreated inferior glenohumeral ligament detachment, yet they are stiff because the middle glenohumeral ligament, the rotator interval, and sometimes subscapularis are excessively tight. Complex releases with revision capsular shift may be required. An example might be Z-plasty subscapularis lengthening combined with an anterior-inferior selective capsular shift.

Other causes of premature osteoarthritis are iatrogenic, such as anterior impingement from a coracoid bone block that is placed too far laterally along the glenoid rim,[2,65,152,159] or impingement on local hardware, such as a screw, and incorrect intra-articular placement of metal anchors.[188] Prevention is the best treatment.

Hardware Problems

Any surgical implant has the potential to break, loosen, and migrate, due to loads across the joint. This complication may occur anytime postoperatively. Zuckerman et al.[188] have emphasized that loose hardware in the shoulder can migrate and may threaten the vital structures of the thorax. They also reported that most of the patients with hardware problems required a new surgery and had significant iatrogenic chondral defects. Moreover, in such revision settings where hardware needs to be removed, the surgeon should be prepared because removing the implant may lead to a significant bone defect that requires treatment and increases the duration of surgery.

Neurovascular

The entire plexus, not just the axillary and musculocutaneous nerves, is at risk during open surgery for anterior instability. Injuries may occur during tissue retraction, especially of the coracobrachialis tendon, during sharp dissection; by direct laceration; and during suture placement. The surgeon should be comfortable locating and dissecting these nerves so that they can be palpated, visualized, and protected during the procedure. Of all the procedures described, the Bristow-Latarjet procedure has the highest reported risk of injury to the axillary and musculocutaneous nerve.[18,24,40,88]

CONCLUSIONS

While arthroscopic capsulolabral repair is preferred by many surgeons for treatment of traumatic recurrent anterior instability, open approaches to repair are still the "gold standard" of care. Moreover, many revision situations require an open approach. Each surgeon should carefully define his or her indications for either approach, based on surgical skill with each procedure and a clear understanding of the spectrum of relevant pathology, which may be encountered in both primary and revision anterior instability surgery. This balanced approach will ensure the highest possible percentage of good to excellent surgical outcomes.

REFERENCES

1. Abboud JA, Soslowsky LJ. Interplay of the static and dynamic restraints in glenohumeral instability. Clin Orthop 2002;400:48.
2. Allain J, Goutallier D, Glorion C. Long-term results of the Latarjet procedure for the treatment of anterior instability of the shoulder. J Bone Joint Surg 1998;80(A):841.
3. Allen AA, Warner JJ. Shoulder instability in the athlete. Orthop Clin North Am 1995;26:487.
4. Altchek D, Warren R, Skyhar M, et al. T-plasty modification of the Bankart procedure for multidirectional instability of the anterior and inferior types. J Bone Joint Surg 1991;73(A):105.
5. Apreleva M, Hasselman CT, Debski RE, et al. A dynamic analysis of glenohumeral motion after simulated capsulolabral injury. A cadaver model. J Bone Joint Surg Am 1998;80:474.
6. Bach B, Warren R, Fronek J. Disruption of the lateral capsule of the shoulder: a cause of recurrent dislocation. J Bone Joint Surg 1988;70(B):274.
7. Bankart ASB. The pathology and treatment of recurrent dislocation of the shoulder joint. Br J Surg 1938;26:23.
8. Barry TP, Lombaro SJ, Kerlan RK, et al. The coracoid transfer for recurrent anterior instability of the shoulder in adolescents. J Bone Joint Surg 1985;67(A):383.
9. Bigliani LU, Kelkar R, Flatow EL, et al. Glenohumeral stability. Biomechanical properties of passive and active stabilizers. Clin Orthop 1996;13 (Review).

10. Bigliani LU, Kurzweil PR, Schwartzbach CC, et al. Inferior capsular shift procedure for anterior-inferior shoulder instability in athletes. Am J Sports Med 1994;22:578.
11. Bigliani LU, Newton PM, Steinmann SP, et al. Glenoid rim lesions associated with recurrent anterior dislocation of the shoulder. Am J Sports Med 1998;26:41.
12. Bigliani L, Pollock R, Soslowsky L. Tensile properties of the inferior glenohumeral ligament. J Orthop Res 1992;10:187.
13. Bigliani LU, Pollock RG, Soslowsky LJ, et al. Tensile properties of the inferior glenohumeral ligament. J Orthop Res 1992;10:187–197.
14. Boardman ND, Debski RE, Warner JJ, et al. Tensile properties of the superior glenohumeral and coracohumeral ligaments. J Shoulder Elbow Surg 1996;5:249.
15. Bodey WN, Denham RA. A free bone block operation for recurrent anterior dislocation of the shoulder joint. Injury 1983;15:184.
16. Bokor DJ, Conboy VB, Olson C. Anterior instability of the glenohumeral joint with humeral avulsion of the glenohumeral ligament. A review of 41 cases. J Bone Joint Surg 1999;81(B):93.
17. Brostrom LA, Kronberg M, Nemeth G. Muscle activity during shoulder dislocation. Acta Orthop Scand 1989;60:639.
18. Bryan WJ, Schauder K, Tullos HS. The axillary nerve and its relationship to common sports medicine shoulder procedures. Am J Sports Med 1986;14:113.
19. Burkart AC, Debski RE. Anatomy and function of the glenohumeral ligaments in anterior shoulder instability. Clin Orthop 2002;400:32.
20. Burkhart SS, DeBeer JF. Traumatic glenohumeral bone defects and their relationship to failure of arthroscopic Bankart repairs: significance of the inverted-pear glenoid and the humeral engaging Hill-Sachs lesion. Arthroscopy 2000;16:677.
21. Burkhart SS, Debeer JF, Tehrany AM, et al. Quantifying glenoid bone loss arthroscopically in shoulder instability. Arthroscopy 2002;18:488.
22. Burkhart SS, Tehrany AM. Arthroscopic subscapularis tendon repair: technique and preliminary results. Arthroscopy 2002;18:454.
23. Burkhead WZ, Richie MF. Revision of failed shoulder reconstruction. Contemp Orthop 1992;24:126.
24. Burkhead WZ Jr, Scheinberg RR, Box G. Surgical anatomy of the axillary nerve. J Shoulder Elbow Surg 1992;1:31.
25. Cameron ML, Kocher MS, Briggs KK, et al. The prevalence of glenohumeral osteoarthrosis in unstable shoulders. Am J Sports Med 2003;31:53.
26. Clare DJ, Wirth MA, Groh GI, et al. Shoulder arthrodesis. J Bone Joint Surg 2001;83(A):593.
27. Cofield R, Irving J. Evaluation and classification of shoulder instability: with special reference to examination under anesthesia. Clin Orthop 1987;223:32.
28. Cole BJ, L'Insalata J, Irrgang J, et al. Comparison of arthroscopic and open anterior shoulder stabilization. A two- to six-year follow-up study. J Bone Joint Surg 2000;82(A):1108.
29. Cole B, Rodeo S, O'Brien S. The developmental anatomy of the rotator interval capsule and the rotator interval defect. An anatomic and histologic analysis of fetal and adult cadaver specimens with clinical implications. In: American Orthopaedic Society for sports medicine specialty day, 1997. San Francisco, 1997.
30. Cole BJ, Rodeo SA, O'Brien S, et al. The anatomy and histology of the rotator interval capsule of the shoulder. Clin Orthop 2001;390:129.
31. Cole B, Warner JJP. Anatomy, biomechanics, and pathophysiology of glenohumeral instability. In: Iannotti J, Williams G, eds. Disorders of the shoulder: diagnosis and management. Philadelphia, Lippincott Williams & Wilkins, 1999:207.
32. Cole BJ, Warner JJP. Arthroscopic versus open Bankart repair for traumatic anterior shoulder instability. Clin Sports Med 2000;19:19.
33. Debski RE, Sakone M, Woo SL, et al. Contribution of the passive properties of the rotator cuff to glenohumeral stability during anterior-posterior loading. J Shoulder Elbow Surg 1999;8:324.
34. Deutsch A, Altchek DW, Veltri DM, et al. Traumatic tear of the subscapularis tendon. Clinical diagnosis, magnetic resonance imaging findings, and operative treatment. Am J Sports Med 1997;25:13.
35. DeWaal Malefijt J, Ooms AJ, VanRens TJ. A comparison of the results of the Bristow-Latarjet procedure and the Bankart/Putti-Platt operation for recurrent anterior dislocation of the shoulder. Acta Orthop Belg 1985;51:831.
36. Diaz JA, Cohen SB, Warren RF, et al. Arthrodesis as a salvage procedure for recurrent instability of the shoulder. J Shoulder Elbow Surg 2003;12:237.
37. Edelson JG. Bony changes of the glenoid as a consequence of shoulder instability. J Shoulder Elbow Surg 1996;5:293.
38. Faber KJ, Homa K, Hawkins RJ. Translation of the glenohumeral joint in patients with anterior instability: awake examination versus examination with the patient under anesthesia. J Shoulder Elbow Surg 1999;8:320.
39. Field LD, Bokor DJ, Savoie FH III. Humeral and glenoid detachment of the anterior inferior glenohumeral ligament: a cause of anterior shoulder instability. J Shoulder Elbow Surg 1997;6:6.
40. Flatow EL, Bigliani LU, April EW. An anatomic study of the musculocutaneous nerve and its relationship to the coracoid process. Clin Orthop 1989;244:166.
41. Fredriksson AS, Tegner Y. Results of the Putti-Platt operation for recurrent anterior dislocation of the shoulder. Int Orthop 1991;15:111.
42. Fuchs B, Jost B, Gerber C. Posterior-inferior capsular shift for treatment of recurrent, voluntary posterior subluxation of the shoulder. J Bone Joint Surg 2000;82(A):16.
43. Galatz LM, Connor PM, Calfee RP, et al. Pectoralis major transfer for anterior-superior subluxation in massive cuff insufficiency. J Shoulder Elbow Surg 2003;12:1.
44. Gallie WE, Le Menuisier AB. Recurring dislocation of the shoulder. J Bone Joint Surg 1948;30(B):9.
45. Gerber C, Fuchs B, Hodler J. The results of repair of massive tears of the rotator cuff. J Bone Joint Surg Am 2000;82(A):505.
46. Gerber C, Hersche O, Farron A. Isolated rupture of the subscapularis tendon. Results of operative repair. J Bone Joint Surg 1996;78(A):1015.
47. Gerber C, Krushell RJ. Isolated rupture of the tendon of the subscapularis muscle. Clinical features in 16 cases. J Bone Joint Surg 1991;73(B):389.
48. Gerber C, Nyffeler RW. Classification of glenohumeral joint instability. Clin Orthop 2002;400:65.
49. Gill TJ, Micheli LJ, Gebhard F, et al. Bankart repair for anterior instability of the shoulder. Long-term outcome. J Bone Joint Surg 1997;79(A):850.
50. Gonzalez-Diaz R, Rodriguez-Merchan EC, Gilbert MS. The role of shoulder fusion in the era of arthroplasty. Int Orthop 1997;21:204.
51. Green M, Christensen K. Magnetic resonance imaging of the glenoid labrum: MR imaging of 88 arthroscopically confirmed cases. Am J Sports Med 1994;22:493.
52. Haaker RG, Eickhoff UM, Klammer HL. Intraarticular autogenous bone grafting in recurrent shoulder dislocation. Mil Med 1993;158:164.
53. Habermeyer P, Schuller U, Wiedemann E. The intra-articular pressure of the shoulder: an experimental study on the role of the glenoid labrum in stabilizing the joint. Arthroscopy 1992;8:166.
54. Harryman DT, Sidles JA, Harris SL, et al. Laxity of the normal glenohumeral joint: a quantitative in vivo assessment. J Shoulder Elbow Surg 1992;1:66.
55. Harryman DT, Sidles JA, Harris SL, et al. The role of the rotator interval capsule in passive motion and stability of the shoulder. J Bone Joint Surg 1992;74(A):53.
56. Harryman DT II, Sidles JA, Clark JM, et al. Translation of the humeral head on the glenoid with passive glenohumeral motion. J Bone Joint Surg 1990;72(A):1334.
57. Hattrup SJ, Cofield RH, Weaver AL. Anterior shoulder reconstruction: prognostic variables. J Shoulder Elbow Surg 2001;10:508.
58. Hauser EDW. Avulsion of the tendon of the subscapularis muscle. J Bone Joint Surg 1954;36(A):139.
59. Hawkins RJ, Angelo RL. Glenohumeral osteoarthrosis: a late complication of Putti-Platt repair. J Bone Joint Surg 1990;72(A):1193.
60. Hawkins RH, Hawkins RJ. Failed anterior reconstruction for shoulder instability. J Bone Joint Surg 1985;67(B):709.

61. Hawkins RJ, Schutte JP, Janda DH, et al. Translation of the glenohumeral joint with the patient under anesthesia. J Shoulder Elbow Surg 1996;5:286.

62. Helfet AJ. Coracoid transplantation for recurring dislocation of the shoulder. J Bone Joint Surg 1958;40(B):198.

63. Hernigou P, Duparc F, Hernigou A. Determining humeral retroversion with computed tomography. J Bone Joint Surg 2002; 84(A):1753.

64. Higgins LD, Warner JJ. Superior labral lesions: anatomy, pathology, and treatment. Clin Orthop 2001;390:73.

65. Hovelius L, Korner L, Lundberg B, et al. The coracoid transfer for recurrent dislocation of the shoulder. Technical aspects of the Bristow-Latarjet procedure. J Bone Joint Surg 1983;65(A):926.

66. Hovelius L, Thorling J, Fredin H. Recurrent anterior dislocation of the shoulder: results after Bankart and Putti-Platt operations. J Bone Joint Surg 1979;61(A):566.

67. Howell SM, Galinat BJ. The glenoid-labral socket: a constrained articular surface. Clin Orthop 1989;243:122.

68. Hutchinson JW, Neumann L, Wallace WA. Bone buttress operation for recurrent anterior shoulder dislocation in epilepsy. J Bone Joint Surg 1995;77(B):928.

69. Iannotti JP, Antoniou J, Williams GR, et al. Iliotibial band reconstruction for treatment of glenohumeral instability associated with irreparable capsular deficiency. J Shoulder Elbow Surg 2002;11:618.

70. Iannotti J, Zlatkin M, Esterhai J. Magnetic resonance imaging of the shoulder. Sensitivity, specificity, and predictive value. J Bone Joint Surg 1991;73(A):17.

71. Itoi E, Lee SB, Amrami KK, et al. Quantitative assessment of classic anteroinferior bony Bankart lesions by radiography and computed tomography. Am J Sports Med 2003;31:112.

72. Itoi E, Lee SB, Berglund LJ, et al. The effect of a glenoid defect on anteroinferior stability of the shoulder after Bankart repair: a cadaveric study. J Bone Joint Surg 2000;82(A):35.

73. Jost B, Koch PP, Gerber C. Anatomy and functional aspects of the rotator interval. J Shoulder Elbow Surg 2000;9:336.

74. Karadimas J, Rentis G, Varouchas G. Repair of recurrent anterior dislocation of the shoulder using transfer of the subscapularis tendon. J Bone Joint Surg 1980;62(A):1147.

75. Karduna AR, Williams GR, Williams JL, et al. Kinematics of the glenohumeral joint: influences of muscle forces, ligamentous constraints, and articular geometry. J Orthop Res 1996;14:986.

76. Kelkar R, Wang VM, Flatow EL, et al. Glenohumeral mechanics: a study of articular geometry, contact, and kinematics. J Shoulder Elbow Surg 2001;10:73.

77. Kido T, Itoi E, Lee SB, et al. Dynamic stabilizing function of the deltoid muscle in shoulders with anterior instability. Am J Sports Med 2003;31:399.

78. Kim SH, Ha KI, Cho YB, et al. Arthroscopic anterior stabilization of the shoulder: two- to six-year follow-up. J Bone Joint Surg 2003; 85(A):1511.

79. Kim SH, Ha KI, Kim SH. Bankart repair in traumatic anterior shoulder instability: open versus arthroscopic technique. Arthroscopy 2002;18:755.

80. Kinnard P, Tricoire J, Levesque R. Assessment of the unstable shoulder by computed arthrography. A preliminary report. Am J Sports Med 1983;11:157.

81. Latarjet M. Technique de la butée coracoïdienne pré-glénoïdienne dans le traitement des luxations récidivantes de l'épaule. Lyon Chir 1958;54:604.

82. Lazarus MD, Harryman DT. Complications of open anterior stabilization of the shoulder. J Am Acad Orthop Surg 2000;8:122.

83. Lazarus MD, Harryman DT. Open repair for anterior instability. In: Waner J, Iannotti J, Gerber C, eds. Complex and revision problems in shoulder surgery. Philadelphia, Lippincott Raven, 1997:47.

84. Lazarus M, Sidles J, Harryman DI, et al. Effect of a chondral-labral defect on glenoid concavity and glenohumeral stability. J Bone Joint Surg 1996;78(A):94.

85. Lee SB, An KN. Dynamic glenohumeral stability provided by three heads of the deltoid muscle. Clin Orthop 2002;400:40.

86. Lephart SM, Myers JB, Bradley JP, et al. Shoulder proprioception and function following thermal capsulorrhaphy. Arthroscopy 2002;18:770.

87. Lephart SM, Pincivero DM, Giraldo JL, et al. The role of proprioception in the management and rehabilitation of athletic injuries. Am J Sports Med 1997;25:130.

88. Levigne C. Résultat à long terme des butées antérieures coracoïdiennes. A propos de 52 cas au recul homogène de 12 ans. Rev Chir Orthop Reparatrice Appar Mot 2000;86(suppl 1):114.

89. Levine WN, Arroyo JS, Pollock RG, et al. Open revision stabilization surgery for recurrent anterior glenohumeral instability. Am J Sports Med 2000;28:156.

90. Lippitt SB, Harris SL, Harryman DT II, et al. In vivo quantification of the laxity of normal and unstable glenohumeral joints. J Shoulder Elbow Surg 1995;3:215.

91. Lippitt S, Vanderhooft J, Harris S. Glenohumeral stability from concavity-compression: a quantitative analysis. J Shoulder Elbow Surg 1993;2:27.

92. Lombaro SJ, Kerlan RK, Jobe FW, et al. The modified Bristow-Latarjet procedure for recurrent dislocation of the shoulder. J Bone Joint Surg 1976;58(A):256.

93. Loomer R, Fraser J. A modified Bankart procedure for recurrent anterior/inferior shoulder instability. A preliminary report. Am J Sports Med 1989;17:374.

94. Lusardi DA, Wirth MA, Wurtz D, et al. Loss of external rotation following anterior capsulorrhaphy of the shoulder. J Bone Joint Surg 1993;75(A):1185.

95. MacDonald PB, Hawkins RJ, Fowler PJ, et al. Release of the subscapularis for internal rotation contracture and pain after anterior repair for recurrent anterior dislocation of the shoulder. J Bone Joint Surg 1992;74(A):734.

96. Magnuson PB, Stack JK. Recurrent dislocation of the shoulder. JAMA 1943;123:889.

97. Magnusson L, Kartus J, Ejerhed L, et al. Revisiting the open Bankart experience: a four- to nine-year follow-up. Am J Sports Med 2002;30:778.

98. Matsen FA III, Lippitt SB, Sidles JA, et al. Practical evaluation and management of the shoulder. Philadelphia, WB Saunders, 1994.

99. Matsen FA III, Thomas SC, Rockwood CA Jr, et al. Glenohumeral instability. In: Rockwood CJ, Matsen FI, eds. The shoulder. Philadelphia, WB Saunders, 1998:233.

100. Matthews LS, Pavlovich LJ Jr. Anterior and anteroinferior instability: diagnosis and management. In: Iannotti J, Williams G, eds. Disorders of the shoulder. Diagnosis and management. Philadelphia, Lippincott Williams & Wilkins, 1999:251.

101. McAuliffe TB, Pangayatselvan T, Bayley I. Failed surgery for recurrent anterior dislocation of the shoulder: causes and management. J Bone Joint Surg 1988;70(B):798.

102. McFarland EG, Caicedo JC, Kim TK, et al. Prevention of axillary nerve injury in anterior shoulder reconstructions: use of a subscapularis muscle-splitting technique and a review of the literature. Am J Sports Med 2002;30:601.

103. McFarland EG, Kim TK, Banchasuek P, et al. Histologic evaluation of the shoulder capsule in normal shoulders, unstable shoulders, and after failed thermal capsulorrhaphy. Am J Sports Med 2002;30:636.

104. McMahon PJ, Lee TQ. Muscles may contribute to shoulder dislocation and stability. Clin Orthop 2002;403(suppl 1):S18.

105. Moeckel BH, Altchek DW, Warren RF, et al. Instability of the shoulder after arthroplasty. J Bone Joint Surg 1993;75 (A):492.

106. Morrey BF, Itoi E, Kai-Nan AN. Biomechanics of the shoulder. In: Rockwood CJ, Matsen FI, eds. The shoulder. 2nd ed. Philadelphia, WB Saunders, 1998:233.

107. Morrey BF, Janes JM. Recurrent anterior dislocation of the shoulder: long-term follow-up of the Putti-Platt and Bankart procedure. J Bone Joint Surg 1976;58(A):252.

108. Neer CS. Involuntary inferior and multidirectional instability of the shoulder: etiology, recognition, and treatment. Instr Course Lect 1985;34:232.

109. Neer CS, Foster CR. Inferior capsular shift for involuntary inferior and multidirectional instability of the shoulder. A preliminary report. J Bone Joint Surg 1980;62(A):897.

110. Neviaser RJ, Neviaser TJ, Neviaser JS. Current rupture of the rotator cuff and anterior dislocation of the shoulder in the older patient. J Bone Joint Surg 1988;70(A):1308.

111. Norris TR. Complications following anterior instability repairs. In: Bigliani L, ed. Complications of shoulder surgery. Baltimore, Williams & Wilkins, 1993:98.

112. Norris TR, Bigliani LU. Analysis of failed repair for shoulder instability: a preliminary report. In: Bateman J, Welsh R, eds. Surgery of the shoulder. Philadelphia, BC Decker, 1984:111.

113. Norris TR, Thomas SC, Rockwood CA Jr. Anterior glenohumeral stability. In: Rockwood CJ, Matsen FI, eds. The shoulder. Philadelphia, WB Saunders, 1990:547.

114. Nove-Josserand L, Levigne C, Noel E, et al. Les lesions isolees du sous-scapulaire. A propos de 21 cas. Rev Chir Orthop 1994;80:595.

115. O'Brien S, Allen AA, Fealy S, et al. Developmental anatomy of the shoulder and anatomy of the glenohumeral joint. In: Rockwood CJ, Matsen FI, eds. The shoulder. 2nd ed. Philadelphia, WB Saunders, 1998:1.

116. O'Brien SJ, Neves MC, Arnoczky SP, et al. The anatomy and histology of the inferior glenohumeral ligament complex of the shoulder. Am J Sports Med 1990;18:449.

117. O'Brien SJ, Pagnani MJ, Fealy S, et al. The active compression test: a new and effective test for diagnosing labral tears and acromioclavicular joint abnormality. Am J Sports Med 1998; 26:610.

118. O'Brien SJ, Warren RF, Schwartz E. Anterior shoulder instability. Orthop Clin North Am 1987;18:395.

119. O'Connell PW, Nuber GW, Mileski RA, et al. The contribution of the glenohumeral ligaments to anterior stability of the shoulder joint. Am J Sports Med 1990;18:579.

120. O'Driscoll SW, Evans DC. Long term results after staple capsulorrhaphy for anterior instability of the shoulder. J Bone Joint Surg 1993;75(A):249.

121. Osmond-Clarke H. Habitual dislocation of the shoulder. The Putti-Platt operation. J Bone Joint Surg 1948;30(B):19.

122. Pagnani MJ, Warner JJP, O'Brien SJ, et al. Anatomic considerations in harvesting the semitendinosus and gracilis tendons and a technique of harvest. Am J Sports Med 1993;12:565.

123. Pavlov H, Warren RF, Weiss CB, et al. The roentgenographic evaluation of certain surgical conditions. Clin Orthop 1985; 184:317.

124. Potzl W, Witt KA, Hackenberg L, et al. Results of suture anchor repair of anteroinferior shoulder instability: A prospective clinical study of 85 shoulders. J Shoulder Elbow Surg 2003;12:322.

125. Reeves B. Experiments on the tensile strength of the anterior capsular structures of the shoulder in man. J Bone Joint Surg 1968;50(B):858.

126. Resch H, Povascz P, Ritter E, et al. Transfer of the pectoralis major muscle for the treatment of irreparable rupture of the subscapularis tendon. J Bone Joint Surg 2000;82(A):372.

127. Richards RR, Beaton D, Hudson AR. Shoulder arthrodesis with plate fixation: functional outcome analysis. J Shoulder Elbow Surg 1993;2:225.

128. Robinson CM, Kelly M, Wakefield AE. Redislocation of the shoulder during the first six weeks after a primary anterior dislocation: risk factors and results of treatment. J Bone Joint Surg 2002;84(A):1552.

129. Rockwood CA Jr. Subluxations and dislocations about the shoulder. In: Rockwood CJ, Green D, eds. Fractures in adults. 2nd ed. Philadelphia, JB Lippincott, 1984:722.

130. Rockwood CA Jr, Jensen KL. X-ray evaluation of shoulder problems. In: Rockwood CJ, Matsen FI, eds. The shoulder. Philadelphia, WB Saunders, 1998:199.

131. Rosenberg BN, Richmond JC, Levine WN. Long term follow-up of Bankart reconstruction: incidence of late degenerative glenohumeral arthrosis. Am J Sports Med 1995;23:538.

132. Rouholamin E, Wootton JR, Jamieson AM. Arthrodesis of the shoulder following brachial plexus injury. Injury 1991;22:271.

133. Rowe CR. Dislocation of the shoulder. In: Rowe C, ed. The shoulder. New York, Churchill Livingstone, 1988:165.

134. Rowe C, Patel D, Southmayd W. The Bankart procedure: a long-term end-result study. J Bone Joint Surg 1978;60(A):1.

135. Rowe CR, Pierce DS, Clarck JG. Voluntary dislocation of the shoulder: a preliminary report on clinical, electromyographic, and psychiatric study of twenty-six patients. J Bone Joint Surg 1979;55(A):445.

136. Rowe C, Sakellarides H. Factors related to recurrences of anterior dislocations of the shoulder. Clin Orthop 1961;20:40.

137. Rowe C, Zarins B. Recurrent transient subluxation of the shoulder. J Bone Joint Surg 1981;63(A):863.

138. Rowe C, Zarins B, Ciullo J. Recurrent anterior dislocation of the shoulder after surgical repair. Apparent cause of failure and treatment. J Bone Joint Surg 1984;66(A):159.

139. Saha A. Dynamic stability of the glenohumeral joint. Acta Orthop Scand 1971;42:491.

140. Savoie FH III, Field LD, Atchinson S. Anterior superior instability with rotator cuff tearing: SLAC lesion. Orthop Clin North Am 2001;32:457.

141. Schippinger G, Vasiu PS, Fankhauser F, et al. HAGL lesion occurring after successful arthroscopic Bankart repair. Arthroscopy 2001;17:206.

142. Shea KP, O'Keefe RM Jr, Fulkerson JP. Comparison of initial pull-out strength of arthroscopic suture and staple Bankart repair techniques. Arthroscopy 1992;8:179.

143. Singson R, Feldman F, Bigliani L. CT arthrographic patterns in recurrent glenohumeral instability. Am J Roentgenol 1987;149:749.

144. Soslowsky LJ, Flatow EL, Bigliani LU, et al. Articular geometry of the glenohumeral joint. Clin Orthop 1992;285:181.

145. Soslowsky LJ, Flatow EL, Bigliani LU, et al. Quantitation of in situ contact areas at the glenohumeral joint: a biomechanical study. J Orthop Res 1992;10:524.

146. Speer K, Deng X, Borrero S, et al. A biomechanical evaluation of the Bankart lesion. J Bone Joint Surg 1994;76(A):1819.

147. Speer K, Hannafin J, Altchek D, et al. An evaluation of the shoulder relocation test. Am J Sports Med 1994;22:177.

148. Stetson WB, Templin K. The crank test, the O'Brien test, and routine magnetic resonance imaging scans in the diagnosis of labral tears. Am J Sports Med 2002;30:806.

149. Sugaya H, Moriishi J, Dohi M, et al. Glenoid rim morphology in recurrent anterior glenohumeral instability. J Bone Joint Surg 2003;85(A):878.

150. Ticker JB, Warner JJP. Selective capsular shift technique for anterior and anterior-inferior glenohumeral instability. Clin Sports Med 2000;19:1.

151. Ticker JB, Warner JJP. Single-tendon tears of the rotator cuff. Evaluation and treatment of subscapularis tear and principles of treatment for supraspinatus tears. Orthop Clin North Am 1997;28:99.

152. Torg JS, Balduini FC, Bonci C, et al. A modified Bristow-Helfet-May procedure for recurrent dislocation and subluxation of the shoulder. Report of two hundred and twelve cases. J Bone Joint Surg 1987;69(A):904.

153. Townley C. The capsular mechanism in recurrent dislocation of the shoulder. J Bone Joint Surg 1950;32(A):370.

154. Trevlyn DW, Richardson MW, Ranelli GC. Degenerative joint disease following extraarticular anterior shoulder reconstruction. Contemp Orthop 1992;25:151.

155. Turkel SJ, Panio MW, Marshall JL, et al. Stabilizing mechanisms preventing anterior dislocation of the glenohumeral joint. J Bone Joint Surg 1981;63(A):1208.

156. Tzannes A, Murrell GA. Clinical examination of the unstable shoulder. Sports Med 2002;32:447.

157. Walch G, Ascani C, Boulahia A, et al. Static posterior subluxation of the humeral head: an unrecognized entity responsible for glenohumeral osteoarthritis in the young adult. J Shoulder Elbow Surg 2002;11:309.

158. Walch G, Boileau P. Morphological study of the humeral proximal epiphysis. J Bone Joint Surg 1992;74(B):14.

159. Walch G, Neyret P, Charret Ph, et al. L'opération de Trillat pour luxation définitive antérieure de l'épaule. Résultats à long terme de 250 cas avec un recul moyen de 11,3 ans. Lyon Chir 1989;85:25.

160. Wall MS, Warren RF. Complications of shoulder instability surgery. Clin Sports Med 1995;14:973.

161. Warner JJ. Management of massive irreparable rotator cuff tears: the role of tendon transfer. Instr Course Lect 2001;50:63.

162. Warner JJP, Allen AA, Gerber C. Diagnosis and management of subscapularis tendon tears. Tech Orthop 1994;9:116.

163. Warner JJ, Beim GM. Combined Bankart and HAGL lesion associated with anterior shoulder instability. Arthroscopy 1997;13:749.

164. Warner JJP, Boardman ND. Anatomy, biomechanics and pathophysiology of glenohumeral instability. In: Warren R, Craig E, Altchek D, eds. The unstable shoulder. Philadelphia, Lippincott-Raven, 1999:51.

165. Warner JJP, Boardman ND. Anatomy, biomechanics, and pathophysiology of glenohumeral instability. In: Warren R, Craig E, Altchek D, eds. The unstable shoulder. Philadelphia, Lippincott-Raven, 1999:51.

166. Warner JJ, Bowen MK, Deng X, et al. Effect of joint compression on inferior stability of the glenohumeral joint. J Shoulder Elbow Surg 1999;8:31.

167. Warner JJP, Caborn DNM, Berger R, et al. Dynamic capsuloligamentous anatomy of the glenohumeral joint. J Shoulder Elbow Surg 1993;2:115.

168. Warner JJP, Deng XH, Warren RF, et al. Static capsuloligamentous restraints to superior-inferior translation of the glenohumeral joint. Am J Sports Med 1992;20:675.

169. Warner JJ, Dirksmeier P. Glenoid fracture nonunion presenting as instability in a young athlete. Arthroscopy 1998;14:738.

170. Warner JJ, Johnson D, Miller M, et al. Technique for selecting capsular tightness in repair of anterior-inferior shoulder instability. J Shoulder Elbow Surg 1995;4:352.

171. Warner JJ, McMahon PJ. The role of the long head of the biceps brachii in superior stability of the glenohumeral joint. J Bone Joint Surg Am 1995;77:366.

172. Warner JJ, Navarro RA. Serratus anterior dysfunction. Recognition and treatment. Clin Orthop 1998;349:139.

173. Warner JJP, Navarro R, Greis P. Office evaluation of the unstable shoulder. Instructional video for the AAOS; Orthopaedic Learning Center, 1995. Rosemont, IL, November 10–12, 1995.

174. Warner JJP, Venegas AA, Lehtinen JT, et al. Management of capsular deficiency of the shoulder. A report of three cases. J Bone Joint Surg 2002;84(A):1668.

175. Warren RF. Subluxation of the shoulder in athletes. Clin Sports Med 1983;2:339.

176. Williams GR. Multidirectional instability. In: Warner J, Iannotti J, Gerber C, eds. Complex and revision problems in shoulder surgery. Philadelphia, Lippincott-Raven, 1997:85.

177. Wilson F, Hinov V, Adams G. Arthroscopic repair for anterior shoulder instability with a Bigliani type I glenoid rim fracture. Arthroscopy 2002;18:E32.

178. Wirth M, Blatter G, Rockwood C. The capsular imbrication procedure for recurrent anterior instability of the shoulder. J Bone Joint Surg 1996;78(A):246.

179. Wirth MA, Rockwood CA. Operative treatment of irreparable rupture of the subscapularis. J Bone Joint Surg 1997; 79(A):722.

180. Wolf E, Cheng J, Dickson K. Humeral avulsion of glenohumeral ligaments as a cause of anterior shoulder instability. Arthroscopy 1995;11:600.

181. Wong KL, Williams GR. Complications of thermal capsulorrhaphy of the shoulder. J Bone Joint Surg 2001;83(A)(suppl 2): 151.

182. Yagishita K, Thomas BJ. Use of allograft for large Hill-Sachs lesion associated with anterior glenohumeral dislocation. A case report. Injury 2002;33:791.

183. Yoneda M, Hayashida K, Wakitani S, et al. Bankart procedure augmented by coracoid transfer for contact athletes with traumatic anterior shoulder instability. Am J Sports Med 1999;27:21.

184. Young DC, Rockwood CA Jr. Complications of a failed Bristow procedure and their management. J Bone Joint Surg 1991; 73:969.

185. Youssef J, Carr C, Walther C, et al. Arthroscopic Bankart suture repair for recurrent traumatic unidirectional anterior shoulder dislocations. Arthroscopy 1995;11:561.

186. Zabinski ST, Callaway GH, Cohen S, et al. Revision shoulder stabilization: 2- to 10-year results. J Shoulder Elbow Surg 1999;8:58.

187. Zarins B, Rowe CR, Stone JW. Shoulder instability. Management of failed reconstructions. Instr Course Lect 1989;38:217.

188. Zuckerman J, Matsen FI. Complications about the glenohumeral joint related to the use of screws and staples. J Bone Joint Surg 1984;66(A):175.

Posterior and Multidirectional Instability: Arthroscopic Solutions

Robert E. McLaughlin   Felix H. Savoie III   Larry D. Field

INTRODUCTION

Posterior and multidirectional instabilities are complex entities that affect the shoulder. Diagnosis and management of these problems can be difficult. Patients affected by these conditions are usually young, active people who are highly motivated to improve, and conservative therapy is usually successful in controlling symptoms. More frequently, however, surgical stabilization is required for these patients to comfortably participate in activities of daily living and sports.

POSTERIOR INSTABILITY

Posterior instability was first described by Rowe and Yee in 1944.[32] Recurrent posterior instability has become a more frequent diagnosis over the last decade, but its treatment has proven less successful than its anterior counterpart. This problem, unlike anterior instability, is due to no one

R. E. McLaughlin: Mississippi Sports Medicine & Orthopaedic Center, Department of Orthopaedic Surgery, University of Mississippi School of Medicine, Jackson, Mississippi.

F. H. Savoie: Mississippi Sports Medicine & Orthopaedic Center, Department of Orthopaedic Surgery, University of Mississippi School of Medicine, Jackson, Mississippi.

L. D. Field: Mississippi Sports Medicine & Orthopaedic Center, Department of Orthopaedic Surgery, University of Mississippi School of Medicine, Jackson, Mississippi.

essential lesion appearing responsible for posterior instability. In addition, many patients with multidirectional instability have a primary posterior component, further confusing the picture. Until recently, diagnosis and treatment of posterior instability was made difficult by the lack of differentiation between unidirectional versus multidirectional conditions, traumatic versus atraumatic versus microtraumatic causes, voluntary versus involuntary instability, and dislocations versus subluxations. Recent advances in arthroscopic examination techniques, and increased understanding of the anatomy of the shoulder stabilizers, have allowed improved comprehension of posterior shoulder instability.

Numerous open operative procedures for treatment of recurrent posterior instability have been reported with failure rates of 30% to 50%. These include bone block (reverse Eden-Hybbinette), glenoid osteotomy, and McLaughlin-type procedures with lesser tuberosity and subscapularis transfer into the reverse Hill-Sachs defect.[16] Posterior capsular procedures include reverse Bankart repair, reverse Putti-Platt procedures with or without the infraspinatus tendon, Neer posterior inferior capsular shift, and the Boyd-Sisk procedures.[5,16] Combination procedures have tended to give better overall results than pure soft-tissue procedures. Overall, however, the success rate reported with open procedures for posterior instability has not approached the success rate reported for anterior instability.[35]

MULTIDIRECTIONAL INSTABILITY

Multidirectional instability (MDI) was originally described by Neer and Foster in 1980.[26] They reported on a population of patients that had recurrent shoulder instability and pain associated with instability in all three directions: posterior, anterior, and inferior. A large redundant inferior capsule was identified intraoperatively in all cases, and they reported good results with an inferior capsular shift procedure based laterally on the humeral head. Their procedure, in which the lateral insertion of the inferior half of the shoulder capsule is shifted superolaterally and the superior half is shifted inferolaterally, simultaneously eliminates excessive anterior, inferior, and posterior capsular laxity (Fig. 3-1). Altchek and Warren developed a T-plasty modification in which the shift was based on a medial capsular plication with a superomedial shift of the capsule (Fig. 3-2). The intermediate and long-term results of their superomedial capsular shift have been good, with excellent outcomes occurring in 75% to 100% of cases.[2]

Caspari developed the first arthroscopic techniques for the treatment of MDI.[8,24] This technique shifts the anterior, inferior, and posterior glenohumeral ligaments superiorly with a multiple suture technique. Arthroscopic repair of multidirectional glenohumeral instability has been gaining favor over the last decade with good short-term results being reported by a number of authors.[1,37,43]

Arthroscopic treatment of both posterior and multidirectional instability has been described, and early results are promising.[3,46] This chapter describes patient evaluation and diagnosis, nonoperative treatment, current arthroscopic techniques, and rehabilitation for the treatment of both disorders.

ADVANTAGE OF ARTHROSCOPIC VERSUS OPEN REPAIR

The use of arthroscopy in the diagnosis and treatment of shoulder pathology has grown rapidly over the last

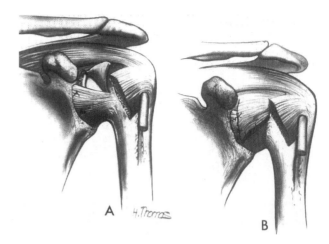

Figure 3-2   Altchek's medially based capsular shift.

decade. There are several advantages to using the arthroscope compared to the open approach. First, arthroscopic surgery is less invasive and produces less musculotendinous damage, aiding in recovery. Second, use of the arthroscope allows for less disturbance of intra-articular anatomy, allowing for more accurate viewing of normal as well as pathological conditions. The entire subacromial space, as well as the intra-articular space, can be visualized with the arthroscope, providing for the simultaneous diagnosis and correction of pathology. In addition, intraoperative modification and final inspection of the repair is also possible. Arthroscopy, therefore, allows pan-articular access to the joint for both diagnosis and stabilization, as well as evaluation, of the repair in the shoulder with minimal soft-tissue morbidity.

ETIOLOGY

The unifying pathomechanical condition of shoulder instability is an increase in glenohumeral translation leading to the development of symptoms. Shoulder stability primarily comes from the glenohumeral ligaments and the rotator interval. Secondary stabilizers include the bony architecture and kinematics, negative intra-articular pressure, glenoid labrum, biceps brachii, rotator cuff muscles, and scapular rotator muscles.

The constraints to posterior instability have been studied by a number of investigators. O'Brien et al. found that the inferior glenohumeral ligament complex (IGHLC), with the posterior inferior capsule, acts as a ligamentous hammock supporting the humeral head and is the primary static stabilizer against posterior instability with the arm in 90 degrees of glenohumeral abduction.[28] The relative contributions of the components of the IGHLC change with flexion/extension or rotation of the arm. With the shoulder in 90 degrees abduction and 30 degrees

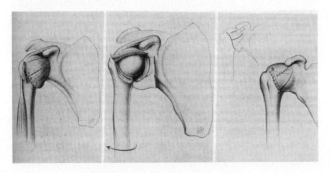

Figure 3-1   Neer capsular shift.

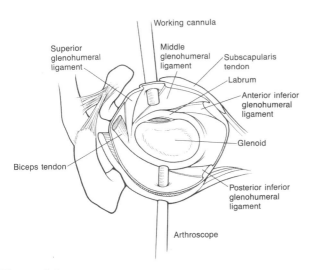

Figure 3-3 Posterior inferior glenohumeral ligament (PIGHL), anterior inferior glenohumeral ligament (AIGHL), superior glenohumeral ligament (SGHL). The rotator interval: area of the capsule between supraspinatus and subscapularis containing the superior glenohumeral ligament and the coracohumeral ligament.

extension, the anterior band of the IGHLC becomes the prime stabilizer against both anterior and posterior translations. When the 90-degree abducted arm is forward flexed to 30 degrees, the posterior band of the IGHLC becomes the primary anterior-posterior stabilizer (Fig. 3-3). Proper function of each of the three components of the IGHLC is believed to be necessary for normal stability in the position of abduction.[29]

Schwartz and Warren noted that damage to both the anterior and posterior capsuloligamentous structures was necessary to allow posterior dislocation of the humeral head.[36] They found that posterior subluxation occurred with cutting posteriorly from 12 o'clock to 6 o'clock and that dislocation occurred only when the anterior superior portion was also cut. Posterior subluxation also occurred when the entire inferior capsule was cut to include the anterior inferior glenohumeral ligament and posterior inferior glenohumeral ligament (PIGHL). Bigliani et al. found that IGHLC stretching occurs with plastic deformation.[7] Ligament failure occurs most commonly at the glenoid insertion and infrequently at the humeral insertion, or midsubstance, of the ligament. Webber and Caspari found that, in patients with posterior instability, the posterior capsule was split horizontally and the labrum was avulsed from the posterior glenoid in the region of the posterior inferior glenohumeral ligament.[42]

In our review of capsular disease, we support the concept that the anterosuperior and posteroinferior capsuloligamentous structures are the primary contributors to posterior shoulder stability and that there is no "essential lesion" responsible for all cases of posterior instability. We believe that laxity develops in the anterosuperior aspect of the shoulder, as well as in the posteroinferior capsular

complex, leading to symptomatic subluxation, also known as the circle concept of posterior instability.

ROTATOR INTERVAL

The rotator interval is also an important structure in maintaining stability of the glenohumeral joint. The rotator interval occupies a triangular space with its apex centered at the transverse humeral ligament over the biceps sulcus and its greatest width located at the base of the coracoid process. The interval space is bordered superiorly by the anterior margin of the supraspinatus tendon and inferiorly by the superior border of the subscapularis tendon, and is usually bridged by the glenohumeral joint capsule. The rotator interval capsule is then structurally enhanced by the coracohumeral ligament (CHL) and superior glenohumeral ligament (SGHL) as it courses from the anterosuperior labrum deep to the substance of the rotator interval capsule and the CHL to insert near the lesser tuberosity (Fig. 3-3).

Harryman et al. have studied the role of the rotator interval in glenohumeral stability in a cadaveric model.[15] They found that sectioning the rotator interval capsule allowed for significantly increased laxity in all three directions: anterior, posterior, and inferior. Imbrication of the rotator interval capsule was shown to decrease inferior and posterior humeral head translation to less than that measured in the intact state.

Several clinical studies have also shown the rotator interval capsule's contribution to stability. Nobuhara and Ikeda reported on a series of patients in whom rotator interval plication was performed for symptomatic glenohumeral instability with good results.[27] Rowe and Zarins identified holes in the rotator interval capsule in 20 of 37 patients undergoing open stabilizations for transient subluxations of the shoulder.[33] Field et al. reported on 15 patients with clinical examination compatible with MDI in whom the only operative finding at open surgical stabilization was an isolated hole or defect in the rotator interval capsule.[11] Closure or imbrication of this rotator interval capsule hole provided for adequate intraoperative stability, and no other stabilization procedures were performed. All of the patients had good or excellent results after an average follow-up of 3.3 years.

LABRUM/BONE DYSPLASIAS

Instability can also be caused by glenoid and/or humeral head dysplasia. When viewing the glenoid en face, its normal shape is similar to a pear, with the lower half being significantly wider than the upper half (Fig. 3-4A). With a large bony Bankart lesion, or even a Bankart lesion without an associated bone fragment but with a significant impression defect, the shape of the glenoid changes to an

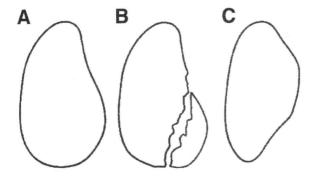

Figure 3-4 (*A*) Outline of pear-shaped glenoid. (*B*) Outline of bony Bankart. (*C*) Deficient anterior inferior glenoid rim.

"inverted pear" (Fig. 3-4, *B* and *C*), where the superior half of the glenoid is wider than the lower half. In a normal glenoid, a "bare spot" is equidistant between the anterior and posterior rims of the glenoid. Locating this bare spot can be useful when estimating the amount of bone loss arthroscopically. Similarly, an "inverted pear" configuration may be created if a large bony Bankart fragment is removed and the capsulolabral complex is repaired to the remaining glenoid. Both situations require a bony solution to avoid creating a serious containment problem for the shoulder.

Two geometric factors exist with regard to containing the humeral head by the glenoid. First, the anterior rim and labrum serve to "deepen the dish" of the glenoid by increasing the length of arc and widening the glenoid. Loss of the anterior rim creates a shallower "dish" and, in effect, a shorter arc of motion with less resistance to shear forces. Therefore, less shear force is required to cause a dislocation. Second is the arc length required to resist axial forces; the bony portion of the glenoid resists axial forces until the anterior rim is reached. At this point, axial forces are resisted by the capsulolabral structures. With an "inverted pear" type glenoid, a shorter arc of bony buttress exists to resist the axial loads than that of a normal glenoid. Subsequently, the repaired glenohumeral ligaments are subjected to higher loads and predisposed to disruption and recurrent instability.

The anterior labrum plays a key role in anterior stability. The role of the posterior labrum, however, is less well defined. In general, Harryman et al. have shown the entire labrum to contribute to shoulder stability, providing 10% of the stabilization by deepening the concavity of the glenoid.[14] We believe that the intact or reconstructed labrum provides a biofeedback to the rotator cuff musculature, stimulating increased contraction and stabilization of the shoulder during activities that potentially could subluxate the glenohumeral joint.

Many authors believe in the importance of distinguishing between patients with acute posterior dislocation versus those with recurrent posterior subluxation.[4,30,39]

Posterior instability can develop from several different entities: congenital laxity or hyperlaxity, chronic overuse, traumatic disclocation/subluxation, or a combination of all of these. Therefore, any previous injuries as well as athletic endeavors should be elicited. Traumatic instability develops from a fall or impact on a flexed, adducted, internally rotated arm. Atraumatic instability usually has a congenital component and is often associated with generalized ligamentous laxity. Recurrence following an acute dislocation is felt to be rare, and symptomatic instability seldom develops. This contrasts patients who develop insidious laxity, which predisposes to recurrent instability.

MULTIDIRECTIONAL INSTABILITY

The primary pathology of multidirectional instability appears to be hyperelasticity of the joint capsule, mainly secondary to dysfunction of the inferior glenohumeral ligament. This laxity can be acquired, congenital, or both. This laxity can progress due to a variety of causes, converting a functionally stable, lax shoulder into one with multidirectional instability.

Neer and Foster described three groups of patients with multidirectional instability. The first group included those with anterior inferior dislocation with posterior subluxation, the second had posterior and inferior dislocation with anterior subluxation, and the third had a recurrent dislocation in all directions.[26]

Additionally, there appear to be two separate populations that develop multidirectional instability. The first group includes those with congenital, generalized hyperelasticity, and the second group is composed of those who develop multidirectional instability due to repetitive activities. In all groups, elimination of the laxity of the capsule is necessary to achieve adequate stability.

HISTORY

A thorough and detailed history is essential in treating patients with shoulder instability. Classification of the instability as acute or chronic, traumatic or atraumatic, anterior, posterior, or multidirectional is of paramount importance. In addition, it is important to ascertain athletic participation because athletes involved in specific sports, namely weightlifting, swimming, throwing, and archery, are more likely to develop instability. Volitional instability must be identified early because these patients tend to do poorly with surgical repair. Volitional instability occurs in two groups. One group represents patients with good muscle control who can subluxate and relocate their shoulder from an early age, which may lead to capsular laxity and subluxation that begins to occur at inopportune times, producing symptoms. The other group represents true voluntary dislocators with psychiatric problems; operative treatment for this population is rarely successful.

Patients with posterior instability usually present in their late teens or twenties. On initial presentation, patients will often complain of mild, unspecific shoulder pain with a feeling of looseness or instability in certain positions, mainly in the flexed, adducted, and internally rotated positions. Many patients associate the onset of symptoms to a specific event, and so a history of trauma with the arm in this position should raise suspicion for posterior shoulder pathology.

Hawkins et al. reported that nearly 40% of their patients with posterior instability reported no pain in the involved shoulder, even though they experienced daily episodes of subluxation.[17] They reported that activities of daily living were unhindered in almost all patients, with most problems reported as sports related. In their study group they reported a low incidence of patients who had instability associated with a history of trauma, which has been contradicted by other studies.[46]

Most patients diagnosed with multidirectional instability present in their late teens or twenties. The presenting symptom is usually pain, most commonly occurring during activities of daily living with the glenohumeral joint in the midrange of function. Symptoms may also include a feeling of instability and transient neurologic symptoms.

Neer feels that patients with multidirectional instability possess two key clinical features. First, their symptoms of pain occur during the midrange of glenohumeral motion. Second, the physical examination shows the ability to subluxate, or dislocate, the joint anteriorly, inferiorly, and posteriorly with reproduction of symptoms in one or more of these directions.[26]

Often, patients with MDI present with an insidious onset of shoulder discomfort. There may be a history of injury, but the degree of trauma is often not considered significant enough to produce the patient's symptoms. In both posterior and multidirectional instability, activity-related complaints are common and range in severity from frank dislocation to subtle episodes of painless instability. Often patients will report a constant dull ache between episodes of intense pain or instability. Intermittently, neurologic symptoms may be the patient's presenting complaint, or it may not occur at all.

It is important to identify the frequency and severity of the symptoms, as well as the force involved in causing the discomfort. If the patient is experiencing multiple dislocations, the method of reduction and effort involved in reducing the shoulder is important to elicit. The position in space of the affected extremity when symptoms occur is also helpful to determine the predominant direction of instability, if one exists. If dislocations occur during sleep, this represents an end-stage disease process, and nonoperative treatment is likely to be ineffective.

PHYSICAL EXAMINATION

The physical shoulder examination for a patient suspected of having shoulder instability begins with inspection. The patient's entire shoulder girdle, as well as the entire involved extremity, needs to be unclothed. Inspecting for muscle atrophy from the front and back is important. The deltoid of patients with MDI may have a squared-off appearance due to inferior subluxation of the humeral head. Scapulothoracic motion should be observed, looking for any excessive scapular protraction or dyskinesia, during both passive and active range of motion for the shoulder. The cervical spine's range of motion needs to be evaluated to rule out referred pain and weakness patterns.

Many patients with MDI show signs of generalized ligamentous laxity, which include metacarpophalangeal hyperextension, genu recurvatum, patellar subluxation, elbow hyperextension, and the ability of the abducted thumb to reach the ipsilateral forearm. Generalized laxity has been reported to occur in 45% to 75% of patients undergoing surgery for MDI.[9] It is important to identify patients with known connective tissue disorders, such as Marfan's syndrome and Ehlers-Danlos syndrome. These patients tend to respond poorly to soft-tissue-only repairs and may need to undergo extensive preoperative testing to rule out any vascular or ocular abnormalities.

The exam begins with a thorough neuromuscular exam of the affected extremity, including range of motion, vascular integrity, and strength in all muscle groups, including scapulothoracic. A sensory exam is carried out in all dermatomes.

Palpation of the shoulder girdle follows. Bigliani et al. reported that two-thirds of the patients they treated with posterior instability had posterior glenohumeral joint-line tenderness, a finding not supported by other authors.[5]

Active and passive range of motion of the shoulder in all directions should be recorded. In assessing patients with posterior instability, a few provocative tests have been described. The first is the jerk test, where the affected arm is placed in forward flexion, adduction, and internal rotation. The examiner then stabilizes the scapula with one hand while providing a posterior and inferior directed force on the elbow. A positive test occurs when the humeral head is able to be subluxed over the posterior glenoid rim to a greater degree than the contralateral side (Fig. 3-5). Often this reproduces the patient's symptoms. Shoulder abduction and external rotation tend to reduce the subluxed humeral head back into the concavity of the joint.

The load and shift test (described later in this chapter) should also be performed. A positive test occurs when the humeral head fails to relocate with the tightening of the posterior ligaments. Increased scapular winging with any provocative test indicates scapulothoracic dyskinesia and should be noted. The Whipple test is also performed, initially unsupported, and then repeated, with the scapula

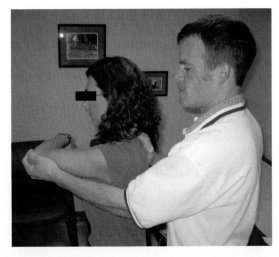

Figure 3-5 Jerk test. The examiner stabilizes the scapula with one hand while providing a posterior and inferior directed force on the elbow. A positive test occurs when the humeral head is able to be subluxed over the posterior glenoid rim to a greater degree than the contralateral side.

supported (Fig. 3-6). A positive test for instability is indicated by painful buckling during the unsupported test and then decreased pain and increased strength when the scapula is stabilized.

The exam continues with an assessment of inferior laxity. With the arm by the patient's side, the examiner places inferior traction on the humerus. A positive test occurs when the skin dimples just inferior to the acromion, and the inferior translation of the humerus is at least 2 to 3 cm. With the arm in adduction and neutral rotation, the superior glenohumeral ligament is the primary stabilizer to inferior translation. However, with the arm externally

rotated, the rotator interval is the primary stabilizer; therefore, the test should be done in both positions.

Testing for inferior laxity should also be performed in the 90-degree abducted position to test for laxity of the inferior capsule. An inferior translation force is applied to the superior proximal humerus in the abducted arm, with inferior subluxation greater than 1 cm considered abnormal.

The exam continues with the patient in the supine position on the exam table. The patient is asked to position the shoulder slightly off the edge of the table. The arm is then placed in 20 degrees of abduction in the plane of the scapula; the examiner then places one hand on the patient's elbow and the other on the proximal humerus and applies a compressive load to the humerus. Anterior- and posterior-directed forces are then applied to the humerus, and the amount of subluxation of the humeral head in the fossa is recorded (Fig. 3-7). This should be done in varying degrees of abduction and external rotation to assess different degrees of tension in the capsular ligament. It is important to remember that up to 50% subluxation of the head in any direction is considered normal. The subluxation is graded according to the following classifications: (a) 1+ indicates that there is excessive translation compared to the contralateral shoulder; (b) 2+ indicates that the humeral head can be subluxated over the rim of the glenoid but spontaneously reduces when the examiner releases pressure; and (c) 3+ indicates frank dislocation of the humeral head over the rim of the glenoid without spontaneous reduction. If subluxation is present, it is important to note whether the patient has a predominant direction of subluxation, which can affect surgical treatment.

A variation of the load and shift tests can be performed with the patient in the sitting position with his or her arm

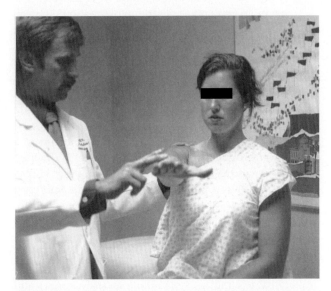

Figure 3-6 Whipple test. The examiner applies a downward force onto the hand with the shoulder flexed to 90 degrees and adducted.

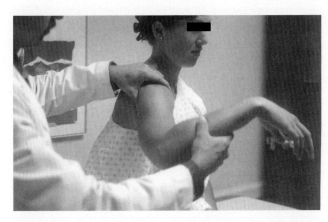

Figure 3-7 Supine anterior-posterior (AP) shift test. The arm is placed in 20 degrees of abduction in the plane of the scapula, and the examiner places one hand on the patient's elbow and the other on the proximal humerus, applying a compressive load to the humerus. Anterior and posterior directed forces are then applied to the humeral, and the amount of subluxation of the humeral head in the fossa is recorded.

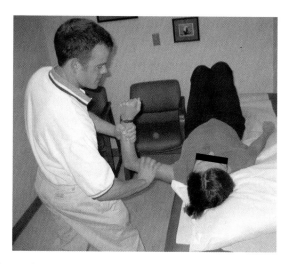

Figure 3-8 Load and shift tests. The examiner sits next to the patient on the affected side and supports the patient's elbow with one hand. The examiner places his or her other hand on the patient's shoulder, with the flat portion of the thumb resting against the posterior humeral head and the index and middle finger over the anterior humeral head, and gently circumducts the patient's arm to relax the shoulder musculature. With the flat portion of thumb, the examiner attempts to sublux the humeral head with an anteriorly directed force. A compressive load is then applied to the humerus, and the shoulder is brought into a position of abduction and external rotation. The degree of initial subluxation, as well as whether the joint relocates after abduction and external rotation, is recorded.

by his or her side (Fig. 3-8). The examiner sits next to the patient on the affected side and supports the patient's elbow with one hand while placing the other hand on the patient's shoulder. The flat portion of the examiner's thumb should rest against the posterior humeral head and the index and middle finger should rest over the anterior humeral head. The examiner gently circumducts the patient's arm to relax the shoulder musculature and, with the flat portion of the thumb, attempts to sublux the humeral head with an anteriorly directed force. A compressive load is then applied to the humerus, and the shoulder is brought into a position of abduction and external rotation. The initial subluxation degree, as well as joint relocation after abduction and external rotation, is recorded. If the anterior capsular structures are intact, the subluxated humeral head should relocate with this maneuver. If not, disruption or attenuation shoulder is suspected. This maneuver should be performed with attempted subluxation in an anterior-superior, straight anterior, and anterior-inferior direction.

The posterior capsuloligamentous structures can be evaluated in a similar manner, performing the same exam with attempted posterior-superior, straight posterior, and posterior-inferior subluxation. The examiner uses his or her index and ring finger to sublux the head, followed by relocation with abduction and external rotation. Labral tears should be suspected when the humeral head relocates into the joint and an audible or palpable clunk or pop is heard.

RADIOLOGIC EVALUATION

Standard anterior-posterior, lateral, and West Point axillary views should be taken of all patients to rule out any uncommon lesions, including Hill-Sachs, reverse Hill-Sachs, bony Bankart, and glenoid dysplasia.

More sophisticated imaging studies, such as computerized arthrotomography (CT arthrogram) and magnetic resonance imaging (MRI), with or without contrast, have been used to better define the pathology in patients with posterior instability or MDI. A patulous capsule can be identified with arthrography, but it usually only confirms the suspected diagnosis. A computed tomography scan is very useful for evaluating suspected glenoid dysplasia or an abnormal version, and should be used in patients with suspected glenoid pathology.

Labral abnormalities can be detected using MRI, but MRI is less effective in detecting a patulous capsule. We feel that MRI alone is not indicated in these patients unless concomitant or alternative pathology is suspected, including labral pathology, biceps, or rotator cuff pathology. In these cases, a magnetic resonance (MR) arthrogram is the study of choice.

NONOPERATIVE MANAGEMENT

The most important concept in the nonoperative treatment of MDI is the idea of the "shoulder at risk." These patients are affected with MDI and function well for years until a minor injury produces a loss of balance of the shoulder musculature. The resultant problems stem from an inability to control the entire shoulder girdle. The instigating incident may be small or large, but the result is an asynchronous firing pattern of the rotator cuff that eventually extends to the larger muscles of the shoulder girdle, producing scapular winging, malposition of the shoulder girdle, secondary impingement, weakness, and pain. The scapula protracts, the humeral head subluxates, and the rotator cuff and trapezius develop irritation as these muscles try to compensate for the lack of normal dynamic serratus and rotator cuff function.

Nonoperative treatment centers initially on dynamic stabilization of the scapulothoracic articulation and pain-free strengthening of the rotator cuff. Active abduction and "empty can" exercises should be avoided until symmetrical scapulothoracic and glenohumeral motion develop. Attentive physical therapy is essential for biofeedback during the early phases of rehabilitation. All exercises must be performed with the scapula retracted to avoid rotator cuff irritation. Because the patient is usually unaware of the malpositioned scapulothoracic articulation, hands-on therapy or taping is required to ensure correct positioning during rehab.

Nonoperative treatment, which includes education and physical therapy, is recommended as the initial treatment for patients with both posterior and multidirectional instability. Therapy for both is designed to strengthen the dynamic stabilizers of the shoulder. Patients must be informed that they need to regain both strength and neuromuscular coordination of the rotator cuff, deltoid, and scapula. Rockwood et al. found that patients with posterior instability responded better to physical therapy than those with anterior instability.[31] Several studies have shown that patients with posterior instability as the result of major trauma did not fare as well with conservative therapy.[12]

Wirth also studied conservative therapy in patients with multidirectional instability and reported satisfactory results in 88% of patients who underwent a specific program of physical therapy.[45]

In addition to a course of physical therapy, an intra-articular shot of corticosteroids and a short course of low-dose oral prednisone combined with nonsteroidal anti-inflammatory medication may be initiated prior to beginning therapy in an attempt to calm the inflammation. We generally recommend this aggressive treatment plan if the patient is experiencing night pain and has palpable swelling. For patients with severe protraction, we prescribe a scapular stabilizing brace and "hands-on" physical therapy.

A minimum of 6 months of adequate therapy is recommended before consideration of surgical intervention.

SURGICAL MANAGEMENT

Posterior Instability

Surgical management for posterior instability has traditionally failed to distinguish between dislocation and recurrent instability. Hawkins et al. reported a high failure and complication rate in a group of 26 shoulders operated on by multiple surgeons for recurrent instability.[17] They employed three different open surgical techniques, including glenoid osteotomy, reverse Putti-Platt, and biceps tendon transfer, with an overall recurrence rate of 50%.

Additional open surgical techniques for posterior instability include staple capsulorrhaphies, biceps tendon transfers, posterior capsular shifts (with or without bone blocks), humeral rotational osteotomies, and posterior glenoid osteotomies. Varying success has been reported using these techniques.[36,41,46] The most promising results have been reported with the use of posterior capsulorrhaphy, with or without posterior bone block or posterior capsular shift, with success rates of 80% to 96% in published studies.[13,34]

Recent success in surgery for posterior instability has been attributed to addressing the capsular redundancy in both the inferior and posterior regions of the glenohumeral joint. In addition, other authors, including ourselves, subscribe to the idea that laxity in the antero-superior capsular

structures needs to be assessed and, if necessary, corrected.[6] Intraoperative evaluation of the structures in the area of the rotator interval has been made easier with the use of the arthroscope.

Operative treatment for multidirectional instability was pioneered by Neer and Foster in the early 1980s and, as previously described, included a lateroinferior capsular shift of the anterior capsule.[27] Altchek and Warren used a similar, medially based capsular shift and reported good results.[2]

This open surgery has emphasized securing soft tissue to bone, direct and indirect tensioning of the capsule, overlapping of the capsule, and positioning and testing the stability of the repair during the procedure. With the advance of arthroscopic techniques, a similar shift is now possible. Arthroscopically, the surgeon can use the same techniques to secure the labrum to bone, directly tension the capsule in multiple quadrants of the shoulder to overlap or thermally address the capsule to alter thickness, and evaluate stability while visualizing the suture repair.

Current debate regarding the use of arthroscopic techniques for shoulder instability has focused on the high recurrence rates reported with earlier repair techniques. Numerous adjunctive soft-tissue techniques, including capsular shrinkage or plication, have been proposed to further constrain the shoulder in an attempt to achieve better results. However, this focus on the soft tissues has diverted critical attention away from recognizing the presence of significant bone deficiency. Such bony injuries include a bony Bankart, compression of the anterior glenoid, or a Hill-Sachs lesion of the humerus. Successfully identifying and addressing these bony deficiencies can allow arthroscopic techniques to equal or better open techniques in regard to recurrence and return to normal function.

All surgical treatment should begin with an exam under anesthesia. After induction of general anesthesia, the affected shoulder is examined with the patient in the supine position. If multidirectional instability is suspected, the predominant direction of the instability, if one exists, should be determined. This is essential to assess because the predominant direction of instability should be corrected first during the operative procedure.

The patient is placed in the lateral decubitus position, with the affected arm placed in 5 to 10 pounds of traction. A standard posterior portal is made, and a complete evaluation of the glenohumeral joint is performed. An anterior portal is established in the rotator interval with an outside-in technique using a spinal needle followed by a trocar. Careful attention is made in creating the anterior portal so as to allow access to the entire anterior and inferior capsule, looking for patulous or redundant tissue. A probe is introduced, and the anterior capsulo-ligamentous structures are inspected, including the anterior labrum, the inferior capsular pouch, and the anterior, middle, and superior IGHLC. In addition, the rotator cuff and posterior labrum are inspected for any pathology.

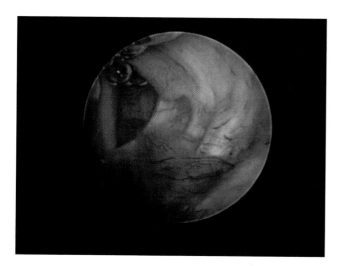

Figure 3-9 Patulous posterior capsule viewed from the anterior portal.

It is also important to evaluate the "drive through sign," the ability to pass the arthroscope easily between the humeral head and the glenoid at the level of the anterior band of the inferior glenohumeral ligament. Although not pathognomonic for instability, it is associated with laxity and should raise suspicion for instability. For this test to be valid, however, the patient needs to be in the beach-chair position. We feel that patients in the lateral position, with proper posterior portal placement, will have a "drive through" sign.

The arthroscope is then moved to the anterior portal, and the posterior capsuloligamentous structures are thoroughly inspected, paying careful attention to identify any labral pathology or redundant posterior capsule (Figs. 3-9 and 3-10). In addition, the anterior labrum can be carefully inspected.

Subluxation of the humeral head should be attempted in all directions with the arthroscope in the anterior as well as posterior portal, and the predominant direction of laxity noted.

RECONSTRUCTION FOR POSTERIOR LAXITY

Three different techniques for repair of the posterior capsuloligamentous structures are used by the authors.

Suretac Technique

The Suretac technique is used for posterior Bankart lesions involving only the attachment of the PIGHL. This is usually combined with a rotator interval plication to restore stability to the shoulder. In this technique, the scope is placed in the anterior portal, and a shaver (with the suction on low)

is used to debride the posterior soft tissues to initiate a healing response and promote tissue scarring in the desired position.

In some cases, it is necessary to reinsert the posterior cannula in a more lateral position to allow access to the glenoid at the proper angle. The same posterior skin incision can be used by withdrawing the cannula into the bursa, pulling the skin laterally, and reinserting the cannula under direct visualization from the anterior portal.

The glenoid neck is abraded in the region of the detachment of the PIGHL and posterior labrum (Fig. 3-11). A pilot hole is then drilled at the glenoid origin of the PIGHL adjacent to the glenoid labrum. The capsuloligamentous complex is then speared with a Kirschner's wire and shifted superiorly to the drilled hole. The wire is then placed into the previously drilled hole, and the Suretac is then placed over the wire and tapped into position, securing the posterior labrum to the posterior glenoid rim (Fig. 3-12). It is important to note that the Suretac technique can be used only when there is a small labral tear with minimal instability in the shoulder. We feel that the Suretac provides "local" fixation only. If the capsuloligamentous structures require shifting, we feel that the Suretac does not provide a fixation

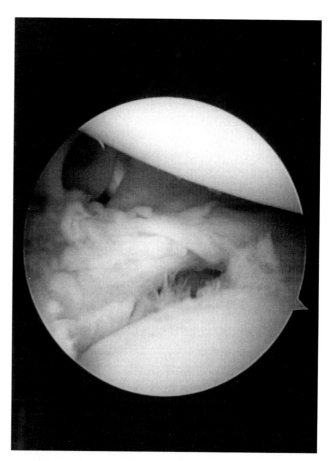

Figure 3-10 Posterior labral avulsion with fraying viewed from the posterior portal.

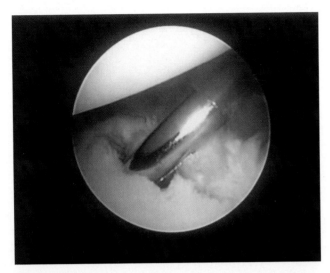

Figure 3-11 Shaver in posterior portal abrading the glenoid neck at 9 o'clock.

secure enough to counteract the shear forces of the shifted capsular complex, and, therefore, should not be used.

The arthroscope is then placed back into the posterior portal, and the rotator interval closed using nonabsorbable No. 2 Ethibond (Ethicon, Somerville, NJ). This is referred to as a rotator interval plication stitch and is designed to restore anterior-superior instability. The shaver is introduced through the anterior portal and the rotator interval capsule abraded to promote a reactive surface for healing. The suction on the shaver is turned off during the abrasion to prevent capsule destruction capsule.

The plication is then performed. With the scope in the posterior portal, a Crawford spinal needle is placed outside-in through the capsule. The skin site for needle introduction is just posterior to the anterior lateral corner of the acromion, with the needle entering the joint just anterior to the anterior edge of the supraspinatus tendon and just lat-

eral to the glenoid rim (Fig. 3-13A). The water inflow is turned off to allow a No.2 Ethibond suture to pass through the spinal needle into the joint. A grabber is introduced through the anterior portal, above the biceps tendon, and used to retrieve the suture end. The suture is brought above the biceps and "parked" in an inferior joint to facilitate retrieval. A suture retriever is placed through the anterior por-

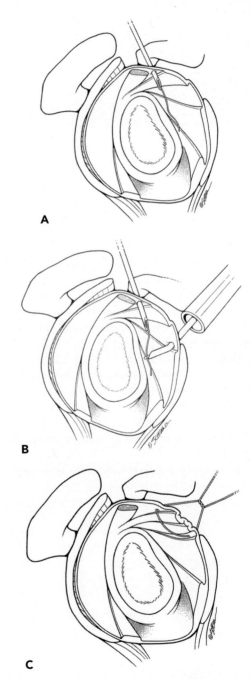

A

B

C

Figure 3-13 (A) Crawford spinal needle passed percutaneously through the capsule anterior to the supraspinatus tendon and biceps tendon. (B) Suture retriever passed through the capsule, piercing the small portion of superior subscapularis tendon, then retrieving the No. 2 Ethibond suture (Ethicon, Somerville, NJ) passed through spinal needle. (C) Tying sutures in the subacromial space, plicating rotator interval.

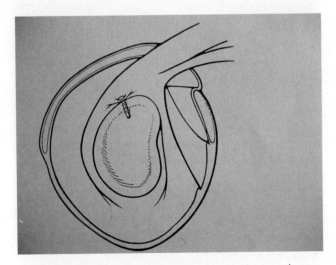

Figure 3-12 Diagram of Suretac in posterior capsule.

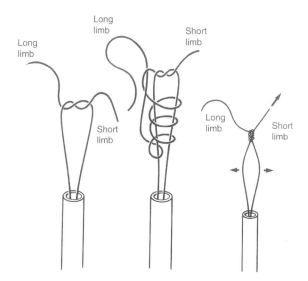

Figure 3-14 Roeder knot technique. Begin by throwing the first half of a square knot, leaving one end long and one end short. The long end is then passed around both limbs of the suture three times and then once around the short limb. The long limb of the suture is then passed through the loop adjacent to the half-square knot. The knot is then compressed by spreading the distal limbs while holding the short limb as a post. The knot is then advanced by pulling on the short limb. It is imperative that the long limb not be pulled until the knot is snug against the soft tissues, because this will lock the knot. The knot is then secured by at least one single half-hitch, with the short limb as a post.

tal to pierce the capsuloligamentous tissue anterior and posterior to the subscapularis tendon. The retriever retrieves the suture and is brought back out of the anterior portal (Fig. 3-13*B*). A switching stick is then introduced through the anterior portal and then pulled back into the bursal space with the trocar. The arthroscopic view is then directed upward, toward the undersurface of the rotator cuff, while the switching stick is pushed against the superior aspect of the cuff in the subacromial bursa, indenting it, thereby using it to guide the trocar to a position posterior and lateral to the stitch in the supraspinatus. The switching stick is then removed and a crochet hook introduced lateral and posterior to the stitch. With the hook facing medially, the device is swept medially and anteriorly, hooking the stitch and retrieving it through the anterior portal. An arthroscopic knot is then tied and tightened to plicate the rotator interval. Adequate plication can be observed and confirmed with the arthroscope in the intra-articular position (Fig. 3-13*C*). An alternative technique is to switch the arthroscope to the subacromial bursa, retrieve the sutures under direct visualization, and then tie them. The arthroscope is then placed back into the joint to evaluate the plication.

For arthroscopic knot tying, we prefer a modification of the Roeder knot (Fig. 3-14.) It is accomplished by first throwing the first half of a square knot, leaving one end long and one end short. The long end is then passed around both limbs of the suture three times, and then once around the short limb. The long limb of the suture is then passed

through the loop adjacent to the half-square knot. The knot is then compressed by spreading the distal limbs while holding the short limb as a post. The knot is then advanced by pulling on the short limb. It is imperative that the long limb not be pulled until the knot is snug against the soft tissues because this will lock the knot. The knot is then secured by at least one single half-hitch, with the short limb as a post.

Inferior Shift

The suture anchor technique is used for more extensive capsule labral avulsions in the posterior inferior quadrant of the shoulder. The posterior portal should be placed more laterally at the start of the procedure to allow access to the glenoid at the proper angle. The debridement and abrasion of the capsule and glenoid are as previously described, but more extensive. The capsule is elevated down around the inferior labrum to the attachment of the anterior band (5 o'clock position) (Fig. 3-15). A pilot hole is drilled at approximately

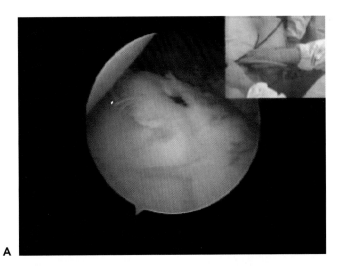

A

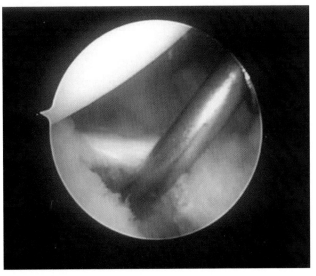

B

Figure 3-15 *(A,B)* Elevating posterior capsule and labrum with small elevator in posterior portal.

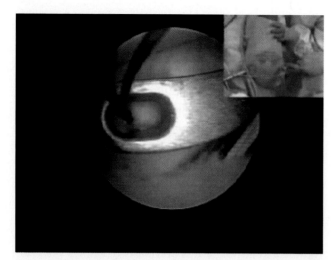

Figure 3-16 The sutures of the anchor are visible at 3 o'clock. The Prolene shuttle suture (Ethicon, Somerville, NJ) is passed through the area of the capsule inferior to the level of the anchor to secure the capsule in a more superomedial position.

the 7 o'clock position on the posterior inferior glenoid, and a suture anchor inserted into the drill hole. A doubled 2-0 Prolene suture (Ethicon) is then placed through the inferior glenohumeral ligament using the Caspari suture punch (Arthroteck, Inc., Warsaw, IN) or Linvatec spectrum suture passer (Linvatec, Largo, FL) at the 5 o'clock or 6 o'clock position (Fig. 3-16). This doubled 2-0 Prolene suture is then used to retrieve one limb of a No. 2 Ethibond suture through the soft tissues (Fig. 3-17). This step is repeated, creating a mattress suture with the No. 2 Ethibond attached to the anchor and through the inferior glenohumeral ligament (IGHL). This suture is then tied arthroscopically, shifting the inferior capsule superiorly and repairing the posterior capsule labral avulsion. A second and third anchor are used as

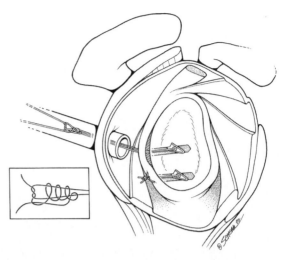

Figure 3-18 Suture anchor technique for reattaching the posterior labrum.

needed to complete the capsular shift (Fig. 3-18). One or two posterior capsular stitches are placed above the capsulolabral repair as needed to reinforce the stability (described in next section). The posterior cannula is backed out of the capsule under direct visualization and reinserted more superior in the capsule, above the repair, before the interval plication stitch is introduced. The camera is then placed back into the posterior portal, and a rotator interval plication stitch is added to further stabilize the shoulder.

Suture Capsulorrhaphy

The suture plication technique is used when there is extensive damage to the posterior and inferior capsulolabral complex or when there are inferior capsular tears near the glenoid attachment of the ligaments. This technique provides the greatest vertical shift of the capsular structures.

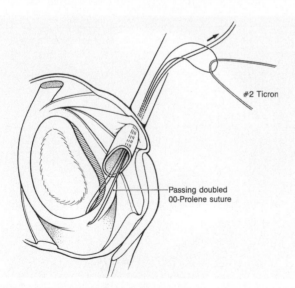

Figure 3-17 Technique for using prolene shuttle to pass a No. 2 Ethibond suture (Ethicon, Somerveille, NJ).

#2 Ticron

Passing doubled 00-Prolene suture

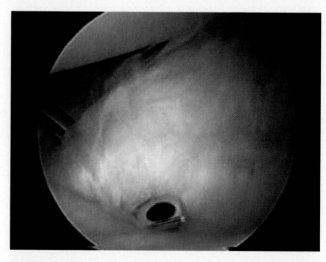

Figure 3-19 Spectrum suture passer (Linvatec, Largo, FL) passed through posterior capsule 1 cm lateral to glenoid neck.

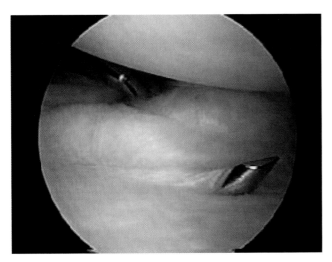

Figure 3-20 The Spectrum suture passer (Linvatec, Largo, FL) is then passed through the posterior labrum superior to the area of the passed-through capsule.

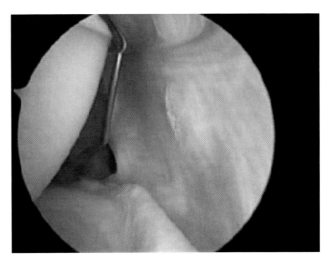

Figure 3-22 Crawford spinal needle passed through the infraspinatus for posterior plication. Viewed from the anterior portal.

The soft tissues and bone of the glenoid are prepared using a shaver inserted through the posterior portal, as previously discussed. Through this portal, the Linvatec spectrum suture passer can be used to pierce the posterior, inferior capsule at the most inferior position possible, incorporating the anterior inferior glenohumeral ligament (AIGHL) as well (Fig. 3-19). The hook is then rotated so that the tip reenters the joint. The capsule is then brought superomedially and placed between the intact labro-glenoid junction at the 6 o'clock position, from inferior to superior, bringing the tip of the hook back into the joint (Fig. 3-20). A doubled 2-0 Prolene suture is then introduced into the joint. This is used to retrieve a No. 2 Ethibond suture through the soft tissue, which is then tied arthroscopically, shifting the inferior capsule superiorly. This is repeated two or three times as needed to complete the repair. Each suture is sequentially placed through the capsule 1 to 2 cm lateral and

1 cm inferior to the area of attachment to the labro-glenoid junction (Fig. 3-21).

In our experience, the posterior capsule in patients with posterior instability may be very tenuous and friable. In these patients, it may be difficult to adequately plicate the posterior capsule due to tissue tearing. In this situation, we place one or two sutures, as described previously, into the inferior capsule and PIGHL because this tissue tends to be more robust. We then augment the plication by passing the suture through the infraspinatus tendon and imbricating the capsule.

A Crawford spinal needle is passed through the skin and into the infraspinatus tendon near the tednond's insertion on the humeral head (Fig. 3-22). The arthroscope remains in the anterior portal and is used to confirm proper placement of the needle. A suture retriever is placed through the posterior portal and used to pierce a portion of the medial infraspinatus and capsule. The water is turned off and a No. 2

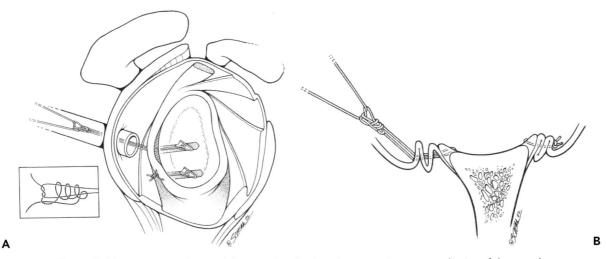

A   **B**

Figure 3-21 *(A,B)* Sagittal view of the capsular plication, demonstrating an accordioning of the capsule.

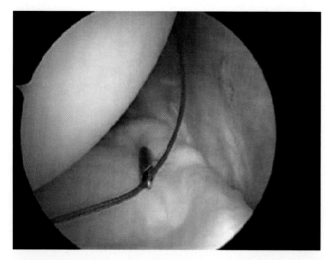

Figure 3-23 Suture retriever passed through the posterior capsule, retrieving a No. 2 Ethibond suture (Ethicon, Somerville, NJ) passed through the spinal needle.

Ethibond suture is passed through the spinal needle into the joint. The suture is retrieved with the retriever and brought back out the posterior portal (Fig. 3-23). A switching stick is placed into the posterior cannula and backed into the bursal space. Using a method similar to the interval plication stitch, the cannula is brought lateral and anterior to the lateral stitch in the infraspinatus, and a crochet hook is used to retrieve the other end of the Ethibond suture. An arthroscopic knot-tying technique is used to tie the suture over the tendon (in the bursal space), plicating the posterior capsule in a lateral-to-medial direction. Adequate plication is confirmed with the arthroscope under direct visualization (Fig. 3-24). This is repeated two or three times, moving more superior on the tendon with each stitch. Stability is assessed after the posterior plication and additional posterior sutures are placed. Once the posterior plication is completed, the arthroscope is

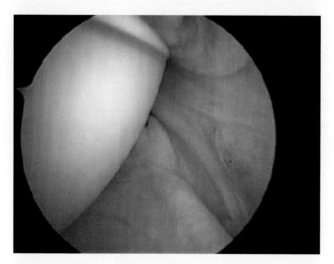

Figure 3-24 The final result of the posterior capsular plication after the suture is tied in the subacromial space. Viewed from the anterior portal.

reinserted above the repair, and the rotator interval closed by the previously described techniques.

Multidirectional Instability

Surgical techniques for multidirectional instability are influenced by the predominant direction of instability, as assessed by the exam under anesthesia. It is paramount to first address the capsular laxity responsible for the predominant direction of instability. If the predominant direction of the instability is posterior, one of the previously mentioned stabilization techniques for posterior instability should be employed. If the predominant direction of the instability is anterior, the anterior portal is made to ensure access to the inferior glenoid and capsule. By using a shaver with the suction on low, or a banana blade through the anterior portal, the anteroinferior capsule is detached from the glenoid. In a similar fashion, the Bankart lesion, if present, is detached. In a right shoulder, a Bankart lesion is detached by beginning at the 1 o'clock position and continuing down the glenoid rim until the posterior band of the glenohumeral ligament has been released to the 7 o'clock position posteroinferiorly. The anteroinferior neck of the glenoid is then aggressively abraded until a bleeding, bony surface is present. The anteroinferior capsule is abraded in a manner similar to the one described for the posterior capsule. Suture anchors are then placed at 5, 3, and 1 o'clock, and the capsule and anterior labrum brought superior and medial by passing and tying the sutures in a manner similar to the one described for a posterior Bankart lesion (Fig. 3-25, *A–C*).

If the anterior labrum is intact and a patulous anterior capsule is in need of plication, a Linvatec or Caspari suture punch is used to shift the anterior capsule superomedial in a manner similar to the one described for the posterior capsule. The first stitch should be placed at 6 o'clock, the second at 4:30, the third at 3 o'clock, and the last at 1 o'clock (Fig. 3-26*A*). Switch the scope around and plicate the posterior capsule. Switch the camera to the back and place an interval plication stitch. If a Bankart lesion is present, or if the anterior labrum is attenuated, suture anchors can be used to provide stable fixation for the shift (Fig. 3-26*B*). Closing of the rotator interval is recommended.

Suture capsulorrhaphy complications for either posterior or multidirectional instability include damage to the axillary nerve and an overtightened capsule. We feel that potential damage to the axillary nerve can be minimized by paying careful attention when plicating the capsule from the 5 o'clock to 7 o'clock position. Deep passes through the capsule with the shuttle device should be avoided because the axillary nerve runs extracapsular, just inferior to the glenoid neck at the 6 o'clock position. In patients with multidirectional instability, it is very difficult to overtighten the capsule, limiting range of motion. With posterior instability, overtightening the capsule can be

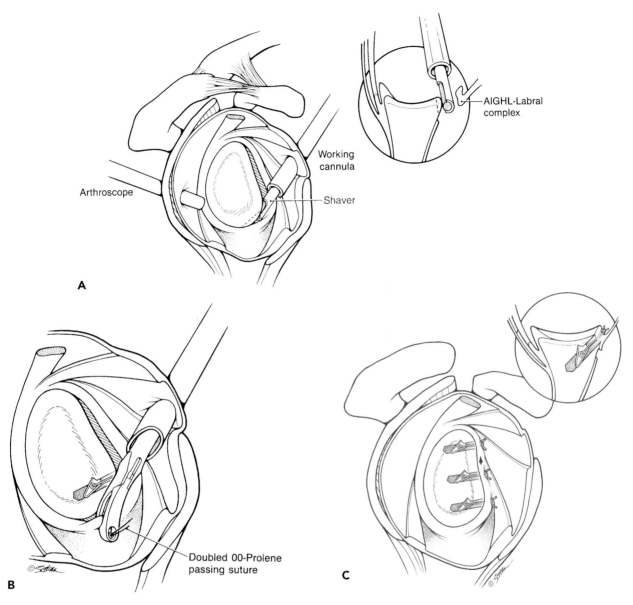

Figure 3-25 (*A*) Lateral and sagittal view of the shaver abrading the anterior inferior glenoid neck. (*B*) Suture punch piercing the capsule inferior to the suture anchor with a Prolene shuttle stitch (Ethicon, Somerville, NJ). (*C*) Final result of suture anchor capsular plication and labral repair.

avoided by internally rotating the shoulder slightly while securing the sutures.

Thermal Capsulorrhaphy

Thermal capsulorrhaphy has gained favor as both an adjunct and stand-alone procedure for the treatment of both posterior instability and MDI.

In 1992, the holmium-yttrium aluminum garnet (YAG) laser was found to shrink the capsular tissue at nonablative energy levels. Basic science studies demonstrated that the thermal effects of laser energy are responsible for the ultrastructural changes in collagen that result in tissue shrinkage. These studies showed that capsular shrinkage can be

achieved using nonablative energy without harmful effects on the viscoelastic properties of the tissue,[18,19] although a decrease in capsular tensile stiffness was noted at higher energy levels.

In 1993, Thabit presented the clinical results of the initial 41 patients treated with laser-assisted capsulorrhaphy for MDI and unidirectional instability. Postoperative Rowe scores averaged 88 to 100 points. All competitive athletes returned to their previous levels of sports participation.[38]

Continued study of the mechanism of laser shrinkage led to the confirmation that heat energy within a specific range produced the changes in the tissue. The optimal range for producing this ultrastructural damage without compromising strength seems to be within 60.0°C to

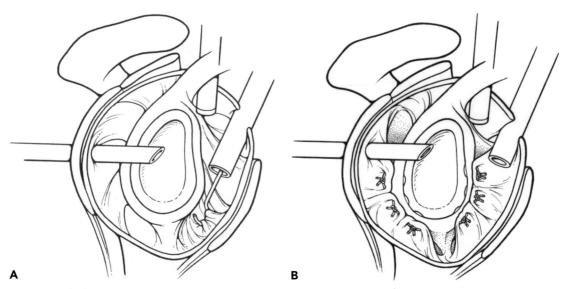

Figure 3-26   (*A*) Spectrum suture passer passed through the anterior inferior capsule. (*B*) Final result of anterior and posterior capsular plication.

$67.5\,^{\circ}\mathrm{C}.^{34}$ A variety of unipolar and bipolar devices, as well as holmium lasers, have been developed to impart heat to the tissue within this range.

All of these devices work by damaging the ultrastructure of the capsule, destroying cells and uncoiling collagen cross-links in a temperature-specific range. If the temperature is too low, there is no effect on the tissue. If the temperature is too high, the entire capsular matrix is destroyed, with devastating clinical results. The cellular response to this heat is a hypercellular reaction producing collagen that is more tightly organized. The clinical effect is a thickened and less elastic capsule, but, from approximately day 5 to day 20, the vascular reaction and cellular invasion of the damaged capsule causes a weakening of the structural properties until the new collagen is produced.[34] Clinically, this means that the shoulder should be protected during this time.

Several unknown factors remain regarding the use of thermal devises to shrink the capsule. The effect of the temperature damage on the proprioceptive and position-sensitive nerve endings is unknown. The need for variable temperature from patient to patient is unknown. The time to fully reform a "normal" capsule is also unknown, as are the long-term shrinkage effects.

Currently, we recommend that thermal capsulorrhaphy be used as an adjunct to capsule suture plication. Suture plication for either posterior or multidirectional instability should be performed as previously described, and the capsule reassessed. Any residual patulous capsule can be treated with thermal capsulorrhaphy. We recommend single radial passes of the probe made from the glenoid side to the humeral side of the capsule. The capsule should be "striped," with areas of virgin capsule left between the areas of thermal capsular shrinkage.

Complications of this procedure include thermal damage to the axillary nerve and capsular necrosis from excessive use of the thermal device. Potential damage to the axillary nerve can be minimized by refraining from using the thermal probe from the 5 o'clock to the 7 o'clock position. Capsular necrosis can be minimized by "striping" the capsule, as mentioned previously.

Glenoid Dysplasia

Glenoid dysplasia must also be recognized and addressed at the time of surgery. Significant retroversion of the glenoid may require correction via osteotomy. Treatment of anterior inferior glenoid deficiency consists of reestablishing the bony buttress to accommodate the axial and shear forces present in the shoulder. This may be achieved through several methods. Allograft bone grafting to the glenoid is not advised because of the graft's propensity to be reabsorbed. The Bristow procedure, with the transfer of the coracoid to the inferior glenoid, is also not recommended because the coracoid's small size fails to reestablish the bony buttress, relying instead on the "sling effect" of the conjoined tendon as the shoulder is brought into abduction and external rotation. A third option is the Latarjet procedure. This procedure differs from the Bristow procedure in that it transfers a much larger portion of the coracoid (2–3 cm of bone) to the conjoined tendon to recreate the bony buttress of the glenoid arc.

REHABILITATION

After surgical stabilization for posterior instability, patients are placed in a gunslinger-type brace (in the operating room), with the shoulder in approximately 45 degrees of abduction, 30 degrees of external rotation, and neutral flexion. Patients stay in this brace for 4 weeks, except to shower, and then slowly progress to passive range of motion.

After surgical stabilization for multidirectional instability, patients are placed in an abduction pillow (in the operating room), with the shoulder in approximately 30 degrees of abduction, neutral rotation, and flexion. They also stay in the sling for 4 weeks, except to shower.

After 4 weeks, they are started on a series of four exercises that are performed ten times, each twice a day. It is imperative that these exercises remain pain free, because painful movements could be a sign of damage to the repair. Exercise one is an external rotation exercise that may be done actively or passively. The patient's hand is positioned across the stomach with the elbow at the side. In a pivoting movement, the patient moves the hand away from the stomach until pointing straight ahead. The patient may use the opposite arm to assist or may do it actively until the arm is facing forward. Exercise two begins with the arm in the same position as in exercise one, with the patient's elbow flexed to 90 degrees and the hand across the stomach. The patient uses the opposite arm to elevate the elbow and forearm in the forward plane away from the body until 90 degrees is achieved. The patient then gently lowers the arm until it is back at the side. The third exercise is the shoulder shrug, which is done with the patient's arms in a resting position. The elbow may be bent or straight; the shoulders are elevated toward the ears and then allowed to return to the resting position. The fourth exercise involves a self-stretching exercise in which the patient sits on a rolling chair and places his or her hands on a waist-high table in front of the patient. Keeping his or her hands on the table, the patient rolls backward, forward flexing the shoulder to a level below the threshold of pain.

Maintenance exercises are begun after 8 to 12 weeks (when range of motion has been restored) and include three exercises, which again must be pain-free. Exercise one uses a bungee cord to strengthen the external and internal rotators. The cord is tied to an immobile object at waist level, and a small rolled towel is placed under the effected upper arm and kept against the patient's body. The elbow is kept at 90 degrees, with the patient's forearm internally rotated across the stomach. The patient then externally rotates against resistance until neutral rotation is reached before slowly returning to the staring position. The second exercise begins with the patient standing back against the wall. The patient holds small weights with arms by the sides and presses back against the wall, holds for 10 seconds, and then relaxes. Exercise three begins with the patient in the same starting position as in exercise two. With arms straight, the patient forward flexes the effected arm until the hand reaches as close to the wall above the head as possible. The patient then brings the arm down slowly to the starting position.

After regaining full range of motion and appropriate strength, strengthening exercises can begin and are to be maintained indefinitely. Again, these must be pain-free.

Increasing strength in internal and external rotation, as well as flexion and extension, is emphasized.

RESULTS

Several reports have documented high success rates for arthroscopic capsular shift in the treatment of MDI. Duncan and Savoie reported preliminary results of arthroscopic capsular shift in ten patients for MDI patients with follow-up from 1 to 3 years.[10] No patients in the study developed recurrent instability. Four athletes returned to sports participation, although no information regarding their preoperative level of activity was reported. Two patients developed pain postoperatively over the posterior suture knot that required removal. All ten patients had a satisfactory rating score, according to the Neer criteria. Treacy and Savoie reported on 25 patients who underwent arthroscopic capsular shift for MDI with an average follow-up of 5 years.[40] Three patients had episodes of instability after the procedure, but none had repeat episodes of dislocation. Eighty-eight percent of patients had satisfactory results, according to the Neer system.

Tauro and Carter reported preliminary results of a modified arthroscopic capsular shift for anterior and anteroinferior instability in four patients with a minimum follow-up of 6 months.[37] No patients developed recurrent instability, although follow-up is short term.

Gartsman reported on 47 patients who underwent arthroscopic capsular plication for MDI.[13] The average follow-up was 35 months, and 94% had good to excellent results. Eighty-five percent of athletes retuned to their desired level of sports participation.

McIntyre reported results of arthroscopic capsular shift in MDI patients, using a multiple suture technique in the anterior and posterior capsule, with follow-up of 32 months.[25] Recurrent instability recurred in one patient (5%), who was treated successfully with a repeat arthroscopic stabilization. Thirteen athletes (93%) returned to their previous level of performance.

Wichman and Snyder reported results of arthroscopic capsular shift for MDI in 24 patients with an average age of 26 and a minimum follow-up of 2 years.[43] Five patients (21%) had an unsatisfactory rating using the Neer criteria. Three of these patients were involved in workers' compensation cases that were not yet resolved, and an additional patient was involved in litigation over a motor vehicle accident.

Lyons et al. reported on laser-assisted capsulorrhaphy for MDI in 26 patients (27 shoulders) with a minimum follow-up of 2 years.[22] Twenty-six of the 27 shoulders remained stable, and 86% of patents returned to their previous level of sports participation.

McIntyre et al. reviewed the results of 20 consecutive shoulders in 19 patients treated with arthroscopic capsular

TABLE 3-1
SUCCESS RATES FOR ARTHROSCOPIC SHIFT FOR MDI

Procedure	Author	Success
Arthroscopic shift for MDI	Duncan et al.	10/10 satisfactory results
Arthroscopic shift for MDI	Treacy el al.	88% satisfactory results
Arthroscopic shift for MDI	Tauro et al.	No recurrent instability
Arthroscopic shift for MDI	Gartsman et al.	94% excellent results
Arthroscopic shift for MDI	McIntyre et al.	93% return to previous level of play
Arthroscopic shift for MDI	Snyder et al.	79% satisfactory results

MDI, Multidirectional instability.

shift for posterior instability.[23] At an average of 31 months postoperatively, they had 15 excellent, 2 good, 1 fair, and 3 poor results. They reported two recurrent dislocations and three subluxations for an overall recurrence rate of 25% (Table 3-1).

Williams et al. reported on a series of 26 patients (27 shoulders) treated with arthroscopic repair for traumatic posterior instability (posterior Bankart lesion) with an average follow-up of 5 years.[44] Symptoms of pain and instability were eliminated in 92% of patients. Two patients required additional surgery.

Wolf reported on a series of 14 patients with recurrent posterior instability treated with arthroscopic capsular plication.[46] Follow-up averaged 33 months, and 12 patients reported excellent results. There was one recurrence of instability, which was remedied by a second operation. All 14 patients were satisfied with their procedure.

Hovis et al. reported on a series of six elite golfers with posterior instability who underwent posterior thermal capsulorrhaphy.[20] At an average of 4.5 years follow-up, all six had returned to their previous level of play.

Antoniou presented results on 41 patients undergoing arthroscopic capsulolabral augmentation for posteroinfe-

rior instability.[3] Patients were followed for an average of 28 months, and 35 (85%) patients had improved stability of the shoulder.

Jorgensen et al. followed 41 patients with posterior instability that were treated with either open or arthroscopic technique.[21] Patients were evaluated for an average of 36 months, and no significant difference was seen in outcome between the two groups. The group treated with the open procedure, however, had a longer hospitalization, slight decrease in external rotation, and more frequent cosmetic complaints (Table 3-2).

CONCLUSIONS

Posterior and multidirectional instability in the shoulder presents a challenge in both diagnosis and treatment. Conservative treatment, including modification of activities and aggressive rehabilitation, usually provides an adequate relief of symptoms. When this fails, arthroscopic treatment can provide comparable results to open procedures, with the added benefit of a minimally invasive procedure.

TABLE 3-2
SUCCESS RATES FOR PATIENTS TREATED FOR POSTERIOR INSTABILITY

Procedure	Author	Success
Posterior capsular shift for PI	McIntyre et al.	25% recurrence
Posterior Bankart repair	Williams et al.	92% successful outcome
Posterior capsular plication for PI	Wolf et al.	86% excellent results
Thermal capsulorrhaphy for PI	Hovis et al.	94% excellent results
Posterior capsular plication for PI	Antoniou et al.	85% successful outcome
Open versus arthroscopic for PI	Jorgensen et al.	equal results, more morbidity open

PI, posterior instability.

REFERENCES

1. Abrams JS, Savoie FH, Tauro JC, et al. Recent advances in the evaluation and treatment of shoulder instability: anterior, posterior and multidirectional. Arthroscopy 2002;9(suppl 2):1–13.
2. Altchek DW, Warren R. T-plasty modification of the Bankart procedure for multidirectional instability of the anterior and inferior type. J Bone Joint Surg 1991;73A:105.
3. Antoniou J, Duckworth DT, Harryman DT III. Capsulolabral augmentation for the management of posteroinferior instability of the shoulder. J Bone Joint Surg Am 2000;82:1220.
4. Antoniou J, Harryman DT. Posterior instability. Orthop Clin North Am 2001;3:463.
5. Bigliani LU, Endrizzi DP, McIlveen SJ, et al. Operative management of posterior shoulder instability. Orthop Trans 1989;13:232.
6. Bigliani LU, Pollock RG, McIlveen SJ, et al. Shift of the posteroinferior aspect of the capsule for recurrent posterior glenohumeral instability. J Bone Joint Surg Am 1995;77:1011.
7. Bigliani LU, Pollock RG, Soslowsky LJ, et al. Tensile properties of the inferior glenohumeral ligament. J Orthop Res 1992;10:187.
8. Caspari RB. Arthroscopic reconstruction of anterior shoulder instability. Tech Orthop 1988;3:59.
9. Cooper RA, Brems JJ. The inferior capsular shift procedure for multidirectional instability of the shoulder. J Bone Joint Surg Am 1992;74:1516.
10. Duncan R, Savoie FH. Arthroscopic inferior capsular shift for multidirectional instability of the shoulder: a preliminary report. Arthroscopy 1993;9(1):24.
11. Field LD, Warren RF, O'Brien SJ, et al. Isolated closure of rotator interval defects or shoulder instability. Am J Sports Med 1995;23:557.
12. Fronek J, Warren RF, Bowen M. Posterior subluxation of the glenohumeral joint. J Bone Joint Surg 1989;71A:205.
13. Gartsman GM, Roddey TS, Hammerman SM. Arthroscopic treatment of multidirectional glenohumeral instability: 2 to 5 year follow-up. Arthroscopy 2001;17(3):236.
14. Harryman DT II, Lazarus MD, Sidles JA, et al. Pathophysiology of shoulder instability. In: McGinty JB, Caspari RB, Jackson RW, et al., eds. Operative arthroscopy, 2nd ed. Philadelphia, WB Saunders, 1996:677.
15. Harryman DT II, Sidles JA, Harris SL, et al. The role of the rotator interval capsule in passive motion and stability of the shoulder. J Bone Joint Surg 1992;74A:53.
16. Hawkins RJ, Belle RM. Posterior instability of the shoulder. Instr Course Lect 1989;38:211.
17. Hawkins RJ, Koppert G, Johnston G. Recurrent posterior instability (subluxation) of the shoulder. J Bone Joint Surg 1984;66A:169.
18. Hayashi K, Markel MD. Thermal modification of joint capsule and ligamentous tissues. Oper Tech Sports Med 1998;6:120.
19. Hayashi K, Thabit G, Vailas A, et al. The effect of nonablative laser energy on joint capsular properties. Am J Sports Med 1996;24:640.
20. Hovis WD, Dean MT, Mallon WJ, et al. Posterior instability of the shoulder with secondary impingement in elite golfers. Am J Sports Med 2002;30(6):886.
21. Jorgesen U, Svend-Hansen H, Bak K, et al. Recurrent post-traumatic anterior shoulder dislocation—open versus arthroscopic repair. Knee Surg Sports Traum Arthros 1999;7(2):118.
22. Lyons TR, Griffith PL, Savoie FH, et al. Laser-assisted capsulorrhaphy for multidirectional instability of the shoulder. Arthroscopy 2001;17(1):25.
23. McIntyre LF, Caspari RB, Savoie FH. The arthroscopic treatment of posterior shoulder instability: two-year results of a multiple suture technique. Arthroscopy 1997;4:426.
24. McIntyre LF, Caspari RB, Savoie FH. The arthroscopic treatment of multidirectional instability: two-year results of multiple suture technique. Arthroscopy 1997;13:418.
25. McIntyre LF. Arthroscopic capsulorrhaphy for multidirectional instability. Oper Tech Sports Med 1997;5:233.
26. Neer CS, Foster CR. Inferior capsular shift for involuntary inferior and multidirectional instability of the shoulder: a preliminary report. J Bone Joint Surg 1980;26A:897.
27. Nobuhara K, Ikeda H. Rotator interval lesion. Clin Orthop 1987;23:44.
28. O'Brien SJ, Neves MC, Arnoczky SJ, et al. The anatomy and histology of the inferior glenohumeral ligament complex of the shoulder. Am J Sports Med 1990;18:449.
29. Papendick LW, Savoie FH. Anatomy-specific repair techniques for posterior shoulder instability. J South Orthop Assoc 1995;3:169.
30. Pollock RG, Bigliani LU. Recurrent posterior shoulder instability: diagnosis and treatment. Clin Orthop Rel Res 1993;291:85.
31. Rockwood CA, Burkhead WZ, Brna J. Subluxation of the glenohumeral joint: response to rehabilitative exercise, traumatic versus atraumatic instability. Orthop Trans 1986;10:220.
32. Rowe CR, Yee LB. A posterior approach to the shoulder. J Bone Joint Surg 1944;26:580.
33. Rowe CR, Zarins B. Recurrent transient subluxation of the shoulder. J Bone Joint Surg Am 1981;63:863.
34. Savoie FH, Field LD. Thermal versus suture treatment of symptomatic capsular laxity. Clin Sports Med 2000;1:63.
35. Savoie FH, Field LD. Arthroscopic management of posterior shoulder instability. Oper Tech Sports Med 1997;5:226.
36. Schwartz E, Warren RF, O'Brien SJ, et al. Posterior shoulder instability. Orthop Clin North Am 1987;18:409.
37. Tauro JC, Carter FM II. Arthroscopic capsular advancement for anterior and anterior-inferior shoulder instability: a preliminary report. Arthroscopy 1994;10:513.
38. Thabit G. The arthroscopically assisted holmium YAG laser surgery in the shoulder. Oper Tech Sports Med 1998;6:131.
39. Tibone JE, Bradley JP. The treatment of posterior shoulder subluxation in athletes. Clin Orthop Rel Res 1993;291:124.
40. Treacy SH, Savoie FH, Field LD. Arthroscopic treatment of multidirectional instability. J Shoulder Elbow Surg 1999;8(4):345.
41. Warren RF, Bowen M. Posterior subluxation of the glenohumeral joint. J Bone Joint Surg Am 1989;71:205.
42. Webber SC, Caspari RB. A biomechanical evaluation of the restraints to posterior shoulder dislocation. Arthroscopy 1985;5:115.
43. Wichman MT, Snyder SJ. Arthroscopic capsular plication for multidirectional instability of the shoulder. Oper Tech Sports Med 1997;5:238.
44. Williams RJ, Strickland S, Cohen M, et al. Arthroscopic repair for traumatic posterior shoulder instability. Am J Sports Med 2003;31(2):203.
45. Wirth MA, Groh GI, Rockwood CA. Capsulorrhaphy through an anterior approach for the treatment of atraumatic posterior glenohumeral instability with multidirectional laxity of the shoulder. J Bone Joint Surg 1998;11(A):1570.
46. Wolf EM, Eakin CL. Arthroscopic capsular plication for posterior shoulder instability. Arthroscopy 1998;14:153.

Posterior and Multidirectional Instability: Open Solutions

4

Suzanne Miller   *Evan L. Flatow*

INTRODUCTION

Posterior and multidirectional shoulder instability are challenging shoulder problems to treat. This is due, in part, to the difficulty we encounter making correct diagnoses. For example, distinguishing between asymptomatic laxity and true symptomatic instability may be difficult. Arthroscopy and magnetic resonance imaging (MRI) have documented a wide variety of labral lesion, ligament variations, and associated rotator cuff injuries, the significance of which are debated. Once diagnosed, posterior and multidirectional instability can be difficult to treat. The frequently large degree of capsular redundancy may be hard to rebalance without asymmetric tightening, and healing in patients with generalized laxity can be unpredictable. Finally, motivational problems, especially voluntary or positional components of the symptoms, are more common with posterior instability and can frustrate attempts at surgical correction.

S. Miller: University of Pittsburgh Medical Center, Center for Sports Medicine, Pittsburgh, Pennsylvania.

E. L. Flatow: Mount Sinai School of Medicine, New York, New York.

PATHOANATOMY

The static stabilizers of the glenohumeral joint include the bony architecture, capsuloligamentous structures, and the labrum. The dynamic stabilizers include the biceps and rotator cuff musculature.

The bony architecture of the glenohumeral joint is such that the two surfaces are almost congruent due to the thicker articular cartilage at the periphery of the glenoid.[33,46] Because the articular surface of the humeral head is three times that of the glenoid, only 25% to 30% of the humeral head is in contact with the glenoid at any one position of the shoulder. This helps explain why the glenohumeral joint has the greatest range of motion of any joint in the human body and thus has a greater tendency to be susceptible to instability. Any change in the contour or orientation of the glenoid can disrupt the normal relationship between the articular surfaces and, subsequently, lead to instability. Some have attributed etiologies, such as anterior humeral head defects (reverse Hill-Sachs lesion), increased proximal humerus retroversion, glenoid abnormalities (hypoplasia and increased retroversion), or glenoid fracture to shoulder instability.[41]

It is unclear how much of a role increased glenoid retroversion accounts for in recurrent posterior subluxation.

Several series have found increased retroversion on computed tomography (CT) imaging in patients with posterior subluxation[10,27] while others have not.[19,43] In one series, localized glenoid hypoplasia was seen as an incidental finding in 18% of a New York population. Criteria for diagnosis was deficiency less than 1.2 cm below the scapular spine on axial CT imaging.[13] Using the same criteria in a prospective manner, the study found that 9 of 12 patients with multidirectional instability had localized hypoplasia at the posteroinferior glenoid. Still, at the present time, most investigators feel that the bony architecture probably plays a relatively small role in instability.

Despite the controversy over bony architecture as the etiology of instability, numerous bony surgical procedures have been described to treat instability. Most are of historical interest. Osseous procedures, including proximal humeral rotation osteotomy and opening-wedge glenoid osteotomy, have had historically poor results with recurrence rates up to 50%.[26] Most of these procedures addressed unidirectional (either anterior or posterior) instability, leaving a large redundant inferior capsular pouch, which may account for high failure rates in patients with posteroinferior or multidirectional instability.

The glenoid labrum also plays a role in glenohumeral stability by increasing the depth of the glenoid and by acting as an anchor for the capsuloligamentous structures. Lippitt[31] reported that the loss of the labrum reduced resistance to inferior and posteroinferior translation is approximately 20%. The superior labrum has also been shown to add inherent stability to glenohumeral translation in the anteroposterior plane of motion. In a cadaveric study, lesions created in the superior labrum anterior posterior, "SLAP tears," led to increases in glenohumeral translation.[40]

The capsuloligamentous restraints to the glenohumeral joint have been studied extensively. The ligaments are thickenings of the capsule and are primarily comprised of type 1 collagen. The stability that the ligaments provide is complex and changes according to arm position and direction of load. When the shoulder is in midrange the capsular ligaments are relatively lax, whereas in extreme positions of internal and external rotation, they become more taught, thus limiting translations and excessive rotation.[48] The anatomy of the inferior glenohumeral ligament is more constant, whereas that of the superior and middle glenohumeral ligaments is more variable. Recently, a biomechanical study,[9] with the arm at 90 degrees of forward flexion, found that the coracohumeral ligament was a contributor to posterior stability with the arm in neutral rotation, and the inferior glenohumeral ligament (IGHL) was an effective contributor to posterior instability in internal humeral rotation.

The material properties of the capsuloligamentous structures have also been investigated. Bigliani et al.,[7] in a ca-

daveric model, found that the IGHL undergoes significant deformation before failure, which supports the clinical finding that repetitive microtrauma can stretch the capsule and lead to instability. This finding may also help explain acquired laxity that allows certain athletes, to function at such extreme ranges of motion with no pain. Warren showed in a cadaver sectioning study that for posterior dislocation to occur there must be injury at the anterior superior portion of the capsule.[52] He termed the injury the "circle concept," meaning that during a severe subluxation or dislocation episode, capsular injury takes place on both the anterior and posterior aspects of the glenohumeral joint.

There are several dynamic stabilizers of the glenohumeral joint. The rotator cuff musculature provides joint compression and acts as a humeral head depressor resisting the upward pull of the deltoid. The biceps also helps to maintain stability[39]; with the shoulder in internal rotation, the biceps stabilizes anteriorly, and, in external rotation, posteriorly.

Currently, capsular laxity is felt to be the primary etiology of recurrent multidirectional or posterior instability and has been the most common finding at surgery in the majority of series.[6,35] This is often seen as a manifestation of recurrent microtrauma in athletes who use their arm in the provocative position. For example, a predominantly posterior instability pattern may manifest in an athlete who spends a lot of time with the shoulder in flexion, adduction, and internal rotation. Injury can occur as both an impact loading mechanism, which can be seen in offensive lineman, weightlifters, and boxers, and as a traction mechanism, seen in the follow-through phases of throwing and swimming. Recently, two series of patients with shoulder contact injuries reported posterior labral detachment 100% of the time with no capsular injury.[32,53] Otherwise, posterior labral detachment has been an uncommon finding in most series.[6]

SURGICAL INDICATIONS AND OTHER OPTIONS

The primary indication for surgery in patients with posterior or multidirectional instability is in patients with prolonged disability or pain due to recurrent dislocation or subluxation who have undergone a trial of nonoperative treatment. It must be emphasized that most patients should improve with a trial of physical therapy that focuses on rotator cuff and scapulothoracic strengthening. For a successful surgical outcome, patients must be able to tolerate postoperative immobilization and follow physical therapy guidelines.

With newer arthroscopic techniques, capsular plication and labral repair are now possible.[1,55] The literature on arthroscopic posterior plication is still relatively new, but success rates reported are in the range of 84% to 90%.[3,34,55]

Stiffness is not usually a common complication after an open procedure to address posterior or multidirectional instability; recurrent instability, however, is.[23,24,29] In addition, with both arthroscopic and open surgical techniques to address multidirectional instability, immobilization of the arm for 6 weeks is fairly standard. Open capsulorrhaphy also allows thickening and overlap of the capsular flaps and frees the external surface of capsule from adjacent structures, allowing more substantial shifting. With this in mind, the indications for arthroscopic treatment are less clear.

In primary cases, open repair can address bony deficiency and osseous abnormalities. In addition, we feel it is advantageous in those who wish to return to contact sports, those with inferior capsular laxity, and those who wish the best success and least chance of recurrence with only one operation.

For revision instability surgery, the current literature regarding results of arthroscopic treatment is sparse. Antoniou reported poor results with arthroscopic posteroinferior shift as a revision procedure. Only 2 of 9 patients had no postoperative instability, and 7 of 9 said that the shoulder felt stiffer. Simple Shoulder Test improved from 5.2 ± 3.9 to 6.9 ± 4.2, which was not significant. Open revision surgery for instability has also had less success than primary cases.[6] When primary surgery has failed, it is often the case that a more extensive procedure is necessary, requiring bone grafting or extra-articular augmentation with either allograft or autograft as an open procedure. Recently, thermal necrosis as a complication of thermal capsulorrhaphy has necessitated open surgery to augment insufficient tissue with either autograft or allograft.

Nonetheless, the decision for open versus arthroscopy capsulorrhaphy is controversial when the bony architecture is "normal" and the capsular tissue is "adequate." The arthroscope is a useful instrument when addressing cases that deal with true multidirectional instability, where an anterior and a posterior shift will be necessary. For example, if the primary pathology or direction of instability is posterior, addressing any anterior laxity or a Bankart lesion might be best done through the arthroscope followed by an open posteroinferior capsular shift. This can potentially lead to decreased morbidity (cosmesis, stiffness) from having both an open anterior and posterior instability procedure. With increasing awareness of superior labral lesions, the arthroscope is also a useful adjunct to treatment, using a combined arthroscopic and open approach. The drawback of this approach is the swelling that occurs after an arthroscopic procedure, making the open procedure more difficult. In addition, if the arthroscopy is performed in the seated position, the open posterior approach would require the surgeon to perform this in the seated position, which is more difficult, or to reposition the patient into the lateral decubitus position.

Contraindications

Voluntary dislocators with underlying psychiatric illness have high rates of failure and are best managed nonoperatively. Patients with locked posterior dislocations can have large defects in the humeral head, which should be managed with muscle transfer or arthroplasty or with osteochondral allografts (see Chapter 5). In addition, active infection and paralysis of the rotator cuff muscles (infraspinatus, teres minor) are contraindications to open instability repair.

PREOPERATIVE PLANNING

History

Careful and thorough history is mandatory because the spectrum of disease is so variable and treatment must be individualized in every case. It is important to determine whether the primary complaint is pain, instability, or both. This is often difficult because complaints can be vague. It is also important to elicit any family history of instability in any joint or any known collagen disorder. Does the patient have a history of subluxations or dislocations in any other joint in the body (patellofemoral, metacarpophalangeal)? Eliciting the timing of the instability and arm position is extremely helpful in making a correct diagnosis. Symptoms with the arm flexed and internally rotated (e.g., pushing open doors) are most likely indicative of posterior instability, whereas pain while carrying heavy bags with the arm in neutral rotation can be a sign of inferior instability. Are the episodes subluxations or dislocations? Was there a traumatic event involved, and what specifically happened? Did the symptom occur after a violent blow in a contact sports situation, or did it occur while reaching for something on a shelf? Voluntary dislocaters with underlying psychiatric illness are very important to identify because surgical treatment in this subset of patients can be less than gratifying. Patients presenting with posterior or multidirectional (posteroinferior) instability have often had anterior instability repairs after being initially misdiagnosed or other procedures to address the posterior instability. Knowledge of the details of previous surgical procedures is imperative. Often hardware, such as staples or screws, have been placed that may need to be removed. The competency of the capsulolabrum must always be questioned when dealing with revision surgery. It is important to restore or correct any abnormal scapulothoracic winging, as this can be a cause of posterior instability. Fortunately, most cases of scapulothoracic winging caused by long thoracic nerve injuries resolve spontaneously. If the winging is persistent, and subsequently causing posterior instability, a pectoralis transfer with or without posterior capsulorhaphy may be necessary to alleviate symptoms.[43]

Physical Examination

When evaluating the shoulder for posterior or multidirectional instability, it is important to examine for generalized ligamentous laxity as well. Testing is considered positive when the patient can perform 3 of 5 tasks, including approximating the thumb to the volar aspect of the forearm, hyperextension of 2nd metacarpophalangeal (MCP) joint greater than 90 degrees, hyperextension of elbow greater than 10 degrees, knee hyperextension, and the ability to touch the palm to the floor with knees straight. Specific to the shoulder, contour should be observed. For example, if there is infraspinatus atrophy, one might suspect a suprascapular nerve palsy. Observation of any prior surgical scars is important for preoperative planning. Active and passive range of motion should be documented and compared side to side. It is especially important to record whether there is any apprehension throughout the range of motion.

Specific subluxation testing has been described by a number of different methods. We feel the "load and shift" test, with patient supine, is most useful in our hands. To test for posterior instability stabilize the medial border of the scapula and direct the patient's humerus posteriorly while flexed to 90 degrees, adducted, and internally rotated.

Another useful posterior apprehension test is the jerk test. With the patient sitting supine, the arm is flexed to 90° and internally rotated. The examiner stabilizes the scapula and axially loads the humerus in a posterior direction while moving the arm across the body. A jerk indicates the head has slid off the glenoid posteriorily. A second jerk may occur when the arm is returned to the original location, indicating relocation.

Often the patient feels pain posteriorly rather than a sense of apprehension. The circumduction maneuver for posterior subluxation is also useful, but one must keep in mind that this can be bilateral and is a normal finding in up to 30% of the population. The test is an active one that can be performed by having the patient flex, adduct, and internally rotate. Subluxation occurs between 90 and 120 degrees, with the head spontaneously reducing between 120 and 180 degrees as the arm is abducted. The key point, regardless of the specific maneuver, is to demonstrate any subluxation that recreates symptoms. On the other hand, patients may guard against the exam so significantly as to leave the examiner unsure. The stability of the contralateral shoulder should be assessed for comparison.

It is also important to test for a sulcus sign by pulling on the humerus in a neutrally positioned arm, which is indicative of an inferior component to the instability.[38] The sulcus should diminish with external rotation of the humerus due to physiologic tightening of the rotator interval tissues, superior glenohumeral ligament (SGHL) and the coracohumeral ligament. If the sulcus does not diminish, one should be suspicious of a rotator interval injury. The neurovascular status of the patient should always be evaluated and documented. This is particularly true in cases of revision surgery where the secondary surgeon is different from the primary surgeon. The patient should be checked for concomitant lesions, such as acromioclavicular joint arthritis, impingement, rotator cuff pathology, or cervical spine problems. Confusing examinations can be clarified with subacromial or acromioclavicular anesthetic injections.

The scapulothoracic joint should also be examined for any winging. Patients with instability often use the scapulothoracic musculature to try and stabilize the glenohumeral joint,[37] which often leads to pain, crepitation, or winging in the scapulothoracic joint. Scapula winging can also be a cause or an exacerbating element of the posterior instability pattern. In some cases, inadequate treatment (strengthening program or muscle transfer) (see chapter 31) may result in failure to achieve a stable glenohumeral joint.

Diagnostic Tests

Plain radiographs can be useful to determine dislocation, humeral or glenoid fractures, bony defects, and old hardware still remaining from prior procedures. Most often in posterior or multidirectional instability, radiographs are usually normal. Usually, plain radiographs in three orthogonal planes are obtained: anteroposterior views in the scapular plane, a lateral view of the scapula ("Y" view), and an axillary view. Additional instability views can be obtained to facilitate preoperative planning. The West Point axillary view is useful to determine whether there are any glenoid rim defects or to see a hypoplastic glenoid. Computed tomography can be useful in assessing the size of reverse Hill-Sachs lesions, glenoid fractures, glenoid size, or version.

Computed tomography arthrography has not correlated well with intraoperative capsular and labral pathology. Magnetic resonance imaging with or without arthrogram is becoming more accurate in assessing the labrum and capsule.

SURGICAL TECHNIQUE

Positions, Special Instruments, and Examination Under Anesthesia

General anesthesia or an interscalene block with supplemental regional anesthesia is administered. Examination under anesthesia is critical because patient guarding while awake often limits the physical examination. The direction of maximal instability should be reconfirmed. An exam of the contralateral shoulder should always be performed because some translation is often within a normal range for an individual and can be equal on both left and right sides. The patient should be placed in the modified beach chair with a bump under the medial border of the scapula. Draping should allow access to the medial border of the scapula posteriorly, the acromioclavicular joint superomedially, and the coracoid anteriorly. A McConnell arm positioner (McConnell Orthopedic Manufacturing Company, Greenville, TX) can be used to maintain arm position.

Open Surgical Procedure

This section will present a modification of the technique of inferior capsular shift originally described for multidirectional instability by Neer and Foster in 1980.[38] The technique was designed to reduce capsular volume on the side of instability and to tighten the capsule on the opposite side of the glenohumeral joint.

We perform the approach on the greatest side of instability, which is determined from a combination of the history, physical exam, and an exam under anesthesia (EUA). The majority of the time, as a confirmatory step, we make our determination after the history and physical exam with the EUA.

The advantages of a lateral, T-based shift are that the surgeon can adjust the degree of takedown around the humeral neck while feeling the extent of the inferior pouch. Second, because the capsule is shaped like a funnel, the larger circumference is positioned laterally. A lateral-based shift provides a greater distance for shifting tissue and more capsular overlap. Third, the axillary nerve is not as close. Fourth, independent adjustment of tension, using a "T" capsulorrhaphy, is allowed medial to lateral and superior to inferior. Finally, humeral capsule avulsions can occur, occasionally, and are best treated laterally. In addition, a recent biomechanical cadaveric study compared glenoid-

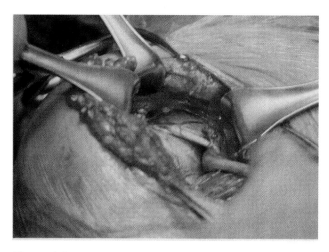

Figure 4-2 After the deltopectoral interval has been developed, the clavipectoral fascia is incised and the strap muscles are bluntly elevated from the underlying subscapularis.

versus humeral-based shifts. Using the glenoid-based shift, a significant loss of external rotation at 45 degrees and 90 degrees of glenohumeral elevation was found.[14]

Anterior Shift

A concealed anterior axillary skin incision, measuring 7 to 8 cm, is made and is used to gain access to the deltopectoral interval (Fig. 4-1). The deltopectoral interval is developed, and the cephalic vein is retracted laterally. Occasionally, 1 cm of the sternal head of the pectoralis may need to be released for visualization. The clavipectoral fascia is incised lateral to the coracoid (Fig. 4-2). A small wedge of the coracoacromial ligament may be removed to better visualize the rotator interval (Fig. 4-3). In revision cases, there can often be extensive scarring in the plane between the clavipec-

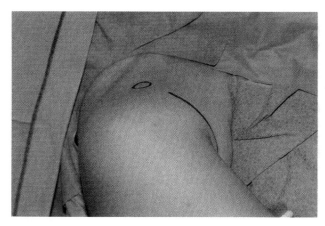

Figure 4-1 A concealed axillary incision begins approximately 3 cm below the coracoid and extends inferiorly for 8 cm into the axillary crease.

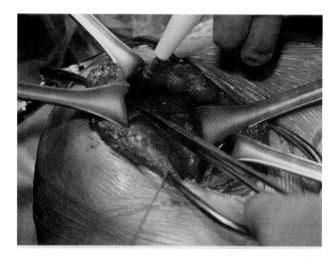

Figure 4-3 A wedge-shaped portion of the coracoacromial ligament is excised for improved exposure on the rotator cuff and upper border of the subscapularis.

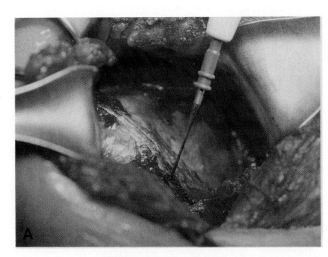 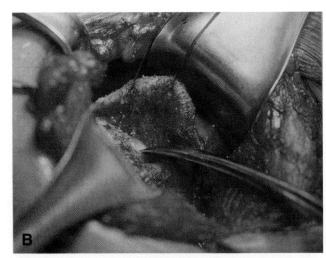

Figure 4-4 The subscapularis tendon is sharply separated from the capsule with a needle tip cautery. More medially, the plane between muscle and capsule may be bluntly developed.

toral fascia and the subscapularis. Staying lateral to the short head of the biceps facilitates identifying the correct plane.

The upper and lower borders of the subscapularis are identified, and the anterior circumflex vessels are ligated and divided. The subscapularis tendon is incised 1 cm medial to the lesser tuberosity, leaving a cuff of tissue for repair (Fig. 4-4). Takedown of the subscapularis is preferred over a subscapularis split for multidirectional instability for two reasons. First, these repairs require external rotation so that the capsule can be dissected off the humeral neck. External rotation tends to close the subscapularis split. Second, to shift the capsule, it must be dissected off of the overlying tendons, which is difficult through a subscapularis splitting approach.

The axillary nerve should be identified and protected throughout the procedure. The capsule is incised laterally, superior to inferior, leaving a 1-cm cuff of tissue for repair, and traction sutures are placed in the free edge. As the humerus is externally rotated and flexed, the capsule is incised around the neck of the humerus (Fig. 4-5). A finger may be placed in the inferior pouch to assess how large it is and how much redundant capsule needs to be released from the humerus before the shift. If pulling up on the sutures on the capsule pushes the finger out and obliterates the pouch, then enough mobilization has been done to accomplish an effective shift (Fig. 4-6). Using the anterior approach to multidirectional instability, the capsule is detached all the way posteriorly so it can be tensioned as the inferior aspect of the capsule is shifted anteriorly.

The horizontal limb of the "T" is made in between the middle and inferior glenohumeral ligaments (Fig. 4-7). If the capsule is thin and redundant medially, a "barrel" stitch may be used to tension it. This can also serve to bunch up tissue at the glenoid rim to reconstruct a bumper to com-

pensate for a deficient labrum (Fig. 4-8). The inferior flap is brought superiorly, and the superior flap inferiorly to overlap the capsule (Fig. 4-9). This is done with the arm in slight external rotation and flexion. Warner[49] has described the concept of "selective shift," wherein the superior flap is tensioned with the arm adducted, and the inferior flap with the arm abducted.

The rotator interval[38] described by Neer and Foster is felt to be enlarged in patients with multidirectional instability. This gap is closed after the shift to prevent inferior subluxation, but not overtensioned, thereby limiting external rotation.

The upper extremity is immobilized in slight abduction and neutral rotation for 6 weeks. During this time, elbow and wrist range of motion are encouraged. At 6 weeks, the brace is discontinued and range-of-motion exercises are begun. At 12 weeks, progressive strengthening is begun.

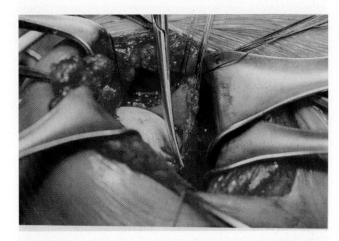

Figure 4-5 Scissors or an elevator may be used to take capsule down around the neck.

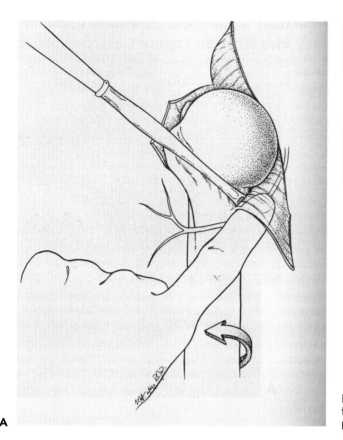

A

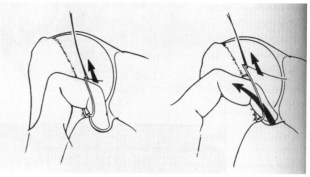

B

Figure 4-6 *(A)* A finger may be used to assess the size of the inferior pouch. *(B)* If the inferior flap has been adequately mobilized, pulling up on it will force the finger out of the pouch.

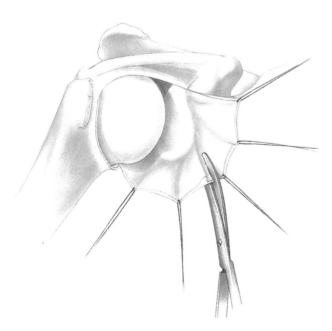

Figure 4-7 The horizontal limb of the "T" is made between the inferior and middle glenohumeral ligaments. The incision comes to, but not through, the labrum.

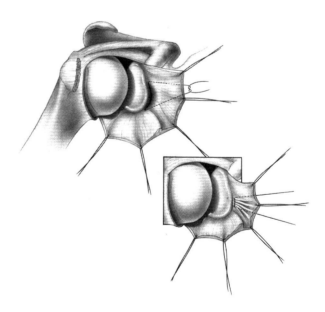

Figure 4-8 If the capsule is thin and redundant medially, a "barrel" stitch may be used to tension it. This can also serve to bunch up tissue at the glenoid rim to reconstruct a bumper to compensate for a deficient labrum.

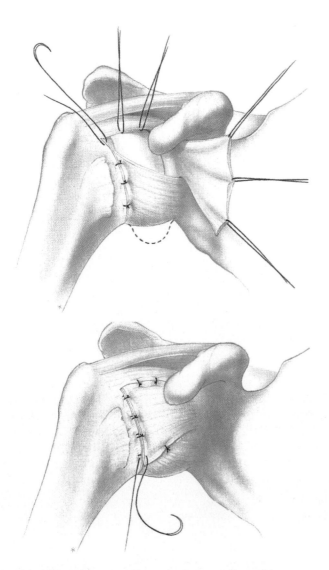

Figure 4-9 The inferior flap is brought superiorly, and the superior flap is brought inferiorly.

Posterior Inferior Capsular Shift

An oblique 10- to 12-cm skin incision angled 40 degrees to 60 degrees from the scapular spine is used. The incision should extend 2 to 3 cm posterior to the posterolateral corner of the acromion. The deltoid is identified and split along a posterior raphe. The deltoid split should be no more than 5 cm from the posterolateral corner of the acromion to protect the axillary nerve (Fig. 4-10). A loose, nonabsorbable figure of eight sutures is placed at the distal end of the split to prevent propagation with retractors and nerve injury. Proximally, the deltoid is detached subperiostally from the spine of the scapula 2 to 3 cm medially and, from the posterolateral corner of the acromion, 1 to 2 cm anteriorly.

The deltoid is retracted superiorly and inferiorly to reveal the infraspinatus superiorly and the teres minor inferi-

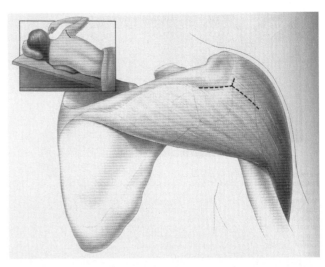

Figure 4-10 The deltoid is taken down from the spine of the scapula for 3 to 4 cm and from the posterior lateral acromion for 1 to 2 cm. The deltoid is split along a raphe for 4 to 5 cm from the posterolateral corner of the acromion.

orly. The infraspinatus must be identified. Two anatomic features of the infraspinatus are the bipennate nature of the muscle and its insertion into a broad facet on the posterior aspect of the greater tuberosity. The teres minor inserts onto a smaller facet on the greater tuberosity just inferiorly (Fig. 4-11). Once identified, the infraspinatus is separated from the posterior capsule medially along both the superior and inferior borders. A finger or peanut is used to bluntly separate the muscle from the capsule initially, and then, as dissection continues laterally, sharp dissection separates the tendon from capsule. Careful medial dissection is required because of the proximity of the suprascapular

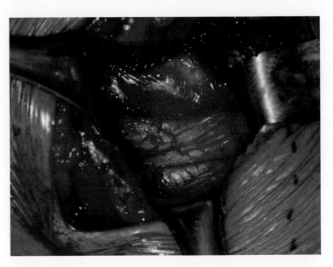

Figure 4-11 The infraspinatus can be differentiated from the teres minor by its bipennate muscle bellies and its insertion into a broad facet on the greater tuberosity.

nerve. After the muscle and capsule are separated, a Penrose drain (Tyco Healthcare Group LP, Mansfield, MA) is passed around the infraspinatus for control. The tendon is then incised approximately 0.5 cm from the insertion into the greater tuberosity, and traction sutures are placed. The tendon can be incised in an oblique fashion from superficial/medial to deep/lateral to develop two flaps (each pinnate of muscle) that can augment the repair.

Once the capsule is exposed, it is incised 1 cm medial to its insertion onto the humeral neck, slightly more medial than the infraspinatus cuff, so that the two cuffs of tissue are easily distinguishable (Fig. 4-12). The incision starts superiorly and progresses inferiorly. Nonabsorbable traction sutures are placed in the capsule for control. Patients with associated inferior or multidirectional instability require greater mobilization of the inferior capsule because these patients will often have a large redundant pouch of capsule inferiorly. Adequate mobilization of the inferior capsule can be determined in a way similar to the anterior approach, described previously, by pulling on traction sutures in the capsule while a finger is in the inferior redundant pouch. With adequate mobilization and superior traction on the inferior capsule, the finger will be pushed out of the pouch. The horizontal limb of the capsule "T" is at the level of the equator of the glenoid and continues medially to the labrum.

At this point, the glenoid and labrum should be inspected. Although rare, a reverse-Bankart lesion may be seen and should be repaired prior to capsular tightening. To repair the reverse-Bankart lesion, the posterior glenoid neck is freshened to bleeding bone, and 2 to 3 drill holes are placed through the glenoid rim. A small Curvtec drill

(Arthrotek, Warsaw, IN) can be used to drill the holes. Anchors may also be used. Number 2 nonabsorbable, braided sutures are passed through each tunnel, and the ends of the suture are then passed through the capsule. The sutures are then tied down on the external surface of the capsule and labrum as a mattress stitch to effectively recreate a buttress.

An examination of the glenoid may also reveal posterior glenoid defects or hypoplasia. In cases where 25% of the posterior glenoid is missing, it may be wise to bone graft the glenoid. Posterior bone graft from the spine of the scapula can be placed to augment the repair in these situations (or in revision capsular shift procedures where the capsule integrity is poor). Although the iliac crest has been described, we prefer the scapular spine because it is harvested via the same incision, decreasing patient morbidity. These augmentations are placed extracapsularly and can be fixed to the glenoid neck with one or two 3.5-mm cannulated screws. It is important to contour the graft to the same radius of curvature as the remaining glenoid so it does not cause impingement of the humeral head. This graft serves to increase the posterior glenoid surface and enhances stability.

The posteroinferior capsular shift is performed with the arm in 10 degrees to 15 degrees of abduction and neutral rotation. The superior flap of the capsule is brought inferiorly and attached with a nonabsorbable braided suture to the lateral cuff of the capsule on the humerus. The inferior flap is then shifted superiorly, tightening the inferior pouch and reattached to the lateral cuff of the capsule (Fig. 4-13, A and B). The infraspinatus is then reattached over the tightened capsule using a No. 2 nonabsorbable suture.

The deltoid raphe split is repaired and the deltoid is reattached medially to the acromion through bone tunnels. The subcutaneous tissue is closed with 3-0 monocryl suture (Ethicon, Somerville, NJ), and a subcuticular 4-0 monocryl suture (Ethicon) is used to close the skin. Steri-strips (3M, St. Paul, MN) and a sterile dressing are applied. The patient's arm is then placed in a brace in 10 degrees to 20 degrees of abduction or slight external rotation for 6 weeks. It is most important to avoid internal rotation in the immediate postoperative period.

Mobilization after the 6 weeks depends on the severity of instability and integrity of the capsular shift. Patients with unidirectional posterior instability resulting from trauma can start active range–of-motion exercises at the 6-week point when the brace is discontinued. Patients with multidirectional instability and generalized laxity should progress with therapy more slowly. Exercises concentrate on active elevation in the scapular plane and external rotation, as well as isometric exercises. Elevation above 150 degrees and internal rotation exercises, which would stress the repair, are delayed for 3 months. The patient is progressed to a full strengthening by 3 months. Sports activities, especially sports involving throwing or swimming, are restricted for 9 months to a year.

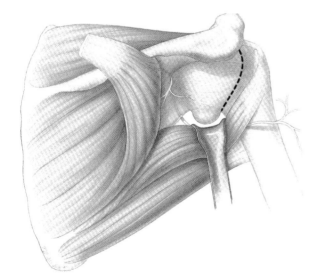

Figure 4-12 The infraspinatus is elevated to expose the capsule. The capsule is incised 1 cm from its lateral insertion. The axillary nerve lies inferior to the capsule along the humeral shaft, and the suprascapular nerve passes along the medial border of the capsule.

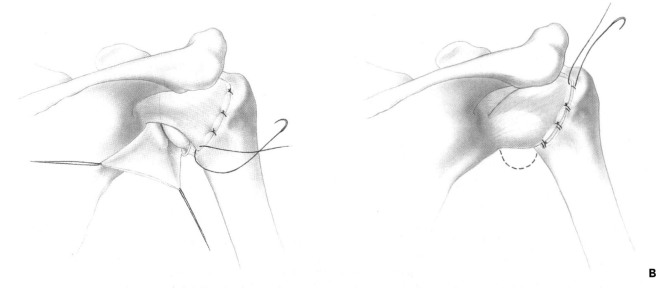

A   **B**

Figure 4-13   (*A*) The superior flap of capsule is mobilized inferiorly and reattached to the lateral cuff of capsular tissue along the humeral neck. (*B*) The inferior flap is brought superior and reattached to the cuff of capsular tissue. This obliterates the inferior pouch and thickens the posterior capsule.

TIPS AND TRICKS

Often the most challenging aspect of posterior repairs is correctly identifying the infraspinatus tendon. The infraspinatus muscle is a bipennate muscle. During the approach, look for three muscle bellies: two will be superior to the infraspinatus and one, the teres minor, will be inferior. Once the bellies are identified, look at the insertions for a difference between the broad facet of the infraspinatus insertions and the smaller, inferior facet of the teres minor to confirm the appropriate interval. Often, in revision surgery, this interval plane may be scarred and difficult to develop. Avoid being too far inferior, where the axillary nerve and posterior humeral circumflex vessels are at risk. If this is the case, the infraspinatus can be taken down, leaving a cuff of tissue at the greater tuberosity, because the subscapularis would have been taken down in an anterior approach.

A key to success is to adequately mobilize the capsule to obliterate inferior redundancy. It is important to mobilize enough inferior capsule off of the humeral neck to perform an effective shift. Using a finger, as described in the procedure section, can be helpful in determining adequate mobilization. This can be particularly challenging in revision surgery, where the capsule can be scarred to the overlying musculature. Often, during an anterior approach, the capsule and subscapularis will need to be taken down and shifted as a unit if they cannot be separated. Sometimes dissection between the capsule and subscapularis is facilitated by starting superior and continuing medially through the rotator interval. Revision shoulders can also present with stiffness and capsular release, or lengthening may need to be performed. If severe stiffness is present, it may be wise to perform releases and see how the patient progresses before undertaking a revision instability operation. This can be performed as either an open procedure or an arthroscopic procedure.

It is important to closely examine the entire glenoid rim and labrum. It is easy to miss anterior Bankart lesions in patients with subtle anterior components of multidirectional instability, especially when using a posterior approach. This is a common cause for failure in a primary instability surgery. A Fukuda retractor (George Tiemann & Co., Hauppauge, NY) can be useful in retracting the humeral head to allow full exposure of the glenoid. Alternatively, the arthroscope can be used as a diagnostic tool before open surgery in identifying any labral abnormalities. Care must be taken to avoid excessive extravasation of fluid, which may make open surgery more difficult.

RESULTS

In 1980, Neer and Foster described the inferior capsular shift for multidirectional instability. The lateral-based T capsulorrhaphy was performed in 40 shoulders for 36 patients. In primary cases, an anterior approach was used in 14 patients and a posterior approach in 15 patients. Five patients required a two-sided approach to repair anterior labral lesions that were found intraoperatively. The procedure was successful in all but one patient who developed instability. Since this time, the procedure has proven successful in 80% to 95% of patients, with recurrence rates in the range of 2.5% to 11% (Table 4-1). Results of open posterior inferior capsular shift for instability has also been a reliable operation (Table 4-2). The literature reports satisfactory results in over 95% of patients, with recurrence rates

TABLE 4-1

RESULTS OF SOFT TISSUE POSTERIOR RECONSTRUCTIONS FOR POSTERIOR INSTABILITY

	# Patients	Follow-up (mo)	Direction Instability	Procedure	Results: Excellent or Good	Prior Surgery	Recurrences	Return to Sport
Misamore[35]	14	45 (26–90)	14 P	Posteroinferior shift posterior approach	93%	0/14	1/14 (7%)	12/14 (86%)
Wirth[54]	10	60 (24–103)	10 P	Posteroinferior shift anterior approach	90%	4/10 3 P	1/10 (10%)	6/10 (60%)
Bigliani[6]	35	5 yrs	13 P 22 MDI	Posteroinferior shift posterior approach	80% 100% P 73% MDI	16/35 8 A, 3P	4/35 (11%)	NA
Tibone[47]	40	2 yrs (2–10 yrs)	40 P	20 posterior staple	50%	13/40	11/40	60% recreational
				20 posteroinferior shift posterior approach		13 A	(27.5%)	50% competitive 28% overhead
Froneck[18]	11		11 P	Posterior approach 5 bone block	91%	4/10 3A, 1P	1/10 (10%)	NA
Hawkins[25]	14	44 (18–98)	14 P	Posterior capsulo-tendinous tensioning	93%	6/14 6 A	1/14 (7%)	10/14 (71%)

A, anterior; MDI, multidirectional instability; P, posterior; yrs, years.

TABLE 4-2

RESULTS OF INFERIOR CAPSULAR SHIFT FOR MULTIDIRECTIONAL INSTABILITY

	Shoulders	Follow-up (mo)	Excellent or Good Results	Prior Surgery	Procedure	Recurrence Rate	Return to Play	Loss of External Rotation
Neer 1980[38]	40		78%	11/40 (27.5%)	14 A x P	1/40 (2.5%)		
Pollock 2000[42]	49	61 (24–132)	91% A 100% P	0/49	34 A 15 P	2/49 (4%)	86% 69% pre level	3% restriction in ER
Bigliani 1994[5]	63	4 yrs (1–9 yrs)	94%	15/63 (24%)	63 A	2/63 (3%)	92% 75% prelevel 50% overhead	7 degrees
Cooper 1992[13]	43	39 (24–71)	86%	16/43 (37%)	43 A	4/43 (9%)	49% 37% Prelevel	
Lebar[30]	10	28 (12–51)	80%	6/10 (60%)	9 A 1 P	1/10 (10%)	20% full active duty	
Altcheck 1991[2]	42		95%			4/42		5 degrees
Bak[4]	26	54 (25–113)	88% A	0/26	26 A	2/26 (8%)	92% 84% prelevel Overhead 76% 57% prelevel	93% <5 degrees
Choi 2002[12]	53	42 (24–73)	92% A 81% P		37 A 16 P	6/53 (11%)	prelevel 82% A 75% P 17% bilateral	NA

A, anterior; P, posterior; yrs, years.

less than 11% in primary repair.[6] When the procedure is performed in a revision setting, the results are not as impressive. In this same series, 11 patients had previous surgical operations (one anterior and six posterior), and the result was satisfactory in only five cases. In the remaining six cases the results were fair in one case and poor in the other five cases. The authors speculate that scarring and, perhaps, unidirectional shortening from other procedures contribute to the difficulty in tissue balancing in revision operations.

COMPLICATIONS

Preoperative

Incorrect Diagnosis

Regardless of the procedure used, for successful instability repair it is of utmost importance to correctly diagnose the direction of instability preoperatively. The diagnosis should then be confirmed with an examination under anesthesia and with intraoperative findings. Not infrequently, patients present with recurrent posterior instability or multidirectional instability after having a surgical procedure done for anterior glenohumeral instability. Unfortunately, misdiagnosis is often the cause of a failed instability operation.[23,24,51,56] In addition, the clinician should rule out other causes of pain in the shoulder, such as the acromioclavicular joint, biceps, or cervical spine. A patient may have a lax shoulder, which is normal for that patient, but have another cause for the pain. Specifically, failure to recognize multidirectional instability has been cited as a common cause of failure. Burkhead[11] reviewed 23 patients with postoperative instability and determined that, in five cases, the cause was missed multidirectional instability. Similarly, Rockwood and Gerber[44] attributed postoperative instability in 68% of patients to failure to recognize multidirectional instability. It is possible to be fooled when examining a globally unstable shoulder, especially if the examination starts with the shoulder in a subluxed position. The best way to ensure where the humeral head is located is to palpate the head and find the point at which it is most medial during anteroposterior translation. This occurs when the humeral head is located; although, in the office setting, this can be difficult due to guarding, which stresses the importance of an EUA.

Scapula Winging

Scapulothoracic winging can be a cause of posterior instability. Scapulothoracic motion and mechanics should be examined preoperatively. If due to a long thoracic nerve palsy, rehabilitation and nonsurgical treatment usually resolves the winging. If nonsurgical treatment fails, a pectoralis muscle transfer may have to be performed. This op-

eration alone may be enough to resolve the posterior instability. After the transfer, if the patient is still asymmetrically unstable, a posterior capsule shift should be performed.

Voluntary Dislocators

Identifying a voluntary subluxator preoperatively is imperative to obtaining a successful outcome after a surgical instability procedure. It is important to distinguish those who subluxate their shoulders in a provocative position versus those who selectively activate muscles to subluxate or dislocate the shoulder with the arm at the side of the thorax. One should be cautious about surgical intervention in those with either presentation, but the latter carries a far worse prognosis. If there is any indication that there is a psychological cause to the shoulder problem, a preoperative psychiatric evaluation should be obtained.

Intraoperative

Neurovascular

Take care and be aware of the axillary nerve, which can be damaged by excessive traction on the deltoid laterally and with blind anterior mobilization of the inferior capsule off of the humeral neck. By minimizing the split of the deltoid to 5 cm from the acromion and placing a stay suture to prevent propagation, the potential for axillary nerve damage is reduced. In posterior repairs, the suprascapular nerve is susceptible to damage as it passes along the medial edge of the capsule on the undersurface of the infraspinatus. Careful blunt dissection of the medial aspect of the infraspinatus from the capsule is necessary to avoid damaging the suprascapular nerve.

Hardware

Prominent, loose, and intra-articular hardware are known complications after procedures using staples or screws for stabilization.[58] The staple has been known to cause damage to the glenoid and erosion of the humeral head cartilage.[28] Often, computed tomography is useful to determine whether hardware is intra-articular (Fig. 4-14). If unsure, a diagnostic arthroscopy can be useful in identifying any intra-articular hardware.

Incomplete Anatomic Repair

Although not commonly present in true multidirectional instability, failure to recognize a labral tear (Bankart lesion) can be a common cause of failure.[16,23,24] Often, the capsulolabrum can be scarred medial to the glenoid (i.e., anterior labroligamentous periosteal sleeve avulsion [ALPSA]) and must be elevated and brought back to its anatomic position.

Surgery for posterior repairs presents its own set of difficulties. There can be posterior erosion or fractures of the

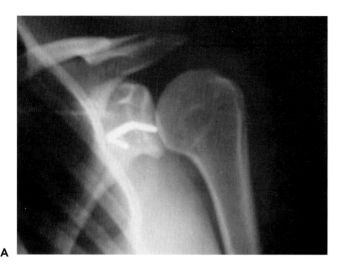

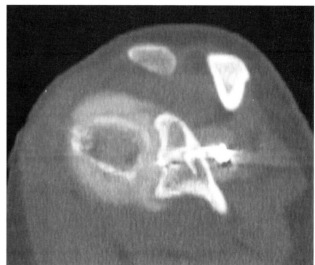

Figure 4-14   (A) A radiograph after an open-wedge osteotomy of the glenoid. (B) A CT scan can be helpful to define any intra-articular hardware.

glenoid rim. If greater than 20% to 25% of the glenoid rim is absent, bone grafting should be considered if revision surgery is planned. Glenoid version and hypoplasia can cause recurrent instability, but, fortunately, these anatomic variants are uncommon.

Postoperative

Recurrent instability following open capsular shift for multidirectional instability is reported to be anywhere from 2.5% to 10%.[2,13,17,38] If a patient with multidirectional instability presents with symptomatic recurrent instability, it is very important to determine whether there was a traumatic event involved.[57] Unless a significant traumatic event has occurred, treatment focusing on rehabilitation (rotator cuff and scapular stabilizers) should precede any surgical intervention because revision instability surgery can be extremely challenging and often less successful than primary surgery.

Lazarus[29] states that the must common direction of persistent instability is inferior and stresses the importance of closing the rotator interval during revision surgery for this subset of patients. If, in a revision setting, the inferior capsule needs to be mobilized, this can often be difficult due to scarring. The capsule may need to be mobilized from both the anterior and posterior direction. The repair can also fail in the anterior or posterior direction. If either the anterior or posterior capsule is too tight, a release may need to be performed. There are cases where releasing scar tissue is enough to relieve symptoms of instability, so, if instability persists, a staged procedure should be considered.

If therapy progresses too rapidly, stretching of the tissues can occur and lead to recurrent instability. This is most commonly seen in the subset of patients with generalized ligamentous laxity. Postoperative rehabilitation needs to be individualized, according to the specific procedure and patient, and adjusted throughout the postoperative course. Full range of motion is usually obtained by 6 months postoperatively. Often in the case of multidirectional instability, one is dealing with an athletic population. Of importance is that repetitive microtrauma, that is, a return to sports too quickly, can lead to failure.

Stiffness

The cause of should stiffness after stabilization procedures must be evaluated with caution. Other etiologies of pain in the shoulder should be ruled out, such as the acromioclavicular joint, cervical spine, or neurologic syndrome (i.e., reflex sympathetic dystrophy or brachial plexopathy), because they may be the cause for loss of motion. In addition, compliance with rehabilitation protocol, as well as compensation and legal issues, should be closely examined. Although not common, stiffness after posterior capsulorrhaphy has been recognized.[50] The loss of motion is usually in flexion, internal rotation, and adduction. Although the etiology is not clear, one can hypothesize that the position of the arm at the time of tensioning and the position of postoperative immobilization may contribute to stiffness. Capsular release has been described as a treatment for this problem.

Arthropathy

Loss of motion after instability surgery has been attributed to the development of degenerative changes.[8,22,45] In cases of multidirectional instability, it is necessary to balance the tissue anteriorly, posteriorly, and inferiorly to avoid overtightening in any one direction. Overtightening in any one direction may lead to degenerative arthritis.

For example, overtightening the shoulder anteriorly may cause posterior subluxation and subsequent posterior wear of the shoulder.[22] Fortunately, this was more commonly reported after medial lateral tightening procedures (i.e., Putti-Platt, Magnuson-Stack, and Bristow), which are now less commonly performed. More recently with anatomic-type reconstructions,[36,38] motion loss is less of a problem, and subsequent arthropathy is less often seen.[2,16]

Subscapularis Failure

Subscapularis failure after an anterior instability repair is another recognized complication.[21] A variety of clinical presentations, such as pain, recurrent instability, and weakness, may manifest after subscapularis rupture. In a physical exam, one may see excessive external rotation on the affected side, a positive liftoff, or a positive belly-press test. Subscapularis tendon repair can be difficult at times due to tenuous or retracted tissue. If direct repair is possible, this is performed using modified Mason-Allen sutures through bone tunnels in the lesser tuberosity. If the subscapularis is unable to be repaired, various options exist. Some have advocated pectoralis transfer, while others have recommended reconstruction with either autograft (hamstrings, plantaris) or allograft (Achilles tendon).

New Injury

Clearly, a new injury in the early postoperative period can damage a repair and lead to recurrent instability. Although recurrent trauma can happen at any time, it is more commonly associated after a repair for unidirectional instability rather than multidirectional instability.[51]

CONCLUSIONS

Patients with posterior or multidirectional instability present much less frequently than those with anterior instability; however, patients with anterior instability are often the most challenging to care for. The inferior capsular shift allows precise correction of capsular laxity and has been shown to be successful.[6] Recently, many surgeons have begun using arthroscopic procedures to repair capsular laxity.[1,4] The appropriate choice for arthroscopic versus open repair remains controversial and requires scientific evaluation. Long-term studies comparing the success of open versus arthroscopic repair are necessary.

REFERENCES

1. Abrams JS, Savoie FH III, Tauro JC, et al. Recent advances in the evaluation and treatment of shoulder instability: anterior, posterior, and multidirectional. Arthroscopy 2002;18(9 suppl 2):1.
2. Altchek DW, Warren RF, Skyhar MJ, et al. T-plasty modification of the Bankart procedure for multidirectional instability of the anterior and inferior types. J Bone Joint Surg Am 1991;73(1):105.
3. Antoniou J, Harryman DT II. Arthroscopic posterior capsular repair. Clin Sports Med 2000;19(1):101.
4. Bak K, Spring BJ, Henderson JP. Inferior capsular shift procedure in athletes with multidirectional instability based on isolated capsular and ligamentous redundancy. Am J Sports Med 2000;28(4):466.
5. Bigliani LU, Kurzweil PR, Schwartzbach CC, et al. Inferior capsular shift procedure for anterior-inferior shoulder instability in athletes. Am J Sports Med 1994;22(5):578.
6. Bigliani LU, Pollock RG, McIlveen SJ, et al. Shift of the posteroinferior aspect of the capsule for recurrent posterior glenohumeral instability. J Bone Joint Surg Am 1995;77(7):1011.
7. Bigliani LU, Pollock RG, Sloslowski LJ, et al. Tensile properties of the inferior glenohumeral ligament. J Orthop Res 1992;10(2):187.
8. Bigliani LU, Weinstein DM, Glasgow MT, et al. Glenohumeral arthroplasty for arthritis after instability surgery. J Shoulder Elbow Surg 1995;4(2):87.
9. Blasier RB, Soslowsky LJ, Malicky DM, et al. Posterior glenohumeral subluxation: active and passive stabilization in a biomechanical model. J Bone Joint Surg Am 1997;79(3):433.
10. Brewer BJ, Wubben RC, Carrera GF, et al. Excessive retroversion of the glenoid cavity: a cause of non-traumatic posterior instability of the shoulder. J Bone Joint Surg Am 1986;68(5):724.
11. Burkhead W, Ritchie M. Revision of failed shoulder reconstruction. Contemp Orthop 1992;24:126.
12. Choi CH, Ogilvie-Harris DJ. Inferior capsular shift operation for multidirectional instability of the shoulder in players of contact sports. Br J Sports Med 2002;36(4):290.
13. Cooper RA, Brems JJ. The inferior capsular-shift procedure for multidirectional instability of the shoulder. J Bone Joint Surg Am 1992;74(10):1516.
14. Deutsch AJ, Barber E, Davy DT, et al. Anterior-inferior capsular shift of the shoulder: a biomechanical comparison of glenoid-based versus humeral-based shift strategies. J Shoulder Elbow Surg 2001;10(4):340.
15. Edelson JG. Localized glenoid hypoplasia: an anatomic variation of possible clinical significance. Clin Orthop 1995;321:189.
16. Flatow EL, Miniaci A, Evans PJ, et al. Instability of the shoulder: complex problems and failed repairs: part II failed repairs. Instr Course Lect 1998;47:113.
17. Flatow EL, Warner JI. Instability of the shoulder: complex problems and failed repairs: part I. Relevant biomechanics, multidirectional instability, and severe glenoid loss. Instr Course Lect 1998;47:97.
18. Fronek JR, Warren RF, Bowen M. Posterior subluxation of the glenohumeral joint. J Bone Joint Surg Am 1989;71A(2):205.
19. Gerber C, Ganz R, Vinh TS. Glenoplasty for recurrent posterior shoulder instability: an anatomic reappraisal. Clin Orthop 1987;216:70.
20. Gerber C, Nyffeler RW. Classification of glenohumeral joint instability. Clin Orthop 2002;400:65.
21. Gries P, Dean M, Hawkins RJ. Subscapularis tendon disruption after Bankart reconstruction for anterior instability. J Shoulder Elbow Surg 1996;5:219.
22. Hawkins R, Angelo R. Glenohumeral osteoarthrosis. J Bone Joint Surg Am 1990;72:1193.
23. Hawkins R, Hawkins R. Failed anterior reconstruction for shoulder instability. J Bone Joint Surg Br 1985;67:709.
24. Hawkins RH, Hawkins RJ. Failed anterior reconstruction for shoulder instability. J Bone Joint Surg Br 1985;67(5):709.
25. Hawkins RJ, Janda DH. Posterior instability of the glenohumeral joint. A technique of repair. Am J Sports Med 1996;24(3):275.
26. Hawkins RJ, Koppert G, Johnston G. Recurrent posterior instability (subluxation) of the shoulder. J Bone Joint Surg Am 1984;66(2):169.
27. Hurley JA, Anderson TE, Dear W, et al. Posterior shoulder instability. Surgical versus conservative results with evaluation of glenoid version. Am J Sports Med 1992;20(4):396.
28. Johnson L. Diagnostic and surgical arthroscopy of the shoulder. St Louis, Mosby-Year Book, 1993.
29. Lazarus M, Guttmann D. Complications of instability surgery. Philadelphia, Lippincott, 1999.
30. Lebar RD, Alexander AH. Multidirectional shoulder instability. Clinical results of inferior capsular shift in an active-duty population. Am J Sports Med 1992;20(2):193.

31. Lippitt S, Vanderhooft E, Harris S, et al. Glenohumeral stability from concavity-compression: a quantitative analysis. J Shoulder Elbow Surg 1993;2:27.
32. Mair SD, Zarzour RH, Speer KP, et al. Posterior labral injury in contact athletes. Am J Sports Med 1998;26(6):753.
33. Matsen FA III, Harryman DT II, Sidles JA. Mechanics of glenohumeral instability. Clin Sports Med 1991;10:783.
34. McIntyre LF, Caspari RB, Savoie FH III. The arthroscopic treatment of posterior shoulder instability: two-year results of a multiple suture technique. Arthroscopy 1997;13(4):426.
35. Misamore GW, Facibene WA. Posterior capsulorrhaphy for the treatment of traumatic recurrent posterior subluxations of the shoulder in athletes. J Shoulder Elbow Surg 2000;9(5):403.
36. Montgomery WI, Jobe F. Functional outcomes in athletes after modified anterior capsulolabral reconstruction. Am J Sports Med 1994;22:352.
37. Neer CI. Shoulder reconstruction. Philadelphia, WB Saunders, 1990.
38. Neer CS II, Foster CR. Inferior capsular shift for involuntary inferior and multidirectional instability of the shoulder: a preliminary report. J Bone Joint Surg Am 1980;62(6):897.
39. Pagnani M, Deng X, Warren RF, et al. Role of the long head of the biceps brachii in glenohumeral instability: a biomechanical study in cadavers. J Shoulder Elbow Surg 1996;5:255.
40. Pagnani MJ, Deng XH, Warren RF, et al. Effect of lesions of the superior portion of the glenoid labrum on glenohumeral translation. J Bone Joint Surg Am 1995;77(7):1003.
41. Pollock RG, Bigliani LU. Recurrent posterior shoulder instability: diagnosis and treatment. Clin Orthop 1993;291:85.
42. Pollock RG, Owens JM, Flatow EL, et al. Operative results of the inferior capsular shift procedure for multidirectional instability of the shoulder. J Bone Joint Surg Am 2000;82A(7):919.
43. Randelli M, Gambrioli P. Glenohumeral osteometry by computed tomography in normal and unstable shoulders. Clin Orthop 1986;208:151.
44. Rockwood C, Gerber C. Analysis of failed surgical procedures for anterior shoulder instability. Orthop Trans 1985;9:48.
45. Samilson R, Prieto V. Dislocation arthropathy of the shoulder. J Bone Joint Surg Am 1983;65A:456.
46. Soslowsky LJ, Flatow EL, Bigliani LU, et al. Articular geometry of the glenohumeral joint. Clin Orthop 1992;285:181.
47. Tibone JE, Bradley JP. The treatment of posterior subluxation in athletes. Clin Orthop 1993;291:124.
48. Warner J, Caborn D, Berger R, et al. Dynamic capsuloligamentous anatomy of the glenohumeral joint. J Shoulder Elbow Surg 1993;2:131.
49. Warner J, Johnson D, et al. The concept of a "selective shift" for anterior inferior instability of the shoulder. Orthop Trans 1994;18:1183.
50. Warner JJ, Iannotti JP. Treatment of a stiff shoulder after posterior capsulorrhaphy: a report of three cases. J Bone Joint Surg Am 1996;78(9):1419.
51. Warren R. Revision shoulder stabilization. J Shoulder Elbow Surg 1995;5:S118.
52. Warren R, Kornblatt I, Marthand R. Static factors affecting posterior shoulder stability. Orthop Trans 1984;8:89.
53. Williams R, Strickland S, Cohen M, et al. Arthroscopic repair for traumatic posterior shoulder instability. Am J Sports Med 2003;31(2):203.
54. Wirth MA, Groh GI, Rockwood CA Jr. Capsulorrhaphy through an anterior approach for the treatment of atraumatic posterior glenohumeral instability with multidirectional laxity of the shoulder. J Bone Joint Surg Am 1998;80(11):1570.
55. Wolf EM, Eakin CL. Arthroscopic capsular plication for posterior shoulder instability. Arthroscopy 1998;14(2):153.
56. Young DC, Rockwood CA Jr. Complications of a failed Bristow procedure and their management. J Bone Joint Surg Am 1991;73(7):969.
57. Zabinski SJ, Simonian P, Warner J, et al. Recurrent instability: surgical failures. In: Warren R, Craig E, Altchek D, eds. Shoulder instability. Philadelphia, Lippincott-Raven, 1998.
58. Zuckerman J, Matsen F. Complications about the glenohumeral joint related to the use of screws and staples. J Bone Joint Surg Am 1984;66:175.

Chronic, Locked Anterior, and Posterior Dislocations

5

Christian Gerber

LOCKED POSTERIOR DISLOCATION

Diagnosis

Chronic, locked posterior dislocation is of diagnostic interest because almost two-thirds of the posterior dislocations are not recognized initially.[3,4,8,14,19] In my experience, 12 of 21 patients with dislocation persisting for more than 4 weeks were referred for treatment without the correct diagnosis.

Posterior dislocations are associated with fractures of the surgical neck of the humerus in almost 50% of the cases. In acute cases, these concomitant fractures, which usually also involve one of the tuberosities,[8] must be identified, because they may be displaced during reduction of the dislocation. Displacement of a fracture-dislocation is almost invariably followed by avascular necrosis and subsequent collapse of the humeral head. In chronic cases, the mild to moderate malunion at the surgical neck level may significantly complicate prosthetic reconstruction of the proximal humerus.

In the typical history of the patient with a traumatic posterior dislocation, the shoulder has undergone a violent injury, most commonly during a motor vehicle accident[3] or during a seizure. Posterior dislocations that have occurred during convulsions often have a somewhat unclear history,

because the patient is completely unaware of the injury and only notices that, for no apparent reason, he or she can no longer externally rotate the arm.

The cause of locked posterior dislocation is a major trauma; there is no particular predisposition to this injury. During convulsions, which precipitate about one-third of all posterior dislocations, the shoulder is more likely to be dislocated posteriorly, because the internal rotators are much stronger than the external rotators. However, anterior dislocations can also be caused by epileptic seizures.

On clinical examination, the coracoid process is prominent, and the proximal humeral shaft is oriented somewhat posteriorly. Active anterior elevation is limited but generally remains around 100 degrees (Fig. 5-1). Active and passive external rotation are always absent (Fig. 5-2). The arm is locked in internal rotation of 10 degrees to 60 degrees.

The anteroposterior and axillary lateral x-ray views always provide diagnostic information (Fig. 5-3). It may be difficult to make the diagnosis solely on the basis of an anteroposterior radiograph, especially if it is not taken with the central x-ray beam parallel to the glenoid fossa. The axillary lateral view is optimal, enabling the examiner to make the diagnosis and estimate the size of the lesion of the humeral head. For a more refined diagnostic workup that includes preoperative planning, computed tomography (CT) is the optimal imaging method. Because the lesions are mostly skeletal, CT provides a more accurate study than that provided by magnetic resonance imaging (MRI).

C. **Gerber:** Professor and Chairman, University of Zurich, Zurich, Switzerland.

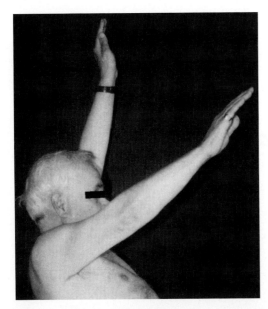

Figure 5-1 Chronic posterior dislocation of the right shoulder 5 years after an epileptic seizure due to a meningioma. Because this patient had to undergo surgery for a brain tumor at age 72, it was decided that no treatment would be undertaken. Five years after the injury, he has approximately 90 degrees of flexion without pain.

Lesions

Several lesions can be created by a locked posterior dislocation. Almost one of two cases is associated with a *fracture of the surgical neck of the humerus* (see Fig. 5-3), which may pose an additional challenge for treatment. *Fractures of the posterior glenoid rim* are rare, but chronic destruction caused by active or passive repetitive rotational movements may necessitate surgical treatment.[3] Posterior *capsular lesions* are probably always present.[3,17,18] Scougall[20] demonstrated in monkeys that these lesions heal spontaneously, and my experience suggests that this pattern also occurs in humans. *Ruptures of the rotator cuff* have been found frequently in experimental posterior dislocations.[17,18] My colleagues and I have observed three cases with concomitant rupture of the rotator cuff, which invariably involved the supraspinatus tendon. However, we did not find that lesions of the posterior cuff were constant features. The *anteromedial humeral head defect*[14] is a constant feature, and it is the key abnormality of locked posterior shoulder dislocation. In the absence of concomitant lesions, reconstruction of the humeral head defect by the restoration of the humeral head surface[6] or by filling the anteromedial humeral head lesion[8,14,15] can restore stability and function of the shoulder without other surgical corrections.

Treatment

Skillful Neglect

Before any treatment is undertaken, it is necessary to establish whether treatment is necessary or whether the natural history may be as favorable as surgical treatment. All patients with posterior dislocations have lost glenohumeral rotation and are therefore definitely limited, but they regain functional anterior elevation. The natural history of locked posterior dislocation is quite favorable. My colleagues and I have observed four untreated patients over

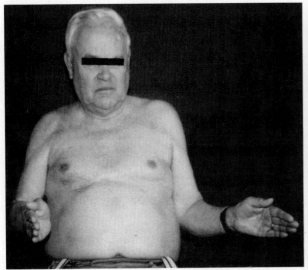
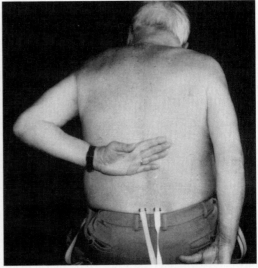

Figure 5-2 Same patient as in Figure 5-1. (*A*) He has a severe loss of external rotation that is partly compensated by thoraco-scapular motion. (*B*) The loss of internal rotation documents that rotational movements in the glenohumeral joint are virtually absent. At this 5-year follow-up visit, these active movements were free of pain, and the patient was satisfied with his shoulder function.

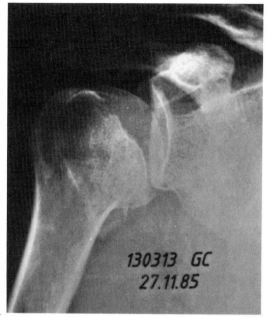
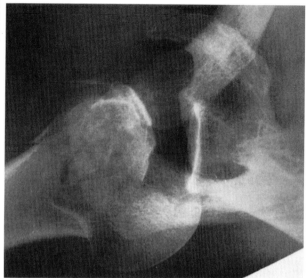

Figure 5-3   Radiologic documentation of a locked posterior dislocation. (*A*) The anteroposterior view allows the physician to recognize the impacted zone of the anteromedial humeral head and the superposition of the humeral head and the glenoid. (*B*) The axillary lateral view allows the physician to recognize the enormous destruction of the humeral head surface and, in this case, the additional, nondisplaced fracture of the surgical neck, which can hardly be seen on the anteroposterior radiograph.

several years (see Figs. 5-1 to 5-3). All of them remained free from pain or had minimal pain, and each had a functional shoulder value of between 60% and 85% of normal, as judged by using the Constant score.[1,2] This is comparable to the function obtained with good shoulder fusion. Twenty shoulders that underwent arthrodesis were reviewed (L. Nagy and C. Gerber, unpublished data), and the overall outcome for these cases was not better than the outcome for untreated, locked posterior dislocations.

On the basis of these observations and the results of treatment of this condition, I think that skillful neglect must be considered, if the patient is old, has limited demands for the affected shoulder, is able to reach the mouth and possibly the front, and has a normal contralateral shoulder. The same conservative approach is warranted if the patient has medical or other concomitant problems suggesting that he or she may be unable to comply with a rehabilitation program. After epileptic seizures, surgery is only considered if the seizures are adequately controlled by medical treatment.

Closed Reduction for Small Defects

If the anteromedial humeral head impression fractures are very small (less than 25% of the cartilage surface), and there is no recent subcapital fracture, a reduction with the patient under general anesthesia may be attempted. If closed reduction is possible, the stability is then tested. If

redislocation does not occur with internal rotation by taking the affected hand to the abdomen, the arm is mobilized in a splint in neutral rotation for 4 weeks, and rehabilitation is then instituted. The arm must not be brought behind the trunk for a minimum of 6 weeks. If closed reduction is possible, a good outcome can be expected without additional surgery. If an open reduction is necessary, it appears logical to ascertain whether the stability is restored. Although transferring the lesser tuberosity with its attached subscapularis tendon into the articular defect is the standard,[16] my colleagues and I prefer to reconstruct the humeral head using autogenous or, more frequently, allograft bone,[6] as used in defects involving 25% to 50% of the articular surface.

Reconstruction of Defects up to Half of the Articular Surface

Indications

The size of the anteromedial humeral head defect dictates the treatment of locked posterior dislocations. McLaughlin[14] first recognized the significance of this lesion and recommended transfer of the subscapularis tendon into the defect to prevent recurrence of glenohumeral instability. Dubousset[3] later recommended reestablishing the contour of the humeral head with autogenous bone graft in conjunction with reconstructing the posterior glenohumeral

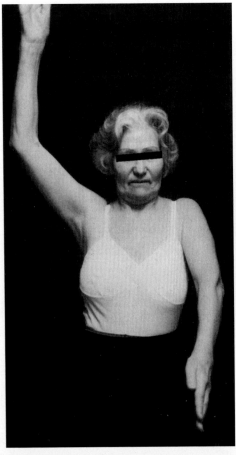

Figure 5-4 Locked posterior dislocation secondary to an epileptic seizure in a 68-year-old woman. Active anterior elevation is only 25 degrees.

depressed cartilage and subchondral buttressing with autologous cancellous bone graft as a joint-preserving alternative to hemiarthroplasty in the acute setting.[5] Subsequently, we reported the results obtained with humeral head reconstruction, using allogenic bone in the chronic setting.[6] We have come to prefer reconstructing the shape of the humeral head, because it seems more logical than other approaches, or prosthetic replacement if humeral head reconstruction is not possible.

We have treated nine posterior dislocations with allogenic reconstruction of humeral head defects of at least 40% of the articular surface. All shoulders had been dislocated for more than 1 month. The diagnosis had initially been missed in each patient, and two individuals had previously been treated with a physical therapy program. Active shoulder flexion averaged 40 degrees (Fig. 5-4) with an average internal rotation contracture present in each case of 40 degrees (Fig. 5-5). Conventional radiography revealed locked posterior dislocations in all cases (Fig. 5-6). The humeral head impaction fracture was measured on horizontal CT scans and found to be between 40% and 55% (Fig. 5-7). The architecture of the remaining humerus was most frequently normal, but it was osteoporotic in long-standing dislocations.

Operative Technique

A deltopectoral approach is used in surgery. Exceptionally, the conjoint tendon may have to be partially released to reach the desired line of incision in the subscapularis tendon.[6] The axillary nerve is identified in every case and protected throughout mobilization of the subscapularis and

capsule. Many modern surgeons recommend transfering the lesser tuberosity with its attached subscapularis tendon into the humeral head defect, if it comprises up to 40% of the humeral head, and, for defects of more than 40% of the articular surface, total shoulder or hemiarthroplasty is recommended.

Chronic posterior dislocations with large anteromedial humeral head defects are, fortunately, rare. Neer and Hughes[16] modified McLaughlin's subscapularis transfer[14] and transferred the lesser tuberosity with its attached subscapularis tendon into the defect. The treatment of lesions involving 25% to 50% of the articular surface with transfer of the lesser tuberosity has repeatedly been reported to yield satisfactory results.[8,16] Hawkins et al.[8] reported good results in nine cases of the subscapularis transfers. Walch et al.[21] reported three excellent, one good, five fair, and one poor outcome after subscapularis transfer in ten patients with anterior head defects of less than 50%. For defects that are larger than 50%, these surgeons attempted rotational osteotomy and reported unsatisfactory results.

My colleagues and I have reported the results of reconstructing the shape of the humeral head by elevating the

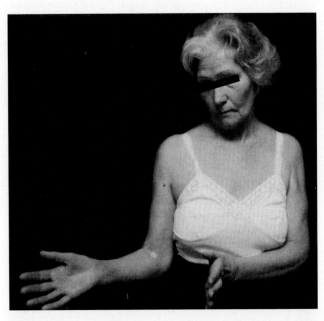

Figure 5-5 Same patient as in Figure 5-4. The arm is locked in 60 degrees of internal rotation.

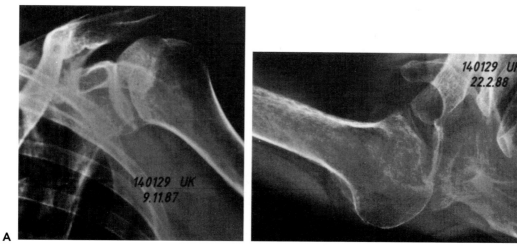

Figure 5-6 (*A*) Anteroposterior and (*B*) axillary lateral views of the patient in Figures 5-4 and 5-5 show the locked posterior dislocation requiring humeral head reconstruction.

the inferior capsule. A vertical capsulotomy leaves the superior glenohumeral ligament and the coracohumeral ligament intact, and adhesions between the capsulolabral complex and the dislocated head are released. Fractures of the posterior glenoid rim are never of sufficient magnitude to warrant glenoid reconstruction. The posterior capsule is stretched into a redundant pouch, but it is not detached from the posterior aspect of the scapular neck. The posterior capsule is not surgically addressed. The procedure is only carried out if minimal internal rotation of the relocated humerus results in recurrence of posterior dislocation.

The defect of the head is tentatively filled with allograft. The allograft is contoured to fit the segmental defect and to restore the original sphericity of the humeral head (Fig. 5-8). The graft is usually fixed with lagged, counter-

sunk 3.5-mm cancellous screws (Synthes, Waldneburg, Switzerland). The anterior capsule is left unrepaired. The superior glenohumeral ligament must remain intact or be repaired, because it has a role in posterior stability of the shoulder. The subscapularis is mobilized from its origin on the anterior surface of the scapula, released from all of its adhesions, and repaired end to end without lengthening or shortening. The arm is kept at the side, with the rotation at 0 degrees, in a removable splint for 6 weeks. Passive external rotation exercises are allowed out of the splint. My

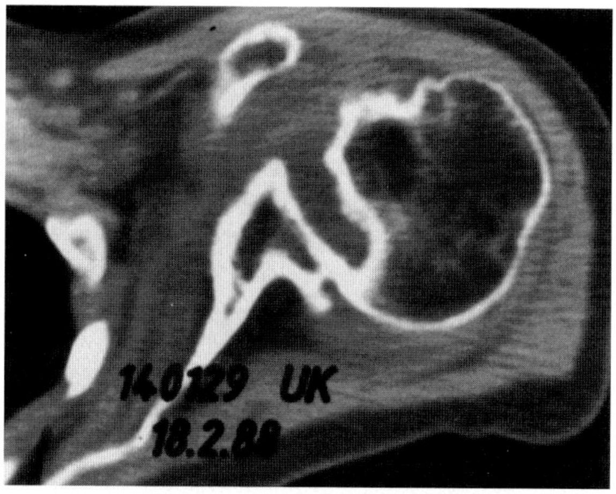

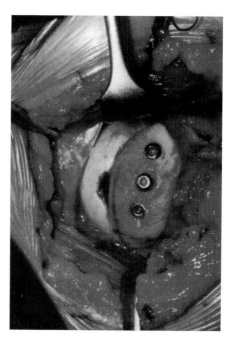

Figure 5-7 To evaluate the size of the humeral head defect, a computed tomography (CT) scan is obtained. It reveals a defect of 40% of the size of the humerus. There is no significant omarthrosis and no osteopenia of the humeral head.

Figure 5-8 Dislocated left shoulder viewed through a deltopectoral approach. A bone graft is sculpted to exactly fit the head surface. It is stabilized in the defect with the use of countersunk screws.

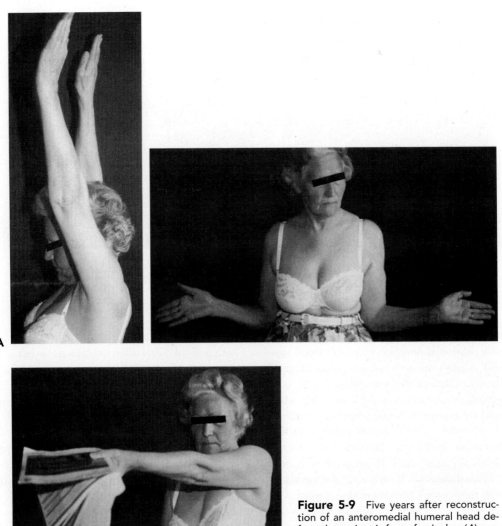

Figure 5-9 Five years after reconstruction of an anteromedial humeral head defect, the patient is free of pain, has (A) normal anterior elevation, (B) external rotation, and (C) strength.

colleagues and I have not encountered problems of function of the subscapularis muscle.

The results of this procedure have been excellent for large anteromedial defects in heads that did not show signs of severe osteoporosis or advanced degenerative joint disease (Figs. 5-8 to 5-11). If the humeral head is already osteoporotic, it will become flattened through the compressive forces acting after relocation of the humeral head, and, in extreme situations, it may virtually collapse. We have had two cases of secondary deformation of the head segment that had been dislocated posteriorly after relocation and reconstruction of the defect with allograft. In each case, the shoulder had been dislocated for more than 1 year, and the humeral head was osteoporotic on retrospective review of the preoperative CT scans (Fig. 5-12).

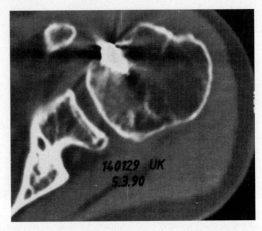

Figure 5-10 Three years after reconstruction, the graft is incorporated, and the head is centered.

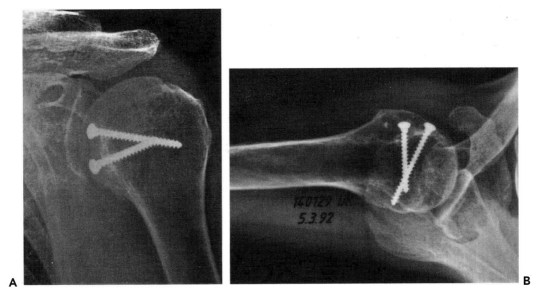

A   B

Figure 5-11   Five years after reconstruction, the humerus is centered in the glenoid fossa, and the graft is incorporated.

Our experience with humeral head reconstruction is probably as good as the results of subscapularis transfer not associated with alteration of the normal anatomy of the proximal humerus. Although it is difficult to recommend the use of allografts, fresh osteochondral allografts have been used to restore joint surfaces with good long-term results in weight-bearing joints.[7,13,18,22] In our series, we obtained a well-vascularized bed, congruity, mechanical graft stability, and incorporation in all cases. Allograft failure[10-12] due to early or late infection, fracture, nonunion at the graft-host junction, or joint instability was not observed, possibly because we tried to avoid implanting allografts in patients with soft, osteopenic bones, a situation that can overload the graft. After a minimum follow-up of 5 years,

the clinical results of humeral head reconstruction with allogenic bone appear comparable with those of currently recommended techniques of treatment.[8,19] For cases with good bone quality of the residual head and without osteoarthrosis, allograft reconstruction may be a valuable alternative. It may also be useful for cases with smaller humeral head defects that are usually treated by subscapularis transfer and for carefully selected cases with larger defects usually considered to require hemiarthroplasty or total joint arthroplasty. This is our preferred method of treatment. It has been successful on long-term follow-up, and, even if the procedure fails, prosthetic reconstruction should be simple because the skeletal anatomy is not distorted by abnormalities of the relation between tubercles and humeral head.

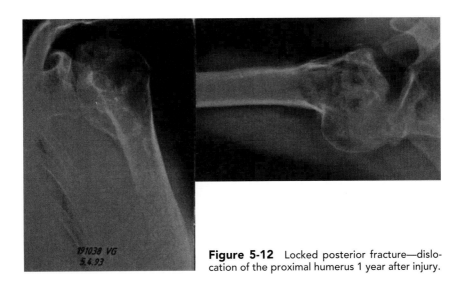

Figure 5-12   Locked posterior fracture—dislocation of the proximal humerus 1 year after injury.

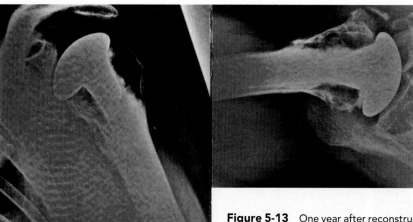

Figure 5-13   One year after reconstruction using a hemiarthroplasty, the tuberosities are not osteotomized, and retroversion of the prosthesis is not abnormal (20 degrees of retroversion). After such a reconstruction, the patient is immobilized in neutral rotation for 6 weeks.

Treatment of Larger Defects

If the defects are larger than 50% of the articular surface, or if the humeral head is very soft, the treatment of choice is hemiarthroplasty, or in selected cases, total joint replacement is indicated. Hawkins et al.[8] reported 16 shoulders in their series that needed treatment with arthroplasty. The overall results were fair, with an average of 140 degrees of flexion and 30 degrees of external rotation for hemiarthroplasty and 152 degrees of flexion and 40 degrees of external rotation for those with total arthroplasty.

If the humeral head cannot be reconstructed, I tend to favor total joint replacement because it allows better restoration of the anatomy and because it may provide better pain relief. Technically, the rules established for total joint replacement are adhered to with few but important exceptions. I try to avoid osteotomy of the tuberosities and prefer to keep the tuberosities at the humeral shaft even if forced to accept a somewhat distorted anatomy of the proximal humerus, as in fracture-dislocations. Formerly, my colleagues and I tried to reconstruct the humerus anatomically with osteotomy and anatomic relocation of the tuberosities. Nonunion, secondary displacement, and unsatisfactory functional results were so common that we abandoned this approach. The tuberosities are left in place, and the humeral head prosthesis is selected to fit the anatomy of the whole proximal humeral complex. Rather than using a third-generation anatomic proximal humeral prosthesis, we may use a nonanatomic prosthesis that can be better for the slightly distorted anatomy (Fig. 5-13). If there has been no subcapital fracture, the head resection is exactly anatomic after the border of the cartilage of the humeral head, and a third-generation humeral replacement (Aequalis, Tornier, France; Replica, Sulzer Medica, Switzerland) is used to perfectly reconstruct the skeletal anatomy that was present before the injury. If there has been a concomitant subcapital fracture, the prosthesis is implanted in 20 degrees of retroversion according to the

normal anatomy. Excessive anteversion is never used. We prefer to release the posterior capsule, subscapularis, and anteroinferior capsule and to reconstruct the humerus as anatomically as possible, rather than to create an abnormal version that persists when the soft tissues have adapted. We think that the skeletal anatomy has to be restored as anatomically as possible, the soft tissues must be released, and the arm may then have to be immobilized in a position of neutral rotation for up to 6 weeks. This allows the soft tissues to adjust their tension, and rehabilitation can be carried out under physiological conditions. This approach has been much more satisfactory than the abnormal versions that we had originally attempted to use to compensate for a tendency to posterior resubluxation (see Fig. 5-13).

LOCKED ANTERIOR DISLOCATION

Chronic, locked anterior dislocation is similar and different from locked posterior dislocation. This type of dislocation always occurs as a major trauma (Figs. 5-14 and 5-15). It

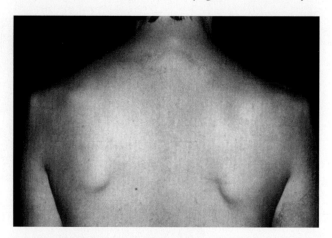

Figure 5-14   Bilateral, locked, anterior dislocation of the shoulder. The patient was unable to give any history about the trauma; this is typical for a convulsive disorder, as in this patient.

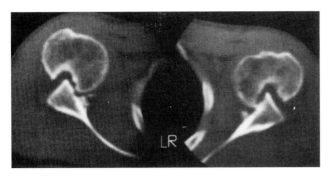

Figure 5-15 Computed tomography (CT) scan of the shoulders of the patient in Figure 5-14. The Hill-Sachs lesions are the key abnormalities, in this case, and are of sufficient magnitude to require operation.

may result from an accident, occur during a manipulation under anesthesia, or be caused by a seizure. The orthopedic surgeon is taught that convulsive disorders cause posterior dislocations, but one half of the locked anterior dislocations that we have seen were caused by seizures. Of all dislocations caused by a convulsive disorder, probably more than one half are anterior. The rarity of the posterior dislocation causes the impression that seizures always lead to posterior dislocations.

Anterior dislocations are only rarely associated with fractures of the surgical neck of the humerus. Because this may occasionally be observed, x-ray analysis is always mandatory before treatment is attempted.[9] Nevertheless, surgical neck fractures are rarer than with posterior dislocations.

Diagnosis

Chronic anterior dislocations are only encountered if the diagnosis of acute dislocation is initially missed. The history reveals that the patient had a relevant injury or a convulsion And, subsequently, observed a loss of function. The patient has often been treated for a "frozen shoulder" syndrome or a contusion of the shoulder. The handicap is moderate, because the position of rotation is more neutral than with posterior dislocations (Figs. 5-16 and 5-17), except for rare cases of unusual types of anterior displacements.

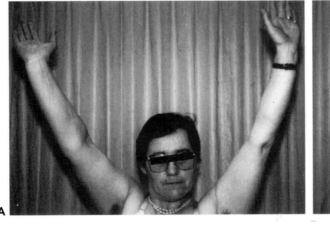
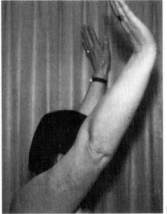
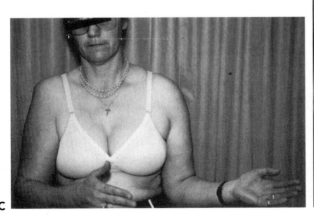
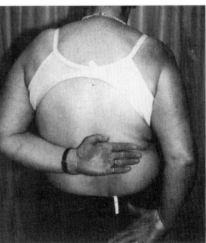

Figure 5-16 (A) Abduction and (B) elevation movements by this patient are virtually symmetrical and are free of pain. The overall function of the patient is satisfactory, despite (C) a severe internal rotation deformity with (C,D) locked internal and external rotations.

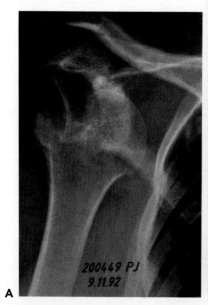

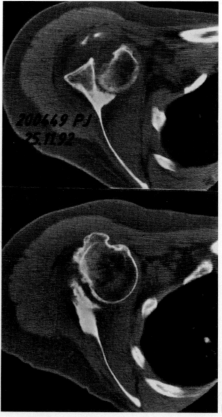

Figure 5-17 (*A*) Plain x-ray film and (*B*) computed tomography (CT) scan of the patient in Figure 5-16. The dislocation was 3 years old when the patient was referred to us. The destruction was considered to be so extensive that surgical reconstruction appeared unlikely to be able to improve the untreated situation.

The diagnosis is easily made if the patient is examined posteriorly, and absence of the prominence of the deltoid is noticed. The shape of the shoulder seen in Figure 5-18 is characteristic of anterior dislocation and is usually not to be confused with other abnormalities. The arm is in slight abduction, and rotation is severely limited, but the internal rotation deformity is usually less severe than with posterior dislocation.

The anteroposterior (see Fig. 5-17) and axillary lateral x-ray views allow diagnosis. A CT scan allows quantitation of the skeletal lesions (see Figs. 5-15 and 5-17) and planning of the treatment.

Lesions

Locked anterior dislocation is characterized by lesions opposite to those seen in locked posterior dislocation, in which the glenoid and capsular lesions appear to be more important than in posterior dislocation. The proximity of the brachial plexus may account for the occasionally neurovascular compromise and constitute an additional aggravating factor if surgical correction is contemplated.

A Hill-Sachs lesion, sometimes of enormous magnitude, may display sclerosis as evidence of the chronicity of the lesion and of the adaptation of the musculoskeletal apparatus. Erosions of the glenoid are much more frequent than with posterior dislocations and may require reconstruction with bone grafts, especially if prosthetic reconstruction is carried out. The anterior capsule is detached from the anterior glenoid rim, and a large Bankart (or Broca-Hartmann) pouch is created to accommodate the volume of the humeral head. With long-standing dislocation, the neurovascular structures become adherent to the subscapularis, and surgical revision carries the risk of injury to nerves and axillary artery and vein.

Treatment

Skillful Neglect

There are no major differences in the treatment concepts for locked posterior or anterior dislocations. Very severe, long-standing destruction with relatively little functional handicap can be treated with skillful neglect, especially if the bony and soft-tissue lesions are so severe that it is highly uncertain that reconstruction can substantially improve the patient's shoulder. If both shoulders are dislocated (Figs. 5-19 to 5-22), the shoulder that has the better potential to be successfully treated is operated on first. As soon as this shoulder is functional, the opposite shoulder is reconstructed.

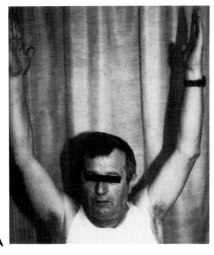

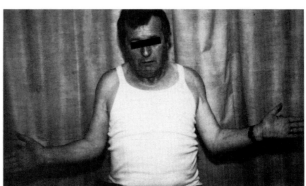

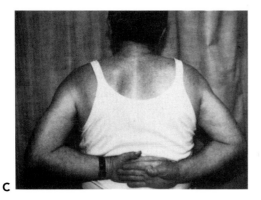

Figure 5-18 (*A*) One year after a prosthetic reconstruction, a patient shows excellent elevation, (*B*) external, and (*C*) internal rotation.

Figure 5-19 Right shoulder of a bilateral, locked dislocation. There are several changes seen on the humerus and the glenoid by (*A*) conventional x-ray film and (*B*) CT scan.

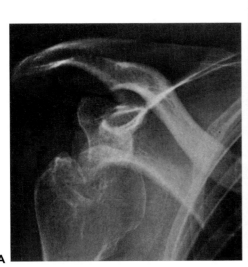

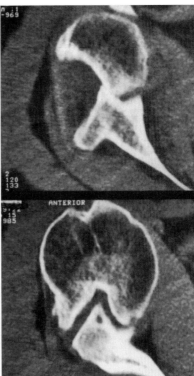

Figure 5-20   Left shoulder of the patient in Figure 5-19. A very large Hill-Sachs lesion is responsible for severe difficulties in reducing dislocations on this side. (*A*) Documentation by x-ray film and (*B*) CT scan shows that reconstruction of the humeral head is mandatory.

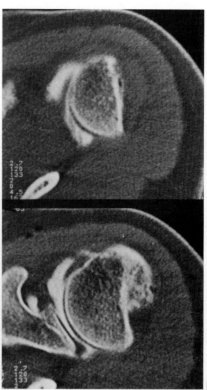

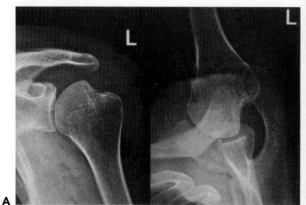

Closed Reduction

My colleagues and I believe that closed reduction is probably never indicated in a truly chronic, locked anterior dislocation, because it may fracture the humerus, and our attempts at closed reduction at the beginning of surgery in patients under general anesthesia were never successful. If

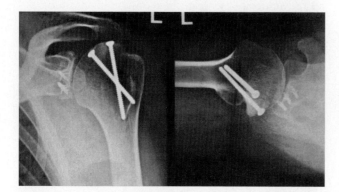

Figure 5-21   Three months after reconstruction of the left shoulder of the patient in Figure 5-20. Using a deltopectoral approach, the humeral head defect has been filled with an allograft to restore the shape of the humeral head, and the anteroinferior capsule has been reinserted to the scapular neck, as in an ordinary anterior capsular repair.

this approach were possible, the same principles for further treatment would apply as for posterior dislocations.

Humeral Head and Anterior Glenoid Reconstruction

For chronic anterior shoulder dislocation, the same treatment principles should be applied as outlined for posterior dislocations. Open reduction of the dislocation should be carried out, and the humeral head defect should be corrected with the implantation of a bone graft using a deltopectoral approach. The entire subscapularis is released, and the humeral head is relocated into the joint. The neurovascular bundle is identified and freed from the subscapularis that must be mobilized. A posterior capsulotomy is performed, and the capsule is almost circumferentially released. The coracoacromial ligament must be incised to allow anterior dislocation of the arm in adduction and extension, as for prosthetic reconstruction. In full external rotation, the humeral head defect is filled with an allograft (i.e., humeral or femoral head segment). The allograft is fixed to the well-vascularized bed with 3.5-mm screws (Synthes).

After reconstruction of the humeral head, the glenoid is reconstructed with a usual anterior capsular repair (see Fig.

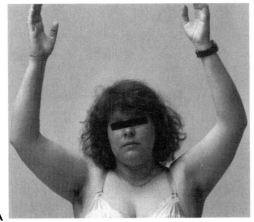
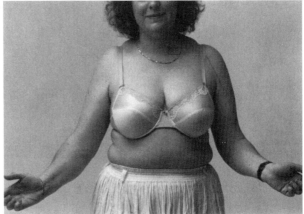
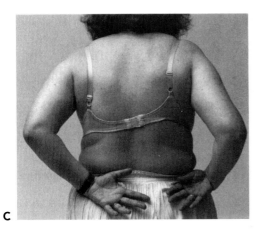

Figure 5-22   Three months after surgery on (*A*) the left shoulder elevation, (*B*) external, and (*C*) internal rotation are already better than on the right side, but it is noticeable how well the right, previously dislocated shoulder functions.

5-21), or an anterior bone block is used to augment the anterior glenoid (Fig. 5-23). If the glenoid is worn, we prefer to use an intra-articular iliac bone graft to formally reconstruct the glenoid cavity and then reinsert the anteroinferior capsule to this bone graft to restore normal anatomy of the glenoid. Postoperatively, the arm is put in a sling for 6 weeks, and external rotation beyond 0 degrees is not allowed for 6 weeks.

This approach has been more satisfactory than rotational osteotomy of the humerus, which has been tried as an alternative to reconstruction of the humeral head. Avascular necrosis has been described after rotational osteotomy, and my colleagues and I have had to perform a later prosthetic reconstruction that was extremely difficult in two cases; therefore, we try to avoid this nonanatomic procedure.

We have only treated four cases of locked anterior dislocation with the previously described approach. One case is too recent to allow definitive conclusions, although the three others have shown a good outcome with elevation over 145 degrees, amplitude of rotation of more than 70 degrees, and a Constant score of more than 70% of an age- and gender-matched normal value.[2] This approach is our preferred method of treatment of such cases.

Prosthetic Reconstruction

If the defect of the humeral head is too large to allow humeral head reconstruction, if the glenoid destruction is so advanced that prosthetic reconstruction of the glenoid seems necessary, if the head is so osteopenic that deformation after relocation is expected, or if an elderly patient has a large humeral head defect, we consider hemiarthroplasty or total shoulder arthroplasty. Reconstruction of the glenoid is often necessary. This is achieved with the use of the resected humeral head. It serves as a bone graft to reconstruct the anterior glenoid. Despite the efforts with bone graft, reconstruction of the glenoid, and ligament reinsertion on the anterior glenoid neck, my colleagues and I have observed recurrence of instability in one case and static anterior subluxation with a poor functional result in another, and we have been unable to determine the reasons for failure in both cases. For prosthetic reconstruction, we would not increase posterior version but instead reconstruct the abnormal version of the glenoid and reconstruct the anterior capsuloligamentous apparatus. Nevertheless, it appears that the results of prosthetic reconstruction of locked anterior instability are less predictable than those of locked posterior instability.

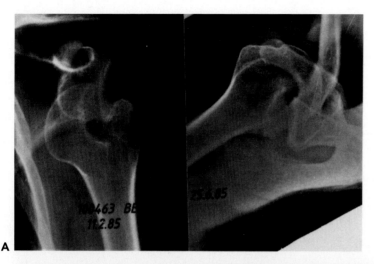

A

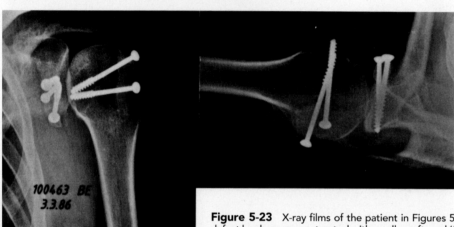

B

Figure 5-23 X-ray films of the patient in Figures 5-14 and 5-15. (*A*) The severe humeral head defect has been reconstructed with an allograft, and (*B*) the anterior glenoid has been augmented with a modified Bristow bone block. The patient was last reviewed 5 years after surgery, and at that time, his shoulder was stable and free of pain but showed mild limitation of external rotation.

SUMMARY

Locked, chronic shoulder instability is, fortunately, rare. The concept of restoring the shape of the humeral head is the mainstay in therapy and the essential step in surgical reconstruction. Although it seems necessary to reinsert the capsuloligamentous apparatus in treating anterior dislocation, this has not been necessary for correcting posterior dislocations.[4,5] Prosthetic reconstruction is demanding, particularly in cases with locked anterior dislocation. The use of nonanatomical first- and second-generation prosthesis is only considered in cases with deformity of the proximal humerus; in such cases, the prosthesis allows a better relation of the prosthetic head segment to the tuberosities (see Fig. 5-13). In all other cases, insertion of a third-generation prosthesis replicates the normal skeletal anatomy. Circumferential soft-tissue release allows the use of physiologic version of the prosthetic components, provided the arm is postoperatively protected in a neutral rotation position for a period of 6 weeks.

REFERENCES

1. Constant CR. Age-related recovery of shoulder function after injury (Thesis). Cork, Ireland, University College, 1986.
2. Constant CR, Murley AHG. A clinical method of functional assessment of the shoulder. Clin Orthop Rel Res 1987;214:160.
3. Dubousset J. Luxation posterieure de l'epaule. Rev Chir Orthop 1967;53:56.
4. Gerber C. Les instabilities de l'epaule. In: Cahiers d'enseignement de la SOFCOT no. 33. Paris, Expansion Scientifique Francaise, 1988:51.
5. Gerber C. L'instabilite posterieure de l'epaule. In: Cahiers d'enseignement de la SOFCOT no. 40. Paris, Expansion Scientifique Francaise, 1991:223.
6. Gerber C, Lambert S. Allograft reconstruction of segmental defects of the humeral head for the treatment of chronic locked posterior dislocation of the shoulder. J Bone Joint Surg 1996;78A:376.
7. Gross AE. Use of fresh osteochondral allograft to replace traumatic joint defects. In: Czitrom AA, Gross AE, eds. Allografts in orthopaedic practice. Baltimore, Williams & Wilkins, 1992:67.
8. Hawkins RJ, Neer CS, Planta RM, et al. Locked posterior dislocation of the shoulder. J Bone Joint Surg 1987;69A:9.
9. Hersche O, Gerber C. Iatrogenic displacement of fracture-dislocations of the shoulder. J Bone Joint Surg 1994;76B:30.

10. Lord CF, Gebhardt MC, Tomford WW, et al. Infection in bone grafts. J Bone Joint Surg 1988;70A:369.
11. Mankin HJ. Complications of allograft surgery. In: Friedlander GE, Mankin HJ, Jell KW, eds. Osteochondral allografts. Boston, Little, Brown, 1983:259.
12. Mankin HJ, Doppelt S, Tomford W. Clinical experience with allograft implantation: the first ten years. Clin Orthop 1983;174:69.
13. McDermott AGP, Langer F, Pritzker KPH, et al. Fresh small-fragment osteochondral allografts: long-term follow-up study on first 100 cases. Clin Orthop 1985;197:96.
14. McLaughlin HL. Posterior dislocation of the shoulder. J Bone Joint Surg 1952;34A:584.
15. Neer CS II. Fractures. In: Neer CS II, ed. Shoulder reconstruction. Philadelphia, WB Saunders, 1990:394.
16. Neer CS II, Hughes M. Glenohumeral joint replacement and postoperative rehabilitation. Phys Ther 1975;55:850.
17. Ovesen J, Nielsen S. Anterior and posterior shoulder instability: a cadaver study. Acta Orthop Scand 1985;57:324.
18. Ovesen J, Sojbjerg JO. Posterior shoulder dislocation: muscle and capsular lesions in cadaver experiments. Acta Orthop Scand 1986;57:535.
19. Rowe CR, Zarins B. Chronic unreduced dislocation of the shoulder. J Bone Joint Surg 1982;64A:494.
20. Scougall S. Posterior dislocation of the shoulder. J Bone Joint Surg 1957;39B:726.
21. Walch G, Boileau P, Martin B, et al. Luxations et fractures-luxations posterieures inveterees de l'epaule: a propos de 30 cas. Rev Chir Orthop 1990;76:546.
22. Zukor DJ, Paitich B, Oakeshott RD, et al. Reconstruction of post-traumatic articular surface defects using fresh small-fragment osteochondral allografts. In: Aebi M, Regazzoni P, eds. Bone transplantation. Berlin, Springer-Verlag, 1989:275.

Rotator Cuff Tears

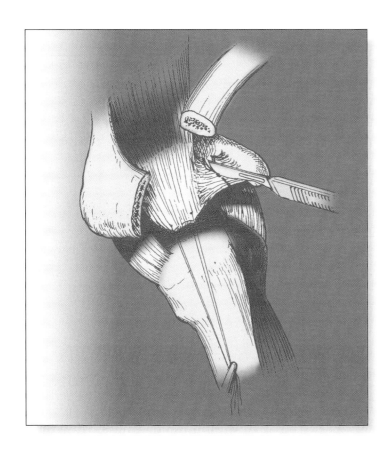

Anterior Superior Rotator Cuff Tears: Repairable and Irreparable Tears

T. Bradley Edwards   **Gilles Walch**   **Laurent Nové-Josserand**   **Christian Gerber**

INTRODUCTION

Shoulder pathology specifically involving the anterior superior rotator cuff is becoming more recognized predominantly because of increasing surgeon awareness. It is now better understood that lesions affecting this part of the rotator cuff are distinct entities that behave differently than the more commonly recognized lesions of the posterior superior rotator cuff. The frequent involvement of the rotator interval and the long head of the biceps tendon mandates that these lesions be treated differently than those lesions limited to the posterior superior rotator cuff.

Tears of the anterior superior rotator cuff are defined as those involving any aspect of the subscapularis tendon and

may involve lesions of the supraspinatus tendon. Additionally, because of their anatomic proximity, anterior superior rotator cuff lesions are frequently coupled with pathology of the rotator interval (superior glenohumeral ligament [SGHL], coracohumeral ligament [CCHL]), and the long head of the biceps tendon. This chapter will provide an overview of anatomy, epidemiology, clinical evaluation, and imaging of anterior superior rotator cuff lesions. Additionally, this chapter will detail our preferred treatment and provide data regarding expected outcomes of treatment of anterior superior rotator cuff tears.

NORMAL ANATOMY

The rotator cuff is a continuous tendinous band that is intimately connected with the glenohumeral articular capsule. It can be divided into three parts: the posterior cuff with the infraspinatus tendon and the teres minor tendon; the superior cuff with the supraspinatus tendon; and the anterior cuff with the subscapularis tendon and the rotator interval. The rotator interval also includes the intra-articular portion of the tendon of the long head of the biceps.

T. B. Edwards: Department of Orthopaedic Surgery, University of Minnesota.

G. Walch: Department of Orthopaedic Surgery, University of Lyon, France.

L. Nové-Josserand: Department of Orthopaedic Surgery, University of Lyon, France.

C. Gerber: Department of Orthopaedics, University of Zurich, Balgrist, Switzerland.

The subscapularis muscle originates in the subscapularis fossa of the scapula. The muscle inserts via a strong tendon on the superior medial aspect of the lesser tuberosity. Many fibers of the subscapularis tendon extend laterally and superiorly to form the medial wall of the bicipital groove and merge with the supraspinatus tendon. The subscapularis tendon and the supraspinatus tendon are thereby intertwined for approximately 1 cm before inserting into the lesser and greater tuberosity, respectively. Inferiorly, the subscapularis tendon becomes less substantial so that its inferior most insertion is almost purely muscular.

The supraspinatus muscle originates in the supraspinatus fossa of the scapula superior to the scapular spine. The muscle inserts via a strong tendon on the superior facet of the greater tuberosity. Many fibers of the supraspinatus tendon extend medially to form the lateral wall of the bicipital groove and merge with the subscapularis tendon.

The rotator interval is composed of the coracohumeral ligament, the superior glenohumeral ligament, the joint capsule, and expansions of the subscapularis and supraspinatus tendons. The coracohumeral ligament is the dominant structure of the rotator interval (Fig. 6-1). It bridges the subscapularis and the supraspinatus tendons and ensures continuity of the rotator cuff. It is triangular, with its base at the coracoid, its apex over the bicipital

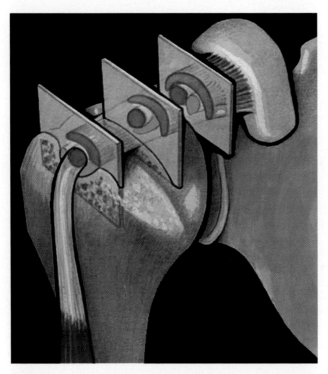

Figure 6-1 Anatomy of the rotator interval. CH, coracohumeral ligament; SGH, superior glenohumeral ligament; LHB, long head of the biceps tendon. (Adapted with permission from Habermeyer P, Walch G. The biceps tendon and rotator cuff disease. In: Burkhead WZ, ed. Rotator cuff disorders. Baltimore, Williams & Wilkins, 1996:142.)

groove, one side inserting mainly into the greater tuberosity, and one side inserting mainly into the lesser tuberosity. It becomes intimately associated with the glenohumeral joint capsule and covers the long head of the biceps tendon.

The superior glenohumeral ligament originates variably from the anterior superior neck of the scapula, either from the cartilaginous labrum, from the osseous scapular neck, or both. It lies deep to the coracohumeral ligament, and at its origin, is separated from it by fatty tissue (Fig. 6-1). Laterally, the superior glenohumeral ligament becomes intertwined with the portion of the coracohumeral ligament that inserts proximal to the tendon of the subscapularis immediately adjacent to the bicipital groove on the lesser tuberosity. Deep fibers from the superior glenohumeral ligament and coracohumeral ligament line the floor of the bicipital groove. These structures (the subscapularis tendon, the coracohumeral ligament, and the superior glenohumeral ligament) are closely related and form a reflection pulley complex that functions as a stabilizer for the long head of the biceps centering it within its groove.[21]

The long head of the biceps tendon takes origin at the supraglenoid tubercle of the scapula. It traverses horizontally over the humeral head reaching the entrance of the bicipital groove where it becomes vertical and extra-articular. Rotation and abduction change the position of the intra-articular portion of the long head of the biceps. As the arm is externally rotated the long head of the biceps translates medially around the curvature of the humeral head, placing increased forces on the medial stabilizing structures as they attempt to maintain the long head of the biceps within the bicipital groove. The ligamentous pulley complex plays a major role in stabilizing the long head of the biceps because insufficient stability is imparted by the osseous constraints of the groove. Hence, the structural integrity of the ligamentous pulley system is mandatory for stability of the long head of the biceps.

PATHOLOGY

For the purposes of this chapter, lesions will be discussed in one of the following categories: isolated lesions of the subscapularis tendon, lesions of the subscapularis and supraspinatus tendons, or associated lesions of the rotator interval and long head of the biceps tendon.

Isolated Lesions of the Subscapularis Tendon

Most subscapularis lesions involve the superior lateral insertion of the tendon at its insertion on the lesser tuberosity. These lesions progress in a medial and inferior direction. The tendon is commonly avulsed directly from bone rather than torn in its midsubstance. Lesions originating at the inferior aspect of the subscapularis tendon have been described but are exceptionally rare. Isolated lesions of the subscapularis tendon can be categorized based on relative size: lesions of the superior third of the subscapularis tendon, lesions of the superior two-thirds of the subscapularis tendon, and complete lesions of the subscapularis tendon.

Superior third lesions of the subscapularis tendon represent an avulsion from the lesser tuberosity. If the ligamentous pulley complex is intact, this lesion is not visible during gross inspection of the rotator cuff. If the ligamentous pulley complex is divided, this type of lesion is identified as a bare area of bone at the superior aspect of the lesser tuberosity. The humeral insertion of the superior glenohumeral ligament may be intact or torn. Minimal tendinous retraction occurs with this type of tear because the inferior two-thirds of the subscapularis tendon remain intact.[21]

Lesions of the superior two-thirds of the subscapularis tendon leave only the inferior muscular insertion intact. With this type of lesion the subscapularis tendon is absent over the entire surface of the lesser tuberosity. In approximately one-half of the cases, this type of tear is not immediately visible during initial open surgical exploration because the lesser tuberosity is obscured by scar tissue hiding the lesion.[7] Tendinous retraction varies according to the extent and chronicity of the lesion.

Complete lesions of the subscapularis consist of an avulsion of both the tendinous and muscular insertions of the subscapularis from the lesser tuberosity. This often occurs with retraction of the musculotendinous unit beyond the glenoid rim into the subscapularis fossa and may result in significant muscular atrophy and fatty degeneration observed on computed tomography (CT) or magnetic resonance imaging (MRI). In younger patients, a midsubstance tendinous rupture with a lateral tendinous stump may be observed in contrast to the typical avulsion from bone.

Lesions of the Subscapularis and Supraspinatus Tendons

A second type of anterior superior rotator cuff lesion involves the supraspinatus tendon, in addition to the subscapularis tendon. In this scenario, tears involving the subscapularis may be classified in much the same way as in isolated lesions of the subscapularis: superior third, superior two-thirds, or complete. Tears of the supraspinatus are usually a superior extension of the subscapularis tear and, hence, preferentially involve the anterior aspect of the supraspinatus tendon. These tears are thought to propagate in a posterior direction and may involve the entire width of the supraspinatus tendon or even extend to involve the infraspinatus tendon.

Lesions of the Rotator Interval and Long Head of the Biceps Tendon

Lesions of the rotator interval and the long head of the biceps tendon are intimately associated with tears of the

anterior superior rotator cuff by virtue of their anatomic locale. Tears of the anterior superior rotator cuff invariably lead to some degree of secondary biceps tendinitis. Biceps tendinitis is a term to describe an alteration in the structure of the tendon and may be atrophic, hypertrophic, frayed, or inflammatory.[21]

Pathology of the anterior superior rotator cuff represents the most common cause of biceps tendinitis and can be classified by the type of underlying lesion. Lesions of the subscapularis can cause inflammation and distension of the ligamentous pulley and bicipital sheath, ultimately destabilizing the biceps within its groove (Fig. 6-2). Degeneration and tearing limited to the rotator interval (coracohumeral ligament and superior glenohumeral ligament) can result in inflammation of the biceps tendon and fraying of its superior aspect from mechanical friction of the tendon against the coracoacromial arch.

Large tears of the rotator cuff, including disruption of the supraspinatus, infraspinatus, and rotator interval, invariably lead to some degree of biceps disease. Once the infraspinatus is disrupted, proximal migration of the humeral head

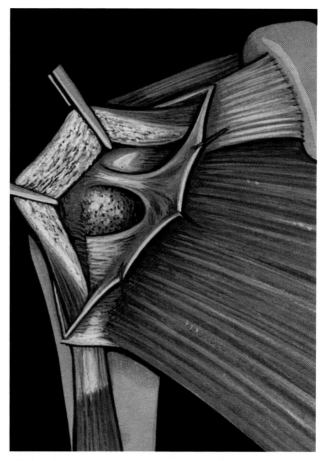

Figure 6-2 Superior one-third lesion of the subscapularis tendon with overlying distension/disruption of the ligamentous pulley, resulting in mechanical abrasion of the biceps tendon on the lesser tuberosity.

ensues, entrapping the biceps tendon between the humeral head and coracoacromial arch, resulting in mechanical abrasion of the tendon with anterior elevation of the arm.

Anterior superior rotator cuff tears with associated rotator interval lesions frequently result in instability of the biceps tendon, in addition to structural changes within the tendon. Instability can occur as subluxation, a transitory or partial loss of contact between the biceps tendon and the bicipital groove, or dislocation, fixed or complete loss of contact between the biceps tendon and the bicipital groove.[20] Biceps subluxation generally occurs in a medial direction via disruption or distension of the ligamentous pulley complex, resulting in fraying of the medial aspect of the biceps tendon.

Dislocation of the biceps tendon can occur with the tendon resting on the lesser tuberosity (partial tear of the subscapularis), the tendon dislocated intra-articularly (complete rupture of the subscapularis), or with the tendon dislocated extra-articularly and resting on the anterior surface of the subscapularis (subscapularis intact, disruption of the rotator interval). When the tendon is resting on the lesser tuberosity, mechanical friction on the tendon will evolve to spontaneous rupture. With complete intra-articular or extra-articular dislocation, absence of mechanical friction often prevents spontaneous rupture.

DIAGNOSIS

The diagnosis of lesions affecting the anterior superior rotator cuff can be difficult, particularly in the case of small lesions limited to the superior portion of the subscapularis tendon and rotator interval. Diagnosis of these lesions requires proper examination and use of appropriate imaging studies.

Epidemiology

Although both sexes are affected, lesions of the anterior superior rotator cuff predominantly affect men. The dominant arm is involved in most cases. In our experience a history of trauma is associated with the onset of symptoms in about 85% of patients. If a trauma involving external rotation and extension of the arm or anterior traumatic dislocation is reported by a patient older than 40 years of age, a subscapularis lesion should be suspected. In cases of less extensive involvement of the subscapularis, there is often little or no trauma. These atraumatic lesions appear to be degenerative in origin.

Clinical History

Three types of presentations are characteristic: chronic and progressive shoulder pain following a traumatic event, pseudoparalytic shoulder, and pain with shoulder stiffness. Roughly, one-half of the patients seek medical advice for chronic and progressively increasing shoulder pain after a defined traumatic event. Pain is constant and aggravated by using the arm at the side or above the head. Night pain is also a common feature. The pattern of pain is not distinctly different from that of isolated supraspinatus tears, with the exception that the patient with a large anterior lesion may also report aggravation of pain with the use of the arm below shoulder level.

Approximately one-third of patients present with a pseudoparalytic shoulder. Passive range of motion is preserved, but active elevation is limited to less than 90 degrees. Pseudoparalysis is typically associated with large multiple tendon rotator cuff tears. Shoulders with pain and stiffness (decrease of active and passive range of motion) are rare. Pain and stiffness are not specific for any type of lesion or severity of injury.

A fourth subset of patients exists with asymptomatic or minimally symptomatic subscapularis tears. These patients are often seen by a physician for another problem and mention their shoulder in passing or may have an acute injury superimposed on a chronic minimally symptomatic subscapularis tear. These tears are generally best left untreated.

Clinical Examination

A thorough shoulder examination should include active and passive ranges of motion. Standard clinical strength testing of the rotator cuff is performed. Of the tests specifically evaluating the anterior superior rotator cuff, Jobe's test is employed to evaluate supraspinatus integrity.[10] Subscapularis involvement is documented with three observations. Increased passive external rotation with the arm at the side is a specific sign for complete subscapularis disruption, provided the contralateral shoulder is normal (Fig. 6-3). The lift-off sign is tested with the arm passively brought into maximal internal rotation behind the

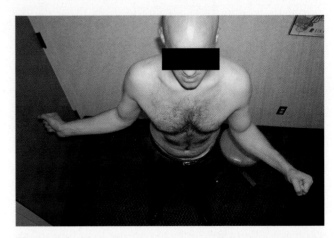

Figure 6-3 Increased external rotation of the shoulder with the arm at the side in a patient with a complete subscapularis disruption.

patient's body.[7] The examiner asks the patient to maintain the position of maximal internal rotation by holding the hand off the back. If this is possible, the subscapularis is largely intact. If the patient cannot maintain this position and the hand drops back toward the back, the test is positive, indicating pathology of the subscapularis (Fig. 6-4). In the complete tear, the hand cannot be held off the back in any capacity, but in partial lesions, the hand may drop toward the back but without dropping to rest on the back. The lift-off sign is less useful in patients experiencing extreme pain with internal rotation and in patients with stiffness, which prevents adequate internal rotation for the test. The belly-press test is positive when the patient is required to flex the wrist and extend the arm to exert force on the lower abdomen with the affected upper extremity (Fig. 6-5). Although the use of clinical tests to detect ruptures of the subscapularis has been extremely reliable for some examiners, partial tears of the subscapularis remain more difficult to di-

agnose than complete tears and may present only with isolated weakness in internal rotation.

Dynamic anterior superior subluxation of the humeral head associated with active elevation of the arm indicates a large tear of the subscapularis and supraspinatus tendons (Fig. 6-6). The patient performs resisted abduction with the examiner observing from behind. Dynamic subluxation occurs during the initial degrees of abduction and may occasionally be palpated under the deltoid rather than be observed.

Pathology involving the long head of the biceps remains an enigma to clinical diagnosis. Although most completely ruptured biceps are easily detectable on clinical examination by the ball-like deformity of the biceps muscle belly present when the arm is elevated to 90 degrees and the elbow is forcibly flexed, more subtle bicipital problems are difficult to diagnose. The palm-up test can be performed with the elbow extended and the forearm supinated. The

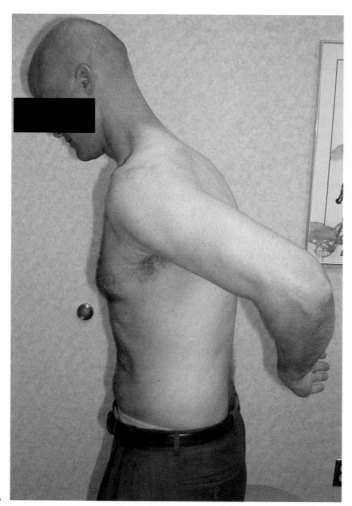

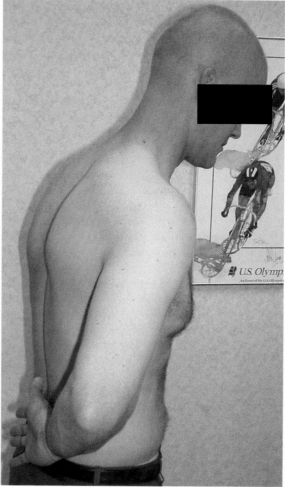

A

B

Figure 6-4 (*A*) Negative lift-off test. The patient is able to keep his hand from resting on his back during shoulder internal rotation. (*B*) Positive lift-off test. The patient cannot lift his hand off of his back.

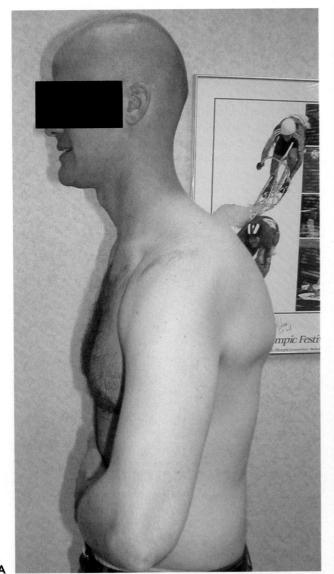
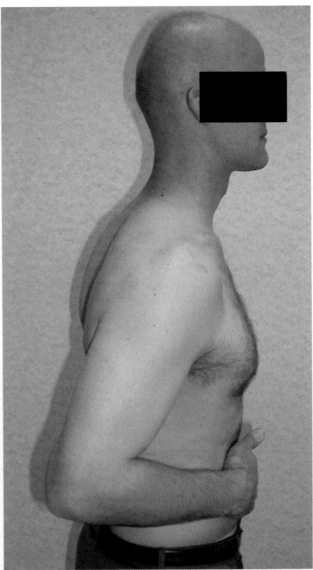

Figure 6-5 (*A*) Negative belly-press test. The patient is able to press on his abdomen while maintaining his wrist in neutral position and his elbow in front of his body. (*B*) Positive belly-press test. As the patient presses his abdomen, the wrist is flexed and the arm is extended.

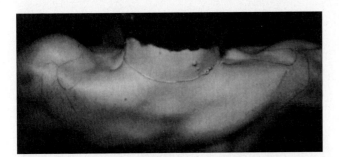

Figure 6-6 On resisted abduction, the left proximal humerus subluxates anteriorly and superiorly, while the right humerus remains centered under the acromion. This dynamic anterior superior subluxation may be visible or palpable and is pathognomonic of combined subscapularis and supraspinatus insufficiency.

patient is asked to elevate the arm against resistance (Speed's test). If pain is elicited along the anterior part of the biceps, the test is positive,. Although other tests have been described (Yergason's test, O'Brien's test), in our experience, none of these tests have been found to be very specific for bicipital lesions. Similarly, dislocation or subluxation of the biceps cannot be reliably detected clinically. A slight clicking sound perceived by the patient and the examiner during rotation is uncommon and may or may not be caused by biceps dislocation.

Similar to the long head of the biceps, pathology of the rotator interval can be difficult to diagnose on clinical examination. A compromised coracohumeral ligament and/or SGHL can only be suspected clinically in patients with abnormal joint laxity. If a positive inferior drawer test in neutral rotation (sulcus sign) does not diminish in external rotation, a lesion of the rotation interval is suspected.

Imaging

Conventional radiography includes anterior posterior views in neutral, internal rotation, and external rotation; a lateral view in the scapular plane; and an axillary view (Fig. 6-7). Ideally, radiography is performed under fluoroscopic and magnification control. The subacromial space between the inferior cortex of the acromion and the humeral head is measured on the anterior posterior neutral rotation view. A subacromial space less than 7 mm indicates an extensive rotator cuff tear involving the posterior rotator cuff (infraspinatus). Cystic lesions or sclerosis of the lesser tuberosity suggest an anterior rotator cuff lesion. Anterior subluxation is often not readily identifiable using conventional radiography, although it may be suspected on axillary views.

Arthrography coupled with subsequent CT is an excellent advanced imaging modality for exploring the anterior superior rotator cuff. Use of a radiopaque contrast medium provides more reliable imaging than air or double-contrast arthrography. Arthrography, performed immediately prior to CT, should include imaging during the injection of the contrast using multiple views. Contrast extravasation into the subacromial bursa is diagnostic of a full thickness rotator cuff tear, which can then be more precisely localized from the various rotational and lateral views.

A subscapularis lesion is suspected if contrast reaches the lesser tuberosity on the anterior posterior view in neutral and, more specifically, in external rotation. This sign, which may be subtle, is positive in 80% of patients with a subscapularis tear. This finding, however, is not apparent in partial ruptures of the superior subscapularis tendon. Failure to visualize the bicipital groove is pathognomonic for a biceps lesion and suspicious for an anterior rotator cuff lesion. This finding, however, is not indicative of the type of biceps lesion, unless the long head of the biceps tendon is visualized medial to the bicipital groove, confirming dislocation (Fig. 6-8). Rupture of the long head of the biceps is confirmed when the bicipital groove is filled with contrast rather than with the tendon.

Although arthrography is useful in the diagnosis of anterior superior rotator cuff lesions, we rarely employ it without a postarthrography computed tomogram. Computed tomographic arthrography offers great diagnostic and prognostic value, allowing diagnosis of subscapularis and long head of the biceps tendon abnormalities, providing an anatomic outline of the subcoracoid space and of

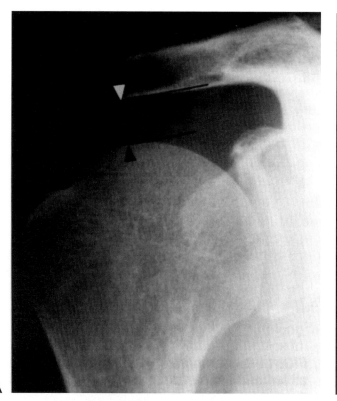
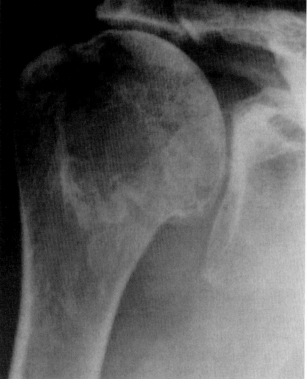

A

B

Figure 6-7 (*A*) Neutral rotation anterior posterior view of the shoulder. The acromiohumeral interval is the shortest distance measurable from the inferior aspect of the acromion and the superior aspect of the humerus. Normally, the acromiohumeral interval ranges from 7 to 14 mm. (*B*) Diminished acromiohumeral interval indicating an extensive rotator cuff tear involving the infraspinatus tendon.

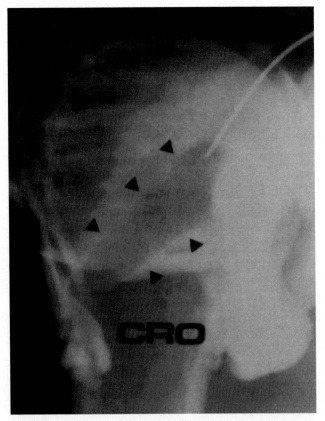

Figure 6-8 Arthrography of the shoulder demonstrating dislocation of the long head of the biceps tendon (*arrows*) and full thickness rotator cuff rupture.

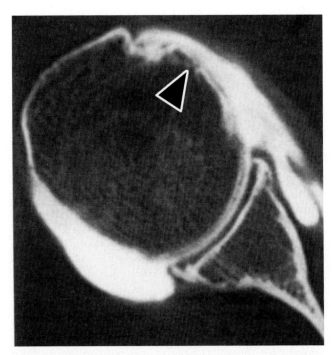

Figure 6-9 Computed tomographic arthrogram of the shoulder. The arrow indicates contrast in contact with the lesser tuberosity at the level of the bicipital groove indicating a tear of the subscapularis tendon. Contrast has filled the bicipital groove confirming rupture of the long head of the biceps tendon.

articular congruence, and allowing evaluation of fatty degeneration of the rotator cuff musculature.

Lesions of the subscapularis tendon are demonstrated by the presence of contrast in contact with the bony surface of the lesser tuberosity, where the subscapularis tendon normally inserts (Fig. 6-9). The size of the lesion is determined by the number of computed tomographic sections on which it is visible. This sign may be difficult to see in very small partial thickness superior lesions or in the rare case of midsubstance tendon rupture.

Dislocation and subluxation of the long head of the biceps tendon are readily identifiable using computed tomographic arthrography (Fig. 6-10). The examiner must be wary of erroneous interpretation of dislocation of the long head of the biceps tendon at the inferior aspect of the groove. This finding is usually the result of recentering of the dislocated tendon, which occurs when the superior part of the subscapularis tendon has ruptured and dye reaches inferiorly into the bicipital groove over the inferior part of the subscapularis muscle fibers that normally insert at the inferior aspect of the lesser tuberosity (Fig. 6-11). Subluxation of the biceps is diagnosed when the biceps is perched on the medial aspect of the lesser tuberosity. The long head of the biceps has the shape of a comma and runs along the

medial wall of the bicipital groove (Fig. 6-12). Subluxation and dislocation of the long head of the biceps virtually always occur with a subscapularis tendon tear. The exception is the rare case in which the biceps is dislocated anterior to an intact subscapularis through a disruption in the rotator interval. Rupture of the long head of the biceps tendon is diagnosed, if the bicipital groove is void and the tendon cannot be visualized intra-articularly (Fig. 6-9).

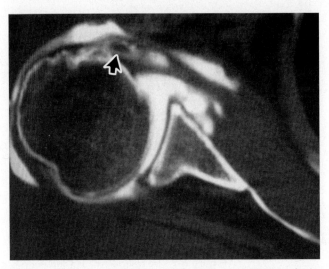

Figure 6-10 Computed tomographic arthrogram of the shoulder. The arrow indicates a dislocated long head of the biceps tendon.

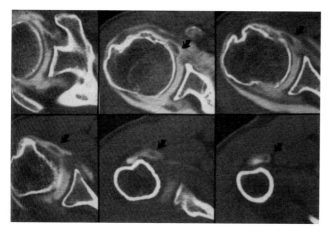

Figure 6-11 Computed tomographic arthrogram of the shoulder showing a superior subscapularis tendon tear with long head of the biceps tendon dislocation. Superiorly (*top row of images*), the subscapularis tendon is ruptured, but inferiorly (*bottom row of images*), the subscapularis, which is nearly purely muscular at this level, inserts normally on the lesser tuberosity. The long head of the biceps tendon traverses the bicipital groove at the inferior level, passing anterior to the muscular portion of the subscapularis insertion (false dislocation of the long head of the biceps tendon anterior to the subscapularis).

Gerber et al.[6] examined the morphology of the subcoracoid space and its potential role for the development of anterior rotator cuff lesions. In a control series of 47 shoulders, the distance between humeral head and tip of the coracoid averaged 8.7 mm with the internally rotated arm at the side and 6.8 mm with internally rotated arm at 90 degrees of elevation. In 40 shoulders with anterior superior rotator cuff lesions, the average coracohumeral distance averaged 8.1 mm, and, in one-third of the cases, it was less than 6 mm. Lesions of the subscapularis tendon and dislocation of the

long head of the biceps tendon were related to a diminished coracohumeral distance. The coracohumeral space became narrower with increasing severity of the subscapularis lesion. The coracohumeral distance averaged 10.6 mm for superior one-third lesions, 7.6 mm for superior two-thirds lesions, and 6.8 mm for complete lesions of the subscapularis. Dislocation of the biceps, especially if intra-articular, is coupled with a reduction of the coracohumeral distance. In some cases, anterior subluxation of the humeral head will lead to glenohumeral static subluxation and coracohumeral contact (coracohumeral impingement; Fig. 6-13).

The degree of fatty infiltration and degeneration of the rotator cuff musculature are major prognosticators of treatment results for rotator cuff tears. Goutallier et al.[8] first recognized this phenomenon using CT of the rotator cuff muscle bellies. Fatty degeneration is classified for each of the rotator cuff muscles: stage 0, characterized by normal muscle and absence of fat; stage 1, characterized by minimal fatty infiltration; stage 2, characterized by less fat than muscle; stage 3, characterized by as much fat as muscle; and stage 4, characterized by more fat than muscle. This classification scheme is depicted in Figure 6-14. It should be emphasized that muscle degeneration assessment is a qualitative analysis of the muscle and does not reflect muscle atrophy.

Although most of our experience with anterior superior rotator cuff imaging lies with computed tomographic arthrography, the modality of choice for evaluating the rotator cuff globally is MRI. Magnetic resonance imaging is highly sensitive and specific in the detection of lesions of the superior and posterior rotator cuff. Complete lesions of the subscapularis are readily identifiable with MRI. Magnetic resonance imaging becomes limited, however, when evaluating incomplete lesions of the superior subscapularis tendon.[16] Additionally, lack of uniformity

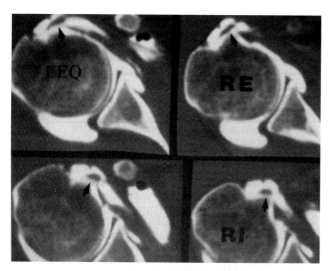

Figure 6-12 Computed tomographic arthrogram demonstrating medial subluxation of the long head of the biceps tendon (*arrows*). Subluxation does not change with external rotation (*top row of images*) or internal rotation (*bottom row of images*).

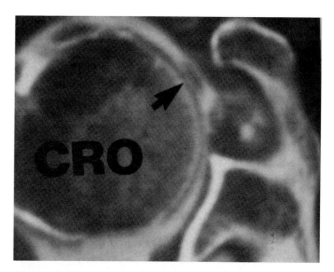

Figure 6-13 Computed tomographic arthrogram demonstrating static anterior humeral head subluxation with resultant coracohumeral impingement. Intra-articular dislocation of the long head of the biceps tendon (*arrow*) also exists.

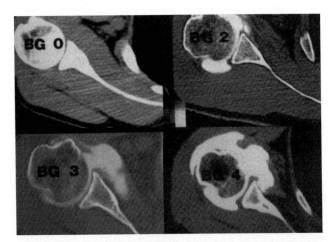

Figure 6-14   Bernageau and Goutallier's staging of fatty degeneration of the subscapularis musculature using computed tomography. Stage 0 (BG 0) is characterized by normal muscle and absence of fat. Stage 1 (not shown here) is characterized by minimal fatty infiltration. Stage 2 (BG 2) is characterized by less fat (dark areas) than muscle. Stage 3 (BG 3) is characterized by as much fat as muscle. Stage 4 (BG 4) is characterized by more fat than muscle.

between different MRI scanners and in the specific protocols employed at different centers makes interpreting anterior rotator cuff and biceps tendon lesions increasingly difficult. For these reasons, if we are clinically suspicious of a lesion involving the anterior rotator cuff, we utilize magnetic resonance arthrography with gadolinium to identify these lesions, using similar criteria to that employed in computed tomographic arthrography (Fig. 6-15).[14]

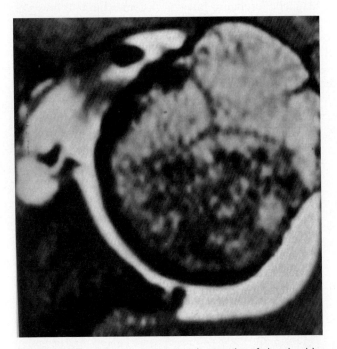

Figure 6-15   Magnetic imaging arthrography of the shoulder demonstrating a tear of the subscapularis tendon and dislocation of the biceps tendon.

Magnetic resonance imaging can also be used to grade fatty degeneration of the rotator cuff musculature. It should be noted, however, that grading of the rotator cuff musculature using magnetic resonance imaging has not correlated to its grading using computed tomography.[3] Additionally, less is known of the prognostic significance of fatty degeneration graded with magnetic resonance imaging compared with computed tomography.

TREATMENT

Treatment of anterior superior rotator cuff lesions can be divided into nonoperative, repair, debridement, and tendon transfer. Additionally, treatment of associated lesions of the long head of the biceps tendon and the rotator interval must be considered. Understanding of proper indications for each of these techniques is critical in optimizing postoperative results.

Indications for Nonoperative Treatment

Nonoperative regimens as the definitive form of treatment are largely reserved for the elderly, debilitated patients in whom an operative procedure is contraindicated secondary to medical problems. Nonoperative treatment consists of nonsteroidal anti-inflammatory agents, activity modification, and, if necessary, periodic corticosteroid injections. Additionally, physical therapy emphasizing the retraining of accessory muscles around the shoulder (latissimus dorsi, teres major) can be employed. Patients who are pain-free with nearly normal shoulder mobility require no treatment.

Indications for Repair

The indications for repairing anterior superior rotator cuff tears are based on multiple criteria. Patient history and clinical examination, specifically the function of the injured shoulder, play a crucial role. Imaging studies obtained prior to operative intervention also play a critical role in selecting the appropriate patient for operative repair.

Patient history, including the patient's age, motivation, activity level, and expectations after surgery, must be evaluated prior to undertaking operative repair. Repair is generally recommended in young active patients with a tear of traumatic etiology. Older patients with a functional affected extremity, who complain only of pain, may be more effectively treated by an arthroscopic debridement. Additionally, a patient must be sufficiently motivated and be willing to participate in 6 months of rehabilitation and convalescence before undergoing repair.

The physical exam will divulge information regarding concomitant involvement of the posterior rotator cuff tendons. Concomitant massive tears of the superior and posterior rotator cuff may contraindicate repair. Additionally, if stiffness is detected on clinical examination, a course of physiotherapy to regain passive mobility should be undertaken before repair is performed.

Secondary imaging studies are important in patient selection for operative treatment. The size of the tear can be evaluated. Significant fatty degeneration of the subscapularis musculature represents a relative contraindication to repair.[8] Last, static anterior subluxation of the humeral head is a poor prognostic indicator and a relative contraindication to repair.

In summary, the ideal candidates for repairing anterior superior rotator cuff tears are physiologically young, motivated patients with a traumatic tear, without clinical or radiographic signs of muscular damage, who are willing to undergo surgical intervention followed by 6 months of rehabilitation. Contraindications to repair are patients unwilling to undergo the procedure and associated rehabilitation, and patients with evidence of fatty degenerated rotator cuff musculature, an associated massive posterior rotator cuff tear, and/or static anterior subluxation of the humeral head. Both arthroscopic and open repair techniques have been described. Although arthroscopic repair of anterior superior rotator cuff tears is technically possible, we believe that arthroscopy gives inadequate visualization of partial tears involving the superior portion of the subscapularis tendon. In these "hidden" lesions of the subscapularis, the overlying bicipital pulley may not be disrupted, making arthroscopic diagnosis difficult; hence, we rarely address repair of subscapularis lesions arthroscopically.

Indications for Arthroscopic Debridement

Certain patients are recognized as poor candidates for anterior superior rotator cuff tear repair. Patients with irreparable tears, patients with severe fatty degeneration of the subscapularis, and patients unwilling to participate in the required rehabilitation and convalescence required following a rotator cuff repair might be better served by arthroscopic debridement. These patients are typically older, lower demand patients who are primarily seeking pain relief from surgical treatment. Patients are not considered candidates for arthroscopic debridement until they have failed an appropriate course (at least 6 months) of nonoperative treatment (previously outlined).

Indications for Tendon Transfer

Certain younger, higher demand patients may present with an irreparable tear of the anterior superior rotator cuff or with a tear combined with severe fatty degeneration of the subscapularis musculature. Pectoralis major tendon transfer is considered in the treatment of this difficult problem and has been described by multiple authors using varia-

tions in technique.[5,15,17,22] Both subcoracoid transfers and transfers passing anterior to the conjoined tendon of the short head of the biceps brachii and the coracobrachialis have been described with acceptable results.

Another group of patients in which pectoralis major transfer has been employed, with some, success is with anterior superior subluxation secondary to a massive anterior superior rotator cuff coupled with an incompetent coracoacromial arch. While difficult to perform, some modest gains in function have been reported following subcoracoid pectoralis major transfer in these patients.[5] Personally, we prefer to employ a reverse-design prosthesis in this challenging patient subset, provided deltoid function is acceptable. The reverse-design prosthesis is a semiconstrained prosthesis with a metal back glenosphere component fixed to the existing glenoid bone via screws and a cup-shaped humeral component (Delta III, Depuy, France). This device allows the humerus to be recentered under the acromion and restores a more nearly normal length tension relationship to the deltoid, allowing the deltoid a mechanically advantageous moment arm to elevate the arm (Fig. 6-16). Use of this prosthesis for this indication has resulted in excellent pain relief and good overhead function.

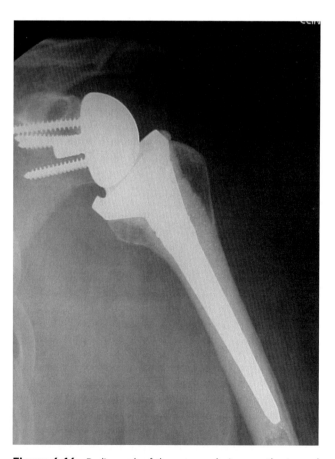

Figure 6-16 Radiograph of the reverse design prosthesis used in the treatment of a massive rotator cuff tear with anterior superior subluxation of the humeral head.

Indications for Treatment of the Long Head of the Biceps Tendon

Of the anatomic structures of the anterior superior rotator cuff, the long head of the biceps tendon is perhaps the most controversial. Few studies of the function of anatomic structures has resulted in more conflicting data than those of the long biceps tendon. Whether the long head of the biceps is an important contributor to glenohumeral stability or simply a vestigial structure with no important function continues to be debated. Although observational studies and vector diagrams have shown the biceps to be a flexor of the glenohumeral joint, depressor of the humeral head, and secondary stabilizer of the shoulder,[9,12] results of electromyographic studies have suggested that these roles are minor or nonexistent.[4,23]

Based on a large clinical experience, we doubt the role of the biceps as an important depressor of the humeral head. We have frequently observed patients with superior humeral head migration and an intact, nondislocated, nonsubluxated biceps tendon, indicating that any action the biceps tendon has as a humeral head depressor is not effective. Additionally, we have treated many older patients with rotator cuff tears with debridement of the tear and biceps tenodesis or tenotomy and have not observed any postoperative increase in superior migration of the humeral head during the first 4 postoperative years.[19] Furthermore, although patients with massive rotator cuff tears have been found to have a larger biceps tendon, we believe this to be secondary to inflammation and fibrosis and do not use induced hypertrophy. Finally, if the biceps tendon plays a role in glenohumeral stability, as suggested by some authors, it is unapparent clinically.[9] We, like most investigators, have witnessed shoulder instability in patients with an avulsion of the anterior portion of the inferior glenohumeral ligament (i.e., Bankart lesion) and a normal biceps tendon, leading us to doubt the biceps tendon's clinical importance as a secondary shoulder stabilizer.

Because the biceps is grossly abnormal in 75% of our patients with subscapularis lesions and the aforementioned explanation of the long head of the biceps tendon's lack of clinically significant function, we choose to systematically concomitantly address the biceps tendon during surgical treatment of tears of the anterior superior rotator cuff. In our experience, tenotomy and tenodesis have been equivalent in terms of pain relief. Tenotomy carries the risk of a cosmetic deformity, although in our experience, this occurs in less than 30% of the older patient population.

We perform biceps tenotomy in patients with anterior superior rotator cuff lesions undergoing arthroscopic debridement. Patients are educated preoperatively regarding the potential postoperative cosmetic deformity. Rarely do we encountered a patient in which the potential for poor postoperative cosmesis is unacceptable. In these patients, we perform an arthroscopic biceps tenodesis. We perform open biceps tenodesis concomitantly in all patients with an intact biceps undergoing an open procedure addressing an anterior superior rotator cuff lesion.

THE AUTHORS' PREFERRED SURGICAL TECHNIQUE

Open Repair

One of two open surgical approaches can be used when addressing tears of the anterior superior rotator cuff: deltopectoral or anterior deltoid-splitting. Classically, the deltopectoral approach is used in the repair of subscapularis tears, providing the best visualization of the entire subscapularis tendon. This is our approach of choice when repairing isolated, complete, or retracted tears of the subscapularis. For tears relegated to the superior subscapularis tendon or in the event that an associated supraspinatus lesion exists, we prefer use of an anterior deltoid splitting approach. Both approaches are performed with the patient in the modified beach-chair position.

For the anterior deltoid-splitting approach, a 7-cm skin incision is made starting just posterior to the acromioclavicular joint extending anteriorly parallel to Langer's lines (Fig. 6-17). The anterior deltoid is split in line with its fibers, and a small flap of the deltoid origin is elevated from the anterior acromion starting just lateral to the acromioclavicular joint, which is not violated. A self-retaining retractor is placed to retract the medial and lateral

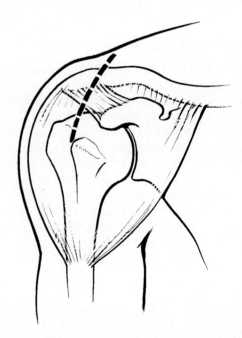

Figure 6-17 Preferred skin incision for the anterior deltoid splitting approach to the rotator cuff. (Adapted with permission from Edwards TB, Walch G. Repair of tears of the subscapularis tendon. Oper Tech Sports Med 2002;10:86.)

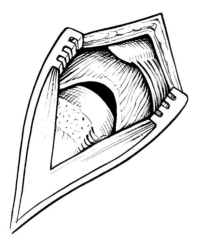

Figure 6-18 Completed exposure of the rotator cuff through an anterior deltoid splitting approach. (Adapted with permission from Edwards TB, Walch G. Repair of tears of the subscapularis tendon. Oper Tech Sports Med 2002;10:86.)

deltoid. A small anterior acromioplasty is performed with an osteotome, enhancing exposure of the subacromial bursa. The subacromial bursa is excised using an electrocautery revealing the underlying rotator cuff and completing the surgical exposure (Fig. 6-18).

When using the anterior deltoid-splitting approach, manual traction is placed on the arm, revealing the rotator interval with the overlying coracohumeral ligament. The rotator interval is opened longitudinally from the glenoid, extending laterally to the bicipital groove. The bicipital groove is opened on its medial aspect to avoid the laterally based vasculature. At this time, the biceps tendon, bicipital pulley, anterior supraspinatus tendon, and superior part of the subscapularis can be inspected. Inspection of the biceps and bicipital pulley is through direct visualization, observing for biceps subluxation or dislocation and tearing or distension of the ligamentous pulley. A biceps tenodesis is systematically performed in all patients with an anterior superior rotator cuff tear, using the technique described later. Inspection of the subscapularis tendon requires palpation of the tendon's lesser tuberosity attachment, using the closed tips of blunt scissors (Fig. 6-19). No "bare bone" should be palpable between the articular surface of the humeral head and the lesser tuberosity; if a bare area exists, this is diagnostic of a subscapularis lesion.

With either the anterior or the deltopectoral approach, the superior margin of the subscapularis tendon must be identified. When using the anterior deltoid-splitting approach, this identification is aided by pushing the humeral head in a posterior direction, using direct force with an instrument, such as a bone tamp, and looking for the tendon from inside the glenohumeral joint. Once the tendon is visualized, a traction suture is placed in the tendon to aid in later reinsertion (Fig. 6-20). In complete tears, a second traction suture is placed inferior to the first.

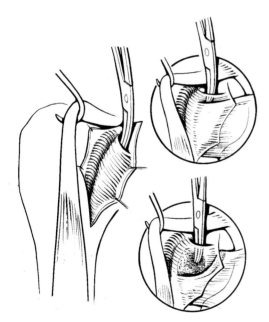

Figure 6-19 Palpation of the superior attachment of the subscapularis tendon on the lesser tuberosity. The presence of bare bone on the lesser tuberosity is diagnostic of a lesion of the subscapularis. (Adapted with permission from Edwards TB, Walch G. Repair of tears of the subscapularis tendon. Oper Tech Sports Med 2002;10:86.)

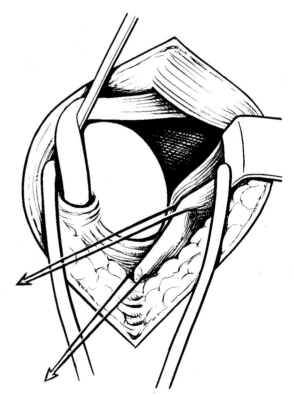

Figure 6-20 Traction sutures placed in the superior subscapularis tendon. (Adapted with permission from Edwards TB, Walch G. Repair of tears of the subscapularis tendon. Oper Tech Sports Med 2002;10:86.)

Lesions of the supraspinatus are generally more readily apparent than those of the subscapularis. Full-thickness lesions are obvious upon excision of the subacromial bursa, as are bursal-sided partial-thickness lesions. Articular-sided partial-thickness lesions can be palpated using the blunt tips of scissors through the opening in the rotator interval. Partial-thickness tears of the supraspinatus tendon, judged to be greater than 50% of the tendon thickness, are disinserted, the tendon edge debrided, and reinserted. Partial-thickness tears of the supraspinatus tendon, judged to be less than 50% of the tendon thickness, are superficially debrided.

In addressing the subscapularis tendon, traction is applied to the previously placed sutures to test the mobility of the subscapularis tendon. In the event that the tendon is retracted and not sufficiently mobile to permit reinsertion, a systematic release of the glenohumeral ligaments and overlying subscapularis bursa is performed to attain the required tendon mobilization. The superior aspect of the tendon is freed from surrounding structures (coracohumeral ligament and superior glenohumeral ligament) by passing scissors along the superior aspect of the tendon to the level of the glenoid. The middle glenohumeral ligament can then be released again, using the scissors. If the tendon is still not sufficiently mobile, the inferior glenohumeral ligament can be divided along with any adhesions within the subscapularis bursa. In these retracted tears, when glenohumeral ligament release is anticipated, a deltopectoral approach is generally utilized, allowing axillary nerve identification and safe inferior glenohumeral ligament (IGHL) release in a plane deep to the subscapularis musculature protecting the nerve (Fig. 6-21). The release of the glenohumeral ligaments carries the theoretical risk of postoperative instability, although we have not seen this occur. Because of the relatively thin nature of the subscapularis tendon, we avoid z-plasty lengthening.

After the subscapularis tendon is sufficiently mobilized, the bare bone area on the lesser tuberosity is prepared for

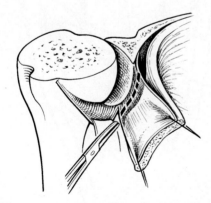

Figure 6-21 Release of the inferior glenohumeral ligament to improve tendon excursion during repair of a retracted subscapularis tear. (Adapted with permission from Edwards TB, Walch G. Repair of tears of the subscapularis tendon. Oper Tech Sports Med 2002;10:86.)

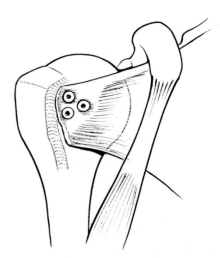

Figure 6-22 Completed repair of the subscapularis tendon using metallic staples. (Adapted with permission from Edwards TB, Walch G. Repair of tears of the subscapularis tendon. Oper Tech Sports Med 2002;10:86.)

tendon reinsertion by removing remaining soft tissue and roughening the surface with a curette. In the past, we have used transosseous sutures for tendon reinsertion; however, we began using metallic capsulorrhaphy staples because of the optimized contact area provided by this device. After witnessing migration of a few of these staples late in the postoperative period after tendon healing, one author now employs suture anchors loaded with two No. 2 polyester sutures to avoid this complication.

After preparing the lesser tuberosity, the previously placed traction sutures are used to reapproximate the subscapularis tendon to the lesser tuberosity. One or more metallic staples are used to reattach the tendon with excellent contact area (Fig. 6-22). Alternatively, one or more suture anchors are placed in the lesser tuberosity. Suture anchors equipped with two sutures provide better surface apposition of the tendon to the lesser tuberosity than anchors equipped with a single suture. The number of staples or suture anchors used depends on the size of the tear, with three or four of each being used for complete detachments. When placing multiple staples or suture anchors, the inferior ones should be placed first, facilitating placement of those located more superiorly.

We perform supraspinatus repair using the double-U technique, described previously.[18] Traction sutures are placed in the torn edge of the supraspinatus tendon. Any tendon appearing unhealthy at the torn edge is debrided sharply. A bone trough is created utilizing an osteotome to score the cortex just lateral to the articular surface in a rectangle shape. A bone tamp is then used to impact the cortical rectangle into the cancellous bone, creating the bony trough.

A No. 2 braided nonabsorbable suture on a large needle is passed transosseously through the lateral cortex of the humerus 1.5 to 2.0 cm distal to the superior aspect of the

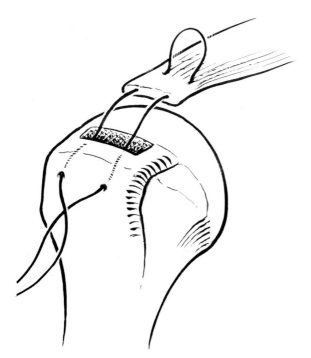

Figure 6-23 Technique for completion of the first "U" suture, providing the first point of fixation in repair of the supraspinatus tendon. (Adapted with permission from Walch G, Edwards TB, Nové-Josserand L, et al. Double U suturing technique for repair of the rotator cuff. Tech Shoulder Elbow Surg 2002;3:136.)

greater tuberosity and into the bony trough. This suture is then placed through the cuff tendon (from inferior to superior), 0.5 cm medial to the free edge. For laminar tendon dissection, the suture is placed through both layers of the tendon. The suture is then passed back through the tendon, back through the trough, and out the lateral cortex, leaving a 1-cm bony bridge (Fig. 6-23).

Next, the same stitch is performed again, but is based on the tendon side. The suture is then passed through the cuff tendon from superior to inferior, approximately 1.0 cm medial to the previously placed suture. The suture is then placed through the bony trough, exiting the lateral cortex 0.5 cm superior to the initial suture. The suture is reintroduced into the humerus, once again leaving a 1-cm bone bridge and then backed out through the trough. Lastly, the suture is placed back through the cuff tendon in an inferior-to-superior direction (Fig. 6-24). In large tears, this process can be repeated in the adjacent tissue before tying any sutures.

With the arm in abduction, the cuff tendons are advanced into the bone trough by pulling the initially placed sutures, which exit from the lateral cortex; the traction stitches can be removed prior to this step. The sutures exiting the lateral cortex are then secured with a square knot and three simple throws that alternate directions. This provides the first point of fixation. The residual suture is *not* cut. The same type of knot is then used to secure the sutures exiting the superior aspect of the cuff tendons, providing the second

point of fixation. Once again, the residual suture is *not* removed. To provide the third point of fixation, the sutures exiting the cuff tendons are tied to the sutures exiting the lateral aspect of the humerus (Fig. 6-25). The residual suture material is then discarded, completing the repair.

A No. 1 braided nonabsorbable suture is then used to close the rotator interval. The stability of the repair and the range of motion is then tested and recorded for later use in postoperative rehabilitation.

Meticulous repair of the deltoid to the acromion utilizing transosseous sutures is imperative if an anterior deltoid-splitting approach has been used. A transosseous suspensory U stitch using a No. 5 nonabsorbable braided suture is utilized. This suture is placed through the deltoid at the aponeurosis from lateral to medial, through the acromion from superior to inferior, back through the acromion from inferior to superior, and finally back through the deltoid from medial to lateral (Fig. 6-26A). The repair is then further secured with additional No. 2 absorbable braided sutures using a simple, interrupted technique (Fig. 6-26B). The wound is closed in layers. The patient is placed in a simple sling (isolated subscapularis repair) or 30-degree abduction sling (subscapularis and supraspinatus repair).

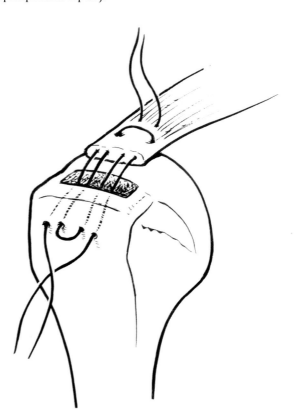

Figure 6-24 Technique for completion of the second "U" suture, providing the second point of fixation in repair of the supraspinatus tendon. (Adapted with permission from Walch G, Edwards TB, Nové-Josserand L, et al. Double U suturing technique for repair of the rotator cuff. Tech Shoulder Elbow Surg 2002;3:136.)

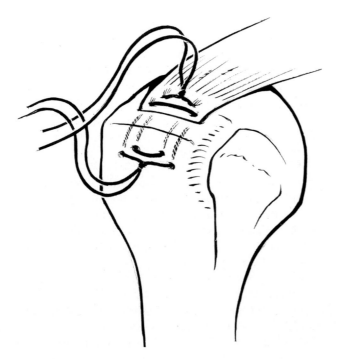

Figure 6-25 The free suture ends (*shown*) are then tied together, providing the third point of fixation in repair of the supraspinatus tendon. (Adapted with permission from Walch G, Edwards TB, Nové-Josserand L, et al. Double U suturing technique for repair of the rotator cuff. Tech Shoulder Elbow Surg 2002;3:136.)

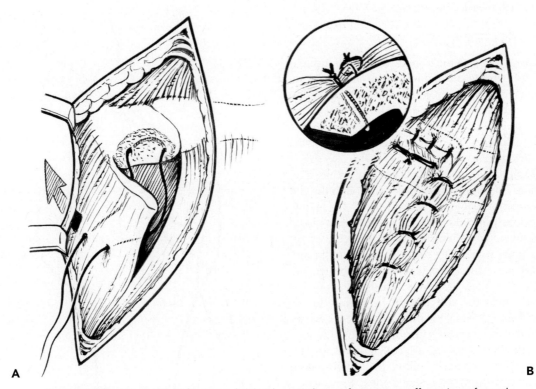

A

B

Figure 6-26 (*A*) and (*B*) Technique of deltoid reattachment for rotator cuff repair performed through an anterior deltoid splitting approach. A No. 2 nonabsorbable braided suture is placed through the deltoid at the aponeurosis from lateral to medial, through the acromion from superior to inferior, back through the acromion from inferior to superior, and finally back through the deltoid from medial to lateral. The repair is then further secured with additional intermuscular sutures using a simple, interrupted technique. (Adapted with permission from Walch G, Edwards TB, Nové-Josserand L, et al. Double U suturing technique for repair of the rotator cuff. Tech Shoulder Elbow Surg 2002;3:136.)

Arthroscopic Treatment

We prefer to perform arthroscopy in the modified beach-chair position utilizing a specialized operating table designed for easy access to the posterior shoulder via a removable panel. Routine glenohumeral diagnostic arthroscopy is performed through a standard posterior arthroscopic portal. Be aware of the anterior superior rotator cuff and the biceps tendon and its stabilizing pulley system. The tendon of the subscapularis is readily visualized anteriorly. It should be noted, however, that, with an intact or merely distended bicipital pulley, tears limited to the superior third of the subscapularis cannot be visualized without sectioning the medial aspect of the pulley.

In the majority of cases, lesions of the bicipital pulley predominately involve the medial aspect. We employ Bennet's techniques, during diagnostic arthroscopy, for visualizing the long head of the biceps tendon and the bicipital pulley system.[1] Flexing the arm to approximately 60 degrees facilitates visualizing the ligamentous pulley and bicipital groove when looking through the posterior arthroscopic portal. A standard 30-degree arthroscope can be positioned anterior within the glenohumeral joint and used to "look around the corner" of the humeral head to evaluate any lesions of the biceps tendon, ligamentous pulley, and subscapularis insertion (Fig. 6-27). Variable amounts of internal rotation and/or use of a 70-degree arthroscope may further facilitate visualization of these structures.

Tears of the subscapularis and supraspinatus tendons are debrided using an arthroscopic shaver placed through an anterior or lateral portal, but only if a full-thickness supraspinatus tear exists. Biceps tenotomy is performed through either an anterior or lateral portal. The biceps tendon is released from its insertion on the superior glenoid labrum using arthroscopic biting forceps, an arthroscopic electrocautery, or an arthroscopic soft-tissue ablator. The arm and elbow are then forcibly extended ensuring retraction of the biceps tendon out of the glenohumeral joint. The entrance to the bicipital groove is visualized arthroscopically after tenotomy confirming tendon retraction. Alternatively, arthroscopic biceps tenodesis can be performed. For details of this technique, refer to the work of Boileau et al.[2]

In an effort to preserve the integrity of the coracoacromial arch, we do not perform an acromioplasty or release of the coracoacromial ligament during arthroscopic debridement. Disruption of the coracoacromial arch can potentially lead to the complication of anterior superior instability.

Pectoralis Major Tendon Transfer

We prefer to perform a subcoracoid pectoralis major transfer based on the technique originally described by Resch et al.[15] The subcoracoid technique probably more closely emulates the force vector produced by an intact subscapularis than the transfer anterior to the conjoined tendon, hence our preference. The patient is placed in the modified beach-chair position, and a standard deltopectoral approach is performed retracting the cephalic vein laterally. The conjoined tendon of the short head of the biceps brachii and the coracobrachialis is identified and retracted medially. The shoulder is externally rotated with the arm at the side exposing the lesser tuberosity. Often the lesser tuberosity is encapsulated by scar tissue, so the subscapularis deficiency may not be obvious until this scar tissue is excised and the bony surface of the lesser tuberosity exposed. A biceps tenodesis is then performed systematically if the long head of the biceps tendon is intact.

For the pectoralis major insertion, we prefer to utilize the entire pectoralis major tendon for the transfer, a procedural modification introduced by Galatz et al.[5] Using a scalpel, the pectoralis major tendon is detached from its insertion on the humerus (Fig. 6-28). Traction sutures of No. 2 braided polyester are placed in the tendon to facilitate later subcoracoid passage. Blunt dissection is then carried out to mobilize the pectoralis tendon medially. The pectoralis major tendon is wrapped in a normal saline soaked sponge to keep it moist.

The musculocutaneous nerve is identified next (Fig. 6-29). Retracting the conjoined tendon laterally, the musculocutaneous nerve is carefully dissected free medial to the coracoid process. The nerve must be visualized to ensure it is protected during the passage of the pectoralis major tendon. The nerve may be as close as 3 cm from the tip of the coracoid process. After the nerve is identified and its protection ensured, dissection can be performed deep to the conjoined tendon to create a passage for the transfer.

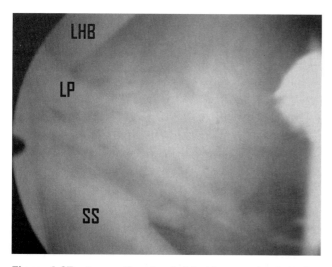

Figure 6-27 A normal long head of the biceps tendon (LHB), ligamentous pulley (LP), and subscapularis tendon (SS) visualized arthroscopically from the posterior portal while "looking around the corner." Note the inability to visualize the superior insertion of the subscapularis tendon as it is obscured from view by the intact ligamentous pulley.

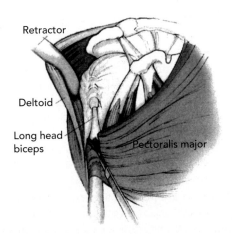

Figure 6-28 The pectoralis major tendon is incised at its insertion. (Adapted with permission from Klepps S, Galatz L, Yamaguchi K. Subcoracoid pectoralis major transfer: a salvage procedure for irreparable subscapularis deficiency. Tech Shoulder Elbow Surg 2001;2:85.)

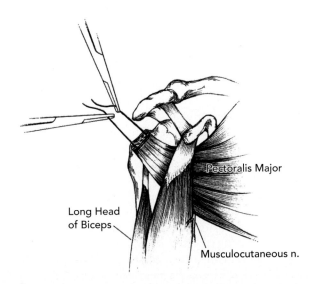

Figure 6-30 After subcoracoid passage of the pectoralis major tendon, the point of attachment for the transfer is selected by observing the amount of passive external rotation possible with the arm at the side of the contralateral upper extremity (assuming the contralateral upper extremity is unaffected) and attempting to fix the transfer so that an identical amount of passive external rotation is permitted on the surgical side. (Adapted with permission from Klepps S, Galatz L, Yamaguchi K. Subcoracoid pectoralis major transfer: a salvage procedure for irreparable subscapularis deficiency. Tech Shoulder Elbow Surg 2001;2:85.)

The size of the subcoracoid passage relative to the pectoralis major is determined by attempting to pass the pectoralis major anterior to the musculocutaneous nerve and deep to the conjoined tendon. If the pectoralis major is too large and places an unacceptable amount of traction on the nerve, we first debulk the muscle of the pectoralis major. If this fails to relieve the tension on the nerve, the first branch of the nerve can be released without any ill effects.[5] Other authors prefer transferring only a portion of the pectoralis major tendon to avoid this problem.[15] In our experience, debulking the pectoralis major and occasionally releasing the first branch of the musculocutaneous nerve has been adequate in dealing with this potential situation.

Once the pectoralis major tendon has successfully been passed beneath the coracoid, securing the tendon to the proximal humerus is next (Fig. 6-30). Both the lesser tuberosity and the greater tuberosity have been proposed as points of attachment.[5,15] We choose the point of attachment by attempting to establish what the "normal" length tension relationship is for each individual patient. This is done by observing the amount of passive external rotation possible with the arm at the side of the contralateral upper extremity (assuming the contralateral upper extremity is unaffected). We then attempt to fix the transfer so that an identical amount of passive external rotation is permitted on the surgical side. Most often, this places the site of attachment on the greater tuberosity; however, in some cases, the lesser tuberosity is preferable, particularly in a patient with a short pectoralis major tendon. The bony surface of the selected point of attachment is then prepared to receive the transfer. We use suture anchors in our fixation method, using the same technique we employ for subscapularis repair, previously described in this chapter. The wound is then closed in layers over a drain, and the patient is placed in a simple sling.

Biceps Tenodesis

We systematically perform a biceps tenodesis when repairing the anterior superior rotator cuff and when transferring the pectoralis major. The bicipital groove is opened using electrocautery on the medial side to avoid the laterally based vasculature. A traction suture is placed in the biceps

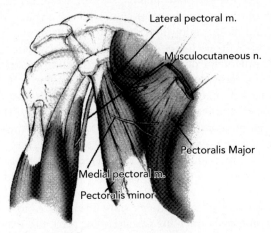

Figure 6-29 Identification of the musculocutaneous nerve during pectoralis major transfer. (Adapted with permission from Klepps S, Galatz L, Yamaguchi K. Subcoracoid pectoralis major transfer: a salvage procedure for irreparable subscapularis deficiency. Tech Shoulder Elbow Surg 2001;2:85.)

tendon just proximal to where it enters the bicipital groove. The proximal attachment of the biceps tendon is visualized and released using scissors. The intra-articular portion of the biceps tendon proximal to the previously placed traction suture is excised. The biceps is retracted distally exposing the bicipital groove. A 6-mm diameter unicortical hole is created in the floor of the groove approximately 1 cm distal to the proximal aspect of the bicipital groove. A curette can be used to enlarge the cortical portion of the hole, if necessary, as is common in the case of an enlarged biceps. The transected end of the biceps tendon is grasped with a small curved hemostat, and, with the shoulder and the elbow flexed, the tendon is placed into the hole. A 9-mm diameter by 25-mm length bioabsorbable interference screw is advanced into the hole until it is flush with the humeral cortex. The traction suture is cut flush with the humerus, completing the tenodesis.

POSTOPERATIVE CARE

We employ essentially the same postoperative regimen for our patients who undergo repair or pectoralis major transfer for tears of the anterior superior rotator cuff. Passive mobility, with the aid of a physical therapist, is initiated on postoperative day 1. Passive external rotation is limited based on intraoperative range of motion and security of the repair. On postoperative day 3, hydrotherapy is initiated after covering the surgical wound with an impermeable dressing. Hydrotherapy consists of submerging the patient in a 34°C pool and commencing passive range of motion exercises like those used by Neer.[13] Hydrotherapy sessions are done daily. Land-based rehabilitation is used as an adjunct to reaffirm mobility gains achieved in the pool. Once the exercises are learned, the patient can largely perform these exercises daily without a physical therapist. After 3 weeks, provided good mobility has been obtained, hydrotherapy sessions are decreased to twice weekly. Rehabilitation consists solely of passive mobilization; no strengthening exercises are performed. A sling is maintained, except when performing therapy exercises for 4 weeks. Active mobility with no resistance is allowed 6 weeks postoperatively. Complete use of the extremity for activities of daily living is allowed at 3 months. Full activity is allowed at 6 months. For more details of this protocol, the reader is referred to the work of Liotard.[11]

In patients undergoing arthroscopic debridement with biceps tenotomy, we also employ a hydrotherapy protocol. In these patients, however, full active mobility is allowed immediately following surgery. The sling is discontinued as soon as the patient is comfortable. As soon as full active and passive mobility are obtained, usually within 2 weeks of surgery, physical therapy can be discontinued. For 3 months following surgery, to minimize the likelihood of cosmetic deformity, we ask these patients to avoid activities that could potentially lead to an eccentric contraction of the biceps.

RESULTS OF SURGICAL TREATMENT

Our results of open repair and arthroscopic debridement for treating anterior superior rotator cuff tears are detailed in the following. Our experience using the pectoralis major transfer is still in progress, thus, we lack the ability to report our long-term results. We, therefore, have elected to provide the reader with a summary of the results for pectoralis major transfer obtained from the available literature.

Open Repair

Our results of open repair in treating anterior superior rotator cuff tears with a minimum 2-year follow-up are depicted in Table 6-1. In this series, the most statistically important prognostic factor was whether or not biceps tenodesis or tenotomy was performed at the time of repair. Tenodesis or tenotomy of the biceps tendon at the time of subscapularis repair was associated with improved subjective and objective results independent of the preoperative condition of the biceps tendon.

Arthroscopic Treatment

Our results of arthroscopic debridement with biceps tenotomy (unless the biceps was already ruptured) in treating anterior superior rotator cuff tears with a minimum 2-year follow-up are depicted in Table 6-2. These patients were selected for arthroscopic treatment based on criteria outlined in the "Indications for Arthroscopic Treatment" section. Pain was the factor most reliably improved with arthroscopic treatment.

Pectoralis Major Tendon Transfer

To our knowledge, four series reporting the results of pectoralis major tendon transfer exist in the literature. Wirth and Rockwood[13] first reported the use of pectoralis major and/or pectoralis minor transfer in the treatment of irreparable subscapularis tears at a minimum 2-year follow-up. Their series of 13 transfers yielded satisfactory results in 10 patients. In all cases, the pectoralis major and/or the pectoralis minor were transferred anterior to the conjoined tendon and attached to the greater tuberosity. They did not stratify their results by type of transfer (pectoralis major versus pectoralis minor versus both).

Resch et al.[11] were the first to report the results of subcoracoid pectoralis major transfer to the lesser tuberosity in the treatment of irreparable subscapularis tears. In their group of 12 patients with minimum 2-year follow-up, the

TABLE 6-1
RESULTS OF REPAIR OF TEARS OF THE ANTERIOR SUPERIOR ROTATOR CUFF

	Number of cases	Follow-up (months)	Constant score—preoperative					Constant score—postoperative					Excellent/good subjective results (%)
			Pain (points)	Activity (points)	Mobility (points)	Strength (points)	Total (points)	Pain (points)	Activity (points)	Mobility (points)	Strength (points)	Total (points)	
Subscapularis only	61	45	4.6	9.5	30.6	10.3	55.0	11.8	17.0	35.2	15.5	79.5	89
Subscapularis and supraspinatus	95	37	3.2	8.4	28.0	8.0	47.6	12.0	17.1	34.5	11.0	74.6	93

TABLE 6-2
RESULTS OF ARTHROSCOPIC DEBRIDEMENT WITH BICEPS TENOTOMY FOR TEARS OF THE ANTERIOR SUPERIOR ROTATOR CUFF

	Number of cases	Follow-up (months)	Constant score—preoperative					Constant score—postoperative					Excellent/good subjective results (%)
			Pain (points)	Activity (points)	Mobility (points)	Strength (points)	Total (points)	Pain (points)	Activity (points)	Mobility (points)	Strength (points)	Total (points)	
Subscapularis only	11	34	4.2	7.4	30.8	6.4	48.8	12.6	18.6	38.8	12.8	82.8	82
Subscapularis and supraspinatus	34	57	3.6	7.4	32.9	7.2	51.1	10.6	15.3	35.8	3.9	65.6	79

Constant score improved from a mean 22.6 points preoperatively to 54.4 points postoperatively. They also reported marked improvement in pain from a mean 1.7 points preoperatively to 9.6 points postoperatively. Similarly, Vidil and Augereau,[12] in their group of five patients with a mean 19-month follow-up, reported improvement in the mean Constant score from 27.5 points to 50.0 points following transfer of the pectoralis major to the lesser tuberosity.

Recently, Galatz et al.,[10] in their group of 14 patients with a mean 17.5-month follow-up, reported their results using a subcoracoid pectoralis major transfer for anterior superior subluxation secondary to massive rotator cuff deficiency. They noted marked improvements in pain (visual analog scores improved from a mean 6.9 points preoperatively to 3.2 points postoperatively) and function (the American Shoulder and Elbow Surgeons functional outcome score improved from a mean 27.2 points preoperatively to 47.7 points postoperatively).

COMPLICATIONS

Complications of surgical treatment of the anterior superior rotator cuff are infrequent. As with all surgical procedures, infection is a potential risk minimized by using a meticulous sterile technique and using perioperative intravenous antibiotics. Additional potential complications are outlined by procedure.

Arthroscopic Treatment

Complications following arthroscopic debridement with biceps tenotomy are rare. Although we do not truly consider it a complication, cosmetic deformity occurs in approximately 30% of older patients who have undergone arthroscopic biceps tenotomy. All patients are educated about this potential outcome preoperatively. For patients who want to avoid possible deformity, arthroscopic biceps tenodesis is offered as an alternative procedure. Additionally, to minimize the likelihood of this deformity, we ask patients to avoid eccentric biceps contractions for the first 3 months postoperatively.

Open Repair

Postoperative stiffness is the major risk following open rotator cuff repair. To avoid this complication, only patients without preoperative stiffness are selected for repair. Early, aggressive physical therapy, consisting of passive mobility based on the hydrotherapy protocol previously described, is instituted.

Repair failure is also a concern, as it is with any rotator cuff repair. Although actual repair failure is tough to define without surgical exploration, clinically evident repair failure has been uncommon. In 61 cases of isolated subscapularis tears undergoing repair with a minimum 2-year follow-up, we have only observed two cases of rerupture documented by secondary imaging studies and two cases of suspected rerupture. We have more frequently witnessed late staple migration, causing one of the authors to favor the suture anchor fixation technique.

If repair is employed through an anterior deltoid-splitting approach in which the deltoid attachment is violated, deltoid detachment becomes a potential complication. Meticulous repair of the deltoid to the acromion utilizing transosseous sutures is imperative. Using this technique, illustrated in Figure 6-25, we have only seen two complications in more than 1000 cases involving the deltoid.

Pectoralis Major Tendon Transfer

In addition to the possible complications following open repair of the anterior superior rotator cuff, pectoralis major tendon transfer carries the risk of musculocutaneous nerve palsy. Although this complication is uncommon and usually transient when it occurs, every effort should be made to avoid it. Avoiding any traction on the nerve with the judicious use of muscle debulking and occasional release of the proximal branches of the nerve are critical in avoiding this complication.

REFERENCES

1. Bennett WF. Subscapularis, medial, and lateral head coracohumeral ligament insertion anatomy: arthroscopic appearance and incidence of "hidden" rotator interval lesions. Arthroscopy 2001;17:173.
2. Boileau P, Krishnan S, Coste JS, et al. Arthroscopic biceps tenodesis: a new technique using bioabsorbable interference screw fixation. Arthroscopy 2002;18:1002.
3. Fuchs B, Weishaupt D, Zanetti M, et al. Fatty degeneration of the muscles of the rotator cuff: assessment by computed tomography versus magnetic resonance imaging. J Shoulder Elbow Surg 1999; 8:599.
4. Furlani J. Electromyographic study of the m. biceps brachii in movements at the glenohumeral joint. Acta Anat (Basel) 1976;96:270.
5. Galatz LM, Connor PM, Calfee RP, et al. Pectoralis major transfer for anterior-superior subluxation in massive rotator cuff insufficiency. J Shoulder Elbow Surg 2003;12:1.
6. Gerber C, Krushell RJ. Isolated rupture of the tendon of the subscapularis muscle: clinical features in 16 cases. J Bone Joint Surg 1991;73B:389.
7. Gerber C, Terrier F, Zehnder R, et al. The subcoracoid space: an anatomic study. Clin Orthop 1987;215:132.
8. Goutallier D, Postel JM, Bernageau J, et al. Fatty muscle degeneration in cuff ruptures. Clin Orthop 1994;304:78.
9. Itoi E, Kuechle DK, Newmann SR, et al. Stabilizing function of the biceps tendon in stable and unstable shoulders. J Bone Joint Surg 1993;75B:546.
10. Jobe FW, Jobe C. Painful athletic injuries of the shoulder. Clin Orthop 1983;173:117.
11. Liotard JP. Rehabilitation following shoulder arthroplasty: experience at a rehabilitation center. In: Walch G, Boileau P, eds. Shoulder arthroplasty. Berlin, Springer-Verlag, 1999:383.

12. Lucas DB. Biomechanics of the shoulder joint. Arch Surg 1973;107:425.
13. Neer CS II, McCann PD, McFarlane EA, et al. Earlier passive motion following shoulder arthroplasty and rotator cuff repair: a prospective study. Orthop Trans 1987;11:231.
14. Pfirrmann CW, Zanetti M, Weishaupt D, et al. Subscapularis tendon tears: detection and grading at MR arthrography. Radiology 1999;213:709.
15. Resch H, Povacz P, Ritter E, et al. Transfer of the pectoralis major muscle for the treatment of irreparable rupture of the subscapularis tendon. J Bone Joint Surg 2000;82A:372.
16. Tung GA, Yoo DC, Levine SM, et al. Subscapularis tendon tear: primary and associated signs on MRI. J Comput Assist Tomogr 2001;25:417.
17. Vidil A, Augereau B. Transfer of the clavicular portion of the pectoralis major muscle in the treatment of irreparable tears of the subscapularis muscle. Rev Chir Orthop 2000;86:835.
18. Walch G, Edwards TB, Nové-Josserand L, et al. Double U suturing technique for repair of the rotator cuff. Tech Shoulder Elbow Surg 2002;3:136.
19. Walch G, Madonia G, Puzzi I, et al. Arthroscopic tenotomy of the long head of the biceps in rotator cuff ruptures. In: Gazielly DF, Gleyze P, Thomas T, eds. The cuff. Paris, Elsevier, 1997:350.
20. Walch G, Nové-Josserand L, Boileau P, et al. Subluxations and dislocations of the tendon of the long head of the biceps. J Shoulder Elbow Surg 1998;7:100.
21. Walch G, Nové-Josserand L, Levigne C, et al. Tears of the supraspinatus tendon associated with "hidden" lesions of the rotator interval. J Shoulder Elbow Surg 1994;3:353.
22. Wirth MA, Rockwood CA Jr. Operative treatment of irreparable rupture of the subscapularis. J Bone Joint Surg 1997;79A:722.
23. Yamaguchi K, Riew KD, Galatz LM, et al. Biceps function in normal and rotator cuff deficient shoulder: an electromyographic analysis. Orthop Trans 1994;18:191.

Massive Tears of the Posterosuperior Rotator Cuff

Laurence D. Higgins   *Jon J. P. Warner*

INTRODUCTION

Tears of the posterosuperior rotator cuff account for the majority of surgically treated massive rotator cuff tears. In Neer's series[81] of 340 rotator cuff tears operated over a 13-year period, 145 were classified as massive. Bigliani et al.[10] operated on 61 massive rotator cuff tears in a 6-year period. During a 12-year period, Ellman[31] performed 50 rotator cuff tear repairs (of which 9 [18%] were massive[51]), reviewed 105 cases (of which 28 had a tear involving the supraspinatus and infraspinatus, and an additional 22 involved the subscapularis[52]), reported that, of 100 consecutive cases during a 5-year period, 27 were massive rotator cuff tears,[39] and reported a series of 50 massive rotator cuff tears operated during a 3-year period. Warner surgically treated 53 massive rotator cuff tears among 213 such injuries undergoing surgery during a 5-year period.[120]

Although the prevalence of these tears may seem low, their impact on patient function and pain is profound. The purpose of this chapter is to consider treatment approaches to massive rotator cuff tears involving the supraspinatus, infraspinatus, and teres minor (i.e., posterior rotator cuff tear). The anatomy, biomechanics, and natural history of these types of rotator cuff tears play a critical role in patient

selection for reconstructive and salvage procedures. Special technical approaches, presented in the form of characteristic cases, highlight some of the problems with surgical repair and offer alternative solutions in cases of massive tears and revision situations.

Anatomically, most massive tears involve the posterior portion of the rotator cuff. Antero-superior rotator cuff tears involving the subscapularis with or without the supraspinatus are discussed in another chapter in this book. Although there is no universal agreement on the definition of massive rotator cuff tears, a consensus appears to be developing. In North America, the definition of Cofield[27] is generally employed, with a massive tear being greater than 5 cm in its maximum diameter. In Europe, tears that encompass two or more of the rotator cuff tendons are considered massive.[39,55,60] This definition is more functional than simply measuring the length of the tear. To accurately measure the extent of the rotator cuff tear, the degenerated rim of tissue is debrided. Because arm position may determine the appearance of the tear's diameter, the length is measured in centimeters when the arm is at the side, and the tendons involved are recorded. Some advocate that the size of the tear not only reflects the anterior to posterior distance but represents the mediolateral retraction of the cuff (by creating an index that is the product of the anterior to posterior dimension multiplied by the medial to lateral retraction).[108] This last gauge is unlikely to provide significant data because the tears are rarely rectangular, and the mediolateral distance is subject to arm position, especially rotation. Because there is

L. D. Higgins: Department of Orthopaedic Surgery, Duke University, Durham, North Carolina.
J. J. P. Warner: Department of Orthopaedic Surgery, Harvard Medical School, Boston, Massachusetts.

no consensus for measureing either pre- or postdebridement of the nonviable tendon stump, no standard exists; however, the authors believe that post-debridement measurements are superior and clinically more meaningful. Furthermore, if the humerus is pushed proximally, the dimensions of the mediolateral distance will increase (and similarly decrease with distal traction). Importantly, the dimension of the tear as a percentage of the size of the humeral head may be a more prognostic indicator because there is significant variation in patient size. Additionally, tissue quality is at least as important as tear size in determining the potential for a secure surgical repair. Acute massive tears may be much larger than 5 cm diameter but have robust, elastic tendon tissue that is easily repaired to its anatomical insertion, while chronic, smaller tears may have thin, friable, inelastic tendon tissue that mobilizes poorly and is repaired only tenuously.[39,56]

As in any surgical procedure, the surgeon must be self-critical about patient selection, surgical treatment, and the ultimate functional outcome to measure the benefits of surgery. The standard outcome of these kinds of rotator cuff tears after surgery is good pain relief but some moderate to severe residual weakness and limitation of upper extremity endurance for work and sport activities. Keeping this in mind, it is possible to remain aware of the potential pitfalls in patient selection and treatment. Successful tendon healing is not always directly correlated with a good clinical outcome; however, powerful shoulder function usually requires an intact tendon repair. The use of arthroscopic repair for massive tears has been evolving and few studies[14,18-21,67,72] document the success of this approach. Galatz et al.[36] reported on the outcome and repair integrity of large and massive rotator cuff tears. Ultrasound documented recurrent tears in 17 of 18 patients at a minimum of 1 year postoperatively, and functional results deteriorated over a 2-year period. Gerber et al.[39] documented repair integrity of 75% 2 years after massive rotator cuff tear repaired with open technique. Thus, it seems that structural integrity after arthroscopic repair is not as assured as with open repair. However, newer techniques of arthroscopic repair promise to bring this method on par with open from the standpoint of tendon healing. Regardless of the operative technique, the patient can anticipate improved function and reduced pain if the preoperative, surgical, and postoperative rehabilitation plans are well formulated and executed.

PREOPERATIVE CONSIDERATIONS

Treatment plans must be formulated on an individualized basis, accounting for functional needs, disability, and patient goals. It is critical that the physician consider whether pain or functional difficulties are the major problem. Coexistent medical conditions may argue against aggressive

reconstructive surgery because of the higher risks of morbidity or mortality. For example, an elderly, frail, female patient with cardiac problems or diabetes mellitus can be treated with a less aggressive surgical approach than an otherwise healthy 50-year-old man, even though they have similar rotator cuff injuries (i.e., similar-sized tears). These patients have different functional needs and goals. The former may have a problem with pain and need functional recovery for activities of daily living only, while the latter may require strength for forceful overhead activities or sports. Surgeons must consider their experience and ability to address these tears with an arthroscopic or open technique and whether salvage procedures are indicated.

PATHOANATOMY AND PATHOMECHANICS

The force potential of each of the four rotator cuff muscles has been determined based on the individual physiological cross-sectional areas.[61,66,69,110,113] Each muscle's leverage can be determined based on a perpendicular drawn from its line of action to the center of rotation of the humeral head.[6] If each muscle's force potential is multiplied by the muscle's leverage, its *functional contribution* can be determined. Tables 7-1 and 7-2 show the supraspinatus's relatively small physiological cross-sectional area and rotational potential compared with the other rotator cuff muscles. This is because of its smaller size and closer insertion to the axis of rotation of the joint. Keating et al.[61] demonstrated that the supraspinatus makes a small (14%) contribution to the overall abduction moment arm. In comparison, the infraspinatus and teres minor, together, contribute 32% and the subscapularis contributes 52%. This illustrates the primary importance of the anterior and posterior components in shoulder joint rotation.

Arm position is critical in determining the role of each muscle. The moment arm of the supraspinatus is largest in the first 30 degrees of abduction. Its mechanical advantage is reduced as the shoulder is abducted above this level.

TABLE 7-1

PHYSIOLOGIC CROSS-SECTIONAL AREAS DETERMINED FOR ROTATOR CUFF TEAR MUSCLES

Muscle	Keating et al. (1993)[61]	Bassettt et al. (1990)[6]
Subscapularis	52%	46%
Supraspinatus	15%	16%
Infraspinatus	33%	38%

TABLE 7-2
ROTATIONAL POTENTIAL OF THE ROTATOR CUFF

Muscle	Keating et al. (1993)[61] (arm at side)	Bassett et al. (1990)[6] (arm 90° abd. +90°ER)
Subscapularis	52% (2.3 cm)*	42% (2.8 cm)
Supraspinatus	14% (2.0 cm)	13% (2.1 cm)
Infraspinatus and teres minor	32% (2.2 cm)	45% (3.1 cm)

abd, abducted; ER, external rotation.
*The numbers in parentheses are average movement arms. The rotational potential is equal to the physiologic cross-sectional area (PCSA) times the force divided by the PCSA times the movement arm.

TABLE 7-3
TENDON EXCURSIONS OF THE ROTATOR CUFF AND DELTOID DURING SCAPULAR PLANE ABDUCTION

Tendon	Excursion (cm)
Deltoid	6.5 ± 0.2
Supraspinatus	3.8 ± 0.2
Infraspinatus and teres minor	3.5 ± 0.2
Subscapularis	0.4 ± 0.2

During simple scapular plane abduction, the tendon excursions of the rotator cuff muscles are minimal compared with the deltoid muscle (Table 7-3).[69] They function more as stabilizers than as prime movers, providing a fixed fulcrum for concentric rotation of the humeral head on the glenoid.[58,92] During early abduction, the deltoid creates a relative upward shearing moment that must be resisted by a force couple with the combined rotator cuff muscles. Disruption of the rotator cuff weakens the stabilizing effect that resists this superior translation.[9,65,83,125,126] In vitro[59,64]

and in vivo[122] studies have shown that the long head of the biceps brachii resists anterior and superior translation of the humeral head on the glenoid, and is often enlarged or "hypertrophied" in patients with large rotator cuff tears.[81,83]

Clinical[18–21,97,99] and experimental[110] observations have shown that even large tears of the rotator cuff can remain well compensated with the appearance of good motion and concentric rotation of the glenohumeral joint (Fig. 7-1). Extension of the tear into the infraspinatus and teres minor or into the subscapularis usually results in complete loss of containment and superior translation of the humeral head.[19–21,38,44,110,118,123] Nevertheless, some patients with symptomatic small tears have very poor function, while others with larger tears retain reasonable function (see Fig. 7-1). Tears that extend inferior to the equator

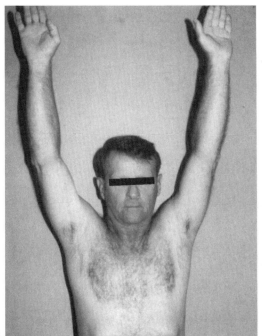
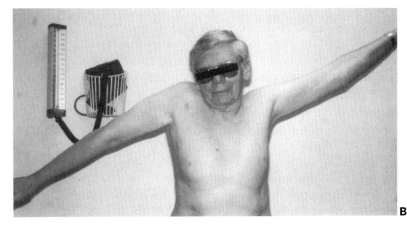

Figure 7-1 (A) A 58-year-old man with bilateral massive rotator cuff tears 1 year after arthroscopic debridement without repair. (B) A 64-year-old man with a chronic right massive rotator cuff tear with pain and poor motion.

result in biomechanical decompensation, with loss of the stabilizing effect of the rotator cuff and, therefore, the fixed fulcrum for rotation of the humeral head on the glenoid.[19,38,44,110] In advanced grades, fatty atrophy plays a significant role and appears to herald the irreparability of the involved tendons and will be discussed later. It should be stressed that atrophy may occur, particularly in the infraspinatus, when the tendon is still intact.[76,80,103,113,129] These findings, and others yet to be elucidated, may help explain the disparity of experience in surgical treatment of massive rotator cuff tears that is found in the literature.[4,7,10,15,18–21,24–26,28,29,31,38,39,42,44,45–47,49,50,68,84–87,91,97,100,106,119,129]

Role of Muscle Atrophy and Fatty Degeneration

The term *massive rotator cuff tear* describes a heterogeneous population of patients with varying degrees of shoulder dysfunction. Goutallier[46] was the first to point out that overall shoulder function and external rotation weakness correlated with the degree of fatty degeneration and muscle atrophy of the infraspinatus muscle, and that such changes were usually chronic and irreversible after surgery[47] Goutallier also recently validated a global fatty degeneration index (GFDI) that predicts the likelihood for recurrent tear after surgery. By using a grading scale from 0 to 4 (in order of severity), the subscapularis, supraspinatus, and infraspinatus are each assigned a score. The mean value for these three muscles determines the GFDI. A GFDI of less than 0.5 was necessary for a retear rate less than 25%, and a GFDI greater than 2 had a 100% retear rate. Of the 220 patients who underwent rotator cuff repair, the highest percentage of recurrent tears were noted in the posterosuperior tears (56% vs. a mean of 36% for all other tears). Although Goutallier has used computed tomography (CT) to assess and grade atrophy, the use of magnetic resonance imaging (MRI) has been similarly investigated.

Warner[124] studied patients with massive rotator cuff tears of similar size and found a correlation between the magnetic resonance imaging (MRI) appearance of atrophy and fatty degeneration and the overall shoulder function and biomechanics (Fig. 7-2). Fuchs et al.[35] compared MRI to CT to assess the validity of MRI as the imaging tool to assign a grade of fatty degeneration according to Goutallier.[46] While interobserver and intraobserver reliability was good for each imaging modality, the correlation between CT and MRI was only fair to moderate. Nevertheless, MRI has replaced CT as the most common imaging modality to assess the rotator cuff.[35,113,120,123]

The amount of muscle atrophy and the acromiohumeral interval are critical preoperative considerations in determining the course of treatment for these patients. If the acromiohumeral interval on a true anteroposterior radio-

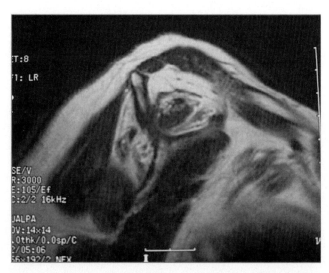

Figure 7-2 Oblique sagittal plane on MRI demonstrates severe fatty degeneration of supraspinatus and infraspinatus muscles.

graph with the arm in neutral rotation is less than 5 mm, and if there is marked muscle atrophy and fatty degeneration on MRI,[88] then surgical repair of the rotator cuff cannot recenter the humeral head in the glenoid, and restoration of strength and function is unlikely. Patients need to be counseled regarding this enhanced risk of tendon retear, if repair is pursued. Furthermore, wanton disregard for this basic tenet of rotator cuff repair and an ill-advised attempt at repair with disruption of the coracoacromial ligament can lead to a disastrous clinical outcome including significant degradation of patients' function and worsening pain. In fact, the occurrence of fixed anterosuperior escape of the humeral head is a difficult and vexing clinical problem, without adequate orthopedic solution.

Surgical relevance of fatty muscle changes have also recently been clarified. Meyer et al.[40,42,74] demonstrated that muscle compliance decreased (the tendon became stiffer and less mobile) in chronic tendon tears, and this precluded direct repair to bone in many cases.[54,75] Warner (unpublished data, 2000) found a correlation between the degree of muscle fatty change on preoperative MRI, and the tendon quality observed intraoperatively. In general, if the fatty muscle change were Goutallier stage 3 or 4, the tendon would be friable and stiff. This was usually associated with inability to repair the tendon to bone.

More recently, Meyer and Gerber[74] described the etiology of fatty muscle atrophy. They observed that when the tendon tears, the pennation angle between the individual muscle fibers decreases, and there is an increased space between muscle fibers that fills with fat. The muscle then becomes retracted and stiff. This was observed to be irreversible after late tendon repair in sheep.

These observations taken together support the conclusion that fatty muscle replacement is a negative prognostic factor for restoration of function and strength after rotator cuff repair.

Role of the Coracoacromial Ligament

The coracoacromial ligament has been shown clinically[4,111] and experimentally[33] to have an important secondary stabilizing role preventing anterosuperior translation when the rotator cuff containment function is lost. In these situations, it acts as a last barrier to unchecked anterosuperior translation of the humeral head, and it must be preserved.[4,15] The type III (hooked) acromion shape is probably a compensatory phenomenon that attempts to reduce superior humeral head displacement in cases of massive rotator cuff tears. Routine acromioplasty may be biomechanically inadvisable in cases of chronic, long-standing massive rotator cuff tears because it may destabilize the coracoacromial ligament with resultant anterosuperior escape[4,102] (Fig. 7-3).

Role of the Long Head of the Biceps

Whether the biceps serves as an important stabilizer of the shoulder in rotator-cuff-deficient shoulders is a matter of continued debate. It is becoming increasingly clear that the biceps does not have an active role in the setting of massive rotator cuff tears, and there may be a passive tenodesis effect as supported by others.[59,64,116,117,128,130] If there is significant biceps disease, most authors advocate tenodesis or tenotomy because this may be a significant pain generator in the setting of cuff disease. Indeed, Walch et al.[116] has provided strong evidence that simple biceps tendon tenotomy may significantly improve pain in patients with irreparable massive rotator cuff tears.

DIAGNOSTIC CONSIDERATIONS

History

Most posterior rotator cuff tears occur in individuals in their 6th through 8th decades of life, and they occur as a result of multiple biological and mechanical factors. The exact cause of full-thickness rotator cuff tear remains a subject of debate; however, the following explanations form the basis of current treatment recommendations. Gradual attrition of the supraspinatus tendon insertion from "outlet impingement" against the anterosuperior acromion and an arthritic clavicle is enhanced by a paucity of blood supply in this region.[81,82,95,98] Intrinsic degeneration in the rotator cuff probably also reduces its structural strength, putting it at greater risk for failure even with trivial trauma.[96]

Some predictions can be made about the size of the tear and quality of tendon tissue based on the history given by the patient. If a patient reports no specific traumatic event and the loss of function and onset of pain as insidious and chronic, then the quality of the tendon tissue is likely poor, and these individuals may also have significant atrophy and fatty degeneration of the spinate musculature.[46,47] Patients who have had multiple steroid injections often have thin, friable tendon tissue, and those with a history of chronic tobacco use also tend to have larger tears and poorer tendon tissue for repair. A chronic, massive rotator cuff tear may also result in disuse osteopenia of the proximal humerus. This can make secure tendon-bone repair more difficult. In some individuals with a long-standing massive rotator cuff tear, there is tendon involution or loss, and the remaining muscle and tendon are inelastic because of scarring and fatty degeneration (Fig. 7-4).[38,44] Surgical

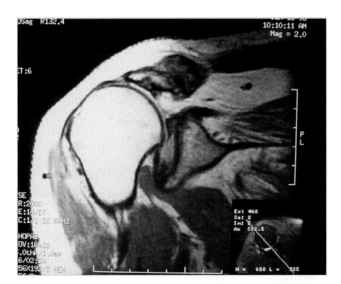

Figure 7-3 MRI demonstrates superior displacement of humeral head with massive rotator cuff tear and fatty degeneration of rotator cuff.

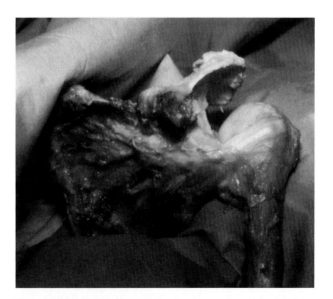

Figure 7-4 A cadaver shoulder from a 78-year-old man demonstrates a chronic massive rotator cuff tear with loss of tendon tissue and atrophy of muscle.

mobilization of the tendons for repair can be very difficult in these cases.[7,31]

When the patient is in his or her fifth or sixth decade and reports a specific traumatic event preceding the onset of shoulder pain and poor function, it is more likely that the quality of the torn tendon and muscle is good, with elastic, easily mobilized tissue. Hersche and Gerber[54] have demonstrated that the duration of the rotator cuff tear is associated with increased stiffness and passive tension of the muscle-tendon unit.

Clinical Appearance

Not all of these patients have a painful arc and positive impingement signs.[82] Massive rotator cuff tears involving the supraspinatus, infraspinatus, and teres minor may often present as a painless pseudoparalysis.

Several physical findings are specific for massive rotator cuff tears involving the posterosuperior tendons. First, in those with a painful and weak shoulder, strength testing may greatly overestimate the true limitations of that individual, because pain inhibition prevents a good effort by the patient.[8] We perform an *impingement test* by injecting 10 to 15 mL of 1% Xylocaine into the subacromial space 10 minutes before examining a patient's strength and active motion.[81,82] Active motion should be assessed with specific attention to scapulothoracic and trunk substitution patterns in individuals with poor glenohumeral motion due to a massive rotator cuff tears (Fig. 7-5). It is imperative to assess any differences between *passive and active motion arcs*, because this gives valuable information about which portions of the rotator cuff are involved. A patient who has a significant lag of active external rotation when the arm is positioned in abduction has a massive tear extending into the infraspinatus and teres minor tendons. The *hornblower's sign*

(signe du clairon) is pathognomonic for a massive rotator cuff tears involving the infraspinatus and teres minor tendons (Fig. 7-6).[38,44,115] The patient is asked to abduct his shoulders while keeping his hands at mouth level. He then externally rotates his shoulders to put his hands on top of his head. The normal side allows this combined abduction and external rotation, and the side with a massive rotator cuff tear is not able to externally rotate with the shoulder in abduction, giving the appearance that the patient is blowing a horn. Alternatively, the patient's hand can be placed in the position of abduction and external rotation and then released (Fig. 7-6). Failure to maintain the arm in this position against gravity confirms the presence of a nonfunctioning posterosuperior rotator cuff. This test can be repeated for external rotation with the arm at the side.

Strength should be at least assessed manually on a 0/5 to 5/5 scale for abduction, internal rotation, and external rotation. Handheld isometric measurement devices (i.e., Isobex, Burgdorf, Switzerland) can also be used to give more quantitative and reproducible measurements of strength. These dynamometers have been validated and provide the best method of simply assessing strength over a 5-second interval.[5]

Radiographic Studies

The *supraspinatus outlet view* is a routine radiograph obtained to clarify the acromial shape as hooked, curved, or flat, and give information about the shape of the supraspinatus outlet (Fig. 7-7A).[2,12,11,13,78,82] Unfortunately, it is not a reproducible view unless carefully controlled by fluoroscopy (Golser, personal communication, 1991; Liotard, personal communication, 1995). Some clinicians routinely use this radiograph, but others do not. The *caudal tilt anteroposterior view*[89] demonstrates the

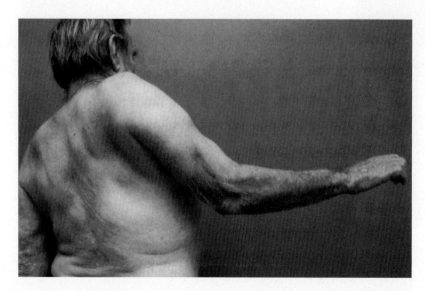

Figure 7-5 A 68-year-old man with a massive rotator cuff tear. On attempted abduction of the arm, there is a compensatory trunk tilt and scapulothoracic substitution.

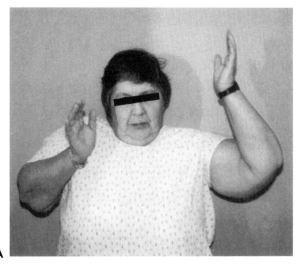
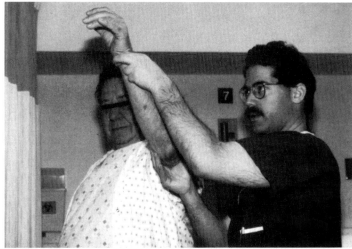
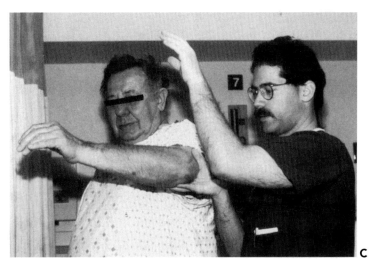

Figure 7-6 (*A*) A 52-year-old woman with a massive rotator cuff tear. She has a positive hornblower's sign, which is pathognomonic for disruption of the infraspinatus. (*B,C*) Demonstration of the hornblower's sign by a modified test that demonstrates a lag of active external rotation with the arm maintained in abduction.

anteroinferior projection of the acromion more accurately (Fig. 7-7). An *anteroposterior view of the acromioclavicular joint* may determine the presence of concomitant acromioclavicular joint disease and that of an inferior osteophyte that may be contributing to outlet impingement (Fig. 7-7).

An *axillary view* is usually obtained to demonstrate the presence of an os acromiale, because this can be present in as many as 19% of patients with large rotator cuff tears, compared with 4% of normal subjects (Fig. 7-7). It is important to identify this ununited acromial apophysis, because it may need surgical stabilization at the time of the rotator cuff repair.

Useful biomechanical information can be obtained from a *true anteroposterior view of the shoulder*. LeClerq[65] described an abduction view obtained with the patient's arm at 30 degrees of abduction and holding a 2-kg weight in the hand. Superior humeral head displacement was diagnostic of a supraspinatus tear. An anteroposterior radiograph ob-

tained with the shoulder in neutral rotation can allow reproducible measurement of the acromiohumeral interval. This measurement correlates with the size of the rotator cuff tear. Normally, the acromiohumeral interval is 7 mm or larger. When it is observed to be less than 3 mm, the shoulder is considered to be statically subluxed superiorly. This is always associated with an infraspinatus tear, and such a massive tear cannot be repaired by conventional means. The humeral head cannot be recentered by repair of the tendons in this situation.

Plain anteroposterior radiographs obtained with the arm actively abducted by at least 30 degrees can provide a reproducible measure of superior translation of the humeral head. The center of the humeral head can be consistently measured relative to the center of the glenoid, and concerns about the obliquity of the x-ray film are not a problem, as can be the case when measuring the acromiohumeral interval (Fig. 7-7).[9,65,125,126]

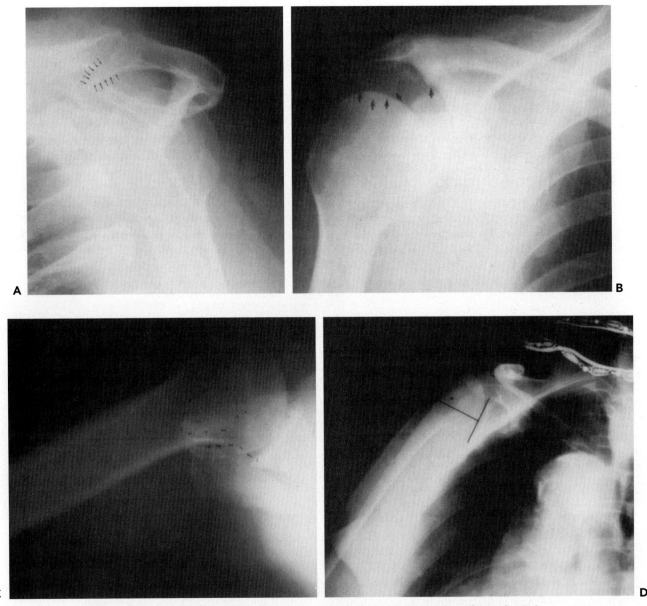

Figure 7-7 (*A*) Large, hooked acromion (*arrows*) on the supraspinatus outlet radiograph. (*B*) Caudal tilt radiograph demonstrates anteroinferior prominence of the acromion and a large inferior osteophyte off the distal clavicle (*arrows*). (*C*) Os acromiale is demonstrated on the axillary view (*dashed lines*). (*D*) Marked superior translation of the humeral head on attempted abduction in a patient with a massive rotator cuff tear.

Adjuvant Imaging Techniques

The arthrogram has traditionally been the gold standard for detection of full-thickness rotator cuff tears, and it remains the most cost-effective diagnostic method.[23] However, it is invasive and can miss partial-thickness and full-thickness tears of the subscapularis tendon. It gives no information about concomitant intra-articular abnormalities, nor can it predict the size of a rotator cuff tear. Furthermore, no information regarding fatty degeneration and atrophy of the rotator cuff is gleaned from this method.

In some European centers, the most cost-effective method used to confirm the presence of a rotator cuff tear is ultrasonography.[56] This technique is not as commonly used in North America because of the variable experiences of radiologists, however, due to its ease of use, ultrasound is increasing in popularity. The application of this technology is user dependent; however, skilled investigators routinely report sensitivities and specificities that exceed 90%. Prickett et al.[94] documented high accuracy (89%) with ultrasound for diagnosing recurrent rotator cuff tears in a series of 44 postoperative patients with persistent shoulder pain. More impressive was an accuracy of 96% in patients with rotator cuff tears without previous surgery.[109]

Magnetic resonance imaging is sensitive, specific, and accurate for the detection of full-thickness and partial-thickness rotator cuff tears.[57,71,76,131] It is an expensive test, however, and its sensitivity, specificity, and accuracy depend on the quality of the images and the knowledge and expertise of the radiologist. In most cases, the authors feel that a careful physical examination usually answers the question about presence and size of a rotator cuff tear; however, MRI provides useful information about the degree of muscle atrophy and fatty degeneration in patients suspected of having massive rotator cuff tears (Fig. 7-2).[46,47,80,125] Shoulder MRI must be performed by a machine with a strong magnet (ideally a 1.5 Tesla magnet) and a dedicated surface coil. To obtain useful information about rotator cuff muscle character, we image to the medial border or the scapula, and we are especially interested in the oblique, sagittal, and axial plane images (Fig. 7-2).

Magnetic resonance imaging and more recently, MRI with arthrography, have been the de facto "gold standard" imaging choice for rotator cuff pathology. Conventional MRI has been improved with the addition of fat-suppressed sequences in the coronal and sagittal oblique plane, increasing overall accuracy.[101,104,114] The addition of gadolinium has enhanced the sensitivity and specificity for partial-thickness and small, full-thickness tears. Meister et al.[71] recently documented the accuracy of coronal oblique T-1 weighted imaging with fat suppression using a gadopentatate arthrogram. For those patients with either a partial- or full-thickness tear seen at arthroscopy (employed as the gold standard), the sensitivity was 84%, and positive predictive value was 93% for MR arthrography.

SURGICAL CONSIDERATIONS

Surgical Philosophy of Repair

In all cases, repair of massive cuff tears remains the goal of surgical treatment. Repairs of the rotator cuff have been highly successful and clearly superior to the natural history of untreated tears.[7,10,23,26,31,32,51,53,81,82,98] There are clinical data that demonstrate that the result of massive rotator cuff tears is inferior to smaller tears.[10,24,31,32,37] Although retear of massive tears may approach 70%, smaller cuff tears have a significantly lower retear rate.[37,51,60] The clinical result of a watertight structural repair is clearly superior than shoulders with a retear. Additionally, the massive tears have a higher frequency of advanced atrophy and cuff degeneration and are associated with poorer quality of the musculotendinous unit.

Arthroscopic management of rotator cuff tears is growing, and its role in the treatment of massive posterosuperior tears is evolving. There is some evidence that surgical morbidity is less than with open rotator cuff repair.[19,21] Indeed, partial arthroscopic rotator cuff repair seems to afford reliable pain relief and some improvement of function in select patients. Our current indication for open rotator cuff repair is for management of revision cases with extensive scarring, associated defects (such as acromial fracture or deltoid deficiency), and need for associated tendon transfers.

Patient Positioning

The patient is positioned on a beach chair and arm positioner (Spider arm positioner, Tenet medical, Calgary, Canada) in an upright, seated position with the head of the bed at about a 45-degree angle (Fig. 7-8). This allows the

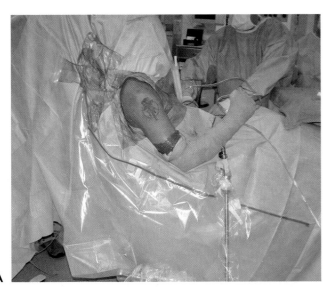
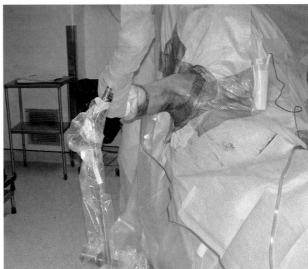

A   B

Figure 7-8   (A) Mechanical arm holder facilitates positioning of arm (*view from side*). (B) Mechanical arm holder positioning arm in abduction (*view from front*).

surgeons to adjust the position so that the front and back of the shoulder are free and the head is supported. Always assess passive range of motion with the patient under anesthesia, because secondary capsular contractures may develop in the setting of chronic rotator cuff tear. In these cases, the shoulder is manipulated before an incision is made, or formal releases are done during the surgery. The hydraulic arm positioner supports the arm while enhancingand maintaining exposure. The use of such a positioner is more secure than a surgical assistant who may fatigue during the surgery.

When a latissimus transfer is performed for salvage reconstruction of the posterosuperior rotator cuff tendons, the patient is positioned in a lateral decubitus position. This procedure is described later in this chapter.

Surgical Approach

The standard incision is an anterior oblique incision in Langer's lines that begins over the top of the acromion and continues to just lateral to the coracoid process (Fig. 7-9A). Avoid incisions that cross laterally over the top of the shoulder, because these cannot be extended if an anterior

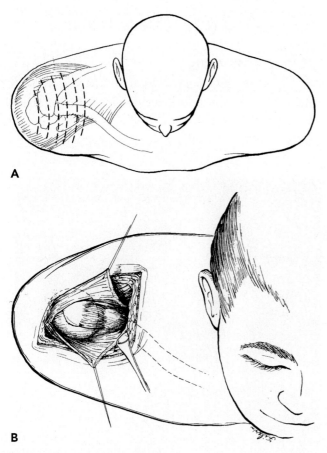

Figure 7-9 (A) Incision within the Langer's lines gives the best cosmesis. (B) Deltoid mobilization.

extension is required for subscapularis tears, and because they create a thick, noncosmetic scar.[16,62] Subcutaneous flaps are mobilized over the acromioclavicular joint and laterally over the palpable lateral extent of the acromion. This is an important step, especially in revision cases in which an injured and retracted deltoid muscle may be adherent to the overlying skin. One approach is to detach the deltoid from the acromion using an electrocautery device, beginning just lateral to the acromioclavicular joint and about 5 mm posterior to the anterior edge. Another approach is to elevate a lateral flap of the deltoid with a scalpel and leave the anterior deltoid attached. In this case, the coracoacromial ligament is left undisturbed.

When the deltoid is detached, it is done by raising a subperiosteal flap off the acromion and splitting the deltoid laterally for a distance of 2 to 3 cm. Extension of the deltoid split further than 5 cm endangers the axillary nerve. The deltoid muscle is split in line with its fibers to the level of the greater tuberosity. By splitting the deltoid laterally, there is better access to the posterior cuff (Fig. 7-9B). Splitting the deltoid too far anteriorly may hinder access to a retracted infraspinatus tear. Subacromial adhesions are then sharply released with either a scissors or an elevator. This ensures that the rotator cuff tendon is more clearly defined with the subsequent dissection, because the rotator cuff can be scarred to the undersurface of the acromion.

In most cases, if the coracoacromial ligament is intact, we prefer to leave it undisturbed because it is an important static restraint to anterosuperior humeral head displacement.[4,81] In patients with significant acromioclavicular joint pain and arthritis, the periosteal incision is extended from the acromion over the distal clavicle, the periosteal-fascial flaps of deltoid and trapezius are elevated, and the distal 10 to 15 mm of clavicle are excised. Sharp dissection is then used to mobilize the subdeltoid interval, because adhesions can connect the deltoid to the proximal humerus. In some individuals with passive loss of motion, especially in revision cases, these two steps can partially improve motion.

A malleable retractor is then inserted underneath the acromion, and a modified acromioplasty is performed with an oscillating saw, taking care to only remove the inferior surface of the acromion and to not detach the origin of the coracoacromial ligament. An extensive bursectomy is then performed by grasping the bursa with a clamp and rotating the arm to expose the anterior and posterior portions of the bursa.

The rotator cuff tear configuration and quality of the tendon tissue can then be defined by placing several sutures into the tendon tissue and rotating the arm to visualize the extent of the tear. External rotation allows inspection of the subscapularis (Fig. 7-10A), and internal rotation brings the infraspinatus and teres minor into view (Fig. 7-10B). The actual tear size is less important than the number of tendons involved, the quality of the tendon tissue, and the degree of tendon retraction. Some massive tears

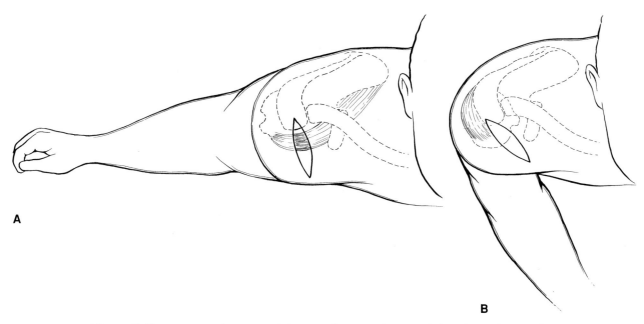

Figure 7-10 (*A*) External rotation of the arm allows visualization of the subscapularis tendon. (*B*) Internal rotation of the arm allows visualization of the infraspinatus tendon.

(>5 cm in diameter) can be easily repaired, although medium (2–3 cm) and large tears (3–5 cm) can be difficult to securely repair because of poor tendon tissue.

In cases with retracted, inelastic musculotendinous units, extensive intra-articular and extra-articular releases are required to lateralize the tendon for repair into the greater tuberosity. The coracohumeral ligament is first divided by pulling on the supraspinatus tendon sutures and cutting soft-tissue extensions to the base of the coracoid process (Fig. 7-11A).[83] If sufficient length is not obtained, the interval between the superior labrum and rotator cuff is sharply divided (Fig. 7-11B). Care should be taken not to

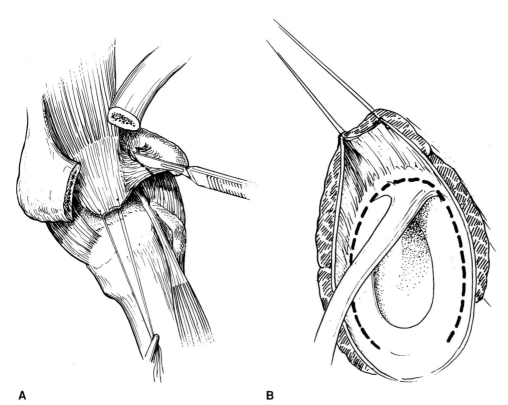

Figure 7-11 Technique of mobilization and repair of a retracted, chronic supraspinatus tendon tear. Acromial and distal clavicle resections are exaggerated to show the technique of tendon release; they are usually less extensive than depicted here. (*A*) Division of the coracohumeral ligament (*dashed line*). (*B*) Intra-articular release of tendon (*dashed line*). The division is between the labrum and the capsule, so the labrum is left on the glenoid. (*continued*)

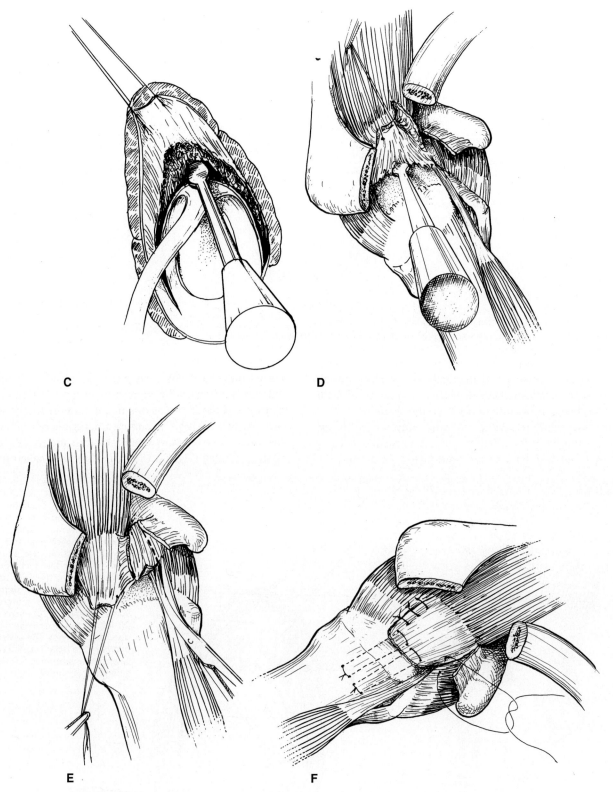

Figure 7-11 *(continued)* *(C,D)* Intra-articular mobilization of the rotator cuff. *(E)* Release of the rotator interval *(dashed line)*. *(F)* Repair of the supraspinatus tendon.

injure the long head of the biceps tendon. A periosteal elevator is then placed into this interval and pushed medially to elevate the supraspinatus off the lateral supraspinatus fossa (Figs. 7-11, *C* and *D*). When performing this maneuver it is important not to advance the instruments more than 2 cm laterally, because there is a risk of injury to the suprascapular nerve.[121] If sufficient mobilization of the supraspinatus tendon is not achieved for its repair, an *interval slide* can be performed by dividing tissue in the rotator interval between the subscapularis and supraspinatus (Figs. 7-11, *E* and *F*).[10] Similar steps can be performed for mobilization of the infraspinatus.[21,108]

When visualization of the retracted tendon is difficult because of medial retraction, the authors have found it helpful to perform an acromioclavicular joint resection in those patients who also have pain related to this joint (Figs. 7-11, *E* and *F*). This allows direct access to the supraspinatus fossa. A specially designed retractor (Subacromial spreader, Protek Company, Switzerland) that allows the humeral head to be distracted inferiorly away from the acromion, can greatly improve the surgeon's view (Figs. 7-12, *A*–*C*). Alternatively, a laminar spreader can be used with the limbs placed on the acromion and the greater tuberosity. The authors do not perform a supraspinatus or infraspinatus slide as described by Debyre,[28] because this poses an unnecessary risk to the suprascapular neurovascular pedicle and shortens the lever arm of the muscle-tendon units.

Improving the Initial Strength of Repair

After mobilizing the cuff tissue sufficiently to reach the greater tuberosity with the patient's arm at the side, the repair can be performed. The ideal repair should have high initial fixation strength, allow minimal gap formation, and maintain mechanical stability until healing of the tendon to bone is complete. Tendon repair to bone may fail more often than suspected.[122] Initial aspects of the repair that can contribute to such failure include suture or knot failure, tendon failure, or suture pullout through bone. Several in vitro studies[22,41] have defined and quantified these weak links in the repair, and our repair methods are based on these observations.

Sutures

Sutures smaller than 1-0 do not provide sufficient strength for repair of large retracted tears. Monofilament absorbable suture materials, such as Maxon or PDS II, lose 50% of their in vitro ultimate tensile strength at 3 to 4 weeks after implantation.[108] Although some surgeons[17] feel that this time course is acceptable for the repair, Gerber and coworkers[29] showed that the elasticity of this suture material permits a large gap to form. These suture materials should not be used for repair of large retracted tears. Braided, nonabsorbable polyester has the best combined ultimate tensile strength and stiffness, and we usually use No. 3 or No. 2 sizes of this type of suture. Currently, several companies offer a new, stronger No. 2 braided, nonabsorbable suture marketed under the trade names of Fiberwire (Arthrex, Naples, FL), Herculine (Linvatec, Largo, FL), Ultrabraide (Smith and Nephew, Mansfield, MA), and Orthocord (Mitek, Johnson and Johnson, Norwood, MA). All of these sutures make it unlikely that the weak link in the tendon-to-bone repair will be the suture itself.

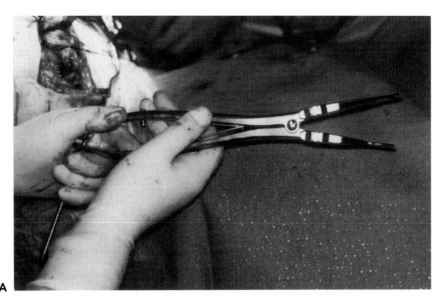

Figure 7-12 *(A)* Acromial distraction device. *(continued)*

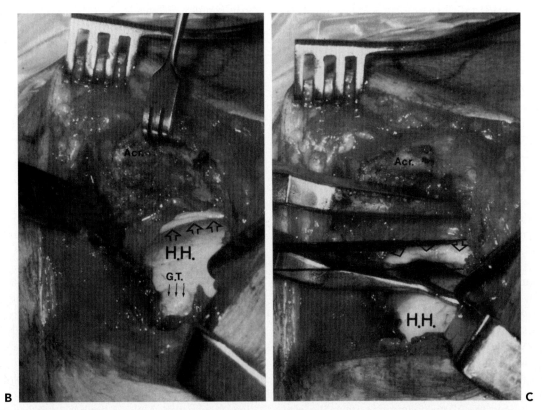

B

C

Figure 7-12 *(continued)* *(B)* Retracted massive rotator cuff tear *(arrows)* is difficult to reach underneath the acromion (Acr.). The humeral head (H.H.) and greater tuberosity (G.T.) are labeled. *(C)* The acromial distractor allows the interval between the humeral head (H.H.) and the acromion (Acr.) to be widened, allowing access to the retracted edge of the rotator cuff tendon *(arrows)* so that it can be mobilized and repaired.

Tendon-Grasping Techniques

Most suture-grasping techniques used for repair are weak or tend to strangulate the tendon tissue.[41] The optimal suture knot technique is the modified Mason-Allen stitch,[41] because it results in twice the holding power of a simple stitch. By grasping fewer fiber bundles, it should cause less strangulation of the tissue than other grasping sutures (Fig. 7-13).[63]

Transosseous Repair

In cases of chronic, long-standing massive rotator cuff tears, the bone of the proximal humerus may be quite osteoporotic, and in these situations, the holding power of the bony cortex may be poor.[73,110] Suture anchor systems relying on cancellous bone fixation can fail at loads one half that of standard transosseous cortical fixation repairs (Fig. 7-14).[41] In these situations, transosseous suture configuration can greatly influence the initial strength of repair. The authors have observed that the pullout strength of transosseous fixation can be increased by a factor of 3,

if the sutures are tied over a bone bridge at least 1 cm in diameter and at least 2 to 3 cm from the tip of the greater tuberosity.[22] This results from the increasing thickness of the cortex distal to the tip of the greater tuberosity (Fig. 7-15A). When there is marked osteopenia, cortical augmentation can further improve holding strength of sutures. Options have included a thin metal plate (Button Plate, Synthes, Paoli, PA) and a small round plastic collar that augments the suture coming out of the lateral bone hole (Cuff Link, Mitek, Johnson and Johnson, Norwood, MA).[22,41,107] These have not caused any significant irritation at their site of insertion. The authors' preference is to orient the transosseous sutures vertically so that the tendon is pulled down from medial to lateral over its bony footprint insertion, and so that the weak link for the transosseous tunnel will be at the lateral hole. The Cuff Link device prevents the suture from cutting through the bony tunnel (Fig. 7-15B). In shoulders with severe bone loss from prior surgery in which it is impossible to tie sutures over a cortical bone bridge, a useful revision technique is to place a bicortical screw and washer into the proximal humerus and then pull the sutures through the bony

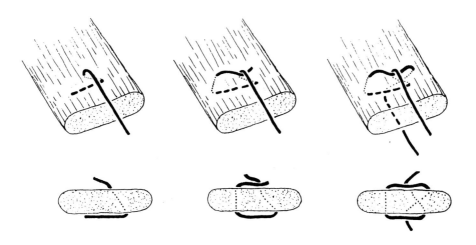

Tendon-Grasping Techniques   ***Details of the Repair***

Figure 7-13   Mason-Allen suture configuration. (Permission from Gerber C, Schneeberger AG, Beck M, et al. Mechanical strength of repairs of the rotator cuff. J Bone Joint Surg 1994; 76B:371.)

trough and tie them around the screw and washer post (Fig. 7-16).

Details of the Repair

Massive rotator cuff tears usually have a configuration in which the tendons pull away from their insertions in medial and inferior directions. In some cases, it may be best to mobilize the supraspinatus and infraspinatus tendons and suture them together in a side-to-side fashion before reattachment to the greater tuberosity. Because the torn edges of a degenerated tendon may delaminate, care should be taken when placing sutures to capture the en-

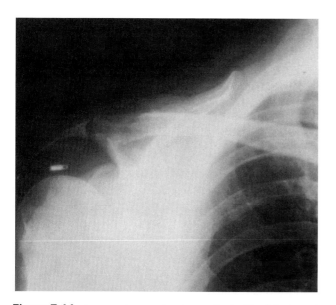

Figure 7-14   Loose suture anchor in a patient with a failed repair of a massive rotator cuff tear.

tire thickness of the tendon with each stitch. Generally, sutures are grouped in pairs with two sets for each tendon, so that two sets of two (total of four) are placed in the supraspinatus and infraspinatus each. A deep bony trough is rarely created. Instead, the authors prefer to remove soft tissue and abrade the bone of the greater tuberosity just medial to the original anatomical insertion. This promotes soft tissue to bone healing but does not remove the structural integrity of the cortical bone of the greater tuberosity. A deep trough risks fracture of the tuberosity and requires further advancement of the tendon into the trough for good bone contact. Using a special suture passer (Concept Rotator Cuff Repair System, Linvatec Corp., Largo, FL), sutures are kept in their pairs and passed into the bony trough and out the lateral cortex of the humerus at least 2 cm distal to the tip of the greater tuberosity (Fig. 7-17).Place two sutures in a Mason-Allen configuration and then pull these through one hole in the greater tuberosity and out of the lateral cortex. A Cuff Link device is placed over this suture to reinforce it. For a massive tear, the authors usually use three sets of two sutures each into three holes in the greater tuberosity.[3]

Tie these sutures down while maintaining the shoulder in abduction using a mechanical arm holder (Spider, Tenet Medical, Calgary, Canada) (Fig. 7-8). The arm is then brought down to the side and moved passively through an arc of motion to determine where the repair comes under tension. The physical therapist uses this information to guide postoperative passive motion therapy.

The deltoid closure is the final and critical step to any rotator cuff repair, because detachment of the deltoid constitutes one of the worst possible complications. The authors place two to three transosseous No. 2, nonabsorbable, braided sutures through the acromion, then fix the deltoid

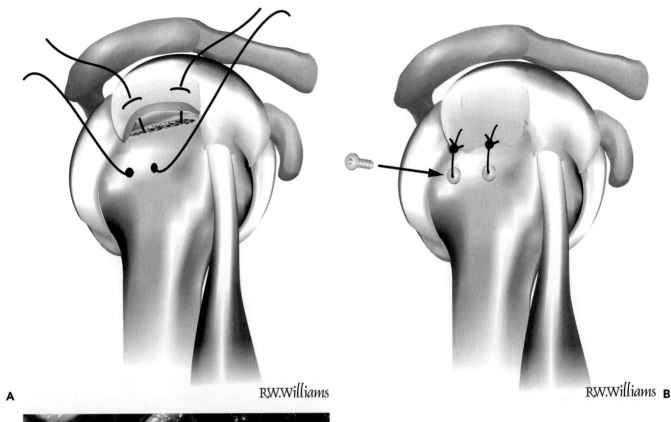

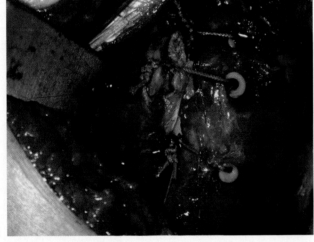

Figure 7-15 (*A*) Added cortical strength if suture exits base for the distal to greater tuberosity. (*B*) Cortical augmentation can be achieved with plastic collar devise that prevents suture pull through bone (see text for explanation). (*C*) Cortical augmentation with plastic collar (Cuff Link, Mitek, Johnson and Johnson, Norwood, MA). See text for explanation.

with Mason-Allen stitches (Fig. 7-18). The lateral deltoid split is then reapproximated, and if an acromioclavicular joint resection has been performed, the trapezius fascia and deltoid fascia are closed in pants-over-vest fashion using nonabsorbable suture.

POSTOPERATIVE TREATMENT

For massive rotator cuff tear reconstruction, the authors routinely use a shoulder immobilizer with an abduction pillow attachment for 6 weeks, despite repairing the ten-

dons to the greater tuberosity with the arm at the side. Abduction of the shoulder reduces constant tension on the musculotendinous unit that has been repaired. Because there is less tension on the suture-tendon-bone repair, it increases the likelihood of healing without disruption. Furthermore, it is reasonable to expect some viscoelasticity of the tendon over the initial 6 weeks after surgery, and this approach allows the musculotendinous unit to stretch gradually without failure at the repair site.

Beginning the first week after surgery, the authors perform passive range of motion under the supervision of a therapist for the first 6 weeks after surgical repair. The au-

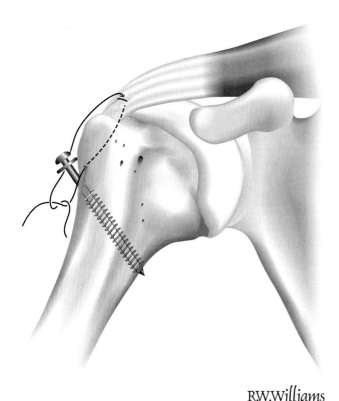

R.W.Williams

Figure 7-16 Biocortical screw used as an anchor when there is deficient proximal bone for rotator cuff fixation in revision cases. It is usually best to use a screw with only distal threads to avoid cutting the sutures when tightening the screw.

thors have not used pendulums or self-assisted range of motion in patients with massive posterosuperior tendon tears. These maneuvers result in active rotator cuff muscle contraction that may compromise the repair in the early healing phase. The authors prescribe the limits of passive motion for the therapist based on intraoperative observations after repair.

At 6 weeks, the patient begins to use the arm for activities of daily living. He or she performs active-assisted motion exercises, but strengthening is delayed until 3 months after surgery. Strengthening with elastic bands is then commenced. Free weights are avoided for at least 4 to 6 months after surgery, because we have seen failures of the repairs caused by excessive overloading. Patients are permitted to swim or swing a tennis racket at 8 months after their surgery. In general, strength gains can continue to be significant over 1 year after the surgery.

Treatment of "Irreparable" Tears

Indications

In the authors' experience, fewer than 5% of all rotator cuff tears remain irreparable after performing all of the previously described steps of tissue mobilization. The term *irreparable rotator cuff tear* is not synonymous with massive ro-

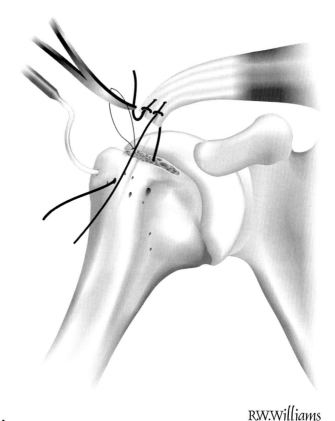

R.W.Williams

A

R.W.Williams

B

Figure 7-17 Technique of suture placement in rotator cuff repair.

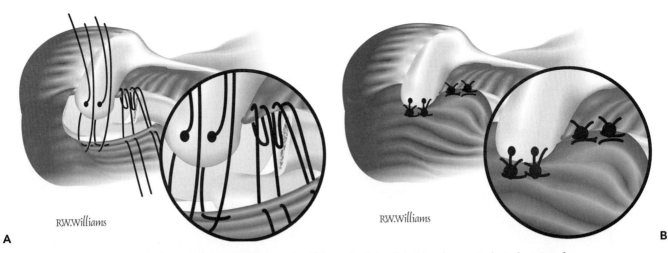

R.W.Williams

R.W.Williams

A   B

Figure 7-18 (A) Placement of sutures and (B) repair of the deltoid and acromioclavicular joint after acromioplasty and distal clavicle resection.

tator cuff tear, because tendon-tissue quality and retraction, as well as the surgeon's skills, are the determining factors for achieving a secure repair.[44] In these cases, the treatment needs to be individualized. In many cases, the surgeon can know by the preoperative evaluation whether the tear is irreparable. For example, patients with radiographic evidence of marked superior translation and pressure changes or erosions on the acromion do not have a reparable tear. These long-standing tears have marked loss of tendon tissue, and

the patients have severe atrophy and fatty replacement of their spinate muscles (Fig. 7-2). Goutllier[46] showed that this chronic muscle degeneration does not recover after surgical repairs. Some of these individuals have poor function but minimal pain, and in these cases, the authors recommend against any surgery. A few have good function and minimal pain, and theyshould not have surgical treatment either (Fig. 7-19). Patients who have pain and poor function associated with arthritis may be best managed by hemi-

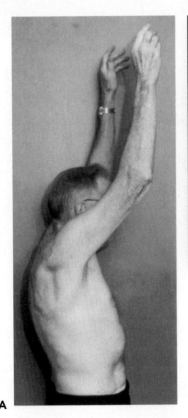

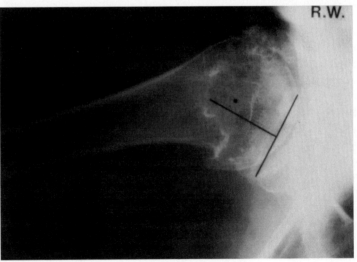

Figure 7-19 (A) An 82-year-old man with symmetrical pain-free motion that allows him to play tennis four times per week. (B) He has radiographic evidence of arthritis and a long-standing rotator cuff tear.

A

arthroplasty replacement, using a large modular head and preserving the coracoacromial ligament as a fulcrum for rotation of the prosthetic humeral head.[4]

Local tendon transfers have been used to close irreparable defects of the cuff. These have included a superior transposition of the upper two thirds of the subscapularis [23,43,44,83] when the supraspinatus cannot be repaired (Fig. 7-20) and superior transposition of the teres minor when the infraspinatus cannot be repaired.[43] The authors avoid such transfers because they weaken the anteroposterior force couple of the rotator cuff. This is important for stability of the humeral head on the glenoid during abduction. If the infraspinatus is torn, the teres minor is the only remaining external rotator, and it does not make sense to risk weakening external rotation to close a cuff defect.

Occasionally a remaining defect in the tendon at the apex of the repair can be closed with autogenous tissue if the long head of the biceps tendon is available. The authors have often found that the long head of biceps is degenerated and can be incorporated into the repair, thus reinforcing the rotator cuff and achieving a biceps tenodesis at the same time.

In patients with pain, poor function, prior infection, and/or bone and soft tissue loss from prior surgery, fusion is an option for treatment, provided that the other shoulder is normal. Such individuals also often have a deltoid injury from prior surgical repair attempts. If the deltoid is normal in these individuals, the option exists for a reverse shoulder prosthesis. This is discussed in more detail in another chapter of this book.

Some elderly patients complaining predominantly of pain may show good pain relief and adequate function following a Xylocaine subacromial injection. An abduction anteroposterior radiograph may show that the humeral head remains centered on the glenoid because of adequate preservation of the rotator cuff-deltoid force couple. Although these individuals have large to massive rotator cuff tears that are potentially reparable, they may prefer not to subject themselves to the surgical morbidity of reconstruction. In these selected cases, the authors have had good short-term success using an arthroscopic debridement technique to relieve pain and improve function.[19,20,32,97] Although strength does not improve, function usually does because of removal of the inhibition from pain caused by mechanical impingement. The appropriate patient for this approach is older than 60 years of age and less active, with preoperative active flexion of at least 120 degrees (after subacromial Xylocaine) and 80% of normal external rotation strength. Debridement fails in individuals with very weak external rotation, a positive hornblower's sign, limited active flexion, and radiographic evidence of superior translation of the humeral head.

In cases of massive rotator cuff tear with associated biceps degeneration, pain is not relieved unless a biceps tenotomy is performed in addition to cuff debridement.

In some cases, an individual may have pain and poor active motion, but good passive motion without any arthritis. These individuals may have had prior surgical attempts that have failed, and they are often seen on MRI to have marked atrophy of the supraspinatus and infraspinatus muscles. Physical examination shows marked external rotation weakness, and a positive hornblower's sign is elicited (Fig. 7-6). The authors have not found any of the tendon grafting techniques to be reliable reconstructive solutions in these

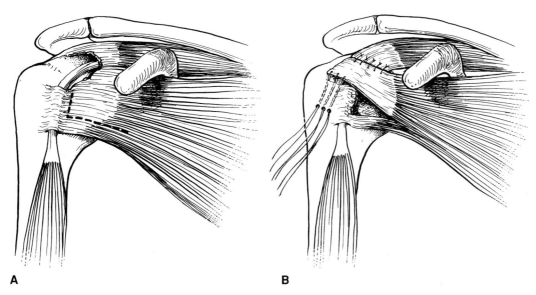

A   B

Figure 7-20   (A) Massive symptomatic rotator cuff tear, closed by (B) subscapularis tendon transposition.

patients.[38,53,90,93] Patients who have marked external rotation weakness but not complete pseudoparalysis are candidates for the latissimus dorsi tendon transfer technique. This extrinsic tendon transfer provides a strong, vascularized tendon that may close the cuff defect and act as a humeral head depressor. With an average follow-up of 5 years, Gerber[38,44] has shown that results of this procedure are long-lasting.[38,44] He has also observed significant pain relief and improved function. The senior author's experience[123] over the past 14 years has also validated this as a viable alternative in carefully selected patients. The subscapularis tendon and deltoid origin must be intact for a patient to be a candidate for this tendon transfer.

Latissimus Dorsi Reconstruction: Surgical Technique

The patient is placed in the lateral decubitus position on a long bean bag. A standard anterosuperior approach to the rotator cuff is made as described previously, and an attempt is made to mobilize and repair the tendon tear. The tendon is mobilized as much as possible, and when it is demonstrated that the supraspinatus and infraspinatus cannot be repaired, the decision for latissimus transfer is made (Fig. 7-21). The authors always prepare the greater tuberosity first and place sutures that will be used to fix the tendon transfer. Several No. 2 nonabsorbable sutures are

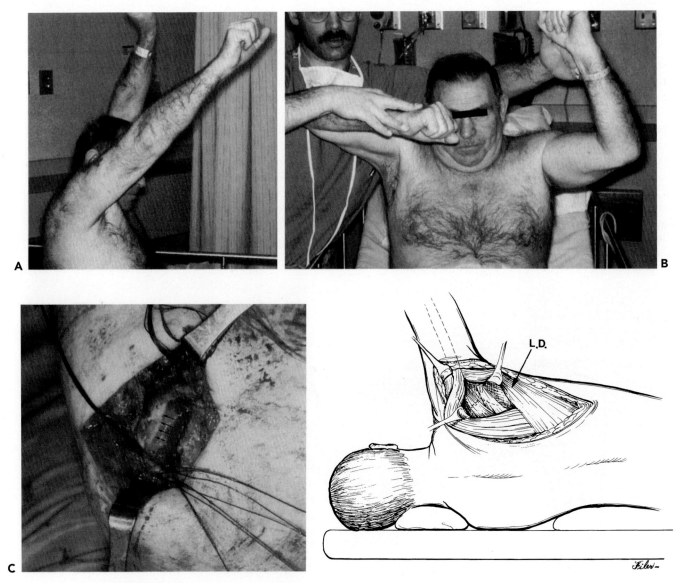

Figure 7-21 (*A*) Patient with a massive rotator cuff tear treated with a latissimus dorsi tendon transfer. Preoperative flexion is limited. (*B*) Preoperative examination demonstrates the hornblower's sign. (*C*) He had a massive rotator cuff tear with a "bald" humeral head (*arrows*). (*D*) The latissimus dorsi (L.D.) is mobilized through a posterior incision.

placed in the teres minor, and several are placed in the subscapularis. After abrading the greater tuberosity, four absorbable anchors loaded with double No. 2, braided, nonabsorbable suture are placed to securely fix the tendon when it is transferred.

The patient's arm is flexed, and a posterior L-shaped incision is made over the posterior joint line and along the palpable border of the latissimus. The muscles of the posterior deltoid, the long head of triceps, the teres major, and the latissimus are carefully identified with dissection. The latissimus muscle is then dissected sharply to free it up from the chest wall and fascia as well as from the teres major. As the latissimus is dissected toward its insertion, the interval between it and the teres major may sometimes be obscured, and care must be taken to separate these two tendons. The authors find it helpful to use a mechanical arm holder placed on the opposite side of the bed, with the arm positioned in abduction and internal rotation (Fig. 7-22). This brings the insertion of the latissimus tendon more posterior and facilitates the dissection. Long thin retractors are used to expose the insertion, and the tendon is then released at the level of its bony attachment to the humerus (Fig. 7-22). Although the radial nerve is relatively close to the plane of dissection, it is not in any danger if the dissec-

tion remains on the latissimus tendon. Dissection then proceeds in a retrograde fashion to define and isolate the neurovascular pedicle and then remove fascial attachments of the muscle to the chest wall and surrounding muscles (Fig. 7-23). Sufficient excursion of the tendon is assured if it can be pulled proximally above the level of the posterior acromion (Fig. 7-24).

The tendon is then prepared prior to its transfer. For the past 10 years, the senior author has utilized fascia lata autograft from the ipsilateral thigh of the patient to reinforce the tendon. It is quite diminutive, and there were some cases early in his experience of tendon rupture after surgery (Fig. 7-25).

The latissimus transfer is then performed. First, a large, curved clamp is passed from the front of the shoulder underneath the acromion and deltoid. The clamp is opened to dilate a soft tissue passage for the tendon. The subdeltoid plane is exposed posteriorly, and dissection is performed to ensure an adequate soft-tissue tunnel for free excursion of the tendon. The sutures in the end of the tendon are then grasped in the clamp, and the tendon is pulled underneath the deltoid and acromion (Fig. 7-26). It is pulled back and forth to make sure it can freely slide in its new position. The tendon is then fixed over the greater tuberosity

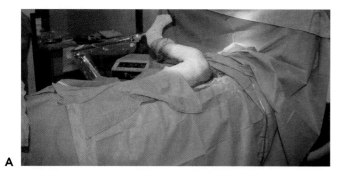
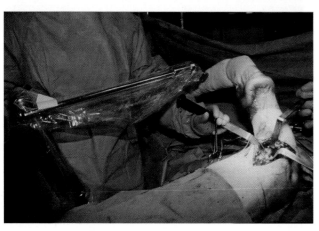
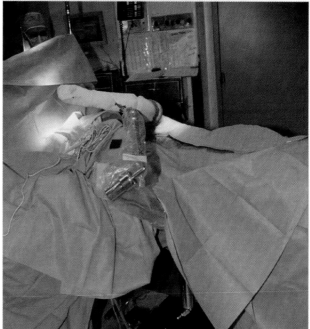

Figure 7-22   (A) The arm is positioned and held with a mechanical arm holder (Spider, Tenet Medical Engineering, Calgary, Canada). Posterior view is demonstrated. (B) The mechanical arm holder is shown from the anterior view (see text for explanation). (C) The arm is held in abduction and internal rotation to dissect the latissimus dorsi tendon insertion. *(continued)*

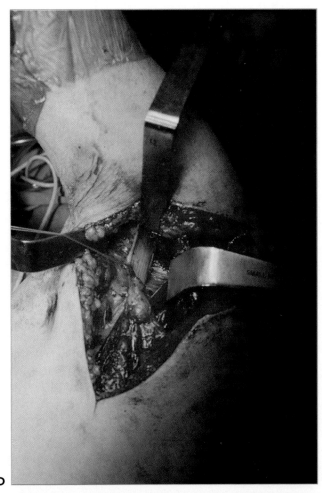

D

Figure 7-22 *(continued)* (D) Close-up view of latissimus dorsi tendon insertion.

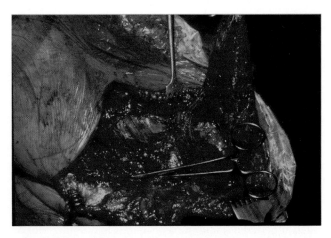

Figure 7-23 Mobilization of the neurovascular pedicle.

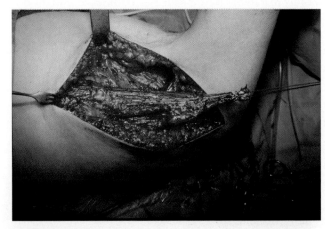

Figure 7-24 After mobilization of the latissimus dorsi tendon, adequate excursion for transfer is demonstrated once the tendon edge can be brought above the posterior acromion.

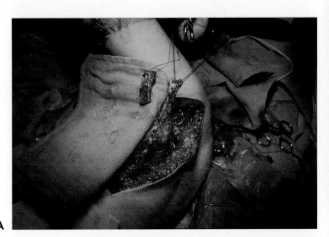

A

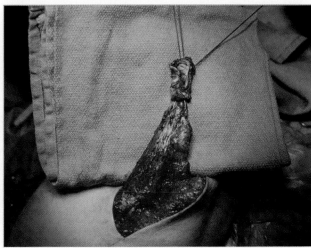

B

Figure 7-25 (A) Fascia lata graft shown with latissimus tendon before augmentation is performed. (B) Fascia lata graft augmentation of latissimus tendon transfer.

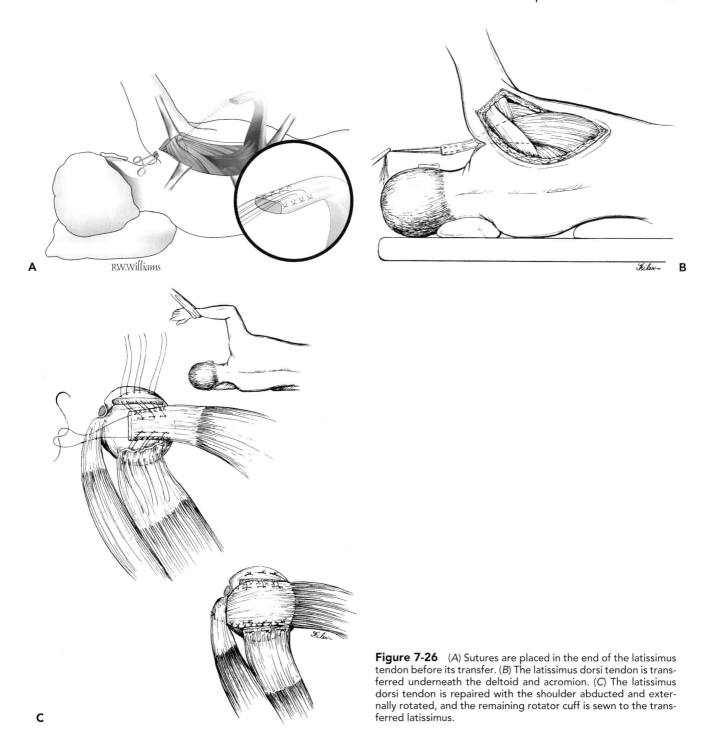

R.W.Williams

A

B

C

Figure 7-26 (*A*) Sutures are placed in the end of the latissimus tendon before its transfer. (*B*) The latissimus dorsi tendon is transferred underneath the deltoid and acromion. (*C*) The latissimus dorsi tendon is repaired with the shoulder abducted and externally rotated, and the remaining rotator cuff is sewn to the transferred latissimus.

using the previously placed anchors along with the sutures in the teres minor and the subscapularis. It is fixed in place with tendon adjusted while the arm is positioned and maintained in about 60 degrees of abduction and 30 degrees of external rotation (Fig. 7-26). This ensures that it has a passive tenodesis effect, as well as proper tension to act as an active external rotator. It is very important to make sure that the latissimus is attached laterally so that its vec-

tor is principally oriented for external rotation. The remaining stump of medial tendon tissue may be sewn into the medial aspect of the latissimus tendon.

The deltoid is then closed as previously described, and the latissimus incision is closed over drains. The shoulder is immobilized on an abduction orthosis that maintains the arm in 60 degrees of abduction and 45 degrees of external rotation (Fig. 7-27).

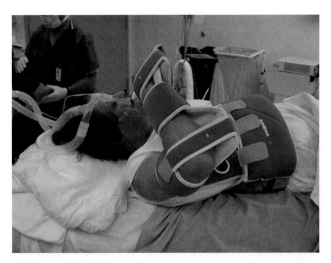

Figure 7-27 Positioning of arm in an abduction orthosis after surgery (see text for explanation).

AFTERCARE

Phase I (first 6 weeks) consists of continuously wearing the brace and passive motion by the therapist, bringing the arm into abduction and external rotation. Adduction and internal rotation are not permitted. This ensures that the tendon moves in its new soft-tissue tunnel and will not become tethered while it heals.

Phase II (second 6 weeks) consists of brace removal and then active-assisted range of motion, as well as passive range of motion. The patient is permitted to use the arm for daily living activities, and water therapy may be commenced to facilitate return of passive motion arcs.

Phase III (12 to 16 weeks) consists of ongoing active-assisted motion; however, a biofeedback program is commenced. The patient is instructed to obtain a cutaneous biofeedback device (Fig. 7-28) and then he or she works with the therapist to activate latissimus contraction during flexion

and external rotation. The authors have observed that the performance of a "J-maneuver" activates the latissimus most reliably. In this maneuver the patient is assisted into flexion of about 90 degrees and then told to pull downward and across the body into adduction. The latissimus will contract. The patient is then asked to maintain this contraction as he or she attempts to flex the arm as it crosses the sagittal plane. The therapist assists in this motion. This method seems to activate the latissimus, and patients gradually learn to flex the arm without first starting with resisted adduction.

In Phase IV (16 weeks and greater), biofeedback continues as long as necessary. It may take up to 1 year for patients to successfully train the tendon transfer to actively assist in arm elevation and external rotation. Strengthening is begun when the patient achieves latissimus contraction during elevation, and the authors try to limit this to elastic bands rather than free weights.

RESULTS

The experiences of the senior author, Gerber, and others have been published.[1,28,77,118,123] Improvement ranges widely depending on the individual patient's pathology; however, it is generally expected that flexion and external rotation improve by a mean of 35 degrees (Fig. 7-29).

FAILED ROTATOR CUFF REPAIRS: REVISION APPROACHES

Most patients remain improved compared with their preoperative morbidity.[23,51] When the repair does fail, revision surgery is considered for individuals who have a poor functional outcome and intolerable pain.[29] The cause of failure may be subdivided into several categories, and the treatment approach should be based on a thorough consideration of these categories (Table 7-4).

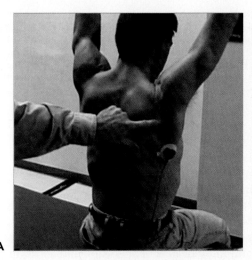 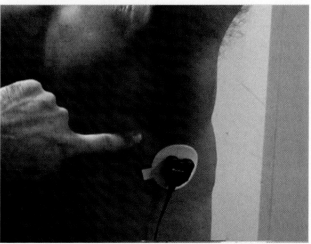

A   B

Figure 7-28 Biofeedback cutaneous electrode in place (see text for explanation).

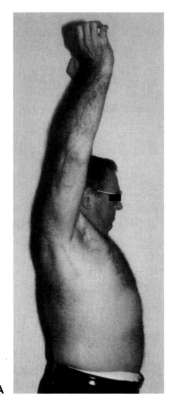

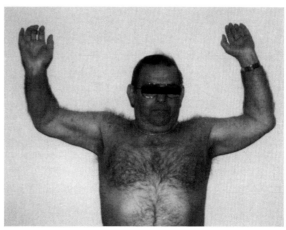

Figure 7-29 Postoperative flexion and external rotation are improved 2 years after latissimus dorsi transfer.

TABLE 7-4	
FAILURE OF ROTATOR CUFF REPAIRS	
Cause	**Potential solution**
FAILURE OF DIAGNOSIS	
Instability	Surgical repair
Suprascapular nerve injury	Surgical release
Adhesive capsulitis	Therapy or manipulation
Missed tendon tear	Revision repair
Glenohumeral osteoarthritis	Conservative or hemiarthroplasty
Acromioclavicular osteoarthritis	Distal clavicle excision
Os acromiale	Repair and bone grafting
Subcoracoid impingement	Coracoidplasty
Marked muscle atrophy	Latissimus transfer
Cervical spondylosis	Treat cervical spine
Visceral causes	Recognize and refer
FAILURE OF SURGICAL TECHNIQUE	
Deltoid injury	Repair or deltoidplasty
Repair of bursal tissue, not cuff	Revision repair
Inadequate acromioplasty	Revision acromioplasty
Acromionectomy	Limited options (fusion ?)
Displacement of bone anchors	Removal and repair
Fracture of greater tuberosity	Revision with screw post anchoring technique
Axillary nerve injury	Exploration and repair
Suprascapular nerve injury	Conservative or latissimus transfer
FAILURE OF POSTOPERATIVE THERAPY	
Stiffness	Therapy, arthroscopic or open releases
Failure of repair	Revision of repair

Patient Selection and Prognostic Factors

In each case of revision surgery, realistic goals should be established for the patient. Several factors predict a poor prognosis:

- Chronic tears of longer than 1 year's duration
- A history of deltoid injury or acromionectomy
- Axillary nerve or suprascapular nerve deficit
- Prior infection
- The presence of an os acromiale (i.e., mesoacromion or basiacromion)
- Marked atrophy or fatty replacement of spinate muscles on MRI
- Acromiohumeral distance of less than 5 mm on an anteroposterior radiograph (<3 mm indicates a very poor prognosis)
- Pseudoparalysis without pain
- Dynamic anterosuperior subluxation of the humeral head on resisted abduction
- Loss of the greater tuberosity from prior surgery
- Poor tendon tissue
- Postoperative shoulder stiffness
- Sympathetic dystrophy or causalgia-type pain
- Concomitant multiple medical illnesses
- Multiple prior steroid injections
- Long history of smoking
- Poor patient compliance and understanding of the problem

Failure of Diagnosis

An incorrect initial diagnosis can cause inappropriate treatment. Suprascapular nerve injury can cause external rotation weakness and pain and can produce atrophy of the spinate. Adhesive capsulitis results in limitation of active and passive motion and can be easily confirmed by an arthrogram showing limited joint volume.

Failure to treat a component of the rotator cuff tear is not uncommon. Typically, a supraspinatus tear may be repaired through an anterosuperior approach with failure to recognize and treat a concomitant subscapularis tendon tear. Instability should be suspected in all young patients with symptoms of a rotator cuff disorder. Other conditions that may be missed and must be treated include osteoarthritis of the glenohumeral joint or acromioclavicular joint, cervical spondylosis with pain referred to the shoulder, reflex sympathetic dystrophy, and visceral causes of pain that may cause shoulder pain, such as subdiaphragmatic abscess, cholecystitis, or a Pancoast tumor.

Role of the Os Acromiale Lesion

An os acromiale is an unfused apophyseal ossification center of the acromion, and it may be present in as many as 19% of individuals with massive rotator cuff tears.[12,30,79] It

is best seen on an axillary x-ray view, although a CT or MR scan can show the anatomy more clearly and give some information about its stability. This lesion does not always require treatment, although it may contribute to impingement through dynamic pull of the deltoid, causing the entire acromion to hinge down through a lose cartilaginous junction (Fig. 7-30).[12,19,78,79,81]

When the os acromiale is small (i.e., preacromion), it can usually be excised and the deltoid origin repaired to the remaining acromion through drill holes. When the os acromiale is large (i.e., mesoacromion or basiacromion), its excision can constitute a complete acromionectomy, and the results of this procedure are usually poor. In these cases, the authors attempt to stabilize the acromion and achieve a fusion across the os acromiale by performing an intercalated dowel-type bone graft with a tension band construct (see Fig. 7-30). The authors do not remove the acromioclavicular joint, because it helps to stabilize the acromion through the acromioclavicular ligaments. Nor do they perform an acromioplasty, because it may also destabilize the acromion. Instead, the acromion is tilted upward so that it diverges away from the humeral head. It is then stabilized with Kirschner wires. A high-speed burr is used to cut a bone trough across the cartilaginous os acromiale, and an iliac crest corticocancellous dowel graft is inserted into this trough. A tension band is then constructed using two cannulated cancellous screws that are placed over the Kirschner wires. These wires are removed, and 18-gauge steel wires are inserted through the screws so that it can be tied down over the bone graft, locking it into place. A cancellous graft is then placed over the superior surface of the acromion. After the os acromiale has been stabilized, the rotator cuff tear is repaired as described previously.

An alternate surgical approach is to use a transacromial approach through the os acromiale to repair the rotator cuff tear and then to stabilize and graft the os acromiale site.

Failure of Surgical Technique

The most difficult problem to treat is injury or detachment of the deltoid origin.[48] This usually results from excessive resection of the acromion or detachment of the deltoid origin repair. In some cases, overzealous retraction can injure the deltoid origin. In the authors' experience, these can be repaired with good, although guarded, results if detected within 3 weeks of the original surgery. The outcome is less certain for chronic cases. A large defect with distal retraction of the deltoid prevents mobilization and advancement proximally back to its origin. In these cases, the authors perform a deltoidplasty by transferring about 1 to 2 cm of the middle deltoid anteriorly on the acromion. This problem is considered in further detail in another chapter of this book.

Other technical errors include the following: inadequate mobilization of tendons resulting in excessive tension at the repair site and in retear; mistaken repair of hypertrophied

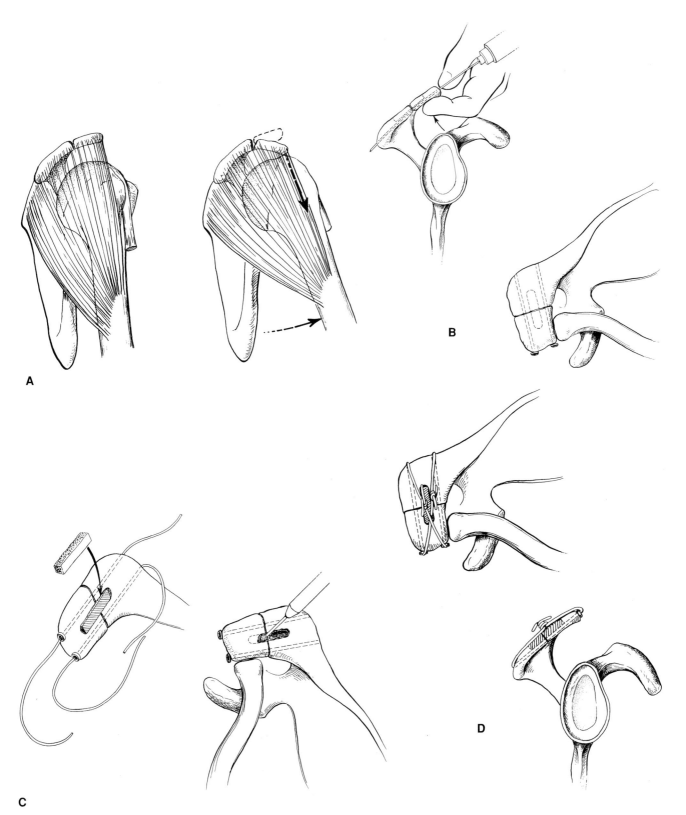

Figure 7-30   Os acromiale repair. (*A*) Impingement created by the pull of the deltoid down on the unstable os acromiale. (*B*) The unstable anterior acromial piece is elevated and then pinned with two pins. Cannulated screws are then used to fix the os acromiale. (*C*) A corticocancellous strut of bone graft is placed across the os acromiale, and 18-gauge wires are threaded through the cannulated screws. (*D*) A tension band construction stabilizes the os acromiale and locks the bone graft into its position on top of the acromion. *(continued)*

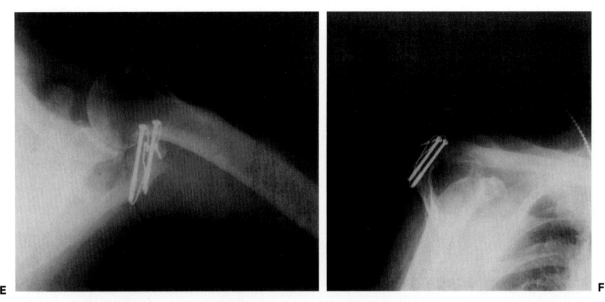

E   F

Figure 7-30 *(continued)* *(E,F)* Axillary and supraspinatus outlet radiographs show the os acromiale fixation.

bursal tissue instead of true rotator cuff tendon, which may be retracted underneath the bursa; inadequate acromioplasty with resulting impingement and failure of the repair; excessive acromioplasty with loss of deltoid lever arm; and injury to the axillary nerve from overzealous retraction or direct trauma from too distal splitting of the deltoid muscle.

Careful examination of deltoid muscle function is important, because sensory testing does not always correlate directly with axillary nerve injury. Injury to the suprascapular nerve from excessive medial dissection into the supraspinatus fossa when mobilizing the tendon[121] should be suspected as a differential diagnosis along with

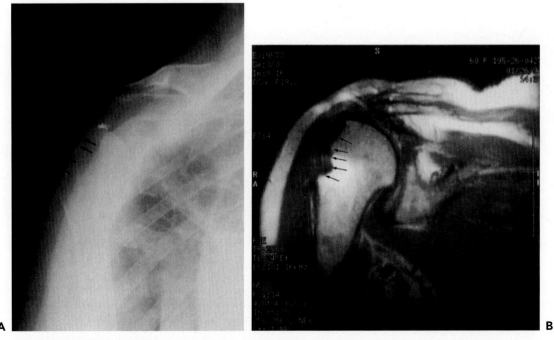

A   B

Figure 7-31 *(A)* Loss of the greater tuberosity *(arrows)* after surgical repair of the rotator cuff but excision of the bone fragment of a greater tuberosity fracture. There is also a loose metal suture anchor. *(B)* MR scan of the same patient demonstrates loss of the greater tuberosity *(arrows)*.

disruption of repair when significant atrophy and weakness of the infraspinatus persists after rotator cuff tear repair. In these cases, the authors routinely obtain electrodiagnostic studies.

Suture anchors can dislodge from osteoporotic bone in the greater tuberosity (Fig. 7-31). The use of suture anchors in this region is ill-advised, because the bone becomes osteoporotic from disuse in chronic cases. Fracture of the greater tuberosity when making a bony trough for the repair (Fig. 7-31) can be treated by the use of a bicortical screw and washer as a post to tie sutures around (Fig. 7-16). Failure of the repair at the tendon (i.e., poor suture configuration) and at the bone (i.e., poor transosseous repair)[22,34,41,107] have already been discussed.

Failure of Postoperative Treatment

Postoperative shoulder stiffness usually results from prolonged immobilization after a surgical repair, although the authors have seen loss of passive external rotation after excessively tight closure of the rotator interval. Although closed manipulation can improve motion in some patients who have failed a supervised therapy program, this places the repair at risk for failure. The authors' approach is to perform arthroscopy and release adhesions in the subacromial space to release a thickened, contracted capsule. This approach is discussed in detail in another chapter of this book.

Overzealous patients or therapists can jeopardize the integrity of a repair. Limits prescribed by the surgeon must be carefully adhered to, and loading of the tendons with resistance exercises should be delayed until 4 to 6 months after most cases of large and massive tendon repairs.

SUMMARY

Careful patient selection through a precise and thorough physical examination allows appropriate and realistic treatment alternatives to be selected for each case of massive posterior rotator cuff tear. Some adjuvant imaging studies may be helpful in addition to plain radiographs, but these should be selected on an individual basis and not employed as general screening examinations. If the surgeon uses a methodical surgical technique, as many as 95% of all rotator cuff tears can be repaired. When there is a truly irreparable rotator cuff tear, we have found transfer of the latissimus dorsi tendon to be a useful treatment option.

REFERENCES

1. Aoki M, Ishii I, Vsui M. Clinical application for measuring the slope of the acromion. In: Post M, Hawkins RJ, Morrey BF, eds. Surgery of the shoulder. St Louis, Mosby-Year Book, 1990:200.
2. Aoki M, Okamura K, Fukushima S, et al. Transfer of the latissimus dorsi for irreparable rotator cuff tears. J Bone Joint Surg 1996; 78B:761.
3. Apreleva M, Ozbayder M, Fitzgibbons PG, et al. Rotator cuff tears: the effect of the reconstruction method on three-dimensional repair site area. Arthroscopy 2002;18:519.
4. Arntz CT, Matsen FA III, Jackins S. Surgical management of complex irreparable rotator cuff deficiency. J Arthroplasty 1991;6:363.
5. Bankes MJ, Crossman JE, Emery RJ. A standard method of shoulder measurement for Constant score with a spring balance. J Shoulder Elbow Surg 1998;7:116.
6. Bassett RW, Browne AO, Money BF, et al. Glenohumeral muscle force and moment mechanics in a position of shoulder instability. J Biomechanics 1990;23:403.
7. Bassett RW, Cofield RH. Acute tears of the rotator cuff: the timing of surgical repair. Clin Orthop 1983;175:19.
8. Ben-Yishay A, Zuckerman III, Gallagher M, et al. Pain inhibition of shoulder strength in patients with impingement syndrome. Orthopedics 1994;17:685.
9. Bernageau J. Roentgenographic assessment of the rotator cuff. Clin Orthop 1990;254:87.
10. Bigliani LV, Cordasco FA, McIlveen SJ, et al. Operative repair of massive rotator cuff tears: long-term results. J Shoulder Elbow Surg 1992;1:120.
11. Bigliani LV, Morrison DS, April EW. The morphology of the acromion and rotator cuff impingement. Orthop Trans 1986;7: 138.
12. Bigliani LV, Norris TR, Fischer J, et al. The relationship between the unfused acromial epiphysis and subacromial lesions. Orthop Trans 1983;7:138.
13. Bigliani LV, Ticker JB, Flatow EL, et al. The relationship of acromial architecture to rotator cuff disease. Clin Sports Med 1991;10: 823.
14. Bishop J, Lo I, Klepps S, et al. Cuff integrity following arthroscopic versus open rotator cuff repair: a prospective study. Presented at the 9th International Congress of Surgery of the Shoulder. Washington, DC, May 2–5, 2004.
15. Bjorkenheim JM, Paavolainen P, Ahovuo J, et al. Surgical repair of the rotator cuff and surrounding tissues: factors influencing the results. Clin Orthop 1988;236:148.
16. Borges AF. The relaxed skin tension lines (RSTL) versus other skin lines. Plast Reconstr Surg 1984;73:144.
17. Bourne RB, Bitar H, Andreae PR, et al. In-vivo comparison of four absorbable sutures: Vicryl, Dexon Plus, Maxon, and PDS. Can J Surg 1988;31:43.
18. Burkhart SS. A stepwise approach to arthroscopic rotator cuff repair based on biomechanical principles. Arthroscopy 2000;16 (1):82.
19. Burkhart SS. Reconciling the paradox of rotator cuff repair versus debridement—a unified biomechanical rationale for the treatment of rotator cuff tears. Arthroscopy 1994;10:4.
20. Burkhart SS. Arthroscopic debridement and decompression for selected rotator cuff tears: clinical results, pathomechanics, and patient selection based on biomechanical parameters. Orthop Clin North Am 1993;24:111.
21. Burkhart SS, Nottage WM, Ogilvie-Harris DJ, et al. Partial repair of irreparable rotator cuff tears. Arthroscopy 1994;10(4):363.
22. Caldwell GL, Warner JJP, Miller MD, et al. Strength of fixation with transosseous sutures in rotator cuff repair. J Bone Joint Surg 1997;79A:1064.
23. Calvert PT, Packer NP, Stoker DJ, et al. Arthrography of the shoulder after operative repair of the torn rotator cuff. J Bone Joint Surg 1986;68B:147.
24. Cofield RH. Rotator cuff disease of the shoulder: clinical concepts review. J Bone Joint Surg 1985;67A:974.
25. Cofield RH. Subscapularis muscle transposition for repair of chronic rotator cuff tears. Surg Gynecol Obstet 1982;154:667.
26. Cofield RH. Tears of the rotator cuff. Instr Course Lect 1981;30: 258.
27. Cofield RH, Parvizi J, Hoffmeyer PJ, et al. Surgical repair of chronic rotator cuff tears. A prospective long-term study. J Bone Joint Surg 2001;83A:71.
28. Debeyre J, Patte D, Elmelik E. Repair of ruptures of the rotator cuff of the shoulder, with a note on advancement of the supraspinatus muscle. J Bone Joint Surg 1965;47B:36.
29. DeOrio JK, Cofield RH. Results of a second attempt at surgical repair of a failed initial rotator cuff repair. J Bone Joint Surg 1984; 66A:563.

30. Edelson JG, Zuckerman J, Hershkovitz I. Os acromiale: anatomy and surgical implications. J Bone Joint Surg 1993;75B:551.
31. Ellman H, Hanker G, Bayer M. Repair of the rotator cuff: end result study of factors influencing reconstruction. J Bone Joint Surg 1986;68A:1136.
32. Ellman H, Kay SP, Wirth M. Arthroscopic treatment of full-thickness rotator cuff tears: 2- to 7-year follow-up study. Arthroscopy 1993;9:195.
33. Flatow EL, Soslowsky LJ, Ticker JB, et al. Excursion of the rotator cuff under the acromion: patterns of subacromial contact. J Shoulder Elbow Surg 1993;2:S22.
34. France EP, Paulos LE, Harner CD, et al. Biomechanical evaluation of rotator cuff fixation methods. Am J Sports Med 1989;17:176.
35. Fuchs B, Weishaupt D, Zanetti M, et al. Fatty degeneration of the muscles of the rotator cuff: assessment by computed tomography versus magnetic resonance imaging. J Shoulder Elbow Surg 1999;8:599.
36. Galatz LM, Ball CM, Teeley SA, et al. The outcome and repair integrity of completely arthroscopically repaired large and massive rotator cuff tears. J Bone Joint Surg 2004;86A:219.
37. Gazielly DJ, Gleyze P, Montagnau C. Functional and anatomic results after rotator cuff repair. Clin Orthop 1994;304:43.
38. Gerber C. Latissimus dorsi transfer for the treatment of irreparable tears of the rotator cuff. Clin Orthop 1992;275:152.
39. Gerber C, Fuchs B, Hodler J. The results of repair of massive tears of the rotator cuff. J Bone Joint Surg 2000;82A:505.
40. Gerber C, Meyer DC, Schneeberger AG, et al. The effect of tendon release and delayed repair on the structure of the involved muscles of the rotator cuff. An experimental study using a new animal model. J Bone Joint Surg Am (In print, 2004).
41. Gerber C, Schneeberger AG, Beck M, et al. Mechanical strength of repairs of the rotator cuff. J Bone Joint Surg 1994;76B:371.
42. Gerber C, Schneeberger AG, Perren SM, et al. Experimental rotator cuff repair: a preliminary study. J Bone Joint Surg 1999;81A:1281.
43. Gerber C, Terrier F, Ganz R. The role of the coracoid process in the chronic impingement syndrome. J Bone Joint Surg 1985;67B:703.
44. Gerber C, Vinh TS, Hertel R, et al. Latissimus dorsi transfer for the treatment of massive tears of the rotator cuff: a preliminary report. Clin Orthop 1988;232:51.
45. Gilcrest EL. The common syndrome of rupture, dislocation, and elongation of the biceps brachii: an analysis of one hundred cases. Surg Gynecol Obstet 1948;58:322.
46. Goutallier D, Postel J-M, Bernageau J, et al. Fatty muscle degeneration in cuff ruptures. Clin Orthop 1994;304:78.
47. Goutallier D, Postel J-M, Gleyze P, et al. Influence of cuff muscle fatty degeneration on anatomic and functional outcome after simple suture of full-thickness tears. J Shoulder Elbow Surg 2003;12:550.
48. Groh GI, Simoni M, Rolla P, et al. Loss of the deltoid after shoulder operations: an operative disaster. J Shoulder Elbow Surg 1994;3:243.
49. Gschwend N, Ivosevec-Radavanovic D, Patte D. Rotator cuff tear-relationship between clinical anatomic-pathological findings. Acta Orthop Scand 1988;107:7.
50. Ha'Eri GB, Wiley AM. Advancement of the supraspinatus muscle in the repair of ruptures of the rotator cuff. J Bone Joint Surg 1981;63A:232.
51. Harryman DT, Mach LA, Wang KA, et al. Repairs of the rotator cuff: correlation of functional results with integrity of the cuff. J Bone Joint Surg 1991;73A:982.
52. Hawkins RJ, Misamore GW, Hobeika PE. Surgery for full thickness rotator cuff tears. J Bone Joint Surg 1985;67A:1349.
53. Heikel HV. Rupture of the rotator cuff of the shoulder: experiences of surgical treatment. Acta Orthop Scand 1968;39:477.
54. Hersche O, Gerber C. Passive tension in the supraspinatus musculotendinous unit after long-standing rupture of its tendon: a preliminary report. J Shoulder Elbow Surg 1998;7:393.
55. Hertel R, Ballmer FT, Lambert SM, et al. Lag signs for diagnosis of rotator cuff rupture. J Shoulder Elbow Surg 1996;5:307.
56. Hodler J, Fretz CJ, Terrier F, et al. Rotator cuff tears: correlation of sonographic and surgical findings. Radiology 1988;169:791.
57. Iannotti JP, Zlatkin MB, Esterhai JL, et al. Magnetic resonance imaging of the shoulder: sensitivity, specificity, and predictive value. J Bone Joint Surg 1991;73A:17.
58. Inman VT, Saunders JR, Abbott LC. Observations on the function of the shoulder joint. J Bone Joint Surg 1944;26:1.
59. Itoi E, Kuechle DK, Newman SR, et al. Stabilizing function of the biceps in stable and unstable shoulders. J Bone Joint Surg 1993;75B:546.
60. Jost B, Pfirrman CW, Gerber C, et al. Clinical outcome after structural failure of rotator cuff repairs. J Bone Joint Surg 2000;82A:304.
61. Keating IF, Waterworth P, Shaw-Dunn J, et al. The relative strength of the rotator cuff muscles. J Bone Joint Surg 1993;75B:137.
62. Kraissel CJ. Selection of appropriate lines for elective surgery. Plast Reconstr Surg 1951;8:1.
63. Krackow KA, Thomas SC, James LC. A new stitch for ligament-tendon fixation: brief note. J Bone Joint Surg 1986;68A:764.
64. Kumar VP, Satku K. The role of the long head of biceps brachii in stabilization of the head of the humerus. Clin Orthop 1989;244:172.
65. LeClerq R. Diagnostique de la rupture du sous-epineoux. Rev Rhum 1950;10:510.
66. Lehtenin JT, Tingart MJ, Apreleva M, et al. Practical assessment of rotator cuff muscle volume using MRI. Acta Orthop Scand 2003;74(6):722.
67. Lo IK, Burkhart SS. Arthroscopic repair of massive, contracted, immobile rotator cuff tears using single and double interval slides: technique and preliminary results. Arthroscopy 2004;20(1):22.
68. Lundberg BJ. The correlation of clinical evaluation with operative findings and prognosis in rotator cuff rupture. In: Bayley I, Kessel L, eds. Shoulder surgery. Berlin, Springer-Verlag, 1982:35.
69. McMahon PJ, Debski RE, Thompson WO, et al. Shoulder muscle forces and tendon excursions during scapular plane abduction. J Shoulder Elbow Surg 1995;4:199.
70. McLaughlin HL. Lesions of the musculotendinous cuff of the shoulder. I. The exposure and treatment of tears with retraction. J Bone Joint Surg 1944;26:31.
71. Meister K, Thesing J, Montgomery WJ, et al. MR arthrography of partial thickness tears of the undersurface of the rotator cuff: an arthroscopic correlation. Skeletal Radiol 2004;33:136.
72. Melillo AS, Savoie FH, Field LD. Massive rotator cuff tears: debridement versus repair. Orthop Clin North Am 1997;28(1):117.
73. Meyer DC, Fucentese SF, Koller B, et al. Association of osteopenia of the humeral head with full-thickness rotator cuff tears. J Shoulder Elbow Surg 2004;13:333.
74. Meyer DC, Hoppeler H, von Rechenberg B, et al. A pathomechanical concept explains muscle loss and fatty muscular changes following tendinous tear and muscle retraction. J Orthop Res (In print, 2004).
75. Meyer DC, Jacob HA, Nyffeler RW, et al. In vivo tendon force measurement of 2-week duration in sheep. J Biomech 2004;37(1):135.
76. Miniaci A, Dowdy PA, Willits KR, et al. Magnetic resonance imaging evaluation of the rotator cuff tendons in the asymptomatic shoulder. Am J Sports Med 1995;23:142.
77. Miniaci A, Mac Leod M. Transfer of the latissimus dorsi muscle after failed repair of a massive tear of the rotator cuff: a two to five year review. J Bone Joint Surg 1999;81A:1120.
78. Morrison DS, Bigliani LU. The clinical significance of variations in acromial morphology. Orthop Trans 1987;11:234.
79. Mudge MK, Wood VE, Frykman GK. Rotator cuff tears associated with os acromiale. J Bone Joint Surg 1984;66A:427.
80. Nakagaki K, Ozaki J, Tomita Y, et al. Alterations in the supraspinatus muscle belly with rotator cuff tearing: evaluation with magnetic resonance imaging. J Shoulder Elbow Surg 1994;3:88.
81. Neer CS II. Shoulder reconstruction. Philadelphia, WB Saunders, 1990:41.
82. Neer CS. Anterior acromioplasty for the chronic impingement syndrome in the shoulder: a preliminary report. J Bone Joint Surg 1972;54A:41.
83. Neer CS, Satterlee CC, Dalsey RM, et al. On the value of the coracohumeral ligament release. Orthop Trans 1989;13:235.
84. Neviaser JS, Neviaser RJ, Neviaser TJ. The repair of chronic massive ruptures of the rotator cuff on the shoulder by use of a freeze-dried rotator cuff. J Bone Joint Surg 1978;60A:681.
85. Neviaser RJ, Neviaser TJ. Transfer of the subscapularis and teres minor for massive defects of rotator cuff. In: Bayley I, Kessel L, eds. Shoulder surgery. Berlin, Springer-Verlag, 1982:60.

86. Neviaser RJ, Neviaser TJ, Neviaser JS. Concurrent rupture of the rotator cuff and anterior dislocation of the shoulder in older patients. J Bone Joint Surg 1988;70:1308.

87. Norwood LA, Barrack R, Jacobson KE. Clinical presentation of complete tears of the rotator cuff. J Bone Joint Surg 1989;71A:494.

88. Nove-Josserand L, Levigne C, Noel E, et al. The acromio-humeral interval. A study of factors influencing its height. Rev Chir Orthop Reparatrice Appar Mot (French) ;82:379.

89. Ono K, Yamamuro T, Rockwood CA Jr. Use of the thirty-degree caudal tilt radiograph in the shoulder impingement syndrome. J Shoulder Elbow Surg 1992;1:246.

90. Ozaki J, Fujimoto S, Masuhara K, et al. Reconstruction of chronic massive rotator cuff tears with synthetic materials. Clin Orthop 1986;202:173.

91. Petersson C. Long-term results of rotator cuff repair. In: Bayley I, Kessel L, eds. Shoulder surgery. Berlin, Springer-Verlag, 1982:64.

92. Poppen NK, Walker PS. Forces at the glenohumeral joint in abduction. Clin Orthop 1978;58:165.

93. Post M. Rotator cuff repair with carbon fiber filament: a preliminary report of five cases. Clin Orthop 1985;196:154.

94. Prickett WD, Teffey SA, Galatz LM, et al. Accuracy of ultrasonography of rotator cuff in shoulders that are painful postoperatively. J Bone Joint Surg 2003;85A:1084.

95. Rathburn JB, Macnab I. The microvascular pattern of the rotator cuff. J Bone Joint Surg 1970;52B:540.

96. Reeves B. Experiments on tensile strength of the anterior capsular structures of the shoulder in man. J Bone Joint Surg 1968;50B: 858.

97. Rockwood CA, Burkhead WZ. Management of patients with massive rotator cuff defects by acromioplasty and rotator cuff debridement. Orthop Trans 1988;12:190.

98. Rockwood CA Jr, Matsen FA III. The shoulder. Philadelphia, WB Saunders, 1990:647.

99. Rockwood CA Jr, Williams GR, Burkhead WZ Jr. Debridement of degenerated irreparable lesions of the rotator cuff. J Bone Joint Surg 1995;77A:857.

100. Romeo AA, Hang DW, Bach BR Jr, et al. Repair of full thickness rotator cuff tears. Gender, age and other factors affecting outcome. Clin Orthop 1999;367:243.

101. Reinus WR, Shady KL, Mirowitz SA, et al. MR diagnosis of rotator cuff tears of the shoulder: value of using T2 weighted fat-saturated images. Am J Roentgenol 1995;164:1451.

102. Soslowsky LJ, Carpenter JE, Buchieri JS, et al. Biomechanics of rotator cuff. Orthop Clin North Am 1997;28:17.

103. Shimizu T, Itoi E, Minagawa H, et al. Atrophy of the rotator cuff muscles and site of cuff tears. Acta Orthop Scand 2002;73:40.

104. Singson RD, Hoang J, San S, et al. MR evaluation of rotator cuff pathology using T2-weighted fat spin-echo technique with and without fat surpression. Am J Roentgenol 1996;166:1061.

105. Stone IK, von Fraunhofer JA, Masterson BJ. Mechanical properties of coated absorbable monofilament suture materials. Obstet Gynecol 1986;67:737.

106. Sugaya H, Moriishi J, Tsuchiya A. Postoperative cuff integrity after arthroscopic full thickness rotator cuff repair: single-row versus dual-row fixation. Presented at the 9th International Congress of Surgery of the Shoulder. Washington, DC, May 2–5, 2004.

107. Sward L, Hughes JS, Wallace WA. The strength of surgical repairs of the rotator cuff. J Bone Joint Surg 1992;74B:585.

108. Tauro JC. Arthroscopic repair of large rotator cuff tears using the interval slide technique. Arthroscopy 2004;20:13.

109. Teefey SA, Rubin DA, Middleton WD, et al. Detection and quantification of rotator cuff tears. Comparison of ultrasonographic, magnetic resonance imaging, and arthroscopic findings in seventy-one consecutive cases. J Bone Joint Surg 2004;86A:708.

110. Thompson WO, Debski RE, Boardman ND III, et al. A biomechanical analysis of rotator cuff deficiency in a cadaveric model. Am J Sports Med 1996;24:286.

111. Ticker JB, Bigliani LU. The coracoacromial arch and rotator cuff tendinopathy. Sports Med Arthrosc Rev 1995;3:8.

112. Tingart MJ, Apreleva M, Zurakowski D, et al. Pullout strength of suture anchors in RCR. J Bone Joint Surg Am 2003;85A (11): 2190.

113. Tingart MJ, Apreleva M, Lehtenin JT, et al. Magnetic resonance imaging in quantitative analysis of rotator cuff muscle volume. Clin Orthop 2003;415:104.

114. Tuite MJ, Asinger D, Orwin JF. Angled oblique sagittal MR imaging of rotator cuff tears: comparison with standard oblique sagittal images. Skeletal Radiol 2001;30:262.

115. Walch G, Boulahia A, Calderone S, et al. The "dropping" and "hornblower's" signs in evaluation of rotator cuff tears. J Bone Joint Surg 1998;80B:624.

116. Walch G, Edwards TB, Nove-Josserand L, et al. Arthroscopic tenotomy of the long head of the biceps in the treatment of rotator cuff tears. Clinical and radiographic results of 307 cases. J Shoulder Elbow Surg (in press, 2004).

117. Walch G, Nove-Josserand L, Boileau P, et al. Subluxation and dislocation of the tendon of the long head of the biceps. J Shoulder Elbow Surg 1998;7:100.

118. Warner JJP. Management of massive, irreparable rotator cuff tears: the role of tendon transfer. Instr Course Lect 2001;50:63.

119. Warner JJP, Allen AA, Gerber C. Diagnosis and management of sub-scapularis tendon tears. Tech Orthop 1994;9:116.

120. Warner JJP, Higgins L, Parsons IM IV, et al. Diagnosis and treatment of anterosuperior rotator cuff tears. J Shoulder Elbow Surg 2001;10:37.

121. Warner JJP, Krushell RJ, Masquelet A, et al. Anatomy and relationships of the suprascapular nerve: anatomical constraints to mobilization of the supraspinatus and infraspinatus muscles in the management of massive rotator-cuff tears. J Bone Joint Surg 1992;74A:36.

122. Warner JJP, McMahon PJ. The role of the long head of biceps brachii in superior stability of the glenohumeral joint. J Bone Joint Surg 1995;77A:366.

123. Warner JJP, Parsons IM IV: Latissimus dorsi transfer: a comparative analysis of primary and salvage reconstruction of massive, irreparable rotator cuff tears. J Shoulder Elbow Surg 2001;10:514.

124. Warner JJP, Waskowitz R, Marks PH, et al. Function in patients with massive rotator cuff tears: with attention to muscle atrophy. Presented at the annual meeting of the American Academy of Orthopaedic Surgeons, San Francisco, CA, February 18–20, 1993.

125. Watson M. Major rupture of the rotator cuff: the results of surgical repair in 89 patients. J Bone Joint Surg 1985;67B:618.

126. Weiner DS, MacNab I. Superior migration of the humeral head. J Bone Joint Surg 1970;52B:524.

127. Wolfgang GL. Surgical repair of the rotator cuff of the shoulder: factors influencing the result. J Bone Joint Surg 1974;56A:14.

128. Yamaguchi K, Riew KD, Galatz LM, et al. Biceps activity during shoulder motion: an electromyographic analysis. Clin Orthop 1997;336:122.

129. Yao L, Mehta U. Infraspinatus muscle atrophy: implications? Radiology 2003;226:161.

130. Yerguson RM. Rupture of the biceps. J Bone Joint Surg 1931;13:160.

131. Zanotti M, Jost B, Lustenberger A, et al. Clinical impact of MR arthrography of the shoulder. Acta Radiol 1999;40:296.

Arthroscopic Repair of Rotator Cuff Tears

8

Laurent Lafosse

INTRODUCTION

The surgical management of rotator cuff tear (RCT) is established by the patient's need for pain relief and improved function and the surgical feasibility based on the surgeon's experience and expertise. The associated symptoms may be explained by subacromial impingement with or without a rotator cuff tear. Historically, French surgeons divided the treatment options into two groups. One group recommended an isolated acromioplasty and obtained satisfactory results in terms of pain, mobility, and function, but without restoring the strength of the shoulder and potentially allowing further increase in the size of the tear and progression of arthritis.[2] The other group proposed isolated tendon tear repair without treating the impingement, a treatment mode that was followed by a high rate of rerupture. Didier Patte was the first surgeon in Europe to combine the two methods and developed the classic anterior release technique called "Grande Liberation Antérieure." This rather aggressive method excised the acromioclavicular articulation and raised four delto-trapezoid flaps, exposing the posterosuperior cuff and the upper third of the subscapularis tendon.

Charles Neer, in the United States, described a less invasive method, which involved an anterior approach to the acromion and cuff starting with an acromioplasty. Potentially, this method allowed simultaneous treatment of impingement and the possibility of tendon repair.[21,22] At the beginning of shoulder arthroscopy, only the acromioplasty was performed arthroscopically. Later on, the rotator cuff repairs were managed by adding a small lateral approach and minimally separating the deltoid fibres to access the

ruptured tendon.[1,8,10,20] In 1988, G. Gartsman published the first results of full arthroscopic rotator cuff repair.[9]

Indications and techniques for management of rotator cuff tears differ among authors. Some manage them only by acromioplasty (mostly arthroscopically).[20,14,23,26] Others always avoid acromioplasty[13] when they repair the cuff. Rotator cuff repair can be done by open, mini-open, or arthroscopic technique. The author started arthroscopic technique in 1992 and, since 2000, has managed all rotator cuff repairs arthroscopically.

PREOPERATIVE ASSESSMENT

When preparing to perform an arthroscopic rotator cuff repair (ARCR), it is necessary to establish a set of preoperative data that includes the following: functional evaluation, clinical evaluation, imaging, and classification of the rotator cuff tear.

Functional Evaluation

A patient questionnaire must be completed, providing the functional information necessary to complete the Constant University of California Los Angeles (UCLA) and American Shoulder and Elbow Surgeon (ASES) shoulder scores.[4,7,25] One should assess the patient's level of pain, limitation in athletic and work activities, and limitation in his or her activities of daily living. If a patient is unclear on how to answer these questions, the physician or office staff should help clarify the questions.

Clinical Evaluation

Atrophy of the deltoid, the supraspinatus, and the infraspinatus muscles should be evaluated. Passive range of

L. Lafosse: Annecy, France.

motion and tenderness of the acromioclavicular and sternoclavicular joints are evaluated to rule out alternate or additional causes of pain and disability other than RCT. The passive and active mobility of both shoulders is measured, beginning with the unaffected side. The supraspinatus strength is tested with the Jobe sign.[16] This may be unreliable due to pain-related weakness. The infraspinatus strength is tested by performing external rotation lag sign with the elbow at the side, and the subscapularis strength is tested by the liftoff test if internal rotation is not limited and by the belly-press test as described by Gerber et al[12] and modified by pushing against the elbow of the patient (Fig. 8-1). Clinical evaluation of symptoms from the long head of the biceps is more difficult. The author uses the abduction rotation external supination (ARES) and abduction rotation internal supination (ARIS) test. In this test the patient does a forced supination against resistance, with the arm positioned in 90 degrees of abduction and 90 degrees of external rotation (ARES) (Fig. 8-2) or internal rotation (ARIS) (Fig. 8-3). In both situations, the biceps must be a normal tendon and must have good anterior (in external rotation) and posterior (in internal rotation) ligaments at the entrance of the groove to be stable. When the biceps is damaged and/or unstable, subluxation of the tendon will occur over the edge of the bony groove and may be painful or weaker than on the other side. Strength is measured by a simple handheld spring scale placed around the wrist with the elbow outstretched.

Imaging

Imaging includes:

1. Radiographs: true A–P, outlet-view, and acromioclavicular. The height of the subacromial space, arthritis by Samuelson score, and the condition of the acromioclavicular articulation are evaluated.

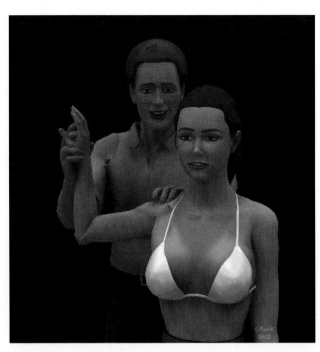

Figure 8-2   ARES: abduction, external rotation supination test.

2. Arthro-CT scan to define the morphology of the tendon tear and to assess muscular atrophy and fatty degeneration.[14] In the author's practice the Arthro-CT has more specificity and sensitivity than MRI.

3. Arthro-MRI is only required for a partial tear that we evaluate with the Codman classification.[3]

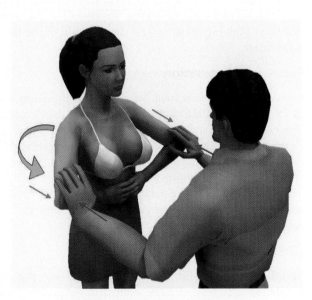

Figure 8-1   Modified subscapularis test.

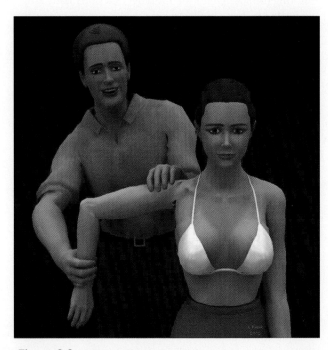

Figure 8-3   ARIS: abduction, internal rotation suprination test.

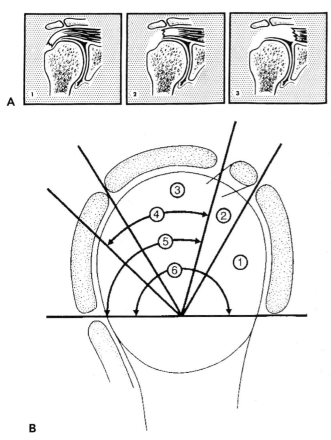

Figure 8-4   Cuff tear classification: (*A*) Sagittal view and (*B*) Coronal view.

Classification of the Rotator Cuff Tear

The author uses the Patte classification,[24] which evaluates the retraction and location of the tear within sagittal and coronal planes (Fig. 8-4). Partial tears are classified as deep, superficial, or intratendinous (Fig. 8-5). A modified Patte classification defines massive tears: at least three involved tendons of which at least one is retracted to the glenoid.

SURGICAL PRINCIPLES

Anesthesia

An interscalene block is performed with or without general anesthesia. The patient is placed in a fully seated, upright

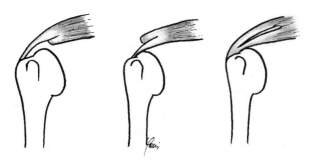

Figure 8-5   Partial cuff tear.

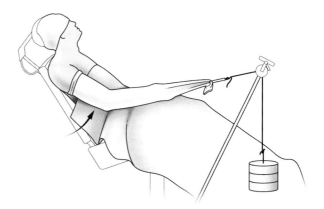

Figure 8-6   Beach-chair position with traction.

position with the arm flexed forward and under traction by weights of about 3 kg (Fig. 8-6). This procedure can be done in the lateral decubitus position, but the author prefers the seated position.

Portals

Five approaches are currently used (Fig. 8-7). The first classical posterior glenohumeral approach is used for the scope, that we translate 3 cm medially as modified by Jan Leudzinger, when AC joint access is planned. A second posterosuperior approach, situated at the posterolateral angle of the acromion, is used for viewing the subacromial space. The two instrument portals are initially localized using a spinal needle working from outside-in, representing the classical lateral acromioplasty portal and another anterior portal near

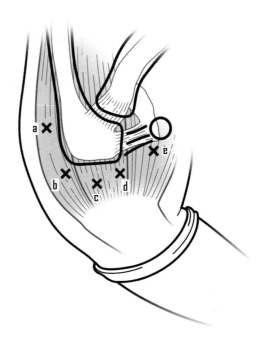

Figure 8-7   Portals.

the coracoacromial ligament. The fifth approach is anterosuperior at the anterolateral corner of the acromion.

Before arthroscopy, 20 cc of 1% lidocaine with epinephrine are injected into the glenohumeral articulation and the subacromial bursa to reduce bleeding.

Diagnostic Arthroscopy

A systematic assessment of the glenohumeral and subacromial space is done both statically and dynamically, and the tissue is probed for stability. After a complete visualization,

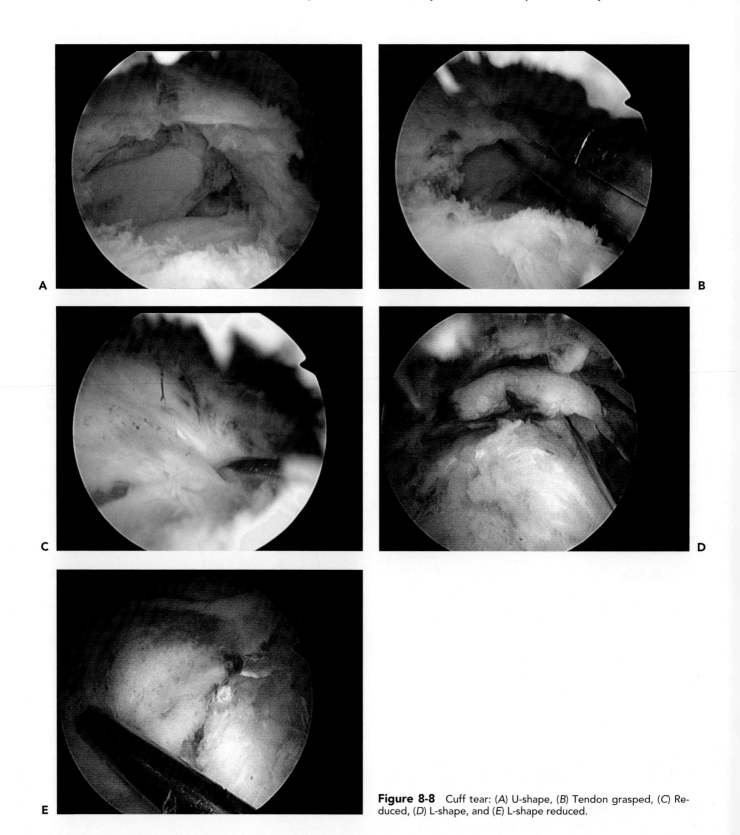

Figure 8-8 Cuff tear: (*A*) U-shape, (*B*) Tendon grasped, (*C*) Reduced, (*D*) L-shape, and (*E*) L-shape reduced.

the degree of cuff retraction and mobilization to the insertion site is tested. When needed a periglenoid capsular and subacromial release is performed so that the tendon can be easily pulled to the tuberosity with the arm by the patient's side. The release is essential to perform the repair without excessive tension. Mobilization is performed from medial to lateral for U-shape tears (Fig. 8-8, *A–C*) or by reducing with traction on the tendon combined with humeral rotation in L-shape tears (Fig. 8-8, *D* and *E*). Special attention is given when delamination occurs to repair both deep and superficial leaves of the tear; this is more commonly seen in massive posterior cuff tear.

The stability of the origin of the long head of the biceps tendon is evaluated with a probe. Its stability within the groove is inspected while the arm is passively moved into internal and external position in order to assess the anterior and posterior pulley. Instability may require repair, tenodesis, or tendon release.

The plan for further treatment is made intraoperatively based on cuff tear size as described by Patte, on the ability to mobilize the cuff to the tuberosity, and on the biceps tendon and muscle quality,.

Release

For large retracted tears the intra-articular capsular and subacromial release is essential to mobilize the tear and decrease the traction on the repair. This is performed with a radiofrequency device (VAPR Mitek, Johnson and Johnson, Norwood, MA).

For posterosuperior cuff tears, the coracoacromial ligament is released from the base of the coracoid at the anterosuperior edge of the glenoid rim with intra-articular assessment. The capsule is released above the labrum from the anterior superior to posterior superior quadrants. Release bursal side scar tissue is removed medially until the cuff muscle is seen.

Special care must be given to the subscapularis release for massive retracted tendons because it usually requires visualization of the axillary nerve and the medial plexus with the axillary artery (Fig. 8-9). This can be a dangerous part of the surgery that should not be done by arthroscopy without advanced expertise.

Acromioplasty

Acromioplasty is systematically performed in addition to the tendon repair, except for massive, partially repairable ruptures where the CA arch is the last structural element to keep superior stability and avoid anterior superior escape of the humeral head. If lack of space impedes the exposure or the passage of the instruments, acromioplasty is performed prior to repair of the tendon. Otherwise it is done after repair to avoid additionalbleeding during the repair. The coracoacromial ligament is released with an electrocautery. A burr is used to remove bone from the acromion starting at the anterior lateral corner and proceeding medial to the AC joint to achieve a flat type I acromion (Fig. 8-10).

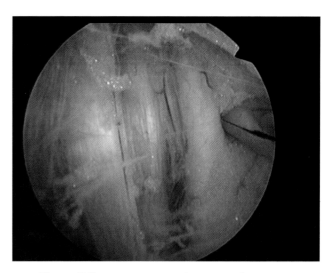

Figure 8-9 Intraoperative arthroscopic plexus view.

AC Joint Resection

When necessary, AC joint resection is done after acromioplasty in three steps:

1. Using the posterolateral portal for visualization, the soft tissue and medial portion of the acromial facet of the AC joint are removed, exposing the distal clavicle. The inferior osteophyte of the distal clavicle is removed.
2. An anterior superior portal is placed into the AC joint, to introduce the burr. Bone is removed from both the acromion and clavicle bone with visualization from the lateral portal. Special care must be taken to remove the posterior and superior clavicle spur, while preserving the attachment of the posterior and superior AC capsular ligaments.
3. A final posterior visualization from the modified posterior portal (previously described) checks the anterior clavicle, ensuring that the superior AC ligament is intact (Fig. 8-11).

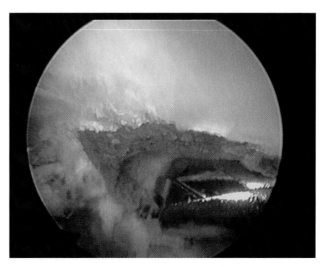

Figure 8-10 Acromioplasty.

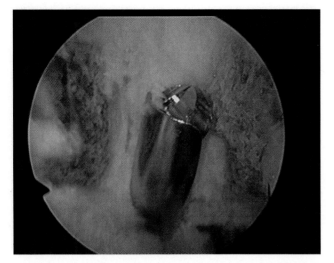

Figure 8-11 AC joint resection.

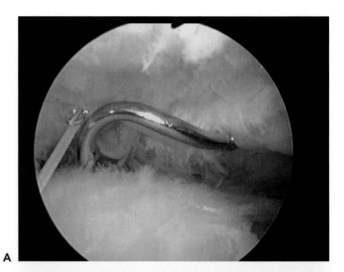

A

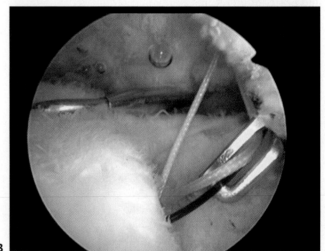

B

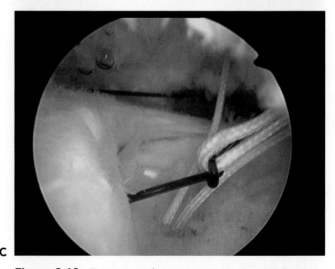

C

Tendon Fixation

Anchors. The type of fixation depends on the bone quality and influences the technique used for anchor insertion. The use of push-in anchors (vs. thread in anchors) enables the surgeon to first pass a suture through the cuff, then load the anchor with the suture and place the anchor in bone. When using screw-in anchors or anchors with two preloaded sutures, an anchor-in first technique is required. The author typically uses metallic implants and reserves the use of absorbable anchors. Tendon attachment is close to articular cartilage when restoring the medial foot print of the rotator cuff or when performing a biceps tenodesis.

Location of the fixation is done according to the lesion, but whenever possible, restoring the normal footprint of the rotator cuff is performed by adding a double row of anchors. One row restores the lateral tendon attachment and the other medial cartilaginous attachment.

Suture No. 2 or No. 3 is always a braided nonabsorbable. PDS sutures break before tendon healing.

Different techniques to pass the braided suture through the tendon using different devices must be available.

■ A two-step technique uses a suture passer (Spectrum, Linvatec, Largo, FL) equipped with a 45-degree curved hook (left-rotated mostly used for a right shoulder and vice versa), loaded with a simple PDS No. 0 pushed through the hook (Fig. 8-12A). The PDS is grasped by forceps and can be pulled out through the same or a different portal easily (the length is as long as necessary), even during or after the suture passer is through the tendon. The PDS is easily used as a shuttle relay for passing a nonabsorbable suture, which is already fixed to an anchor (Fig. 8-12B). This avoids any twist or soft-tissue interposition when many sutures are used (Fig. 8-12C).

Figure 8-12 Two-step technique suture passing. (*A*) Spectrum hook. (*B*) Both PDS and braided suture grasped. (*C*) Suture retrieved through anterior portal.

■ Direct braided suture passing is done in two ways:
1. A needle loaded with the suture is grasped by a second retriever (Fig. 8-13), and the instrument from a second instrument portal is used to grasp the suture. Alternatively, the same instrument can be used in the same portal by a straight-shaped (Fig. 8-14) or a curve-shaped instrument (Fig. 8-15) once the tendon is perforated. A special on-shuttle instrument allows for this to be done in one step (Fig. 8-16). The diffi-

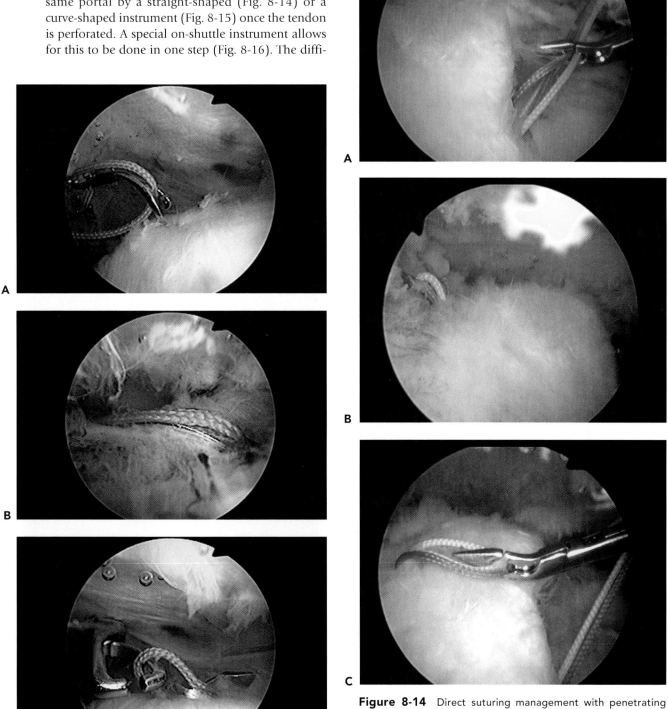

A

B

C

Figure 8-13 Direct suturing management with suture leader. (*A*) Coming from front. (*B*) Going through the tendon. (*C*) Grasper taking the overloaded suture.

A

B

C

Figure 8-14 Direct suturing management with penetrating grasper. (*A*) Catching suture. (*B*) Going through tendon. (*C*) Catching suture back.

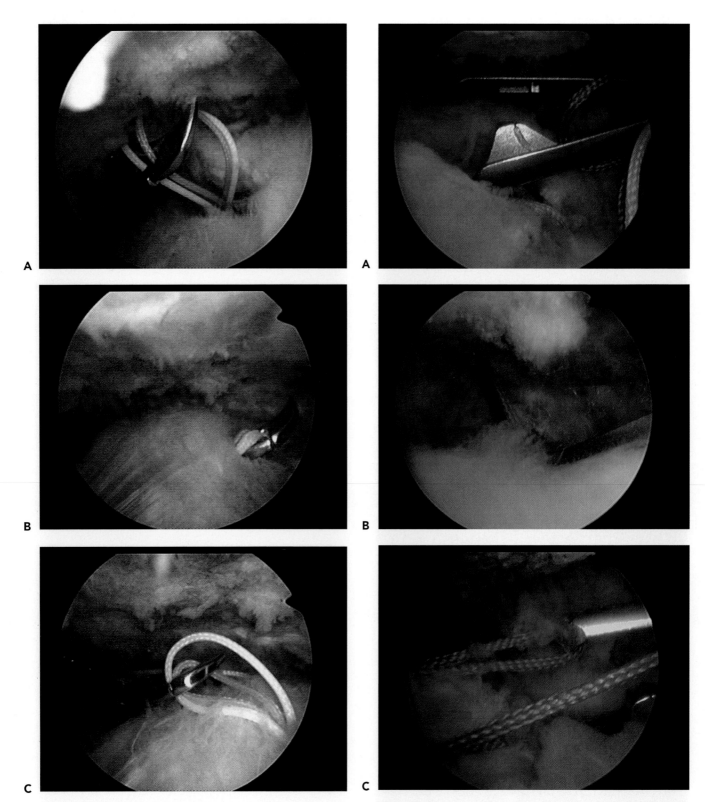

Figure 8-15 Direct suturing management with Clever hook. (*A*) Catching suture. (*B*) Going through tendon. (*C*) Catching suture back.

Figure 8-16 Direct suturing with ExpresSew device (Surgical Solutions, Carlsbad, CA). (*A*) Catching suture. (*B*) Going through tendon. (*C*) Catching suture back.

culty lies in releasing the suture from the instrument, without pulling it out of the tendon, and grasping it with the same instrument.

2. A suture is retrieved by using a perforating grasper already passed through the tendon. The difficulties with this technique are anticipating the position of the retriever and preparing to bring the suture to the retriever (Fig. 8-17).

The key to the tendon perforation is the access and the direction of the device to perforate the tendon as perpendicular as possible to the direction of the fibers. An in-line device must come from the top or the bottom of the tendon. A curved device should come in perpendicular to the tendon (from either the anterior or posterior portal for the supraspinatus tendon), except for the ExpresSew (Arthrex), which has a different-shaped needle that can perforate the side of the tendon.

Different stitches are possible (Fig. 8-18):

- Simple stitch
- U shape by perforating the cuff from the superficial to the deep layer and back by twisting the perforating hook in one pass of the instrument, to realize a guy rope attachment
- A mattress suture by performing successive passage of the suture through the cuff

The knot used is either a sliding knot called "easy knot"(Fig. 8-19, A and B)[17] or successive half loops, when the suture does not slide in the anchor. The difficulty of successive half hitches is to keep the first half hitch tight while making the second tight. A flat "double first half loop" as first knot is commonly used (Fig. 8-19, C–F). Whichever knot is used, it is essential that the surgeon is comfortable with it and trained before being in the operating room.

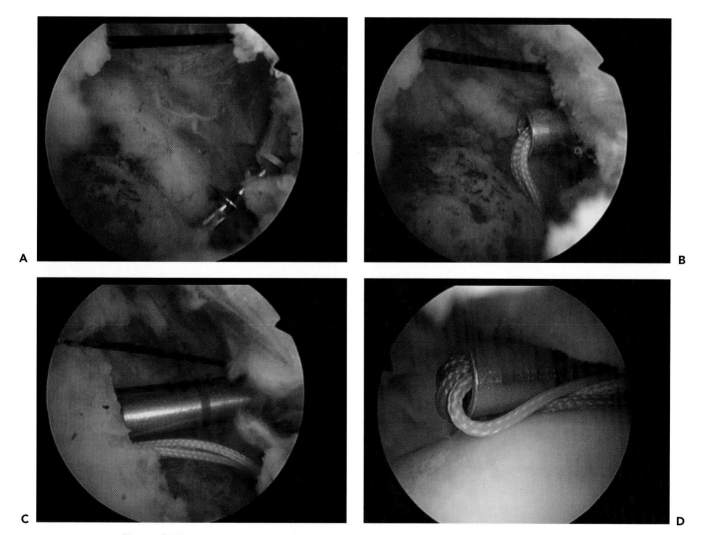

Figure 8-17 Direct suturing by retrieving with Clever hook. (*A*) Lateral anchor from bursal view. (*B*) 2 sutures, 4 post. (*C*) All punched with the screw handle. (*D*) Intra-articular view. *(continued)*

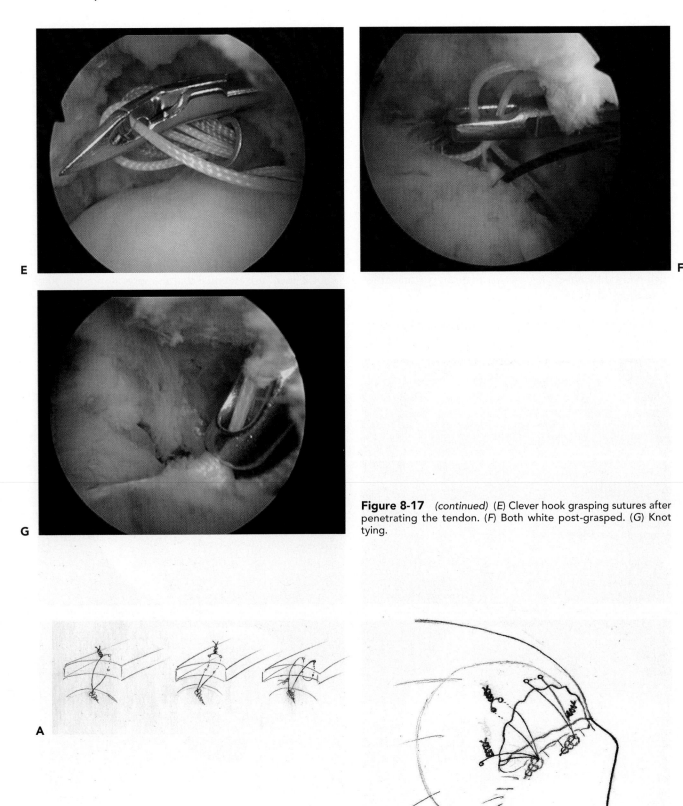

Figure 8-17 *(continued)* (*E*) Clever hook grasping sutures after penetrating the tendon. (*F*) Both white post-grasped. (*G*) Knot tying.

Figure 8-18 (*A,B*) Three different stitches: S (simple), U (horizontal mattress), and Guy-rope.

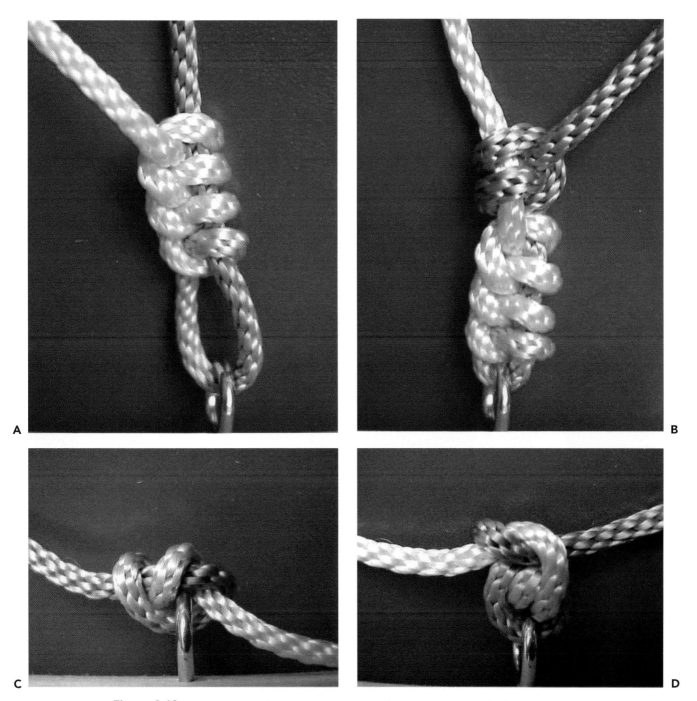

Figure 8-19   Knots. (*A*) Easy knot: step one. (*B*) Easy knot: step two. (*C*) Flat knot: step one. (*D*) Flat knot: step two. *(continued)*

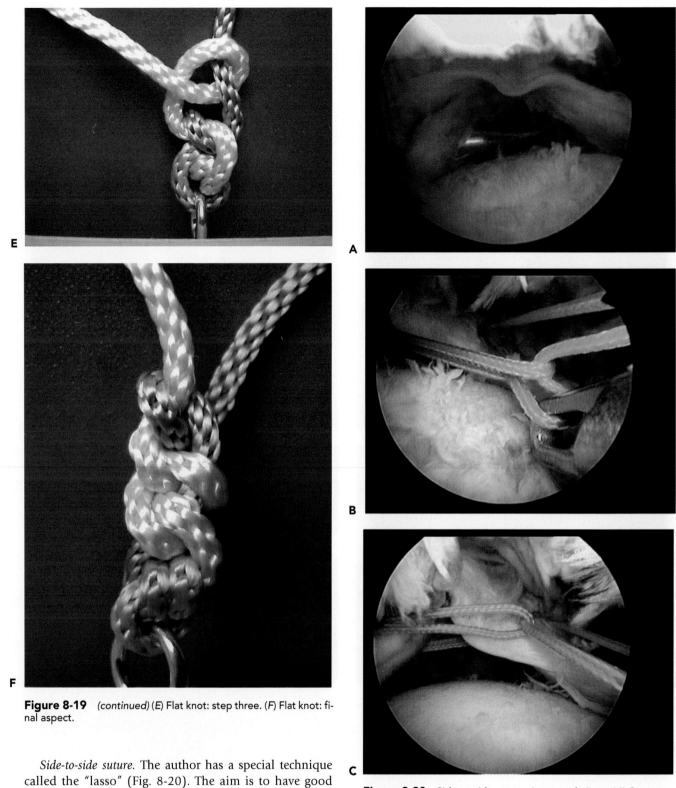

E

F

A

B

C

Figure 8-19 *(continued)* (E) Flat knot: step three. (F) Flat knot: final aspect.

Figure 8-20 Side-to-side suture: Lasso technique. (A) Step one. (B) Step two. (C) Step three. *(continued)*

Side-to-side suture. The author has a special technique called the "lasso" (Fig. 8-20). The aim is to have good strength of the suture when tightened. Once a double braided suture is passed through the two tendons or two edges of the same tendon, then one of the free ends of the same suture is passed through the loop located on the other side. The suture through the loop is tied to the other side of the suture. When the suture is pulled through the loop, it

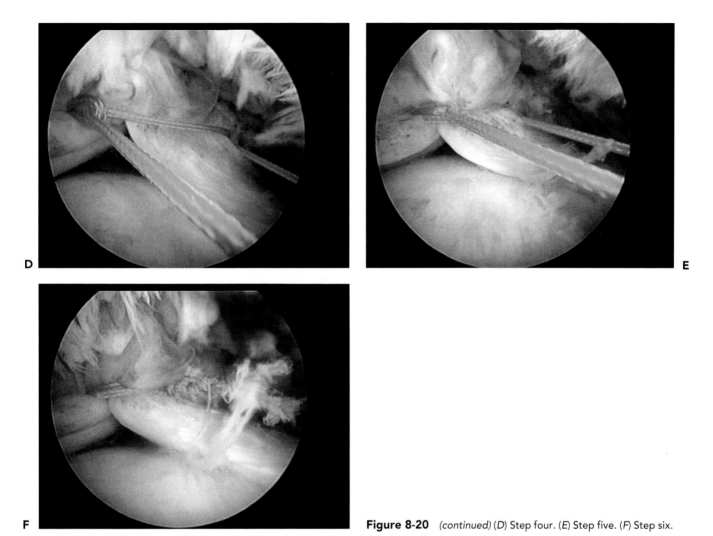

D

E

F

Figure 8-20 *(continued) (D)* Step four. *(E)* Step five. *(F)* Step six.

gives a perfect method for tightening the suture on the tendons.

Cannula. In most circumstances the author avoids the use of cannula in the subacromial space because it extends to the size of the portals and does not avoid fluid leaking, especially when the sutures pass through the diaphragm of the cannula. A cannula is used for the lateral portal when several anchors are used so as not to entrap the deltoid fibers or when the device used for going through the tendon charges the suture outside the shoulder. Instrument portals are switched often and extra portals added to adapt to the lesion and have perfect access for the scope and the instruments. Fluid pressure is kept low, and surgery must be performed in an efficient manner because swelling will make the repair very difficult after 180 minutes.

Based on the lesion and the anchor situation, visualization during the repair may be first done from the glenohumeral joint for subscapularis repairs or from the subacromial side for posterior superior tears.

At the end of the surgery the quality of the repair is checked and judged from the subacromial and the glenohumeral joint (reduction, tension, tightness).

SURGICAL TECHNIQUE

Partial Tear

Superficial Tear: "Guy-Rope" Technique

The guy-rope technique (Fig. 8-21) is currently used for partial superficial tears only. A posterior subacromial portal and a lateral instrumentation portal, the greater tuberosity is abraded and a hole is drilled as lateral as possible into the border of the greater tuberosity. A metallic anchor (Mitek super quick GIV anchor) or a screw (Mitek Fastin anchor) loaded with a double suture is placed laterally through the strong cortical bone of the great tuberosity. Through an anterior portal a pig-tail suture passer (Lin-

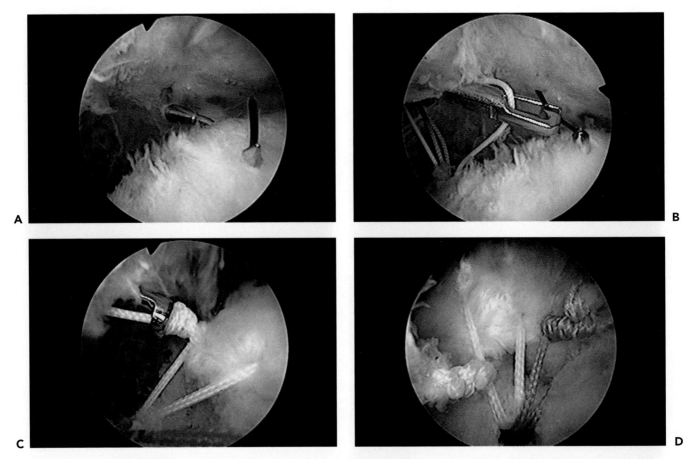

Figure 8-21 Superficial cuff tear: Guy-rope technique. (A) Step one. (B) Step two. (C) Step three. (D) Step four.

vatec), equipped with a 45-degree curved hook (left-rotated for a right shoulder and vice versa), is loaded with a single strand of PDS No. 0. The instrument is passed through the cuff from the superficial to the deep layer and then back again, twisting the hook, resulting in a U suture (Fig. 8-21A). The PDS end is grasped at the same time as one of the two sutures, is loaded on the anchor by a forceps, and is pulled out through the lateral portal. The PDS is used as a shuttle relay for passing the nonabsorbable suture (Fig. 8-21, B and C). A sliding knot on the anterior strand of the thread is pushed on the cuff and pulled laterally to the anchor to bring the tendon to the greater tuberosity. The knot is then secured by changing traction on the threads, and two additional half loops are pushed along the posterior thread. The second suture is passed through the tendon in the same way to obtain a double "Guy-Rope" technique (Fig. 8-21D).

Intratendinous Tear

Only an acromioplasty is performed for this lesion because it is thought that relief of the impingement prevents further tendon damage.

Deep Tear

Articular surface rotator cuff tears most often affect the supraspinatus. A common pathology associated with this condition is secondary biceps tendon instability when the tendon tear is located at the level of the posterior biceps pulley. This lesion is best visualized with internal rotation of the shoulder as the biceps tendon subluxates over the lateral wall of its groove (Fig. 8-22, A and B).

The aim of the supraspinatus repair is to rebuild the juxta-cartilaginous tendon's insertion. To reattach the supraspinatus, after cleaning the bursa and acromioplasty, the repair is managed by intra-articular visualization. A small anterosuperior portal close to the anterior corner of the acromion is placed near the rotator interval at the anterior part of the supraspinatus above the biceps groove guided. A Fastin screw anchor (Mitek) is inserted in the previously abraded area of the tuberosity, close to the cartilage and to the posterior border of the biceps groove (Fig. 8-22C). Two techniques are possible to pass the four sutures through the tendon. A Linvatek suture passer can be introduced by the lateral portal used for the acromioplasty, perforating the cuff from outside to inside; the PDS is then gently grasped at the same time as one of the four

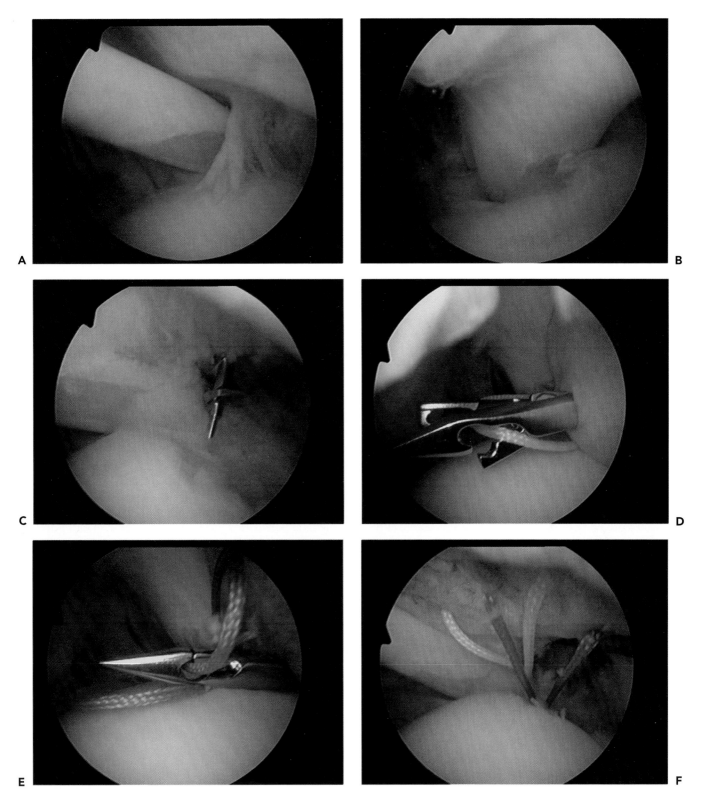

Figure 8-22   Articular cuff tear: Paragliding technique. (*A*) Step one. (*B*) Step two. (*C*) Step three. (*D*) Step four. (*E*) Step five. (*F*) Step six. (*continued*)

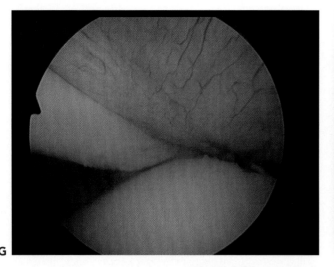

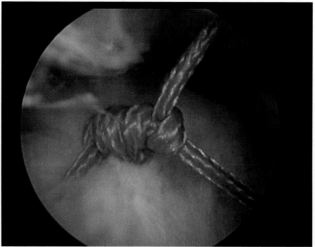

G   H

Figure 8-22 *(continued)* (*G*) Step seven. (*H*) Step eight.

sutures with a smooth U-shaped grasper through the antero-lateral portal. The PDS is used as a shuttle relay to pull the braided suture through the supraspinatus. Alternately, the bird-beak suture passer can be used to perforate the cuff from the top through the anterosuperior postal, retrieving the suture (Fig. 8-22, *C–G*). The four threads are successively passed and pulled on the tendon like ropes on a parachute. Visualization of the knot may be done on subacromial space, but secure tension is necessary to ensure good application of the cuff over the bone (Fig. 8-22*H*).

It is important to avoid strangulation of the biceps with the suture fixation. When the biceps pulley reconstruction is not secure or anatomical, or when biceps degenerative changes are visible, then a tenodesis of the biceps is performed.

Full Thickness Tear

With a full thickness tear, reattachment of the tendons establishes an anatomical footprint of the tendon using two rows of suture: one row medially at the cartilage-bone interface and the other row on the lateral aspect of the great tuberosity (Fig. 8-23).

Supraspinatus

After removal of the bursa scar and mobilization of the tendon, the repair starts with medial fixation. The anchor is passed through an accessory small portal (about 2–3 mm) situated at the lateral border of the acromion to reach the greater tuberosity as perpendicularly as possible. The repair is done with visualization of the biceps tendon as described for partial deep cuff tear, or from subacromial, if biceps is torn or fixed to the groove (tenodesis) (Fig. 8-24). Bone suture fixation is done with either a screw (Fastin [Mitek] or OBL 5 [Smith & Nephew]) or an anchor through the an-

terosuperior portal. The easiest way to pass the suture through the cuff at the proximal part of the tendon is to use the spectrum (Linvatek) from the anterior portal. The device is passed from superfical to deep in the tendon. The PDS is grasped with a green and white suture on the same time and then relayed through the cuff with the PDS. The same technique is used to pass successively the two other threads passing the cuff in distances of about 5 mm from each other. These sutures are not tied at this point, but pulled through an anterior portal to keep them out of the surgical field.

A second anchor is then placed laterally, and the sutures are passed as a simple stitch or a U stitch for a guy-rope technique, as described previously. The Spectrum instruments are often used for U stitch, and a grasper may be used for simple stitch.

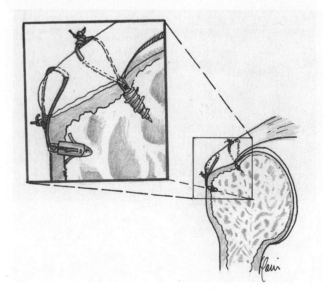

Figure 8-23 Footprint fixation.

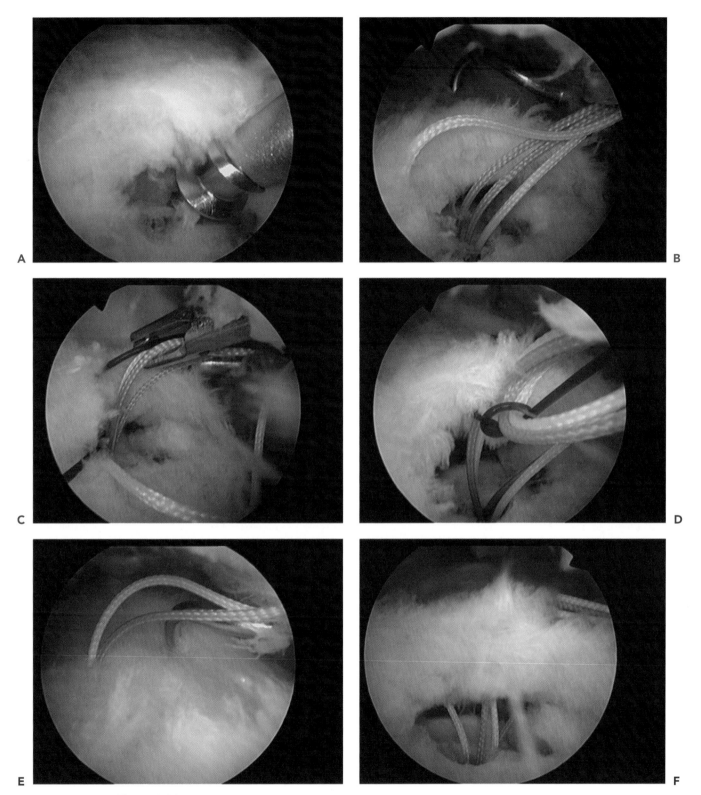

Figure 8-24 Supraspinatus U-shape footprint repair. (*A*) Step one. (*B*) Step two. (*C*) Step three. (*D*) Step four. (*E*) Step five. (*F*) Step six. (*continued*)

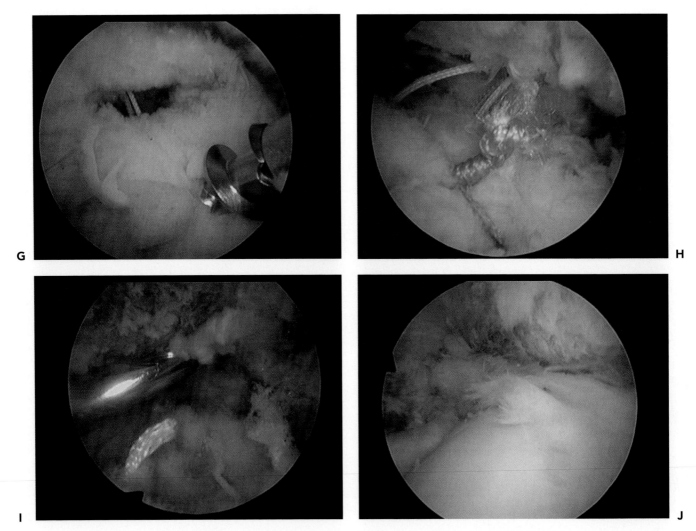

Figure 8-24   *(continued)* *(G)* Step seven. *(H)* Step eight. *(I)* Step nine. *(J)* Step ten.

Knots are tied first with the lateral fixation followed by the medial sutures. Acromioplasty is managed at the end only when visualization and access in the subacromial space is good, and control of the repair is done from the bursal side (Fig. 8-24*I*) and the articular side (Fig. 8-24*J*).

Extended Infraspinatus Tear

Tears that extend into the infraspinatus tendon are often L or V shaped (Fig. 8-25). These tears require a reverse approach for the tendon-to-bone reinsertion. The arm is placed closer to the side of the body. The visualization is through the anterolateral portal. The tendon is pulled from posterior to anterior and to a lesser degree from medial to lateral. The first anchors are placed at the posterolateral border of the greater tuberosity following the same principles of a supraspinatus repair but using two posterior portals for the instruments. In case of a laminated tear, the deeper flap one is fixed first to the medial part of the tuberosity. Before tendon fixation to bone, a tendon-to-tendon suture repair is necessary between the split in the infraspinatus tear to close the "L" portion of the tear. The side-to-side sutures between supraspinatus and infraspinatus are performed after the tendon-to-bone to perform an anatomical repair with lateral view and both anterior and posterior portal for instrumentation.

Subscapularis

Tear of the Upper Third

Subluxation, or dislocation, of the long head of the biceps tendon (LHB) is often associated to this pathology. When the LHB is in its normal position in the groove then one needs to be careful to neither create instability by damaging the medial pulley nor create an impingement between the LHB and the knots tied for subscapularis fixation. The entire operation is performed in the anterior portal and a lateral portal or alternatively located at the rotator interval near the LHB (Fig. 8-26). The scope is placed near the bicipital groove and is oriented inferior. To expose the sub-

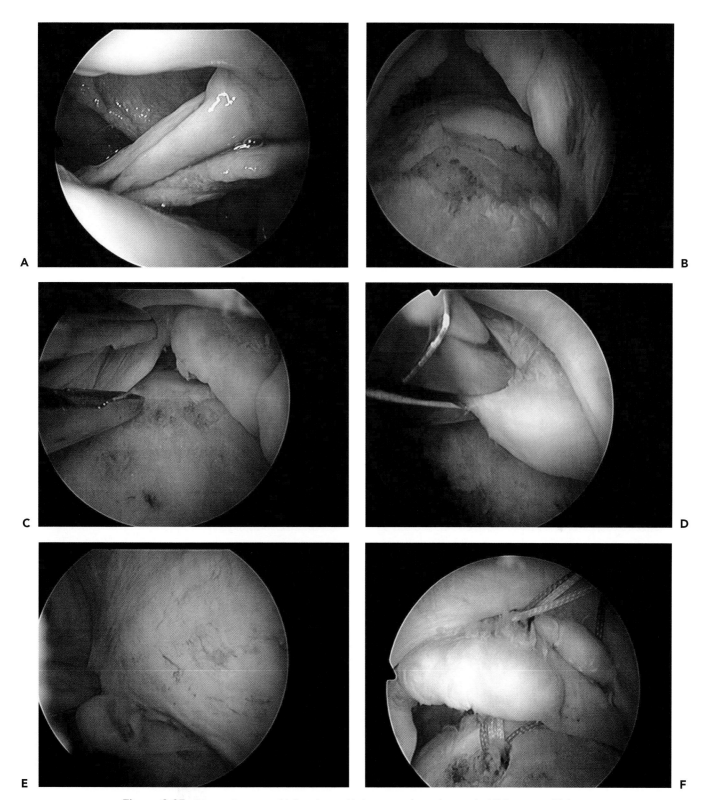

Figure 8-25 Supraspinatus and infraspinatus V-shape tear footprint repair. (*A*) Step one. (*B*) Step two. (*C*) Step three. (*D*) Step four. (*E*) Step five. (*F*) Step six. (*continued*)

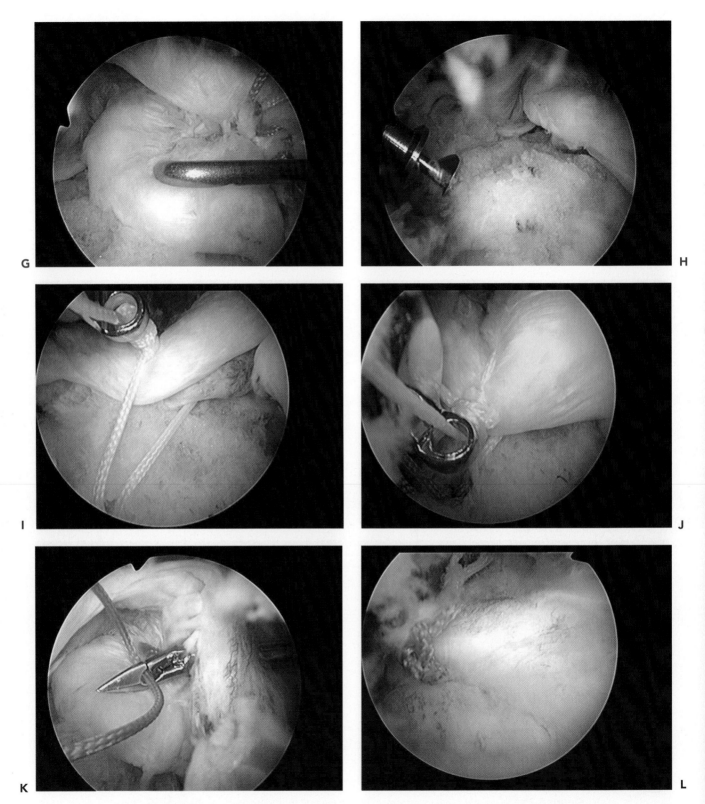

Figure 8-25 *(continued)* (*G*) Step seven. (*H*) Step eight. (*I*) Step nine. (*J*) Step ten. (*K*) Step eleven. (*L*) Step twelve. (*continued*)

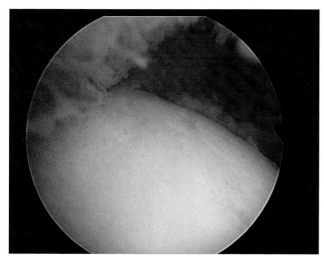

M

Figure 8-25 *(continued)* *(M)* Step thirteen.

scapularis, the arm must be positioned with more flexion than usual. After abrasion of the lesser tuberosity, an anchor is inserted just in from the biceps groove, and the braided suture is passed through the subscapularis tendon in the same manner as used for the other tendon repairs. The suture retriever may be passed through the cannula or the anterosuperior portal, based upon the location of the tendon. A "U" and a simple suture is used on an anchor with a double suture. While pulling at the strands, the knot is tightened and the arm is internally rotating the arm to help reduce the tear.

Intermediate Tendon Retraction

The technique of successively placing two to three anchors beginning at the inferior part of the tear and moving superiorly is related to an open technique of transosseus tendon repair using sutures in bone.

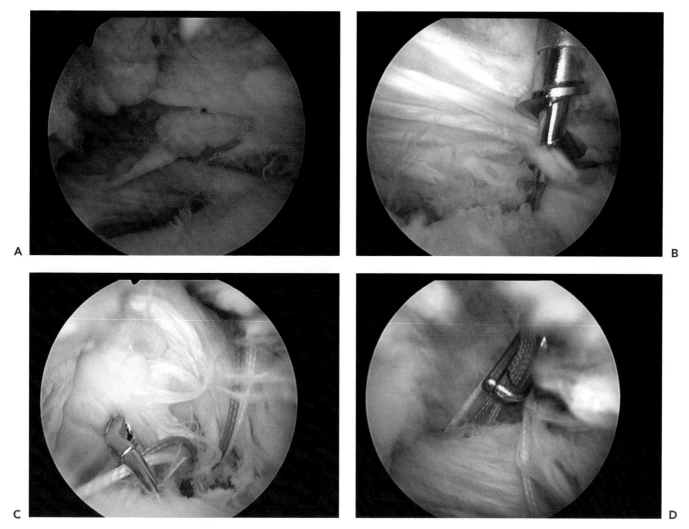

A   **B**   **C**   **D**

Figure 8-26 Subscapularis one-third superior tear. *(A)* Step one. *(B)* Step two. *(C)* Step three. *(D)* Step four. *(continued)*

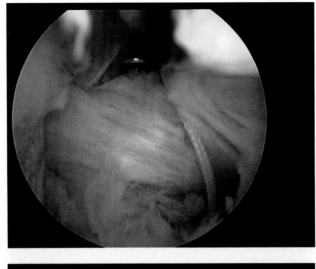

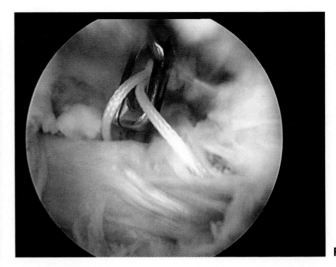

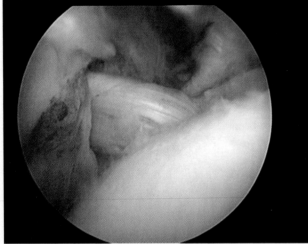

Figure 8-26 *(continued)* *(E)* Step five. *(F)* Step six. *(G)* Step seven.

Extended Rupture

First, a release is done through the anterior portal that is near the rotator interval. The same procedure is used for the subcoracoid release and is facilitated with slight forward flexion of the arm. When there is an isolated tear of the subscapularis, the scope is in the glenohumeral joint. When the tear involves the supraspinatus, the scope is placed in the subacromial space through the posterolateral portal. The suture hook is inserted via the anterior approach while the passed PDS end is removed through the anterolateral portal. The technique is identical to the one described in the intermediate lesions, and the repair is performed from inferior to superior.

The Long Head of the Biceps Tendon

The long head of the biceps tendon (LHB) (Fig. 8-27) can be compromised at its base (SLAP lesion) or by degenerative changes within its substance. Long head of the biceps tendon damage can occur secondary to instability at the groove. Instability is often associated with tears of the up-

per subscapularis or leading edge of the supraspinatus. In a type II SLAP lesion, reattachment to the glenoid is performed using suture anchors. If a tendinopathy is present, either a simple tenotomy is preferred for elderly patients, or arthroscopic tenodesis into the bicipital groove is performed for younger or more active patients. Two approaches are sufficient: an anterior lateral portal for visualization, and an anterior superior portalfor direct access to the biceps groove. After slight abrasion of the proximal groove, a screw loaded with two sutures is inserted on the entrance of the groove. The spectrum hook is passed twice through the LHB with PDS No. 1 as a shuttle relay to pass the braided suture. The tendon is then cut and the sutures tied, fixing the end of the cut LHB into the entrance of the groove. The advantage of this technique is that the tendon can heal into the groove, avoiding the biceps muscle deformity associated with retraction of the tendon.

Massive Ruptures

The authors define *massive tear* as a minimum of three tendons involved, with at least one retracted to the glenoid. In such cases, even in retracted tears, the ability to mobilize

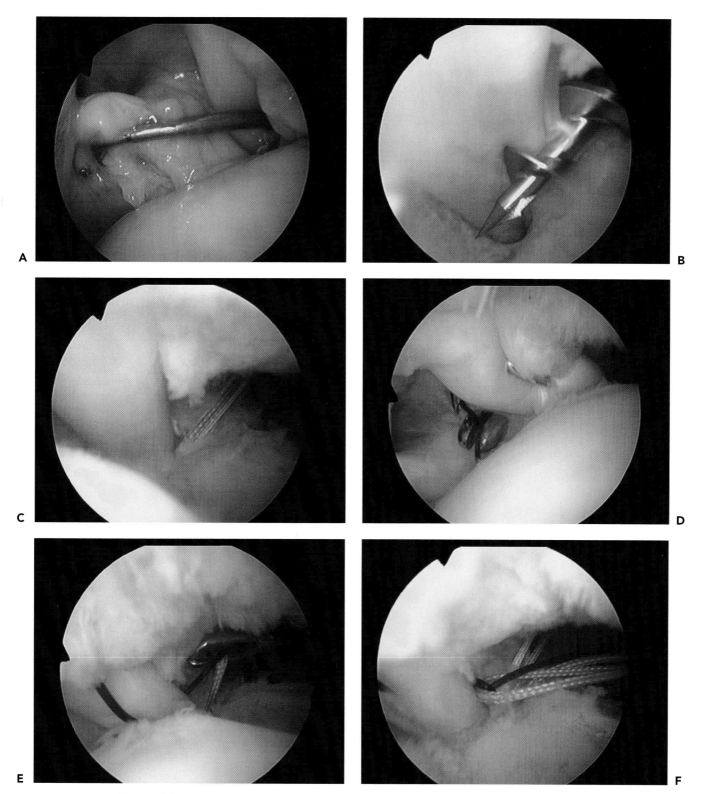

Figure 8-27   Long head biceps tenodesis with suture on anchor fixation. (*A*) Step one. (*B*) Step two. (*C*) Step three. (*D*) Step four. (*E*) Step five. (*F*) Step six. (*continued*)

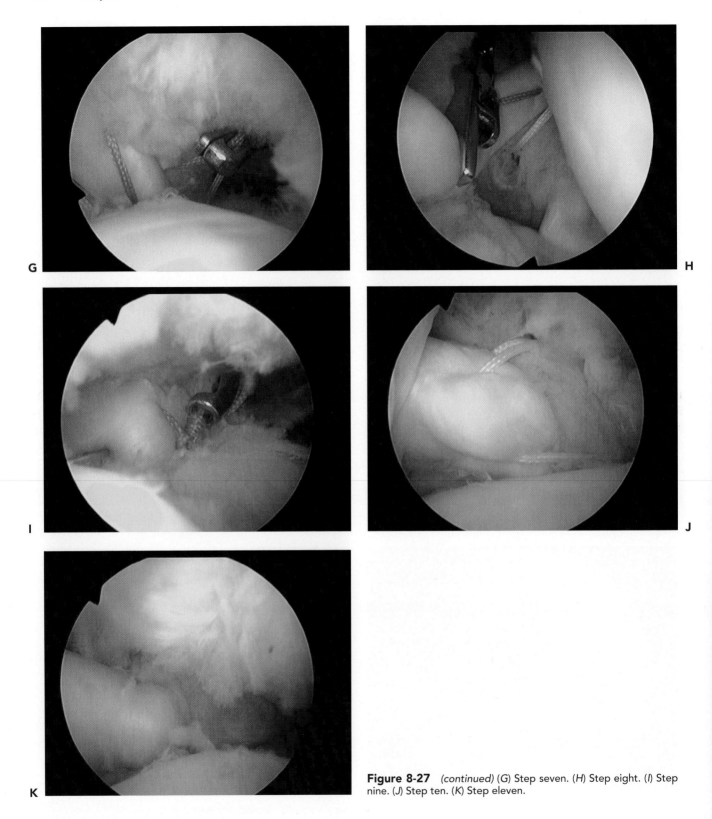

Figure 8-27 *(continued)* (*G*) Step seven. (*H*) Step eight. (*I*) Step nine. (*J*) Step ten. (*K*) Step eleven.

and reduce the tendon to the tuberosity defines the ability to proceed with the repair. What initially appears to be an irreparable tear can, in some cases, be reduced after an extensive release. The geometry of the tear must be understood, and the atrophy of the muscles should not be moderate or severe.

The repair is performed in the following order: biceps, subscapularis, infraspinatus, and supraspinatus. When necessary, the side-to-side repair is done at the end to complete the repair. If a complete repair is not possible, then that portion of the tear that can be performed is completed. When possible, a side-to-side suture can result in a gain in function with every suture placed.

Revision Surgery

Revision Surgery in Arthroscopic Operated Rotator Cuffs

The results of primary surgery do not always correspond to the preoperative expectations. In selected cases revision is performed because of poorly placed or loose anchors or after postoperative retears. If the rerupture has happened shortly after the operation, secondary to a clear event, then the chance to repair the tendon with an arthroscopic repair is high. When this occurs a timely decision to reoperate is required.

Revision Surgery After Open Operated Rotator Cuffs

As with open rotator cuff repairs, reoperation of failed repair by arthroscopic revision is difficult and is often caused by subacromial adhesions that result in a "captured cuff" than by postoperative cuff ruptures. When reoperation is performed for rerupture, visualization of the tear is difficult due to the adhesions, but it can be performed. Often the results are very good, with quick restoration of an initially painful and immobile shoulder as a result of the release of adhesions and mobilization of the tendon.

Tricks and Pitfalls

Working in the subacromial space is difficult because of scarring and because of inflamed tissues often swollen by the saline fluid. These tissues may have excessive bleeding after initial shaving; therefore, the systematic use of an electrocautery device along with the shaver is indispensable. The work has to be done quickly, without excessive intra-articular pressure. Scopes should be placed in multiple portals to see the bursa and scar from different angles. When the postoperative radiographs demonstrate an anchor dislodged from bone into the soft tissues, it should be extracted as soon as possible to prevent possi-

ble impingement or articular cartilage damage. When knots become snared or sutures become entangled, it is best to cut the suture and start with a new suture and anchors. This can happen even with the most experienced surgeon.

POSTOPERATIVE CARE

Closure of the portal is accomplished with a resorbable intracapsular suture. The arm is held in a 30-degree abduction brace for 6 weeks. Passive motion in forward elevation and external rotation is started immediately after surgery and is limited based upon the quality of the tendon and the repair. The range of motion is achieved more easily than for open surgery, and the risk for long-term stiffness is less with the arthroscopic technique. It is crucial not to perform exercises that create pain by aggressive physiotherapy, because the tendon repair can rerupture. The brace is removed for nursing and resting as often as it is wished. The rehabilitation is done by passive mobilization during the first 3 months postoperatively. Active exercises are often done by the patient himself, because they start activities of daily living without being disturbed by pain. Clinical follow-up and x-rays are done at 6 weeks and 3 months. At 6 months an arthro-CT is performed to assess the quality of the tendon repair, as well as the muscular atrophy and fatty degeneration. Guided by these objective findings the rehabilitation can be modified.

RESULTS

Material and Methods

The author has evaluated 116 shoulders in 115 patients and operated for full thickness rotator cuff tears from 1998 to 2001. In this series, there were 63 (55%) men and 52 (45%) women with a median age of 57 years (range 36–80 years). There were 13 anterosuperior lesions (six large subscapularis tears), 40 superior, 36 posterosuperior, and 27 massive rotator cuff tears.

The patients were evaluated preoperatively and postoperatively according to the criteria of the Constant and Murley Score (CMS).[4] Preoperatively, all patients had a standard set of radiographs, arthrography, and arthro-CT scan. Postoperatively, all had standard radiographs; 89 patients had an arthrogram and 17 of these had an additional CT scan. Preoperative and postoperative images were measured for humeral head–acromion distance (HAD), arthrographic signs of retear, tear retraction, and, when CT scan available, for fatty degeneration (FD) of the muscles according to the criteria of Goutallier and Bernageau.[14]

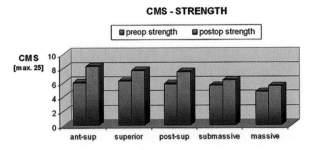

Figure 8-28   CMS score preoperative and postoperative.

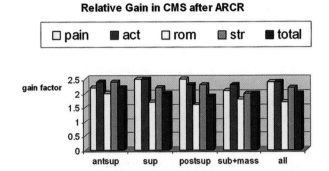

Figure 8-30   Gain of CMS/location.

Clinical Outcomes

Average follow-up was 26 months (24–60 months). There were no infections for frozen shoulders. Revision surgery was performed for retear, biceps problems, and captured cuff problems.

The CMS increased from 40.3 of that of a normal shoulder preoperatively to 80.1 postoperatively. All parameters of CMS were improved (Fig. 8-28). The postoperative scores correlated with the high patient satisfaction. The correlation of the site of the tear with the relative gain in CM score (gain in CMS/preoperative CMS) is shown in Figure 8-29. Anterosuperior tears showed the greatest improvement with an average increase of 43.6%. The average increase for superior lesions was 41.1%, for posterosuperior lesions was 39.5%, and for massive lesions was only 36.4%.

The best improvement in pain was found in the posterosuperior lesions, the greatest improvement in activities of daily living were with superior lesions, and the best outcome in mobility and strength were with anterosuperior lesions. The influence of the intraoperative state of the LHB on its treatment was studied in the anterosuperior lesion.

Eighty-seven of the 116 patients had a postoperative arthrogram or arthro-CT; 42 (48.3%) were watertight, and 45 (51.7%) had a positive arthrogram. The presence of complete healing based upon the presence of a leak or arthrogram was different among the different lesions (Fig. 8-30).

A negative arthrogram is clearly a complete healing of

the tendon, but a leak of contrast can be correlated to a recurrent tear or to nonwatertight repair. In some shoulders this may still represent partial healing or almost complete healing in a case when the rotator interval was not closed. Our arthrogram data are difficult to evaluate because of incomplete recording of the intraoperative estimate of the cuff repair or the nature of the rotator interval closure.

Correlation between clinical results and postoperative arthrograms demonstrates that patients with a leak of contrast (51.7%) had a greater gain in all CMS variables than those with a watertight cuff, but both patient groups had similar absolute postoperative Constant scores (Fig. 8-31). This further supports our opinion that a leak on a postoperative arthrogram is not always correlated to a clinically significant recurrent tear. Conversely, a poor clinical result, in which recurrent surgery was necessary, was always correlated with a massive leak of contrast on arthrogram and a massive retraction at the second surgery. In some cases revision surgery was required for persistent untreated biceps pathology or a cuff capture due to adhesions, and in these cases there was a negative arthrogram.

CONCLUSION

Over 2 decades have passed since the introduction of diagnostic and simple ablative arthroscopy of the shoulder as the

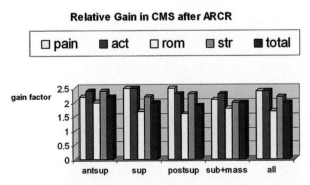

Figure 8-29   Gain of CMS after ARCR.

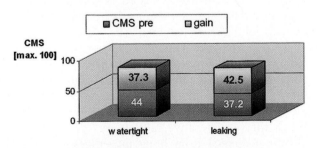

Figure 8-31   Gain of CMS/leakage.

treatment of choice for impingement syndrome. The techniques for arthroscopic rotator cuff repair have evolved in this time. After more than 10 years of experience with arthroscopic repair of an RCT, it seems to the author that it is a very valuable and successful method. Nevertheless, it is still an extremely difficult surgery, even for certain small-sized tears. The difficulties arise from the limited size of the subacromial space, the quality and nature of the degenerative tendon tissue, and the retraction and tissue tension due to changes in the muscles that occur with chronic tears. The quality of the anatomical and clinical results continues to encourage the performance and perfection these techniques.

REFERENCES

1. Altcheck DW, Warren RF, Wickiewicz TL, et al. Arthroscopic acromioplasty: technique and results. J Bone Joint Surg 1990;72A:1198.
2. Augereau B, Apoil A. La réparation des grandes ruptures de la coiffe des rotateurs de l'épaule. Rev Chir Orthop 1988;74(suppl 2):95.
3. Codman CA. The shoulder. Boston, Thomas Todd (private publisher), 1934.
4. Constant CR, Murley AMG. A clinical method of functional assessment of the shoulder. Clin Orthop 1987;214:160.
5. Cordasco FA, Backer M, Craig EV, et al. The partial-thickness rotator cuff tear: is acromioplasty without repair sufficient? Am J Sports Med 2002;30(2):179.
6. Debayre J, Patte D, Elmelik E. Repair of ruptures of the rotator cuff of the shoulder. With a note on advancement of the supraspinatus muscle. J Bone Joint Surg (Br) 1965;47B:36.
7. Ellman H, Hanker G, Bayer M. Repair of the rotator cuff: end result study of factors influencing reconstruction. J Bone Joint Surg 1986;68A:1136.
8. Esch JC, Ozerkis LR, Helgager JA, et al. Arthroscopic subacromial decompression: results according to the degree of rotator cuff tear. Arthroscopy 1988;4:241.
9. Gartsman GM, Bennett JB, Blair ME, et al. Arthroscopic subacromial decompression: an anatomical study. Am J Sports Med 1988;16:48.
10. Gartsman GM. Arthroscopic acromioplasty for lesions of the rotator cuff. J Bone Joint Surg 1990;72A:169.
11. Gartsman GM, Khan M, Hammerman SM. Arthroscopic repair of full thickness rotator cuff tears. J Bone Joint Surg 1998;80A:832.
12. Gerber C, Krushell RJ. Isolated rupture of the tendon of the subscapularis muscle: clinical features in 16 cases. J Bone Joint Surg (Br) 1991;73B:389.
13. Goldberg BA, Lippitt SB, Matsen FA III. Improvement in comfort and function after cuff repair without acromioplasty. Clin Orthop 2001;390:142.
14. Goutallier D, Postel JM, Bernageau J, et al. Fatty muscle degeneration in cuff rupture. Clin Orthop 1994;304:78.
15. Hoe-Hansen CE, Palm L, Norlin R. The influence of cuff pathology on shoulder function after arthroscopic subacromial decompression: a 3- and 6-year. J Shoulder Elbow Surg 1999;8(6):585.
16. Jobe FW, Moynes DR. Delineation of diagnostic criteria and a rehabilitation program for rotator cuff injuries. Am J Sports Med 1982;10:336.
17. Lafosse L. Arthroscopic repair of supra-spinatus full thickness tear: 15 cases. In: Gazielly DF, Gleyze P, Thomas T (eds).The cuff. Amsterdam, Elsevier, 1997:287.
18. Lafosse L. Reinsertion arthroscopique d'une rupture étendue du sous scapulaire. Congres La Baule SFA, Vidéo Flash, 2001.
19. Levy HJ, Gardner RD, Lemak LJ. Arthroscopic subacromial decompression in the treatment of full-thickness rotator cuff tears. Arthroscopy 1991;7:8.
20. Liu SH. Arthroscopically assisted rotator cuff repair. J Bone Joint Surg (Br) 1994;76B:592.
21. Neer CS II. Anterior acromioplasty for the chronic impingement syndrome of the shoulder. J Bone Joint Surg 1972;54A:41.
22. Neer CS II. Impingement lesions. Clin Orthop 1983;173:70.
23. Norlin R. Arthroscopic subacromial decompression versus open acromioplasty. Arthroscopy 1989;5:321.
24. Patte D. Classification of rotator cuff lesions. Clin Orthop 1990;254:81.
25. Richards RR, An KN, Bigliani LU, et al. A standardized method for the assessment of shoulder function. J Shoulder Elbow Surg 1994;3(6):47.
26. Rockwood CA, Williams GR, Burkhead WZ. Debridement of degenerative, irreparable lesions of the rotator cuff. J Bone Joint Surg 1995;77A:739.
27. Zvijac JE, Levy HJ, Lemak LJ. Arthroscopic subacromial decompression in the treatment of full-thickness rotator cuff tears: a 3- to 6-year follow-up. Arthroscopy 1994;1:518.

Arthroscopic Rotator Cuff Repair

James C. Esch   **Bradford S. Tucker**

INTRODUCTION

Shoulder arthroscopy has improved our understanding and treatment of rotator cuff tears. It facilitates easy viewing from different angles, as opposed to open treatment, which, when performed through a small incision, has a limited exposure, in part, because of the acromion. This arthroscopic viewpoint has led to the recognition of several common rotator cuff tear patterns.[13] Tear pattern recognition, suture anchors, and tissue-passing instruments enable the surgeon to mobilize and repair a torn rotator cuff to its bony footprint with consistency. Associated pathology within the shoulder joint—articular cartilage, glenoid labrum, and biceps tendon problems—can also be treated. The authors rely on the arthroscope to repair all rotator cuff tears.

RADIOGRAPHY AND MAGNETIC RESONANCE IMAGING

The surgeon must carefully examine routine anteroposterior (AP), axillary, and arch radiographs. The glenohumeral space and acromiohumeral distance are carefully evaluated on the AP view for arthritis, aseptic necrosis, and calcifications. The axillary view is routinely obtained because it tells the surgeon whether an os acromiale is present. The arch view shows acromiale shape and thickness. Additionally, a weight-bearing "push-up" AP view,

J. C. Esch: Department of Orthopaedics, University of California, San Diego, School of Medicine, San Diego, California.
B. S. Tucker: Department of Surgery, Atlantic City Medical Center, Atlantic City, New Jersey.

in which upward pressure is placed on the humerus, can be obtained to evaluate narrowing of the acromiohumeral space (Fig. 9-1).

Magnetic resonance imaging (MRI) imparts the best image of a torn rotator cuff, showing the subscapularis tendon and status of the deltoid muscle. The size and shape of supraspinatus and infraspinatus tendon tears are revealed (Fig. 9-2), as is any atrophy within the rotator cuff muscles. Smaller scanners and newer software afford excellent images in a convenient office setting (Fig. 9-3). These scans can also be reviewed on a computer. The Orthopedic surgeon should personally review the MRI scan.

SURGICAL OPTIONS, INDICATIONS, AND DECISION MAKING

The office radiographs and MRI complement the patient's history of symptom onset, discomfort, and loss of function. Discuss with the patient the ease or difficulty of repair, the extent of rehabilitation, and the expected result. Surgery provides good pain relief. Weakness, however, is slower to recover and will recover incompletely if there is significant muscle atrophy. Patients with significant pain are usually unaware of any accompanying weakness. The patient should have a clear idea of the goals and problems of surgery. Despite these caveats, some patients will have unrealistic expectations for surgical correction of their symptoms. Point out to the patient that an MRI obtained after surgery may show incomplete healing of the rotator cuff repair.[6]

Small to large tears of the supraspinatus and infraspinatus tendons can be repaired by standard arthroscopic repair techniques. Tear size and configuration dictate the specific

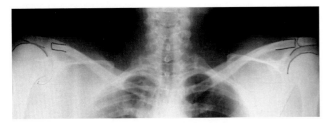

Figure 9-1 Radiograph of narrowed acromial humeral space.

surgical technique. Usually, repair requires a combination of a margin convergence and a tendon-to-bone repair using suture anchors. Margin convergence involves suturing the anterior and posterior leaves of the tear in a sequential side-to-side manner, starting medially and proceeding laterally until the tear converges toward the bony footprint. The free edge is then attached to the footprint with suture anchors. The value of an arthroscopic rotator cuff repair is a secure arthroscopic repair through smaller incisions, without disruption of the deltoid muscle attachment. The final repair is "decompressed" by smoothing the undersurface of the acromion.

Arthroscopic repair of a massive cuff tear is unpredictable. Surgical visualization and mobilization determine whether a massive tear is repairable, partially repairable, or irreparable. A tear is not deemed irreparable until it is evaluated at the time of arthroscopy. Many tears that appear irreparable preoperatively can be mobilized by capsular techniques and interval slides,[13] enabling a partial or complete repair of a once "irreparable" tear (Fig. 9-4). The authors do not treat any rotator cuff tears by open techniques.

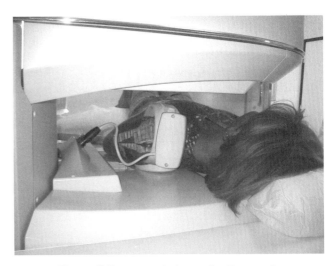

Figure 9-3 Tri-city Orthopaedics E-scan unit.

If the tear is indeed irreparable, debride the bursal tissue and preserve the coracoacromial arch. Some surgeons prefer to make the undersurface of the acromion smooth by removing a large anterior spur so that the undersurface of the acromion is flatter, but the insertion of the coracoacromial ligament onto the undersurface of the acromion must be preserved. If the coracoacromial ligament is removed, the humeral head may "escape" anterior, leading to anterosuperior shoulder instability. This creates a disastrous complication, especially in the patient who can lift the arm overhead even though there is a massive rotator cuff tear. Partial repair of the rotator cuff tear—namely, the subscapularis or infraspinatus tendons while leaving a defect in the supraspinatus tendon—is helpful,[18] improving pain and function by restoring the rotator cuff cable and force couples necessary for arm elevation.[13]

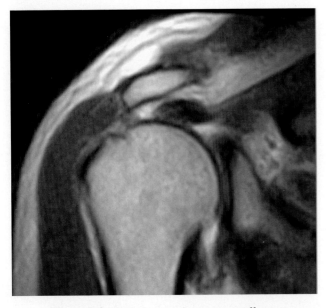

Figure 9-2 MRI of a complete rotator cuff tear.

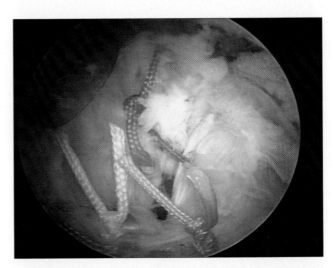

Figure 9-4 A massive rotator cuff repaired with sutures.

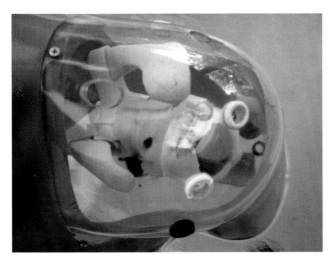

Figure 9-5 "Alex" shoulder model with a cuff repair (Pacific Research).

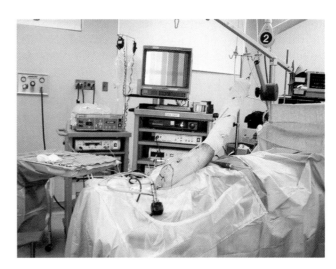

Figure 9-7 Operating room setup, anesthesiologist is at the foot of the table.

SURGICAL TECHNIQUE

The surgeon must balance skill versus ego in arthroscopic rotator cuff repair. The surgeon must be in control of the operating theater. Detailed knowledge of the proper tools, suture management, and knot-tying techniques is essential. The skills required for the specific steps can be honed using the "Alex" shoulder model (Fig. 9-5). The surgeon must have not only a favorite plan, Plan A, but also a Plan B and even a Plan C. A surgeon learning arthroscopic rotator cuff repair can easily bail out of the arthroscopic procedure at any time and proceed to an open repair of the rotator cuff through a mini deltoid-splitting incision.

Control of Bleeding

Controlling bleeding is essential for a good repair. Some tips for efficient control of bleeding include flowing fluid in through the arthroscope, controlling outflow through

the shaver blades, and being aware of the nuances of an arthroscopic fluid management system (Fig. 9-6). The anesthesiologist lowers and safely monitors the systolic blood pressure in the range of 90 to 100 mmHg. Use electrocautery to stop any troublesome bleeding vessels. Nonsteroidal anti-inflammatory drugs (NSAIDs) and other drugs that can cause bleeding must be discontinued at least 7 days before surgery.

Patient Positioning

Arthroscopic cuff repair can be done in the seated position. The authors place the patient in the lateral decubitus position. Turn the operating table so that the anesthesiologist is at the foot (Figs. 9-7 and 9-8). Prepare and drape the shoulder after the arm is suspended with 10 to 15 lb of weight. Perform a glenohumeral arthroscopy in a systematic fash-

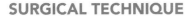

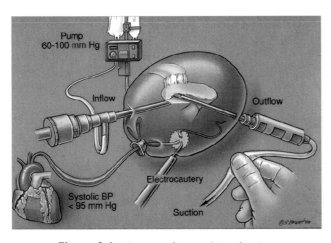

Figure 9-6 Concepts for good visualization.

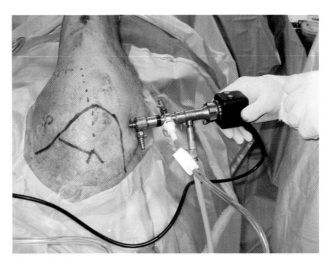

Figure 9-8 Posterior portal with fluid inflow through the arthroscope.

ion using a standard posterior portal and an anterior portal created with the Wissinger rod technique through the rotator interval. Treat any cartilage and labrum pathology. Examine the rotator cuff tear and evaluate the cuff footprint.

Portal Placement

Create three portals for the rotator cuff repair. Enter the subacromial bursa from the posterior portal for initial viewing. Create the lateral portal three fingerbreadths lateral to the acromion (Fig. 9-9). Remove the bursa, debride the torn cuff, and abrade the bony footprint through this portal. Make the anterior subacromial portal by entering the bursa just lateral to the coracoacromial ligament. This enables the cannula to be easily moved but does not disrupt the coracoacromial arch. Excise bursa as necessary for visualization. Use electrocautery as necessary to control bleeding. Create additional portals as necessary. Insert suture anchors through a miniportal off the edge of the acromion. The additional superior portal behind the acromioclavicular joint can be used for a suture-retrieving device to pass sutures through the edge of a crescent-shaped tear.[5]

The authors prefer the lateral subacromial portal—the "50-yard line" view (see Fig. 9-9)—for optimal viewing of the rotator cuff. Place 7- to 8.5-mm plastic cannulas in the anterior and posterior portals for use in passing tools and suture. Move the tools, suture, and even the arthroscope as needed. Do not become limited to one portal.

Preparing the Site and Beginning the Repair

Remove the bursa tissue as necessary for visualization of the cuff repair. Find a tissue plane that can see the extent of the cuff tear. Free up any adhesions between the cuff or

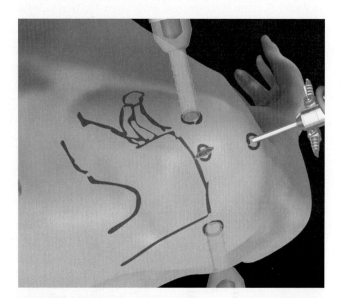

Figure 9-9 The arthroscope is in lateral portal, providing the "50-yard-line" view. Note the anchor insertion portal adjacent to the acromion.

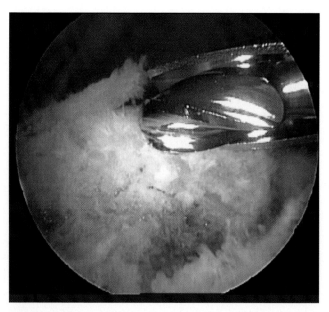

Figure 9-10 A shaver or burr decorticates the cuff footprint to create a bed for healing.

bursa and the overlying acromion. Use a shaver-blade or high-speed burr to remove any remaining rotator cuff at the greater tuberosity insertion. Gently debride the surface of the bone to provide bleeding for repair of the cuff to bone (Fig. 9-10). Gently shave the edges or layers of the rotator cuff edges, but do not excise any significant pieces of the torn cuff that are mechanically sound.

Determine Tear Configuration

The next step involves determining the configuration and repairability of the cuff. Use probes or grasping forceps to assess how to repair the rotator cuff. Use grasping forceps in both hands while an assistant holds the arthroscope. First determine the feasibility of a repair and then, if feasible, the steps necessary to achieve it. Diagram the final repair on paper, even though changes may occur during the procedure.

Rotator cuffs tear in a crescent-, L-, or U-shaped fashion. Crescent-shaped tears (Fig. 9-11) can be repaired directly to the bony footprint under minimal tension with double-loaded suture anchors placed though a miniportal off the edge of the acromion (Fig. 9-12). The sutures can be passed though the free edge of the tear by means of an ArthroPierce (Smith & Nephew Endoscopy, Andover, MA) inserted superiorly behind the acromioclavicular joint from the supraclavicular fossa portal, while viewing from the lateral portal (Figs. 9-13 and 9-14). This allows a good bite of tissue. The ArthroPierce can also pass through the free edge of the tear from the posterior portal. Alternatively, the sutures can be passed with a suture-passing device (Fig. 9-15) from the lateral portal, viewing from the posterior portal. Other options include a curved CuffSew (Smith & Nephew Endoscopy),

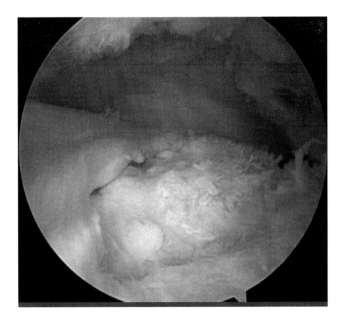

Figure 9-11 Bursal-side view of a complete crescent-shaped tear.

device, a suture punch, a crescent hook, and other devices that shuttle suture through the tendon.

L-shaped tears run parallel to the anterior edge of the supraspinatus, and U-shaped tears are located in the infraspinatus-supraspinatus interval; both tend to be highly mobile in the anterior to posterior direction. With L-shaped tears, the posterior leaf is more mobile than the anterior leaf (capsule in the rotator interval), whereas both leaves are mobile with U-shaped tears. Therefore, repair L- and U-shaped tears initially by a side-to-side margin convergence using a free suture, creating, in effect, a small crescent-shaped tear. Then attach the free edge of the tear to

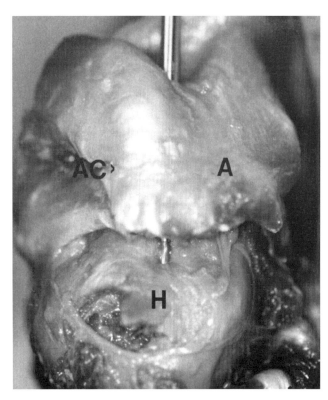

Figure 9-13 Drawing of ArthroPierce (Smith & Nephews Endoscopy, Andover, MA) inserted behind the acromioclavicular joint (AC) and medial to the acromion (A). It passes through the cuff to the anchor in the bone of the humerus (H).

the bone using the suture anchor technique. Sometimes it becomes necessary to place the sutures through the torn cuff only *after* the suture anchors have been appropriately positioned in the bony footprint, because the footprint will be covered during margin convergence, and access to it will

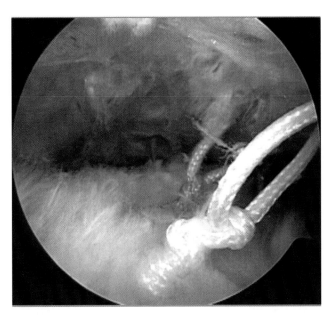

Figure 9-12 Crescent-shaped tear repaired to bone.

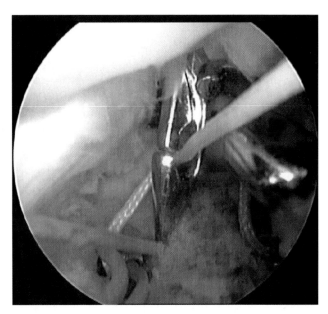

Figure 9-14 ArthroPierce from superior portal through the cuff retrieving suture.

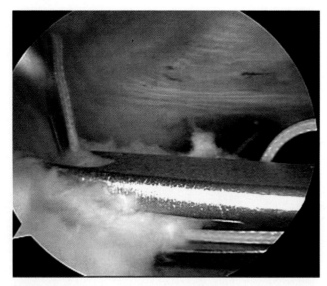

Figure 9-15 ExpresSew (Surgical Solutions, Valencia, CA) device from the lateral portal passing suture through the cuff.

be lost. Include any layering of the torn rotator cuff into the suturing technique, just as in open surgery.

Mobilization Techniques for Retracted Tendons

If necessary in large tears, insert an elevator to release the capsule from the undersurface of the rotator cuff to remove tension from the final repair.[22] The surgeon may be able to mobilize the tendon for a complete repair, do a partial repair, use an aggressive "interval-slide" technique, or deem the tear irreparable.

The surgeon may be unable to mobilize the cuff and call the tear irreparable. A bursectomy can afford pain relief. This is preferable in older patients with pain. The authors prefer a biceps tenotomy, if the biceps tendon is intact.

A second option, which is the authors' preference, is to do a partial repair of the tear. This requires either closing the apex of the tear with side-to-side sutures and/or moving the posterior limb (infraspinatus tendon) to as close to its normal attachment as possible (Fig. 9-16). A biceps tenotomy or tenodesis is also done.

A third option is to mobilize the supraspinatus tendon by releasing its anterior and posterior attachments.[14,17] The anterior release is in the rotator interval along the course of the biceps tendon cutting the coracohumeral ligament and rotator interval tissue. The posterior release is in the supraspinatus-infraspinatus interval just behind the scapular spine. This enables the surgeon to have a 1- to 2-cm strip of tendon to advance to the greater tuberosity. The authors rarely do this because the supraspinatus muscle is atrophied, and the suprascapular nerve can be damaged. These mobilization techniques can work by a tenodesis effect even if the muscle has atrophy.

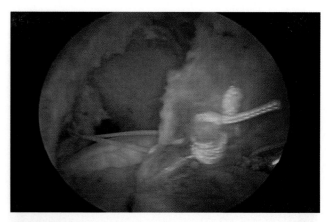

Figure 9-16 Partial repair of the infraspinatus to prevent further tearing at its insertion. The supraspinatus was not repairable.

Margin Convergence

Figure 9-17 illustrates the initial margin convergence suture just 5 mm from the apex of the tear. This proximity prevents extension of the tear. From the posterior portal, pass a relatively straight CuffSew device loaded with a No. 2 braided polyester suture through the tear limbs from posterior to anterior. Unload the suture from the anterior portal and withdraw the CuffSew from the posterior portal. Load the knot pusher on this posterior suture limb. This is the "post" limb for the arthroscopic knot. Use a suture-grabbing device or crochet hook in the posterior portal to withdraw the anterior suture limb (Fig. 9-18). This is the "loop" strand for the arthroscopic knot. Next, tie a sliding knot (Fig. 9-19). Pull on the postsuture limb while guiding and manipulating the knot with the knot pusher as it brings the tissue of the torn cuff together. Secure the knot with three half-hitches, changing posts after each loop. Cut the knot. Repeat as necessary.

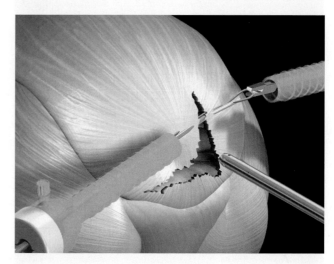

Figure 9-17 Margin convergence with a single-pass CuffSew (Smith & Nephew Endoscopy) tool.

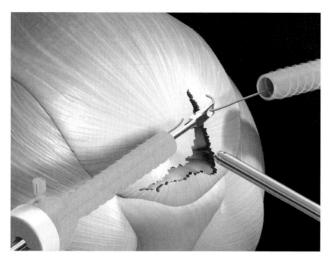

Figure 9-18 Retrieving the suture with a suture-grasping forceps.

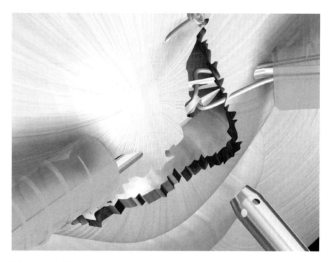

Figure 9-20 A suture handoff from the Straight CuffSew (Smith & Nephew Endoscopy) to the ArthroPierce (Smith & Nephew Endoscopy).

Subsequent margin convergence sutures are placed by grasping and moving the tissue to an optimal position without creating a large dog-ear at the repair site. The authors prefer a "suture handoff" technique—the CuffSew-to-ArthroPierce handoff technique—for accurate placement of the sutures on either side of the repair (Fig. 9-20). To perform this handoff, use a straight CuffSew device to pass a

No. 2 braided suture from the anterior portal through the tear. Then "hand it off" to an ArthroPierce passed through the predetermined point in the posterior limb of the tear from the posterior portal. The posterior suture strand is the post limb of the arthroscopic knot. The anterior strand is the loop limb. Tie a sliding arthroscopic knot plus three half-hitches, reversing posts. Insert as many sutures as necessary to approximate the edges of the tear.

Completing the Repair with Suture Anchors

Insert the suture anchors into bone, carefully watching them enter and remain below the surface of the bone. Use an 18-gauge needle off of the edge of the acromion to get the correct angle for insertion of the suture anchor into the bony footprint. The authors prefer to insert the anchor through a cannula into the subchondral bone near the articular cartilage (Figs. 9-21 and 9-22). Insert one to three anchors at this time, depending on the size of the tear. Visualize the proper steps and arrangements for suture repair. Mark the sutures with hemostats. They can be left in this portal or changed as desired.

Pass the suture through the edge of the cuff in the appropriate position for repair. The authors' preference is to pass the ArthroPierce through the tissue and retrieve the suture (Fig. 9-23). Pass the first suture by inserting the ArthroPierce through the posterior attachment of the infraspinatus or supraspinatus portion of the rotator cuff and retrieving one of the sutures from the most posterior anchor; pull this suture out through the posterior portal. Load the knot pusher on this posterior suture limb. This is the post-limb for the arthroscopic knot. Use a suture-grabbing device or crochet hook in the posterior portal to withdraw the other suture limb from the anchor. This is the loop strand for the arthroscopic knot. Tie a sliding knot and pull on the postsuture limb while guiding and manipulating the

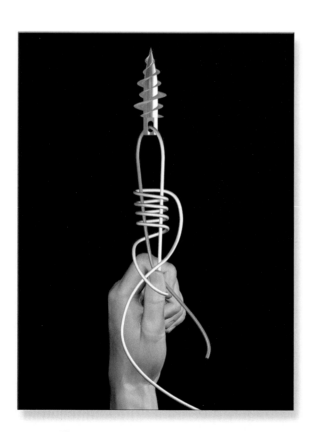

Figure 9-19 Hangman's sliding knot.

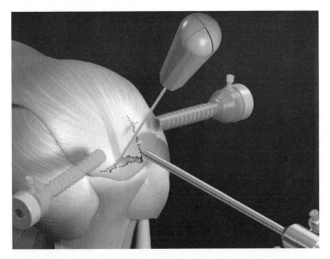

Figure 9-21   Drawing of a suture anchor inserted into cuff footprint through a separate portal.

knot into place as it brings the tissue of the torn cuff together. Secure the knot with three half-hitches, changing posts after each loop. Cut the knot. Repeat these simple sutures as necessary.

Tie the arthroscopic knots in the appropriate portal so that they will easily slide, avoiding friction of the suture on the bone or anchor eyelet. Pay attention to the depth and orientation of the anchor and its eyelet in the bone. Do not bury the suture anchor deeper than the recommended insertion depth. This can lead to early clinical failure because the suture cuts through the bone, resulting in gap formation at the insertion zone (seen in a bovine model)[4] or as the deep anchor becomes superficial, again resulting in gap formation at the insertion zone (seen in a human cadaver

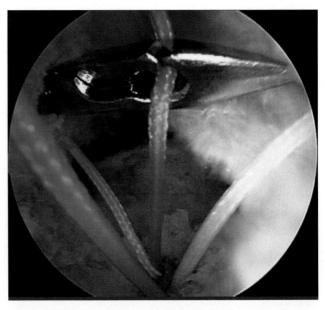

Figure 9-23   Retrieving the suture off of the anchor with the ArthroPierce (Smith & Nephew Endoscopy).

model)[19] during cyclic loading. The authors often tie knots from the lateral portal, with the arthroscope in the posterior portal, preferring a sliding knot with three half-hitches, alternating posts. If the suture does not easily slide, tie alternating half-hitch knots with the first two or three loops on the same post. If the first simple half-hitch does not lie down easily, use a small needle holder to stabilize the first throw while the second throw is put down the cannula (Fig. 9-24). Bring the needle holder through an adjacent portal or the one used for anchor insertion. This knot-stabilizing maneuver is similar to placing a finger on the ribbon when tying a bow on a package.

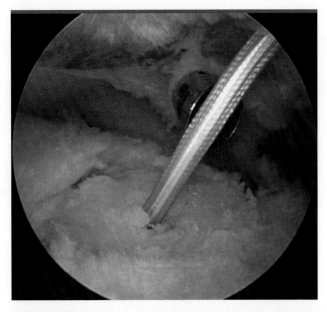

Figure 9-22   Photograph of a suture anchor inserted into the cuff footprint.

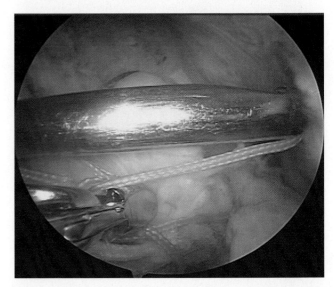

Figure 9-24   Stabilizing the half-hitched knot with a hemostat-type device.

When possible, reinforce the primary tendon-to-bone repair by placing a suture medial to the repair, through intact tendon tissue, and then tie this suture to an anchor that is placed on the greater tuberosity lateral to the first row of anchors. This creates a tension band repair on the first row of sutures (Fig. 9-25A). First, place an anchor on the greater tuberosity from the lateral portal while viewing from posterior. Pass the sutures from this anchor out through the anterior portal. Move the arthroscope back to the lateral portal. Place one suture limb through the intact supraspinatus tendon medial to the previous sutures by passing an ArthroPierce from the posterior portal proximal through the supraspinatus tendon to grasp the suture that is in the anterior portal. Pull this suture out through the posterior portal. The second limb is passed in a similar retrograde fashion through the infraspinatus: pass an ArthroPierce through the infraspinatus and grasp the suture on the greater tuberosity anchor. Tie the suture from the posterior portal. Repeat this with the second suture on the anchor.

RESTORE THE CUFF FOOTPRINT

Biomechanical evidence indicates that the initial fixation strength of a double-layer repair exceeds that of isolated single-layer repairs with either suture anchors or tran-

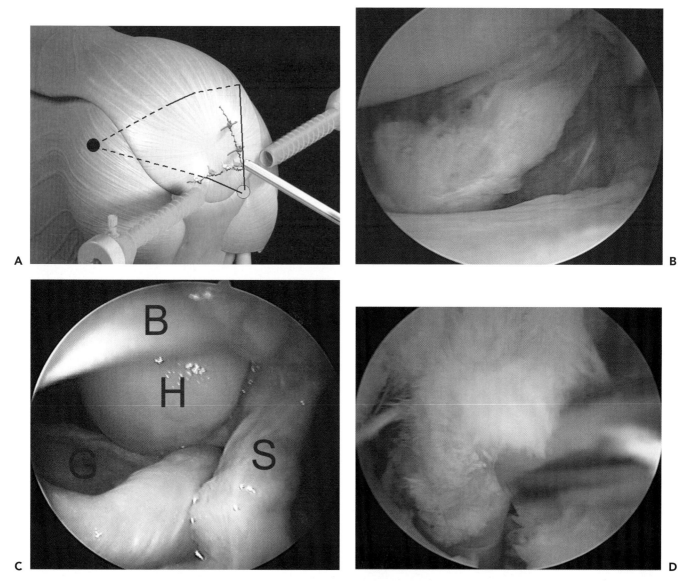

Figure 9-25 (*A*) The final repair is augmented with a tension band suture from the anchor (*gray dot*) through the cuff with the knot (*black dot*) tied from the posterior portal. (*B*) Subscapularis tear as seen from the posterior portal. (*C*) View of a normal subscapularis (S) insertion into the lesser tuberosity of the humerus (H). The biceps (B) tendon is above. (*D*) View of subscapularis tear from anterosuperior portal (same patient as in Fig. 9-25A). (*continued*)

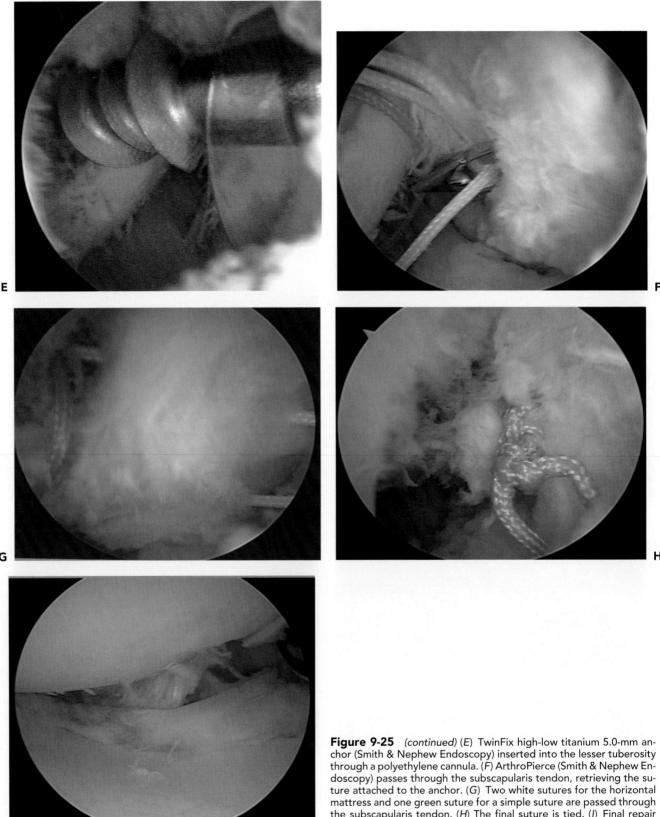

Figure 9-25 *(continued)* (*E*) TwinFix high-low titanium 5.0-mm anchor (Smith & Nephew Endoscopy) inserted into the lesser tuberosity through a polyethylene cannula. (*F*) ArthroPierce (Smith & Nephew Endoscopy) passes through the subscapularis tendon, retrieving the suture attached to the anchor. (*G*) Two white sutures for the horizontal mattress and one green suture for a simple suture are passed through the subscapularis tendon. (*H*) The final suture is tied. (*I*) Final repair seen from posterior portal.

sosseous tunnels.[20] The double-layer repair gives a larger repair area but does not restore the normal footprint. This double-row technique provides better potential for healing and, ultimately, greater strength of repair.[1]

Burkhart[3] recommends that the suture anchors be 1 cm apart with two sutures per anchor. The authors prefer simple sutures for most cuff repair unless a double-row technique is used. In this case, use a mattress suture in the medial row next to the articular cartilage. The mattress and Mason Allen sutures tend to tighten and constrict the tissue rather than afford better fixation. Gerber believes that a better repair is obtained with the Mason Allen suture.[8]

Revision Rotator Cuff Surgery

The same techniques for primary rotator cuff surgery apply to the patient with a failed previous rotator cuff repair. It does not make any difference if the primary repair was done by arthroscopy or open surgery. An aggressive excision of adhesions and subacromial bursectomy may be necessary in some patients. The surgeon must be careful not to remove any more acromion than necessary to create a smooth undersurface.

Subscapularis Tears

Frayed, loose remnants of the tendon are debrided through a low anterior portal at the superior margin of the subscapularis (Fig. 9-25B). The view from this portal allows more complete visualization of the tendon and footprint, and aids in arthroscopic repair.

If the tendon is readily visualized and deemed appropriate for repair, the anterior working portal needs to be modified to increase the working space in this area. The shaver is introduced into the joint through the anterior working portal, and the portal is retracted outside the capsule. The capsule is then debrided around the portal to create a hole approximately 1.5 cm in diameter in the rotator interval capsule. This portal enables viewing of the subscapularis tendon into the lesser tuberosity. The surgeon needs to be familiar with a view of the normal subscapularis tendon from this portal (Fig. 9-25C).

The frayed margins of the subscapularis tendon are once again gently debrided back to healthy tissue (Fig. 9-25D). Tendon excursion is then assessed using arthroscopic graspers. The anticipated repair site about the lesser tuberosity is also assessed. Visualization is again aided by placing the arthroscope into the high anterior portal, with a working cannula placed posteriorly. Once the bony bed repair site is determined, a burr is used to gently prepare it.

A TwinFix titanium 5.0-mm doubly loaded suture anchor (Smith & Nephew Endoscopy) is placed through the low anterior portal into the inferior portion of the bony bed

(Fig. 9-25E). The sutures are then retrieved out the posterior portal, with one limb left near the leading edge of the subscapularis tear. A straight ArthroPierce is used in the low anterior portal to pierce the inferior margin of the torn tendon, and the suture is retracted through the tendon (Fig. 9-25F). The second limb of the suture is withdrawn through the tendon to create a horizontal mattress suture pattern. Next, the second suture in the anchor is placed through the tendon in a more superior position in similar fashion (Fig. 9-25G). The sutures are tied with sliding arthroscopic knots backed up with four alternating throw, alternating post-locking stitches.

Depending on the magnitude of the tear, a second suture anchor may be required. It is placed approximately 1 cm superior to the first anchor. The two sutures are placed through the torn tendon in like fashion. It is usually helpful for suture management to place the sutures already passed through the tendon outside the low anterior cannula, exiting through the same portal.

Once the anchors and sutures have been passed, they are tied (Fig. 9-25H). The arm is held in internal rotation while the sutures are tied arthroscopically and cut beginning inferiorly and proceeding superiorly. The repair is then evaluated for integrity by probing and visualizing the repair as the arm is taken through a gentle range of motion (Fig. 9-25I). This maneuver also aids in determining postoperative passive external rotation.

If the long head of the biceps tendon has pathology, a decision should be made as to debridement, tenotomy or tenodesis, and the procedure performed.

POSTOPERATIVE CARE

Control of pain immediately after surgery is important. Ice packs, especially for the first 3 days, and NSAIDs and narcotics as needed are the mainstays of pain control. The authors inject 0.25% bupivacaine with epinephrine into the subacromial space, around the portals, and around the suprascapular nerve from the supraclavicular fossa portal. Healing of the rotator cuff to bone is necessary for optimal function.[10] Immobilize the shoulder in an UltraSling (dj Orthopedics, Inc., Carlsbad, CA) for 4 to 8 weeks, depending on the size of the tear. Passive shoulder exercises are begun immediately, with passive supine forward elevation from 0 degrees to 90 degrees and external rotation to 10 degrees. Active assistive motion is allowed between 6 and 8 weeks, and active motion is allowed at 8 to 12 weeks. As a rule, the authors tend to go slow rather than fast with these repairs. No weightlifting is allowed until 4 to 6 months after surgery.

Some patients will experience postoperative stiffness, especially with smaller tears. If this is present 12 weeks postoperatively, a Dynasplint (Dynasplint Systems, Severna Park, MD) is used for gentle home stretching.

RESULTS

In a review of 51 shoulders in 48 patients more than 2 years postoperatively,[11] surgery had improved the pain scores in all patients, with 48 of 51 shoulders (94%) getting a satisfactory rating by the patient. Three patients with larger and massive tears reported unsatisfactory results secondary to shoulder weakness. Average time to return to work among those who were employed was 3.2 months, with an average recovery of 5.1 months. Smaller tears recovered faster than medium or large tears. Postoperative supraspinatus strength was significantly better for small and medium tears than for larger and massive tears. University of California Los Angeles (UCLA) scores for all tears significantly improved from the preoperative average of 10.3 (±2.4) to 32.1 (±4.3) postoperatively (Fig. 9-26). Small tears had an average score of 35, medium tears of 33.2, and large tears of 30. Excellent results on postoperative UCLA scores were achieved in 26 (51%) patients and good results in 17 (33%) patients. Fair results were seen in 7 shoulders (14%), and 1 shoulder (2%) had a poor result. The average overall Western Ontario Rotator Cuff (WORC) score was 86.8% (±17.1) of normal (Fig. 9-27).[12] Scores for smaller and medium tears were significantly better than for large or massive tears. Scores for motion, lifestyle, and physical symptoms were slightly higher than those for work and sports recreation. The only complication of this study was that two screws (out of 75) were loose postoperatively. One patient with a massive tear experienced superior migration of the humeral head and degenerative changes of the glenohumeral joint. One patient had symptomatic AC arthrosis at his most recent follow-up.

Metcalf performed a meta-analysis that compared open and arthroscopic rotator cuff repairs.[15] There was no significant difference in the overall results between open, arthroscopic, and mini-open techniques with regard to

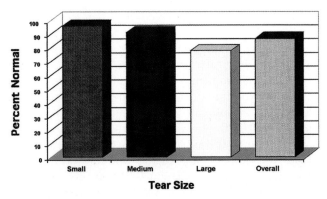

Figure 9-27   Bar graph showing average Western Ontario Rotator Cuff (WORC) scores for tear sizes.

pain relief, range of motion, percentage of good and excellent results, satisfaction percentage, and strength. The results depend more on the surgeon's expertise than on repair technique (Table 9-1). The patient populations from different surgeons could not be assumed to be similar with regard to demographics, method of documentation, tear size, prior treatment, and social and medical comorbidities. The number of shoulder functions in patients with rotator cuff tears has been shown to be inversely associated with social and medical comorbidities.[9]

COMPLICATIONS

Complications of arthroscopic rotator cuff surgery are similar to those associated with open surgery, such as infection, stiffness, incomplete healing, loosening of an anchor, and injury to the deltoid muscle. The potential of deltoid muscle detachment is much less because the deltoid is not taken down for exposure.

Intraoperatively, the surgeon should know proper suture and knot management so that the surgery proceeds in a timely fashion. Excessive operative time may lead to excessive swelling, which can make visualization, and therefore repair, difficult. Additionally, it can increase swelling in the area of the trachea, if the patient is in the lateral position, making extubation difficult.

For certainty of placement, the anchors should be visualized going into the bone rather than being placed transtendon.

CONCLUSION

Short-term studies have demonstrated excellent results for arthroscopic rotator cuff repairs. Arthroscopy offers the advantages of a minimally invasive approach, smaller incisions, easy access to the glenohumeral joint for treatment of intra-articular disease, less tissue dissection, and less po-

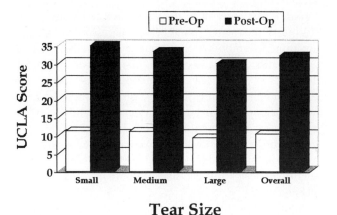

Figure 9-26   Bar graph showing mean preoperative (pre-op) and postoperative (post-op) University of California Los Angeles (UCLA) rating scale scores.

TABLE 9-1
SUMMARY OF ROTATOR CUFF REPAIR RESULTS

Author	Mean age (yr)	Mean follow-up (mo)	Results % Good or excellent	% Satisfactory	Mean ROM	% Pain relief	Strength (out of 5)
Kersey and Esch[7] (arthroscopy)	68	53	84	94	170	92	4.8
Murray et al.[16] (arthroscopy)	58	39	96	98	170	93	4.9
Wilson et al.[21] (arthroscopy)	52	48	91	90	141	91	4.7
Burkhart et al.[2] (arthroscopy)		42	95	100	141	84	4.6
Gartsman et al.[7] (arthroscopy)	61	30	84	90	149	78	4.3
Mean arthroscopic repair[5]	56	46	90	92	147	87	4.6
Mean open repair[5]	55	58	81	89	146	78	4.2
Mean mini-open repair[5]	58	35	87	93	150	86	4.5

MO, months; ROM, range of motion; yr, years.

tential injury to the deltoid muscle. Arthroscopy has improved our diagnostic assessment and recognition of the major tear patterns of the rotator cuff that require different repair techniques. With the development of various arthroscopic suture-passing instruments and techniques, it is now possible for the surgeon to consistently accomplish a secure repair of the rotator cuff with relative ease.

REFERENCES

1. Apreleva M, Ozbaydar M, Fitzgibbons PG, et al. Rotator cuff tears: the effect of the reconstruction method on three-dimensional repair site area. Arthroscopy 2002;18(5):519.
2. Burkhart SS, Danaceau SM, Pearce CE. Arthroscopic rotator cuff repair: analysis of results by tear size and by repair technique-margin convergence versus direct tendon-to-bone repair. Arthroscopy 2001;17:905.
3. Burkhart SS, Wirth MA, Simonich M, et al. Knot security in simple sliding knots and its relationship to rotator cuff repair: how secure must the knot be? Arthroscopy 2000;16(2):202.
4. Bynum CK, Lee S, Mahar A, et al. Failure mode of suture anchors as a function of insertion depth. Unpublished data.
5. Ciccone WJ II, Miles JW III, Cheon SJ, et al. The use of the supraclavicular fossa portal in arthroscopic rotator cuff repair. Arthroscopy 2000;16:399.
6. Galatz LM, Ball CM, Teefey SA, et al. Complete arthroscopic repair of large and massive rotator cuff tears: correlation of functional outcome with repair integrity. Presented at AAOS 2002 annual meeting
7. Gartsman GM, Khan M, Hammerman SM. Arthroscopic repair of full-thickness tears of the rotator cuff. J Bone Joint Surg Am 1998; 80:832.
8. Gerber C, Schneeberger AG, Perren SM, et al. Experimental rotator cuff repair: a preliminary study. J Bone Joint Surg Am 1999; 81 (9):1281.
9. Harryman DT II, Hettrich CM, Smith K, et al. A prospective multipractice investigation of patients with full-thickness rotator cuff tears. J Bone Joint Surg Am 2003;85:690.
10. Harryman DT II, Mack LA, Wang KY, et al. Repairs of the rotator cuff. Correlation of functional results with integrity of the cuff. J Bone Joint Surg Am 1991;73:982.
11. Kersey RC, Esch JC. Arthroscopic repair of complete, isolated rotator cuff tears. Presented at the annual meeting of the Arthroscopy Association of North America, Seattle, WA, April 2000.
12. Kirkley A, Litchfield RB, Jackowski DM, et al. The use of the impingement test as a predictor of outcome following subacromial decompression for rotator cuff tendonosis. Arthroscopy 2002; 18:8.
13. Lo I, Burkhart SS. Current concepts in arthroscopic rotator cuff repair. Am J Sports Med 2003;31:308.
14. Lo IK, Burkhart SS. Arthroscopic repair of massive, contracted, immobile rotator cuff tears using single and double interval slides: technique and preliminary results. Arthroscopy 2004;20(1):22.
15. Metcalf MH, Savoie FH III, Smith KL, et al. Meta-analysis of the surgical repair of rotator cuff tears: a comparison of arthroscopic and open techniques. Presented at AAOS 2003 annual meeting
16. Murray TF Jr, Lajtai G, Mileski RM, et al. Arthroscopic repair of medium to large full thickness rotator cuff tears: outcome at 2- to 6-year follow-up. J Shoulder Elbow Surg 2002;11:19.
17. Tauro JC. Arthroscopic repair of large rotator cuff tears using the interval slide technique. Arthroscopy 2004;20(1):13.
18. Tippett JW. Partial repair of rotator cuff tears greater than five centimeters. Presented at AANA 1998 annual meeting
19. Tucker BS, Upasani VV, Mahar A, et al. Effects of suture anchor depth on failure mode in cadaver humerus. Unpublished data.
20. Waltrip RL, Zheng N, Dugas JR, et al. Rotator cuff repair: a biomechanical comparison of three techniques. Am J Sports Med 2003; 31(4):493.
21. Wilson F, Hinov V, Adams G. Arthroscopic repair of full thickness tears of the rotator cuff: 2- to 14-year follow-up. Arthroscopy 2002;18:136.
22. Zuckerman JD, Leblanc JM, Choueka J, et al. The effect of arm position and capsular release on rotator cuff repair: a biomechanical study. J Bone Joint Surg Br 1991;73:402.

The Stiff Shoulder

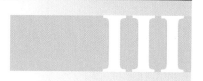

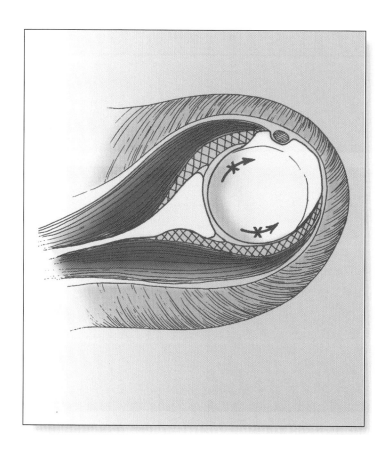

Idiopathic and Diabetic Stiff Shoulder:

Decision-Making and Treatment

Frances Cuomo   Evan L. Flatow   Jason A. Schneider   Julie Y. Bishop

INTRODUCTION

Frozen shoulder is one of the most common, yet poorly understood disorders of the glenohumeral joint. This is primarily due to the inability of physicians to agree on the exact definition of frozen shoulder syndrome, difficulty defining and differentiating it clearly from other conditions with similar symptoms and findings but with distinctly different etiologies, and confusing terminology. Frozen shoulder syndrome comprises a group of conditions with different underlying etiologies. Initially, periarthritis of the shoulder was used as an all-encompassing term to describe painful shoulders for which the symptoms could not be explained on the basis of arthritis of the glenohumeral joint.[36] Codman described the disorder known as *frozen shoulder* as a "condition difficult to define, difficult to treat, and difficult to explain from the point of view of pathology."[28] The terms *adhesive capsulitis* and *periarthritis* of the shoulder are used, at times, with a meaning synonymous with frozen shoulder. In this

chapter, a working definition of frozen shoulder is suggested: frozen shoulder is a condition of uncertain etiology characterized by significant restriction of both active and passive shoulder motion that occurs in the absence of a known intrinsic shoulder disorder.[153]

Previous authors have defined primary frozen shoulder as an idiopathic condition and secondary frozen shoulder as one associated with a known intrinsic, extrinsic, or systemic pathology.[75] Although this is most likely a worthwhile distinction, it is probably inappropriate to include all intrinsic, extrinsic, and systemic etiologies as secondary frozen shoulder. Intrinsic disorders, such as rotator cuff pathology, should be considered separately because they represent a known underlying disorder or condition that results in the clinical picture of frozen shoulder. Extrinsic disorders, such as cervical radiculopathy or intrathoracic conditions, and systemic disorders, such as diabetes mellitus or hypothyroidism, should be considered together yet separate from the intrinsic disorders because they more closely resemble the primary or idiopathic condition. This schema is shown in Figure 10-1.

In this chapter, primary frozen shoulder, as well as secondary frozen shoulder due to the systemic cause of diabetes mellitus, will be discussed by reviewing pathophysiology, evaluation, operative and nonoperative management, and complications. Secondary frozen shoulder associated with intrinsic conditions and secondary etiologies, classified as extrinsic or other systemic causes, will not be discussed because, in these situations, treatment

F. Cuomo: Beth Israel Medical Center, Insall Scott Kelly Institute for Orthopaedics, New York, New York.

E. L. Flatow: Department of Orthopaedic Surgery, Mount Sinai Medical Center, New York, New York.

J. A. Schneider: Beth Israel Medical Center, Insall Scott Kelly Institute for Orthopaedics, New York, New York.

J. Y. Bishop: Department of Orthopaedic Surgery, Mount Sinai Medical Center, New York, New York.

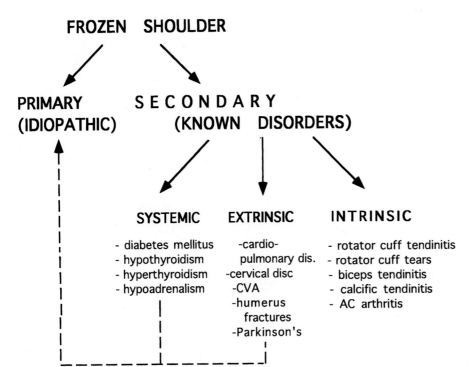

FROZEN SHOULDER

PRIMARY (IDIOPATHIC)

SECONDARY (KNOWN DISORDERS)

SYSTEMIC
- diabetes mellitus
- hypothyroidism
- hyperthyroidism
- hypoadrenalism

EXTRINSIC
-cardio-pulmonary dis.
-cervical disc
-CVA
-humerus fractures
-Parkinson's

INTRINSIC
- rotator cuff tendinitis
- rotator cuff tears
- biceps tendinitis
- calcific tendinitis
- AC arthritis

Figure 10-1 Proposed pathways for the development of frozen shoulder syndrome.

approaches are directed primarily at correction of the underlying disorder, which is critical to the alleviation of the symptoms of frozen shoulder. Exclusion criteria for primary frozen shoulder, therefore, include patients with glenohumeral arthritis, fractures, dislocations, cervical spondylosis, neuromuscular disease, and referred pain from an intrathoracic source. Intrinsic shoulder pathology, such as subacromial impingement, calcific tendonitis, and postsurgical stiffness, therefore, is also excluded from this review and will be discussed elsewhere in the book.

SURGICAL ANATOMY AND BIOMECHANICS

When discussing frozen shoulder syndrome, it is important to include the overall shoulder girdle complex. The shoulder girdle complex consists not only of the glenohumeral joint but also of the acromioclavicular, sternoclavicular, and scapulothoracic articulations. Scapulothoracic and glenohumeral movements occur simultaneously as the arm is used away from the side.[56] The normal glenohumeral to scapulothoracic ratio is 2:1, with the majority of elevation attributed to the glenohumeral joint.

The inherently loose articulation of the normal shoulder is a necessary anatomic feature that permits the large range of motion required for normal shoulder function. The glenohumeral joint is enclosed entirely by the joint capsule. The capsule of the shoulder is normally a loose structure whose surface area is almost twice that of the humeral head.[61] The stability of the shoulder is maintained further by osseous, static, and dynamic stabilizers. It is a nonconstrained articulation with the larger humeral head having nearly perfect congruity with the smaller osseous glenoid. To enhance the surface area of this loose articulation, the fibrous glenoid labrum is attached around the periphery of the glenoid. The dynamic stabilizers of the joint consist of the rotator cuff musculature and the long head of the biceps tendon. The rotator cuff muscles' primary function is to create compression of the convex humeral head into the matched concavity of the glenoid fossa. The capsuloligamentous structures are the primary static stabilizers and are responsible for the stability of the joint, mainly at the extreme positions of rotation and translation because they are normally lax during most shoulder rotations. The capsule attaches around the perimeter of the glenoid and extends across to attach to the anatomic neck of the humerus, except inferiorly, where the attachment is about 1 cm distal to the articular margin. There are numerous areas within the capsule that are thickened secondary to attachment or confluence with local structures. The tendons of the rotator cuff adjacent to the joint capsule thicken the capsule anteriorly, superiorly, and posteriorly. In addition, the superior, middle, and inferior glenohumeral ligaments will present further areas of thickening of the joint capsule.[11,12,14,34,40] The inferior capsule, however, is not supported by adjacent muscles and tendons, thereby leaving a lax double-fold of capsule, which forms the inferior or axillary recess. This potential axillary pouch space, formed by the redundant capsule fold, is normally present while the arm is at the side, but the pouch disappears and the capsule becomes taut as the arm is brought up to the forward elevation or abduction allowed by the stretch of the inferior capsule. Superiorly, there is a triangular-shaped region between the anterior border of the supraspinatus tendon and the superior border of the subscapularis tendon known as the *rotator interval*. The ligamentous components of this region are the superior glenohumeral ligament and the coracohumeral ligament. Classic descriptions of the coracohumeral ligament describe it as a dense fibrous structure originating on the lateral surface of the coracoid process at its base and inserting into the greater and lesser tuberosities adjacent to the bicipital groove.[34]

At arthroscopy or arthrography, several normal recesses may be identified in the normal shoulder. Anteriorly, a synovial recess called the *rotator cleft* is often present between the superior and middle glenohumeral ligaments, also known as the *subscapular bursa*. There is also a posterior outpouching of the capsule, deep to the infraspinatus muscle, known as the *infraspinatus bursa*. There is an inferior recess of redundant capsule forming a pouchlike fold when the arm is at the side. The synovial membrane is also a structure implicated in the frozen shoulder process. This structure lines the capsule and is in continuity with the surrounding bursae and recesses. The synovium invests the long head of the biceps and passes deep to the transverse humeral ligament in the bicipital groove. The biceps tendon sheath may extend for a distance of 5 cm beyond the transverse ligament into the bicipital groove. The tendon sheath extends distally, especially when the arm is in abduction. This arm position is where the least amount of biceps tendon is intra-articular.[85,86]

During normal motion of the shoulder, the tightening and loosening of the glenohumeral ligaments and capsule encircling the humeral head is accompanied by lengthening and shortening of the rotator cuff and deltoid muscle.[142] These structures, working in concert, allow for the normal 2:1 glenohumeral to scapulothoracic ratio necessary for the elevation of the arm. In the pathologic state of frozen shoulder syndrome, Nicholson noted that the scapula usually moved excessively in upward rotation to compensate for the loss of glenohumeral motion. On clinical examination, he consistently found the inferior glide of the humerus to be the most restricted of the accessory movements of the shoulder.[98] Numerous investigators have described the pathologic findings associated with the frozen shoulder in an attempt to offer explanation for the observed microscopic capsular changes.[28,75,77,78,87,91,92,107,117,132] Much of our current understanding of the pathology of frozen shoulder is due to the work of J. S. Neviaser, who coined the term "adhesive capsulitis" to describe an avascular, tense capsule that was markedly adherent to the humeral head and associated with decreased joint volume and synovial fluid. The histologic changes were consistent with chronic inflammation, fibrosis, and perivascular infiltration in the subsynovial layer, with the synovial layer remaining uninvolved.[92]

Simmonds theorized that a chronic inflammatory reaction caused by a degeneration of the supraspinatus tendon resulted in the capsular changes seen in frozen shoulder. He described a local hyperemia within the joint capsule, as observed earlier by Neviaser.[132] He thought that the tight, fibrotic characteristics of the capsular tissue extended out into the soft tissues around the shoulder.

From intraoperative findings of gross contracture of the rotator cuff, McNab postulated that the primary lesion was in the cuff itself, with subsequent contracture of the capsule and coracohumeral ligament. He confirmed a region of constant hypovascularity in the supraspinatus tendon, called the *critical zone* by Codman,[28] and theorized that this was responsible for the initial cuff degeneration.[117] The localized degeneration of collagen was then theorized to induce an autoimmune response. McNab felt that the round cell infiltrate found in the capsule at open surgical release of the shoulder could be interpreted as an autoimmune response.[117] Further reports have failed to identify any statistically significant clinical or laboratory evidence for an immunologic basis for this condition.[75,85] Lundberg confirmed the absence of intra-articular adhesions in his operative observations at cinearthrography.[74,75] Although at histologic examination synovial cells were found to be largely unchanged, Lundberg did report finding a more compact, dense collagen layer within the shoulder capsule. The glycosaminoglycans distribution in the shoulder capsule had the characteristics of a repair action.[73]

Ozaki and associates described the role of contracture of coracohumeral ligament and the rotator interval in the pathogenesis of frozen shoulder. These investigators found fibrosis, hyalinization, and fibrinoid degeneration in these structures.[117] Neer also reported the importance of coracohumeral ligament contracture, but he stressed that it was unlikely that any one anatomic structure or pathologic process was responsible for causing the entire symptom complex associated with frozen shoulder.[89-91] The normal rotator interval contains elastic membranous tissue that, as a result, enhances the range of motion of the glenohumeral joint. The coracohumeral ligament helps to strengthen this region and acts as a suspensory ligament of the humeral head. The long head of the biceps is located beneath the rotator interval. In patients with chronic severe adhesive capsulitis, the pathologic findings in the coracohumeral ligament and in the rotator interval are extremely important. These structures are contracted and can be converted into a thick fibrous cord that holds the humeral head tightly against the glenoid fossa and restricts glenohumeral movement in all directions.

Much of the information regarding the gross and microscopic pathologic findings has been derived from operative observation and autopsy studies. DePalma described the fibrous capsule, synovial tissue, and rotator cuff as thickened, fibrotic, and contracted around the humeral head. The folds in the capsule and the synovial membrane along the inferior aspect of the humeral head were obliterated.[33]

Recent arthroscopic evaluation of patients with arthrographically documented adhesive capsulitis is believed by some authors to involve four stages of the disease. Stage 1, the preadhesive stage, is seen in patients with minimal or no motion limitation. There is a fibrinous synovial inflammatory reaction that is only detectable by arthroscopy. This reinforces the need to obtain arthroscopic evaluation of any patient who is treated by decompression for an impingement syndrome. In stage 2, acute adhesive synovitis, there is proliferative synovitis and early adhesion formation. The adhesions are seen well in the dependent folds extending to the humeral head. Stage 3, the stage of maturation, has less synovitis with loss of the axillary fold. Stage 4, the chronic stage, has adhesions that are fully mature and markedly restrictive.[97]

PATHOPHYSIOLOGY

The syndrome of frozen shoulder was first described by Duplay in 1896. He introduced the term "scapulo-humeral periarthritis" and felt that the initiating lesion was an obliteration of the subdeltoid bursa.[36] Since then, numerous pathologic mechanisms have been proposed to explain the cause of frozen shoulder syndrome, all of which still remain largely theoretical. Myer suggested that the initiating lesion was a breakdown on the intra-articular portion of the biceps tendon.[88] His observations were supported subsequently by Pasteur[111] and Lippman[68] and, more recently, by De-Palma.[32] Codman, however, felt that the changes in the biceps tendon were of little etiological significance.[28]

McLaughlin, one of the earliest investigators to describe the changes in the rotator cuff, stressed the importance of contracture of the subscapularis in the development of the syndrome.[81,82] Bateman reported his observations on the development of a hypertrophic inflammatory synovitis associated with intra-articular adhesions.[5] Several investigators have proposed an autoimmune basis for frozen shoulder.[7,21,22,23,50] Although some clinicians have reported a high incidence of HLA B27 in patients with frozen shoulder,[22] others have not confirmed this association.[61,100,124,137] In later studies, serum immunoglobulin A (IGA) levels were found to be significantly lower in patients with frozen shoulder, while the immune complex and C-reactive protein levels were increased.[7,21,23] In general, however, sufficient evidence to support an immunologic therapy has been lacking.

A relationship to myofascial pain syndrome has been proposed. A syndrome of active trigger points about the shoulder, specifically within the subscapularis muscle, has been suggested as a possible cause of frozen shoulder syndrome.[138] Trigger points are defined as locally tender, self-sustaining, hyperirritable foci located in the skeletal muscle or its associated fascia. The trigger points are also characteristically related to a zone of referred pain when the trig-

ger is stimulated. Once activated, perpetuating factors may be responsible for the chronicity of pain. Another characteristic of the myofascial pain syndrome is palpable bands of muscle fibers that undergo a local twitch response when the trigger point is stimulated with a snapping palpation.[14,133,149]

Travell and others theorized that the subscapularis trigger points exert an influence on the sympathetic vasomotor activity, leading to hypoxia of the periarticular tissues. It is further theorized that the hypoxia leads to a local proliferation of fibrous tissue about the shoulder capsule, resulting in the clinical picture of frozen shoulder syndrome.[88,138] A biochemical basis for frozen shoulder has been proposed. Lundberg, in his analysis of the capsule on patients with frozen shoulder, found an increase in glycosaminoglycans and a decrease in glycoprotein content. These biochemical changes in the capsule, however, are consistent with the process of fibrosis, and they may represent the effect of frozen shoulder rather than its cause.[73,75]

Neurologic dysfunction has been postulated as a cause of frozen shoulder syndrome. In 1959, Kopell proposed suprascapular compression neuropathy as a possible cause of frozen shoulder, but electromyography and nerve conduction studies have not supported this theory.[63] Others have suggested that frozen shoulder is a result of autonomic dysfunction and represents a form of reflex sympathetic dystrophy.[123] Sufficient evidence to support these hypothesis has not been provided.

Bunker et al. prospectively studied 50 patients with the diagnosis of primary frozen shoulder. These authors were able to identify increased serum lipid levels in these patients compared to age- and sex-matched control subjects. The fasting serum triglyceride and cholesterol levels were significantly elevated in the frozen shoulder group. Increased serum triglyceride levels have also been found in patients with diabetes and with Dupuytren's disease, suggesting that hyperlipidemia may be the common thread that links these three disorders.[24,25]

Various endocrine disorders are associated with frozen shoulder. In particular, patients with diabetes manifest a much greater incidence of frozen shoulder than their nondiabetic counterparts.[17] Frozen shoulder has also been reported to occur with increased incidence among patients with thyroid disorders, hypoadrenalism, and corticotrophin deficiency.[13,39,148,26]

Trivial trauma has been postulated to be an important factor, particularly when it is followed by a prolonged period of immobilization.[32,115] This does seem to be the sequence of events in some patients who develop frozen shoulder. The association of frozen shoulder with major trauma to the shoulder or other parts of the upper extremity is recognized. The association with minor trauma, which may be forgotten, is difficult to document and may be overlooked.[28,82] Most patients who sustain minimal trauma, even when combined with a period of immobilization, do not develop frozen shoulder. This has led some investigators to conclude that there are some patients who possess a "constitutional" predisposition for the development of frozen shoulder. Support for this theory is provided by the significant incidence of bilateral frozen shoulders.[22,75,101,119,151]

The role of psychologic factors has been considered in the development of frozen shoulder. Some investigators have suggested that a certain personality structure, coupled with untoward life events and inappropriate response to stress, may serve as a predisposing or precipitating factor for the development of frozen shoulder.[29,39,71,123] Coventry chose the term *periarthritic personality* to describe one component of a three-part theory on the pathogenesis of frozen shoulder in a group of patients with painful stiff shoulders. He observed that most patients had "a peculiar emotional constitution in which they were unable to tolerate pain, expected others to make them well, and refused to take personal initiative in their recovery."[29] Other studies, however, have found no evidence for a characteristic personality disorder.[101,151] It would, therefore, appear that a specific periarthritic personality type is difficult to identify. The role of psychologic factors should be considered, at best, a secondary factor in the management of these patients.

Fibromatosis has also been implicated in causing frozen shoulder syndrome. The pathomechanics are believed to be found in fibrous tissue contracture formed in response to cytokines, lymphocytes, or monocyte products. Platelet-derived growth factor is a potent mytogenic polypeptide for mesenchymal cells. Immunocytochemistry was performed with monoclonal antibodies on the rotator ligament excised from 12 patients with resistant frozen shoulder. Bunker and Anthony report that the pathologic process is active fibroblastic proliferation accompanied by some transformation to a smooth muscle phenotype (myofibroblasts). The fibroblasts lay down collagen, which appears as a thick nodular band or fleshy mass. These appearances are reportedly very similar to those seen in Dupuytren's disease of the hand, with no inflammation and no synovial involvement. The contracture acts as a checkrein against external rotation, causing a loss of both active and passive movement.[24]

Frozen shoulder associated with a known underlying disorder is considered to be secondary, and this group includes intrinsic, extrinsic, or secondary disorders. Intrinsic shoulder abnormalities include rotator cuff tears, tendonitis of the long head of the biceps tendon, calcific tendonitis, and acromioclavicular arthritis. Extrinsic disorders, which represent pathologic conditions apart from the shoulder region, include ischemic heart disease and myocardial infarction[83,151]; pulmonary disorders including tuberculosis,[59] chronic bronchitis, emphysema,[130] and tumor[31]; cervical disc disease and radiculopathy[4,60,151]; cerebral vascular hemorrhage[16,19]; previous coronary artery by-

pass graft surgery[133]; previous breast surgery; lesions of the middle humerus[134]; and central nervous system disorders, such as Parkinson's disease.[122] Systemic disorders represent generalized medical conditions that are known to occur in association with frozen shoulder. Such conditions and poor prognostic indicators include diabetes mellitus, hypothyroidism, hyperthyroidism, and hypoadrenalism.

EPIDEMIOLOGY AND NATURAL HISTORY

Epidemiologically, the exact prevalence and incidence of frozen shoulder are not known; however, the cumulative risk of at least one episode of frozen shoulder has been estimated to be a minimum of 2%.[75] It is most frequently found in patients between the fourth and sixth decades of life, and it is more common in women than men.[4] The nondominant extremity appears to be more commonly involved, with most reported cases described as affecting the left side.[32,68,75] Bilateral involvement occurs in 6% to 50% of cases, although only 14% of these bilateral cases manifest simultaneously.[4,7,23,75,123] When a history of bilateral involvement is identified, the possibility of a constitutional predisposition should be explored.[5,75,123] With adhesive capsulitis, the same shoulder is rarely involved again.[7,8]

There is significant controversy over the natural history of frozen shoulder with respect to both objective and subjective outcomes. Historically, frozen shoulder has been touted as a condition in which "recovery is always sure and maybe confidently expected."[28] Several investigators using a variety of treatment methods have reported a high percentage of affected patients achieving full range of motion.[28,42,68] In addition, they have found complete or near complete symptomatic relief.[42,50] More recent investigations have questioned the early optimistic reports, finding measurable restriction at follow-up in 39% to 76% of patients[20,27,83,87,119] and persistent symptoms in up to 45%.[7,115]

The time course of adhesive capsulitis has been described as classically lasting 18 to 24 months.[7] Recent studies have challenged this commonly held belief. Reeves noted that the mean duration of symptoms was 30 months.[119] Patients describing themselves as functionally recovered tend to underestimate their loss of motion.[20] Reeves described some shoulder motion restriction in over 50% of patients in a 5- to 10-year follow-up, but functional impairment was identified in only 7%.[119] Clark found that 42% of patients had persisting limitations of motion after 6 years of follow-up.[27] Binder, in a prospective study, noted that 90% of patients did not regain the minimum range of motion when matched for age and sex with a controlled group 6 months after diagnosis. He also reported that 40% of patients failed to regain a minimum range of motion when matched for age and sex with a controlled group when followed for a minimum of 3 years.[7] In a retrospective study of a carefully selected group of frozen shoulder patients performed by Schaffer et al., almost half remained symptomatic many years after the onset of symptoms, and up to 56% had residual restriction in one or more planes.[130]

Despite the subjective and objective outcome of this disorder, there seems to be widespread agreement with regard to the seeming lack of significant or frequent functional disability documented at cessation of treatment. Regardless of objective restriction or the presence of symptoms, few patients are reportedly functionally restricted to any significant degree.[7,27,69,119] The lack of correlation between subjective and objective findings has been noted consistently.[7,9,20,27,50,87] Symptomatic patients frequently have no measurable restricted range of motion in any plane. Conversely, those patients with the most significant motion were often pain-free. However, whether this difference is from the patient adapting to the restricted motion or due to the restricted motion not being present in daily living activities is an unresolved issue. According to Neer, however, the presence of such restriction depends upon the functional demands of the patient.[91] Even in the active patient, the presence of 150 degrees of active elevation, 50 degrees of external rotation, and internal rotation to the eighth thoracic vertebras is probably sufficient for normal function. In Schaffer's report of an older population whose functional demands were surely less than the demands just stated, the degree of restriction tolerated in any plane was certainly even greater. The authors state that the preeminent importance of forward flexion and elevation in daily activities superseded the findings of restriction predominantly in the abducted and externally rotated positions, which resulted in little functional impairment.[130]

In general, the natural history of frozen shoulder is uncertain, and additional randomized, prospective studies are needed. The difficulty of performing these studies, however, is because of the ethical dilemma of assigning patients to an untreated group.

DIABETES MELLITUS

Patients with diabetes mellitus, in particular, manifest a much greater incidence of frozen shoulder than their nondiabetic counterparts. The incidence of frozen shoulder in diabetic patients is approximately 10% to 20%, but may be as high as 36%.[17,67,75,151] Bridgman found that the incidence of frozen shoulder in 800 diabetic patients was 10.8%, compared with 2.3% in 600 nondiabetic controls.[17] Diabetic patients have a significantly higher incidence of bilateral involvement, with bilateral presentation in as many as 77% of those cases.[127] Generally, frozen shoulder is noted more frequently in patients with long-standing insulin-dependent diabetes mellitus (IDDM).[2,103,108,125] It is

generally believed that the long-term use of supplemental insulin and fluctuating levels of glucose increase the risk of developing shoulder stiffness.[84] The high blood-glucose levels are thought to accelerate aging of certain body proteins, which trigger a series of chemical reactions in proteins. This eventually leads to cross-linking between adjacent molecules, such as long collagen chains.[2,84,128] This makes the collagen more resistant to degeneration and more likely to accumulate.

The frozen shoulder in patients with diabetes is reported to be more persistent and resistant to treatment than an idiopathic frozen shoulder. Regardless of the treatment, the patient with diabetes often has residual loss of motion. Several studies have demonstrated that patients who present with diabetic frozen shoulder do not respond well to either nonsurgical stretching or manipulation under anesthesia (MUA). Manipulation under anesthesia is only partially effective in IDDM, and is more effective for those who have a shorter duration of symptoms. In many cases, the patients are left with persistent pain and loss of motion and function.[43,58,84] Arthroscopic release has recently resulted in better outcomes than MUA. Patients overall did significantly better, but still some patients were resistant to treatment, and movement limitation persisted.[79,103]

EVALUATION

Frozen shoulder syndrome entails a complex of symptoms rather than a specific diagnostic entity; therefore, a careful clinical history and physical examination is crucial to making the diagnosis. Patients often complain of a gradual loss of function associated with discomfort of varying levels of intensity about the shoulder. Minimal or no trauma is often reported. The symptoms usually begin insidiously and are often worse at night. The examiner should inquire about whether or not there is pain that interrupts sleep. Overhead and internal rotation or behind-the-back activities become especially difficult to perform because motion is diminished. These symptoms closely resemble those found in rotator cuff pathology, thereby mandating a careful physical examination to consider frozen shoulder as the primary condition or one that is secondary to a specific shoulder problem. The patient should be asked to describe how the shoulder condition limits function, as well as the duration of pain. The physician needs to inquire about risk factors, especially diabetes and thyroid disorders, because these may adversely affect the outcome. The patient should be asked about specific occupational duties because frozen shoulder is more common in patients with sedentary occupations than in manual laborers.

As the shoulder stiffens, there is progressive loss of glenohumeral motion. The most significant loss is usually in external rotation with lesser loss of abduction and internal rotation.[19] The patient may report functional restrictions such as difficulty using the arm above the chest level, reaching to the side, or putting on a coat. Loss of internal rotation is exhibited by functional restrictions in dressing or performing personal hygiene activities. There may be discomfort over the acromioclavicular joint, which can be secondary to increased scapulothoracic motion. Pain at the end point of restricted shoulder motion is characteristic.

Physical Examination

A thorough physical examination not only of the affected glenohumeral joint but also of the opposite shoulder, cervical spine, and trunk should always be performed to exclude any associated abnormality or pathology. The clinical hallmark of frozen shoulder syndrome is the glenohumeral joint's limited active and passive ranges of motion. When the scapula is stabilized by the examining physician's hand, it should become apparent that the primary limitation is in the shoulder joint. Pain may be absent when the shoulder is moved within its free range, depending upon the stage of presentation. Both active and passive motion losses must be recorded and compared because concomitant conditions, such as a rotator cuff tear, can result in active motion in a shoulder that is also stiff due to adhesions. The examiner must be careful to identify and control compensatory motions to measure only pure glenohumeral motion. Patients with glenohumeral stiffness often exhibit relatively good motion due to increased scapulothoracic motion or trunk lean. Active shoulder elevation is measured in the plane of the scapula with the patient seated and is referenced to the patient's thorax, not to a line vertical to the floor. This eliminates compensatory movement, such as associated trunk tilt or increased scapulothoracic contribution to overall motion. External rotation, as well as internal rotation along the thoracic and lumbar vertebrae, is measured with the arm at the side. A firm end point is often expected, with pain at the extremes of motion. There has been little consensus about the degree of restriction of shoulder motion needed to make the diagnosis of frozen shoulder.[7,8] In general, external rotation, abduction, and internal rotation are the most affected.

Passive motion should then be evaluated with the patient in the supine position, restricting excessive scapulothoracic movement and eliminating lumbar or trunk tilt, thereby providing a more accurate assessment of pure glenohumeral motion. Passive forward elevation, external rotation at the side, and internal and external rotation at 90 degrees of abduction as well as a cross chest adduction are measured.

Localized areas of tenderness, especially about the rotator cuff, biceps tendon, and acromioclavicular (AC) joint, should be assessed, in addition to a complete neurologic exam. Specific patterns of motion are also noted with regard to the etiology of the stiffness. For example, primary adhesive capsulitis is usually associated with global motion

loss, whereas postsurgical or posttraumatic stiffness may present with loss of motion in all planes, or it may be a more discreet limitation of motion affecting some planes while relatively sparing others. Recognizing these different motion-loss patterns are important in determining etiology, as well as planning the nonoperative, and possibly operative, treatment program. Motion loss often correlates with the location of a capsular contracture. Isolated areas of pathology within the capsule will have varying clinical presentations. For example, limited external rotation with the arm in the abducted position is usually associated with scarring in the anteroinferior region of the capsule, as opposed to limited external rotation in the adducted shoulder, which is associated with contracture in the anterosuperior capsular region in the rotator interval.[90,92,107] Limited internal rotation in adduction and abduction is associated with scarring in the posterior capsule, which is also reflected in loss of horizontal cross-chest adduction.[49] Extra-articular contractures, such as those ensuing from subdeltoid or subacromial bursitis and the impingement process, as well as subscapularis entrapment, can also cause scarring between tissue planes and contribute to global motion loss.

Upon completing the physical examination, the most helpful additional test that can be performed within the office setting is the lidocaine injection test. This is limited not only to the subacromial space, but it can also be applied to the AC joint, depending upon the presence or absence of the impingement signs as well as AC joint tenderness and pain on cross-chest adduction. In the case of a subacromial disorder, an injection of 10 cc of 1% lidocaine into this region will reveal true active motion as opposed to pain-inhibited motion. When the pain is eliminated, one must record the postinjection increase in motion, which helps to differentiate loss due to impingement versus true motion loss from soft-tissue contracture. In an individual with limited motion secondary to pain from rotator cuff pathology, an increase in forward elevation will be noted, as well as relief of pain. This is in contrary to the patient with a true soft-tissue contracture in which limited passive and active motion will persist, despite anesthetic in the subacromial space.

Laboratory and Imaging Studies

Routine hematologic testing should include a complete blood cell count, chemistry profile, rheumatoid factor test, and serology. These results, however, are usually normal. Although no specific test is diagnostic, the erythrocyte sedimentation rate is elevated in as many as 20% of patients.[7,8] There remains ongoing controversy about the significance of the reported increased levels of immune complexes in patients with adhesive capsulitis.[22,23,61] Bulgen et al. reported on 40 patients with clinical signs of frozen shoulder who had shown an increase in immune complex levels, including C-reactive protein and impaired cell-mediated immunity. Tests to measure these values 8 months following the onset of the shoulder disorder revealed a tendency for the values to return to normal levels.[23] Fasting serum triglyceride and cholesterol levels have also been found to be significantly elevated in those patients with frozen shoulder syndrome, compared to age- and sex-match controlled subjects.[25]

With the exception of disuse osteopenia, radiographic findings are usually negative. Significant findings, however, may aid in identifying underlying intrinsic disorders, and a complete set of radiographs consisting of scapular anteroposterior films in neutral, external, and internal rotation, as well as supraspinatus outlet and axillary views should be obtained. These views provide excellent visualization of the proximal humerus and surrounding soft tissues. A normal glenohumeral joint is often confirmed through plain radiography in patients with primary frozen shoulder. Disuse osteoporosis is often evident, especially in patients who present with the clinical features of reflex sympathetic dystrophy. Minor degenerative changes of the humeral head in the area of the greater tuberosity, or a narrowing of the subacromial space, have also been reported with incidences of 19% and 12%, respectively.[20]

Technetium scanning has been used to evaluate the frozen shoulder. Findings of increased uptake, although nonspecific, are probably secondary to hypervascularity. Wright et al. noted a favorable association between an increased pertechnetate uptake about the shoulder and rapid response to corticosteroid injections.[151] Binder et al. observed that over 90% of their patients had an increased uptake on the diphosphonate scans, with 29% having more than a 50% increase in uptake compared with the opposite shoulder. These authors, however, could not find any association between the bone scan findings and the duration of symptoms, the initial severity of the disease, the arthrographic findings, or the eventual recovery.[9]

The early descriptions of the characteristic shoulder arthrography findings in frozen shoulder syndrome by Neviaser have allowed a better understanding of the underlying shoulder joint pathology, without having to resort to surgical exposure. He described, as typical, the combination of a decreased joint volume, an irregular joint outline, and variable filling in the bicipital tendon sheath at arthrography.[96] The reduction in the shoulder joint capsule capacity to less than 10 to 12 cc and the variable lack of filling of the axillary fold and subscapular bursa are the currently accepted characteristic findings.[1,51,72,95,96] Since the time of this classic description, arthrography has been used as a standard diagnostic technique to confirm frozen shoulder. This technique reveals at least a 50% reduction of shoulder joint volume and a box-like appearance of the joint cavity.[9,123] The shoulder joint volume capacity of patients with frozen shoulder is noted to be only 5 to 10 mL as compared with that of normal shoulders, which is 20 to 30 mL.[41,42,61,72,123] The findings during arthrography include a tight, thickened capsule[42,61,95] and loss of the axillary recess, the subcoracoid folds, and the subscapular bursa.[51,72,92,115] Binder et al. noted that, although arthrography is useful in the diagnosis of frozen shoulder, arthrographic findings do not indicate the type of onset (i.e., primary or secondary) or the rate or extent of recovery.[9] Other authors confirm that such findings have also not been shown to have any predicted value in terms of disease severity or prognosis.[57,72]

Lundberg, as well as other authors, have used arthrography to document joint capsule tearing during manipulation under anesthesia.[1,75] Tears of the capsule allow dye to escape into the extracapsular space; however, no tears of the rotator cuff tendons, following manipulation under anesthesia, were noted in an extensive study by Lundberg.[75]

TREATMENT

Pain relief and motion and function restoration are the overall goals in treating frozen shoulder syndrome patients. A basic understanding of the disease course is imperative when formulating a treatment plan. Reeves described this condition as consisting of three phases. The painful phase, characterized by diffuse shoulder pain and progressive stiffness, lasts 3 to 9 months and is reportedly followed by the stiffening, or frozen, phase. During the stiffening phase, the pain is diminished and a more comfortable but severely restricted range of motion exists, which usually lasts 4 to 12 months. In the final phase, the thawing phase, motion and function gradually improve over the next 12 to 42 months, although to a variable degree.[119] Ideally, efforts should be directed toward preventing this syndrome by identifying the patients at risk and initiating early intervention. This is best accomplished by emphasizing early motion in potential secondary cases (after trauma and surgery) whenever possible. Unfortunately, most patients present with an already painful stiff shoulder. The clinician must design a treatment plan that is individualized and based on the severity and chronicity of the patient's symptoms, as well as previous therapeutic efforts. As in other medical conditions where the pathophysiology is poorly understood, many different forms of treatment are used empirically in the management of frozen shoulder syndrome. Treatment is continuously modified, depending on the individual's response to a particular treatment modality.

The first objective in the treatment of patients with frozen shoulder syndrome is pain relief. This is essential because it permits patients to more readily participate in an exercise program aimed at restoring motion and recovering function. Efforts to obtain pain relief by rest, analgesia, or transcutaneous electrical nerve stimulation (TENS) are useful in the early stages of this syndrome.[8,123] The routine use of narcotics should be avoided because they carry a risk of dependency, and nonsteroidal anti-inflammatory medication can be equally effective, although there have been no controlled studies to document their efficacy compared with placebo.[35,55,120] Nonsteroidal anti-inflammatory medications are often used empirically, but, when questioned, patients found the nonsteroidal agents less helpful than nonsalicylate analgesics.[8] Oral corticosteroids have also been recommended for the treatment of frozen shoulder, but there exists little evidence to support their routine use.[8,11,12,37,93]

Many medical practitioners prefer the intra-articular injection of steroids accompanied by local analgesics and gentle active motion, especially in the freezing stage of frozen shoulder.[20,51,72] Local intra-articular and subacromial corticosteroid injections have been used to relieve pain, but less frequently to improve motion in patients with frozen shoulder.[3,20,30,65,93,116,126] They may be particularly helpful in the early phase of the condition, when pain prevents the patient from actively participating in rehabilitation. Holligworth reported that injecting a corticosteroid directly into the anatomic site of the lesion produces pain relief and at least 50% range-of-motion improvement in 26% of cases studied.[53] Adversely, Quigley[115] and Neviaser[94] report the belief that steroids cannot affect established scars, contractures, or adhesions, although Quigley felt that they may reduce pain if administered in conjunction with manipulation.

Paired injections have also been used, as shown in a study by Richardson, who reported the results of a blind, controlled multicenter study of 37 patients afflicted with frozen shoulder syndrome. These patients received two injections of 25 mg of prednisolone acetate, one into the bursa and one into the glenohumeral joint, on the initial visit and again at 2 weeks, and then were compared with controls receiving injections of normal saline. Richardson also noted the inability of most physicians to successfully inject into the markedly retracted shoulder joint.[121] Several authors believe that an arthrogram is better used to determine the anatomical landmarks for subsequent intra-articular injections, although a technically satisfactory arthrogram could not be achieved in 12% of their patients.[146]

Murnaghan et al. also compared regional infiltration of the shoulder joint capsule with 25 mm of hydrocortisone acetate with injections of 2% lidocaine in the absence of a control group. The authors found both treatments to be beneficial, but the hydrocortisone failed to offer any significant advantage.[86]

The use of intra-articular injections, in summary, has theoretical merits and is reported with various results, but, in general, the evidence is equivocal. In patients with moderately stiff shoulders for whom pain is a major impediment to exercise, an intra-articular injection repeated on one or two occasions seems to be justified.[87] Steroid injections have not been shown to improve the return rate of shoulder motion.[75,116] Although steroid injections have been reported to be beneficial in some regard, their use should be limited due to the potentially deleterious side effects on the connective tissue.

Nonoperative Treatment

Patients with frozen shoulder should be placed on an exercise program aiming to regain range of motion (Fig. 10-2). Indications for treating frozen shoulder, in general, are based on the chronicity and etiology of the stiffness. Nonoperative treatment is indicated in those primary or secondary frozen shoulders with stiffness of less than 6 months and/or no previous treatment. Each patient should begin an active-assisted range-of-motion exercise program complying with gentle, passive, stretching exercises. These exercises should be performed four to five times daily and should include forward elevation, internal and external rotation, and cross-body adduction. They can be performed standing or sitting, but are most readily performed in the supine position. It is most important to perform four to five short sessions per day, each lasting 5 to 10 minutes, rather than one long session, because the shoulder will become stiff again in between each session. It is important to perform these exercises gently, and it should be stressed that, at each session, the arm should be pushed slightly past the point of pain; otherwise, no range-of-motion progress can be expected. Forward elevation may be assisted, using the opposite arm or a pulley to pull the arm up over the head; external rotation is aided with a cane while the patient is lying supine and holding the arm at the side; and external rotation is performed by pulling the arm behind the back with the assistance of the opposite arm or a towel. Using the opposite extremity, the affected limb is stretched to its limit and slightly beyond, held in place for a count of 5 to 10 seconds, and then brought to a resting position. Periods of rest in between each session are necessary to relieve muscle tension and pain.

To encourage continued exercises, daily bar charts can be used to document progress and to highlight small improvements in range of motion that the patient might otherwise not notice, especially by patients who are easily discouraged. Local modalities consisting of heat at the initiation of the exercise session and ice at its conclusion may be helpful to increase flexibility and reduce inflammation, respectively. These modalities are certainly not curative, but can aid in decreasing discomfort, which will allow greater ease in performing the exercises.

Forward elevation of the shoulder is performed with the extremity grasped either at the wrist or behind the elbow while in the plane of the scapula and pushed upward gradually. This is best performed supine to keep compensatory factors, such as trunk tilt, to a minimum. A pulley can also be used to accomplish this motion, which is best performed with the patient seated with back toward the pulley. Similarly, cross-body adduction is performed as the affected ex-

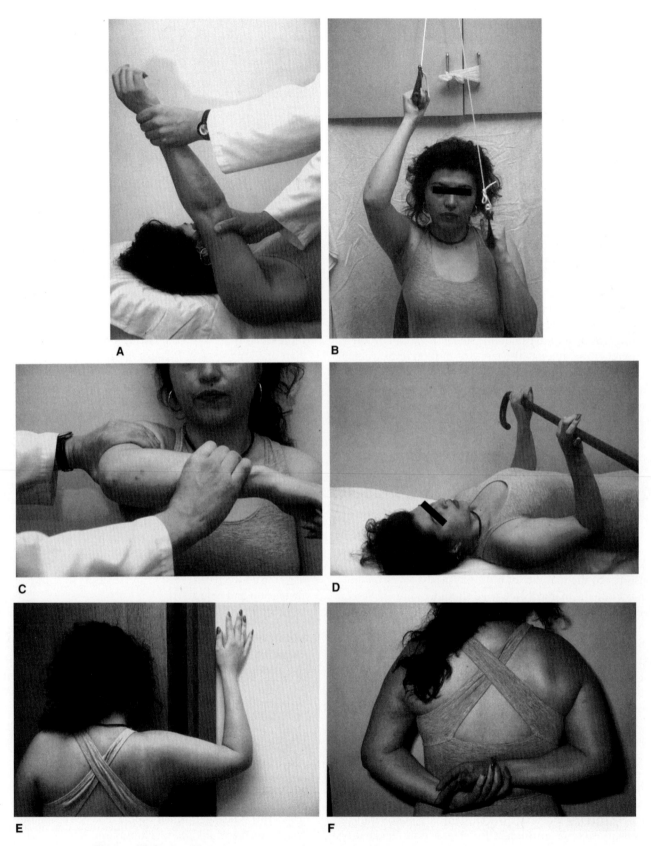

Figure 10-2 Stretching exercises. (*A,B*) Forward elevation. (*C*) Cross-body adduction. (*D,E*) External rotation. (*F*) Internal rotation. (*continued*)

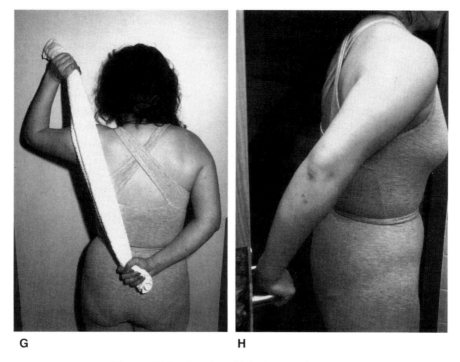

G   H

Figure 10-2   *(continued)* (*G–H*) Internal rotation.

tremity is pulled across the chest toward the contralateral shoulder. This maneuver assists in stretching the posterior portion of the capsule, which is of utmost importance in obtaining internal rotation. External rotation is performed supine, with the elbow close to the body. The hand holds a stick, with the elbow flexed to 90 degrees, which is then used to rotate the affected extremity away from the body. Internal rotation is performed by pulling the wrist of the affected extremity into extension, first behind the back, and then by bringing the hands up between the shoulder blades. It may also be assisted with a towel or by grasping a door handle behind the back and performing a deep knee bend. It should be noted that, in the early stages of the exercise program, one should start with simple stretching, such as Codman's pendulum exercise, to gently loosen and relax the shoulder. The patient bends at the waist, balances with the good arm, and allows the stiff side to swing with gravity in a circular motion, with the hand turned inward and then outward. Overly forceful stretching exercises are contraindicated in the early phases of the frozen shoulder syndrome and may exacerbate symptoms. Consistent reassurance from the physician promotes continued compliance.

The physical therapist plays a major role as a teacher, explaining to the patient that symptom resolution takes time and that pain decreases as motion improves. Whenever possible, the therapy program should be performed on a weekly basis under the supervision, or in addition to, a physical therapist. The patient should understand that the success or failure of therapy depends, in large measure, on performing the exercises as directed, not only with the therapist but by

him- or herself four to five times daily. In a closely supervised physical therapy program, most patients will improve with time, although it may take months. Thus, in most cases, more invasive treatment is generally not required.

Capsular Distention

The method of capsular distention, referred to as distention orthography or brisement, has been advocated for expanding the contracted capsule.[1,38,41,54,72,106] In this procedure, fluid is injected into the glenohumeral joint in sufficient enough volume to generate a high-enough pressure to cause capsular disruption, which becomes evident when there is a significant decrease in the pressure necessary to continue the injection. This procedure has been performed in a variety of ways: with contrast as part of an arthrogram[41,72,106,119]; with saline and local anesthesia, such as hydraulic distention[38]; and with arthroscopy.[54] As with all other methods of treatment for frozen shoulder syndrome, the reported results have been variable and difficult to interpret because the procedure is often combined with other procedures, such as manipulation or corticosteroid injections, and the experience has been limited. The addition of these other variables makes it difficult, if not impossible, to compare reports. An article by Rizk examined 16 patients with adhesive capsulitis of the shoulder treated in an open trial of capsular distention with intra-articular injection of 30 cc of fluid containing 8 cc of 1% lidocaine, 2 cc of corticosteroid, and 20 cc of radio contrast material. A capsular tear during arthrography occurred in all cases, usually occurring at the subscapular bursa or subacromial bursa documented by extravasation in either of these areas. Rupture at the distal bicipital sheath occurred in two patients and was not associated with pain relief. Thirteen of 16 patients experienced immediate pain relief and increased shoulder mobility. This improvement was maintained over a follow-up interval of 6 months. Given these results, the authors felt that disrupting the constructed capsule by hydraulic distention seemed to be the mechanism for achieving symptomatic relief in adhesive capsulitis.[123]

Manipulation Under Anesthesia

No aspect of shoulder adhesive capsulitis is more varied or controversial than treatment. Manipulation under general anesthesia has been shown to result in rapid return to normal range of motion in some cases, but several authors have found that, although manipulation shortens the time during which the shoulder range of motion is extremely restricted, the overall course of the disease remains unchanged.[75,87] Timing of manipulation is also controversial, but advocates suggest manipulating patients who do not obtain 90 degrees of passive forward elevation and show no progress after 3 to 6 months of supervised physical therapy. This procedure has been successful in improving the range of motion of frozen shoulders that have not responded to a rehabilitation program or exhibited progression of stiffness while undergoing conservative treatment.[50–52,69,97,110,137] Manipulation should be performed in a gentle, controlled manner to avoid complications. Complications that have been reported include humeral fracture, glenohumeral dislocation, rotator cuff tears, and radial nerve injuries. Manipulation is contraindicated in those patients with severe osteopenia, in which fracture is a high risk; in those with reflex sympathetic dystrophy; and in patients whose stiffness is secondary to a previous surgery or fracture. Manipulation is ill-advised in these situations due to increased risk of fracture; disruption of the soft-tissue repair; nerve injuries, such as brachial plexus traction; palsies; and postmanipulation instability. Patients who will be unable or unwilling to cooperate with the required postmanipulation exercise program are also contraindicated for this procedure. It is important to emphasize that treatment of primary adhesive capsulitis should not be considered while the patient is experiencing severe pain in addition to motion loss, because this may represent the inflammatory phase of the disease. Neviaser and Neviaser have pointed out that any surgical treatment in this stage will likely exacerbate the patient's motion loss by increasing capsular injury. It is important to wait until pain is present only at the end range of motion, indicating that the active inflammatory process has resolved. Any type of operative or manipulative intervention during this inflammatory phase has the potential to worsen symptoms.[97]

Manipulation can be performed under either general or regional anesthesia. The anesthetic technique is an extremely important aspect of the overall treatment. There must be complete muscle paralysis during the procedure. The advantages of regional anesthesia are that regional anesthesia allows direct observation of the recovered motion by the patient and the more effective, immediate use of continuous passive motion and physical therapy. It also has the benefit of eliminating the subsequent pain interfering with therapy in the immediate postoperative period. Therefore, it is recommended that an interscalene regional block with a long-acting agent, such as bupivacaine, be used. The block may be administered either as a single percutaneous injection or by the placement of indwelling interscalene catheter.[18,114] If a single block is performed, it may be repeated in the morning on the first and second postoperative days for continued pain relief and ease of therapy. This will greatly decrease the patients' requirement for narcotics while increasing their tolerance to physical therapy and continuous motion. Use of 0.5% bupivacaine as a single block will provide anesthesia for approximately 12 hours. If an interscalene catheter is used, a continuous slow drip of bupivacaine is administered.

The patient is placed supine along the edge of the operating table with the scapula stabilized along its axillary border, allowing more isolated and controlled glenohumeral movement of the involved extremity. Forward elevation manipulation is carried out first. The humerus is grasped close to the axilla to diminish the lever arm effect. With gradual traction and flexion, there is usually a palpable and audible release of adhesions. This maneuver usually results in rupture of the inferior portion of the capsule.[63,96] The arm is then stretched across the patient's chest into adduction to stretch the posterior capsule and aid in returning internal rotation. The arm is then brought down to the side of the body while holding it in the supracondylar area of the distal humerus to avoid spiral fracture of the humerus; a two-finger pressure only is placed on the forearm rotating the humerus externally, taking care to avoid injury to the elbow ligaments. This maneuver releases anterior capsular adhesions. The arm is then manipulated at 90 degrees of scapular plane abduction with further external rotation performed in this plane to stretch the anteroinferior capsule. Continuing with the arm in scapular plane abduction, internal rotation is performed holding the arm at the proximal humeral level to release the posterior capsule. The arm is then stretched across the patient's chest into adduction to further release the posterior capsule. Further stretch of the inferior capsule is obtained with increased abduction in the scapular plane. While maintaining internal rotation, the arm is lowered to the patient's side with the elbow extended and the forearm pronated to complete the posterior capsule release. All rotational maneuvers must be performed carefully, holding the arm in the supracondylar or proximal humeral areas to decrease the risk of fracture. The object of a manipulation under anesthesia is for the recovered motion to be symmetric with the uninvolved side.

Postmanipulation rehabilitation is of paramount importance in maintaining the motion gained. Immediately following manipulation, the patient is met in the recovery room by the therapist to initiate the therapeutic exercise program. It is particularly helpful if regional anesthesia has been used, because a long-acting block permits exercise without discomfort. Continuous passive-motion machines have also been used after manipulation, but there have been no long-term controlled studies to verify their efficacy. In the authors' experience, these machines help continue motion within a somewhat functional range, but fail to stress the shoulder to the extreme limits of overhead elevation as well as external rotation. They are also cumbersome and difficult to set up with regard to external rotation and in changing positions from the bedside to a seated position.

After discharge from the hospital, the premanipulation exercise program is continued but under a more frequent basis. If good range of motion was obtained initially but is then lost, Harryman has suggested repeating the procedure, especially within the first 3 to 4 weeks after the initial manipulation.[47] However, this has not been necessary in our experience.

A prospective clinical study was performed by Bulgen et al. examining the evaluation of three treatment regimens for frozen shoulder, including intra-articular steroids, mobilization, and ice therapy and compared this to no treatment at all. In this prospective study of 42 patients followed for 8 months, the authors stated that there was little long-term advantage in any of the treatment regimes but that the steroid injections may have had a benefit with regard to pain and range of movement in the early stages of the condition.[20]

Manipulation of the shoulder has been advocated as a safe and effective means of enabling these patients to return to functional motion about the shoulder area. Haggart et al. looked at 97 patients treated with manipulation of the shoulder. They found that 95% had excellent or good results with 4 to 9 years of follow-up.[44] Harmon reported 400 manipulated shoulders.[46] On three separate follow-up studies 2 to 3 years post-manipulation, he found that there was full, painless motion in 64% to 94% of the patients. In a study by Hill and Bogumill, 9 of 12 patients (75%) with frozen shoulder syndrome had full, painless range of motion of the shoulder at the time of follow-up postmanipulation, whereas 3 of 12 (25%) continued to complain of minimal aching about the shoulder joint after vigorous activity but did not feel that this was impairing their ability to function. All of the patients felt they were able to perform satisfactorily at their job, during activities of daily living, and during recreational activities. Five out of six of the patients (83%) were not working prior to their shoulder prob-

lems but returned to work within an average of 3 months after the manipulation. Those patients who were working prior to their shoulder problems were back to work within 1 month of manipulation. These authors state that manipulation was a safe means of treating adhesive capsulitis and significantly shortened the course of the disease. Manipulation allowed these patients to return to a normal life style and to work much sooner than the reported natural history of this condition indicated.[52]

It should be noted that patients with diabetes mellitus are extremely resistant to treatment, and often MUA has no effect on the course of adhesive capsulitis. Several studies that report good results with manipulation in the general population often report on multiple diabetic patients who develop recurrence or are resistant to manipulation.[44,110] Janda and Hawkins evaluated patients with diabetes mellitus who underwent manipulation. During the postmanipulation course, the gains in motion made at the time of manipulation and the relief of pain achieved began to diminish at 2 weeks, gradually returning to premanipulation levels at 4 weeks. The level of pain and the limitation of motion were noted to continue during the entire period of follow-up. The authors believed that manipulation had little or no effect on the patient outcome and that it may prove wise to avoid manipulation in such patient because it may have no recognizable advantages.[58]

Arthroscopic Release

Although conservative management with or without manipulation under anesthesia is a generally effective treatment strategy for frozen shoulder syndrome, considerable interest has been shown in arthroscopic surgical procedures for this disorder. Arthroscopy is more frequently being used not only in the evaluation of frozen shoulder but in the treatment as well. Arthroscopy may provide some diagnostic information (e.g., labral tears or rotator cuff tears), that is not identified during the clinical evaluation.[54,80] Arthroscopy not only helps identify associated pathology, but also permits its treatment, including debridement of intra-articular adhesions, subacromial decompression, removal of calcific deposits, and treatment of acromioclavicular arthritis. Arthroscopy has also been used as a means of capsular distention.[54,147]

Although most patients with primary frozen shoulder syndrome respond to physical therapy in nonoperative measures, some will require closed manipulation to achieve and maintain sufficient improvement in motion. A small percentage of those patients will continue to have motion loss that is refractory even to manipulation of the shoulder under anesthesia. Perhaps the most significant benefit of arthroscopy in the treatment of frozen shoulder is the releasing of contracted structures in those patients with resistant cases. It is usually performed in association with some type of manipulation. This procedure allows precise, selective capsular release, thereby avoiding the potential morbidity associated with an open procedure. It has the advantage of allowing for more immediate and aggressive active and passive range of motion exercises than after open release.

Historically, arthroscopy has been of little therapeutic value in patients with adhesive capsulitis of the shoulder. However, the role of arthroscopy in the treatment of frozen shoulder is increasing. Several recent studies have evaluated the usefulness of arthroscopic capsular release, showning that arthroscopic capsular release is a safe and effective form of management of refractory frozen shoulder.[6,45,99,102,103,112,129,140,144]

The primary indication for arthroscopic capsular release is a failed attempt at conservative management. It has also been used in the postoperative shoulder, such as after rotator cuff repair. In these patients, subacromial decompression and a selective capsular release can be performed, lessening the chance of fracture or re-tear of the rotator cuff. Patients with full thickness rotator cuff tears may also be candidates for arthroscopic capsular release, which may decrease the chance for tears that can occur with closed manipulation, provided the source of stiffness is felt to be intracapsular. This procedure should be avoided in patients who are sensitive to significant fluid shifts and in those in whom extensive extra-articular adhesions are suspected, such as posttraumatic or selected surgical procedures.[47,141] The latter patients are often better treated with an open release. Arthroscopic release is also abandoned, if the surgeon cannot identify a discrete subscapularis tendon superiorly. If this structure cannot be identified, the procedure must be converted to an open release because failure to curtail the arthroscopic release in this situation can result in the division of the subscapularis tendon as well as the anterior capsule. Arthroscopy, whether as an adjunct to manipulation or in the form of arthroscopic release, is reserved for patients with frozen shoulder whose symptoms do not improve with an adequate course of physical therapy and home exercise program. In general, the senior authors do not suggest arthroscopic treatment before pursuing a minimum 6-month course of stretching exercises in which the patient has plateaued with regard to motion over a 2-month period.

The operative technique involves three basic components: anesthesia, preferably by interscalene regional anesthesia; manipulation of the shoulder, performed either before, during, or after the third portion of component of this triad; and arthroscopic release. The interscalene block has been safe and well tolerated in the senior author's experience, as well as in the experience of others.[18]

The procedure is performed with the patient in the beach-chair position for both an anterior or posterior capsule release. A lateral decubitus position is also used by some surgeons who prefer the added joint distraction produced when traction is applied to the arm in this position.

The arthroscope is inserted through a standard posterior viewing portal and carefully slid intra-articularly over the humeral head because more inferior passage is difficult to insert the arthroscope into a stiff shoulder where capsular contracture and decreased joint volume are problematic. Articular injury from forcefully inserting the arthroscope is certainly a concern. Chondral damage can be avoided by gently inserting the arthroscope over the humeral head rather than taking a more inferior approach. Some surgeons have recommended using a 3.9-mm diameter arthroscope, such as that used for small joint arthroscopy in the wrist, although the senior authors have used the standard 30 degree 5.5-mm arthroscope without difficulty. The problem of entering a stiff joint with the arthroscope can be completely avoided by manipulation prior to arthroscopic insertion, thereby increasing the available space.[93,105,118] If the joint has been previously manipulated, it should be lavaged of blood. A systematic inspection is then undertaken to determine the site and severity of information as well as to visualize the location of the ruptured structure after manipulation. The biceps tendon is the first anatomic landmark that should be identified. It marks the upper edge of the rotator interval, which is formed by the anterior edge of the supraspinatus and the superior border of the subscapularis tendon.[49] This region is usually composed of a thick band of scar tissue, which may obscure the normally visible upper edge of the subscapularis tendon.

A standard anterior working portal is then established, through which a variety of instruments can be passed. This portal is placed just beneath the biceps tendon, and the capsular scar tissue is divided with the use of an electrocautery device and a motorized shaver. The capsular division begins superiorly, just inferior to the biceps tendon, and continues inferiorly until the discrete upper edge of the subscapularis is encountered. This is the area of the rotator interval, including the coracohumeral ligament and anterosuperior capsule, which is aggressively divided and debrided with a shaver. Electrocautery may be used through the anterior portal to detach the coracohumeral ligament from its coracoid attachment. This is especially important if resistance to external rotation with the arm at the side persists after closed manipulation. Both Neer[90] and Ozaki[107] have shown that such a release performed through an open approach is successful in restoring external rotation in shoulders with refractory frozen shoulder syndrome.

With partial release having been performed, the humeral head moves more easily inferiorly and laterally, allowing more space in the joint for the arthroscope to be moved about. At this point, the option to perform a manipulation to restore motion in all planes is available if partial release has not been obtained prior to manipulation or prior to manipulation and in conjunction with the release of the rotator interval region. Electrocautery can be used to incise the anterior glenohumeral ligaments, which allows the motorized shaving instrument to more efficiently excise the tissue. The release proceeds from superior to inferior, including the inferior axillary portion of the capsule. The arm is frequently manipulated during the procedure, using the same maneuver as described previously to assess the adequacy of the release. External rotation in adduction is usually restored with almost no force. If there continues to be minimal or no improvement of motion in the remaining planes, the remainder of the anteroinferior capsule is released. Capsular release is performed from the midcapsular region and extended inferiorly to obtain external rotation in abduction. Some surgeons have expressed concern about the risk to the axillary nerve with capsular release, and this certainly warrants caution.[114] The subscapularis can act as a buffer in the adducted position because it is interposed between the anteroinferior capsule and the axillary nerve when the arm is in the adducted position. Avoid releasing in the axillary pouch region with this technique. A restriction in cross-body adduction and internal rotation generally indicates further constriction in the posterior capsule warranting posterior capsular release. In these cases, the viewing and working portals are switched and a posterior capsular release is performed in a similar fashion.

A small subset of patients may have an isolated posterior capsular contracture characterized by motion loss primarily limited to internal rotation, cross-chest or horizontal adduction, and flexion, with relative preservation of external rotation. This type of posterior capsular contracture has been implicated in impingement-type pain and may result in nonoutlet-type impingement caused by increased anterosuperior translation during shoulder elevation and internal rotation. This condition is treated with posterior capsular release to restore lost motion and normal kinematics.[143]

The posterior capsular release is performed with the arthroscope placed through a cannula in the anterosuperior portal, and the posterior portal is used as the operative portal. Again, either with electrocautery or a motorized shaver, posterior capsular release is performed from just posterior to the biceps tendon down to the posterior inferior rim of the glenoid. The arthroscopic release of the posterior capsule must be performed just at the glenoid rim; the infraspinatus is quite superficial, and there is risk of dividing the infraspinatus tendon if the capsular division is performed more laterally. Division of the infraspinatus would potentially weaken external rotation by creating a tear within the tendon.

Inspection of the subacromial space is then performed by releasing bursal adhesions. If impingement secondary to the coracoacromial ligament is noted, incision or excision of the hypertrophic ligament may be performed. Associated lesions, such as calcific deposits and acromioclavicular arthritis, which may have been the underlying cause of the development of stiffness, should be simultaneously addressed arthroscopically. Acromioplasty may also be performed, if this is deemed to be the etiology of the stiffness,

with the caution that excessive surgical debridement can possibly produce more adhesions. The goal is to obtain motion that is symmetric with the contralateral or unaffected side. One must understand that the arthroscopic technique performed is tailored to fit the precise pathology encountered in each patient.

Arthroscopic release in conjunction with manipulation is not indicated in the treatment of every stiff shoulder. For example, shoulders with stiffness because of scarring between the subscapularis, strap muscles, and the deltoid (i.e., from previous surgery) cannot be adequately addressed with this form of treatment and are candidates for open release when they remain sufficiently symptomatic. Moreover, patients with severe osteoporosis are not suitable candidates either, based on the risk of fracturing the humerus during manipulation.

Segmuller et al.[129] reviewed the results of patients who underwent an arthroscopic release of the inferior capsule, reproducing, in a controlled fashion, a traumatic disruption of the inferior capsule commonly caused by manipulation with the patient under anesthesia. The authors reviewed a purely arthroscopic treatment of what they termed *adhesive capsulitis*. The outcome of 26 shoulders was assessed with an average follow-up of 13.5 months. The release was performed in a lateral decubitus position with the arthroscope in the posterior portal. In all cases, the arthroscope was unable to pass into the anterior portion of the joint, and the posterior inferior portal was established under direct vision, with the needle used as a guide. This portal was placed into the inferior recess approximately 5 cm inferior to the posterior corner of the acromion. A cutting diathermy knife was used to divide the inferior capsule from the 3 o'clock position anteriorly to 9 o'clock position posteriorly. Capsular biopsies were also performed. Traction was then released and the arm brought into full abduction, with an occasional minor breakdown of adhesions reported. After traction was reestablished, the arthroscope is used to obtain hemostasis and explore the anterior aspect of the joint. In patients with limited internal rotation, the middle glenohumeral ligament was divided. Invariably, a proliferative synovitis was found just in the area beneath the biceps tendon insertion, and a limited synovectomy was performed. Subsequently, the subacromial space was inspected, and, at the end of the procedure, 1 cc of celestone and 10 cc of 0.5% bupivacaine with epinephrine were instilled into both the glenohumeral and subacromial spaces. In the recovery room, the patients received intensive physiotherapy, and daily physiotherapy was continued further after discharge from the ambulatory surgery. According to the constant scoring system, 87% of patients had achieved a good or excellent result when compared with the contralateral normal shoulder score. A total of 88% of patients were very satisfied with the procedure, and no operative complications had occurred.[129]

Pollock et al. reported on the use of arthroscopy in the treatment of resistant frozen shoulder, combining the technique of manipulation under interscalene regional anesthesia followed by arthroscopic examination and debridement of the glenohumeral joint in the subacromial space. The authors state that the addition of the arthroscope allowed identification and treatment of the associated pathology, such as impingement lesions and secondary subacromial space inflammation, calcific deposits, and acromioclavicular arthritis. Range of motion was also increased by arthroscopically guided sectioning of the coracohumeral ligament. The treatment regime yielded overall satisfactory results in 25 of 30 shoulders (83%). The authors note that a subgroup of diabetic patients faired less well than other groups with only 64% satisfactory results.[114]

Warner et al. reported the results of arthroscopic release of 23 patients with idiopathic adhesive capsulitis with the use of interscalene regional anesthesia, followed by repeated nerve blocks or continuous infusion through an interscalene catheter. The authors reported significant improvement in range of motion, including a mean flexion improvement of 49 degrees, external rotation improvement of 42 degrees, and mean internal rotation improvement of eight spinous process levels. The authors did combine the release with varying amounts of closed manipulation throughout the procedure, which was felt to require much less force than when performed alone.[140]

Treatment of the resistant frozen shoulder was reviewed with regard to manipulation versus arthroscopic release by Ogilvie-Harris. Arthroscopy was performed in 40 patients with persistent pain, stiffness, and functional loss for at least one year without improvement, despite conventional nonoperative treatment for frozen shoulder syndrome. In the first 20 patients, manipulation was performed in conjunction with an arthroscopy either before or after. In the second 20 patients, the contracted structures were divided through arthroscopic release. The arthroscopic division was performed in four sequential steps:

1. Resection of the inflammatory synovium in the interval between the subscapularis and supraspinatus (i.e., rotator interval)
2. Progressive division of the anterior superior glenohumeral ligament and anterior capsule
3. Division of the subscapularis tendon but not muscle
4. Division of the inferior capsule

The results were assessed independently on the basis of pain, stiffness, and function. With follow-up varying from 2 to 5 years, it was noted that patients treated with arthroscopy and manipulation did as well as the patients treated with arthroscopic division alone with regard to range-of-motion restoration. However, the patients in the arthroscopic division group had significantly better pain relief and restoration of function. Fifteen of 20 patients treated with arthroscopic division had an excellent result

compared to 7 of 18 patients treated with arthroscopy and manipulation. Initially, diabetic patients did not perform as well, but the outcome was similar to patients without diabetes in the long term. The authors state that, if, after suitable waiting time (at least one year) and adequate nonsurgical treatment, the patient continued to report significant pain, loss of motion, and functional impairment, arthroscopic division of the rotator interval and anterior structures offered the patient a better chance of a long-term, excellent result. The authors stressed that patients with diabetes, in particular, should be considered for this form of management in preference to treatment by manipulation.[104]

Ogilvie-Harris also reviewed arthroscopic release of patients with diabetic frozen shoulder. They performed arthroscopic release on 17 patients who failed to respond to conservative management and considered arthroscopic release to be an effective treatment for the resistant diabetic frozen shoulder.[103] They progressively released the anterior structures from superior to inferior. Starting from the interval area, they released the anterior superior glenohumeral ligament, the intra-articular portion of the subscapularis, the anterior capsule, and the inferior capsule. Postoperatively, physiotherapy was carried out daily to maintain the range of motion. At a follow-up of 1 to 5 years, the patients were significantly improved in regard to pain, range of motion, and function.

Open Release

Open surgical release is reserved for patients who fulfill one or more of the following criteria: (a) significant osteopenia, a previous fracture with posttraumatic stiffness, such that closed manipulation might carry an increased risk of fracture through either the osteoporotic bone or through the previous fracture site; (b) failed closed manipulation or failed arthroscopic release, despite compliance with the postoperative rehabilitation program; (c) attempted manipulation or arthroscopic release that was unsuccessful in regaining range of motion; (d) previous surgical repairs that prohibit manipulation or at risk for disruption (i.e., previous rotator cuff repair); or (e) cases in which the adhesions are felt to be primarily extra-articular in nature. In general, the goal of this procedure is to release contracted structures so that the range of motion can be increased while maintaining glenohumeral stability. The objective is to release both intra- and extra-articular contracted structures. The advantage of an open surgical release is that it can free up both sides of the joint without risk of soft tissue or bony injury.

Open releases generally have been successful, but experience and reports of large series have been limited.[62,70,76,90,91] Although the major advantage of this procedure is that it affords the surgeon the opportunity to accurately locate and release contracted structures under direct vision, the major disadvantage of an open release is postoperative pain, which can interfere with initiating motion. When performing an open release, it is critical to identify the tissues that are contracted and determine how the release should increase range of motion. The structures usually released include the subacromial and subdeltoid bursal adhesions[62,107] and the coracohumeral ligament and rotator interval.[62,66,89,91,107] A complete perilabral capsular release is also performed circumferentially or selectively around the glenoid, and the subscapularis,[8,104] which is often lengthened and then released 360 degrees and securely repaired to maintain anterior stability. After these structures are released, the surgeon should address the degree of motion regained and the necessity for further dissection.

After either general or interscalene block anesthesia, a deltopectorial incision is used, and the open procedure is begun by releasing adhesions between the deltoid, acromion, coracoacromial ligament, coracoid, and strap muscles from the underlying rotator cuff. Extensive scarring through all layers of the dissection is identified. Adhesions between the deltoid and the humerus are sharply released. This must be done with care because the axillary nerve travels approximately 3 cm distal to the lateral border of the acromion on the undersurface of the deltoid. This dissection is made easier with the shoulder in the abducted position, which allows the deltoid to become lax and more easily retracted. Dissection in this area may be done sharply or bluntly, taking care to stay lateral to the coracoid in an attempt to avoid injuring the musculocutaneous nerve. The dissection continues gently under the deltoid to avoid entering the muscle laterally and injuring the axillary nerve. Internally rotating the arm while gently retracting the deltoid muscle will allow release of the subdeltoid adhesions in an anterior to posterior manner until the deltoid can move freely over the proximal humerus when the arm is rotated. Within the subacromial space, the coracoacromial ligament is either incised or excised, and the subacromial space may be filled with dense scar adhesions between the rotator cuff and the acromion, which will most likely require sharp release.

The conjoined tendon is then separated and retracted medially from the scarred area, and joined to the underlying subscapularis. This can usually be accomplished with the combination of blunt and sharp dissection. It is essential to keep the dissection lateral to the base of the coracoid process to prevent injury to the neurovascular structures, especially the musculocutaneous nerve.

The coracohumeral ligament and rotator interval are then released by identifying the superior border of the subscapularis and dissecting the supraspinatus and subscapularis from the coracoid bluntly or sharply, as needed. The rotator interval is released extending from the humerus to the coracoid.[90,91,107] As dissection proceeds from superficial to deep within these tissue layers, the shoulder may be gently manipulated at this point to regain further motion.

If there is still marked limitation of external rotation due to scarring in the interval between the subscapularis and the capsule, the option of splitting the subscapularis between its fibers and elevating it off of the capsule, versus a coronal plane lengthening of the subscapularis tendon, is available. The coronal Z-plasty of the subscapularis tendon is begun by incising the superficial fibers of the tendon vertically at its lesser tuberosity insertion. The subscapularis is then separated from the underlying remaining tendon and capsule and reflected medially. The superficial half of the tendon remains attached to the muscle, with the remaining deep half divided at the glenoid and remaining attached to the lesser tuberosity. The deepened or remaining tendon and capsule are then incised from the labrum medially. The orientation of the coronal dissection can be guided by determining the thickness of the scarred tendon and capsular tissue once the rotator interval region has been opened. The subscapularis is usually entrapped in scar tissue. To achieve full mobility, it may be necessary to visualize and dissect the axillary nerve. With the nerve adequately visualized and protected, the subscapularis can be released circumferentially on its superior, inferior, deep, and superficial surfaces.

At this point, if abduction and internal rotation are still limited, the inferior and posterior capsules can be released. This can be done selectively or circumferentially, depending on the degree and pattern of stiffness. The release is performed just lateral to the labrum and proceeds from the anterior superior to anteroinferior and then from posterior inferior to posterosuperior, as needed. If the posterior capsule needs to be released, it is most easily visualized by placing a humeral head retractor to displace the humeral head posteriorly within the joint along with a blunt retractor beneath the inferior capsule to protect the axillary nerve. After the release of all contracted structures, the lateral end of the superficial subscapularis is sutured to the deep end of the tendon and capsule with the arm in the maximum external rotation that would allow secure closure of the Z-plasty with nonabsorbable suture. Each centimeter of length gained from the lengthening increases external rotation by approximately 20 degrees (Fig. 10-3). Range of motion is assessed again to determine where there is tension on the soft-tissue repair and, thus, define a "safe zone" for early passive range of motion and rehabilitation.

Ozaki et al. studied the results of an open release of recalcitrant chronic adhesive capsulitis of the shoulder and the role of contracture of the coracohumeral ligament and rotator interval. Seventeen patients who failed to improve with standard nonoperative measures underwent open release through an anterolateral incision. Release concentrated on the hypertrophied coracohumeral ligament and contracted tissues within the rotator interval at operation. The major cause of restricted glenohumeral movement was found to be contracture of these structures. Histologic study revealed fibrosis, hyalinization, and fibrinoid degeneration

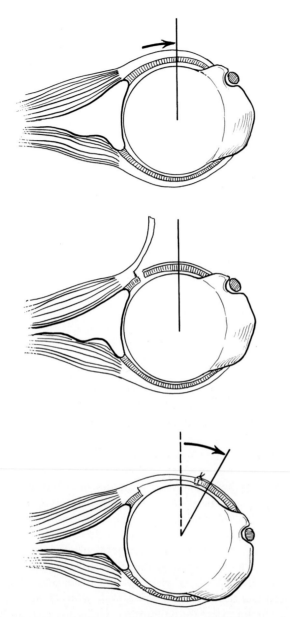

Figure 10-3 Contracted subscapularis and anterior capsule (*top*) limit external rotation. This condition is treated by incising the subscapularis from the lesser tuberosity laterally (*middle*) and suturing it to the medial end of the capsule, which is transected close to the glenoid (*bottom*). This release results in substantial lengthening of these structures. Each centimeter of length gained increases external rotation by approximately 20 degrees.

in the contracted connective tissues, as well as fibrosis of the subsynovial tissue and absence of the synovial cell layer on the joint side of the rotator interval. Once release has been performed within the rotator interval, the glenohumeral joint was then gently manipulated through a full range of motion also mobilizing the biceps tendon within its groove. Immediately postoperatively, active mobilization of the shoulder was begun. At an average follow-up of 6.8 years, 16 patients were reported as having full range of motion,

with one presenting with a slight limitation of motion. The authors stated that they felt the essential changes in the tissue at the time of surgery that produce chronic adhesive capsulitis—such as fibrosis, hyalinization, and fibrinoid degeneration of the contracted connective tissues, a decrease in the number of synovial cells, in addition to the absence of the synovial cell layer on the joint side of the rotator interval—may be related to an intrinsic disorder of collagen. They report that this procedure is logical and simple, and they recommend an open operative release of the contracted structures, especially the hypertrophied coracohumeral ligament and rotator interval, in patients in whom the shoulder does not respond to nonoperative therapy.[107]

Postoperative Treatment

An organized and aggressive postoperative therapy program is extremely important to maintain the motion gained during surgery. Immediately after arthroscopic release, the patient should be met in the recovery room by the therapist to initiate the exercise program. A repeat manipulation can be performed later the same day, if a long-acting block has been administered, or on the following day, if an indwelling catheter has been placed; however, we find this unnecessary. Continuous passive motion machines can be used but have failed to prove their efficacy. The patient is encouraged to use the arm for daily living activities, so a sling is not worn. Exercises are performed four to five times a day for approximately 10 to 15 minutes at a time with a self-assisted and pulley-assisted stretching exercise program. Supervised physical therapy on an outpatient basis is begun three to five times per week in the early postoperative period, and then slowly decreased as time and motion progress.

When a soft-tissue repair has been performed, as with the Z-plasty lengthening in the front of the shoulder, passive motion is again initiated, but restricted with regard to internal rotation behind the back and excessive external rotation, which may place undue tension on the subscapularis repair. Intraoperatively, the position at which resistance is felt and the repair is observed to be under tension is noted and used to guide the postoperative limits of motion. After 4 to 6 weeks, an aggressive active range-of-motion program is begun with continued stretching for both the arthroscopic and open releases. The strengthening phase of the postoperative regimen is delayed until nearly full and pain-free motion has been achieved, which requires approximately 3 months.

COMPLICATIONS

The majority of complications encountered with the treatment of frozen shoulder are iatrogenic. Potential complications of manipulation include fractures of the humerus, dislocation of the glenohumeral joint, rotator cuff tears or tear extension, and injuries to the brachial plexus. Additional complications after arthroscopic or open release include axillary nerve injury, as well as recurrent stiffness secondary to extensive surgical dissection.

The primary objective in treating frozen shoulder is to increase the range of motion. This should be taken into account when deciding on a rational approach for the treatment of the complications incurred while managing this problem. Iatrogenic fractures of the proximal humerus and shaft present an exceptionally difficult problem. These necessitate stabilization with internal fixation in such a way as to permit early shoulder range of motion and prevent the ensuing stiffness, which is so likely to occur after fracture immobilization.

Rotator cuff tears or tear extensions that occur after manipulation are also possible causes of failure. Although this may rarely occur, these tears usually heal spontaneously, provided that they are not superimposed on an impingement tear.[92] Extending any previously existing impingement tears would necessitate repair, which may either be performed at the time of manipulation with special attention to postoperative range of motion to prevent recurrent stiffness, or, after successful maintenance of motion, the patient could be reevaluated and a treatment program established and directed during rotator cuff repair.

The long overhead suspension of the arm after manipulation, which has been advocated by some surgeons, can be a source of neurologic injury.[94] Traction injuries of the brachial plexus and peripheral nerves have been reported after closed manipulation of the shoulder.[10] These injuries are usually neuropraxias that can recover spontaneously over time. It is crucial to maintain passive motion while the nerves are recovering to avoid recurrent stiffness. Although a sling should be used to prevent excessive traction on the plexus while it is recovering, it should be removed for physical therapy and home exercise sessions. The patient and the physical therapist need to be made aware of the problem so that extremes of range of motion, particularly forward elevation and abduction, are avoided to prevent further nerve injury. The diagnosis of middle and lower plexus injuries can be made almost immediately with somatosensory-evoked potentials. Diminished sensory nerve action potentials at 5 days after the injury may also be helpful in diagnosing an early plexopathy. Definitive electrodiagnostic studies can be performed three weeks after the injury to evaluate the extent of nerve damage and the potential of recovery.

AUTHORS' PREFERRED TREATMENT

The senior authors' approach has always been to make a thorough initial assessment, obtaining a complete history of shoulder symptomatology as well as other associated medical conditions, which may contribute to the cause of frozen shoulder. After a careful preliminary diagnostic workup, as previously discussed, the senior authors insist upon accurate scapular anteroposterior, lateral, and axillary radiographs of the shoulder. If any symptomatology seems to be related to the cervical spine, then radiographs of this area are also reviewed. An underlying cause is always sought and an attempt is made to determine whether the presentation is that of a primary or secondary frozen shoulder. If a secondary frozen shoulder is diagnosed, concurrent treatment of the precipitating factor is also started when possible.

After range of motion is recorded, an assessment is made as to whether or not pain is restricted just to the extreme of motion or throughout the entire range. If pain is persistent throughout, analgesics, such as anti-inflammatory medications, are added to the treatment regime. We have not found the use of intra-articular steroid injections to be beneficial in our patients. A careful explanation is given to the patient regarding the effect of immobilization of the arm against the side and the importance of light use and passive exercises. The authors also explain that the aim of reestablishing external rotation and elevation is to eliminate the pain caused by stiffness.

At the time of the initial visit, we begin gentle pendulum exercises and a stretching program. These exercises are to be performed three to five times daily and, and then advanced according to the amount of stiffness and pain. Passive forward elevation is performed by assisting the arm on the unaffected side up over head of the patient, who is in a supine or seated position. This may also be done with a pulley as well, which helps the patient extend the arm up to a solid object that is just beyond reach, after which the patient lowers himself or herself and sustains a moderate stretch, adjusted to tolerance, for 5 to 10 seconds. External rotation stretch is performed in the supine position with the elbow flexed to 90 degrees, rotating the arm out to the side with a stick or cane. Internal rotation is performed with either the assistance of a cane or the opposite arm behind the back, at which time the affected side is pushed into hyperextension and then pulled up behind the back flexing the elbows. Adduction is also performed by pulling the involved extremity across the chest with the assistance of the uninvolved side. Short, 5- to 10-minute exercise sessions are repeated throughout the day. At first, there is little attempt made to progress strengthening exercises because the main focus should be on stretching until an acceptable range of motion has been achieved. A supervised physical therapy program can also be instituted in conjunction with the home exercise program. This is the best instituted program for those patients with severe stiffness and a long history of shoulder pain, often after failed treatment. This nonoperative stretching approach can be continued as long as improvement continues to occur. It is important for the physician to supervise the program, checking the range of motion at intervals and discussing goals of therapy with the therapist and patient until complete range of motion is recovered and the patient is comfortable.

At the next visit, usually 6 to 8 weeks later, the patient is again examined and progress recorded. The exercises are reviewed and refined as needed. As pain subsides more aggressive stretching can be instituted. If other etiologies of the frozen shoulder syndrome become apparent as treatment progresses, then confirmation and treatment of this source is begun. For example, if impingement-type pain seems to be present in the overhead position, a subacromial lidocaine, and possibly steroid injection, for diagnosis and treatment can be given. Unless a rotator cuff tear is suspected or other concern regarding diagnosis and pathology is present, an MRI is rarely used in a diagnostic workup of frozen shoulder syndrome.

If the patient with a significant deficiency in motion reaches a plateau, in which, over a 4- to 6-month period, no further improvement in range of motion occurs, an arthroscopic release with a closed manipulation is our treatment of choice.

Each patient is treated with an indwelling interscalene catheter and then sedated to comfort in the operating suite. The procedure is then performed with the patient seated in the "beach chair" position (T-MAX beach chair, Tenet Medical Engineering, Calgary, Canada) with the arm supported using the pneumatic arm positioner (The Spider, Tenet Medical Engineering). The patient is appropriately bolstered and padded and then sterilely prepped and draped. Introduction of the trocar through the posterior capsule generally requires extra force due to the capsular contraction and decreased joint volume. A gentle atraumatic entry is performed with insertion at the top of the humeral head to avoid chondral damage to the articular surfaces. A 1:300,000 dilution of epinephrine is used in the arthroscopy fluid. The senior authors perform arthroscopy prior to manipulation, the joint volume is decreased and initial maneuverability is difficult, thus the anterior capsule is addressed first. The biceps tendon is identified; however, the upper border of the subscapularis may be obscured by thickened scar tissue. An anterior portal is then established just inferior to the biceps tendon, and the shaver is introduced initially. Significant synovitis may be present (Fig. 10-4), so a gentle debridement is performed followed by lightly touching the inflamed regions of synovitis with the electrocautery. Specialized instruments for capsular resection consisting of straight and angled forceps are then introduced through the anterior portal. The capsular resection begins anteriorly and first proceeds inferior to the biceps tendon. The cannula is withdrawn until it is just outside the capsule, and the resection forceps are used as a dissecting instrument to free the capsule (Fig. 10-5). Resection proceeds inferiorly until the upper border of the subscapularis is visualized. The forceps are used to dissect between the capsule and subscapularis, and resection of the anteroinferior capsule is completed down to the bottom of the glenoid

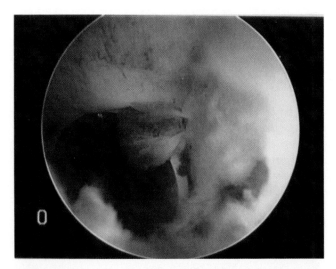

Figure 10-4 Initial observation of the glenohumeral joint revealing typical synovial inflammation and diminished joint space. An anterior portal has been established.

(Fig. 10-6). At this point, the humeral head has started to move laterally and inferiorly, already increasing the joint volume and providing more room to manipulate the arthroscope. The tips of the forceps should always be visible before closing to resect capsular tissue, especially in the inferior aspect of the capsule. Resection with the forceps, instead of with the electrocautery, involves less risk of inadvertent heat injury or transection of the axillary nerve. The resection forceps are then placed into the rotator interval and the anterior superior capsular resection is completed and the rotator interval capsule is resected. Care must continually be taken to visualize all structures before resection, especially assuring that subscapularis tendon is not transected when performing the anteroinferior release. When releasing the

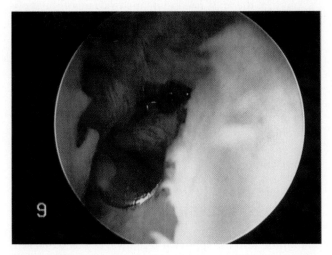

Figure 10-5 After the anterior cannula is established, the instruments are introduced into the joint, and the cannula is then withdrawn until it is just outside the capsule. The forceps are used to free and resect a strip of capsule.

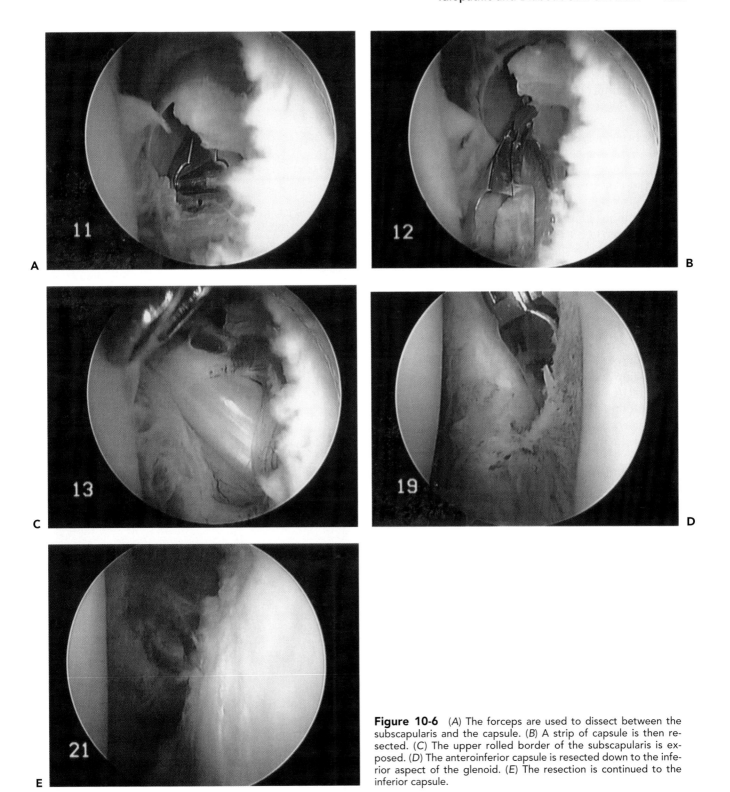

A

B

C

D

E

Figure 10-6 (*A*) The forceps are used to dissect between the subscapularis and the capsule. (*B*) A strip of capsule is then resected. (*C*) The upper rolled border of the subscapularis is exposed. (*D*) The anteroinferior capsule is resected down to the inferior aspect of the glenoid. (*E*) The resection is continued to the inferior capsule.

rotator interval, care must be taken to avoid carrying the resection into the tendon of the supraspinatus.

In the cases of idiopathic frozen shoulder, a global capsular resection is routinely performed, followed by a posterior capsular resection. Switching sticks are utilized, and the arthroscope is placed in the anterior portal while the work-

ing, operative portal is placed posteriorly. The posterosuperior capsule is resected next, starting just posterior to the biceps origin and continuing down to the posterior cannula. The capsule is lifted away from the rotator cuff after dissection with the tips of the forceps and sectioned approximately 1 cm peripheral to the labrum. Muscle fibers of the rotator cuff muscles will become visible, but the resection forceps should always be between the cuff and the capsule. Thus, again, care must be taken to avoid resecting biceps root, labrum, or cuff. Next, the posteroinferior capsule is resected. The posterior cannula is again withdrawn until just outside the capsule, and the tips of the forceps are used to dissect between the capsule and cuff. The switching sticks are again used and the arthroscope is moved to the posterior portal. An accessory posteroinferior portal is then created 3 to 4 cm below the posterior portal. First, a spinal needle is placed, then a blunt trochar is passed, and this is replaced with the blunt-tipped capsular resection forceps. The capsule resection is continued until the posteroinferior resection track meets the anteroinferior resection and a complete 360-degree resection has taken place (Fig. 10-7). As long as the tips of the forceps are always visible, injury to the axillary nerve or any vessels will be avoided. After this, any residual synovitis is debrided, and the electrocautery is used to obtain hemostasis.

The arthroscope is removed from the joint, the arm is removed from the arm holder, and range of motion is assessed. Manipulation is performed in all planes to assure that complete motion has been restored. Often at this point, motion is restored with almost no manipulative force. While performing the manipulation, any audible or palpable signs of further release of tissue are carefully sought after. If there continues to be any residual restrictions, the arthroscope can be placed back into the joint, and that area can be addressed. Intra-articular injections of corticosteroids at the time of surgery are not used.

The postoperative protocol is as important as the procedure itself. The patient is admitted for at least 2 days of intensive physical therapy. Continuous regional anesthesia via the indwelling interscalene catheter facilitates physical therapy in the postoperative period because it allows initial pain-free range of motion. The patient is encouraged to be out of the sling and may use the arm for light tasks. Formal physical therapy occurs under direct supervision twice a day, but the patient is also strongly encouraged to perform stretches several times a day as well. The use of the indwelling interscalene catheter also offers a psychological benefit to the patient: immediately after surgery, the patient sees the motion gains that have been achieved and realizes that it is possible to achieve this motion. Patients have also been found to cooperate more with their therapist when their initial sessions are less painful. The patient is transitioned to oral narcotics, and the catheter is removed postoperative day 2 or 3, depending on the pain levels and ability to maintain the motion gains. Upon discharge, patients are instructed to perform their stretches four times a day on their own and go to therapy 5 days a week for 2 weeks. At that time, they return to the office for a follow-up visit. If they are having difficulty maintaining their motion gains, at 4 to 6 weeks after surgery, a manipulation under anesthesia and corticosteroid injection are considered.

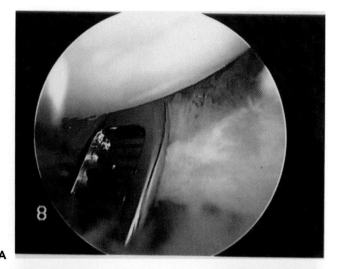

A

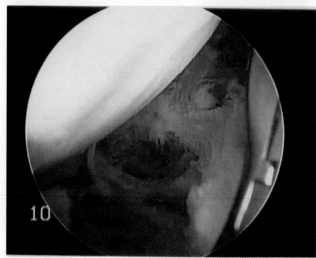

B

Figure 10-7 After switching the arthroscope to the anterior portal and resecting the posterosuperior capsule, a second posteroinferior portal is created. (A) Again, the capsular resection forceps are used to dissect and resect the posteroinferior capsule, always staying within 1 cm of the inferior labrum to avoid neurovascular damage. (B) The resection is continued until the posteroinferior track meets the anteroinferior track. A 360-degree resection is completed, as the underlying muscle is clearly visible.

REFERENCES

1. Andren L, Lundberg BJ. Treatment of rigid shoulders by joint distension during arthrography. Acta Orthop Scan 1965;36:45.
2. Arkkila PE, Kantola IM, Viikari JS, et al. Shoulder capsulitis in type I and II diabetic patients: association with diabetic complications and related diseases. Ann Rheum Dis 1996;55:907.
3. Barry H, Ferndandes I, Bloom B, et al. Clinical study comparing acupuncture, physiotherapy, injection, oral anti-inflammatory therapy in shoulder cuff lesions. Curr Med Res Opin 1980;7:121.
4. Baslund B, Thomsen BS, Jensen EM. Frozen shoulder: current concepts. Scan J Rheum 1990;19:321.
5. Bateman JE. The shoulder and neck, 2nd ed. Philadelphia, WB Saunders, 1978.
6. Beaufils P, Prevot N, Boyer T, et al. Arthroscopic release of the glenohumeral joint in shoulder stiffness: a review of 26 cases. Arthroscopy 1999;15:49.

7. Binder A, Bulgen DY, Hazleman BL. Frozen shoulder: a long-term prospective study. Ann Rheum Dis 1984;43:361.
8. Binder A, Hazleman BL, Parr G, et al. A controlled study of oral prednisolone in frozen shoulder. Br J Rheumatol 1986;25:228.
9. Binder AI, Bulgen DY, Hazleman BL, et al. Frozen shoulder: an arthrographic and radionuclear scan assessment. Ann Rheum Dis 1984;43:365.
10. Birch R, Jessop J, Scott G. Brachial plexus palsy after manipulation of the shoulder. J Bone Joint Surg (Br) 1991;73:172.
11. Bland JH, Merrit JA, Boushey DR. The painful shoulder. Semin Arthritis Rheum 1977;7:21.
12. Blockey NJ, Wright JK, Kellgren JH. Oral cortisone therapy in periarthritis of the shoulder: a controlled trial. Br Med J 1954;1:1955.
13. Bowman CA, Jeffcoate WJ, Patrick M, et al. Bilateral adhesive capsulitis, oligoarthritis and proximal myopathy as presentation of hypothyroidism. Br J Rheum 1988;27:62.
14. Bowen MK, Deng XH, Warner JP, et al. The effect of joint compression on stability of the glenohumeral joint. Trans Orthop Res Soc 1992;17:289.
15. Bradley JP. Arthroscopic treatment for frozen capsulitis. Oper Tech Orthop 1991;1:248.
16. Braun RM, West F, Mooney V, et al. Surgical treatment of the painful shoulder contracture in the stroke patient. J Bone Joint Surg (Am) 1971;53:1307.
17. Bridgman JF. Periarthritis of the shoulder and diabetes mellitus. Ann Rheum Dis 1972;31:69.
18. Brown AR, Weiss R, Greenberg C, et al. Interscalene block for shoulder arthroscopy: comparison with general anesthesia. Arthroscopy 1993;9:295.
19. Bruckner FE, Nye CJ. A prospective study of adhesive capsulitis of the shoulder (frozen shoulder) in a high risk population. Q J Med 1981;50:191.
20. Bulgen DY, Binder A, Hazleman BL, et al. Frozen shoulder: a prospective clinical study with an evaluation of three treatment regimens. Ann Rheum Dis 1983;43:353.
21. Bulgen DY, Binder A, Hazleman BL, et al. Immunological studies in frozen shoulder. J Rheum 1982;9:893.
22. Bulgen DY, Hazleman BL, Voak DL. HLA-B27 and frozen shoulder. Lancet 1976;1:1042.
23. Bulgen DY, Hazleman BL, Ward M, et al. Immunological studies in frozen shoulder. Ann Rheum Dis 1978;37:135.
24. Bunker TD, Anthony PP. The pathology of frozen shoulder. A Dupuytren-like disease. J Bone Joint Surg (Br) 1995;77:677.
25. Bunker TD, Esler CAN. Frozen shoulder and lipids. J Bone Joint Surg (Br) 1995;77:864.
26. Choy EH, Corhill M, Gibson T, et al. Isolated ACTH deficiency presenting with bilateral frozen shoulder. Br J Rheum 1991;30:226.
27. Clarke GR, Willis LA, Fish WW, et al. Preliminary studies in measuring range of motion in normal and painful stiff shoulders. Rheum Rehabil 1975;14:39.
28. Codman EA. Rupture of the supraspinatus tendon and other lesions in or about the subacromial bursa. In: The shoulder. Boston, Thomas Todd, 1934.
29. Coventry MB. Problem of painful shoulder. JAMA 1953;151:177.
30. Dacre JE, Beeney N, Scott DL. Injections and physiotherapy for the painful stiff shoulder. Ann Rheum Dis 1989;48:322.
31. Demaziere A, Wiley AM. Primary chest wall tumor appearing as frozen shoulder: review and case presentations. J Rheumatol 1991;18:911.
32. DePalma AF. Loss of scapulohumeral motion (frozen shoulder). Ann Surg 1952;135:193.
33. DePalma AF. Surgery of the shoulder, 2nd ed. Philadelphia, JB Lippincott, 1973:455.
34. Depalma AF, Gallery G, Bennett GA. Variational anatomy and degenerative lesions of the shoulder joint. In: Blount WP, ed. Instruction course lectures. Ann Arbor, MI, American Academy of Orthopaedic Surgeons, 1949:255.
35. Duke O, Zeclear E, Grahame R. Anti-inflammatory drugs in periarthritis of the shoulder: a double blind, between-patient study of naproxen versus indomethacin. Rheumatol Rehabil 1981;20:54.
36. Duplay ES. De la periarthrite scapulohumerale et des raideurs de l'epaule qui en son la Consequence. Arch Gen Med 1872;20:513.
37. Ehrlich M, Carp SP, Berkowitz SS, et al. ACTH and cortisone in periarthritis of the shoulder (frozen shoulder). Ann Rheum Dis 1951;10:485.
38. Fareed DO, Gallivan WRJ. Office management of frozen shoulder syndrome: treatment with hydraulic distension under local anesthesia. Clin Orthop 1989;242:177.
39. Fleming A, Dodman S, Beer TC, et al. Personality in frozen shoulder. Ann Rheum Dis 1975;35:456.
40. Flood V. Discovery of a new ligament. Lancet 1829:671.
41. Gilula L, Schoenecker PL, Murphy WA. Shoulder arthrography as a treatment modality. Am J Roentgenol 1978;131:1047.
42. Grey RG. The natural history of "idiopathic" frozen shoulder. J Bone Joint Surg Am 1978;60:564.
43. Griggs SM, Ahn A, Green A. Idiopathic adhesive capsulitis. A prospective functional outcome study of nonoperative treatment. J Bone Joint Surg 2000;82:1398.
44. Haggart GE, Dignam RJ, Sullivan T. Management of the "frozen" shoulder. JAMA 1956;161:1219.
45. Hannafin JA, Chiaia. Adhesive capsulitis: a treatment approach. Clin Orthop 2000;372:95.
46. Harmon PH. Methods and results in the treatment of 2,580 painful shoulders. Am J Surg 1958;95:427.
47. Harryman DT. Shoulders: frozen and stiff. Instr Course Lect 1993;42:247.
48. Harryman DT, Sidles JA, Clark JM, et al. Translation of the humeral head on the glenoid with passive glenohumeral motion. J Bone Joint Surg 1990;72:1334.
49. Harryman DT, Sidles JA, Harris SL, et al. The role of the rotator interval capsule in passive motion and stability of the shoulder. J Bone Joint Surg 1992;74:53.
50. Hazleman BL. The painful stiff shoulder. Rheumatol Phys Med 1972;11:413.
51. Helbig B, Wagner P, Dohler R. Mobilization of frozen shoulder under general anesthesia. Acta Orthop Belg 1983;49:267.
52. Hill JJ, Bogumill H. Manipulation in the treatment of frozen shoulder. Orthopedics 1988;11:1255.
53. Hollingworth GR, Ellis R, Hattersley TS. Comparison of injection techniques for frozen shoulder pain: results of a double-blind, randomized study. Br J Med 1983;287:1339.
54. Hsu SY, Chan KM. Arthrographic distension in the management of frozen shoulder. Int Orthop 1991;15:79.
55. Huskisson EC, Bryans R. Diclofenac sodium in treatment of the painful stiff shoulder. Curr Med Res Opin 1983;8:350.
56. Inmann VT, Sauders JB, Abbott LC. Observations on the shoulder. J Bone Joint Surg 1944;26:1.
57. Itoi E, Tabata S. Range of motion and arthrography in the frozen shoulder. J Shoulder Elbow Surg 1992;1:106.
58. Janda DH, Hawkings RJ. Shoulder manipulation in patients with adhesive capsulitis and diabetes mellitus: a clinical note. J Shoulder Elbow Surg 1993;2:36.
59. Johnson JT. Frozen shoulder syndrome in patients with pulmonary tuberculosis. J Bone Joint Surg 1959;41A:877.
60. Kamieth H. Rontgenkefunde der Halswerbesaule und der Schulter bie der Periarthritis Humerscapularis undihre einordnung in die pathogenese diser Erkankung (Radiography of the cervical spine in shoulder periarthritis). Z Orthop 1965;100:162.
61. Kessel L, Bayley I, Young A. The upper limb: the frozen shoulder. Br J Hosp Med 1981;25:334.
62. Kieras DM, Matsen FA III. Open release in the management of refractory frozen shoulder. Orthop Trans 1991;15:801.
63. Kopell AP, Thompson WA. Pain and the frozen shoulder. Surg Gynecol Obstet 1959;109:279.
64. Kraft GH, Johnson EW, Laban MM. The fibrositis syndrome. Arch Phys Med Rehab 1968;49:155.
65. Lee M, Haq AM, Wright V, et al. Periarthritis of the shoulder, a controlled trial of physiotherapy. Physiotherapy 1973;59:312.
66. Leffert RD. The frozen shoulder. Instr Course Lect 1985;34:199.
67. Lequesene M, Dang N, Bensasson M, et al. Increased association of diabetes mellitus and capsulitis of the shoulder and shoulder-hand syndrome. Scand J Rheumatol 1977;6:53.

68. Lippman RK. Frozen shoulder: periarthritis: bicipital tenosynovitis. Arch Surg 1943;47:283.

69. Lloyd-Roberts GG, French PR. Periarthritis of the shoulder: a study of the disease and its treatment. Br Med J 1959;1:1966.

70. Lusardi DA, Wirth MA, Wurtz D, et al. Loss of external rotation following anterior capsulorrhaphy of the shoulder. J Bone Joint Surg 1993;75:1185.

71. Lorenz TH, Musser MJ. Life, stress, emotions, and the painful shoulder. Ann Arthritis Med 1952;37:1232.

72. Loyd JA, Loyd HM. Adhesive capsulitis of the shoulder: arthrographic diagnosis and treatment. South Med J 1983;76:879.

73. Lundberg BJ. Glycosaminoglycans of the normal and frozen shoulder joint capsule. Clin Orthop 1970;69:279.

74. Lungberg BJ. Pathomechanics of the frozen shoulder and the effect of brisement force. In: Bayley J, Kessel L, eds. Shoulder surgery. Berlin-Heidelberg, Springer-Verlag, 1982:109.

75. Lundberg BJ. The frozen shoulder: clinical and radiographical observations. The effect of manipulation under general anesthesia: structure and glycosaminoglycan content of the joint capsule. Acta Orthop Scand Suppl 1969;119:1.

76. MacDonald PB, Hawkins RJ, Fowler PJ, et al. Release of the subscapularis for internal rotation contracture and pain after anterior repair for recurrent anterior dislocation of the shoulder. J Bone Joint Surg 1992;74:734.

77. Macnab I. Rotator cuff tendonitis. Ann Coll Surg Engl 1973;53:271.

78. Macnab I. Rotator cuff tendonitis. In: McKibbon GT, ed. Recent advances in orthopaedics. Edinburgh, Churchill Livingstone, 1975.

79. Massoud SN, Pearse EO, Copeland SA. Operative management of the frozen shoulder in patients with diabetes. J Shoulder Elbow Surg 2002;11:609.

80. McGraw JW, Turba JE. Frozen shoulder. Treatment by arthroscopy and manipulation. Orthop Trans 1989;12:661.

81. McLaughlin HL. Lesions of the musculotendinous cuff of the shoulder. J Bone Joint Surg 1944;26:31.

82. McLaughlin HL. On the "frozen shoulder." Bull Hosp Joint Dis Orthop Inst 1951;12:283.

83. Mintner WT. The shoulder-hand syndrome in coronary disease. J Med Assoc 1987;56:45.

84. Moren-Hybbinette I, Moritz U, Schersten B. The clinical picture of the painful diabetic shoulder-natural history, social consequences and analysis of concomitant hand syndrome. Acta Med Scand 1987;221:73.

85. Mosley HF. Shoulder lesions. Springfield, IL, Charles C. Thomas, 1945:66.

86. Murnaghan GF, McIntosh D. Hydrocortisone in painful shoulder: a controlled trial. Lancet 1955;269:798.

87. Murnaghan JP. Frozen shoulder. In: Rockwood CAJ, Matsen FA, eds. The shoulder. Philadelphia, WB Saunders, 1990:837.

88. Myer AW. Chronic functional lesions of the shoulder. Arch Surg 1937;35:646.

89. Neer CS, Satterlee CC, Dalsy R, et al. On the value of the coracohumeral ligament release. Orthop Trans 1985;34:199.

90. Neer CS, Satterlee CC, Dalsy R, et al. The anatomy and potential effects of contracture of the coracohumeral ligament. Clin Orthop 1992;280:182.

91. Neer CS II. Frozen shoulder. In: Neer CS, ed. Shoulder reconstruction. Philadelphia, WB Saunders, 1990:422.

92. Neviaser JS. Adhesive capsulitis of the shoulder: study of pathological findings in periarthritis of the shoulder. J Bone Joint Surg 1945;27:211.

93. Neviaser JS. Adhesive capsulitis of the shoulder (the frozen shoulder). Med Times 1962;90:783.

94. Neviaser JS. Adhesive capsulitis and the stiff and painful shoulder. Orthop Clin North Am 1980;11:327.

95. Neviaser JS. Arthrography of the shoulder joint. J Bone Joint Surg 1962;44:1321.

96. Neviaser RJ. Painful conditions affecting the shoulder. Clin Orthop 1983;173:63.

97. Neviaser RJ, Neviaser TJ. The frozen shoulder: diagnosis and management. Clin Orthop 1987;223:59.

98. Nicholson GG. The effects of passive joint mobilization on pain and hypomobility associated with adhesive capsulitis of the shoulder. J Orthop Sports Phys Ther 1985;6:238.

99. Nicholson GP. Arthroscopic capsular release for stiff shoulders: effect of etiology on outcomes. Arthroscopy 2003;19:40.

100. Noy S, Dekel S, Orgad S, et al. HLA-B27 and frozen shoulder. Tissue Antigens 1981;17:251.

101. Oesterreicher W, Van Dam G. Social and psychological researches into brachialgia and periarthritis. Arthritis Rheum 1964;7:670.

102. Ogilvie-Harris DJ, Biggs DJ, Fitsialos DP, et al. The resistant frozen shoulder. Manipulation versus arthroscopic release. Clin Orthop 1995;319:238.

103. Oglvie-Harris DJ, Myerthall S. The diabetic frozen shoulder: arthroscopic release. Arthroscopy 1997;13:1.

104. Ogilvie-Harris DJ, Wiley AM. Arthroscopic surgery of the shoulder. J Bone Joint Surg 1986;68:201.

105. Ogilvie-Harris DJ, Wiley AM. Arthroscopic surgery of the shoulder: a general appraisal. J Surg 1976;19:203.

106. Older MW, McIntyre JL, Lloyd GJ. Distention arthrography of the shoulder joint. Can J Surg 1976;19:203.

107. Ozaki J, Nakagawa Y, Sakurai G. Recalcitrant chronic adhesive capsulitis of the shoulder: role of contracture of the coracohumeral ligament and rotator interval in pathogenesis and treatment. J Bone Joint Surg 1989;71A:1511.

108. Pal B, Anderson J, Dick WC, et al. Limitation of joint mobility and shoulder capsulitis in insulin and non-insulin dependent diabetes mellitus. Br J Rheumatol 1986;25:147.

109. Parker RD, Froimson AL, Winsburg DD, et al. Frozen shoulder. Part I. Chronology, pathogenesis, clinical picture and treatment. Orthopedics 1989;12:869.

110. Parker RD, Froimson AI, Winsburg DD, et al. Frozen shoulder. Part II. Treatment by manipulation under anesthesia. Orthopedics 1989;12:989.

111. Pasteur F. Su rune forrme nouvelle de periarthralgia et d'ankylose de l'epaule. J Radiol Electrol Med Nucl 1934;18:327.

112. Pearsall AW, OSbahr DC, Speer KP. An arthroscopic technique for treating patients with frozen shoulder 1999;15:2.

113. Placzek JD, Roubal PJ, Freeman C, et al. Long-term effectiveness of translational manipulation for adhesive capsulitis. CORR 1998;356:181.

114. Pollock RG, Duralde XA, Flatow EL, et al. The use of arthroscopy in the treatment of frozen shoulder. Clin Orthop 1994;304:30.

115. Quigley TB. Checkrein shoulder, a type of "frozen" shoulder: diagnosis and treatment by manipulation and ACTH or cortisone. Clin Orthop 1982;164:4.

116. Quin CE. "Frozen shoulder": evaluation and treatment with hydrocortisone injections and exercises. Ann Phys Med 1965;8:22.

117. Rathbun JB, Macnab. The microvascular pattern of the rotator cuff. J Bone Joint Surg 1970;52B:540.

118. Reeves B. Arthroscopic changes in frozen and post-traumatic stiff shoulder. Proc Royal Soc Med 1966;59:827.

119. Reeves B. The natural history of the frozen shoulder syndrome. J Rheumatol 1975;4:193.

120. Rhind V, Downie WW, Bird HA, et al. Naproxen and indomethacin in periarthritis of the shoulder. Rheumatol Rehabil 1982;21:51.

121. Richardson AT. Ernest Fletcher lecture: the painful shoulder. Proc R Soc Med 1975;68:731.

122. Riley D, Lang AE, Blair RD, et al. Frozen shoulder and other shoulder disturbance in Parkinson's disease. J Neurol Psychiatry 1989;52:63.

123. Rizk TE, Pinals RD. Frozen shoulder. Semin Arthritis Rheum 1982;11:440.

124. Rizk TE, Pinals RS. Histocompatibility type and racial incidence in frozen shoulder. Arch Phys Med Rehabil 1984;65:33.

125. Rosenbloom AL, Silverstein JH. Connective tissue and joint disease in diabetes mellitus. Endocrinol Metab Clin North Am 1996;25:473.

126. Roy S, Oldham R. Management of painful shoulder. Lancet 1976;1:1322.

127. Sattar MA, Lugman WA. Periarthritis: another duration-related complication of diabetes mellitus. Diabetes Care 1985;8:507.

128. Scarlat MM, Harryman DT. Management of the diabetic stiff shoulder. Instr Course Lect 2000;49:283.

129. Segmuller HE, Taylor DE, Hagan CS, et al. Arthroscopic treatment of adhesive capsulitis. J Shoulder Elbow Surg 1995;4:403.

130. Shaffer B, Tibone JE, Kerlan RK. Frozen shoulder: a long term follow-up. J Bone Joint Surg (Am) 1993;74:738.
131. Shaw DK, Deutsch DT, Bowling RJ. Efficacy of shoulder range of motion exercise in hospitalized patients after coronary artery bypass graft surgery. Heart Lung 1989;18:364.
132. Simmonds FA. Shoulder pain, with particular reference to the "frozen shoulder." J Bone Joint Surg (Br) 1949;31:426.
133. Simmons DB. Myofascial pain syndromes: where are we? Where are we going? Arch Phys Med Rehabil 1988;69:209.
134. Smith CR, Binder AI, Paice EW. Lesions of the midshaft of the humerus presenting as shoulder capsulitis. Br J Rheumatol 1990;29:386.
135. Steinbrocker I, Argyros TG. Frozen shoulder: treatment by local injection of depot corticosteroids. Arch Phys Med Rehabil 1974;55:209.
136. Stodell MA, Sturrock RD. Frozen shoulder. Lancet 1981;2:527.
137. Thomas D, Williams RA, Smith DS. The frozen shoulder: a review of manipulative treatment. Rheumatol Rehabil 1980;19:173.
138. Travell JG, Simmons DG. Myofascial pain and dysfunction: trigger point manual. Baltimore, Williams & Wilkins, 1983:410.
139. Warner JP. Frozen shoulder: diagnosis and management. Am Acad Orthop Surg 1997;5:130.
140. Warner JP, Allen A, Marks PH, et al. Arthroscopic release for chronic refractory adhesive capsulitis of the shoulder. J Bone Joint Surg 1996;78:1808.
141. Warner JP, Allen AA, Marks P, et al. Arthroscopic release of refractory capsular contracture of the shoulder. Video presentation, American Academy of Orthopaedic Surgeons, 62nd annual meeting, Orlando, FL, 1995.
142. Warner JP, Coborn DNM, Berger R, et al. Dynamic capsuloligamentous anatomy of the shoulder joint. J Shoulder Elbow Surg 1993;2:115.
143. Warner JP, Ianotti JP. Treatment of a stiff shoulder after posterior capsulorrhaphy. J Bone Joint Surg 1996;78:1419.
144. Watson L, Dalziel R, Story I. Frozen shoulder. A 12-month clinical outcome trial. J Shoulder Elbow Surg 2000;9:16.
145. Watson JR. Simple treatment of the stiff shoulder. J Bone Joint Surg 1963;45B:207.
146. Weiss JJ, Ting YM. Arthrography assisted intra-articular injection of steroids in the treatment of adhesive capsulitis. Arch Phys Med Rehabil 1978;59:285.
147. Wiley AM. Arthroscopic appearance of frozen shoulder. J Arthrosc Rel Surg 1991;7:138.
148. Wohlgethan JR. Frozen shoulder in hyperthyroidism. Arthritis Rheum 1987;30:936.
149. Wolfe F. Fibrositis, fibromyalgia and musculoskeletal disease: the current status of fibrositis syndrome. Arch Phys Med Rehabil 1988;69:527.
150. Wright MG, Richards AJ, Clark MB. 99-M pertechnetate scanning in capsulitis. Lancet 1975;2:1265.
151. Wright V, Haq AM. Periarthritis of the shoulder: I. Aetiological considerations with reference to personality factors. Ann Rheum Dis 1976;35:213.
152. Young A. Immunological studies in the frozen shoulder. In: Bayley J, Kessel L, eds. Shoulder surgery. Berlin-Heidelberg, Springer-Verlag, 1982:110.
153. Zuckerman JD, Cuomo F. Frozen shoulder. In: Matsen FA, Fu F, Hawkins RJ, eds. The shoulder: a balance of mobility and stability. Rosemont, IL, American Academy of Orthopaedic Surgeons, 1993:253.

Acquired Shoulder Stiffness: Posttraumatic and Postsurgical

11

Thomas F. Holovacs   *Jon J. P. Warner*

WHAT IS THE PROBLEM?

Definition and Classification

In contrast to primary adhesive capsulitis, *acquired* shoulder stiffness is a condition in which limitation of active and passive range of motion occurs after a well-defined traumatic event or a surgical procedure, and it is often associated with prolonged immobilization of the shoulder.[30,34,37,51,52,59,70,80,87,91,97] It can follow a number of posttraumatic and postsurgical scenarios. These include trauma with or without fracture and distortion of the articular surfaces and tuberosities, stiffness occurring after anatomical instability procedures (i.e., Bankart procedure and capsular shift), stiffness after rotator cuff repair, stiffness after nonanatomic instability shoulder stabilization procedures (i.e., Bristow, Putti-Platt, Magnuson-Stack), and stiffness after any shoulder procedure, open or arthroscopic.

Approach to management of acquired shoulder stiffness requires an appreciation of the pathology and likely natural history in each clinical scenario. Although treatment of idiopathic adhesive capsulitis is usually conservative, many experts agree that nonsurgical approaches to acquired

T. F. Holovacs: The Harvard Shoulder Service, Massachusetts General Hospital, Boston, Massachusetts.
J. J. P. Warner: The Harvard Shoulder Service, Massachusetts General Hospital, Boston, Massachusetts.

shoulder stiffness are not only less likely to be successful, but they may also result in eventual arthrosis in some cases.

Normal and Abnormal Anatomy/Mechanics of the Shoulder

The glenohumeral joint is inherently lax to allow for the wide range of multiplanar motion necessary for work, daily living, and sports participation. The glenohumeral ligaments act largely as passive restraints to excessive ranges of rotation and translation. So the relative capsular laxity in the midranges of motion is a feature of normal shoulder motion. In fact, joint compression created by muscle contraction is the major stabilizing force through much of the midrange rotations for the glenohumeral joint.

Although many cases of acquired shoulder stiffness result from global capsular contracture, scarring or shortening of specific regions of the capsule has been shown to lead to specific patterns of motion limitation.[26,33,43,85] When the shoulder is in an adducted position, the rotator interval, which is composed of the coracohumeral and superior glenohumeral ligaments, becomes involved and typically limits flexion, extension, and external rotation. The anteroinferior capsuloligamentous complex is a restraint for external rotation in abduction, whereas the posteroinferior capsule limits internal rotation and forward flexion. These patterns are important to recognize when considering the regions of the capsule that may require surgical release to recover motion.

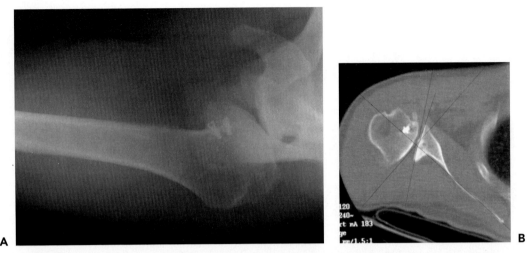

Figure 11-1   A 35-year old physician with painful loss of motion and arthritis after multiple surgeries for anterior instability. (*A*) Plain axillary radiograph demonstrates posterior subluxation and bone loss. (*B*) CT scan confirms posterior glenoid erosion.

Of great clinical relevance are experimental observations,[32,34] when the shoulder is rotated, of soft-tissue contractures that cause increased translation of the humeral head on the glenoid socket in a direction opposite to the location of the capsular contracture. For example, a Putti-Platt procedure shortens the anterior soft-tissues and causes the humeral head to translate posteriorly when external rotation is attempted. The consequence of this can be an increased joint-reactive load on the posterior glenoid and eventual development of articular erosion and arthritis.[4,32,34] This has been termed *capsulorrhaphy arthropathy*[32] (Fig. 11-1).

Anterior or posterior capsular contractures can also cause increased superior humeral head translation when a patient attempts to bring the shoulder into forward flexion[32,82] (Fig. 11-2). These altered mechanics compress the rotator cuff against the acromial surface as the humeral head is pushed superiorly by the contracture. This has been termed "nonoutlet"-type impingement, and it explains why many patients feel impingement-like symptoms when they have a stiff shoulder.[31,32,90] Arthroscopic release[89] and experimental capsular sectioning[33] have been shown to restore normal glenohumeral kinematics (Fig. 11-2).

Scapulothoracic pain can also be a confounding initial presentation in these patients. Because the shoulder complex is an intercalated series of joints, loss of glenohumeral motion usually causes a compensatory increase in scapulothoracic motion. Many patients present with secondary scapular winging, and some will complain of pain in the periscapular region.[87]

Finally, in osteoarthritis, global thickening and scarring are typical features of the joint capsule and may be the consequence of dysfunctional synoviocytes.[75] Moreover, it is our opinion that, in long-standing cases of motion loss,

there may be adaptations in the muscle architecture of the rotator cuff through fatty replacement and fibrous infiltration that reduce muscle compliance and further add to motion loss.

Pathogenesis

Acquired Capsular Contracture/Shortening

Idiopathic adhesive capsulitis is characterized by inflammation and subsequent scarring of the joint capsule, as well as by decreases in intra-articular volume and capsular compliance limiting motion in all planes.[87] Inflammation of the joint capsule and subsequent scarring may also occur as an *acquired* entity, that is, after trauma or surgery. It is not clear whether the cause of posttraumatic or postsurgical capsulitis is different from that of idiopathic adhesive capsulitis or whether some patients simply develop adhesive capsulitis in the context of trauma or surgery. Age, length of immobilization, and endocrine, neurologic and psychologic disorders, all recognized as important in the pathogenesis of idiopathic adhesive capsulitis, also seem to play a role in the development of shoulder stiffness after trauma or surgical treatment.[35]

Three different basic forms of acquired shoulder stiffness can be defined (Fig. 11-3):

- *Capsular contracture* (posttraumatic or postsurgical): stiffness after arthroscopic capsular shift, open Bankart repair, or open rotator cuff repair.
- *Extra-articular adhesions between tissue planes*: stiffness after Bristow, Putti-Platt, or Magnuson-Stack procedures.
- *Skeletal or articular incongruity*: proximal humeral malunion with displaced tuberosities, or stiffness associated with posttraumatic arthritis.

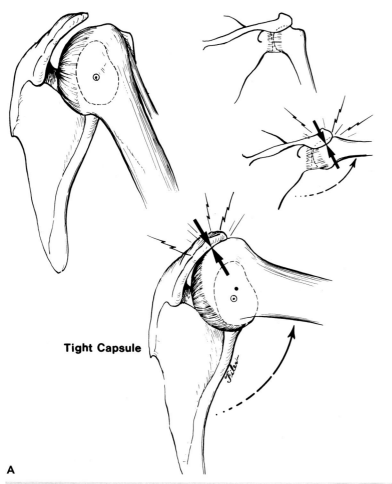

Tight Capsule

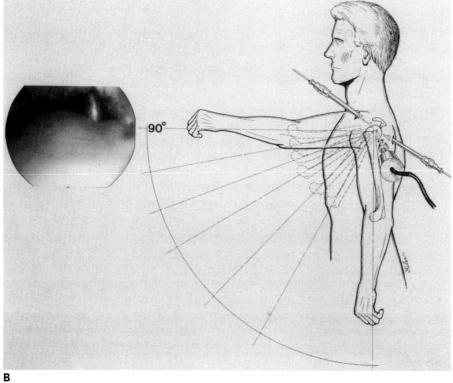

Figure 11-2 Nonoutlet impingement secondary to posterior capsular contracture. (*A*) A tight posterior capsule causes the humeral head to translate anteriorly and superiorly when the shoulder is flexed. This causes nonoutlet impingement. (*B*) An arthroscopic impingement test demonstrates impingement at 90 degrees of flexion in this patient with a posterior capsular contracture. *(continued)*

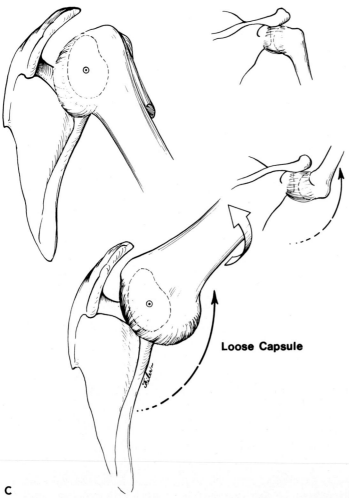

Loose Capsule

C

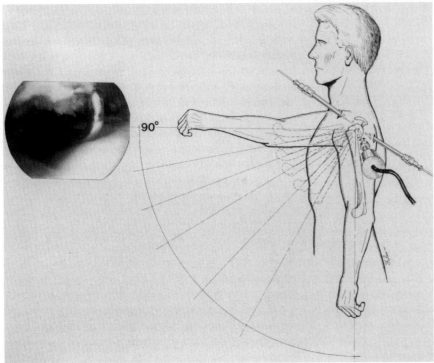

90°

D

Figure 11-2 *(continued)* *(C)* After release of the posterior capsule, the humeral head remains centered on the glenoid during flexion. *(D)* An arthroscopic impingement test after posterior capsular release demonstrates less superior movement of the humeral head during flexion to 90 degrees.

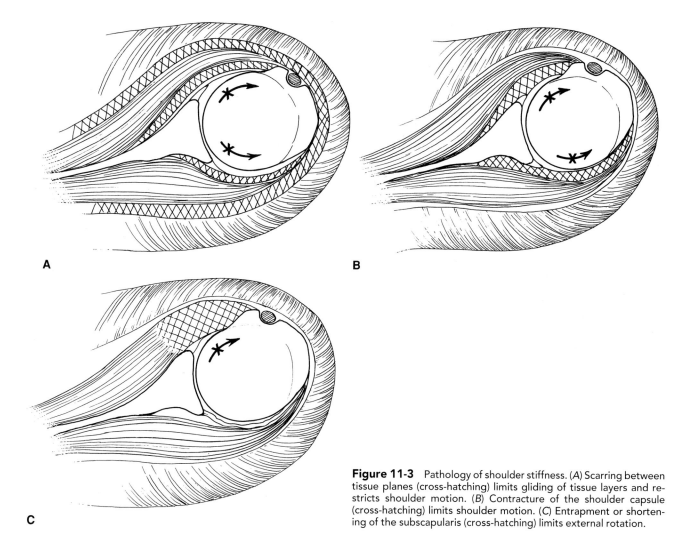

A

B

C

Figure 11-3 Pathology of shoulder stiffness. (*A*) Scarring between tissue planes (cross-hatching) limits gliding of tissue layers and restricts shoulder motion. (*B*) Contracture of the shoulder capsule (cross-hatching) limits shoulder motion. (*C*) Entrapment or shortening of the subscapularis (cross-hatching) limits external rotation.

Although features of these three general categories can overlap in the same patient, this classification system is useful for developing a logical therapeutic approach.

Some specific examples include:

- *Calcific tendinitis*: Stiffness after surgical excision of calcific tendinitis of the rotator cuff reportedly affects 6–20% of patients. The pathologic mechanism is unknown but the clinical symptoms are similar to those of adhesive capsulitis.[54] In many cases, a conservative approach similar to that utilized for idiopathic frozen shoulder is successful.
- *Post-thermal capsulorrhaphy*: Reports on thermal capsulorrhaphy suggest that stiffness is a common complication of this procedure.[22] Patients who have undergone this procedure often present with the same symptoms as patients with idiopathic adhesive capsulitis, although the etiology is different. This procedure creates thermal injury to capsular tissue through an internal burn, which then results in a degree of inflammation; scarring also occurs as an obligatory repair mechanism. Why some patients develop this complication and others do not is un-

clear. Miniaci[58] has proposed that it is related to transient axillary nerve neuritis in some way.
- *Post-rotator cuff repair*: A recent meta-analysis[91] of greater than 500 surgical cases reported in literature concluded a 4% incidence of measurable symptomatic loss of motion in patients undergoing rotator cuff surgery; however, it seems that this underreports the actual incidence of this complication. Even so, the need for surgical management of stiffness after rotator cuff repair seems to be rare.
- *Stiffness after anatomical instability repair*: There is no documented reported incidence of stiffness after capsular shift repair or arthroscopic or open Bankart repair for traumatic or atraumatic shoulder instability. Several articles have postulated that these patients were analyzed as a cohort of all patients presenting with refractory stiffness[17]; however, virtually none of these series inferred anything but extremely rare incidences of symptomatic loss of motion after instability surgery. This most certainly represents underreporting, because many individuals may note loss of rotation after instability surgery but

may either not be symptomatic initially or only become symptomatic if postsurgical capsulorrhaphy arthropathy eventually recurs.

■ *Stiffness after nonanatomical instability repairs*: Stiffness may occur from extra-articular procedures that shorten tendons around the shoulder or asymmetrically shorten the anterior capsule. For example, a Putti-Platt procedure shortens both the anterior capsule and the subscapularis. A Magnuson-Stack procedure reduces external rotation by attaching the subscapularis insertion lateral to the bicipital groove with the arm in external rotation, which is the procedure's aim. A Bristow or Latarjet procedure can shorten the subscapularis, especially if there is prolonged immobilization, because the subscapularis is scarred to the transferred conjoined tendon and coracoid process. All of these procedures can result in asymmetric motion loss, which has been shown to place the glenohumeral joint at risk for early osteoarthritis. Furthermore, loss of external rotation can actually coexist with untreated instability because inferior capsular laxity may remain untreated with these operations. This creates the paradoxical situation of a patient who complains of loss of motion but still has a sense of apprehension about instability episodes.

■ *Extra-articular adhesions between tissue planes (scarring of gliding surfaces)*: Another requirement for normal shoulder mobility is free gliding between tissue planes. In the normal shoulder, the rotator cuff glides underneath the coracoacromial arch and the deltoid muscle. Trauma and prolonged immobilization or surgical procedures can lead to scarring between the deltoid and the proximal humerus, the rotator cuff and the acromion, and the rotator cuff and the joint capsule. Furthermore, prominent implants used to stabilize proximal humeral fractures may lead to scarring of the subdeltoid bursa (Fig. 11-4).

■ *Skeletal or articular incongruity*: Smooth, normally shaped articular surfaces, properly oriented to each other, represent the osteoarticular requirement for normal glenohumeral range of motion. Skeletal deformity is always associated with soft-tissue scarring.

Displaced fractures of the proximal humerus treated conservatively or in which anatomic reduction could not be achieved or maintained can be associated with stiffness resulting from not only soft-tissue contracture but also skeletal deformity. Intra-articular fractures with loss of the normal relationship between the humeral head and tuberosities are usually associated with poor function, partly because of stiffness but also because of malpositioning of the tuberosity. Extra-articular deformities are usually better tolerated.

Stiffness resulting from articular incongruity (and capsular contracture) is one of the leading features of osteoarthritis. Except for selected cases in the early stage of the degenerative process in which only the soft-tissue contrac-

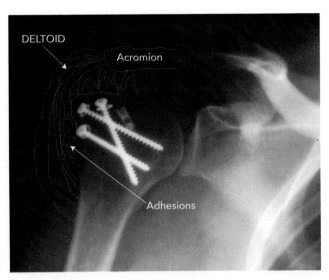

Figure 11-4 Adhesions between deltoid and rotator cuff after fracture repair and prolonged immobilization in a sling.

ture needs to be addressed, correction of the articular deformity, through corrective osteotomy or replacement arthroplasty, is required in the majority of the cases. In the case of replacement arthroplasty, stiffness can be the result of nonanatomic reconstruction, such as oversizing and improper orientation of the components, and tuberosity-related problems, such as nonunion or malunion.

The muscular imbalance seen in patients with brachial plexus birth palsy has been shown to lead to an age-related articular deformity if the condition is not addressed early. Once humeral head flattening and glenoid dysplasia have developed, soft-tissue release alone, either arthroscopically or as an open procedure, cannot increase mobility.[93]

Bony block procedures to treat instability, such as the Bristow, Latarjet, and Trillat procedures, are techniques that distort the skeletal and soft-tissue anatomy. Subscapularis entrapment or impingement and articular incongruity may lead to limitation of motion after these procedures.[91]

Clinical Evaluation

An accurate history and physical examination are prerequisites to proper treatment of the refractory stiff shoulder. Patients with adhesive capsulitis frequently report no inciting traumatic event whatsoever. These patients describe the insidious and unremitting onset of shoulder pain, which predates stiffness and is unresponsive to physical therapy. Acquired shoulder stiffness, on the other hand, occurs as a result of a well-defined event, such as prolonged immobilization following trauma and anatomic (capsular shift) or nonanatomic (Putti-Platt) surgical *over*tightening for glenohumeral instability.[34,70,82,87] Prior surgery or trauma must be clarified. For example, if a patient had a fracture and then developed stiffness after prolonged immobilization, this might indicate that there are adhesions between tissue planes as well as a capsular contracture. Radiographic imaging would then determine whether there is bony incongruity around the joint.

Medical conditions, such as diabetes, must also be considered.[66,87] Patients who develop a stiff shoulder without trauma or even after trauma or surgery may have this as a confounding variable. Finally, a patient who develops a stiff shoulder after rotator cuff surgery may also have a re-rupture of the rotator cuff, which may affect decision making because both stiffness and rotator cuff insufficiency must be addressed.

Symptoms

As described in the preceding text, symptoms may vary among patients. Some patients complain not only of motion loss but also of impingement-type pain with pain radiating into the deltoid area. The mechanism, as described previously, is one of nonoutlet impingement. Others may also have periscapular pain due to transfer overload onto the scapulothoracic articulation as a compensation for glenohumeral motion loss. Still others with very severe motion loss may have minimal complaints of pain and be willing to tolerate their motion loss. These individuals are particularly challenging because, if the severe loss of external rotation is left untreated, they may be the most at risk for eventual capsulorrhaphy arthropathy. Indeed, this is one of the few groups of patients in whom we often advise surgical contracture release prior to developing symptoms of pain. If the patient waits many years for pain to develop, irreversible articular damage will have already occurred due to the mechanical overload of the posterior joint (Fig. 11-1).

Physical Examination

Begin the physical examination of the shoulder by inspecting the ipsilateral and contralateral shoulders for signs of prior trauma/surgery, atrophy, and deformity. The patient should always be examined while viewing the exposed shoulder and torso from the front and back. *Active* motion of the shoulder girdle is assessed using a goniometer with the patient seated. Document active flexion, elevation in the scapular plane, and abduction, as well as internal/external rotation, both at the side and in abduction. Assess passive mobility in the same planes of motion, first with the patient seated and, then, supine (to stabilize the scapula and minimize scapulothoracic substitution). It should be noted that scapulothoracic substitution might give the appearance of good shoulder motion when glenohumeral motion is actually quite restricted. Patients with shoulder stiffness have active and passive motion loss that is equal. If there is active motion loss but passive motion is preserved, one should think of rotator cuff insufficiency. Weakness associated with passive motion loss may also indicate a rotator cuff tear or nerve injury.

Patterns of motion loss are very important to recognize. Primary adhesive capsulitis tends to present with global motion restriction, whereas postsurgical or posttraumatic stiffness may present with a more discrete or isolated motion loss.[26,87] For example, a patient may have good flexion but marked loss of external rotation after a Putti-Platt or Bristow procedure, which has selectively shortened the anterior capsule and subscapularis. Another example, diminished external rotation in *adduction*, indicates contracture of the anterosuperior capsule and the rotator interval, while limited external rotation in *abduction* is associated with scarring in the anteroinferior capsule. Furthermore, limitation of internal rotation in either adduction or abduction may be associated with posterior capsular scarring. These preoperative observations are important because they indicate which portions of the capsule may need to be addressed, if a surgical release is required.

In addition to passive limitation of motion, many patients will complain of symptoms that suggest rotator cuff impingement. Although these patients may have pain with flexion, the impingement symptoms that seem to suggest rotator cuff disease are actually secondary due to alterations in joint mechanics as a result of the capsular contracture. This is "nonoutlet" impingement, which occurs without altering the architecture of the coracoacromial arch and, instead, is due to a tight capsule that pushes the humeral head in a superior direction when flexion is attempted[31,32,90] (Fig. 11-2). Periscapular pain may also develop due to the scapulothoracic muscles stretching to compensate for the limited glenohumeral joint motion.

Imaging Studies

Plain radiographs are always essential to rule out arthrosis, associated fracture malunion, and loose or misplaced metal implants and hardware.

Arthrography has been advocated by many to confirm a decreased joint capacity.[66] However, it has been shown that there is no direct correlation between arthrographic findings and motion loss.[40] Therefore, its use is often limited to an adjunctive role, such as ruling out a concomitant rotator cuff tear.

Magnetic resonance imaging (MRI) and contrast-enhanced computed tomography (CT) are limited in use, aiding in the diagnosis of additional shoulder pathology, such as locating a rotator cuff tear or the exact position of hardware that may be impinging on the articular surface.

Acquired Capsular Contracture/Shortening

Acquired capsulitis means the development of shoulder stiffness after a traumatic incident, surgical treatment without tissue or bone repair, i.e., decompressing calcifying tendinitis, or after arthroscopic or open surgery. Examples of this last category might include arthroscopic thermal capsulorrhaphy, Bankart and capsular shift procedures, Bristow procedure, Putti-Platt procedure, rotator cuff repair, and other shoulder reconstructions.

After trauma or surgery of the shoulder, some patients develop severe pain that cannot be explained by the underlying condition. This type of shoulder stiffness seems similar to the idiopathic form of the disease. Some patients may have the diabetes risk factor. The symptoms usually do not occur immediately after trauma or surgery, but 2 to 6 weeks. The patient's pain is constant and is especially severe at night. Attempts at regaining motion rapidly with physical therapy may lead to exacerbating the chronic discomfort. Regular pain medication prescribed after the traumatic event or operation, or subacromial infiltration with a local anesthetic, does not help to control the pain. On physical examination, any manipulation of the shoulder is extremely painful to the patient. At this stage, loss of passive range of motion may be discrete, but passive rotation amplitude, especially in abduction, is already decreased and is very painful. Active range of motion is limited by pain as well as by soft-tissue shortening.

Acquired capsular contracture, with or without concomitant scarring between tissue planes, is usually seen after fractures or surgery. The prolonged immobilization often required for healing injured or repaired structures plays an important role in developing this type of stiffness. Scarring between the tissue plains of the gliding surfaces can cause global motion restriction and pain. Global motion restriction is a common feature of fractures of the proximal humerus. If open reduction is indicated to achieve anatomic reduction, subdeltoid scarring can be very important, especially if postoperative immobilization is required. Prominent humeral prosthetic implants impair gliding in the subdeltoid space.

Unlike in patients in the acute inflammatory stage, pain is usually present, especially in the end-range of motion, but motion limitation is the main complaint. Pain mimics the symptoms of subacromial impingement, limits active range of motion, and is localized on the lateral side of the arm. Depending on the underlying problem, specific patterns of motion restriction are observed.

Persistent motion loss after rotator cuff repair may be the result of inadequate operative technique or inadequate postoperative rehabilitation, and it is more likely to happen in patients demonstrating preoperative stiffness.[20,21,91] It is very important to ensure that the patient who has a rotator cuff repair has a supple shoulder. This can be established through physical therapy prior to surgery, closed manipulation, operative release of adhesions during surgery.

Incorrect operative technique includes poor release, especially of the coracohumeral ligament, or tight closure of the rotator interval in internal rotation, leading to loss of external rotation and flexion.[33,43] Repair by excessively advancing the musculotendinous unit is characterized by loss of internal rotation, if the posterosuperior rotator cuff

is at issue, or by a decrease in external rotation, as seen after subscapularis repair.[92] Indeed, some loss of external rotation is mandatory when repairing a chronic subscapularis tendon tear, because the motion loss means the repair is intact.

Failure to address associated pathologic processes, such as acromioclavicular arthropathy or biceps tendon disease, as well as complications, such as deltoid insufficiency or nerve injury, will usually result in postoperative pain and increased risk of stiffness. Adequate mobilization immediately after the surgical procedure is important to maintain glenohumeral flexibility.

Optimized postoperative pain management is also mandatory to allow efficient physical therapy, especially in patients with low pain tolerances.[20] Stiffness after rotator cuff repair can occur in the presence of a recurrent rupture as well. In this situation, limited active and passive range of motion is associated with weakness.

Stiffness is a potential complication of all capsuloligamentous procedures to treat instability. Traditional procedures, such as the Putti-Platt and Magnuson-Stack procedures, are designed to restrict external rotation by shortening the anterior capsule and the subscapularis tendon.[53] The Bankart or capsular shift procedure, considered to address the soft-tissue disorder specifically and, therefore, to restore stability without motion limitation, can also be associated with severe limitation of external rotation if the capsule is overtightened.[83]

Skeletal or Articular Incongruity

Stiffness in the presence of a skeletal or articular deformity is typically found after bone block procedure to treat instability, malunited fracture of the proximal humerus, nonanatomic replacement arthroplasty, and neglected residual plexus birth palsy.

Stiffness after instability procedures using a bone block affects mobility either by entrapping the subscapularis tendon (Bristow and Trillat procedures) or by resulting in articular incongruence (Eden-Hybbinette and Latarjet).[1,25,67,96] An open approach that releases the subscapularis or corrects the articular deformity is required.[55,87,96]

Stiffness after shoulder arthroplasty, while not rare, is usually painless and well tolerated by patients. It may be the consequence of inadequate capsular releases and subscapularis mobilization or poor compliance with a postoperative therapy program. Malpositioning of the humeral component may also result in poor recovery of motion and painful shoulder stiffness. Another chapter of this books discusses this in greater detail.

Arthroscopic release for patients with stiffness resulting from major structural distortion does improve range of motion, but it is not as successful as it is for patients with idiopathic stiffness. When stiffness is associated with nonanatomic reconstruction after replacement arthroplasty, a complex open approach involves global soft-tissue release and implant revision with or without tuberosity osteotomy.

Treatment

Any rational treatment approach to this difficult clinical problem must be based on the understanding that the natural history of the disorder depends, in part, on its cause. For example, external rotation loss after an anterior shoulder stabilization procedure may be relatively resistant to conservative treatment, whereas motion loss after prolonged immobilization for a traumatized shoulder may be responsive to conservative management.

Physical Therapy

The mainstay of initial management for shoulder stiffness is physical therapy. The primary indication for operative treatment is failure to restore normal motion after a prolonged trial of physical therapy. Absolute measures of improvement vary, yet physical therapy is considered to be a failure if passive range of motion is not restored to within 80% of the contralateral, unaffected shoulder, and/or the patient continues to have pain and functional impairment. With this in mind, certain scenarios are unlikely to respond to therapy, including cases where there is a known distortion of soft-tissue anatomy from prior surgery, such as Bristow, Putti-Platt, or Magnuson-Stack procedures for instability.

The recommended duration of physical therapy treatment varies from 3 to 36 months.[30,37,66,70,87,89,91] It is important to differentiate between primary and secondary causes of stiffness; however, the latter is more often resistant to conservative treatment.[87,91] In postoperative or posttraumatic stiffness cases, operative treatment is recommended if physical therapy has failed to meet the previously mentioned criteria after 6 to 12 months. Indeed, some patients may recover most or all of their motion after 1 year of conservative management. Alternatively, patient dissatisfaction with the progress of physical therapy can justifiably hasten operative intervention.

Experiment studies have demonstrated that soft-tissue contracture causes increased translation of the humeral head on the glenoid socket in a direction opposite to the contracture during attempted shoulder motion.[32] Anterior and posterior capsular contractures have been shown to increase translation in the superior direction. This can result in rotator cuff compression as the humeral head is pushed superiorly by the contracture and induces a "nonoutlet"-type impingement. Furthermore, an asymmetric anterior contracture tends to cause the humeral head to move posteriorly on the glenoid with attempted external rotation. This has been associated with the development of arthritis and has been termed *capsulorrhaphyarthropathy*. For these reasons, most shoulder surgeons perceive acquired shoulder stiffness as a condition that merits aggressive treatment.[2,30,35,44,46,52,60,62,65,68,72,76,79]

Anesthesia/Analgesia Management

When conservative treatment fails to restore motion, closed manipulation, arthroscopic release, or open surgical release is indicated. Adequate anesthesia is a prerequisite for a successful overall treatment, for both the arthroscopic and open surgical approach. Our prior experience, and the experience of others,[16,91] has demonstrated the effectiveness of regional anesthesia using an interscalene block and indwelling catheter after surgery, allowing anesthesia not only for painless surgery but also for complete muscle paralysis, which is necessary for safe introduction of the arthroscope into a contracted joint and then release of capsular contractures. The interscalene indwelling catheter remains in place during the procedure and for 48 hours following the procedure. Supplemental sedation of general anesthesia can then be used, if desired. Alternatively, if general anesthesia is utilized, complete muscle paralysis is necessary. Postoperative pain control can alternatively be achieved with an intra-articular catheter, which administers long-acting local anesthetic into the joint. Commercial devices that accomplish this are available. Though others have used this approach with success, we have not found oral, intravenous, or intramuscular pharmacologic management of pain to be sufficiently adequate to allow for early postoperative motion in most patients.

Closed Manipulation Under Anesthesia

Closed manipulation under anesthesia has historically been advocated as the next step after conservative therapy failure.[66] The clinician must decide on the likelihood of extra-articular scarring in addition to capsular contracture and then tailor the surgical treatment to address these factors. In a relatively acute case of motion loss after surgery or trauma for which therapy has failed to regain motion, closed manipulation may be attempted. Many surgeons, however, believe this approach is usually unsuccessful and some form of surgical release is required.[34,52,55,70,96] Although closed manipulation may be attempted, it is important to inform the patient that an arthroscopic or open release may be necessary. Furthermore, rare complications of humeral fracture or nerve injury may occur with forceful manipulation of the shoulder.[19,46,57]

Closed manipulation is performed with the patient under anesthesia and with complete muscle relaxation. Formal contraindications to this approach include marked osteopenia, recent soft-tissue repair, malunion, or known extra-articular contracture (i.e., Bristow procedure).[19,29,36,42,46,57,71,81]

Closed manipulation is performed by a method similar to that described by Neviaser and Harryman.[30,66] The scapula is stabilized with one hand while the humerus is grasped with the other hand just above the elbow. The shoulder is first externally rotated and then abducted in the coronal plane. The shoulder is externally rotated in abduction and then internally rotated while maintaining abduction. It is then flexed and finally brought back into adduction and internally rotated. Motion is usually restored in all planes, along with a palpable and audible yielding of soft tissue.

Arthroscopic Release

Arthroscopic capsular release for the stiff shoulder was described in the early 1990s as an alternative to closed manipulation, permitting a controlled, precise means to selectively and incrementally release the capsule and often, the extra-articular adhesions.[31,37,70,89,91]

The main indication for arthroscopic capsular release is shoulder stiffness due to capsular contracture, recalcitrant to nonoperative means.[87] This occurs most commonly in primary adhesive capsulitis, but it may also occur postsurgically or posttraumatically. Posttraumatic stiffness without bony incongruity, stiffness after rotator cuff repair, and stiffness after Bankart or capsular shift surgery are all conditions that can be managed effectively with arthroscopic release.

The presence of osteoarthritis is not an absolute contraindication to arthroscopic release as long as the humeral head remains round and congruent in the glenoid fossa. Indeed, release of a capsular contracture can mitigate the pain of osteoarthritis when combined with debridement.

Stiffness after surgery for instability may represent a special case. In such circumstances, where there is severe loss of external rotation, the patient remains at risk for developing arthritis due to excessive joint-compressive force, which is directed across the posterior joint as a result of the anterior soft-tissue contracture. In these patients, we recommend release of their contracture, if therapy has been unsuccessful for more than 1 year after their instability repair surgery.

Arthroscopic capsular release may be performed with the patient in the beach-chair position or lateral decubitus position. We prefer the former because it allows greater mobility of the arm, simple and accurate assessment of passive range of motion, and simple conversion to an open approach, if necessary.

Technique of Arthroscopic Capsular Release

After positioning the patient on the operating room table in the beach-chair position, assess and document passive range of motion under anesthesia. This allows easy and direct comparison to the range of motion achieved after the capsular release.

We have stopped performing closed manipulation prior to introduction of the arthroscope because this usually results in incomplete return of motion and causes hemorrhage into the joint from partial capsular rupture. This makes visualization difficult. Furthermore, arthroscopic release allows for less forceful restoration of joint motion;

thus, it does not risk rupture of rotator cuff tendons (especially in patients who may have stiffness after rotator cuff repair), and there is less risk of fracture.

The entire upper extremity is prepared in a sterile fashion such that the entire shoulder girdle (including the medial border of the scapula) will be in the operative field after draping. We use a mechanical arm-holder to maintain the position of the arm and shoulder without requiring an extra surgical assistant (Fig. 11-5).

The posterior arthroscopic portal is slightly higher (0.5 cm) than routine. An 18-gauge spinal needle is then inserted into the joint, and sterile saline is introduced into the contracted intra-articular space. Usually, only 10 to 15 cc of saline is permitted, and its backflow out of the needle confirms proper placement. The saline also fills the small space of the joint so that the arthroscope can be introduced, with backflow through the scope sheath confirming proper placement. Furthermore, increased intra-articular pressure pushes the articular surfaces away from one another and reduces the risk of articular damage when introducing the arthroscope.

An incision is then made and the arthroscope is inserted in the same orientation of the spinal needle, carefully guiding it over the humeral head. In severe cases of capsular contracture, only the superior portion of the anterior joint is visible because of the capsular contracture. However, the biceps and intra-articular subscapularis tendons, along with the intervening rotator interval, are typically visible. An 18-gauge spinal needle is then introduced into the joint just underneath the biceps, and a 6-mm cannula is intro-

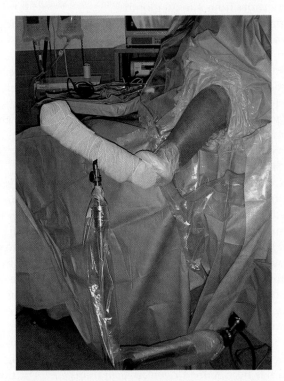

Figure 11-5   Beach-chair positioner with articulated arm holder (T-Max Beach Chair and Spider Arm Holder, Tenet Medical Engineering, Calgary, Canada).

duced into the superior joint. A radiofrequency device and motorized shaver are then used to remove any synovium that might obscure visualization.

Anterior Capsular Release

The first step is to release the contracture of the rotator interval capsule, anatomically comprised of the superior glenohumeral and the coracohumeral ligaments. This is the superior portion of the joint just underneath the long head of the biceps tendon. The upper border of the subscapularis is often obscured by scar tissue. Although any sharp instruments may be used, we prefer to use a radiofrequency device with a hook-tip and begin by cutting tissue just underneath the long head of the biceps (Fig. 11-6A). This region

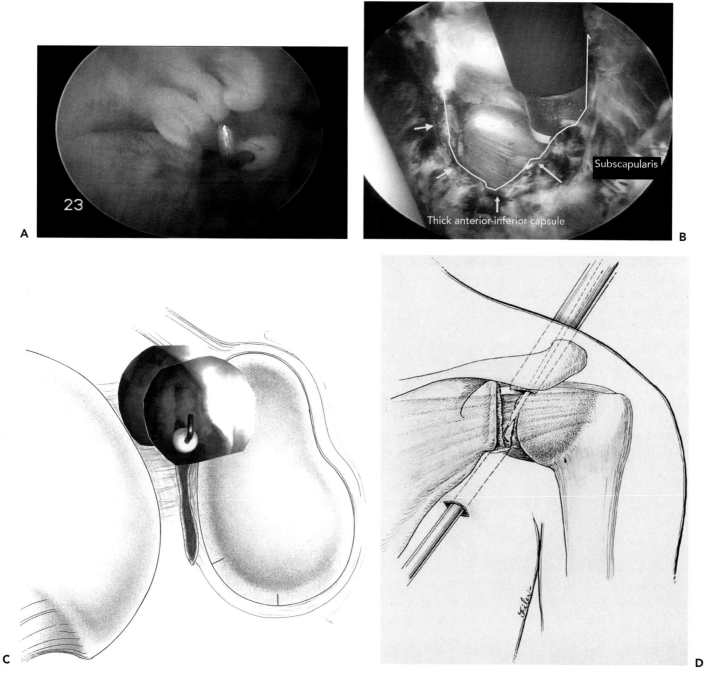

Figure 11-6 (A) Hook-tip radiofrequency device used to cut capsular contracture (Vapr Hook Tip, Mitek, Johnson and Johnson, Norwood, MA). (B) Release of upper subscapularis with hook tip radiofrequency device. (C,D) Release of inferior capsule to 6 o'clock position. (C reprinted with permission from Holovacs TH, O'Holleran JD, Warner JJP. Arthroscopic capsular release for stiff shoulder. In: Craig EV, ed. The shoulder. Master techniques in orthopaedic surgery, 2nd ed. Philadelphia, Lippincott Williams & Wilkins, 2004:172.)

of the capsule is released so that the upper border of the subscapularis is exposed (Fig. 11-6B). If necessary, the thickened capsular tissue may be released to the base of the coracoid process.

The anterior capsular release then continues inferiorly, dividing the capsular scar off of the subscapularis muscle. Compared to normal capsular tissue, which is usually no more than 2 mm thick, the capsular tissue in these cases may be up to a centimeter thick. Gentle external rotation of the arm may also help by placing the capsular scar under tension, allowing for easier release. The release is continued to the 6 o'clock position (Fig. 11-6, C and D). As long as subscapularis muscle is visualized, the axillary nerve is not at risk.

Posterior Capsular Release

In patients with persistent loss of internal rotation, a posterior capsular release is required. This is performed by placing the arthroscope through the anterior cannula and then using a switching stick to remove the arthroscopic sheath and insert a 6-mm cannula posteriorly. The fluid inflow is through the anterior cannula (Fig. 11-7A).

A radiofrequency device with a hook tip is introduced through the posterior portal while visualizing the posterior capsule from the anterior portal. The posterior capsule is then released from a point just behind the long head of biceps tendon insertion to about the 8 o'clock position on the glenoid rim (Fig. 11-7B). The posterior capsule will be observed to be markedly thickened compared with its normal 1-mm thickness, and the muscle of the in-

fraspinatus will be seen as the end point of the capsular release.

Following the arthroscopic release, a gentle manipulation of the shoulder is performed using the sequence described previously. Usually, supple resistance-free motion encounters little resistance.

We routinely perform a subacromial bursoscopy to determine if there is a component of subacromial bursitis that must be addressed. In cases where subacromial and subdeltoid scarring are expected (prior rotator cuff repair, fracture repair), placement of the arthroscope in this position releases these adhesions. A routine subacromial decompression is then performed, although, in some patients, dense scarring may make this a difficult procedure. In such cases, the shaver or radiofrequency device may be kept in one position while the humerus is rotated to bring adhesions to the tip of the device. Care is taken to free up the space completely lateral to the acromion between the deltoid and proximal humerus (Fig. 11-8, A and B).

Aftercare

Immediate cryotherapy (Cryocuff, Aircast Co., Rutherford, NJ) is preferred by our senior surgeon, and this is utilized frequently during the early phase of treatment to reduce pain and swelling. In the recovery room, when the patients are awake, they are shown their postoperative passive range of motion, which helps them understand that their motion has been recovered and it is their job to maintain this gain.

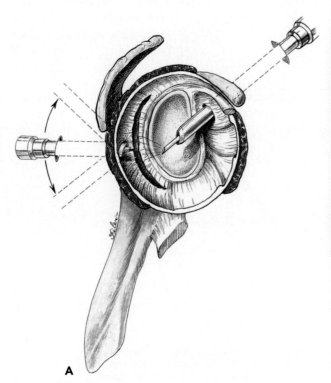

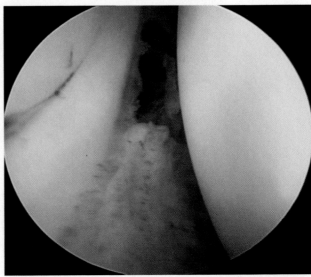

Figure 11-7 (A) Arthroscopic posterior capsular release. Portal placement (see text for explanation). (B) Arthroscopic posterior capsular release technique. (A reprinted with permission from Holovacs TH, O'Holleran JD, Warner JJP. Arthroscopic capsular release for stiff shoulder. In: Craig EV, ed. The shoulder. Master techniques in orthopaedic surgery, 2nd ed. Philadelphia, Lippincott Williams & Wilkins, 2004:172.)

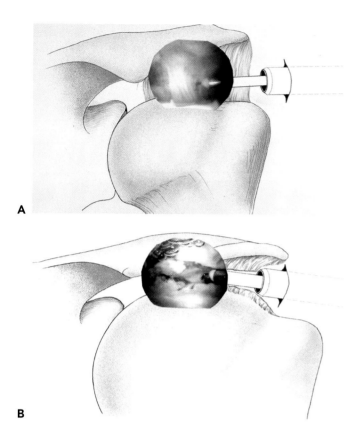

A

B

Figure 11-8 (*A*) Subacromial adhesions in a stiff shoulder after rotator cuff repair can be very dense and run from the acromion into the rotator cuff. (*B*) Arthroscopic release of subacromial adhesions accomplished with a radiofrequency device.

The patients remain in the hospital for 48 hours, during which time they receive analgesia from a continuous inflow of bupivacaine through the interscalene catheter. After placing the interscalene catheter, the patient receives a bolus of 30 to 40 cc of a combination of 1.5% mepivacaine and 0.5% bupivacaine, usually in a combination of 20 cc of each. The infusion is then usually 0.1% bupivacaine run at a variable rate ranging from 10 to 20 cc per hour, depending on the individual patient's degree of pain. Physical therapy is performed twice each day while in the hospital, with the therapist instructed to passively move the shoulder into all planes. Some surgeons advocate using a continuous passive-motion machine, although we have not found this to be more effective than skilled physical therapy and do not utilize this approach. The patients are discharged on the afternoon of the second postoperative day without a sling and are instructed to begin immediate physical therapy and to try to use their shoulder for daily living activities.

Supervised physical therapy is performed 5 days each week for the first 2 weeks and then usually 3 days per week for the next 2 weeks. Afterward, therapy is individualized to each patient's needs. We also use water therapy whenever possible, which we have found, as have others,[47,48,78] that

the zero gravity environment of a warm water environment facilitates more rapid restoration of motion. Strengthening, using elastic bands and weights, is begun whenever there is supple range of motion available.

Open Surgical Release

Patients with shoulder stiffness resulting from contracture of the *extra-articular* soft tissues, such as after a Bristow or Putti-Platt procedure, are not appropriate candidates for arthroscopic capsular release. In such cases, contracture involves both the capsule and the subscapularis tendon.[30,44,52,55,62] Open surgical release of extra-articular adhesions is the treatment of choice, and, in some cases, a Z-plasty lengthening of the capsule and subscapularis tendon is required. If there is a question about feasibility of the arthroscopic approach, an initial arthroscopic attempt at release can be performed and converted to open, if necessary. This is best facilitated if the patient is in a beach-chair position.

A regional interscalene block of anesthesia is used with a catheter and with or without supplemental general anesthesia. Prior incisions may dictate and affect the approach, but the preferred incision is deltopectoral. Typically, there is extensive scarring at all tissue plains and levels of dissection, so a layer by layer dissection is performed. The deltopectoral interval is developed, and the adhesions between the deltoid and the humerus are released (Fig. 11-9*A*). This must be done with care, because the axillary nerve may be at risk if exposure and lysis of adhesions are not meticulous. The axillary nerve can often be palpated on the deep surface of the deltoid muscle, approximately 3 to 5 cm below the lateral border of the acromion. To facilitate this dissection, the shoulder is abducted to relax the deltoid, and a blunt retractor is then placed underneath the deltoid and over the humeral shaft. Adhesions can then be sharply divided (Fig. 11-9*B*).

After the subdeltoid interval is completely free and the humerus glides freely underneath the deltoid, the dissection proceeds medially. The subacromial space may be restricted by dense scar tissue between the rotator cuff and the acromion. This scar is released by gently retracting the deltoid with the arm in abduction and then sharply dividing scar tissue off the undersurface of the acromion. Great care must be taken with deltoid retraction, because overzealous retraction can injure the muscle at its origin or insertion.

The conjoined tendon is then identified, and the lateral border developed. The strap muscles are separated from the underlying subscapularis and retracted medially. This may be done by a combination of blunt and sharp dissection, provided that the surgeon is mindful of the musculocutaneous nerve. Keeping the dissection lateral to the coracoid process can prevent injury to the neurovascular structures.

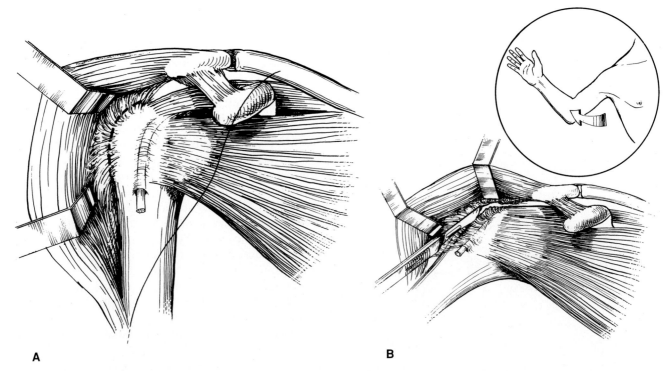

A

B

Figure 11-9   (A) Extensive adhesions between the deltoid and proximal humerus limit rotation. (B) Abduction and external rotation relax the deltoid and allow it to be retracted so that the subdeltoid adhesions can be divided.

The superior border of the subscapularis tendon is next identified, and the rotator interval is released from the humerus to the coracoid.[61,73] With each step, as the dissection releases adhesions between tissue layers, the shoulder is gently manipulated to regain motion. Any significant limitation of external rotation remaining is usually caused by a shortened subscapularis from prior surgery. In these cases, coronal Z-plasty lengthening of the subscapularis and capsule is performed. This is done by dividing the scarred subscapularis tendon in the coronal plane so that the superficial half of the tendon remains attached to the muscle while the remaining deep half is divided at the glenoid and remains attached to the lesser tuberosity (Fig. 11-10).

The subscapularis is usually entrapped in scar, and it must be completely released so it can move normally with humerus rotation. To fully mobilize this muscle-tendon unit, it is usually necessary to visualize and dissect the axillary nerve. Place a vessel loop around the axillary nerve, and then globally release the subscapularis on its superior, inferior, deep, and superficial surfaces (Fig. 11-11).

If abduction and internal rotation are still limited, the inferior and posterior capsule can be released through the joint via the deltopectoral approach. A global capsulotomy is then performed by displacing the humeral posteriorly with a humeral head retractor while protecting the axillary nerve with a blunt retractor placed underneath the inferior capsule. The capsule is then released, under direct vision,

from an inferior–to-posterosuperior direction. The retractors are then removed and the shoulder is placed through a range-of-motion exercise to determine motion gains. The humeral head is then re-located, and the arm is positioned in the maximum external rotation allowing a secure closure of the Z-plasty of the anterior capsule and subscapularis tendon using large, nonabsorbable, braided sutures. Subscapularis mobilization greatly increases excursion of this muscle-tendon unit, but repair of the tendon to the length of the capsule attached to the humerus is usually necessary to gain maximum external rotation. It is typically possible to gain at least 40 degrees of external rotation, but the result depends on the quality of the tendon and capsular tissue (Fig. 11-12, A and B).

Range of motion is assessed to determine where there is tension on the soft-tissue repair and define a "safe zone" for early passive range of motion. This information is communicated to the physical therapist, who assists the patient in the immediate postoperative period.

Aftercare

The therapy program is similar to that described previously for arthroscopic release, except that motion is passive until soft-tissue repairs are healed, typically 4 weeks. Water therapy is very helpful and usually begins in the first week after surgery because the zero gravity environment of a pool allows for range of motion without stressing soft-tissue repairs.

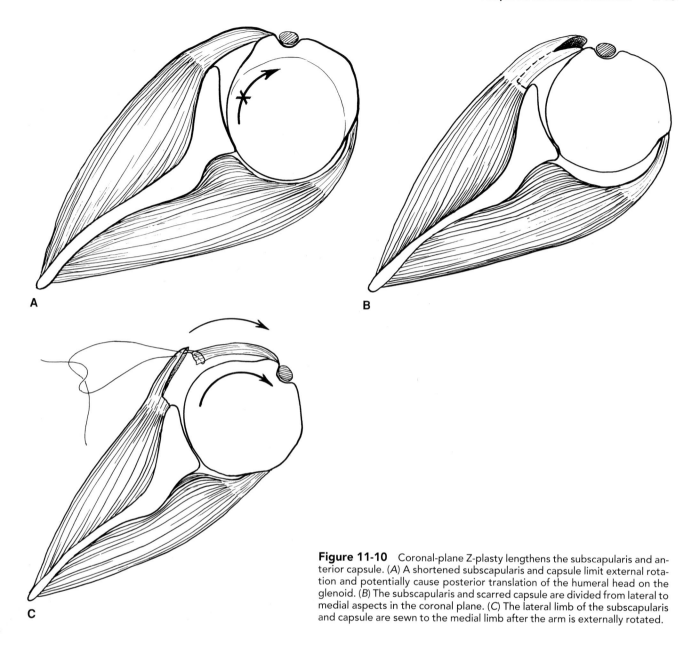

Figure 11-10 Coronal-plane Z-plasty lengthens the subscapularis and anterior capsule. (*A*) A shortened subscapularis and capsule limit external rotation and potentially cause posterior translation of the humeral head on the glenoid. (*B*) The subscapularis and scarred capsule are divided from lateral to medial aspects in the coronal plane. (*C*) The lateral limb of the subscapularis and capsule are sewn to the medial limb after the arm is externally rotated.

CLINICAL EXPERIENCE

Closed manipulation can be an effective treatment alternative for cases of idiopathic adhesive capsulitis,[66] but its success in treating postsurgical and posttraumatic stiffness is limited by the extent and location of adhesions. The clinician must decide on the likelihood of extra-articular scarring, in addition to capsular contracture, and then tailor the surgical treatment to address these factors. In relatively acute cases of motion loss after surgery or trauma for which therapy has failed to regain motion, closed manipulation may be attempted; however, this is usually unsuccessful, and some form of surgical release is required.[34,52,55,70,96] Although closed manipulation may be attempted, it is im-

portant to inform the patient that an arthroscopic or open release may be necessary.

Since the introduction of arthroscopic capsular release in the early 1990s as an alternative method for treating refractory stiff shoulder, it has become an accepted method of treatment for adhesive capsulitis, with definite advantages over open approaches.[31,89] This technique represents a specific treatment for patients with intrinsic capsular contracture refractory to nonoperative measures.[31,37,70,89,91] It allows a global approach to the capsular scar tissue release and even some adhesion release between tissue planes. Results of Warner[89] and Harryman[30,31] have demonstrated that, in the case of refractory adhesive capsulitis due to trauma or of idiopathic cause, the expected outcome is bet-

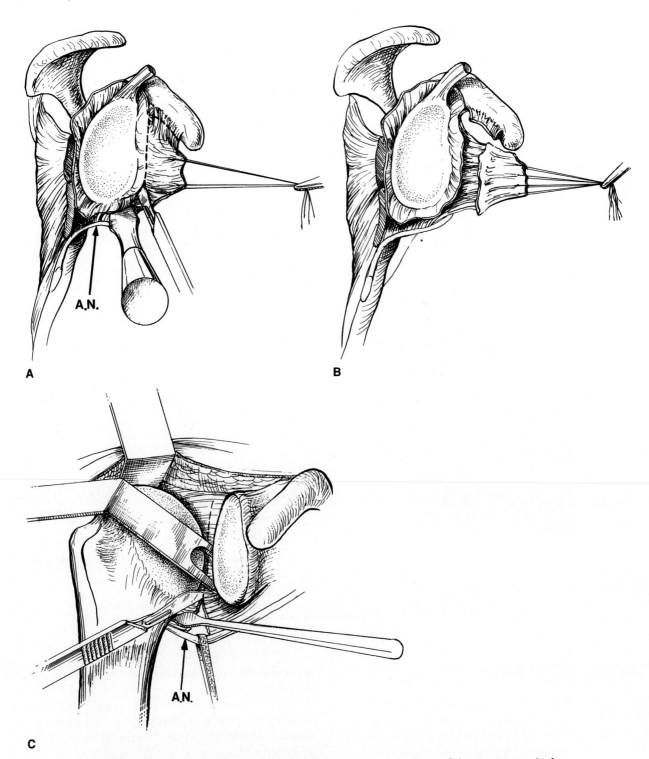

Figure 11-11 Mobilization of a subscapularis contracture and release of the posterior and inferior capsule. (*A*) The axillary nerve (AN) is protected with a retractor while the inferior and anterior parts of the capsule are divided (*dashed line*). The coracohumeral ligament (*shorter dashed line*) is also divided. (*B*) The subscapularis is mobilized medially after its global release. (*C*) A vessel loop has been placed around the AN, and a retractor protects it as the inferior and posterior capsule is divided. *(continued)*

ter than 90% good to excellent. Pain relief is very likely, and motion improves to normal ranges. All of the patients in their study had refractory motion loss, despite ongoing

physical therapy over many months, and they were at an end point of their tolerance for the functional limitations and pain. Clearly, a small percentage of individuals with shoulder stiffness in this setting will require operative management to regain motion, and the morbidity of this approach is small.

In the setting of severe trauma or postsurgical stiffness, the results are less predictable.[23,24, 37,90,91] In such cases, there may be concomitant injury to the joint or more extensive soft-tissue damage, which may limit motion recovery. As a general rule, patients should be made aware of this; however, it is still a reasonable option in this setting for treating motion loss refractory cases.

There is also probably a role for arthroscopic release in conjunction with management of arthritis and the stiff shoulder in young patients. This condition is considered in detail in another chapter in this text.

In patients who have a known extra-articular contracture, or who fail to have improvement of motion with an arthroscopic release, a formal open release is appropriate, and the results are probably mostly determined by the

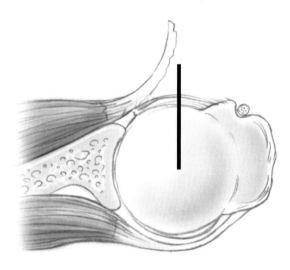

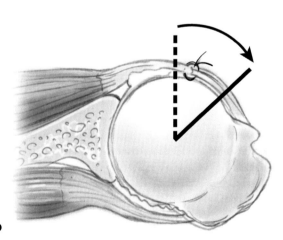

Figure 11-11 *(continued)* *(D)* "Z-plasty" lengthening of anterior soft tissue requires separation of a superficial layer dissected from the humeral insertion of the subscapularis to the glenoid rim. The deep layer is then developed by detaching it along the glenoid rim. The shoulder is then externally rotated and the two layers are sewn end to end.

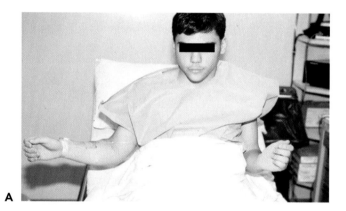

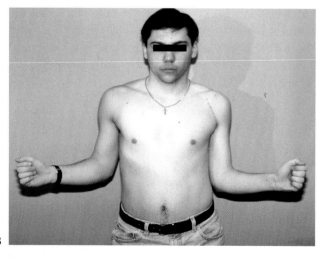

Figure 11-12 *(A)* A 20-year-old man with severe loss of external rotation after a Putti-Platt procedure. *(B,C)* Four months after open Z-plasty lengthening procedure of subscapularis and capsule. *(continued)*

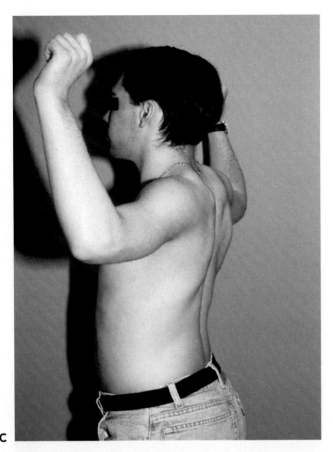

C

Figure 11-12 (continued)

quality of the articular surfaces and the surrounding soft-tissue envelope.[34,44,52,55]

CONCLUSIONS

Postoperative pain management and physical therapy are critical components for a good outcome, and we have found interscalene regional analgesia, as well as water therapy, to be very effective adjuncts to maintaining and improving motion after release of the stiff shoulder.[12,16,45,47,48]

REFERENCES

1. Allain J, Goutallier D, Glorion C. Long-term results of the Latarjet procedure for the treatment of anterior instability of the shoulder. J Bone Joint Surg Am 1998;80:841.
2. Barry H, Fernandes I, Bloom B, et al. Clinical study comparing acupuncture, physiotherapy, injection and oral anti-inflammatory therapy in shoulder cuff lesions. Curr Med Res Opin 1980;7:121.
3. Ben-Yishay A, Zuckerman JD, Gallagher M, et al. Pain inhibition of shoulder strength in patients with impingement syndrome. Orthopedics 1994;17:685.
4. Bigliani LU, Kelkar R, Flatow EL, et al. Glenohumeral stability: biomechanical properties of passive and active stabilizers. Clin Orthop 1996;330:13.
5. Bigliani LU, Morrison DS, April AW. The morphology of the acromion and its relation to the rotator cuff tear. Orthop Trans 1986;10:228.
6. Binder A, Bulgen DY, Hazleman BL. Frozen shoulder: a long-term prospective study. Ann Rheum Dis 1984;43:361.
7. Boileau P, Trojani C, Walch G, et al. Shoulder arthroplasty for the treatment of the sequelae of fractures of the proximal humerus. J Shoulder Elbow Surg 2001;10:299.
8. Boone DC, Azen SP. Normal range of motion of joints in male subjects. JBJS 1979;61A:756.
9. Bowman CA, Jeffcoate WJ, Patrick M, et al. Bilateral adhesive capsulitis, oligoarthritis and proximal myopathy as presentation of hypothyroidism. Br J Rheum 1988;27:62.
10. Bradley JP. Arthroscopic treatment for frozen capsulitis. Op Tech Orthop 1991;1:248.
11. Bridgeman JF. Periarthritis of the shoulder and diabetes mellitus. Ann Rheum Dis 1972;31:69.
12. Brown AR, Weiss R, Greenberg C, et al. Interscalene block for shoulder arthroscopy: comparison with general anesthesia. Arthroscopy 1993;9:295.
13. Bulgen DY, Binder A, Hazelman BL, et al. Immunological studies in frozen shoulder. J Rheum 1982;9:893.
14. Bulgen DY, Binder AL, Hazelman BL, et al. Frozen shoulder: prospective clinical study with an evaluation of three treatment regimens. Ann Rheum Dis 1984;43:353.
15. Clarke GR, Willis LA, Fish WW, et al. Preliminary studies in measuring range of motion in normal and painful stiff shoulder. Rheumatol Rehabil 1975;14:39.
16. Cohen NP, Levine WN, Marra G, et al. Indwelling interscalene catheter anesthesia in the surgical management of stiff shoulder: a report of 100 consecutive cases. J Shoulder Elbow Surg 2000;9(4):268.
17. Cole BJ, L'Insalata J, Irrgang J, et al. Comparison of arthroscopic and open anterior shoulder stabilization: a two- to six-year follow-up study. J Bone Joint Surg Am 2000;82:1108.
18. Constant CR, Murley AHG. A clinical method of functional assessment of the shoulder. Clin Orthop 1987;214:160.
19. DePalma AF. Loss of scapulohumeral motion (frozen shoulder). Ann Surg 1952;135:193.
20. Gazielly DF, Gleyze P, Montagnon C. Functional and anatomical results after rotator cuff repair. Clin Orthop 1994;304:43.
21. Gazielly DF, Gleyze P, Montagnon C, et al. Functional and anatomical results after surgical treatment of ruptures of the rotator cuff: part I. Preoperative functional and anatomical evaluation of ruptures of the rotator cuff. Rev Chir Orthop Reparatrice Appar Mot 1995;81:8.
22. Gerber A, Warner JJP. Thermal capsulorrhaphy to treat shoulder instability. Clin Orthop 2002;400:105.
23. Gerber A, Warner JJP. Stiff shoulder: post-traumatic stiffness and post-surgical stiffness. In: McGinty JB, Burkhart SS, Jackson RW, et al., eds. Operative arthroscopy. Philadelphia: Lippincott Williams & Wilkins, 2003:558.
24. Gerber C, Espinosa N, Perren TG. Arthroscopic treatment of shoulder stiffness. Clin Orthop 2001;390:119.
25. Gerber C, Terrier F, Ganz R. The Trillat procedure for recurrent anterior instability of the shoulder. J Bone Joint Surg Br 1988;70:130.
26. Gerber C, Werner CM, Macy JC, et al. Effect of selective capsulorrhaphy on motion of the glenohumeral joint. J Bone Joint Surg 2003;85(1):48.
27. Goldberg BA, Scarlat MM, Harryman DT. Management of the stiff shoulder. J Orthop Sci 1999;4:462.
28. Griggs SM, Ahn A, Green A. Idiopathic adhesive capsulitis: a prospective functional outcome study of nonoperative treatment. J Bone Joint Surg 2000;82:1398.
29. Haines JF, Hargadon EJ. Manipulation as the primary treatment of frozen shoulder. J R Coll Surg Edinb 1982;27:5.
30. Harryman DT III. Shoulder: frozen and stiff. Instr Course Lect 1985;42:199.
31. Harryman DT, Matsen FA, Sidles JA. Arthroscopic management of refractory shoulder stiffness. Arthroscopy 1997;13:133.
32. Harryman DT III, Sidles JA, Clark JM, et al. Translation of the humeral head on the glenoid with passive glenohumeral motion. J Bone Joint Surg 1990;72A:1334.

33. Harryman DTIII, Sidles JA, Harris SL, et al. The role of the rotator interval capsule in passive motion and stability of the shoulder. J Bone Joint Surg 1992;4A:53.
34. Hawkins RJ, Angelo RL. Glenohumeral osteoarthritis: a late complication of the Putti-Platt repair. J Bone Joint Surg 1990;72A:1193.
35. Hazelman BD. The painful stiff shoulder. Rheumatol Phys Med 1972;11:413.
36. Helbig B, Wagner P, Dohler R. Mobilization of frozen shoulder under general anesthesia. Acta Orthop Belg 1983;49:267.
37. Holloway GB, Schenk T, Williams GR, et al. Arthroscopic capsular release for the treatment of refractory postoperative or post-fracture shoulder stiffness. J Bone Joint Surg 2001;83:1682.
38. Holovacs TF, O'Holleran J, Warner JJP. Arthroscopic capsular release for refractory shoulder stiffness. In: Craig EV, ed. Master techniques in orthopaedic surgery, shoulder. Philadelphia, Lippincott Williams & Wilkins, 2003:171.
39. Hsu SYC, Chan KM. Arthroscopic distension in the management of frozen shoulder. Int Orthop 1991;15:79.
40. Itoi E, Tabata S. Range of motion and arthrography in frozen shoulder. J Shoulder Elbow Surg 1992;1:106.
41. Jaberg H, Warner JJP, Jakob RP. Percutaneous stabilization of unstable fractures of the humerus. J Bone Joint Surg 1992;74:508.
42. Janda DH, Hawkins RJ. Shoulder manipulation in patients with adhesive capsulitis and diabetes mellitus: a clinical note. J Shoulder Elbow Surg 1993;2:36.
43. Jost B, Koch P, Gerber C. Anatomy and functional aspects of the rotator interval. J Shoulder Elbow Surg 2000;9:336.
44. Kieras DM, Matsen FA III. Open release in the management of refractory frozen shoulder. Orthop Trans 1991;15:801.
45. Kinnard P, Truchon R, St-Pierre A, et al. Interscalene block for pain relief after shoulder surgery. Clin Orthop 1994;304:22.
46. Leffert RD. The frozen shoulder. Instr Course Lect 1985;34:199.
47. Liotard JPL, Edwards TB, Padey A, et al. Hydrotherapy rehabilitation after shoulder surgery. Tech Shoulder Elbow Surg 2003;4(2):44.
48. Liotard JP, Walch G. Nonsurgical management of shoulder stiffness. In: Warner JJP, Ianonotti JP, Gerber C, eds. Complex and revision problems in shoulder surgery. Philadelphia, Lippincott-Raven, 1997:149.
49. Lloyd-Roberts GG, French PR. Periarthritis of the shoulder: a study of the disease and its treatment. Br Med J 1959;1:1569.
50. Lundberg BJ. Glycosaminoglycans of the normal and frozen shoulder joint capsule. Clin Orthop 1970;69:279.
51. Lundberg J. The frozen shoulder: clinical and radiographical observation. The effect of manipulation under general anesthesia: structure and glycosaminoglycan content of the joint capsule. Acta Orthop Scand Suppl 1969;119:1.
52. Lusardi DA, Wirth MA, Wurtz D, et al. Loss of external rotation following anterior capsulorrhaphy of the shoulder. J Bone Joint Surg 1993;75A:1185.
53. Matsen FA, Thomas SC, Rockwood CA. Glenohumeral instability. In: Rockwood CA, Matsen FA, eds. The shoulder. Philadelphia, WB Saunders, 1998:689.
54. Mole D, Kempf JF, Gleyze P, et al. Results of endoscopic treatment of non-broken tendinopathies of the rotator cuff: part II. Calcifications of the rotator cuff. Rev Chir Orthop Reparatrice Appar Mot 1993;79:532.
55. MacDonald PB, Hawkins RJ, Fowler PJ, et al. Release of the subscapularis for internal rotation contracture and pain following anterior repair for recurrent anterior dislocation of the shoulder. J Bone Joint Surg 1992;74A:734.
56. McLaughlin HL. On the frozen shoulder. Clin Orthop 1961;20:126.
57. McLaughlin HL. On the frozen shoulder. Bull Hosp Joint Dis 1951;12:383.
58. Miniaci A, McBirnie J. Thermal capsular shrinkage for treatment of multidirectional instability of the shoulder. J Bone Joint Surg 2003;85(12):2284.
59. Murnagham JP. Frozen shoulder. In: Rockwood CA Jr, Matsen FA III, eds. The shoulder. Philadelphia, WB Saunders, 1990:422.
60. Murnagham JP. Primary adhesive capsulitis of the shoulder. Orthop Trans 1983;7:137.
61. Neer CS II. Frozen shoulder. In: Neer CS II, ed. Shoulder reconstruction. Philadelphia, WB Saunders, 1990:422.
62. Neer CS, Satterlee CC, Dalsey R, et al. The anatomy and potential effects of contracture of the coracohumeral ligament. Clin Orthop 992;28:182.
63. Neviaser JS. Adhesive capsulitis of the shoulder: study of pathological findings in periarthritis of the shoulder. J Bone Joint Surg 1945;27:211.
64. Neviaser JS. Arthrography of the shoulder joint. J Bone Joint Surg 1942;44:1321.
65. Neviaser RJ. Painful conditions affecting the shoulder. Clin Orthop 1983;173:63.
66. Neviaser RJ, Neviaser TJ. The frozen shoulder: diagnosis and management. Clin Orthop 1987;223:59.
67. Niskanen RO, Lehtinen JY, Kaukonen JP. Alvik's glenoplasty for humeroscapular dislocation: 6-year follow-up of 52 shoulders. Acta Orthop Scand 1991;62:279.
68. Ozaki J, Kakagawa Y, Sakurai G, et al. Recalcitrant chronic adhesive capsulitis of the shoulder: role of contracture of the coracohumeral ligament and rotator interval in pathogenesis and treatment. J Bone Joint Surg 1989;71A:1511.
69. Pal B, Anderson J, Dick WC, et al. Limitation of joint mobility and shoulder capsulitis in insulin and non-insulin dependent diabetes mellitus. Br J Rheumatol 1986;25:147.
70. Pollock RG, Duralde XA, Flatow EL, et al. The use of the arthroscopy in treatment of resistant frozen shoulder. Clin Orthop 1994;304:30.
71. Quigley TB. Indication for manipulation and corticosteroids in the treatment of stiff shoulder. Surg Clin North Am 1975;43:1715.
72. Reeves B. The natural history of the frozen shoulder syndrome. Scand J Rheumatol 1975;4:193.
73. Reeves B. Arthrographic changes in frozen and post-traumatic stiff shoulder. Proc R Soc Med 1966;59:827.
74. Rhind B, Downie WW, Bird HA, et al. Naproxen and indomethacin in periarthritis of the shoulder. Rheumatol Rehabil 1982;21:51.
75. Rinaldi N, Barth T, Leppelmann-Jansen P, et al. Normal synoviocytes and synoviocytes from osteoarthritis and rheumatoid arthritis bind extracellular matrix proteins differently. Immun Infekt 1995;23:62.
76. Rizk TE, Christopher RP, Pinals RS, et al. Adhesive capsulitis (frozen shoulder): a new approach to its management and treatment. Arch Phys Med Rehabil 1983;64:29.
77. Shaffer B, Tibone JE, Kerlan RK. Frozen shoulder: a long-term follow-up study. J Bone Joint Surg 1992;74A:738.
78. Speer KP, Cavanaugh JT, Warren RF, et al. A role for hydrotherapy in shoulder rehabilitation. Am J Sports Med 1993;21:850.
79. Steinbrocker O, Argyros TG. Frozen shoulder: a long-term follow-up study. J Bone Joint Surg 1992;74A:738.
80. Stodell MA, Sturrock RD. Frozen shoulder. Lancet 1981;2:257.
81. Thomas D, Williams RA, Smith DS. The frozen shoulder: a review of manipulative treatment. Rheumatol Rehabil 1980;19:173.
82. Ticker J, Beim G, Warner J. Recognition and treatment of refractory posterior capsular contracture of the shoulder. Arthroscopy 2000;16:27.
83. Ticker JB, Warner JJP. Selective capsular shift technique for anterior and anterior-inferior glenohumeral instability. Clin Sports Med 2000;19:1.
84. Waldburger M, Meier JL, Gobelet C. The frozen shoulder: diagnosis and treatment. Prospective study of 50 cases of adhesive capsulitis. Clin Rheumatol 1992;11:364.
85. Warner J, Deng X, Warren R, et al. Static capsuloligamentous restraints to superior-inferior translation of the glenohumeral joint. Am J Sports Med 1992;20:675.
86. Warner J, Johnson D, Miller M, et al. Technique for selecting capsular tightness in repair of anterior-inferior shoulder instability. J Shoulder Elbow Surg 1995;4:352.
87. Warner JJP. Frozen shoulder: diagnosis and management. J Am Acad Orthop Surg 1997;5:130.
88. Warner JJP. Shoulder arthroscopy in the beach-chair position: basic set-up. Op Tech Orthop 1991;2:147.
89. Warner JJP, Allen AA, Marks PH, et al. Arthroscopic release for chronic refractory adhesive capsulitis of the shoulder. J Bone Joint Surg 1996;78:1808.

90. Warner JJP, Allen AA, Marks PH, et al. Arthroscopic release of post-operative capsular contracture of the shoulder. J Bone Joint Surg 1997;79:1151.

91. Warner JJP, Greis PE. The treatment of stiffness of the shoulder after repair of the rotator cuff. Instr Course Lect 1998;47:67.

92. Warner JJP, Higgins L, Parsons M, et al. Diagnosis and treatment of anterosuperior rotator cuff tears. J Shoulder Elbow Surg 2001;10:37.

93. Waters PM, Smith GR, Jaramillo D. Glenohumeral deformity secondary to brachial plexus birth palsy. J Bone Joint Surg 1998; 80:668.

94. Wiley AM. Arthroscopic appearance of frozen shoulder. Arthroscopy 1991;7:138.

95. Wohlgethan JR. Frozen shoulder in hyperthyroidism. Arthritis Rheum 1987;30:936.

96. Young DC, Rockwood CA Jr. Complications of a failed Bristow procedure and their management. J Bone Joint Surg 1991; 73:969.

97. Zuckerman JD, Cuomo F. Frozen shoulder. In: Matsen FA, Fu FH, Hawkins RJ, eds. The shoulder: a balance of mobility and stability. Rosemont, IL, American Academy of Orthopaedic Surgeon Publications, 1992:253.

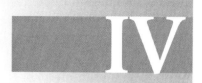
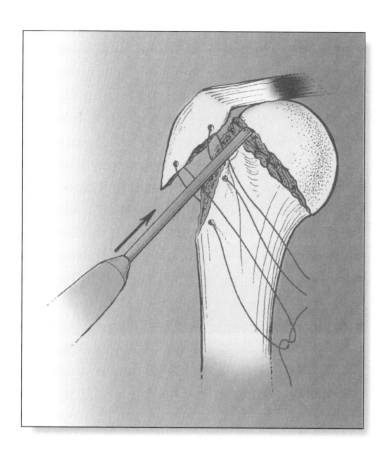

Two-Part Proximal Humerus Fractures

12

Julie Y. Bishop   Evan L. Flatow

PATHOLOGY

Risk Factors

Most fractures of the proximal occur in older, often female patients, with osteoporotic bone.[38] Their cortical bone is thin, osteoporotic, and brittle, and the cancellous bone is very porous. This particular population is at high risk for poor postoperative compliance because many have poor coordination, often live alone without help, and may have limited understanding of the importance of careful protection followed by rehabilitation. Proximal humerus fractures also occur in the high-energy trauma group. Although this may result in such fractures at any age, young patients typically experience these fractures[38] because their cortical and cancellous bones are of excellent quality. They are often better able to comprehend and comply with the post-fracture rehabilitation protocol.

There are additional factors to consider when choosing a treatment plan and predicting outcomes in two-part proximal humerus fractures. Concomitant injuries, such as associated dislocations, nerve injuries, or rotator cuff tears, must all be considered when formulating a treatment plan. The young patient with a high-energy proximal humerus fracture and associated polytrauma will often require a different treatment plan than the treatment plan associated with an isolated fracture. Patient factors, such as alcoholism, ability to comply with postoperative care, and systemic injuries (e.g., brain injury, metabolic bone disease, parkinson, renal osteodystrophy, or any other forms of osteopenia)[26] may affect outcomes and should influence the treatment choice. Functional demands, activities of daily living, patient expectations, and patient mental status must all be determined prior to treatment. Failure to properly assess these patient risk factors could certainly lead to poor results and, at times, devastating outcomes.

Mechanism of Injury

The most common mechanism of injury for proximal humerus fractures is a fall onto an outstretched hand from a standing height.[49,50,57] In most cases, severe trauma does not play a significant role. Instead, trauma need only be minor to moderate because of the osteoporosis that may be present. In younger patients, high-energy trauma, such as a motor vehicle accident, is the more typical injury. Strong muscular contraction has also been proposed as a mechanism, especially for the greater tuberosity fractures,[27] but this is usually seen with electric shock or seizure.[47,89]

Although, in theory, a direct blow to the upper arm could shatter the proximal humerus, most fractures are believed to result from indirect violence.[16,28] However, it is surprising that little is known about how this actually occurs. Howard and Eloesser[39] constructed an elaborate cadaver model to investigate these mechanisms. Contact with the acromion and glenoid rim, as well as traction from the rotator cuff, has been thought to initiate the fracture planes.[16,28] The lower incidence of isolated greater tuberosity fractures in older patients, then, may represent a result of age-related weakening of the cuff tendons, resulting in a diminution of their contribution to an avulsion force.[38]

J. Y. Bishop: Department of Orthopaedic Surgery, Mount Sinai School of Medicine, New York, New York.
E. L. Flatow: Department of Orthopaedic Surgery, Mount Sinai School of Medicine, New York, New York.

Once the fragments separate, muscle forces contribute to their displacement (Fig. 12-1A). The shaft is generally drawn anteriorly and medially by the pectoralis major.[23] The greater tuberosity may be pulled posteriorly by the infraspinatus and superiorly by the supraspinatus.[22,74] At other times, however, an intact rotator interval between the supraspinatus and subscapularis may limit greater tuberosity displacement. The subscapularis tends to retract medially as an isolated lesser tuberosity fragment or to rotate internally as a head segment, to which only the lesser tuberosity remains attached.[74]

Concomitant Injuries

Proximal humerus fractures may be isolated or may be a part of a multitrauma.[86] All patients must be examined for any evidence of other fractures and injuries, especially the neck or the chest wall. In the polytrauma patient, a dramatic shoulder injury can obscure other findings. The entire upper extremity should be palpated, in particular, to rule out any concomitant wrist fractures. Rib fractures have also been reported in association with proximal humerus fractures.[33] If the patient has amnesia, bilateral injuries, or a posterior fracture-dislocation, the physician must rule out a seizure disorder or electric shock.

A detailed neurovascular exam of the upper extremity is essential in all fractures of the proximal humerus (Fig. 12-1B). Axillary artery and brachial plexus injuries have been reported,[33,35,58,96,106] with increasing frequency in fracture dislocations.[83] The axillary artery and its lateral branches, the anterior humeral circumflex arteries, and the posterior humeral circumflex arteries are the relevant vessels when determining proximal humerus fractures. Arterial injuries that accompany proximal humerus fractures often involve the axillary artery near the origin of the circumflex arteries for several reasons: (a) this region is close to the surgical neck, whose sharp spikes are often drawn toward the artery by the pull of the pectoralis major; (b) the two circumflex origins and the lateral continuation of the axillary artery represent a "tethered trifurcation" that is unable to fall away from bone edges easily; and (c) glenohumeral dislocation dumps the head segment into this area and stretches the axillary artery across it. The finding of asymmetric radial pulses may be a subtle clue to axillary artery injuries. If vascular injury is suspected, an angiogram is indicated,.

Isolated axillary nerve injuries and mixed brachial plexus injuries are the most common neurologic injuries found after proximal humerus fractures.[7,106] Although nerve lesions occur at a higher frequency with four-part proximal humeral fractures,[7,75] a meticulous neurologic

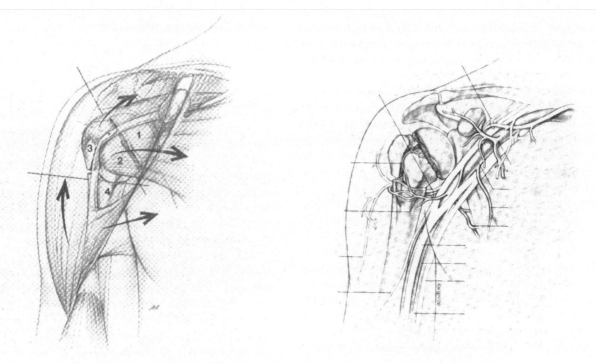

A

B

Figure 12-1 (*A*) Displacement of fracture fragments results from the pull of muscles attaching to the various bony components. The subscapularis inserts on the lesser tuberosity and can cause medial displacement, whereas the supraspinatus and infraspinatus insert on the greater tuberosity can cause superior and posterior displacement. The pectoralis major inserts on the humeral shaft and displaces it medially. (*B*) The brachial plexus and axillary artery lie adjacent to the coracoid process and can be injured with fracture of the proximal humerus.

exam should always be performed. Neurologic injuries associated with closed reduction methods are difficult to distinguish from those injuries that occur at the time of fracture or surgery due to the acutely injured, swollen, and painful shoulder. Thus, again, emphasizing the importance of the initial examination. Sensation should be tested over the deltoid muscle in the axillary nerve distribution, although this may be an unreliable finding. Testing for deltoid activity may be painful; however, the ability of the patient to actively set the deltoid muscle in an isometric contraction should be assessed. In addition to axillary nerve function, the motor function and sensory distribution of the musculocutaneous nerve, as well as other peripheral nerves, should be specifically examined.

Closed injury to the brachial plexus or peripheral nerves requires documentation and may be treated expectantly. Electromyography is usually reserved for late evaluation of lingering neurologic deficits. Neurologic injury should not delay the definitive management of the fracture because most nerve injuries are neuropraxias and will resolve sufficiently to allow adequate function.[5] Complete lesions that do not resolve can be evaluated and treated appropriately between 3 and 6 months after the injury.

IMAGING

Classification

Classifying proximal humerus fractures has evolved in the recent past; however, controversies still exist in the choice of the best classification system and, most importantly, the implications for treatment that they may have. The Neer classification system, proposed in 1970,[73] is still widely used by most orthopedic surgeons for the diagnosis and treatment of proximal humerus fractures. This classification was based on Codman's contribution, that fractures occur along the anatomic lines of epiphyseal union, and on 26 years of clinical experience treating proximal humerus fractures. This system emphasizes the degree of displacement rather than the pattern of fracture lines. It is easy because it requires a knowledge of anatomy, not the memorization of a complex classification scheme. Fractures are classified by displacement of any of the four principal fragments. If no segment is displaced more than 1 cm or rotated more than 45 degrees, the fracture is considered a one-part fracture, regardless of the number or location of fracture lines. A two-part fracture has a single displaced segment. The most common two-part fractures are surgical neck (the shaft is separated from the head and both attached tuberosities) and greater tuberosity fractures (Fig. 12-2). Lesser tuberosity two-part fractures are rare, while anatomic neck fractures are almost never seen in isolation. Neer also categorized two-part fracture-dislocations with either anterior or posterior dislocation of the articular segment.

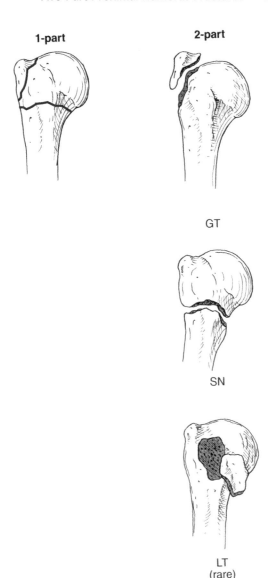

Figure 12-2 Simplified Neer classification of 1- and 2-part fractures. A segment is considered displaced in the presence of more than 1-cm displacement or greater than 45 degrees of angulation. GT, greater tuberosity; SN, surgical neck; LT, lesser tuberosity.

Accurate Radiographs

Accurate, careful radiographs are essential to plan treatment and to determine the prognosis of a two-part proximal humerus fracture. All too often, a surgeon receives inadequate oblique views from the emergency department and orders a computed tomography (CT) scan, as if this will substitute for carefully repeating and obtaining high-quality, plain radiographs. As inconvenient as it is, personally positioning the patient is usually the best way to obtain the proper information.

Clear delineation of the fracture pattern is best accomplished with the radiographic trauma series. This consists of an anteroposterior (AP) view of the scapula, a lateral "Y-view" of the scapula, and an axillary view (Fig. 12-3). The lateral "Y-view" can be useful in evaluating the facets of the greater tuberosity, which has three facets into which the tendons of the supraspinatus, the infraspinatus, and the teres minor insert. Recognizing these facets on radiographs can be helpful in determining the extent of involvement of the greater tuberosity in a fracture. The axillary view is useful for correctly identifying a fracture-dislocation and for evaluating the articular surfaces of the glenoid and humerus. This view is often omitted even though its importance has been stressed by several authors over the years.[5,8,18,73,94] The arm can be held in gentle abduction of about 30 degrees by a knowledgeable person so that further displacement of the fracture does not occur. However, the senior author's preference is the velpeau axillary view, in which the arm stays in the sling, the patient leans back, and the beam is aimed down the shoulder, as the plate is placed below the shoulder. This view has the advantage of not shifting the fracture pattern because a portion of the motion required for abduction of the shoulder in the routine axillary view may occur through the fracture site.[20] In this fashion, three orthogonal views may be taken without removing the arm from the sling.

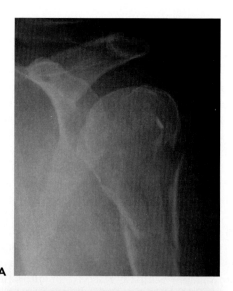

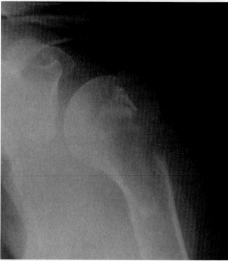

Figure 12-4 (*A*) Anteroposterior view of the shoulder with the arm in internal rotation. Assessment of the degree of displacement of the greater tuberosity is difficult. (*B*) The arm has been externally rotated 20 degrees, and a true anteroposterior view of the scapula is taken, with subsequent better visualization of greater tuberosity displacement. (Reprinted with permission from Flatow EL. Fractures of the proximal humerus. In: Bucholz RW, Heckman JD, eds. Rockwood and Green's fractures in adults, 5th ed. Philadelphia, Lippincott Williams & Wilkins, 2001:997.)

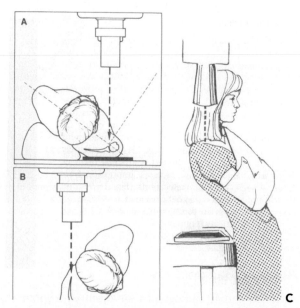

Figure 12-3 Trauma series. The trauma series consists of anteroposterior and lateral x-rays in the scapular plane as well as an axillary view. These views may be done with the patient sitting, standing, or prone. (*A*) For the anteroposterior x-ray in the scapular plane, the posterior aspect of the affected shoulder is placed against the x-ray plate, and the opposite shoulder is tilted forward approximately 40 degrees. (*B*) For the lateral (or Y-view of the scapula), the anterior aspect of the affected shoulder is placed against the x-ray plate, and the other shoulder is tilted forward approximately 40 degrees. The x-ray tube is placed posteriorly along the scapular spine. (*C*) The velpeau axillary view is preferred after trauma when the patient can be positioned for this view, because it allows the shoulder to remain immobilized and avoids further displacement of the fracture fragments.

If the fracture is several weeks old and is relatively stable, the surgeon may choose to take the AP view of the scapula in slight external rotation: this gives a clear view of the greater tuberosity (Fig. 12-4). It is easily accomplished by loosening the sling, gently rotating the arm to about 20 degrees of external rotation while checking for bone crepitus, and letting the patient hold onto an intravenous pole or table edge (Fig. 12-5). Recently, the senior author's work on the reliability and reproducibility of evaluating radiographs of the greater tuberosity was presented.[81] It was found that the anteroposterior (AP) ER view as well as the AP 15-degree caudad projections best profiled the greater

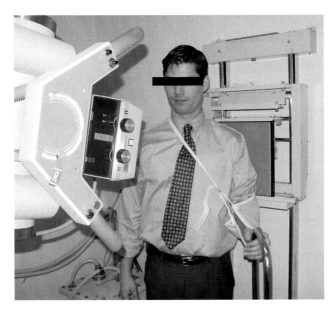

Figure 12-5   Positon for anteroposterior view of the scapula in external rotation, which gives a clear view of the greater tuberosity. The sling is loosened, the arm is gently rotated to 20 degrees of external rotation, letting the patient hold onto an intravenous pole or table edge while the radiograph is taken. This view should not be used, if there is a substantial risk of fracture displacement from this small amount of rotation.

tuberosity and were more accurate in their assessment of overall fracture displacement (average error of 5.1 mm). They were also the most accurate views at the level of displacement (5–10 mm), where surgery may be indicated (average error, 1.8 and 2.2 mm). Overall, multiplane radiographic imaging, which includes these views as well as the normal trauma series, will improve the diagnostic imaging accuracy and aid in determining the appropriate treatment.

Computed Tomography Scans

Although accurate radiographs allow the experienced surgeon to consistently identify displaced segments, CT is occasionally helpful to assess tuberosity displacement and articular surface involvement.[94] The head may be split or have a significant impression defect, both of which may be well visualized on CT. Morris et al.[70] have reported on a series of patients in which CT was helpful in judging the amount of displacement of tuberosity fractures. Posterior and medial retraction of the greater tuberosity is best seen on a transverse cut of a CT scan (or, of course, the axillary radiograph). Usually, the tuberosity fragment overlapping the articular surface is present. Computed tomography imaging has also been advocated in evaluating more complex fractures, which will be discussed in subsequent chapters.[5,19,45,91,94] However, while CT has proven to be a useful adjunct, one must be aware that CT evaluation is certainly not meant to be a substitute for ideal radiographs.

Of note, CT scan evaluation of fracture patterns has been assessed in relation to interobserver and intraobserver reliability of the Neer classification system. The effect of CT on increasing reliability and reproducibility was assessed by Bernstein et al.[4] The mean kappa coefficient for intraobserver reliability was 0.64 with only radiographic evaluation and 0.72 (substantial) with radiographs and CT scans. The intraobserver reliability increased while the interobserver reproducibility did not change with the addition of CT scans.

Thus, overall, a CT scan should be ordered only when good radiographs fail to show the fracture pattern clearly. Computed tomography scans are most helpful in checking for dislocations, in ruling out glenoid fractures, and in assessing posterior retraction of the greater tuberosity.

Magnetic Resonance Imaging

Although magnetic resonance imaging (MRI) scans are not often needed in the evaluation of two-part proximal humerus fractures, some nondisplaced greater tuberosity fractures may be impossible to see on radiographs. Magnetic resonance imaging, thus, may be helpful because the fracture line can be well visualized.[105] These radiographically occult fractures often have associated marrow edema, which can be identified on the MRI (Fig. 12–6).[62,64] Occult fractures that

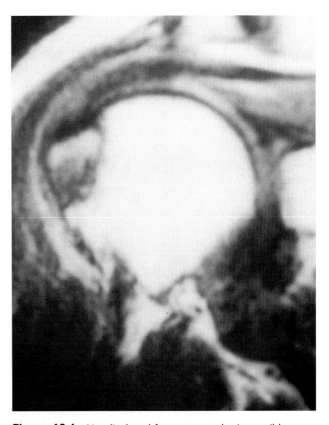

Figure 12-6   Nondisplaced fractures may be impossible to see on radiographs; magnetic resonance imaging has been helpful in these cases because the fracture line is well seen, as in this case.

are imaged acutely can have a linear or curvilinear signal that is seen within diffuse edema. Images taken within a later time frame may allow resolution of the fracture line with the persistence of edema.[64] These findings have then led some to conclude that MRI can prevent unnecessary arthroscopy in patients with a clinically suspected traumatic rotator cuff tear, which is actually a subtle greater tuberosity fracture that is not visable on plain radiographs.[84]

SURGICAL NECK FRACTURES

The principle involved in treating minimally displaced fractures is early protection combined with gradual mobilization. Although, in theory, more than 1 cm of displacement makes the surgical neck "displaced," in practice, in most elderly patients, surgeons accept almost any degree of displacement as long as there remains some solid bone contact. Angulation is well compensated for by shoulder motion or can be adjusted by small manipulations after a week or so, after the fracture becomes sticky. Elderly patients with reduced demands (i.e., more likely to accept a stiff shoulder), with poor health, and who are poor rehabilitation candidates are more likely to receive nonoperative treatment. In young patients, less than 50% shaft diameter displacement and less than 45-degree angulation in the dominant arm are acceptable indications for nonoperative treatment, although, in some individual cases, surgery may be considered for less displacement or angulation.

Most patients are placed in a sling for the first week to 10 days and are instructed to pull a shirt over it at night. Swathes rarely stay on and are uncomfortable. Hand, wrist, and elbow motion begins immediately. On the next visit, the physician holds the patient's elbow and flexed forearm in one hand and palpates the tuberosities and biceps groove with the other while the patient leans over. If the proximal and distal humerus "move as a unit," the patient is started on gentle pendulum range of motion. If, on the other hand, a slip or give is felt in association with some bone crepitus or catching, the patient is left immobilized for another week and is then reassessed. At 3 or 4 weeks, if radiographs are unchanged and the bone again feels solid, gentle assistive exercises (pulley elevation, external rotation with a stick, extension with a stick) are begun, along with formal physical therapy. At 6 weeks, there is rapid progression to terminal stretches and light resistive exercises.

Koval et al. followed 104 patients with minimally displaced proximal humerus fractures for at least 1 year after treatment in this fashion.[51] Ninety percent of these patients had no pain, and most patients achieved 90% of their contralateral shoulder motion. Motion was better when formal physical therapy had been started early.

There are only a few, rare indications for surgical treatment of a minimally displaced proximal humerus fracture: ipsilateral neurovascular injury requiring exploration, repair, or protection; an open fracture; or multiple trauma requiring mobilization as fast as possible.

Closed Reduction

If a two-part surgical neck fracture is displaced at initial presentation, closed reduction may often be attempted. This can usually be performed if there is an unimpacted fracture without bone contact. A hematoma block can often be helpful, or this maneuver can be performed in the operating room, with the option of operative intervention, if a stable reduction cannot be attained. It is imperative, when using the C-arm image intensifier in the operating room, to drape the patient so that the arm is entirely free to move. The image intensifier must be able to easily project a true anteroposterior and axillary view of the fracture site. The arm is then adducted and flexed 90 degrees, thus relaxing the pectoralis. A translation force (usually posteriorly and laterally, because the typical fracture is anteriorly angulated and is anteromedially displaced) is applied to reduce the deformity, while longitudinal traction is applied. After a reduction is felt, a gentle attempt to reimpact the bones is made. If the fracture is reducible and stable, treatment as outlined for minimal displacement is continued for 4 weeks rather than 7 to 10 days (Fig. 12-7). If the fracture is reducible but unstable, percutaneous pins should be considered. If a reduction cannot be achieved, open reduction and internal fixation are considered. Interpositioning the biceps tendon, capsule, or subscapularis may prevent closed reduction. Significant comminution at the surgical neck fracture site may preclude a stable closed reduction.

Closed Reduction and Percutaneous Pinning

Technique

Closed reduction and percutaneous pinning of unstable two-part proximal humerus fractures is a well-known technique for treating these kinds of fractures and, typically, should be reserved for patients with good bone quality and a fracture that can be reduced closed but is unstable and cannot maintain the reduction.[3,41] It does offer some theoretical advantages over open techniques because it limits soft-tissue trauma and any associated morbidity. It does not add an additional risk to the vascular supply of the humeral head articular segment; however, there is an inherent risk to the surrounding neurovascular structures during the pinning process.[87] Lateral pins should be distal enough to avoid injuring the anterior branch of the axillary nerve; however, the pin must be placed above the deltoid insertion to avoid injuring the radial nerve. Anterior pins may risk injuring the musculocutaneous nerve, cephalic vein, and the biceps tendon. Also, multiple images should be taken to avoid penetrating the humeral head cartilage. Finally, this technique demands a compliant patient who will agree to maintain the immobilization of his or her arm

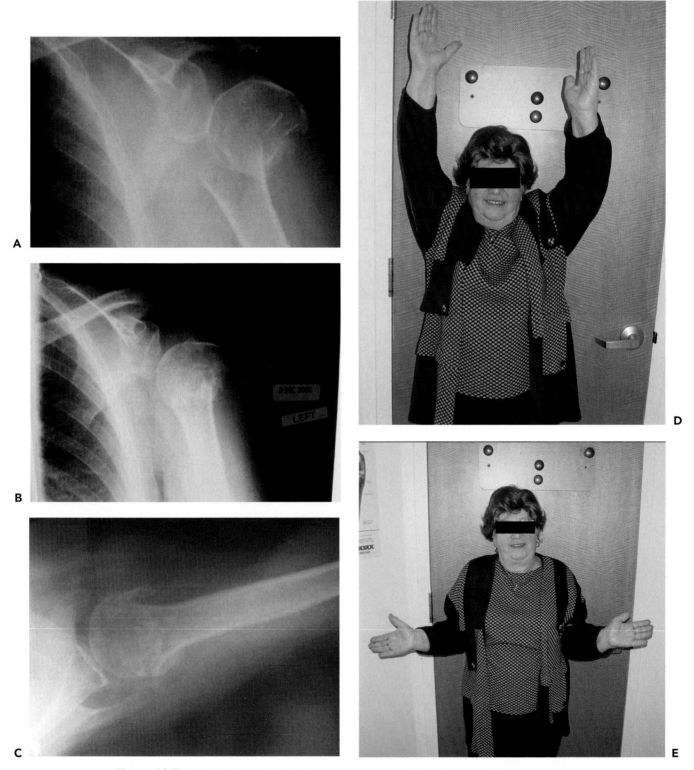

Figure 12-7 Displaced surgical neck fracture in a 76-year-old female. (*A*) Initial injury anteroposterior view. (*B,C*) Three months after closed reduction in the operating room. Fracture is healed on the anteroposterior and axillary views. (*D,E*) Patient has regained symmetrical motion in forward elevation and external rotation 3 months after closed reduction.

and who is available for close follow-up of the pin positions and skin condition.

For percutaneous pins insertion, the patient is placed on a radiolucent table, with the arm and shoulder off the side, as detailed previously. Again, the C-arm image intensifier must be carefully positioned so that anteroposterior and axillary views are easily obtained. Only then should the patient be sterilely prepped and draped. If obtaining the reduction is difficult, a 2.5-mm terminally threaded pin may be used as a "joystick" when inserted through the greater tuberosity into the humeral head. This "joystick" can then be used to reduce the head to the shaft. Once a good reduction is achieved, 2.5-mm terminally threaded Schantz pins are drilled up into the humeral head from down along the lateral metaphysis. These pins are first started at a more perpendicular angle, then, as they penetrate, the drill should drop to the correct angle. As they approach the head, these pins are advanced by hand without power, for a safer feel. The normal 20 degrees of retroversion of the humeral head should be considered when inserting the pins. Although two or three pins in this direction may be adequate, the construct will be stronger if two more pins are inserted downward from the greater tuberosity into the head and then exit the cortex on the opposite side of the shaft (Fig. 12-8). Significant pressure should not be exerted, because this may cause the pin to bend and slip. These pins are always used if there is a concomitant greater tuberosity fracture. Studies have been performed to examine the immediate stability of percutaneous pinning techniques and have found that the most stable construct consists of two pins inserted down from the greater tuberosity into the head and two pins inserted up from the shaft.[6,72]

Aftercare

The arm remains immobilized for 3 weeks. Movement is prevented until the pins are removed, particularly the pins placed through the greater tuberosity into the medial cortex of the shaft. The pins are closely watched for any signs of migration or superficial skin infection, so serial radiographs are taken. The pins are then removed with the aid of local anesthesia (the pins are cut beneath the skin) after approximately 3 weeks. During the first 3 weeks, only hand and elbow motion are allowed. Once the pins are removed, gentle pendulums are begun, as well as pulley elevation, and external rotation with a stick.

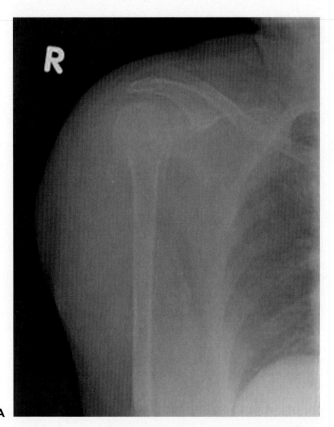

A

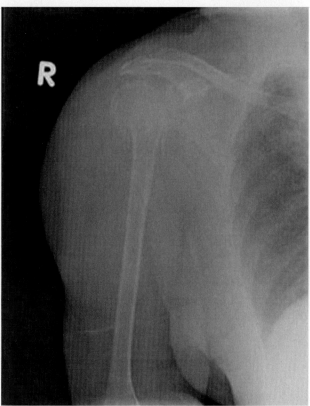

B

Figure 12-8   Displaced surgical neck fracture that was unstable after closed reduction in the operating room. (*A,B*) Initial injury films, anteroposterior and axillary views. *(continued)*

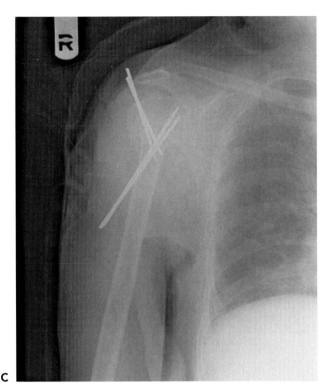

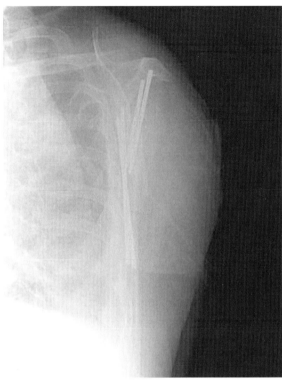

C

D

Figure 12-8 *(continued)* *(C,D)* Radiographs after closed reduction and percutaneous pin fixation of the surgical neck. (Courtesy of J. Gladstone.)

Open Reduction and Internal Fixation

Principles

Surgical neck fractures with poor bone quality, extensive comminution at the fracture site, and a poorly compliant patient make closed percutaneous pinning a suboptimal choice for fixation. In these situations, it is often best to proceed directly to open reduction and internal fixation (ORIF). Many devices have been proposed for fixation, including intramedullary nails or rods, plates and screws, wires or cables, nonabsorbable sutures, and various combinations of each. Many attempts have been made to identify the most stable construct for repairing proximal humerus fractures. Plates and screws have performed well in cadaver tests,[15] perhaps because the bone quality is better than in actual clinical cases. One study found that plates and intramedullary nails of roughly equal strength were both better than tension-band wiring.[88] If plates are used, screw placement is important: one study showed that screw fixation in the humeral head is strongest when placed centrally and engaging the subchondral plate.[55] More recently, locking plates have been available, and, although promising, no results are yet available (Fig. 12-9).

Open reduction with minimal soft tissue dissection should always be a closely adhered to principle. However, this approach is more important in the valgus-impacted three-or four-part fracture, where preservation of vascularity to the articular segment through retained soft-tissue at-tachments is of utmost importance.[37] Extensive surgical dissection, soft-tissue stripping, reduction, and stabilization can further devascularize the humeral head and add further to the risk of avascular necrosis. Although the vascularity of the humeral head is rarely compromised in surgical neck fractures, the operative goal should always include the need to minimize extensive dissection while attempting to reduce and stabilize the fracture.

Techniques of Fixation

If open reduction is undertaken, a deltopectoral approach is performed. After the superficial exposure, identify the coracoid and strap muscles because medial dissection to these structures may result in damage to the neurovascular structures. The long head of the biceps should be identified because this structure may be interposed in the fracture, preventing reduction. The fracture site should be carefully inspected for any other soft-tissue interposition, after which the stability of the reduction and the possible need for longitudinal fixation can be assessed. Internal fixation is accomplished with heavy, nonabsorbable (No. 5) sutures. The suture is passed around the cuff insertion to drill holes in the lateral shaft and around the subscapularis insertion to drill holes in the medial shaft. Sutures through the strong rotator cuff tendon insertion are usually more secure than other types of fixation in osteoporotic bone. Wires or cables may provide greater immediate stability but

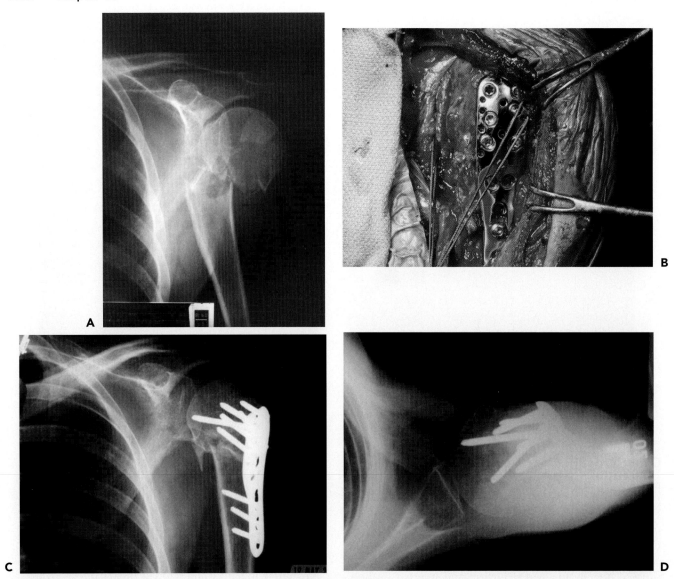

Figure 12-9 A 48-year-old female who presented with a displaced surgical neck fracture 3 weeks after injury. (*A*) Anteroposterior radiograph is shown. (*B*) Closed reduction was not possible due to tissue interposition. Open reduction via a deltopectoral approach with a proximal humerus locking plate was performed. (*C,D*) Radiographs taken 8 weeks after surgery show anatomical reduction and fracture healing.

may irritate the subacromial space. Wires may also break or migrate; therefore, heavy nonabsorbable sutures are preferred when possible.

For surgical neck fractures that can be reduced and impacted, the heavy suture technique incorporating the rotator cuff may be all that is needed for fixation. Surgical neck comminution, without any additional cracks at the tuberosity-head junction, often requires intramedullary rod supplementation. Two Enders nails may be placed at the greater tuberosity-articular surface interface through small stabs in the cuff tendon (Fig. 12-10). They can be separate or incorporated into the tension-band loop, especially if small holes are drilled into the top of the Enders rod.[20] The figure-of-eight suture can be passed through the eyelets of the nail and can thus also help to prevent superior migration.[20] The shoulder is then put through a range-of-motion exercise to assess the stability of the fixation. If

stable, the incisions in the cuff are closed and the wound is then closed over Hemovac suction drains (Bard Medical Division, Covington, GA).

Aftercare

Unless some lack of stability is noted intraoperatively, early passive range of motion is instituted after ORIF, including pulley elevation in the scapular plane, external rotation with a stick, pendulum motion, and hand-and-elbow range of motion. Progression to full stretches is rapid. Strengthening is added at 6 weeks.

Results

One author for this chapter and others reported satisfactory results with the approach outlined, but motion is often

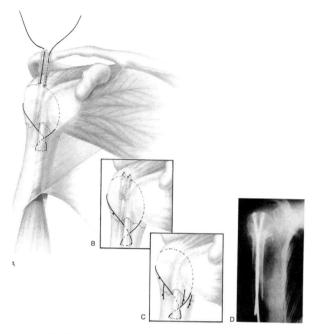

Figure 12-10 Operative repair of surgical neck two-part fracture. (*A*) Reduction of a surgical neck fracture with the insertion of two Enders rods for longitudinal stability. (*B*) A heavy nonabsorbable suture can be passed through the rods as well as through the rotator cuff and the proximal shaft. (*C*) A figure-of-eight suture can be used alone if there is minimal comminution and good longitudinal stability of the fracture. (*D*) AP radiograph of an operative repair of a displaced surgical neck fracture with two Enders rods and heavy suture.

only 80% to 85% of that of the uninjured side.[20] In addition, people rarely come back for treatment of surgical neck malunions, and, when they do, our treatment results are no worse than those of acute repair. For these reasons, the senior author has become less aggressive in the treatment of surgical neck fractures. Surgery is reserved for young athletes who need full motion, or for those with grossly displaced, unimpacted fractures.

GREATER TUBEROSITY FRACTURES

Greater tuberosity fractures were well described by Taylor in 1908,[99] and they were often treated with abduction traction, spica casts, or braces, with the aim of bringing the head up to meet the tuberosity.[44,68,53] Keen[46] appears to have been the first to perform open reduction and internal fixation of an acute fracture in 1907; however, he credited Bardenhauer with having developed the concept in 1886 and Muller with having done the first repair of an old fracture in 1898.[66] McWhorter reported in 1925 on two cases in which he excised the fragment and performed a primary rotator cuff repair.[66] Most authors, however, do prefer to save the tuberosity, by a variety of fixation methods, which will be discussed in the following.

It is important to point out that tuberosity fractures are frequently misdiagnosed on emergency department radio-

graphs. The fragments are often small and comminuted, and they may seem unimportant to examiners who do not realize that they contain the attachment of most of the rotator cuff.[95] Small fragments may also be interpreted as calcium deposits[10] (Fig. 12-11*A*). Therefore, as already emphasized, careful imaging and interpretation is imperative. The greater tuberosity is displaced superiorly by the supraspinatus and/or posteromedially by the infraspinatus and teres minor (Figs. 12-11, *B* and *C*). Superior displacement is best appreciated on the AP view or the outlet view. Posterior and medial retraction is best seen on the axillary view, or, if necessary, a transverse cut of a CT scan (Fig. 12-11*D*).

Nonoperative Treatment

Early reports on the nonoperative treatment of greater tuberosity fractures gave little data on the amount of displacement of those fractures.[31,93,99] McLaughlin found that fractures of the greater tuberosity that healed with more than 1 cm of displacement resulted in permanent disability, whereas those with .5 cm or less of displacement did well.[65] Those patients who had displacement between .5 and 1 cm had a prolonged recovery, some with permanent disability and pain, and 20% needed a reconstructive procedure.[65] Oliver et al. reported a 69% satisfaction rate when 79 fractures (including displaced and nondisplaced) were treated nonoperatively. Patients who had a displaced frac-

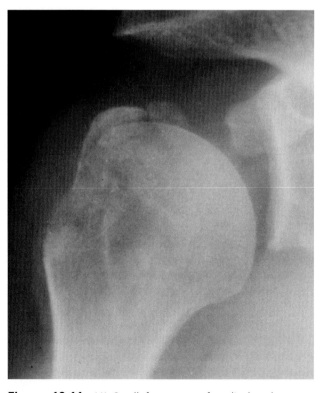

Figure 12-11 (*A*) Small fragments of a displaced greater tuberosity fracture that may be misidentified as calcific tendonitis. *(continued)*

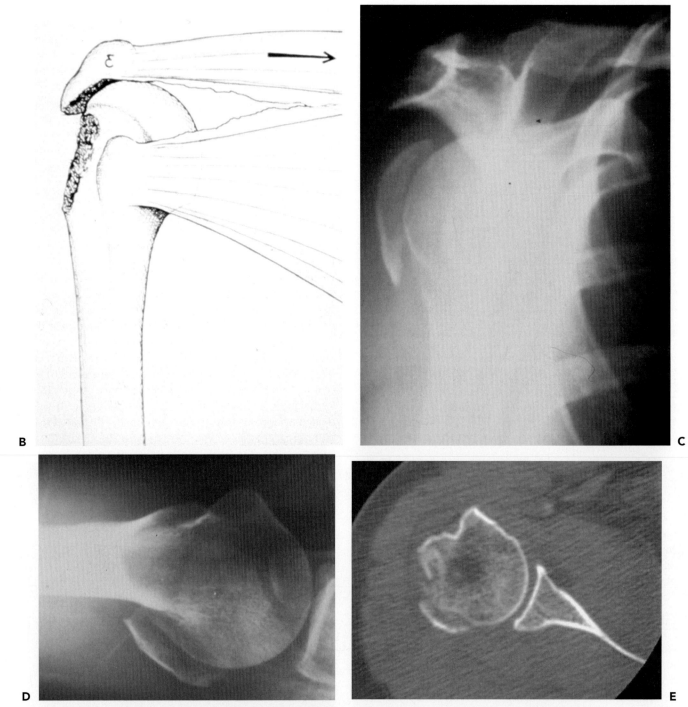

Figure 12-11 *(continued)* *(B)* Greater tuberosity fractures are displaced superiorly by the supraspinatus and posteromedially by the infraspinatus and teres minor. *(C)* Posterior displacement is seen on this outlet view. *(D)* Posterior and medial displacement is best visualized on the axillary view or, if necessary, on *(E)* an axial cut on the computed tomography scan.

ture and received nonoperative care had the worst outcome, with significant functional impairment.[104]

Currently, nonoperative treatment is rarely used for displaced greater tuberosity fractures, unless age or infirmity argues against surgical management. If this approach is chosen, the same principles and techniques discussed for the care of minimally displaced fractures are used. The senior author prefers nonoperative treatment if there is less than 5 mm of superior or 10 mm of posterior displacement in young and active patients, and will accept up to 10 mm of superior displacement in the nondominant arm in sedentary patients.

Management of Concomitant Dislocation

Fractures of the greater tuberosity frequently occur with anterior glenohumeral dislocation.[17,67,92] In this scenario, however, attention is often focused on the dislocation, and the tuberosity fragment may not be appreciated. Furthermore, when there is an associated glenohumeral dislocation, the tuberosity fragments are often drawn across the glenoid by the stretched rotator cuff and may be mistaken for glenoid fracture fragments. From 7% to 15% of glenohumeral dislocations have an associated greater tuberosity fracture.[11,90,102] Bilateral cases have also been reported.[60] Thus, as stated, careful examination of radiographs is necessary, not only to see the greater tuberosity fragment, but to assess for any other fractures.

Once the fracture pattern is appropriately recognized and assessed, a gentle reduction in the emergency room can be undertaken. A shattered proximal humerus can be the unfortunate result of forceful attempts in the emergency room to reduce the fracture-dislocation. When in doubt, an attempt in the operating room while using intra-articular anesthetic injection, interscalene block, or general anesthesia with the image intensifier available may be considered. In rare or long-standing cases, open reduction of the dislocation may be required.[40] Fortunately, once reduced, such dislocations rarely recur.[65]

With reduction of the glenohumeral dislocation, the tuberosity may or may not reduce into its bed (Fig. 12-12).[30,86] Usually it will reduce, guided by the remaining intact portion of the rotator interval that tethers the supraspinatus (attached to the greater tuberosity) to the subscapularis (attached to the lesser tuberosity).[30,31] If it remains displaced, only then should open reduction and internal fixation be considered. Repair in such patients restores dynamic stability by reattaching the muscles of the rotator cuff.[65]

Operative Indications

It should be recognized that Neer was required by the *Journal of Bone and Joint Surgery* to come up with some criteria for displacement, thus 1 cm and 45 degrees were arbitrary and were intended as concepts rather than as rigid guidelines for treatment. The senior author has found that often small degrees of superior tuberosity displacement can cause symptoms. Recently, a biomechanical model has shown that small amounts of residual displacement may alter the balance of forces required to elevate the arm at the glenohumeral joint.[9] Thus, knowing the excellent results of early repair,[22] which are better than the results of malunion repair,[85] a more aggressive approach has been taken with greater tuberosity fractures. In an active, healthy patient, more than 10 mm of posterior retraction or 5 mm of superior displacement will lead to early repair consideration.

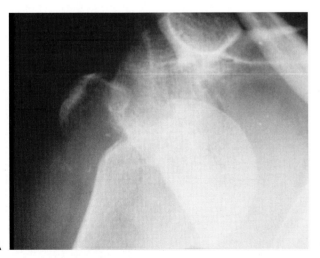
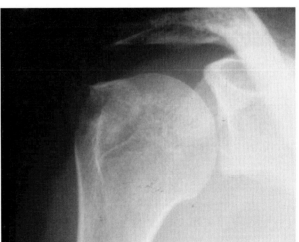

A   **B**

Figure 12-12 (*A*) Two-part anterior fracture-dislocation with a displaced greater tuberosity fracture. (*B*) After closed reduction, the greater tuberosity fracture reduced and healed without further displacement.

Closed Reduction and Pinning

More recently, arthroscopically guided percutaneous repair has been performed, with one series showing excellent results at early follow-up.[25] Concomitant arthroscopic treatment of an acute traumatic glenohumeral dislocation and greater tuberosity fracture has been described.[24] Both the Bankart lesion and tuberosity fracture were repaired using arthroscopic techniques. However, the authors did note that insufficient bone stock, significant displacement, or retraction may necessitate open repair. When comparing open versus pinning for two-part greater tuberosity fractures, Williams and Wong[103] felt that often the deforming forces of the rotator cuff and comminution of the tuberosity fragment lend these fractures more toward open reduction and internal fixation. As the technique of closed reduction and percutaneous pinning becomes more popular, especially in the treatment of certain three- and four-part fractures, it is certainly a reasonable alternative, with comparable results to open fixation (Fig. 12-13). Often, the pins are initially placed to facilitate percutaneous placement of cannulated screws.[13,71,79,80,98] In the case of tuberosity fragmentation or small avulsion pieces, where screw fixation is not possible, two pins, placed to engage the medial cortex, can be utilized after reduction. In this instance, the principles of percutaneous pinning are followed, closely watching the pins postoperatively and removing them at 3 to 4 weeks.

Open Reduction and Internal Fixation

Open reduction and internal fixation have been achieved with pins[98] and screws,[71,80] but transosseous sutures have generally been preferred for comminuted fractures of the greater tuberosity (Fig. 12-14).[42,79] Some authors have preferred to utilize screw fixation, especially in young patients, when the tuberosity is one large piece. However, many have noted that the bone is soft and often comminuted and have preferred to use sutures that incorporate the rotator cuff tendon insertion into the repair.[22,,43,77,79] There are some authors who prefer sutures exclusively.[2,76] Overall, most series

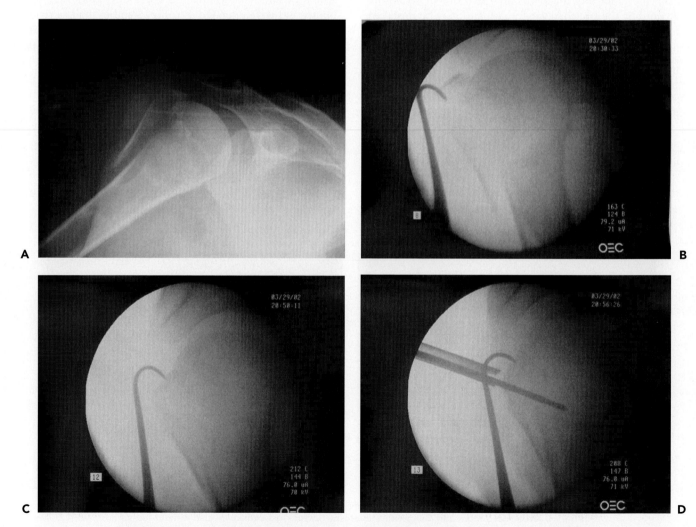

Figure 12-13 (A) Displaced greater tuberosity fracture. (B,C) Reduction of the greater tuberosity fragment. (D) While holding the reduction, the first pin is placed in a superior to inferior direction. (continued)

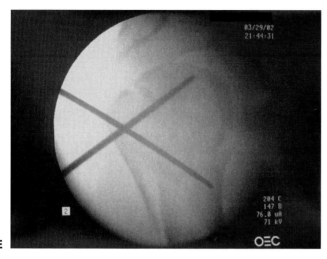
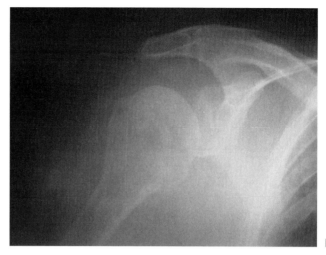

Figure 12-13 *(continued)*   *(E)* Two pins are placed for optimal stability. Pins are removed after 3 to 4 weeks and gentle motion is started. *(F)* AP radiograph 1 year after surgery is shown.

have shown good results.[22,79] Levy found worse results with the smaller tuberosity fragments, perhaps because these functioned more like a cuff avulsion.[54] The senior author has found that his results with greater tuberosity fractures have been surprisingly good, with near-normal motion and strength in most patients, more similar to the results of rotator cuff repair than to the care of other types of fractures.[22]

Greater tuberosity fractures are essentially bony rotator cuff avulsions, and a superior cuff approach through a deltoid split allows convenient retrieval of posteriorly retracted segments and solid repair. On rare occasions, if there is a long metaphyseal spike, then a deltopectoral approach will be used. The repair incorporates the strong rotator cuff tendon, which often is more secure than the osteoporotic bone.

A 6- to 7-cm incision is made in the skin creases superiorly, then flaps are elevated. A 3- to 4-cm split in the deltoid is made in the direction of its fibers from the anterolateral corner of the acromion distally. A stay suture is placed to prevent propagation of the split. The hemorrhagic bursa and inflamed soft tissue should then be cleared to clearly visualize the bony edges of the fracture fragment and its bed on the proximal humerus. Traction sutures can then be placed in the cuff with heavy sutures to facilitate mobilization. The fragment is cleaned and then secured into its bed by transosseous heavy (No. 2 and No. 5) permanent braided sutures that are placed anteriorly, laterally, and posteriorly in the fragment (Fig. 12-14). The rotator interval should be closed as well because this can stabilize the fragment against posterior and superior retraction. The deltoid is meticulously repaired, and a layered closure is effected.

Rehabilitation

Patients with greater tuberosity fractures are immediately begun on passive elevation in the plane of the scapula, external rotation with a stick, and pendulum exercises. No ac-

tive motion is allowed until 6 weeks and until radiographs show early bone healing. Internal rotation is avoided for 3 months, but full-elevation terminal stretches and light active-to-resistive exercises may begin at 6 weeks. Full strengthening and stretching are pursued at 3 months.

LESSER TUBEROSITY FRACTURES

Two-part lesser tuberosity fractures are rare, but they have been reported.[1,21,34,59,61,63,97] They occur more often in association with two- or three-part proximal humerus fractures or as a part of a posterior fracture dislocation. Through a comprehensive search, Ogawa et al. found 70 reported cases in the literature.[78] Of these, 18 were chronic, suggesting that these injuries are often overlooked. The average age at the time of fracture was 35, and the male to female ratio was approximately 3:1. Isolated avulsions can occur after a fall with an abducted and externally rotated humerus.[32] When the arm is in this position, the tension in the subscapularis muscle is at a maximum, which can possibly cause an avulsion of the lesser tuberosity when additional force is applied through the trauma. Displacement tends to be medial because of the pull of the subscapularis, but the fragment may rotate and may be prominent against the coracoid as the shoulder internally rotates. Just as in tendinous subscapularis avulsions, medial dislocation of the biceps can occur, and patients may have a lift-off sign on physical examination.[82]

The trauma series of radiographs, and possibly the addition of CT scans, can aid in determining the size and displacement of the lesser tuberosity fragment (Fig. 12-15). Morris et al. have found that plain radiographs are often inadequate in assessing the lesser tuberosity fragment position when compared to surgical findings. Thus, they felt that CT evaluation improves the accuracy of the initial as-

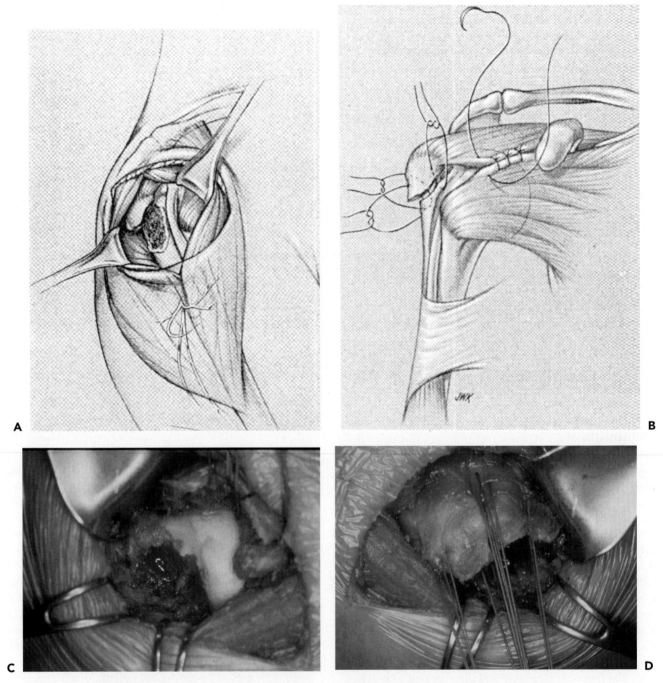

A

B

C

D

Figure 12-14   (A,B) Diagram depicting suture repair of the greater tuberosity. (Reprinted with permission from Flatow EL, Cuoma F, Madley MG, et al. Open reduction and internal fixation of two-part displaced fractures of the greater tuberosity of the proximal part of the humerus. J Bone Joint Surg Am 1991;73:1213.) (C) A superior deltoid-splitting approach is utilized; the defect is easily seen by rotating the head under the split. (D) The tuberosity is mobilized into the wound with heavy sutures and then secured into its bed by transosseous, nonabsorbable sutures.

sessment.[70] One study found that the fragment is most often projected at the caudal edge of the glenoid on the AP radiographs.[101] However, they found that the axillary view showed the fragment clearly in all cases. It has been suggested that the lesser tuberosity fragment can be easily mistaken for calcific tendonitis or an osseous Bankart lesion.[21]

Thus, a careful radiographic view and CT, if necessary, should be performed when this diagnosis is suspected. Magnetic resonance imaging may be helpful in evaluating the subscapularis tendon in relation to the fragment and for ruling out any possible associated soft-tissue injury, i.e., a biceps injury or labral tear.[78]

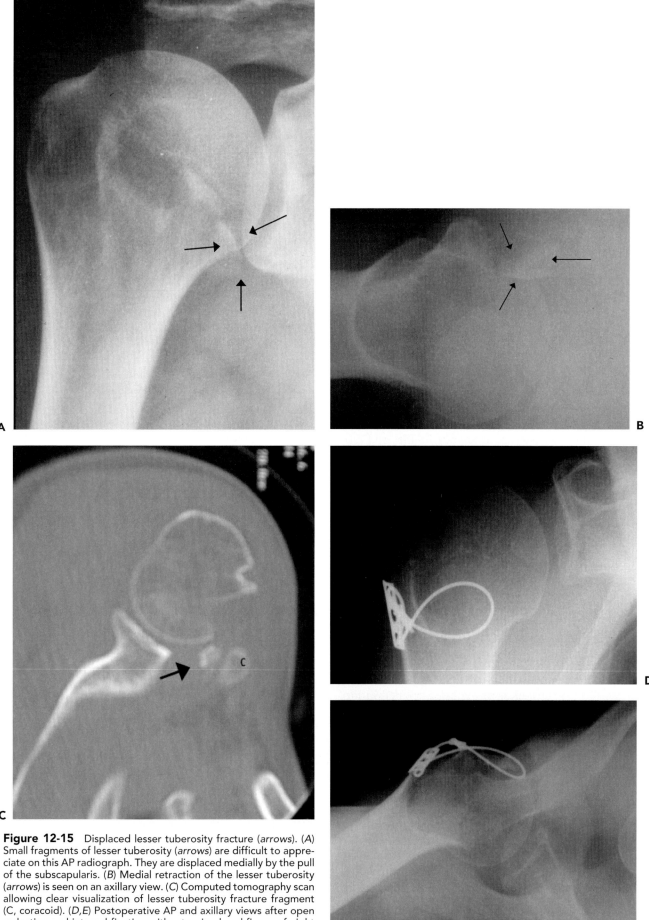

Figure 12-15 Displaced lesser tuberosity fracture (*arrows*). (*A*) Small fragments of lesser tuberosity (*arrows*) are difficult to appreciate on this AP radiograph. They are displaced medially by the pull of the subscapularis. (*B*) Medial retraction of the lesser tuberosity (*arrows*) is seen on an axillary view. (*C*) Computed tomography scan allowing clear visualization of lesser tuberosity fracture fragment (C, coracoid). (*D,E*) Postoperative AP and axillary views after open reduction and internal fixation with a tension band figure-of-eight cable.

Treatments have included nonoperative management,[14] excision of the fragment with subscapularis repair,[52,53] and open reduction and internal fixation.[32,82]

Nonoperative Management

There is more of a tradition of nonoperative management for lesser tuberosity fractures. Historically, it was believed that there are redundant internal rotators and that simple sling immobilization would draw the fragment back toward its bed. As we have become more sophisticated in our assessment of the subscapularis after Gerber's descriptions, more surgeons have become aggressive with respect to repairing displaced fractures of the lesser tuberosity. In the case of a chronic lesser tuberosity fracture, it may be reasonable to first attempt physiotherapy with specific strengthening exercises.[78] If disabling symptoms persist, however, open reduction and internal fixation are indicated.

Management of Concomitant Dislocation

Lesser tuberosity fractures tend to occur in conjunction with posterior glenohumeral dislocations, but this injury is far less commonly seen than two-part anterior fracture dislocations. Posterior dislocations are rare injuries and can occur from directly, from trauma, or indirectly, via a seizure or electrical shock.[12,36] Management is similar in that the dislocation is addressed first, after which the lesser tuberosity is reevaluated to see whether it requires repair. Again, the reduction maneuver must be undertaklen with care. The biceps tendon has been reported to sublux posteriorly, thus preventing reduction,[29] which most commonly occurs when the fractured tuberosity fragment includes the bicipital groove. In these types of cases, an open reduction may be necessary.

Operative Management

In acute cases of lesser tuberosity fractures, the long-term outcomes of open reduction and internal fixation have been excellent.[78] Three-fifths of the cases reported in the literature were treated with open reduction and internal fixation.[78] Operative treatment is especially indicated when the superior aspect of the tuberosity is fragmented and there is a possibility of a dislocating biceps tendon. However, simple excision of the lesser tuberosity fragment has not been shown to be adequate treatment.[53,69,97,100]

The senior author prefers to fix all displaced lesser tuberosity fractures, using 5 to 10 mm of displacement as a guideline. As stated, displacement can best be evaluated on the axillary view, augmented with CT scans, if necessary.

A standard deltopectoral approach is used, with care taken in mobilizing the subscapularis and lesser tuberosity, because there may have been scarring to the axillary nerve medially. Releasing the anterior capsule and freeing it of all attachments to the coracoid may be necessary to mobilize the tuberosity, which is repaired into its freshened bed with a tension band figure-of-eight cable (Figs. 12-15, *D* and *E*). A much smaller-sized lesser tuberosity fragment can be excised,[53] but the subscapularis tendon must be repaired directly to the proximal humerus. If malunion or nonunion of a large, lesser tuberosity fragment occurs, it may act as a block to internal rotation and may also involve the articular surface of the humeral head.

Rehabilitation

Patients with lesser tuberosity fractures immediately begin pure forward flexion to about 90 degrees in full internal rotation. Gentle passive external rotation just to neutral is also performed. At 6 weeks, external rotation to 45 degrees and full elevation are allowed with pulleys if bone healing appears present on radiographs. At 3 months, full stretching and strengthening are instituted.

ANATOMIC NECK FRACTURES

Anatomic neck fractures are almost never seen in isolation and are extremely rare. In a simpler modification of the Neer classification[48] (see Fig. 12-2), the senior author has actually deleted the anatomic neck fracture from this classification because it is so rare. The author knows of only one early open reduction and internal fixation of an isolated anatomic neck fracture (Fig. 12-16). Because there are really no data or follow-up studies on fixation of this type of fracture, it is difficult to give solid recommendations. However, if screw fixation is utilized, studies have shown that screw fixation in the humeral head is strongest when placed centrally and engaging the subchondral plate.[56] Fractures that cannot be anatomically reduced and secured should undergo hemiarthroplasty because the risk of nonunion and avascular necrosis would be expected to be quite high.

CONCLUSION

The majority of two-part proximal humerus fractures can be managed successfully with nonoperative treatment. However, there are certain fracture patterns that necessitate surgery, and there are several keys to a satisfactory outcome in these cases. The correct diagnosis must be made initially with accurate radiographs and any appropriate additional studies. Any concomitant injuries must be recognized and treated in a timely fashion. Although various methods for fixing proximal humerus fractures exist, each fracture is unique, and one should discriminate and use sound judgement to determine the appropriate

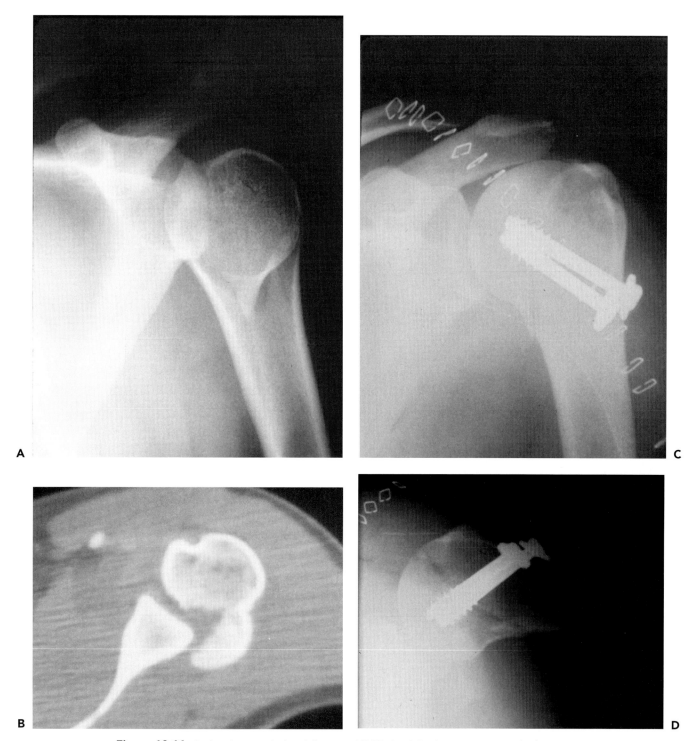

Figure 12-16   Isolated anatomical neck fracture. (*A*) AP view is inadequate to assess displacement. (*B*) A computed tomography scan shows the dislocation of the head with anatomical neck displacement. (*C,D*) AP and axillary views after osteosynthesis. (Courtesy of Edward Yang, M.D.)

treatment for each case. Finally, the postoperative rehabilitation protocol must be followed carefully. A well-supervised regimen is essential for a successful overall outcome, because even a perfect reduction will be a poor result if motion is not restored.

REFERENCES

1. Andreasen AT. Avulsion fracture of the lesser tuberosity of the humerus. Lancet 1941;1:750.
2. Baker DM, Leach RE. Fracture dislocation of the shoulder—report of three unusual cases with rotator cuff avulsion. J Trauma 1965; 5:659.
3. Bernirschke SK, West GG, Henley MD, et al. Percutaneous pin fixation of surgical neck fractures of the humerus. Orthop Trans 1992;16:231.
4. Bernstein J, Adler LM, Blank JE, et al. Evaluation of the Neer system of classification of proximal humeral fractures with computerized tomographic scans and plain radiographs. J Bone Joint Surg Am 1996;78:1371.
5. Bigliani LU. Fractures of the proximal humerus. In: Rockwood CA, Green DP, eds. Fractures in adults, 3rd ed. Philadelphia, JB Lippincott, 1990:871.
6. Bixler BA, Naidu SH, Capo JA, et al. Percutaneous pinning of proximal humerus fractures: a biomechanical study. Orthop Trans 1996;20:865.
7. Blom S, Dahback LO. Nerve injuries in dislocations of the shoulder joint and fractures of the neck of the humerus. A clinical and electromyographical study. Acta Chir Scand 1970;136(6):461.
8. Bloom MH, Obata WG. Diagnosis of posterior dislocation of the shoulder with use of velpeau axillary and angle up roentgenographic views. J Bone Joint Surg 1967;49A:943.
9. Bono CM, Renard R, Levine RG, et al. Effect of displacement of fractures of the greater tuberosity on the mechanics of the shoulder. J Bone Joint Surg Br 2001;83(7):1056.
10. Brickner WM. Certain afflictions of the shoulder and their management. Int Clin 1924;2:191.
11. Cave EF. Shoulder girdle injuries. In: Fractures and other injuries. Chicago, Year Book, 1958:250.
12. Checchia SL, Santos PD, Miyazaki AN. Surgical treatment of acute and chronic posterior fracture-dislocation of the shoulder. J Shoulder Elbow Surg 1998;7(1):53.
13. Chen C, Chao E, Tu Y, et al. Closed management and percutaneous fixation of unstable proximal humerus fractures. J Trauma 1998;45(6):1039.
14. Chun JM, Groh GI, Rockwood CA Jr. Management of two-part fractures of the proximal humerus. Orthop Trans 1993;17:936.
15. Clare DJ, Hersh CK, Athanasiou K, et al. Biomechanical fixation strength in surgical neck fractures of the proximal humerus. Orthop Trans 1998;22:339.
16. Codman EA. The shoulder: rupture of the supraspinatus tendon and other lesions in or about the subacromial bursa. Boston, Thomas Todd, 1934.
17. Codman EA. The shoulder: rupture of the supraspinatus tendon and other lesions in or about the subacromial bursa. Boston: Thomas Todd, 1934.
18. Cofield RH. Comminuted fractures of the proximal humerus. Clin Orthop 1988;230-49–57.
19. Connor PM, D'Alessandro DF. Role of hemiarthroplasty for proximal humerus fractures. J South Orthop Assoc 1995;4:9.
20. Cuomo F, Flatow EL, Madday M, et al. Open reduction and internal fixation of two- and three-part displaced surgical neck fractures of the proximal humerus. J Shoulder Elbow Surg 1992;1:287.
21. Earwaker J. Isolated avulsion fracture of the lesser tuberosity of the humerus. Skeletal Radiol 1990;19:121.
22. Flatow EL, Cuoma F, Madley MG, et al. Open reduction and internal fixation of two-part displaced fractures of the greater tuberosity of the proximal part of the humerus. J Bone Joint Surg Am 1991;73:1213.
23. Garceau GJ, Cogland S. Early physical therapy in the treatment of fractures of the surgical neck of the humerus. Indiana Med 1941; 34:293.
24. Gartsman GM, Taverna E, Hammerman SM. Arthroscopic treatment of acute traumatic anterior glenohumeral dislocation and greater tuberosity fracture. Arthroscopy 1999;15(6):648.
25. Geissler WB, Petrie SG, Savoie FH. Arthroscopic fixation greater tuberosity fractures of the humerus. Arthroscopy 1994;10:344.
26. Gerber C, Warner JJ. Alternatives to hemiarthroplasty for complex proximal-humeral fractures. In: Warner JJ, Iannotti JP, Gerber C, eds. Complex and revision problems in shoulder surgery. Philadelphia, Lippincott-Raven, 1997:215.
27. Gibbons AP. Fracture of the tuberculum majus by muscular violence. BMJ 1909;2:1674.
28. Gold AM. Fractured neck of the humerus with separation and dislocation of the humeral head (fracture-dislocation of the shoulder, severe type). Bull Hosp Jt Dis 1971;32:87.
29. Goldman A, Shermon O, Price A, et al. Posterior fracture dislocation of the shoulder with biceps interposition. J Trauma 1987;27 (9):1083.
30. Gratz CM. Anterior subglenoid dislocation with fracture of the greater tuberosity of the humerus. Surg Clin North Am 1930;10: 549.
31. Greeley PW, Magnuson PB. Dislocation of the shoulder accompanied by fracture of the greater tuberosity and complicated by spinatus tendon injury. JAMA 1934;102:1835.
32. Haas SL. Fracture of the lesser tuberosity of the humerus. Am J Surg 1944;63:253.
33. Hardcastle PH, Fisher TR. Intrathoracic displacement of the humeral head with fracture of the surgical neck. Injury 1981;12: 313.
34. Hartigan JW. Separation of the lesser tuberosity of the head of the humerus. N Y Med J 1895;61:276.
35. Hayes JM, Van Winkle GN. Axillary artery injury with minimally displaced fracture of the neck of the humerus. J Trauma 1983;23: 431.
36. Hayes PL, Klepps S, Bishop J, et al. Posterior shoulder dislocation with lesser tuberosity and scapular spine fractures. J Shoulder Elbow Surg 2003; in press.
37. Hersche O, Gerber C. Iatrogenic displacement of fracture-dislocation of the shoulder. A report of seven cases. J Bone Joint Surg Br 1994;76(1):30.
38. Horak J, Nilsson B. Epidemiology of fractures of the upper end of the humerus. Clin Orthop 1975;112:250.
39. Howard NJ, Eloesser L. Treatment of fractures of the upper end of the humerus: an experimental and clinical study. J Bone Joint Surg 1934;32:1.
40. Ilahi OA. Irreducible anterior shoulder dislocation with fracture of the greater tuberosity. Am J Orthop 1998;27:576.
41. Jaberg H, Warner JJ, Jakob RP. Percutaneous stabilization of unstable fractures of the humerus. J Bone Joint Surg Am 1992;74: 508.
42. Jakob RP, Kristiansen T, Mayo K, et al. Classification and aspects of treatment of fractures of the proximal humerus. In: Bateman JE, Welsh RP, eds. Surgery of the shoulder. Philadelphia, BC Decker, 1984:330.
43. Johansson O. Complications and failures of surgery in various fractures of the humerus. Acta Chir Scand 1961;120:469.
44. Jones R. On certain fractures about the shoulder. Ir J Med Sci 1932; 78:282.
45. Jurik AG, Albrechtsen J. The use of computed tomography with two- and three-dimensional reconstructions in the diagnosis of three- and four-part fractures of the proximal humerus. Clin Radiol 1994;49:800.
46. Keen WW. Fractures of the tuberculum majus. Ann Surg 1907;45: 938.
47. Kelly JP. Fractures complicating electroconvulsive therapy and chronic epilepsy. J Bone Joint Surg Br 1954;36:70.
48. Klepps SJ, Hazrati Y, Flatow EL. Classification of proximal humerus fractures. In: Levine WN, Marra G, Bigliani LU, eds. Fractures of the shoulder girdle. New York, Marcel Dekker, 2003.
49. Kocher MS, Feagin JA Jr. Shoulder injuries during alpine skiing. Am J Sports Med 1996;24:665.

50. Kocher T. Beitrage Zur Kenntnis Einiger Praktisch Wichtiger Frac-turformen. Basel, Carl Sallmann, 1986.
51. Koval KJ, Gallagner MA, Marsicano JG, et al. Functional outcome after minimally displaced fractures of the proximal part of the humerus. J Bone Joint Surg Am 1997;79:203.
52. Kunkel SS, Monesmith EA. Isolated avulsion fracture of the lesser tuberosity of the humerus: a case report. J Shoulder Elbow Surg 1993;2:43.
53. LaBriola JH, Mohaghegh HA. Isolated avulsion fracture of the lesser tuberosity of the humerus: a case report and review of the literature. J Bone Joint Surg Am 1975;57:1011.
54. Levy AS. Greater tuberosity fractures of the humerus. Orthop Trans 1998;22:594.
55. Liew ASL, Johnson JA, Patterson SD, et al. The effect of screw po-sition on fixation in the humeral head. Orthop Trans 1998;22:98.
56. Liew ASL, Johnson JA, Patterson SD, et al. The effect of screw po-sition on fixation in the humeral head. Orthop Trans 1998;22:98.
57. Lind T, Kroner K, Jensen J. The epidemiology of fractures of the proximal humerus. Arch Orthop Trauma Surg 1989;108:285.
58. Lindholm TS, Elmstedt E. Bilateral posterior dislocation of the shoulder combined with fracture of the proximal humerus: a case report. Acta Orthop Scand 1980;51(3):485.
59. Lorenz H. Die isolerte Fractur des Tuberculum minus humeri. Dtsch Z Chir 1901;58:593.
60. Marke DC, Blasier RB. Bilateral anterior dislocation of the shoul-ders with greater tuberosity fractures. Orthopaedics 1994;17:945.
61. Markel DC, Donley BG, Blasier RB. Percutaneous intramedullary pinning of proximal humeral fractures. Orthop Rev 1994;23:667.
62. Mason BJ, Kier R, Bindleglass DF. Occult fractures of the greater tuberosity of the humerus: radiographic and MR imaging find-ings. Am J Roentgenol 1999;172(2):469.
63. McAuliffe TB, Dowd GS. Avulsion of the subscapularis tendon: a case report. J Bone Joint Surg Am 1987;69:1454.
64. McCauley TR, Disler DG, Tam MK. Bone marrow edema in the greater tuberosity of the humerus at MR imaging: association with rotator cuff tears and traumatic injury. Magn Reson Imaging 2000;18(8):979.
65. McLaulgin HL. Dislocation of the shoulder with tuberosity frac-ture. Surg Clin North Am 1963;43:1615.
66. McWhorter GL. Fractures of the greater tuberosity of the humerus with displacement. Surg Clin North Am 1925;5:1005.
67. Meyerding HW. Fracture-dislocation of the shoulder. Minn Med 1937;20:717.
68. Miller SR. Practical points in the diagnosis and treatment of frac-tures of the upper fourth of the humerus. Indust Med 1940;9:458.
69. Miura Y, Hattori T, Kunishima Y, et al. Isolated fracture of the lesser tuberosity of the humerus: a case report. J Joint Surg (Japan) 1990;9:955.
70. Morris MF, Kilcoyne RF, Shuman W. Humeral tuberosity fractures: evaluation by CT scan and management of malunion. Orthop Trans 1987;11:242.
71. Muller Me, Allgower M, Willeneger H. Manual of internal fixation. New York, Springer-Verlag, 1970:297.
72. Naidu SH, Bixler B, Capo JT, et al. Percutaneous pinning of prox-imal humerus fractures: a biomechanical study. Orthopedics 1997;20:1073.
73. Neer CD II. Displaced proximal humeral fractures. I. Classifica-tion and evaluation. J Bone Joint Surg Am 1970;52:1077.
74. Neer CS. Four-segment classification of displaced proximal humerus fractures. AAOS Instr Course Lect 1975;24:160.
75. Neer CS, McIlveen SJ. Recent results and technique of prosthetic replacement for 4-part proximal humeral fractures. Orthop Trans 1986;10:475.
76. Neer CS II. Fractures about the shoulder. In: Rockwood CA, Green DP, eds. Fractures in adults. Philadelphia, JB Lippincott, 1984:675.
77. Neer CS II, McIlveen SJ. Remplacement de la tete humerale avec reconstruction des tuberosities et de la coiffe dans les fractures de-placees a 4 fragments. Rev Chir Orthop Reparatrice Appar Mot 1988;74(suppl 2):31.
78. Ogawa K, Takahashi M. Long-term outcome of isolated lesser tuberosity fractures of the humerus. J Trauma 1997;42(5):955.
79. Oliver H, Dufour G, Duparc J. Fracture of the trochiter. Rev Chir Orthop Reparatrice Appar Mot 1976;62:113.
80. Paavolainen P, Bjorkenheim JM, Slatis P, et al. Operative treat-ment of severe proximal humeral fractures. Acta Orthop Scand 1983;54:374.
81. Parsons BO, Klepps SJ, Miller S, et al. The reliability and repro-ducibility of radiographs of greater tuberosity fractures: a cadav-eric study. Presented at AOSSM speciality day, AAOS, New Or-leans, 2003.
82. Paschal SO, Hutton KS, Weatherall PT. Isolated avulsion fracture of the lesser tuberosity of the humerus in adolescents. J Bone Joint Surg Am 1995;77:1427.
83. Pasila M, Jaroma H, Kiyiluoto O, et al. Early complications of pri-mary shoulder dislocations. Acta Orthop Scand 1978;49(3):260.
84. Reinus WR, Hatem SF. Fractures of the greater tuberosity pre-senting as rotator cuff abnormality: magnetic resonance demon-stration. J Trauma 1998;44(4):670.
85. Rodosky MW, Duralde XA, Connor PM, et al. Operative treat-ment of malunions of proximal humerus fractures. Orthop Trans 1997;21:624.
86. Rose SH, Melton LJ, Morrey BF, et al. Epidemiologic features of humeral fractures. Clin Orthop 1982;64:24.
87. Rowles DJ, McGrory JE. Percutaneous pinning of the proximal part of the humerus. An anatomic study. J Bone Joint Surg Am 2001;83A(11):1695.
88. Ruch DS, Kuzma GR. Biomechanical rigidity following fixation of proximal humerus fractures. Orthop Trans 1998;22:599.
89. Salem MI. Bilateral anterior fracture-dislocation of the shoulder joints due to severe electric shock. Injury 1983;14:361.
90. Savoie FH, Geissler WB, Vander Griend RA. Open reduction and internal fixation of three-part fractures of the proximal humerus. Orthopaedics 1989;12:65.
91. Schai P, Imhoff A, Preiss S. Comminuted humeral head fractures: a multicenter analysis. J Shoulder Elbow Surg 1995;4:319.
92. Schlaepfer K. Uncomplicated dislocations of the shoulder: their rational treatment and late results. Am J Med Sci 1924;167:244.
93. Sever JW. Fracture of the head of the humerus: treatment and re-sults. N Engl J Med 1937;216:1100.
94. Sidor ML, Zuckerman JD, Lyon T, et al. The Neer classification system for proximal humeral fractures: an assessment of interob-server reliability and intraobserver reproducibility. J Bone Joint Surg 1993;75A:1745.
95. Simpson NS, Schwappach JR, Toby EB. Fracture-dislocation of the humerus with intrathoracic displacement of the humeral head: a case report. J Bone Joint Surg Am 1998;80:889.
96. Stableforth PG. Four-part fractures of the neck of the humerus. J Bone Joint Surg Br 1984;66:104.
97. Stangl FH. Isolated fracture of the lesser tuberosity of the humerus. Minn Med 1933;16:435.
98. Stevens JH. Fracture of the upper end of the humerus. Ann Surg 1919;69:147.
99. Taylor HI. Isolated fracture of the greater tuberosity of the humerus. Ann Surg 1908;54:10.
100. Tohyama H, Ogino T, Minami A, et al. Old isolated fracture of the lesser tuberosity of the humerus. Rinsho Seikeigeka 1990;25:657 (in Japanese).
101. Van Laarhoven HAJ, te Slaa RL, van Laarhoven EW. Isolated avul-sion fracture of the lesser tuberosity of the humerus. J Trauma 1995;39:997.
102. Wentworth ET. Fractures involving the shoulder joint. N Y State J Med 1940;40:1182.
103. Williams GR Jr, Wong KL. Two-part and three-part fractures: open reduction and internal fixation versus closed reduction and percutaneous pinning. Orthop Clin North Am 2000;31(1):1.
104. Young TB, Wallace WA. Conservative treatment of fractures and fracture-dislocations of the upper end of the humerus. J Bone Joint Surg Br 1985;67:373.
105. Zanetti M, Weishaupt D, Jost B, et al. MR imaging for traumatic tears of the rotator cuff: high prevalence of greater tuberosity frac-tures and subscapularis tendon tears. Am J Roentgenol 1999;172(2):463.
106. Zuckerman JD, Flugstad DL, Teitz CC, et al. Axillary artery in-jury as a complication of proximal humeral fractures: two case reports and a review of the literature. Clin Orthop 1984;189:234.

Three-Part Fractures: Open Reduction and Internal Fixation, or Arthroplasty?

Maxwell C. Park   *Walter G. Stanwood*   *Louis U. Bigliani*

INTRODUCTION

Before the advent of the Neer classification,[58] Dr. Neer described the treatment of surgical neck fracture-dislocations where "the head fragment remained extruded" from the glenohumeral joint.[61] In this series, the most common treatment was excision of the humeral head. "Replacement prosthesis" was listed as a treatment option being developed at the time. Two years later, Dr. Neer reported on his first series of patients treated with hemiarthroplasty; he outlined the indications for hemiarthroplasty, including "fracture with dislocation of the head fragment."[60] He wrote:

> Upon exploring the shoulder if it is seen that a reasonable amount of the articular surface is intact and retains soft tis-

sue attachments, [gentle] reduction of the fracture and preservation of the head is the procedure of choice. Rarely, the anatomic head is dislocated and deprived of soft tissue attachments, or is fragmented. In this instance reduction is followed by avascular necrosis and traumatic arthritis. Resection is indicated.

In these few sentences, Dr. Neer touched on the key considerations for treating complex proximal humerus fractures: (1) extent of injury, with dislocation suggesting more trauma; (2) bone quality, as it relates to the size of the fragments; (3) soft tissue and blood supply, as it relates to avascular necrosis (AVN) of the humeral head; and (4) gentle technique during open reduction, suggesting minimal dissection. These salient considerations will be discussed in this chapter as they relate in particular to three-part fractures of the proximal humerus.

Proximal humerus fractures account for 4% to 5% of all fractures and most commonly affect elderly patients with osteoporotic bone.[1,22,36,71] Eighty-five percent of proximal humerus fractures are nondisplaced or minimally displaced[56,58] and are adequately treated with early, protected mobilization. Therefore, the incidence of displaced proximal humerus fractures, particularly three-part

M. C. Park: Center for Shoulder, Elbow and Sports Medicine, New York Orthopaedic Hospital, College of Physicians and Surgeons, Columbia University, New York, New York.

W. G. Stanwood: Center for Shoulder, Elbow and Sports Medicine, New York Orthopaedic Hospital, College of Physicians and Surgeons, Columbia University, New York, New York.

L. U. Bigliani: Center for Shoulder, Elbow and Sports Medicine, New York Orthopaedic Hospital, College of Physicians and Surgeons, Columbia University, New York, New York.

patterns requiring surgical intervention, is relatively low.[30,41] Three- and four-part fractures represent 13% to 16% of all proximal humeral fractures.[36] When encountered, they can be difficult to treat, even in the most experienced hands.

PATHOLOGY

Risk Factors

Elderly patients are at high risk for proximal humerus fractures,[50] and females are twice as likely as males to sustain these injuries.[71] Osteoporosis, as it relates to elderly women, is a major consideration in understanding these statistics. Osteoporosis, along with humeral head viability, is one of the most critical considerations when scrutinizing the ultimate treatment decision for complex proximal humerus fractures.

Mechanisms of Injury

The most common mechanism of injury is a fall onto an outstretched arm from a standing height or less[50,64,86] or a direct blow to the shoulder itself.[4] This relatively low-energy trauma is most often associated with the elderly population with osteopenic bone. Higher energy trauma, such as a motor vehicle accident, accounts for more of these fractures in the younger and male populations and presents a greater likelihood of a concomitant dislocation.[4,29,68] Polytrauma is more common in the younger population.[71] Another mechanism of injury, as first described by Codman, involves extreme rotation of an abducted arm, which can cause fracture as the humeral head impinges against the acromion.[11] Less commonly, convulsions can cause fracture-dislocations[4,68]; the dislocations can be anterior[74] or posterior.[5,18,67,79] When the mechanism is trivial and a proximal humerus fracture is sustained, consider a pathological etiology.

Concomitant Injuries

Stableforth reported an incidence of 6.1% for brachial plexus injury in proximal humerus fractures.[88] The brachial plexus is particularly susceptible with fracture dislocations; inspection and palpation should reveal loss of normal shoulder contour. Any displacement at the surgical neck can injure the axillary nerve as it passes underneath the glenohumeral joint; the axillary nerve is the most commonly injured nerve in the setting of proximal humerus fractures.[4,6] When encountering a proximal humerus fracture, the surgeon must palpate the deltoid for voluntary contractions to assess axillary nerve injury.

Given its close proximity to the shoulder joint, the axillary artery is the most commonly injured vascular structure with proximal humerus fractures.[4] Vascular injuries occur predominantly in the third part of the axillary artery, where it is tethered to the humerus by the anterior and posterior humeral circumflex arteries.[4,88] When vascular damage is present, it is often associated with severe medial shaft displacement through the surgical neck.[96] A cool extremity with asymmetrical brachial or radial pulses raises suspicion for significant arterial injury requiring emergent intervention.

"Transitory Subluxation"

Occasionally, inferior subluxation occurs after proximal humerus fractures and results from a global atony of the deltoid muscle.[4] This is generally self-limited and has not been shown to affect outcome.[59] Support the arm in a sling, and promote recovery through gentle isometric exercises.[4] If subluxation persists after 4 weeks, then rule out an axillary nerve palsy.

RISK OF AVASCULAR NECROSIS

Avascular necrosis rates of the humeral head are 12% to 25% in three-part fractures.[24] The anterior circumflex artery helps supply the anterior rotator cuff, and the posterior circumflex and suprascapular anastomoses supply the posterior cuff.[72] The anterolateral branch of the anterior circumflex humeral artery provides the primary blood supply to the humeral head.[23,47] This artery reaches the bicipital groove at the surgical neck and may be compromised at this level in surgical neck fractures. The anterolateral branch is conceivably more at risk with higher energy trauma (e.g., three-part fracture worse than two-part fracture, dislocation worse than without dislocation). Schai et al. stated that the blood supply of the humeral head comes mainly through muscular insertions at the tuberosities and through vessels entering the bone distal to the anatomical neck, and that the major blood supply of the humeral head is maintained through the intact lesser tuberosity.[76] The anterolateral branch, before entry into the humeral head (arcuate artery), runs along the lateral aspect of the bicipital groove.[23] Seggl and Wieglein[78] and Brooks et al.[8] noted the importance of numerous branches of the anterior and posterior humeral circumflex arteries supplying the humeral head via soft tissue traversing the medial anatomical neck. In a case report by Gerber et al., AVN of the humeral head was absent after posttraumatic rupture of the anterior and posterior humeral circumflex arteries, suggesting the clinical relevance of the intraosseous blood supply by anastomoses of the deep brachial artery.[25] Appreciating the significance of vascular anatomy perfusing the humeral head can improve surgical techniques and thus may improve outcomes for the treatment of three-part fractures.

IMAGING AND SPECIAL TESTS

Accurate Radiographs

Radiographic trauma series should be obtained for all patients with proximal humerus fractures.[58,64] This series includes three views: (1) anteroposterior, (2) scapular-lateral, and (3) axillary. When arm abduction necessary for axillary radiographs cannot be tolerated, obtain a Velpeau axillary radiograph.[7] The trauma series provides the ability to assess fracture displacement and angulation in three planes. Park et al. highlighted the inherent difficulty with obtaining adequate radiographs for making this assessment.[64] In particular, with respect to the surgical neck fracture, the apex of the humeral head is often not tangent to the radiograph and is either internally or externally oriented depending on the radiograph plate and beam, thus misrepresenting the true head-shaft angle.[64] However, the trauma series remains the most practical diagnostic tool available to the shoulder surgeon, despite studies questioning the reliability and reproducibility of classifying proximal humerus fractures with radiographs.[80,81]

Computed Tomography (CT) Scans

Computed tomography (CT) scans can aid in assessing fracture lines involving the articular surface, which would have implications for operative management. Some authors find CT indispensable when the number of fragments cannot be reliably defined.[76] Three-dimensional reconstructions provide additional information with regard to capital impaction, fracture displacement, and dislocation.[43] A head-splitting fracture or large (greater than 40%) humeral head impression fracture are patterns adverse to operative reduction.[12] CT scans, in general, can be used as an adjunct to a proper radiographic trauma series to better appreciate the extent of comminution. When indicated, CT scans with 2-mm cuts should be obtained. However, addition of CT scans to the workup offers little value in improving reproducibility of the Neer classification.[2,83,84]

Magnetic Resonance Imaging (MRI)

Magnetic resonance imaging (MRI) is not routinely used to assess proximal humerus fractures, nor has its significance in this setting been proven in the literature. However, MRI can document the status of the rotator cuff. Codman realized the importance of the rotator cuff tendons in keeping proximal humerus fractures in "mutual apposition."[11] He emphasized "how tenaciously the short rotators with their periosteal prolongations cling to all the fragments and tend to hold them together." The rotator cuff can be used as a fixation point in open-reduction and internal fixation (ORIF).[64] In addition, cuff disruption may predispose the humeral head to AVN, if no other remaining perfusion is present af-

ter a severe surgical neck fracture. If available to the shoulder surgeon, MRI may facilitate preoperative planning, insofar as rotator cuff status can be reliably assessed. However, in the majority of cases, an MRI is usually not necessary.

Other Studies

As discussed previously, concomitant brachial plexus and axillary artery injuries in the setting of proximal humerus fractures should always be clinically assessed. Angiography is indicated when a cold extremity with asymmetrical pulses presents in the setting of a severely displaced surgical neck fracture, raising the suspicion for arterial compromise. When a brachial plexus injury is present, electromyography (EMG) is appropriate approximately 3 weeks after the time of injury; if persistent and not self-limited, signs of injury are best characterized with EMG during this subacute period.

NONOPERATIVE TREATMENT

Indications

In theory a three-part fracture without soft-tissue interposition might be reduced and treated nonoperatively; in most cases, however, the patho-anatomy poses a challenge to reduction and results in an unstable fracture. The muscles attached to the fragment determine the displacement patterns. For the three-part fracture with greater tuberosity (GT) displacement, the subscapularis internally rotates the humeral head; for the three-part lesser tuberosity fracture (LT), the supraspinatus externally rotates the head. The pectoralis major internally rotates and medializes the shaft. The biceps tendon may be interposed between the fracture fragments. Repeated attempts at closed reduction are not recommended, especially in the elderly population, because the bone quality may be poor and further comminution may occur.[4] Also, repeated manipulation has been associated with neurological deficit and heterotopic ossification.[59]

If a patient cannot tolerate anesthesia due to medically related comorbid conditions, then operative treatment is precluded and closed management must be pursued. In addition, if a patient cannot participate in postoperative physical therapy, operative management may be unwise. If a pathological fracture secondary to tumor or metastases is present, nonoperative management may be unreliable, and surgical repair may be advantageous.

Results in the Literature

Numerous studies reported acceptable results for the conservative treatment of three- and four-part fractures in elderly patients.[38,48,99–102] Zyto reported on nine elderly patients with three-part fractures available for retrospective review at 10 years, the longest follow-up in the literature for this fracture pattern.[100] The mean Constant score[13] was 59, and disability was reported as none in four patients, mild in three, and moderate in two; no patients had severe disability. All patients could accept their shoulder condition. However, death occurred in 66% of their original cohort (average age 66 years), which consisted of 58 patients. Zyto concluded that nonoperative treatment of displaced three-part fractures in elderly patients should be considered as an acceptable treatment option. In a retrospective review, Ilchmann et al. showed that seven patients (average age 73 years) with three-part fractures treated conservatively had better scores than eight patients (average age 62 years) treated with tension-band osteosynthesis; they used their own clinical outcomes measure which graded pain, function, and motion.[38] The conservatively treated group had better average scores for pain and function. They reported one patient with AVN in the conservative group and three in the tension-band group. They concluded that satisfactory results can be achieved with closed treatment of three-part fractures.

Not only have the results shown that closed treatment is acceptable, but several recent studies have proven that the operative treatment is not any better.[77,101–103] Zyto et al. compared 18 patients with three-part fractures treated nonoperatively to 19 patients treated with tension-band constructs.[101] Overall, the average age was 74 years. At least 30% contact between the head and shaft were required, and no manipulation was performed. There were no significant differences between conservatively and surgically treated patients after more than 3 years follow-up, and there were no differences in function. Another study by Zyto et al. found no differences between their three-part fractures treated conservatively and surgically with internal fixation; at 3 years follow-up, 96% of their patients, with a mean age of 73 years, accepted their shoulder situation.[102] In two separate studies, Schai et al. showed that patients treated conservatively had similar mean Constant scores[13] to those treated with ORIF[76,77]; in the more recent multicenter study, the patients with three-part fractures treated conservatively and with osteosynthesis had similar Constant scores that were not significantly different—78 and 83, respectively.

Although the previous studies suggest that nonoperative treatment for three-part fractures is acceptable,[38,48,99–103] many studies have reported unsatisfactory results with conservative management associated with pain, malunion, and AVN.[28,59,61,66,89] Rasmussen et al. reviewed 42 patients with displaced two-, three-, and four-part proximal humerus fractures treated conservatively.[66] The median age was 77 years and the median follow-up was 2 years. There was a statistically significant difference between those with two-part fractures and the rest of the cohort, with the former group doing better. There were 17 three-part fractures, and only 7

patients (41%) had excellent or satisfactory results.[66] In 1970, Neer reported on 39 three-part fractures in patients with an average age of 55.3 years.[59] These patients, after closed reduction under anesthesia, were treated with a Velpeau bandage, a hanging cast, or overhead ulnar-pin traction. Only one patient had an excellent result, and two had satisfactory results. Failures were attributed to malunion, nonunion, and AVN of the humeral head. Other complications included neurologic deficit and heterotopic ossification, both thought to have been exacerbated by repeated attempts at reduction. Neer concluded that nonoperative treatment was inadequate and advocated ORIF for displaced three-part fractures.

In general, unless a patient cannot tolerate anesthesia, the authors recommend joint preservation via operative repair for three-part fractures. If severe comminution or osteoporosis exists and limits fixation, consider hemiarthroplasty. In most cases, humeral head replacement in the setting of three-part fractures provides opportunity for shoulder salvage, if ORIF is not possible.

OPEN REDUCTION AND INTERNAL FIXATION

Advantages

The advantages of ORIF in the properly selected patient include joint preservation and the opportunity for salvage via hemiarthroplasty, should the need arise. Other authors raise the concern over prosthesis longevity and favor ORIF for complex fractures of the proximal humerus.[24]

The relative benefit of ORIF over hemiarthroplasty is emphasized by recalling the potential multiple causes for failure after humeral head replacement. These include: (1) greater tuberosity detachment, (2) prosthetic loosening, (3) nerve injury, (4) glenoid erosion, (5) prosthesis malposition, (6) dislocation, (7) heterotopic bone formation, and (8) deep infection.[12] In addition, multiple studies[31,44,57,97,103] investigating hemiarthroplasty for complex proximal humerus fractures have had less satisfactory outcomes when compared to Neer.[59] In a recent study, Zyto et al. reviewed 27 patients who had sustained displaced three- or four-part fractures of the proximal humerus and were treated with hemiarthroplasty.[103] Seventeen patients had three-part fractures, and ten had four-part fractures. The median age was 71 years. The mean follow-up period was 39 months. The median Constant score[13] was 51 for the three-part fractures and 46 for the four-part fractures. The median range of motion for all the patients in flexion was 70 degrees; internal rotation, 50 degrees; and external rotation, 45 degrees. Nine patients still had moderate or severe pain. Eight patients had moderate or severe disability. They concluded that their results were disappointing and that further studies on open reduction and fixation were justified.

Disadvantages

The disadvantages of ORIF for three-part fractures include the inherent risks of AVN, nonunion, and malunion. According to Hagg et al., open reduction doubles the risk of AVN compared to closed treatment.[28] In addition, hardware use presents iatrogenic risks such as failure, migration, impingement, pain, and reoperations.[14–16,20,30,33,39,40,59,63,86,90] Metallic fixation is not well tolerated in comminuted or severely osteoporotic bone and may be better managed with cuff-incorporating sutures.[64]

In the three-part fracture with osteoporotic bone or significant comminution and severe displacement or dislocation with soft-tissue injury, a hemiarthroplasty obviates the risk of AVN and surgical neck nonunion. Satisfactory results with hemiarthroplasty for complex fractures of the proximal humerus have been reported.[12,17,27,54,59,85,88,91] However, except for the series by Neer[59] and Compito et al.,[12] active motion has often been less than 100 degrees of forward elevation, the chief benefit being pain relief. Notably, the average ages for these two reports were 55.3 years and 62 years, respectively.

As shown in multiple series, the outcome after hemiarthroplasty for complex shoulder fractures tends to be worse with increasing patient age.[26,27,31,44,57,97,103] Elderly patients with osteoporotic bone and fragile soft tissues tend to be the very patients that require hemiarthroplasty. This highlights the most significant issue in managing three-part fractures, further justifying more attention to improving current joint-preserving techniques and developing new methods as well. Recently, a low-profile fixed, angled plate with locking screws has gained popularity, with its theoretical advantage of having multiple fixed points of purchase within the plate (Fig. 13-1, A–D). However, a randomized prospective study using this device has yet to be published.

Closed Reduction and Percutaneous Pinning

Percutaneous pins have become popular as a minimal fixation device for proximal humerus fractures[10,16,32,33,40,69,86,96] (Fig. 13-2, A–C). The primary benefit from closed reduction and percutaneous pinning is the minimally invasive nature of the procedure; the technique relies on ligamentotaxis and sufficient bone. In theory, the blood supply to the humeral head is at less risk because no soft-tissue dissection is required for this technique. As with other fixation techniques, bone with purchase is essential to allow for early motion. However, soft-tissue interposition precludes this technique, and technically, this procedure is demanding with a steep learning curve.[40] Herscovici et al. reviewed 36 patients with an average age of 50 years treated with percutaneous pinning for 37 proximal humerus fractures; there were 21 two-part, 16 three-part, and 4 four-part fractures.[33] The average age for the three-part fracture group was 56 years. Some of the fixation devices did not have ter-

minal threads. They emphasized wide pin spread to maximize stability. There were eight complications in this group. All five patients treated with K-wires had loosening and failure of fixation; two patients had malunion of less than 15 degrees, and one developed osteomyelitis. The remaining ten patients had an average shoulder score of 70.4 (range, 27–100), with an average forward elevation of 108 degrees. All 4 four-part fracture patients did not respond to fixation; there were three cases of AVN, and two of varus deformity greater than 57 degrees. They concluded that threaded pins should be used, and that stable fixation allowing early motion with good results can be expected in patients with two- and three-part fractures.

Soete et al. reported on 31 patients with a mean age of 68 years who underwent transitory percutaneous pinning for displaced proximal humerus fractures.[86] There were 7 two-part, 20 three-part, and 4 four-part fractures. They used 2.5-mm terminally threaded pins. The mean follow-up was 45 months. They reported a high satisfactory rate for three-part fractures, with an average functional score of 55 out of 65. Complications included infection, loss of reduction, and AVN; there were no cases of significant pin migration. The mean Constant score of 83% was not as high as that reported by Resch et al., whose cohort (average age of 54 years) had a mean Constant score of 91% for three-part fractures.[69] Soete et al. attributed this to the comparably high mean age of their patients. Ease of pin removal was considered an advantage. They concluded that percutaneous pinning is a good technique for proximal humerus fractures, pointing out that the shoulder can tolerate moderate residual deformity. They emphasized that this technique preserves whatever blood supply remains.

Disadvantages of this technique include pin migration, loss of reduction, and infection.[33,40,51,82] Given the increasing use of this technique,[10,16,32,33,40,69,86,96] recent studies have emerged emphasizing the potential technical risks involved. Hernigou and Germany found unrecognized pin joint penetration in 8 of 30 patients during fixation of unstable surgical neck (SN) fractures.[32] Rowles and McGrory recommended that lateral pins should be distal enough to avoid the axillary nerve (anterior branch) and favored multiple fluoroscopic views to avoid joint penetration.[73] They found no truly safe zone anteriorly, because the cephalic vein, the long head biceps tendon, and the musculocutaneous nerve were at imminent risk. The greater tuberosity pins should be placed with the arm in external rotation to move the axillary nerve and the posterior humeral circumflex artery farther away from the surgical neck, while aiming for a point 20 mm or more from the inferior aspect of the humeral head. The patho-anatomy, such as hematoma and fracture displacement, may alter the anatomical relationships reported in this study.

In summary, closed reduction and percutaneous pinning theoretically minimize AVN as soft tissue dissection is minimized, and reports show satisfactory results for three-

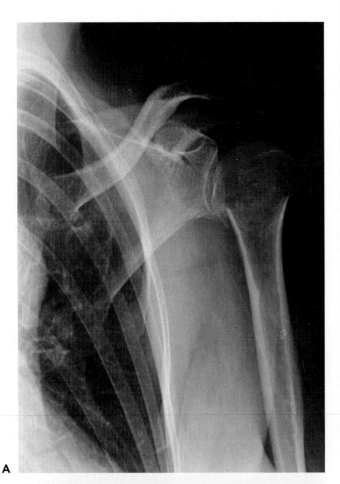

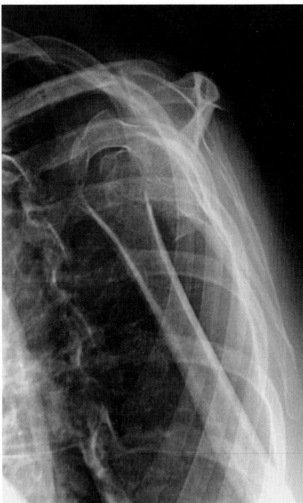

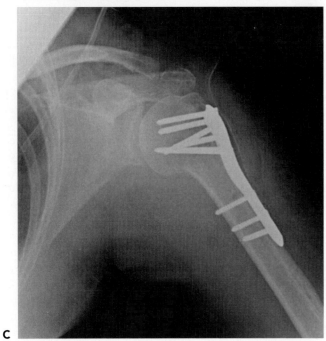

Figure 13-1 (*A*) Preoperative anteroposterior (AP) radiograph revealing a three-part fracture; greater tuberosity displacement is evident on this view. (*B*) Preoperative scapular-lateral radiograph of the same fracture; the surgical neck is displaced. (*C*) Postoperative AP radiograph showing satisfactory reduction using a low-profile fixed, angled plate with locking screws. (*continued*)

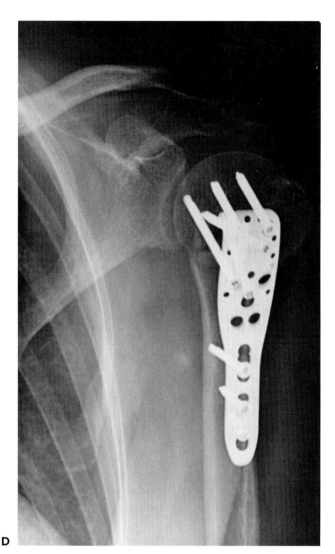

D

Figure 13-1 *(continued)* *(D)* Postoperative AP internal rotation view. The plate is below the greater tuberosity, thus avoiding impingement.

part fractures. However, the procedure is technically demanding, and failures of fixation can occur, especially in patients with osteoporotic bone. The patho-anatomy must be appreciated to avoid iatrogenic injury.

ORIF: Principles, Techniques, and Aftercare

The key to successful ORIF of three-part fractures is selecting the proper patient. First, recognizing the three-part fracture pattern is crucial. The AVN rates after operative treatment for three- and four-part fractures are 12% to 25% and 41% to 59%, respectively.[24] In terms of patho-anatomy, only one intact tuberosity differentiates three- and four-part fractures. Should the soft tissue to the intact tuberosity be compromised, a four-part equivalent pattern may be created with respect to potential for AVN, particularly in the elderly population with fragile soft tissues.

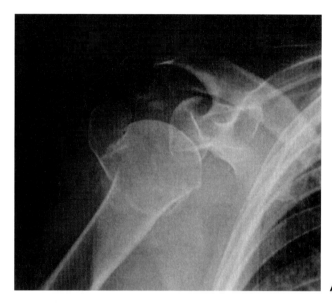

A

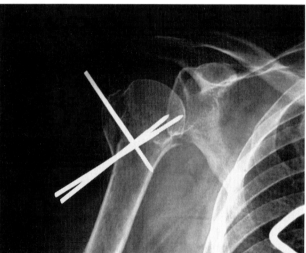

B

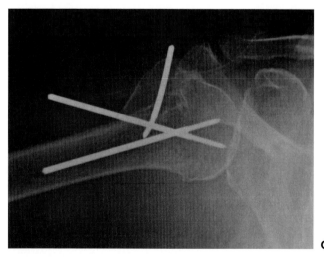

C

Figure 13-2 *(A)* Preoperative anteroposterior (AP) radiograph revealing a three-part valgus impacted surgical neck and greater tuberosity fracture. *(B)* Postoperative AP radiograph showing satisfactory reduction with three percutaneous pins; the greater tuberosity is adequately below the humeral head. *(C)* Postoperative axillary radiograph from the same patient.

Once a three-part fracture has been correctly identified, the two essential factors in the decision for ORIF are: (1) bone quality and (2) humeral head viability—bone quality for fixation and stability to allow early motion, and humeral head viability via intact soft tissues to minimize the risk of AVN. Soft tissue status is affected by the mechanism and pattern of injury, and the iatrogenic trauma of surgery. The patient must be able to comply with therapy.[3,15,16,21,30,37,52,53,59,64,94] Better outcomes have been reported in younger patients who have sufficient bone.[15,20,42,3,59,69,75]

The assessment of bone quality and humeral head viability begins with the history, physical examination, and radiographic trauma series. The age and sex of the patient can lead to the expectation of osteoporosis, with elderly women at highest risk.[50,71] The mechanism of injury is a gauge of potential bony comminution and soft-tissue injury, for example, in a fracture-dislocation. A medical history (e.g., steroid use or previous fractures) can also help the surgeon assess the likely bone quality of the patient. The personality of the patient will have potential effect on postoperative physical therapy compliance; a noncompliant patient is a contraindication to surgery.[16,94] The physical exam can give a measure of the traumatic energy encountered by the patient. Deformity and asymmetrical shoulder contour raises the suspicion of glenohumeral dislocation, which represents the maximal displacement of fracture fragments and is often accompanied by comminution and soft-tissue injury. The brachial plexus is particularly susceptible to fracture dislocations. Asymmetrical pulses are an ominous sign for severe arterial injury. As per Neer, a radiographic trauma series is required to classify these fractures and to guide treatment.[58,59] Radiographs in three orthogonal views also give a direct visual measure of the patient's bone quality and the degree of displacement or comminution. Computed tomography and MRI may give additional information regarding bone quality and soft-tissue injury.

Once the history, physical examination, and radiographic studies have confirmed the potential to reconstruct a stable reduction, with a viable humeral head, the technical aspects of open reduction must be considered. Ideally, ORIF should be performed acutely,[59,60] and there must be adequate bone to allow for a stable reconstruction that can tolerate early motion postoperatively.[15,30,52,64] For this reason, the surgeon and the operating team must always be prepared to perform humeral head replacement in the event that the head is found to be avascular, or the bone will not allow fixation for early postoperative motion.

Many operative techniques have been used to treat displaced proximal humerus fractures, including plates,[20,30,34,35,39,63,93,94,98] pins,[10,16,32,33,40,69,86,96] staples,[19] screws,[14] intramedullary nails,[15,45,49,55,62,65,90,92] wires,[9,14,30,59] sutures,[16,21,59,64] and combinations of these devices.[14–16,30,45] Current trends in surgical technique include limiting soft-tissue dissection around the fracture fragments, minimizing the use of hardware required for stable fixation, and using percutaneous pinning techniques as discussed previously.[15,33,40,45,64,69,86,90] The ultimate goal is to create a stable construct with minimal risk for AVN.

ORIF utilizes the deltopectoral approach for three-part fractures, allowing surgical neck and tuberosity exposure. The rotator interval can be extended to facilitate exposure of the fracture site and the articular surface; the interval is closed anatomically before closure to avoid loss of external rotation. It is important that the suture for approximation of the interval should be placed laterally only.

In cases of three-part fractures with sufficient bone quality and minimal comminution, as often occurs in younger patients, rigid fixation, such as plates, can be employed.[20,53,75] More recent reports, emphasizing minimal dissection, show the successful use of plates in the elderly population.[94] Care must be taken to avoid creating a construct with proud hardware that might impinge on the acromion, and the anterolateral branch of the anterior humeral circumflex artery must be preserved during extensive dissections to avoid AVN.[23,46,68,87] Hardware-related problems, such as migration, failure, impingement, and reoperations, are disadvantages to rigid metallic fixation.[20,63,94]

In the majority of three-part fractures, the authors prefer using heavy nonabsorbable polyester sutures or 18-gauge figure-of-eight wires; these must incorporate the rotator cuff[64] (Fig. 13-3, A–D). The rotator cuff is an essential fixation point, especially in elderly patients with soft bone.[3,4,11,15,21,30,64] Modified Enders rods can be used for comminuted surgical neck fractures to achieve longitudinal and rotational stability[15]; Williams et al. showed that the addition of Enders rods to interfragmentary wire sutures alone, in cadaveric humeri, improves resistance to torsional load by a factor of 1.5.[95]

However, the authors' recent study shows that suture fixation without hardware can provide adequate stability for early motion.[64] The benefits of minimal dissection are used with this technique, and hardware complications are avoided. The technical surgical goal is to create a nondisplaced or minimally displaced fracture pattern that is stable. The greater tuberosity must be reduced anatomically to avoid impingement. Anterior acromioplasty is not a routine part of this procedure, but should be performed if mechanical subacromial impingement is present. Notably, slight residual surgical neck deformity does not preclude a satisfactory outcome[33,40,52,64,86]; however, an anatomical reduction should always be attempted in proximal humerus fractures at risk for AVN.[23]

Once the fracture has been reconstructed, including any rotator cuff tears, the shoulder is taken through a gentle range of motion as tolerated to assess stability. This intraoperative range of motion dictates the immediate postoperative physical therapy regimen. The three-phase protocol

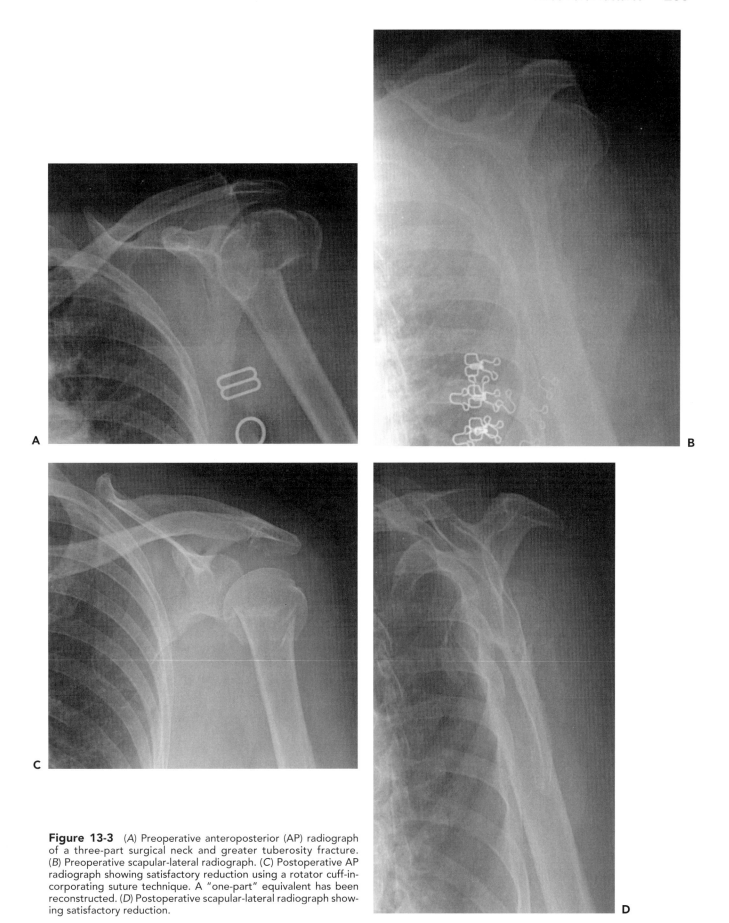

Figure 13-3 (*A*) Preoperative anteroposterior (AP) radiograph of a three-part surgical neck and greater tuberosity fracture. (*B*) Preoperative scapular-lateral radiograph. (*C*) Postoperative AP radiograph showing satisfactory reduction using a rotator cuff-incorporating suture technique. A "one-part" equivalent has been reconstructed. (*D*) Postoperative scapular-lateral radiograph showing satisfactory reduction.

described by Hughes and Neer[37] is initiated within the first postoperative week, depending on pain control. Pendulums are started immediately; in addition, supine assisted forward flexion to 120 degrees and external rotation with a stick to 30 degrees is instructed. Usually, 6 weeks postoperatively, after clinical and radiographic evidence of early healing is present, gentle stretching and pulley-assisted elevation are initiated; isometric strengthening of the rotator cuff and deltoid is encouraged. Between 8 to 12 weeks, more aggressive stretching and strengthening is allowed, using rubber bands and light weights, for example. Patients are graduated to a home program on an individual basis during different phases at the discretion of the surgeon and physical therapist.

Results of ORIF

Numerous studies report satisfactory ORIF results for three-part fractures, both when the mean age was less than 60 years[15,20,53,59,75] and when the mean age was 60 years and over.[16,30,35,64,94] Ostensibly, elderly patients with osteopenic three-part fractures are not precluded from successful results with joint-preserving ORIF. Two recent studies represent the spectrum of devices used for these fractures—sutures[64] and plates.[94]

Wanner et al. reported on 60 patients with displaced two-, three-, and four-part proximal humerus fractures treated with two one-third tubular plates.[94] Thirty-three (55%) of these patients had three-part fractures. The overall average age was 62 years, and the average follow-up was 17 months. Inclusion criteria included the patient's predicted ability to participate in postoperative physical therapy. All patients were operated on within 72 hours after admission. Minimal dissection and anatomical reduction was emphasized in their technique. When poor bone quality was encountered and the screws did not tighten adequately, bone cement was injected into the plate screw holes (n = 9). For complex fractures where stable fixation was not achieved by the two plates, additional osteosutures were used (n = 6). This study showed 88% excellent to satisfactory results that were independent of age (cutoff, 60 years) and fracture-type (two-, three-, or four-part). There were hardware-related problems among the three-part fracture group: two patients had subacromial impingement of the lateral plate, and one had loosening; all these patients required a second operation. There were no cases of AVN in the three-part group. The constructs allowed for early motion in compliant patients. Their results for patients with four-part fractures were not significantly different than for two- or three-part fractures, and they recommend that these patients, too, should be treated with ORIF, provided there is adequate compliance and low comorbidity.

More recently, Park et al. reported on the clinical and radiographic outcomes for two- and three-part fractures treated solely with rotator cuff-incorporating heavy nonab-

sorbable sutures.[64] There were 27 patients (28 shoulders) with an average age of 64 years. The average follow-up was 4.4 years. Extensive dissection was not required for this technique. The rotator cuff is a mandatory point of fixation, especially in patients with osteoporotic bone. The goal was to create a nondisplaced to minimally displaced construct. Overall, 89% of patients had excellent or satisfactory results, and the average American Shoulder and Elbow Surgeons (ASES) score[70] was 87 (range, 35–100). All six patients with three-part fractures achieved excellent results. There were no cases of AVN, and all hardware-related complications were obviated. Four patients had varus or valgus malunion not exceeding 20 degrees; three had excellent results. The three patients with unsatisfactory results failed to progress with physical therapy in a timely manner. This study showed that sutures incorporating the rotator cuff can provide stability sufficient to allow early motion. Although the goal is to reconstruct a "one-part" equivalent, some residual deformity does not preclude an excellent outcome. A compliant patient is crucial for a successful result.

In summary, these studies[64,94] highlight the important factors in achieving successful outcomes in patients treated with ORIF for three-part fractures. Bone quality is critical for reconstruction; when bone is osteoporotic, additional fixation is essential (e.g., bone reinforcement with cement,[94] incorporating the rotator cuff[3,64]) to creating a construct stable enough to tolerate early motion. Limiting soft-tissue dissection and bone stripping preserves any residual blood supply to the humeral head. An anatomical reduction should be strived for, although some surgical neck residual deformity does not preclude an excellent outcome. Compliance with therapy determines the ultimate success in outcome.

PRACTICAL RULES FOR DECIDING BETWEEN ORIF AND HEMIARTHROPLASTY

The key factors when contemplating ORIF are (1) bone quality and (2) humeral head viability. These factors should be assessed using information extracted from the history, physical examination, and radiographic studies. "Bone quality" factors include the extent of osteoporosis and the degree of comminution; these can be assessed primarily from the patient's age, gender, mechanism of injury, and radiographs. Factors for "humeral head viability" include the extent of the primary injury (e.g., presence of dislocation) and the surgical technique in relation to the periarticular soft tissues. In most cases, ORIF can be performed for three-part fractures. Blood supply to the humeral head comes from periarticular soft tissues, with a major contribution along the bicipital groove; an intraosseous supply may exist as well. Therefore, as long as either the soft tissues are viable and contiguous with the head *or* the bone has sufficient purchase to create a stable construct, ORIF is always a potentially successful joint-preserving intervention—especially with improved surgical techniques. In the rare case where *both* severe osteoporosis and an avascular humeral head (whether a result of the injury, the limitations of a particular surgical technique, or a combination thereof) exist, hemiarthroplasty should be considered to allow the earliest possible motion.

REFERENCES

1. Bengner U, Johnell O, Redlund-Johnell I. Changes in the incidence of fracture of the upper end of the humerus during a 30-year period: a study of 2,125 fractures. Clin Orthop Rel Res 1988;231:179.
2. Bernstein J, Adler LM, Blank JE, et al. Evaluation of the Neer system of classification of proximal humeral fractures with computerized tomographic scans and plain radiographs. J Bone Joint Surg [Am] 1996;78(9):1371.
3. Bigliani LU. Proximal humerus fractures. In: Post M, Bigliani LU, Flatow EL, et al., eds. The shoulder: operative technique. Baltimore, Williams & Wilkins, 1998.
4. Bigliani LU, Flatow EL, Pollock RG. Fractures of the proximal humerus. In Rockwood CA Jr, Matsen FA, eds. The shoulder, 2nd ed, vol 2. Philadelphia, WB Saunders, 1998.
5. Blasier RB, Burkus JK. Management of posterior fracture dislocations of the shoulder. Clin Orthop 1988;232:199.
6. Blom S, Dahlback LO. Nerve injuries in dislocations of the shoulder joint and fractures of the neck of the humerus: a clinical and electromyographical study. Acta Chir Scand 1970;136:461.
7. Bloom MH, Obata WG. Diagnosis of posterior dislocation of the shoulder with use of Velpeau axillary and angle up roentgenographic views. J Bone Joint Surg [Am] 1967;49:943.
8. Brooks CH, Revell WJ, Heatley FW. Vascularity of the humeral head after proximal humeral fractures: an anatomical cadaver study. J Bone Joint Surg [Br] 1993;75:132.
9. Bungaro P, Pascarella R, Rollo G, et al. Osteosynthesis with percutaneous wiring in fractures of the proximal humerus. Chir Organi Mov 1998;83:381.
10. Chen CY, Chao EK, Tu YK, et al. Closed management and percutaneous fixation of unstable proximal humerus fractures. J Trauma 1998;45(6):1039.
11. Codman EA. Fractures in relation to the subacromial bursa. In: Codman E, ed. The shoulder: rupture of the supraspinatus tendon and other lesions in or about the subacromial bursa, 1st ed. Boston, Thomas Todd, 1934.
12. Compito CA, Self EB, Bigliani LU. Arthroplasty and acute shoulder trauma. Reasons for success and failure. Clin Orthop 1994;307:27.
13. Constant CR, Murley AHG. A clinical method of functional assessment of the shoulder. Clin Orthop 1987;214:160.
14. Cornell CN, Levine D, Pagnani MJ. Internal fixation of proximal humerus fractures using the screw-tension band technique. J Orthop Trauma 1994;8(1):23.
15. Cuomo F, Flatow EL, Maday MG, et al. Open reduction and internal fixation of two- and three-part displaced surgical neck fractures of the proximal humerus. J Shoulder Elbow Surg 1992;1(6):287.
16. De la Hoz Marin J, Hernandez Cortes P, Tercedeor Sanchez J. Surgical treatment of three-part proximal humeral fractures. Acta Orthop Belg 2001;67(3):226.
17. Dimakopoulos P, Potamis N, Lambris E. Hemiarthroplasty in the treatment of comminuted intra-articular fractures of the proximal humerus. Clin Orthop 1997;341:7.
18. Din KM, Meggitt BF. Bilateral four-part fractures with posterior dislocation of the shoulder: a case report. J Bone Joint Surg Br 1983;65:176.
19. Doursounian L, Grimberg J, Cazeau C, et al. A new internal fixation technique for fractures of the proximal humerus—the Bilboquet device: a report on 26 cases. J Shoulder Elbow Surg 2000;9(4):279.
20. Esser RD. Treatment of three- and four-part fractures of the proximal humerus with a modified cloverleaf plate. J Orthop Trauma 1994;8:15.
21. Flatow EL, Coumo F, Maday MG, et al. Open reduction and internal fixation of two-part displaced fractures of the greater tuberosity of the proximal part of the humerus. J Bone Joint Surg Am 1991;73(8):1213.
22. Gallagher JC, Melton LJ, Riggs BL, et al. Epidemiology of fractures of the proximal femur in Rochester, Minnesota. Clin Orthop 1980;150:163.
23. Gerber C, Hersche O, Berberat C. The clinical relevance of posttraumatic avascular necrosis of the humeral head. J Shoulder Elbow Surg 1998;7(6):586.
24. Gerber C, Warner JJP. Alternatives to hemiarthroplasty for complex proximal-humeral fractures. In: Warner JJP, Iannotti JP, Gerber C, eds. Complex and revision problems in shoulder surgery. Philadelphia, Lippincott-Raven, 1997.
25. Gerber C, Lambert SM, Hoogewoud HM. Absence of avascular necrosis of the humeral head after post-traumatic rupture of the anterior and posterior humeral circumflex arteries. J Bone Joint Surg Am 1996;78:1256.
26. Goldman RT, Koval KJ, Cuomo F, et al. Functional outcome after humeral head replacement for acute three- and four-part proximal humeral fractures. J Shoulder Elbow Surg 1995;4(2):81.
27. Green A, Barnard WL, Limbird RS. Humeral head replacement for acute four-part proximal humerus fractures. J Shoulder Elbow Surg 1993;2:249.
28. Hagg O, Lundberg B. Aspects of prognostic factors in comminuted and dislocated proximal humeral fractures. In Bateman JE, Welsh RP, eds. Surgery of the shoulder. Philadelphia, BC Decker, 1984.
29. Hartsock LA, Estes WJ, Murray CA, et al. Shoulder hemiarthroplasty for proximal humeral fractures. Orthop Clin North Am 1998;29(3):467.
30. Hawkins RJ, Bell RH, Gurr K. The three-part fracture of the proximal part of the humerus. J Bone Joint Surg Am 1986;68(9):1410.
31. Hawkins RJ, Switlyk P. Acute prosthetic replacement for severe fractures of the proximal humerus. Clin Orthop 1993;289:156.
32. Hernigou P, Germany W. Unrecognized shoulder joint penetration during fixation of proximal fractures of the humerus. Acta Orthop Scand 2002;73(2):140.
33. Herscovici D Jr, Saunders DT, Johnson MP, et al. Percutaneous fixation of proximal humeral fractures. Clin Orthop 2000;375:97.
34. Hessman M, Baumgaertel F, Gehling H, et al. Plate fixation of proximal humeral fractures with indirect reduction: surgical technique and results utilizing three shoulder scores. Injury 1999;30(7):453.
35. Hintermann B, Trouillier HH, Schafer D. Rigid internal fixation of fractures of the proximal humerus in older patients. J Bone Joint Surg Br 2000;82(8):1107.
36. Horak J, Nilsson BE. Epidemiology of fracture of the upper end of the humerus. Clin Orthop 1975;112:150.
37. Hughes M, Neer II CS. Glenohumeral joint replacement and postoperative rehabilitation. Phys Ther 1975;55:850.
38. Ilchmann T, Ochsner PE, Wingstrand H, et al. Non-operative treatment versus tension-band osteosynthesis in three- and four-part proximal humeral fractures. Int Orthop 1998;22(5):316.
39. Instrum K, Fennel C, Shrive N, et al. Semitubular blade plate fixation in proximal humeral fractures. J Shoulder Elbow Surg 1995;7:462.
40. Jaberg H, Warner JJP, Jakob R. Percutaneous stabilization of unstable fractures of the humerus. J Bone Joint Surg Am 1992;74:508.
41. Jakob RP, Kristiansen T, Mayo K, et al. Classification and aspects of treatment of fractures of the proximal humerus. In Bateman J, Welsh RP, eds. Surgery of the shoulder. St. Louis, CV Mosby, 1984.
42. Jakob RP, Miniaci A, Anson PS, et al. Four-part valgus impacted fractures of the proximal humerus. J Bone Joint Surg Br 1991;73(2):295.

43. Jurik AG, Albrechtsen J. The use of computed tomography with two- and three-dimensional reconstructions in the diagnosis of three- and four-part fractures of the proximal humerus. Clin Radiol 1994;49:800.

44. Kay SP, Amstutz HC. Shoulder hemiarthroplasty at UCLA. Clin Orthop 1988;228:42.

45. Khodadadyan-Klostermann C, Raschke M, Fontes R, et al. Treatment of complex proximal humeral fractures with minimally invasive fixation of the humeral head combined with flexible intramedullary wire fixation: introduction of a new treatment concept. Langenbecks Arch Surg 2002;387(3–4):153.

46. Kuner EH, Siebler G. Dislocation fractures of the proximal humerus: results following surgical treatment: a follow-up study of 167 cases (in German). Unfallchirurgie 1987;13:64.

47. Laing PG. The arterial supply to the adult humerus. J Bone Joint Surg Am 1956;38:1105.

48. Leyshon RL. Closed treatment of fractures of the proximal humerus. Acta Orthop Scand 1984;55:48.

49. Lin J, Hou SM, Hang YS. Locked nailing for displaced surgical neck fractures of the humerus. J Trauma 1998;45:1051.

50. Lind T, Kroner TK, Jensen J. The epidemiology of fractures of the proximal humerus. Arch Orthop Trauma Surg 1989;108:285.

51. Maurer F. Sequestered bone infection after Kirschner wire osteosynthesis of humeral head fracture (German). Acktuelle Traumatol 1993;23:380.

52. McLaughlin HL. Injuries of the shoulder and arm. In: McLaughlin HL, ed. Trauma. Philadelphia, WB Saunders, 1959.

53. Moda SK, Chadha NS, Sangwan SS, et al. Open-reduction and fixation of proximal humerus fractures and fracture-dislocations. J Bone Joint Surg Br 1990;72(6):1050.

54. Moeckel BH, Dines DM, Warren RF, et al. Modular hemiarthroplasty for fractures of the proximal part of the humerus. J Bone Joint Surg 1992;74(6):884.

55. Monin S, van Innis F. Fractures of the proximal end of the humerus treated by the Kapandji centro-medullary nailing technique: a review of 21 cases. Acta Orthop Belg 1999;65:176.

56. Moriber LA, Patterson RL Jr. Fractures of the proximal end of the humerus. J Bone Joint Surg Am 1967;49:1018.

57. Movin T, Sjoden GO, Ahrengart L. Poor function after shoulder replacement in fracture patients. A retrospective evaluation of 29 patients followed for 2–12 years. Acta Orthop Scand 1998;69 (4):392.

58. Neer II CS. Displaced proximal humeral fractures. Part 1: classification and evaluation. J Bone Joint Surg Am1970;52:1077.

59. Neer II CS. Displaced proximal humeral fractures. Part 2: treatment of three-part and four-part displacement. J Bone Joint Surg Am 1970;52:1090.

60. Neer II CS. Indications for replacement of the proximal humeral articulation. Am J Surg 1955;89:901.

61. Neer II CS, Brown Jr TH, McLaughlin HL. Fracture of the neck of the humerus with dislocation of the head fragment. Am J Surg 1953;85:252.

62. Ogiwara N, Aoki M, Okamura K, et al. Ender nailing for unstable surgical neck fractures of the humerus in elderly patients. Clin Orthop 1996;330:173.

63. Palmer SH, Handley R, Willett K. The use of interlocked "customized" blade plates in the treatment of metaphyseal fractures in patients with poor bone stock. Injury 2000;31(3):187.

64. Park MC, Murthi AM, Roth NS, et al. Two-part and three-part fractures of the proximal humerus treated with suture fixation. J Orthop Trauma 2003;17(5):319.

65. Rajasekhar C, Ray PS, Bhamra MS. Fixation of proximal humeral fractures with the Polarus nail. J Shoulder Elbow Surg 2001; 10(1):7.

66. Rasmussen S, Hvass I, Dalsgaard J, et al. Displaced proximal humeral fractures: results of conservative treatment. Injury 1992;23(1):41.

67. Reckling FW. Posterior fracture-dislocation of the shoulder treated by a Neer hemiarthroplasty with a posterior surgical approach. Clin Orthop 1986;207:133.

68. Rees J, Hicks J, Ribbans W. Assessment and management of three- and four-part proximal humeral fractures. Clin Orthop 1998; 353:18.

69. Resch H, Povacz P, Frohlich R, et al. Percutaneous fixation of three- and four-part fractures of the proximal humerus. J Bone Joint Surg Br 1997;79:295.

70. Richards RR, An Kai-Nan, Bigliani LU, et al. A standardized method for the assessment of shoulder function. J Shoulder Elbow Surg 1994;3(6):347.

71. Rose SH, Melton LJ III, Morrey BF, et al. Epidemiologic features of humeral fractures. Clin Orthop 1982;168:24.

72. Rothman RH, Parke WW. The vascular anatomy of the rotator cuff. Clin Orthop 1985;41:176.

73. Rowles DJ, McGrory JE. Percutaneous pinning of the proximal part of the humerus: an anatomic study. J Bone Joint Surg Am 2001;83:1695.

74. Salem MI. Bilateral anterior fracture-dislocation of the shoulder joints due to severe electric shock. Injury 1983;14:361.

75. Savoie FH, Geissler WB, Vander Griend RA. Open reduction and internal fixation of three-part fractures of the proximal humerus. Orthopedics 1989;12(1):65.

76. Schai P, Imhoff A, Preiss S. Comminuted humeral head fractures: a multicenter analysis. J Shoulder Elbow Surg 1995;4(5):319.

77. Schai P, Imhoff A, Staubli AE. Differentialdiagnostik und Therapie der mehrfragmentaren Humeruskopffraktur—eine Analyse aus drei klinischen Studien. Z Unfallchir Versicherungsmed 1993;86 (1):27.

78. Seggl W, Weiglein A. Die arterielle Blutversorgung des Oberarmkopfes und ihre prognostische Bedeutung bei Luxationen, Frakturen und Luxationsfrakturen des Oberarmkopfes. Acta Chir Austriaca 1991;23(suppl 92):1.

79. Shaw JL. Bilateral posterior fracture-dislocation of the shoulder and other trauma caused by convulsive seizures. J Bone Joint Surg Am 1971;53:1437.

80. Sidor ML, Zuckerman JD, Lyon T, et al. The Neer classification system for proximal humeral fractures: an assessment of interobserver reliability and intraobserver reproducibility. J Bone Joint Surg Am 1993;75(12):1745.

81. Siebenrock KA, Gerber C. The reproducibility of classification of fractures of the proximal end of the humerus. J Bone Joint Surg Am 1993;75(12):1751.

82. Siebler G, Walz H, Kuner E. Minimal osteosynthesis of fractures of the head of the humerus: indications, technique, results (German). Unfallchirurg 1989;92:169.

83. Sjoden GOJ, Movin T, Aspelin P, et al. 3D-radiographic analysis does not improve the Neer and AO classifications of proximal humeral fractures. Acta Orthop Scand 1999;70(4):325.

84. Sjoden GOJ, Movin T, Guntner P, et al. Poor reproducibility of classification of proximal humeral fractures. Additional CT of minor value. Acta Orthop Scand 1997;68(3):239.

85. Skutek M, Fremerey RW, Bosch U. Level of physical activity in elderly patients after hemiarthroplasty for three- and four-part fractures of the proximal humerus. Arch Orthop Trauma Surg 1998;117(4–5):252.

86. Soete PJ, Clayson PE, Costenoble VH. Transitory percutaneous pinning in fractures of the proximal humerus. J Shoulder Elbow Surg 1999;8(6):569.

87. Speck M, Lang FJH, Regazzoni P. Proximal humeral multiple fragment fractures: failures after T-plate osteosynthesis (in German). Swiss Surg 1996;2:51.

88. Stableforth PG. Four-part fractures of the neck of the humerus. J Bone Joint Surg Br 1984;66:104.

89. Svend-Hansen H. Displaced proximal humeral fractures. Acta Orthop Scand 1974;56:359.

90. Takeuchi R, Koshino T, Nakazawa A, et al. Minimally invasive fixation for unstable two-part proximal humeral fractures: surgical techniques and clinical results using J-nails. J Orthop Trauma 2002;16(6):403.

91. Tanner MW, Cofield RH. Prosthetic arthroplasty for fractures and fracture-dislocations of the proximal humerus. Clin Orthop 1983;179:116.

92. Wachtl SW, Marti CB, Hoogewoud HM, et al. Treatment of proximal humerus fracture using multiple intramedullary flexible nails. Arch Orthop Trauma Surg 2000;120(3–4):171.

93. Wanner GA, Romero J, Hersche O, et al. Dislocated proximal humerus fracture: results after stabilization with a double plate. Langenbecks Arch Chir Suppl Kongressbd 1998;115:1211.

94. Wanner GA, Wanner-Schmid E, Romero J, et al. Internal fixation of displaced proximal humeral fractures with two one-third tubular plates. J Trauma 2003;54(3):536.

95. Williams GR, Copley LA, Iannotti JP, et al. The influence of intramedullary fixation on figure-of-eight wiring for surgical neck fractures of the proximal humerus: a biomechanical comparison. J Shoulder Elbow Surg 1997;6(5):423.

96. Williams GR Jr, Wong KL. Two-part and three-part fractures: open reduction and internal fixation versus closed reduction and percutaneous pinning. Orthop Clin North Am 2000;31(1):1.

97. Wretenberg P, Ekelund A. Acute hemiarthroplasty after proximal humerus fracture in old patients: a retrospective evaluation of 18 patients for 2–7 years. Acta Orthop Scand 1997;68(2):121.

98. Yamano Y. Comminuted fractures of the proximal humerus treated with hook plate. Arch Orthop Trauma Surg 1986; 105:359.

99. Young TB, Wallace WA. Conservative treatment of fractures and fracture dislocations of the upper end of the humerus. J Bone Joint Surg Br 1985;67(3):373.

100. Zyto K. Non-operative treatment of comminuted fractures of the proximal humerus in elderly patients. Injury 1998;29(5): 349.

101. Zyto K, Ahrengart L, Sperber A, et al. Treatment of displaced proximal humeral fractures in elderly patients. J Bone Joint Surg Br 1997;79(3):412.

102. Zyto K, Kronberg M, Brostrum L-A. Shoulder function after displaced fractures of the proximal humerus. J Shoulder Elbow Surg 1995;4(5):331.

103. Zyto K, Wallace WA, Frostick SP, et al. Outcome after hemiarthroplasty for three- and four-part fractures of the proximal humerus. J Shoulder Elbow Surg 1998;7(2):85.

Four-Part Proximal Humeral Fractures: ORIF

Erwin Aschauer   *Herbert Resch*

PATHOLOGY

Risk Factors

Fractures of the proximal humerus are very frequent injuries. About 4% of all fractures occur in this region,[14] and women are affected twice as frequently as men.[31] In comparison with proximal femoral fractures, the frequency is about 70% to 100%.[14,31] "Most of these fractures result from a fall on the outstretched arm in older people." These patients have osteoporotic bones, which are very fragile. Poor bone quality often leads to complex fractures, so it is not surprising that the severity of the injuries increases with age.[7] Court-Brown et al. reported in an epidemiological study that no less than 70% of the patients having three- or four-part fractures are older than 60 years, and more than 50% are older than 70 years.

Because free range of motion is so important for shoulder function during the different activities of everyday life, proper treatment of these difficult fractures requires careful consideration of the principles of soft-tissue treatment, as well as the principles of fracture treatment.

E. Aschauer: General Hospital Salzburg, Department for Trauma and Sport Traumatology, Salzburg, Austria.

H. Resch: General Hospital Salzburg, Department for Trauma and Sport Traumatology, Salzburg, Austria.

In severely displaced proximal humerus fractures, parts of the periosteum are disrupted, and, in some cases, there is no more connection between the fragments at all. Together with the periosteum, the blood vessels are destroyed, creating a risk of avascular necrosis of fragments, especially of the humeral head.[24] In the past, this was the reason to do a prosthesis in acutely displaced humeral head fractures; nowadays, we have acquired better knowledge of the blood supply of the humeral head and have new techniques at our disposal[2,12,13,20,22,27–29] to preserve periosteum and blood vessels during the operation.[5,9,25,27,33] Moreover, we believe that a secondarily implanted prosthesis, because of humeral head necrosis after primary osteosynthesis, has no worse outcome than that of prosthesis placed for an acute fracture.

Mechanisms of Injury

Proximal humerus fractures usually result from falling on the outstretched arm or a direct blow to the shoulder. The fracture pattern is determined by the interaction of the external forces applied to the arm and the internal forces of the intrinsic shoulder muscles. The upper arm is connected to the body by the thoracohumeral muscle (pectoralis major, latissimus dorsi) and the scapulohumeral muscles (deltoid, supraspinatus, infraspinatus, subscapularis, teres major, teres minor, biceps, and triceps). All of these muscles have an influence on the mechanism of injury and fracture type and can cause secondary displacement as well. The resulting force vector on the cuff to the intact humeral head would be directed downward and medially. The pectoralis major muscles, teres major and latissimus dorsi, pull the humeral shaft medially into internal rotation. The deltoid, biceps, and triceps muscles raise the arm against gravity (Fig. 14-1). Normally, the effects of the muscles on the different fragments after the fracture can be first seen some days after the injury. The reason is loss of muscle tension during early posttraumatic period. Knowledge of these facts is important to choose the right kind of treatment, conservative or operative, and, when operative, which implant.

Furthermore, position and fragment distances can indicate whether there are any periosteal connections. The muscles are usually fully tensioned at the moment of the fall, causing a fracture. Due to the muscle pull, the greater and lesser tuberosity will be displaced in three- and four-part fractures. Later, no more change of this position is possible, only the angulation of the shaft fragment will look different on the first x-ray. The tuberosities remain the same as they were at the moment of the accident.

Based on the principle of mechanisms of fractures you can distinguish between two kinds of fractures: avulsion fractures and impacted fractures (valgus fractures). Avulsion fractures are caused by the interaction of fall energy and the effects of the rotator cuff muscles on the humeral head. The main fracture line can be found along the surgical neck, where there is a weak transitional zone between cortical and cancellous bone. If there are no more fracture lines, a two-part fracture will result. Additional displace fracture planes features of tuberosities lead to three-part fractures. The rotator cuff does not lose its effect immediately after the fracture, which leads to typical displacements. In case of subcapital two-fragment fractures, a varus position will take place (Fig. 14-2A). Subcapital fracture and fracture of the lesser tuberosity lead to a mixed varus and externally rotated position of the humeral head (Fig. 14-2B). Fracture of the greater tuberosity, in addition to a subcapital fracture, leads to varus and internal rotation (Fig. 14-2C). The strength of the rotator cuff very often tears the periosteum, so these fractures are unstable and have a tendency to medially displace the shaft fragment. Because of the destroyed periosteum, the greater tuberosity goes up into the subacromial space; the lesser tuberosity mostly will be displaced medially. In four-part fractures, both tuberosities are broken over and the rotator cuff has no effect on the head anymore.

In impacted fractures, the axial force of the glenoid to the articular part of the humeral head pushes the head fragment down onto the metaphysis. The tuberosities break out and are pushed aside laterally and to the front. If the impaction of the head fragment is not too severe, the lesser tuberosity can remain on the head, resulting in a three-part valgus fracture. In most cases, however, both tuberosities are fractured (four-part valgus fracture), and there are two main fracture lines: one along the surgical neck and a second along the anatomic neck. The tuberosities remain in periosteal connection with the shaft fragment.

Avulsion Fractures

Surgical Neck Fractures
Often varus displacement of the head fragment takes place only days after injury. Depending on the condition of the periosteum on the medial side, the head fragment is displaced medially in different degrees (sometimes after a few days). In many cases, the head is in an excentric position, that is, situated dorsally to the axis of the humeral shaft. On an anteroposterior (AP) x-ray, this excentric malposition leads to an overlapping of anatomic structures and looks like impaction. An additional axial or trans-scapular view can avoid this misinterpretation (Fig. 14-3, A and B). It is typical to see this phenomenon only a few days after the injury, when the tension of the muscles comes back again.

Surgical Neck Fracture and Fracture of the Greater Tuberosity
Because of the fracture of the greater tuberosity, the supraspinatus and infraspinatus muscle no longer effect the humeral head. The only remaining muscle moving the

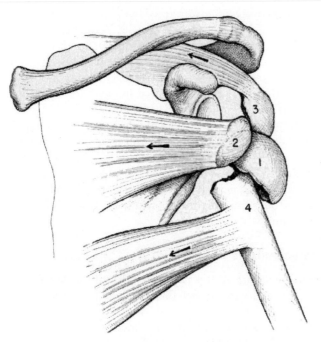

Figure 14-1 The typical displacements of the fragments occurring in four-part-fractures due to the effects of the rotator cuff: the shaft fragment is medialized through the pull of the pectoralis major muscle, the articular fragment falls into the defect of broken-out tuberosities and becomes impacted, the supraspinatus muscle pulls the greater direction cranially and dorsally, and the subscapular muscle leads to a medial displacement of the lesser tuberosity.

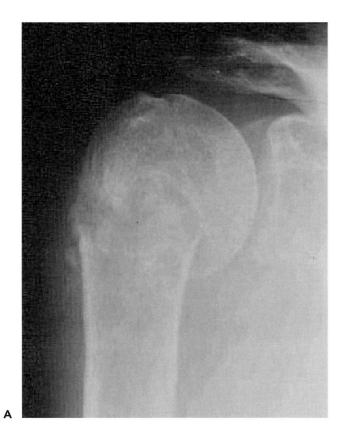

A

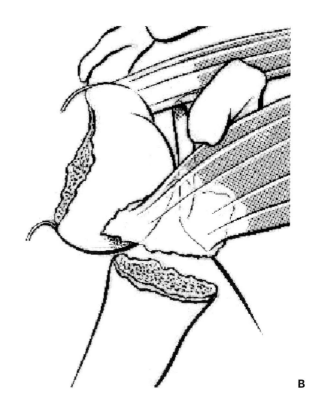

B

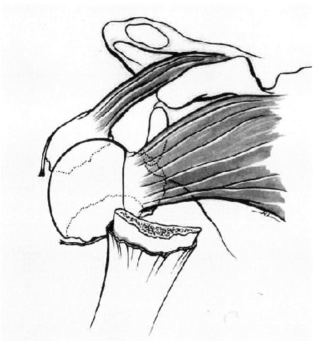

C

Figure 14-2 (A) Varus position of the head fragment in subcapital fractures according to the direction of the rotator cuff vector. (B) Mixed varus and externally rotated malposition in cases with additionally broken out lesser tuberosity because of loss of the effect of the subscapular muscle. (C) Varus and internal rotation in subcapital fractures combined with fracture of the greater tuberosity because of pull of the subscapular muscle.

humeral head is the subscapularis, which rotates the head internally without any resistance. The extent of the rotation depends on the condition of the periosteum between the head and the shaft. When all periosteal connections are disrupted, the head is rotated internally to the maximal extent and looks like a ball—perfectly circular—on the AP

x-ray. Corresponding to the lack of any connections, the humeral shaft is displaced medially to the head, caused by the pull of the pectoralis major. The greater tuberosity also has no more connection to the shaft and is displaced upward and dorsally by the pull of supraspinatus and infraspinatus.

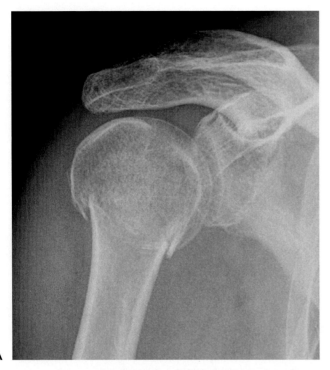
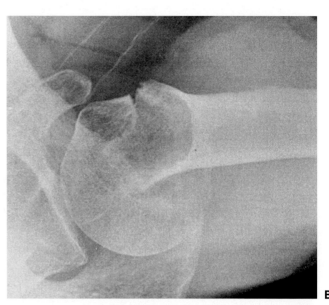

A
B

Figure 14-3   (A) This anteroposterior (AP) view looks like an impacted subcapital fracture, but (B), on the axial view, you can see that there is only an antecurvation of the fracture and no real impaction.

Surgical Neck Fracture and Fracture of the Lesser Tuberosity

After fracture of the lesser tuberosity, the subscapulary muscle has no more effect on the humeral head. The supraspinatus and infraspinatus pull the head in varus and external rotation. A completely destroyed periosteum leads to grotesque rotations of the head, and the pectoralis major displaces the shaft medially.

Impacted Valgus Fractures

Four-Part Fracture

The impact of the glenoid pushes the humeral head down toward the metaphysis, breaks the tuberosities out, and pushes them aside. The tuberosities remain at the right height, and their periosteal connections are not torn. The rotator cuff has no effect on the humeral head at all. The only connection between the head and shaft may be on the medial side in the form of remaining periosteum (so-called hinge periosteum). This periosteum is very important; it makes reduction easier and maintains the blood supply of the head. This periosteum is always intact if no lateral displacement occurs between the articular head fragment and the shaft. Biomechanical studies on cadavers have shown that the periosteum can bear 6 mm of lateral displacement and 9 mm of medial displacement[26,29] (Fig. 14-4, A and B). Normally, the impaction is not exactly axial; instead, a simultaneous tilt of the head frag-

ment to the dorsal takes place, so rotation is possible. This all creates a distorted picture on the x-rays, so it is not easy to find the correct diagnosis. The dorsal tilt, however, ensures that the dorsomedial periosteum remains, even with lateral displacement.

Concomitant Injuries

The mechanism leading to a fracture of the proximal humerus, in most cases, is a fall on the outstretched arm from standing—or even less—height, particularly with older people. The injury only needs to be moderate in degree because osteoporosis is usually present. In this group of patients, proximal humeral fractures commonly occur as single injuries without any associated fractures.

With younger people, the severity of injury is usually more serious. The resulting fractures are often more complicated, more displaced, and sometimes dislocated. In addition, there is more soft-tissue damage, such as contusions, disruptions of tendons and muscles, or even lesions of nerves and blood vessels. Many fractures of the proximal humerus occur in patients with multiple traumas. In those cases, the upper arm injury is not the main problem, and attention is focused on more life-threatening problems. It is not unusual, howevr, to later detect the fracture by chance on a chest x-ray.

Electric shocks or convulsive episodes can cause shoulder dislocations and fracture dislocations. The dislocations can be both anterior and posterior and are easily overlooked.

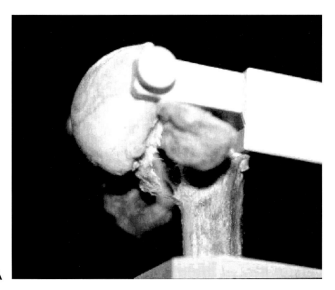

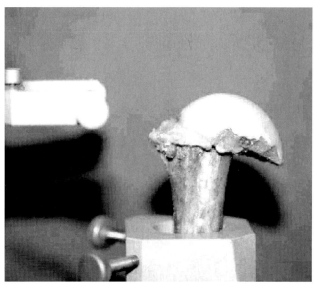

Figure 14-4 (*A*) A biomechanical study detected that in cases of displacement of the head to the medial the periosteum is stripped off the shaft and can bear 9 mm of medialization, after 15 mm it is disrupted in all cases. (*B*) On the other hand, displacement to the lateral leads to disruption of the periosteum between 6 and 11 mm because it is stretched over the edge of the shaft fragment.

Another ethiology for fractures of the proximal humerus is metastatic disease. In weakened bones, fractures can occur without trauma while performing trivial daily activities.

Dislocation Versus Impacted Valgus

In contrast to impacted valgus fractures, severely displaced humeral head fractures ("true" four-part fractures) have a worse prognosis because there are only very few or no soft-tissue links at all (i.e., destroyed hinge periosteum).

The extreme variant of this fracture type is the four-part fracture dislocation. The head fragment is displaced far away from the shaft fragment and reduction—open as well as percutaneous—is very difficult to obtain. The risk of avascular necrosis of the head fragment is high, so prosthetic replacement is the treatment of choice in most cases. With younger people, however, an attempt—whether closed or open—should be made to reduce the fracture to obtain the original anatomy of the humeral head. If a necrosis does develop, a good functional outcome can be expected with secondary prosthetic replacement because the tuberosities are healed in good position.

In some elderly patients, when the condition of the patient does not allow the implantation of a prosthesis, percutaneous treatment can be performed under regional anesthesia.

Head Splits

Impression and head-splitting fractures lead to a prosthesis implant in a high percentage of cases. Treatment of the im-

pression of the articular surface of the humeral head depends on the size of the defect. Small defects up to 20% of the head's surface can be managed with reduction and immobilization of the arm. One can manage larger defects, especially those located in the anterior head (Hill-Sachs defects), by transferring the lesser tuberosity into the defect.

Head splits are usually associated with fractures of the tuberosities or the surgical neck. If the patient has a good bone stock, open reduction and internal fixation can be attempted, but it is a difficult procedure with a high rate of secondary redisplacement. With younger people, however, it is worth trying.

SPECIAL TESTS

Accurate Radiographs

Accurately performed x-rays are essential for visualizing the fracture type, making the correct diagnosis, and planning treatment. The Neer trauma series includes a true AP, an axillary, and an additional lateral trans-scapular view.[24] To perform a true AP view in the scapular plane, the contralateral shoulder has to be rotated out approximately 40 degrees so that the glenoid surface comes into the sagittal plane (a true AP view). The lateral trans-scapular view, also called *tangential* or *Y-view* is performed in many hospitals as second view but does not enable correct fracture assessment, particularly regarding lesser tuberosity displacement.[35] It can be done in either a sitting, standing, or prone position without removing the arm from the sling.

A good axillary view is essential. No other view can show the situation on the lesser tuberosity in a comparably exact manner. Furthermore, it allows the interpretation of the axis and the relation between the head and shaft as well as between the head and glenoid. The x-ray is performed on the sitting patient with the arm abducted. Being careful in abducting and resting the patient's arm, it is possible to do this in almost all cases. An alternative technique is the Velpeau axillary view. It is not necessary to remove the arm from an already applicated sling, and the arm can remain close to the chest. The patient is seated and tilted backward in a 45-degree angle over the table. The x-ray plate lies below on the table, and the tube comes from above in a vertical direction. Howerver, incorrect or oblique views will misrepresent the fracture and create confusion.

Conclusions from Radiographs to Periosteum Condition

If there is no displacement in the horizontal plane on either the AP or axillary view, then the periosteum on the medial side is intact. In subcapital fractures with misrepresented impaction (AP view) but true anterior angulation (axillary view), the periosteum on the medial and in the front is disrupted. In these cases, there is a high risk of secondary displacement of the shaft because of the pull of major pectoralis muscle medially. If there is such a displacement on the primary x-ray, you can expect an increase in the following days.

Lateral displacement of the greater tuberosity without change of height (typical of impacted fractures) leaves the periosteal connection between shaft and greater tuberosity intact. Depending on the degree of lateral displacement, the periosteum is stripped some distance from the shaft ("long rein"), and the tuberosity follows the posterior pull of the infraspinatus. After the reduction of the head fragment, the greater tuberosity will come close to the shaft again (AP view) but will remain in a posterior position. If there is proximal (superior) displacement of the greater tuberosity, periosteal connections between shaft and tuberosity are destroyed, and the tuberosity follows the pull of the rotator cuff under the acromion (typical in avulsion fractures) (Fig. 14-5).

Medial displacement of the lesser tuberosity is possible in cases of the disruption of the periosteum between shaft and tuberosity (avulsion fractures). In impacted fractures the periosteum remains intact, and the apparent medial displacement of the lesser tuberosity on the axillary view is caused by impaction of the head fragment underneath the tuberosity.

CT scans

If good radiographs are available, an additional CT scan does not usually provide any further useful information.[37] Sometimes a CT scan is helpful in preoperative planning,

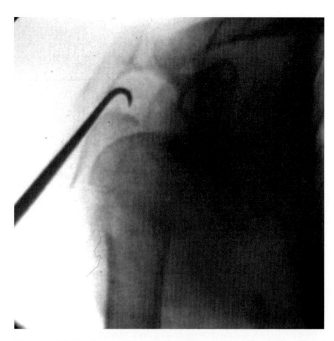

Figure 14-5 If there is no periosteal connection on the lateral side, the greater tuberosity will be displaced into the subacromial space following the pull of the supraspinatus muscle. It must be brought down to the original height using a percutaneously inserted hook.

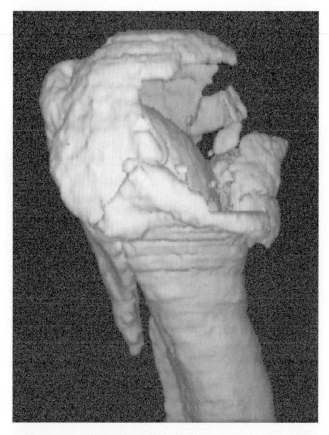

Figure 14-6 An example of an excellent three-dimensional reconstructed CT scan showing an impression fracture.

especially for percutaneous treatment. The nature of the fracture is best demonstrated with three-dimensionally CT reconstruction.[29] It is useful to understand the fracture type, the relation between fragments, and the conclusions concerning soft-tissue connections. Also, evaluating the amount of articular involvement with a head-splitting or impression fracture is possible (Fig. 14-6).

MRI

Magnetic resonance imaging is inferior to CT scan in visualizing bony structures. It may be helpful in diagnosing concomitant injuries of muscles, tendons, or intra-articular structures. An attempt to visualize the blood supply of the head by using gadolinium has not been successful so far.

Other Studies

Conventional tomography was used to verify nonunions in the past, but CT is now the initial procedure of choice. With the help of an image intensifier it is possible to perform a dynamic examination to check the stability of fractures and implanted material.

NONOPERATIVE TREATMENT

Indications

About 85% of all fractures of the proximal humerus are not displaced or are minimally displaced, so good results after conservative treatment can be expected.[9] Displacement, instability, or concomitant dislocation requires an operative treatment to achieve good shoulder function. The shoulder, with its large capsule, allows a wide range of motion,[30] so it can compensate for some displacement between the head and shaft fragment. Up to 30-degree angulation in the lateral plane and horizontal displacement, and up to half of the width of the shaft, may be tolerated. However, displacement tuberosity, in relation to the head fragment, that is more than 3 mm should be treated operatively. Often you can see the tuberosities in place, but the head fragment depressed. Impression fractures of the head and head-splitting fractures may yield poor results after conservative treatment.

Closed reduction of displaced four-part fractures is not a realistic option because the muscles of the rotator cuff that pull away the fragments will render such attempts impossible.

In some cases, conservative treatment may be preferred because the patient is not able to tolerate an operation or the patient does not agree to the operation.

Results in Literature

In literature, many different methods of treatment of proximal humerus fractures are reported, and much controversy exists. Fortunately, most fractures are not displaced or are minimally displaced, so, in general, a satisfying result can be expected. Four-part fractures are mostly displaced, and most authors agree that conservative treatment of these cases leads to poor or bad results.[21,24,39,40] However, controversy exists regarding the best kind of operative treatment of displaced four-part fractures.

In a comparative study by Zyto, the results of conservative treatment, open reduction with internal fixation, and implantation of an acute fracture prosthesis were quite the same.[44] While conservative treatment has not changed much over recent years, newly designed types of shoulder prosthesis have slightly improved the results of replacement. Open reduction and plating also improved as an option with the new generation of plates, especially locking plates and better soft-tissue preserving techniques. Finally, the best alternative may be closed reduction and percutaneous fixation of the fragments, which has gained popularity. For all of these reasons nonoperative treatment is less frequently used for complex, displaced proximal humerus fractures. However, it remains the best method for minimally displaced fractures.

Early functional treatment is the best conservative method. After initial immobilization in a sling, early motion should begin on days 7 to 10 with a gentle range-of-motion exercises. This treatment method can take place in all undisplaced, stable fractures. In minimally displaced fractures, the fracture must be clinically stable before starting exercises. In practice, a test under control of the image intensifier can show whether the fragments move as a unit. The sling may be discarded after 3 weeks. Early functional treatment is essential to achieve good results, because the greatest amount of improvement in the range of motion is possible between 3 and 8 weeks after injury.[3]

OSTEOSYNTHESIS

Indications: Role of Dislocation, Head Split in Decision

Operative treatment is indicated in most cases of four-part fractures. Undisplaced four-part fractures suited for conservative treatment are not very common. In case the head fragment or the tuberosities are displaced, operation is always the treatment of choice. In order to protect the blood supply of the fragments, especially the humeral head, surgical technique that emphasizes soft-tissue preservation is imperative. Based on this consideration, closed reduction and percutaneous fixation are favored. Using a special technique and a new device, the "humerus block" (discussed later), excellent results can be achieved even in severely displaced four-part fractures.

In principle, fracture dislocations do not contraindicate an attempt at closed reduction. If closed reduction fails, an open reduction, via a small approach, can be performed, but the fixation can still be done in a minimally invasive manner. Impression fractures of the head may occur in combination with dislocation, and up to 20% loss of the articular surface is allowed with closed reduction and will usually lead to an adequate result. This enables the patient to take up most activities of daily life in a restricted manner. With older individuals, this "less-than-perfect" result is acceptable, especially when the fracture is in the nondominant arm. The goal of the treatment is to obtain an anatomic reduction of the shoulder along with a stable situation. Larger impression fractures should be treated with open surgery, often with an acute humeral head prosthetic replacement.

Head-split fractures can hardly be treated with closed reduction because it is very difficult to manipulate two parts of the head and fix both to the shaft fragment. Open reduction and internal fixation—minimally invasive—are the treatments of choice. The most important step in the surgery of displaced four-part fractures is the reduction and fixation of the tuberosities to the humeral head. Fixing the insertion of the rotator cuff at the wrong place will lead to a poor functional result.

Advantages of Osteosynthesis Versus Humeral Head Replacement

In comparison to prosthetic replacement, reduction and osteosynthesis offer many benefits to the patient. The operation is much less invasive and can be performed even in frail, older individuals with cardiac disease or similar problems. Postoperative complications are rare, and rehabilitation is easier and shorter. Avascular necrosis of the humeral head may occur in some cases, but usually only part of the head is involved. In such cases, the clinical result may still be very satisfactory. When humeral head replacement is needed for avascular necrosis after minimal percutaneous fixation, the result can be much better than in the acute situation, provided that the tuberosities are healed in a good position. Particularly in younger patients, head-preservation should be the goal in all cases because the survival time of a prosthetic implant is limited and the revision of a shoulder prosthesis is sometimes a difficult procedure.[15,16]

Closed Reduction and Minimally Invasive Osteosynthesis

Minimally invasive surgery for humeral head fractures started in 1962, when Lorenz Bohler first described the technique of percutaneously inserting pins for fixation of unstable surgical neck fractures.[4] Later, this treatment was also recommended by other authors for minimally displaced three-part fractures.[15,16,36] Svend Hansen and Stableforth published unsatisfactory results but did not report anything about the exact technique of their methods.[39,40] Our own experience has shown that percutaneous treatment does not increase the rate of avascular head necrosis and leads to excellent or good results, in most cases. Therefore, it is a method of treatment favored in our clinic. There are two problems for the surgeon to resolve: achieving anatomic reduction by percutaneous technique[21] and fixing the achieved situation in a stable manner percutaneously.[24] The second question becomes very important for older patients with osteoporotic bone. Similar to proximal femur fractures, a dynamic component of the osteosynthesis is very helpful and guarantees rapid healing.

A thorough understanding of the anatomic relationship among the numerous fragments is important for the blood supply of the humeral head as well as benefiting from the so-called ligamentotaxis effect of intact soft-tissue connections.[15] Therefore, it is essential to study the nature of the fracture in detail before entering the operating room. An intact periosteum greatly facilitates reduction. But to make use of this help, it is absolutely necessary to know where the periosteum is still intact and where it must be destroyed. A careful study of the preoperative x-ray will help determine the integrity of the periosteum. For example, if a fracture occurs but there is no wide distance between the fragments, it can be assumed that the periosteum is intact. On the other hand, the greater the distance between the fragments, the greater the probability that the periosteum is disrupted. In cases where the head fragment is displaced medially or laterally in relation to the shaft, the periosteum on the medial side may be injured in two different ways. If a medial displacement of the head occurs, the periosteum will be stripped from the shaft fragment, but, up to a certain amount of displacement, it will not be destroyed (Fig. 14-7A). The vessels within the periosteum will also survive, and a continuing blood supply of the head fragment can be expected. There is neither the danger of avascular necrosis of the humeral head nor the risk of the bone failing to heal. If the head is displaced laterally, however, the periosteum is stretched over the sharp edge of the shaft fragment and will be destroyed before medial displacement (Fig. 14-7B). Based on anatomic and biomechanic studies, the rupture of the periosteum begins, on average, after 9 mm with medial displacement and after 6 mm with lateral displacement. After 15 mm with medial displacement and 11 mm with lateral displacement, the periosteum on the medial side is completely destroyed in all cases[11,26,29](Fig. 14-4, A and B). The periosteum on the lateral side is not as important for the blood supply of the head, but is useful while reducing the greater tuberosity because, like a rein, the periosteum

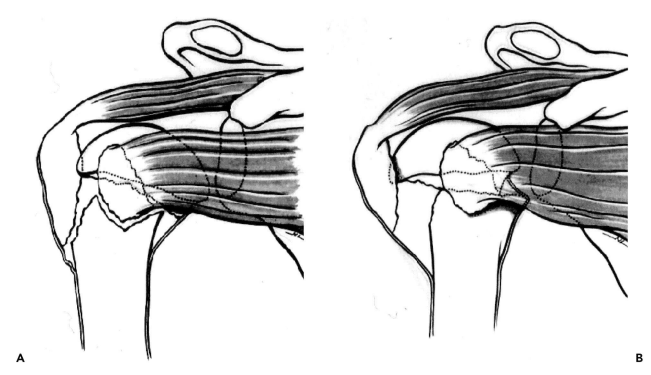

A   B

Figure 14-7   (*A*) If the head fragment is medially displaced, the periosteum will be stripped off the shaft fragment. Up to 15 mm of medial displacement can be tolerated. (*B*) Lateral displacement stretches the periosteum over the proximal edge of the shaft fragment and will lead to a total disruption of the medial periosteum much earlier.

pulls the greater tuberosity in place automatically, in many cases as soon as the head fragment is raised to the correct height. Carefully performing preoperative examination of the fractured head is mandatory; visualization on at least two x-ray planes—anterior-posterior and axial—is essential for correct fracture assessment. The nature of the fracture is best demonstrated with a three-dimensional CT reconstruction. These impressive images show the situation the surgeon otherwise has to create in his or her brain. Three-dimensional reconstructions may be helpful, but are not necessary in all cases.

Indication of Percutaneous Treatment of Humeral Head Fractures: Four-Part Fractures

Minimally invasive treatment of four-part fractures is a preferable method for all cases. It is usually possible to attempt the percutaneous method; however, one should be prepared to convert to an open procedure if adequate reduction cannot be achieved. Even if an open reduction is necessary, the fixation may still be accomplished in most cases with pins and screws. We see no strict contraindications, only lesser indications, such as humeral head fractures with severe lateral displacement of the articular fragment (true four-part fractures, according to the Neer classification) and severely displaced fracture dislocations.

In these cases, poor results may occur, but, in many cases, good results can be expected nevertheless.

Operative Technique

Usually, the operation is performed under regional anesthesia. The patient is placed in the supine position with the upper body inclined at an angle of about 30 degrees and the patient's head is supported on a headrest. The arm is draped completely free to permit full mobility in all planes. The image intensifier is located cranially. The C-arm is set to create a right angle between the central beam and the humeral shaft and head (Fig. 14-8). This setup allows a second, axillary view of the fractured humeral head by abducting the arm at any time during the operation. For hand protection, special radioresistant gloves should be worn during the operation. The operation starts with the reduction of the humeral head fragment. This is performed percutaneously with the aid of an elevator inserted through a small skin incision. To find the right entry point, the humeral head, in the lateral view, is divided into three thirds. The boundary between the anterior and the middle third is the best approach because the anterior fracture line of the greater tuberosity is always situated about 5 to 10 mm behind the bicipital groove. Using this fracture gap, the elevator can be quite easily placed under the articular fragment to raise it to the correct height (Fig. 14-9, *A* and *B*).

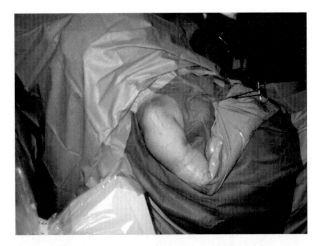

Figure 14-8 The position of the patient is the supine position. The upper body is inclined in an angle of 30 degrees. The arm is draped completely free to allow full motion of the shoulder during the operation. The C-arm comes from cranial and is set to create a 90-degree angle between the central beam and the upper arm. Abducting the arm in axial view can easily be performed.

The fixation of the head fragment to the shaft in this position is achieved by means of K-wires that are locked in a special fixation device, the so-called "Humerus block." First, the Humerus block is fixed to the proximal humerus shaft with one screw, which requires a skin incision of about 3 to 4 cm. Then, a drill guide aids in placing two K-wires right across the block, through the lateral cortex and up into the head fragment until the points reach the subchondral bone; this is important, especially with older patients, because the subchondral zone is where there is good bone quality. At last, the K-wires are locked separately in the block with two small, special screws (Fig. 14-10). The two wires cross in both planes and lead to an angular and rotational stable fixation of the head fragment because of the three-point fixation—block, lateral cortex, and subchondral bone of the head (Fig. 14-11). During the whole procedure, an assistant must hold the arm adducted in neutral position. Often, a spontaneous reduction of the tuberosities can now be observed, because periosteal connections remain. The tuberosities can now be easily fixated

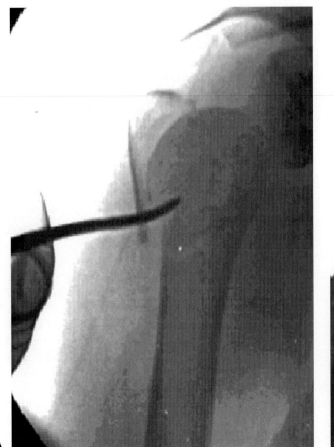
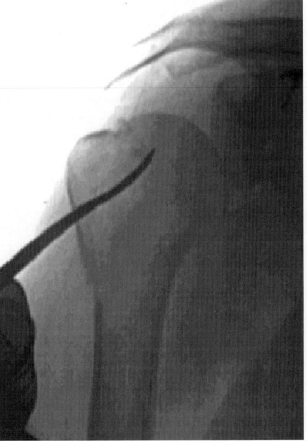

A   B

Figure 14-9 (A) A percutaneously inserted elevator is placed under the articular fragment using the anterior fracture gap of the fracture of the greater tuberosity, which is about 5 to 10 mm behind the intertubercular groove. The boundary between the anterior and the middle third of the humeral head would be the correct entry point. (B) With the tip of the elevator under the subchondral bone the head fragment can easily be raised up to the original height.

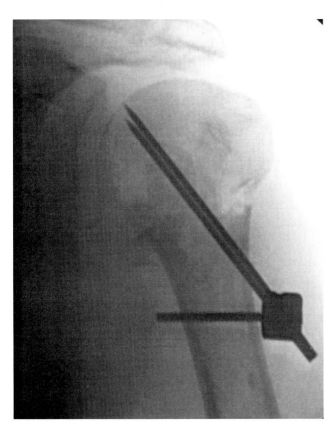

Figure 14-10 The completely implanted device, called "Humerus block" on an x-ray at the end of the operation.

with cannulated screws. If the tuberosities remain displaced they have to be reduced as well. This can also be done percutaneously by inserting small hooks through the first incision that was made to reduce the head fragment. It is remarkable that the remaining dislocation of the greater tuberosity after the reduction of the head fragment is not

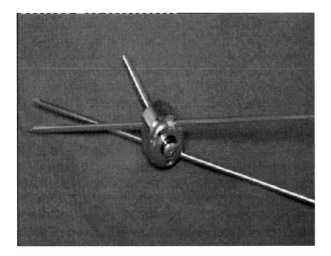

Figure 14-11 The grip of the two K-wires in the subchondral bone and the lateral cortex together with the fixation of the humerus block to the shaft, produces a rigid fixed-angle and rotationally stable head/shaft construct.

cranial, but dorsal (Fig. 14-12, A–C). If only the anteroposterior view is used, it can miss posterior displacement of the greater tuberosity. For this reason, the C-arm of the image intensifier should be shifted slightly to create AP views in different angles, and, most important of all, create an axillary view. Rotating the arm internally will show the posterior aspect of the reduced, or perhaps not reduced, greater tuberosity. The insertion point of the screws fixing the greater tuberosity is normally the borderline between the middle and posterior thirds of the humerus head. Two screws are necessary for rotation stable fixation. With younger people, when a dynamic setting of the head fragment along the K-wires is not desirable, directing one screw to the head and one to the shaft fragment increases the stability of the osteosynthesis. For the reduction and fixation of the lesser tuberosity additional small incisions are needed. A small hook positioned in the subscapular tendon or the biceps tendon can bring the lesser tuberosity down and lateral. The quality of reduction can be checked in the axial view only. The height of step-off in the axial view shows the amount of the displacement and is caused mainly by medialization, (Fig. 14-13, A and B). In most cases sufficient stability can be reached with one screw.

Concerning the treatment and the expected results, there is a difference between valgus impacted four-part fractures and severely displaced four-part fractures (true four-part fractures and four-part fracture dislocations). In valgus impacted fractures, the articular fragment is pushed down and gets impacted into the metaphysis with or without additional medial or lateral displacement. The greater tuberosity is displaced laterally by being driven out from the depressed head fragment, but remains in the correct longitudinal position. On AP radiographs, this situation might be misinterpreted as superior displacement of the greater tuberosity. The lesser tuberosity is displaced to the anterior and also remains in its correct longitudinal position. The pull of the subscapular muscle leads to a slight medial displacement. The fact that the tuberosities are in correct longitudinal position proves that the periosteum between the shaft and the tuberosities is intact. Lack of significant horizontal displacement shows that the periosteum is not destroyed on the medial side. This is important not only because of the blood supply and subsequently low risk of avascular necrosis of the head fragment but also because the periosteal connections can be used as a mechanical hinge (so-called hinge periosteum) during reduction. The only thing to do is to raise the articular fragment. The reduction of the head with little medial or lateral displacement is done by the hinge periosteum automatically. The laterally tilted greater tuberosity comes close to the head due to the pull of the now tensioned rotator cuff; the intact periosteum between the tuberosity and shaft causes anatomic reduction at once in many cases (Fig. 14-14, A and B); although, sometimes, a hook is needed to eliminate the remaining slight posterior displacement.

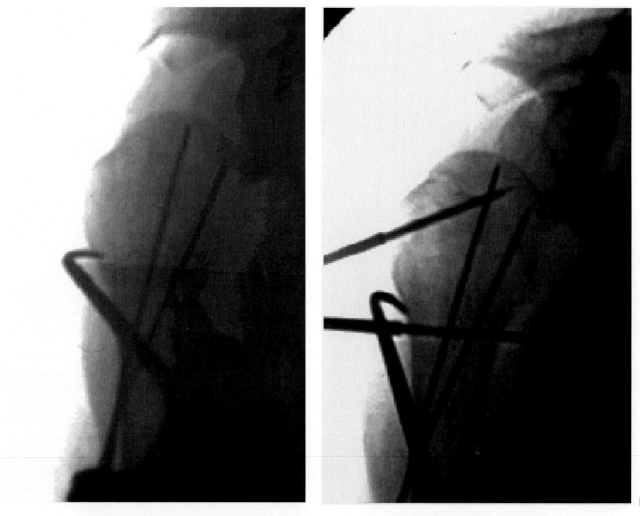

A   B

Figure 14-12 (A) Sometimes the greater tuberosity remains dorsally displaced. A percutaneously inserted hook can eliminate this failure—the position of the hook shows that the direction of the reduction is from dorsal to ventral. (B) Cannulated moulders fix the greater tuberosity temporarily. They allow a radiographic check as well as a clinical examination if there would be enough stability. (continued)

In severely displaced humeral fractures, the articular fragment is situated a wide distance from the shaft fragment, and very little to no soft-tissue connections are left (destroyed hinge periosteum). The extreme variant of this fracture type is the four-part fracture dislocation. The greater the amount of displacement, the higher the rate of avascular necrosis will be. Closed as well as open reduction is very difficult. The most important thing for proper shoulder function after healing is to fix the tuberosities in their correct positions. Otherwise, the muscles affecting the upper arm are not well balanced. However, the fixation of tuberosities in their right position is only possible when the articular fragment is reduced. So the reduction and fixation of the head fragment in anatomic position is the key to success in the head-preserving surgery of four-part fractures of

the humeral head. The technique of closed reduction and fixation is more complicated. Sometimes the greater tuberosity must be fixed to the head before it is possible to achieve a good reduction of the head fragment to the shaft. Particularly difficult situations can force the surgeon to convert to open technique, but only concerning the reduction—for fixation the same implants can be used. Comminuted greater tuberosities cannot be fixed with screws alone, and transosseous sutures or wire cerclages may be needed, which can only be performed by an open procedure. With younger patients an attempt is always justifiable, sometimes in combination with the transfer of a bone graft on a vascular pedicle from the acromion. However, older patients may also benefit from the attempt at minimally invasive head-preserving surgery.

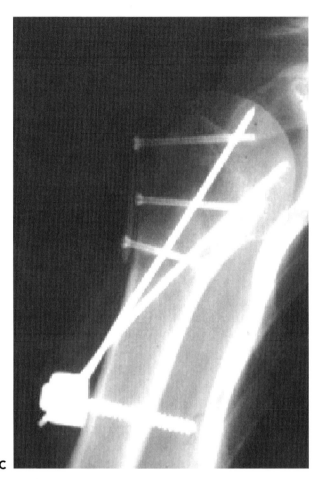

C

Figure 14-12 *(continued)* *(C)* If the results are satisfying to the surgeon, he or she will change the moulders against cannulated screws over the guidewire.

Results

Positive results can be expected if minimally invasive reconstruction of the humeral head is performed after sufficient preoperative assessment and planning, with correct operative technique, and accepting no more than 3 mm remaining displacement of the fragments (Fig. 14-15, *A* and *B*). The average Constant score of patients with valgus impacted four-part fractures treated, according to this technique, is 91% in valgus impacted fractures and 87% in all four-part fractures.[29] Lateral displacement of the head fragment decreases the quality of the outcome. The rate of avascular necrosis for all patients with four-part fractures treated with minimally invasive repair is about 11%. Major complications, such as nerve palsy and infection, are rare. The migration of pins is prevented by the locking screws in the "Humerus block." The major problem encountered is perforation of the points of the K-wires through the surface of the humeral head: if the head sinks back with the fixed tuberosities along the wires. This dynamic effect may help bone healing, but it can also irritate the glenoid. If this oc-

curs, the K-wires should be withdrawn a few millimeters under the surface of the head in a second operation. Sometimes cessation of the early functional treatment and immobilization are enough. Immobilization of the shoulder in a sling is allowed for a few weeks because stiffness is infrequent since there is no open approach. Usually, all patients operated on with this technique get a special device (a shoulder bandage) that ties the arm to the body and is to be worn up to 3 weeks. Exercises can be started as early as 1 day after the operation by just temporarily removing the bandage, but rotation must be avoided. The removal of the Humerus block is performed usually after 4 to 6 weeks; the small titanium screws can remain in the bone.

Other semirigid minimally invasive techniques, like "Helixwire"[18] or "Zifko Nails,"[43] are not suitable for four-part fractures but will suffice in simple subcapital fractures. The principle of the Helixwire is that a spiral-shaped wire is inserted through the cortex of the shaft and then turned until it reaches the subchondral bone. This wire provides stability against horizontal displacements but less rotational stability. Anatomic reduction and fixation of the articular fragment in four-part fractures, and particularly the fixation of the tuberosities, is not possible (Fig. 14-16, *A* and *B*). Zifko nails are inserted through a cortical window above the olecranon and fossa and then driven up to the subchondral bone of the head. Neither the anatomic position of the head nor the realignment of broken tuberosities in four-part fractures are taken into consideration. Both of these techniques, thus, have limited indications for severe fractures.

Open Reduction and Internal Fixation

Principles

The goal of open reduction and internal fixation in severe fractures of the humeral head is anatomical reduction because the rotator cuff needs exact insertion points at the head to guarantee trouble-free function. The second problem of open reduction is exposing the fragments as far as required to achieve anatomic position and at the same time, preserving the soft tissues as much as possible so as not to destroy the connections between the fragments that are important for their blood supply. Finally, an absolutely stable construct must result because the external immobilization of the shoulder after an open procedure will lead to stiffness.

Operative Technique

The positioning of the patient and the type of anesthesia are similar to those for minimally invasive techniques. An image intensifier is also useful in open procedures. The standard approach is the deltopectoral approach, preserving both the origin and the insertion of the deltoid muscle.

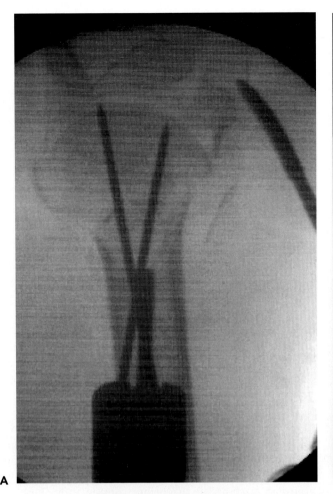
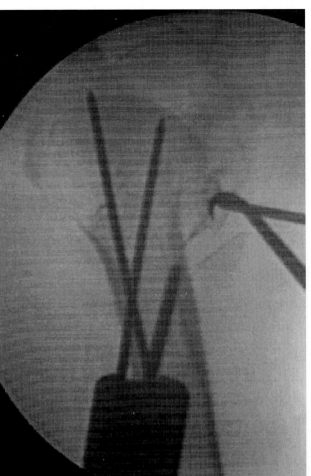

A

B

Figure 14-13 (*A*) The displacement of the lesser tuberosity is best seen on an axial view. It is reduced by means of a hook—this action is watched via the image intensifier. (*B*) After eliminating the step-off, the tuberosity is fixed with one cannulated screw.

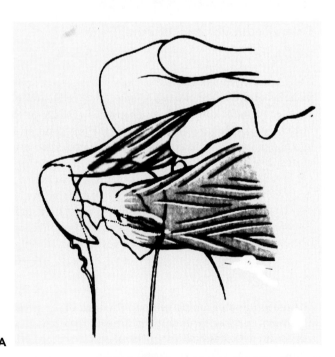
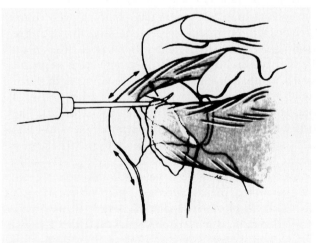

A

B

Figure 14-14 (*A*) The impacted head fragment pushes the tuberosities aside, but they are in correct longitudinal position. (*B*) Raising the head fragment leads to an automatic reduction of the tuberosities, in most cases. Concerning the greater tuberosity the tensioned rotator cuff leads to this reduction together with the intact lateral periosteum (rein).

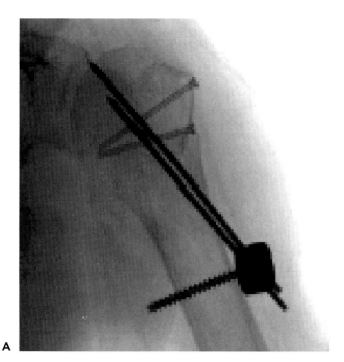

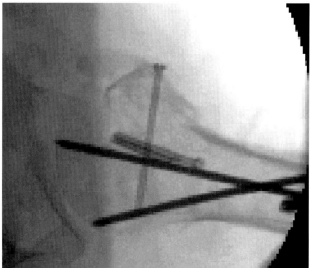

A

B

Figure 14-15   (*A,B*) A postoperative x-ray of a severely displaced four-part fracture treated percutaneously with Humerus block and cannulated screws. It is a nice result that led to a very good clinical outcome and a satisfied patient.

Proper deltoid function allows rapid postoperative rehabilitation.

The skin incision is below the clavicle and extends across the coracoid process and then follows the deltopectoral sulcus down to the area of insertion of the deltoid muscle. The cephalic vein should be preserved and retracted laterally. Occasionally, retracting it medially is easier.[9] The dissection of the deltoid and the pectoralis muscle is done bluntly with just the fingers or a suitable instrument. The fracture then appears between the divided muscles. The biceps tendon helps with the orientation and identification of the fragments. The deltoid muscle is retracted laterally only as far as needed to expose the greater tuberosity. If a larger exposure is necessary, the insertion of the deltoid muscle can be elevated and the upper part of the tendon of the major pectoralis muscle can be incised. All structures should be handled very carefully so as to not disrupt soft-tissue links with blood vessels (Fig. 14-17). The fragments are reduced by means of elevators and hooks. Temporary fixation with K-wires, cerclages, or sutures restores the humeral head. For definitive stabilization, different implants are in use.

Minimal osteosynthesis with two or three K-wires brought in from the lateral cortex of the shaft fragment, combined with figure-eight wires to fix the tuberosities, is only promising in minimally displaced fractures with intact periosteum. To increase stability, the figure-eight wires should cross the intertubercular groove and run through the shaft fragment as far proximally as possible to increase an-

gular stability and to catch the tuberosities intraosseously or subtendinously. In cases of metaphyseal comminution it is not possible to bring the articular fragment up to the original height because an unstable situation would be created. Shortening of the overall humeral length is not a problem, but attention must be paid so that the tuberosities is fixed in relation to the head and not to the shaft. Otherwise, cuff tension is inadequate and an impingement syndrome may result.[9] If the head fragment shows a tendency towards horizontal displacement, additional intramedullary fixation is added by using two rush rods.

The recently developed Humerus block (AO) gives adequate angular and rotational stability. For the fixation of the tuberosities, thin cannulated titanium screws guarantee a stable fixation without danger of further fragmentation. This screw system is based on a new technology. The hole is not drilled, but created by a cannulated moulder, so no bone defects do not result. The surrounding bone is hardened through compression and thus the screws get an excellent grip. With some of these moulders the head is restored, and if the radiographic results are satisfactory, the moulders are replaced with the cannulated screws over the guide wire (Fig 14-18).

Conventional plates for treatment of four-part fractures will fail in many cases for lack of angular stability. In the past the "T-plate" and the "Cloverleaf-shaped plate" were widely used. It was incorrectly assumed that plating leads to a very high rate of avascular necrosis of the head.[17] However, it is likely that the surgical manipulations,

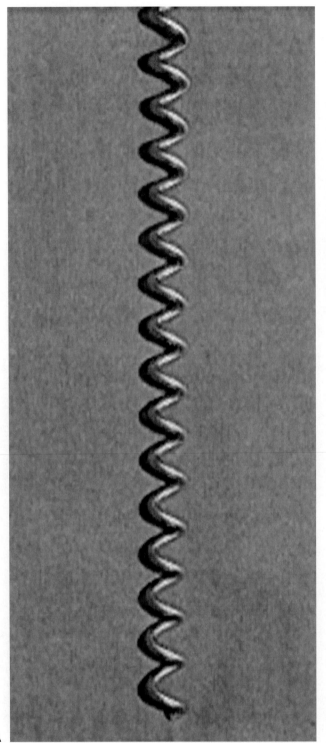

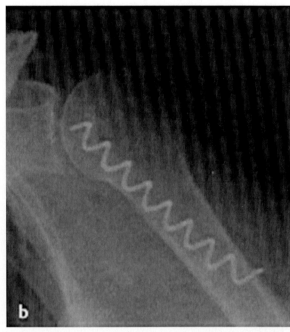

Figure 14-16 (*A*) The "Helix wire." (*B*) A three-part fracture treated with helix wire: the head fragment is reduced, the greater tuberosity remained dorsally displaced and is seen in the bone defect on the lateral side.

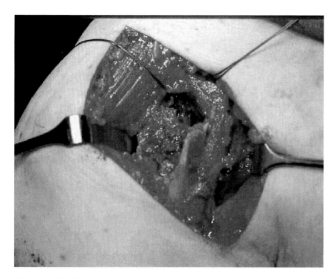

Figure 14-17 The preparation must be performed very carefully with emphasis on soft-tissue preservation. It is better to use "Langenbeck" hooks and never "Hohmann" hooks.

rather than implant, are responsible. Responsive indirect techniques of reduction are crucial for the rate of head necrosis.[12] Because of the absence of angular and longitudinal stability of the screws in the proximal holes, secondary loss of fixation occurs very frequently, especially in connection with early functional after-treatment.[38] Tilting and loosening are natural consequences (Fig. 14-19, *A* and *B*).

Angular stability can be improved by using two plates. Hertel recommended the stabilization of valgus impacted four-part fractures by implanting two plates. One plate is positioned behind the intertubercular groove and pushes the greater tuberosity toward the articular fragment previously raised. Thus, the tuberosity helps support the head. Screws are inserted through the tuberosity into the head as well as into the shaft fragment. A second plate fixes the head and lessens tuberosity from the anterior. So the head and both tuberosities are angularly and rotationally fixed to the shaft.

Another technique for making a conventional plate angularly stable is to bend it in a 90-degree angle to create an angled plate with a short side that is hammered into the head fragment. The insertion point of the short side is behind the intertubercular groove—like other plates—and about in the middle of the head. The long side is fixed to the shaft with screws. Directing the first screw up into the head increases the stability of the head fixation. This technique is also very suitable to treat subcapital nonunions (Fig. 14-20). Szyszkowitz tried to get more stability with conventional plates applying bone cement in the drill holes.[41]

A new generation of implants with locking screws promises positive results due to stable fixation and a less invasive technique of implantation. Actually, they should not be named plates because another biomechanical prin-

ciple has been realized (Fig. 14-21). The implant is not fixed on the bone, and there is no possibility to reduce the fracture by getting the bone closer to the implant while fastening the screws. The "fixed-angle proximal humerus plate" is a rigid device that stabilizes a previously reduced fracture much like an internal fixator. In older patients the disproportion between the rigid implant and the weak bone might increase the risk of cutting out.[1]

Technique

The exposure of the fracture is performed only as far as necessary to get a sufficient view to identify the fragments.

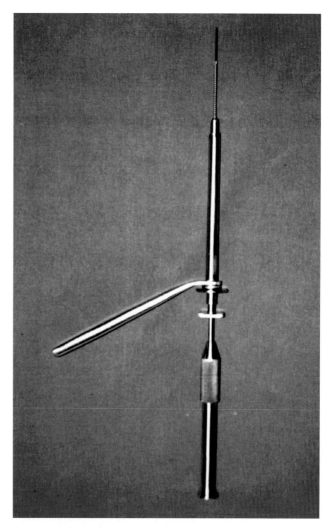

Figure 14-18 For percutaneous fixation of the tuberosities we use a special screw system. First a combination of a guidewire and a moulder is drilled in to fix the reduced fragment. With some of these moulders the humeral head can be restored, like with K-wires. Then step by step the moulders are removed and exchanged against screws over the guidewires. Using a moulder instead of a drill the hole is created without bone defect, so an excellent grip of the screws can be accepted. Using a tube that is equipped with a handle, this system also allows placing the screws percutaneously in regions with thick soft tissue covering.

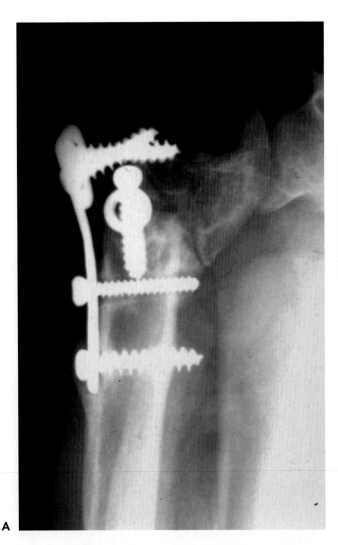

A

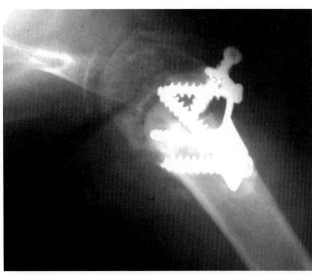

B

Figure 14-19 (*A,B*) Loosening of plate and screws after fixation of a proximal humerus fracture with a conventional plate. Because of lack of angular stability these implants are not suitable to fix unstable fractures.

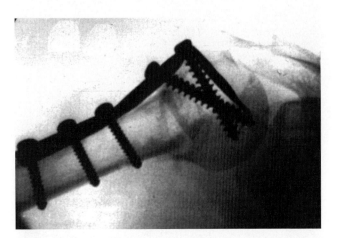

Figure 14-20 A blade-plate construct provides fixed-angle stability to proximal humerus fractures. This can be used in acute fractures as well as in nonunions.

Detachment of the deltoid muscle, as well as skeletonization or periosteal stripping of the tuberosities must be avoided. After analyzing the directions of displacements, reduction is achieved by simple axial tension on the 60-degree abducted arm. In that position the deltoid muscle is most relaxed. Remaining horizontal displacements are eliminated by additional pressure against the directions of deformities. The fragments can also be directed by means of K-wires in the manner of joy-sticks. The assistant has to keep a firm hold on the reduced fragments until the plate is definitely secured. Defects below the raised articular fragment are filled up by reduced tuberosities in order to avoid bone grafting. The greater tuberosity is situated directly below the cranial end of the plate and will be fixed with the fixed-angle screws later on. The locking plate is mounted laterally on the humeral head and shaft, behind the intertubercular groove. To achieve proper alignment with the axis of the humerus, it is temporarily fixed to the head by a

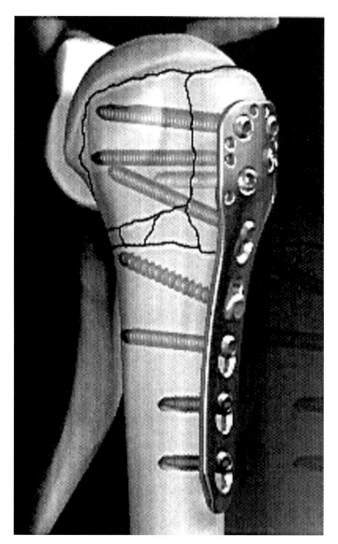

Figure 14-21 The angular stable plate for the proximal humerus developed from the AO. The screws are locked in the plate with threaded heads.

the often very small head fragment. Seidl recommended the use of the so-called "Cup Washer" in combination with the "Seidl Nail" that he designed. A spider-like device is modeled to the surface of the head and catches the tuberosities as well as the rotator cuff.[34] He himself reported good results in 85% of his patients. Other authors, however, strongly disagreed.[42]

An additional feature of the AO unreamed humerus nail is a spiral-blade that is to be inserted through the proximal end of the nail.[12] It is hammered in and fixes the head fragment while the tuberosities have to be fixed to the head separately.

Recently, short proximal humerus nails have been developed. They have multiple locking holes in different planes at the proximal end. The developers maintain that the articular fragment and tuberosities can be fixed in a more stable manner by using these locking screws. Due to the shortness of these nails distal locking is possible by

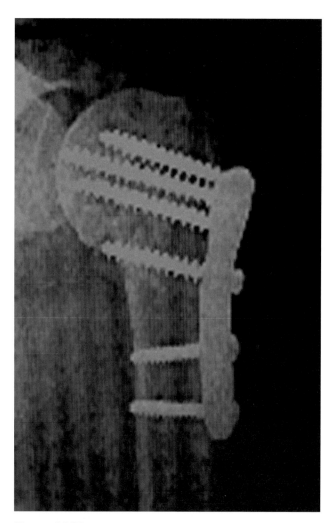

Figure 14-22 A nice early postoperative result after osteosynthesis with an angular stable plate. Cutting out of the screws in osteoporotic situations is a big problem.

K-wire that is inserted through a separate hole and should be placed in the rotating center of the head. Then the plate is fixed to the shaft with one cortical screw in the oval hole. Slight height corrections can still be done. All screws are equipped with a threaded head so that they become locked after fastening. A special drill guide that is fixed in the inside thread of the hole is required. The proximal screws diverge into the humeral head and guarantee a rigid fixation (Fig. 14-22). Fragments that are not fixed to the implanted device are now taken with strong sutures. Splintering of the osteoporotic head is possible in older patients, therefore the points of the screws should end a few millimeters from the cartilage so as not to perforate the articular surface.

Conventional locking nails are only appropriate for limited duties in treatment of four-part fractures because of difficulties concerning the fixation of the tuberosities and means of an integrated target device. The restoration of the humerus head is done by open surgery.

Open reduction and internal fixation should allow functional treatment. Postoperatively, the arm is positioned in slight abduction and external rotation beside the upper body. Exercises begin on the first postoperative day with passive motion in the scapular plane up to 90-degree abduction. Continuous passive motion devices may be very helpful. Depending on the level of pain, the rehabilitation program is continued with rapidly intensifying assisted and active exercises without restrictions concerning the range of motion. X-rays in two perpendicular views are made 5 to 7 days after the operation to check the position of fracture and implant.

Results of Osteosynthesis Concerning the Effect of Avascular Necrosis

The avascular necrosis of the humeral head is a common complication in four-part fractures. The quality of the results depends very strongly on the occurrence of partial or total head necrosis.[6,32] The frequency of head necrosis is related to the fracture type and on the kind of treatment, especially the manipulation of the soft tissue and has been reported to range from 26% to 75%.[16,19,23,24,32] Compared with three-part fractures, the risk of avascular necrosis is about two to three times higher.[10]

In the past the high risk of avascular necrosis led to the opinion that a primary prosthetic replacement for acute fractures would be better than osteosynthesis. But the results of acute shoulder replacement could not support that position. Furthermore, new operative techniques and implants have allowed preservation of the blood supply of the fragments. Another trend is a reduction in the amount implanted materials—plates are smaller and additional cerclages are obsolete. An AO multicenter study from 1998 reported about 61% minimally invasive and 22% open surgery, but only 17% humeral head replacement. Although these numbers include all proximal humerus fractures, the minimally invasive treatment of four-part fractures is gaining ground. The new "Humerus block" combines two important characteristics to accomplish a positive outcome. In the first instance it is minimally invasive as well as stable enough to allow early exercising. A second advantage when using this implant and technique is that the risk of humeral head necrosis is reduced to 11%.

Practical Rules for Deciding Between Osteosynthesis and Humeral Head Replacement

Humeral head replacement for acute proximal humerus fractures has significant surgical morbidity for elderly patients. Perfect results are infrequent, because the tuberosity healing is unpredictable. In half of the cases, they will pull off or resorb. Moreover, the rehabilitation period is lengthy and intense, which is strenuous for older patients. For this reason, we prefer percutaneous osteosynthesis for minimally displaced four-part fractures (valgus impacted fractures), even in elderly patients. In severely displaced fractures, an attempt with closed reduction and fixation is justified, but the surgeon may have to resort to open surgery—using the same implants for repair. In younger patients, fracture dislocations are treated by attempting closed surgery.

Using other implants, such as plates, internal fixators, or nails which pursue other philosophy of biomechanics, will not lead to better results but to more complications.

So the absolute indications for primary fracture prosthesis of the humeral head are only a few: fracture dislocations with older patients, fractures with severe lateral displacement of the head, and impression of the head affecting more than 50% of the articular surface. Performing a humeral head prosthesis because of avascular necrosis after osteosynthesis is much easier, provided that the tuberosities are healed in correct position.

REFERENCES

1. Bartsch S, Hullmann S, Hillrichs B, et al. Die Osteosynthese der dislozierten Humeruskopffraktur mit der winkelstabilen proximalen Oberarm–Platte. Aktuelle Traumatologie 2001;2:64.
2. Bertoft ES, Lundh I, Ringquist I. Physiotherapie after fractures of the proximal end of the humerus. Scand J Rehab Med 1984;16:11.
3. Birrer K, Kübler N, Babst R. Gewebeschonende winkelstabile Plattenosteosynthese proximaler Humerusfrakturen. Erste Erfahrungen mit einer kanülierten Winkelplatte. Hefte zu Der Unfallchirurg Jahrestagung der DGU 2000;64:S350.
4. Böhler J. Percutane Osteosynthese mit dem Röntgenbildverstärker. Wiener klinische Wochenschrift 1962;26:485.
5. Brooks CH, Revell WJ, Heatley FW. Vascularity of the humeral head after proximal humeral fractures: an anatomical study. J Bone Joint Surg 1993;75B:132.
6. Brunner U, Ruchholtz A, Trupka A, et al. Three- and four-part fractures of the proximal humerus in adults: factors to influence the outcome after ORIF. J Shoulder Elbow Surg 1995;4:63.
7. Court-Brown CM, Garg A, McQueen MM. The epidemiology of proximal humeral fractures. Acta Orthop 2001;72:365.
8. Esser RD. Open reduction and internal fixation of three- and four-part fractures of the proximal humerus. Clin Orthop 1994;299:244.
9. Habermeyer P, Schweiberer L. Schulterchirurgie, Urban & Schwarzenberg, 1995.
10. Hägg O, Lundberg B. Aspects and prognostic factors in comminuted and dislocated proximal humeral fractures. In: Bateman J, Welsh RP, eds. Surgery of the shoulder, St. Louis, Mosby, 1984.
11. Hausberger K, Resch H, Maurer H. Blood supply of intraarticular fractures of the humeral head: an anatomical and biomechanical study. 14th Congress of the European Society for Shoulder and Elbow Surgery, Lisbon, 2000.
12. Hessmann MH, Rommens PM. Osteosynthesetechniken bei proximalen Humerusfrakturen. Chirurg 2001;72:1235.
13. Hintermann B, Trouillier HH, Schäfer D. Rigid internal fixation of fractures of the proximal humerus in older patients. J Bone Joint Surg (Br) 2000;82B:1107.
14. Horak J, Nilsson BE. Epidemiology of fracture of the upper end of the humerus. Clin Orthop 1975;112:250.
15. Jaberg H, Jakob RP. Trümmerfraktur des proximalen Humerus. Der Orthopäde 1987;16:320.

16. Jakob R, Miniaci A, Anson PS. Four-part valgus impacts fractures of the proximal humerus. J Bone Joint Surg 1991;73B:295.
17. Kuner EH, Siebler G. Luxationsfrakturen des proximalen Humerus—Ergebnisse nach operativer Behandlung. Unfallchirurgie 1987;13:64.
18. Laminger KA, Traxler H. Osteosynthese proximaler Humerusfrakturen—Die Behandlung instabiler Frakturen am proximalen Humerusende durch elastische intramedulläre Wendeln. Unfallchirurgie 1999;23:183.
19. Leyshon RL. Closed treatment of fractures of the proximal humerus. Acta Orthop Scand 1984;55:48.
20. Lill H, Josten C. Konservative oder operative Versorgung der Humeruskopffraktur beim alten Menschen? Chirurgie 2001;72:1224.
21. Mills ED, Horne G. Fractures of the proximal humerus in adults. J Trauma 1985;25:801.
22. Mückter H. Entwicklung eines Osteosyntheseverfahrens zur winkel-und rotationsstabilen Versorgung kopfnaher Brüche des Oberarmes. Mat-Wiss Werkstofftechnik 1999;30:814.
23. Neer CS II. Displaced proximal humerus fractures, part I. classification and evaluation. J Bone Joint Surg (AM) 1970;52A:1077.
24. Neer CS II. Displaced proximal humerus fractures, part II. treatment of three-part and four-part displacement. J Bone Joint Surg (Am) 1970;52A:1090.
25. Resch H, Beck E, Bayley J. Reconstruction of valgus impacted humeral head fractures— indication, technique and long-term results. J Shoulder Elbow Surg 1995;4:73.
26. Resch H, Aschauer E, Povacz P, et al. Closed reduction and fixation of articular fractures of the humeral head. Tech Shoulder Elbow Surg 2000;3:154.
27. Resch H, Hübner C, Schwaiger R. Minimally invasive reduction and osteosynthesis of articular fractures of the humeral head. Injury 2001;32(suppl 1):S-A25.
28. Resch H, Povacz P, Schwaiger R. Osteosynthesis of intra-articular fractures of the proximal humerus. Surg Tech Orthop Traumatol 2000;55B:170.
29. Resch H, Hübner C. Percutaneous treatment of proximal humeral fractures. In: Levine WN, Marra G, Bigliani L, et al., eds. Fractures of the shoulder girdle. New York, Marcel Decker, 2003.
30. Rockwood CA, Matsen FA. The shoulder. Philadelphia, WB Saunders, 1990.
31. Rose SH, Melton LJ, Mooney BF, et al. Epidemiologic of humeral fractures. Clin Orthop 1982;168:24.
32. Ruchholz S, Trupka A, Wiedemann E, et al. Einflussgröben in der operativen Behandlung instabiler 3- und 4 Fragmentfrakturen. Deutsche Gesellschaft für Unfallchirurgie, Abstracts. 1994;S 26, Demeter Gräfelfing
33. Seggl W, Weiglein A. Die arterielle Blutversorgung des Oberarmkopfs und ihre prognostische Bedeutung bei Luxationen, Frakturen und Luxations-Frakturen des Oberarmkopfes. Act Chir Austriaca 1991;23:1.
34. Seidel H, Gahr RH, Hein W. Nagelung proximaler Oberarmschaft- und Oberarmkopffrakturen. Dynamische Osteosynthese. New York, Springer, Berlin Heidelberg, 1995:S209.
35. Sidor ML, Zuckerman JD, Lyon T, et al. Classification of proximal humerus fractures: the contribution of the scapular lateral and axillary radiographs. J Shoulder Elbow Surg 1994;3:24.
36. Siebler G, Kuner EH. Late results after surgical treatment of proximal humerus fractures in adult persons. Unfallchirurgie 1985;11:119.
37. Sjöden GOJ, Movin T, Güntner P, et al. Poor reproducibility of classification of proximal humeral fractures. Acta Orthop Scand 1997;68(3):239.
38. Speck M, Lang FJH, Regazzoni P. Proximale Humerusmehrfragmentfraktur— Misserfolge nach T-Platten-Osteosynthesen. Swiss Surg 1996;2:51.
39. Stableforth PG. Treatment of four-part proximal humeral fractures. J Bone Joint Surg (Br) 1984;66B:104.
40. Svend Hansen H. Displaced proximal humeral fractures. Acta Orthop Scand 1974;45:359.
41. Szyszkowitz R, Seggl W, Schleifer P, et al. Proximal humeral fractures: management techniques and expected results. Clin Orthop 1993;292:13.
42. Togninalli D, Remiger A. Antegrade or retrograde intramedullary nailing in diaphyseal or sub-capital humeral fractures in the adult. Swiss Surg 1998;4:193.
43. Zifko B, Poigenfürst J, Pezzei CH. Die Markdrahtung instabiler proximaler Humeruskopffrakturen. Orthopäde 1992;21:115.
44. Zyto K, Wallace WA, Frostick SP, et al. Outcome after hemiarthroplasty for three- and four-part fractures of the proximal humerus. J Shoulder Elbow Surg 1998;7:85.

Hemiarthroplasty for Management of Complex Proximal Humerus Fractures: Preoperative Planning and Surgical Solution

Ariane Gerber *Jon J. P. Warner*

INTRODUCTION: THE PROBLEM

Proximal humerus fractures that require surgical treatment account for only 20% of fractures in this region because most are satisfactorily managed with nonoperative methods. A small percentage of the fractures involve severe comminution or occur in the setting of poor quality bone, which precludes stable fixation and thus requires endoprosthetic treatment. These cases can be very technically

A. Gerber: Department for Orthopaedic Surgery, Department for Trauma and Reconstructive Surgery, Medical School-Charité, Berlin, Germany.

J. J. P. Warner: Partner's Department of Orthopaedic Surgery, Massachusetts General and Brigham and Women's Hospitals, Harvard Medical School, Boston, Massachusetts.

challenging, owing to loss of available anatomic landmarks. Indeed, many poor outcomes can be directly attributed to surgical errors in placement of the prosthesis. Typically, the humeral head placed is either too large or too small, and the prosthetic height is either too short or too long. Excessive retroversion is not uncommon as a factor seen in failed treatments[1–4,6,7] (Fig. 15-1).

In these cases, there is loss of anatomic reference points due to distortion of the proximal humeral anatomy. Together, with the anatomic fact that there is a wide range of proximal humeral anatomy, it is not surprising that placement of a humeral component in a manner which restores normal articular position may be a difficult feat.[5,14,19] Factors to consider include variable humeral head diameter, neck-shaft inclination, retroversion, and offset of the humeral head center relative to the shaft axis. Thus, the goal

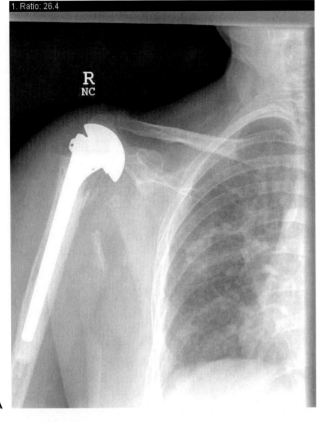

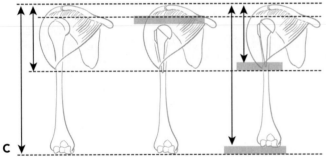

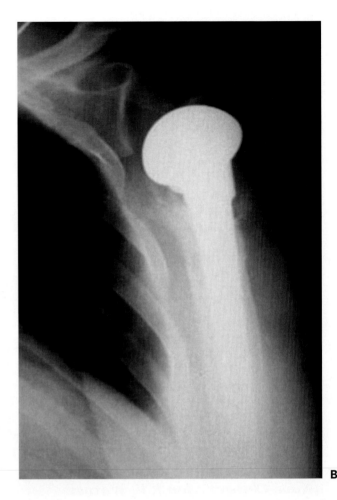

Figure 15-1 (*A*) Too long a prosthesis reconstruction. (*B*) Too short a prosthesis reconstruction. (*C*) Shortening of the humerus reduces deltoid tension, and this results in inferior subluxation of the prosthesis.

of reconstruction is to restore the anatomic relationships between the humeral head component and the tuberosities. This should affect forces across the joint, which will allow not only for tuberosity healing and proper soft-tissue tensioning, but also for less wear and tear on the glenoid. Indeed, misplacement of the humeral component has been associated with accelerated glenoid wear.[18]

Another critical technical problem is secure tuberosity fixation and healing, and loss of tuberosity fixation and poor function are, unfortunately, not uncommon (Fig. 15-2).

Other factors that can contribute to a poor outcome include advanced patient age and poor bone quality, patient comorbid factors, such as poor general health, poor social supports for postoperative care, and supervised therapy program.

Even in the best surgical hands the expected clinical outcome is largely limited to pain relief but not restoration of function. Although Neer[16] reported reliable restoration of shoulder motion, the best contemporary studies[13,20,21] show that less than 50% of patients can expect to be able to raise their arms over their heads after hemiarthroplasty for acute fracture. Indeed, recent studies[11,12,20,21] have demonstrated that surgeon experience and hospital volume closely correlate to expected outcome, with lower volume centers having a poorer outcome and higher complication rate. It therefore would seem that many of the variables affecting patient outcome after this surgery are directly controlled by the surgeon.

The purpose of this chapter is to review our current approach to preoperative patient selection, planning, surgical technique, and postoperative care for a successful outcome using hemiarthroplasty to manage acute proximal humerus fractures that cannot be surgically reconstructed by fixation methods. Few publications consider all steps critically important, and most usually concentrate on the surgical techniques. We believe that patient selection followed by accurate preoperative planning prepares the surgeon to achieve a predictable and consistently good outcome.

Indications for Hemiarthroplasty

Patient Selection

In many cases of complex proximal humerus fracture osteosynthesis, either by closed means or through formal open reduction, internal fixation may be the best choice, especially in young patients with good quality bone. The goal is to maintain anatomic relationships between the humeral head and tuberosities. Even in the case of avascu-

lar necrosis, the prognosis may remain quite good, and subsequent arthroplasty reconstruction, if necessary, can be more easily performed than if a malunion were the problem.[9] Our indications for immediate hemiarthroplasty for proximal humeral fracture include severe comminution of the articular segment, impression fracture greater than 40% of the articular surface, four-part fracture in an older individual, two- or three-part fracture with poor bone quality in some older individuals.[10,16]

Prior to performing surgery, it is very important to establish that the patient has good social support for postoperative recovery and understands the immediate postoperative commitment to physical therapy following surgery.

Preoperative Planning: Anatomical Basis

Patient Assessment

First, a thorough preoperative history and clinical examination should be performed to evaluate the patient's

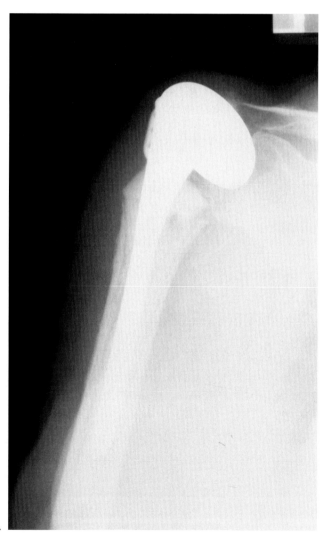

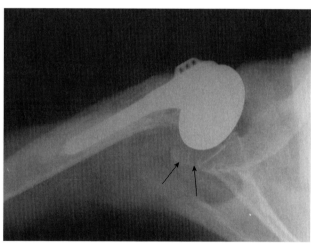

Figure 15-2 (A) AP view demonstrates no observable greater tuberosity. (B) Axillary x-ray shows remnant of greater tuberosity in a posterior displaced position (arrows).

overall health status and identify any medical comorbidities. Their ability to perform a strict postoperative rehabilitation program should also be assessed. Furthermore, associated injuries, like neurovascular injuries of the injured arm, should be documented prior to surgery.

Radiographic Assessment

Conventional radiographic evaluation with orthogonal views must include an anteroposterior radiograph and axillary radiograph. This is essential to accurately classify the fracture configuration and document humeral head and tuberosity positions. The anteroposterior view gives information about the amount of displacement of the greater tuberosity and the extent of metaphyseal comminution of the fracture. The axillary view is essential to evaluate the presence of an associated glenohumeral dislocation and to appreciate the amount of displacement of the lesser tuberosity. In selected cases, a CT scan may add information about fragment displacement and associate injury to the glenoid.

Little is written about preoperative planning for surgical reconstruction with hemiarthroplasty. Although many arthroplasty designs are available and some utilize a variety of jigs for placement, the emphasis of many techniques is based on intraoperative decision making and visual approximation of anatomy. We believe that this is one reason why many surgical results reflect nonanatomic reconstruction, which may be the inevitable cause of failure of the procedure.

The objectives of prosthetic replacement of the humeral head for fractures are to determine the proper size and position of the prosthetic head, despite loss of anatomic references, and to perform a stable osteosynthesis of the tuberosities. Indeed, accurate placement of the prosthesis in terms of reestablishing proper head height, retroversion, and tuberosity offset strongly correlates with tuberosity healing and ultimate functional outcome.[1,2,13]

Anatomic studies have shown that there is a large variability of proximal humeral anatomy among individuals and between both shoulders in the same individuals.[1-3] The data obtained in those cadaveric studies create the basis for design of most modern third-generation implants. However, in the setting of a complex proximal humerus fracture, arthroplasty reconstruction is based on mean values of inclination, retroversion, medial, and lateral offsets and is therefore always an approximation of normal individual anatomy. Whereas head size and head height can reliably be determined with preoperative planning, definition of retroversion remains an unsolved problem.[14] Most authors recommend a hemiarthroplasty implant for the fracture at a mean retroversion of 20 degrees to 30 degrees. Considering that individual retroversion can range from 10 degrees to 60 degrees, an error in rotation can theoretically

be up to 30 degrees to 40 degrees.[5-7] This is of great importance, because malrotation of the implant seems to be a significant factor for early failure of fixation of the tuberosities.[6,7]

If arthroplasty is indicated, we always obtain bilateral long arm radiographs in the anteroposterior plane so that the humeral length can be determined. A magnification marker is utilized so that comparison views of the contralateral shoulder can act as an accurate reference for length. The size of the contralateral humeral head can be templated to determine the proper size of the humeral head. This will ensure that proper tuberosity offset can be obtained because the humeral head size is accurate. The proper length of the prosthesis is determined by measuring the length of the contralateral normal side and then subtracting the length of the fractured humerus. This will give the length required to place the humeral component at the proper height (Figs. 15-3 and 15-4): The distance *a* (distance between the proximal end of the shaft and the top of the prosthesis) determined in the drawing can then be mea-

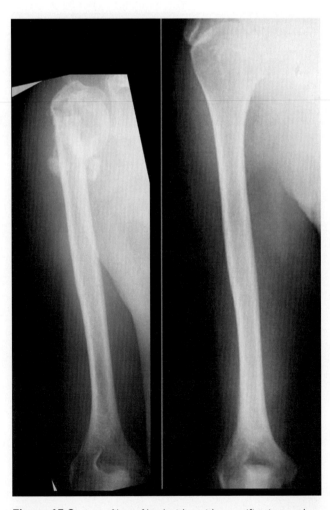

Figure 15-3 Long films of both sides with magnification markers or scanograms are required to determine humeral length.

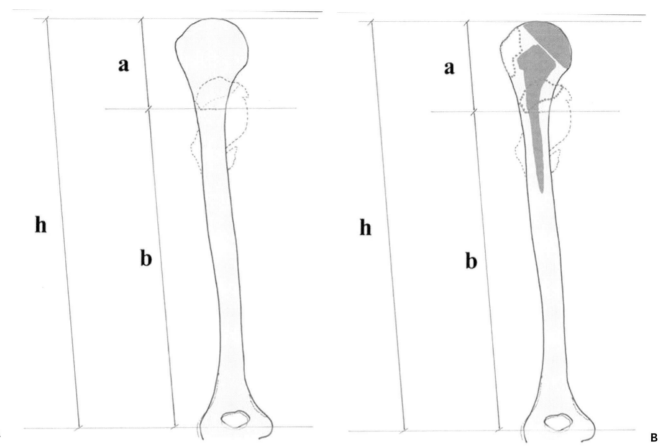

Figure 15-4 The length of the normal shoulder (h) is measured and corrected for magnification compared to the contralateral (fractured) side. The length of the humerus on the fractured side from the elbow to the diaphyseal edge of the fracture is (b). The height of the prosthesis to restore correct length is then (a), where (h) − (b) = (a).

sured intraoperatively (Fig. 15-5) and is required for reconstruction of humeral length h (Fig. 15-6). In addition, the surgeon can anticipate if bone loss will require an associated bone graft to restore tuberosities to the proper position. Allograft can then be available or the patient's iliac crest can be sterilely prepared, if necessary. This method has been used by Boileau et al., though they utilized an intraoperative jig for the reconstruction and demonstrated an accuracy to within 1 cm of the contralateral side.[3]

Positioning of the component in the proper version is an intraoperative decision as described in the following text.

Implant Selection

Little consideration has been given to selection of implants for hemiarthroplasty in the setting of acute fracture. Recent observations have suggested that geometry and surface contour of the proximal stem may affect tuberosity healing.[15] Too thick a proximal humeral stem may result in pull-off of tuberosities by over-lateralizing them and preventing healing due to over-tensioning. To thin a proximal humeral stem may result in medialization of tuberosities also with

poor healing (Fig. 15-7). This is reflected in multiple stem designs and, to date, no one design seems to improve on overall results. Kralinger et al.[13] have noted, in a retrospective and uncontrolled study, that stems with a rough proximal coating had higher rates of tuberosity union.

Some stem designs provide fins that may be taken as useful landmarks for positioning of the tuberosities and in maintaining reduction (Fig. 15-8), whereas others are designed with low profile to allow the tuberosities to fit closely onto the stem and against bone graft (Fig. 15-7).

SURGICAL TECHNIQUE

Anesthesia

Surgery can be performed under general or regional block anesthesia or a combination of both. Regional anesthesia will allow for improved postoperative pain control, but is not essential to the surgical procedure. What is essential, however, is complete muscle paralysis because this allows for easier reconstruction of the tuberosities and rotator cuff.

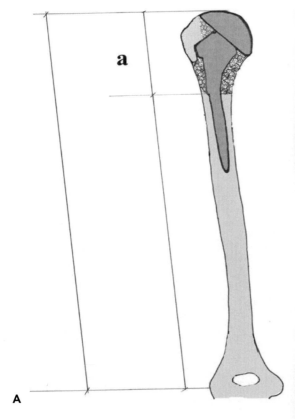

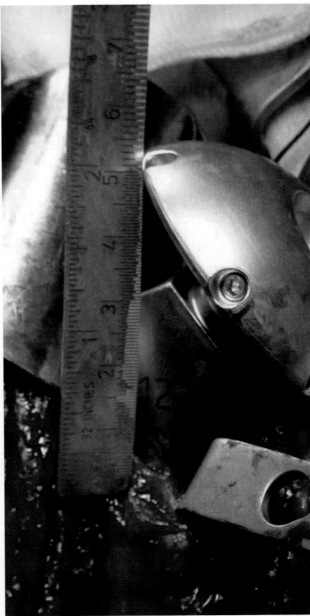

Figure 15-5 The distance to be restored, (a) is then measured intraoperatively to confirm proper head height. Bone grafting is planned preoperatively based on this measurement.

B

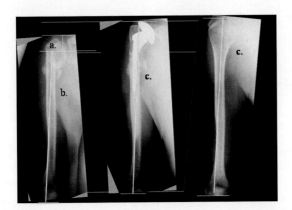

Figure 15-6 Restoration of correct length allows for secure tuberosity reconstruction and healing.

Positioning

The patient placed in the beach-chair position using a beach chair device or a long bean bag that is contoured so that the front and back of the shoulder are freely exposed and the shoulder and arm can be manipulated to allow for access to the tuberosities and shaft. It is important that full adduction and extension of the arm are possible to allow good access to the humeral shaft. Furthermore, positioning should allow intraoperative radiographic assesment with an image intensifier, if required. We routinely employ an articulate arm holder that takes the place of an assistant and allows for reproducible positioning (Fig. 15-9).

If it is anticipated, based on preoperative radiographic assessment, that bone grafting will be required, the iliac

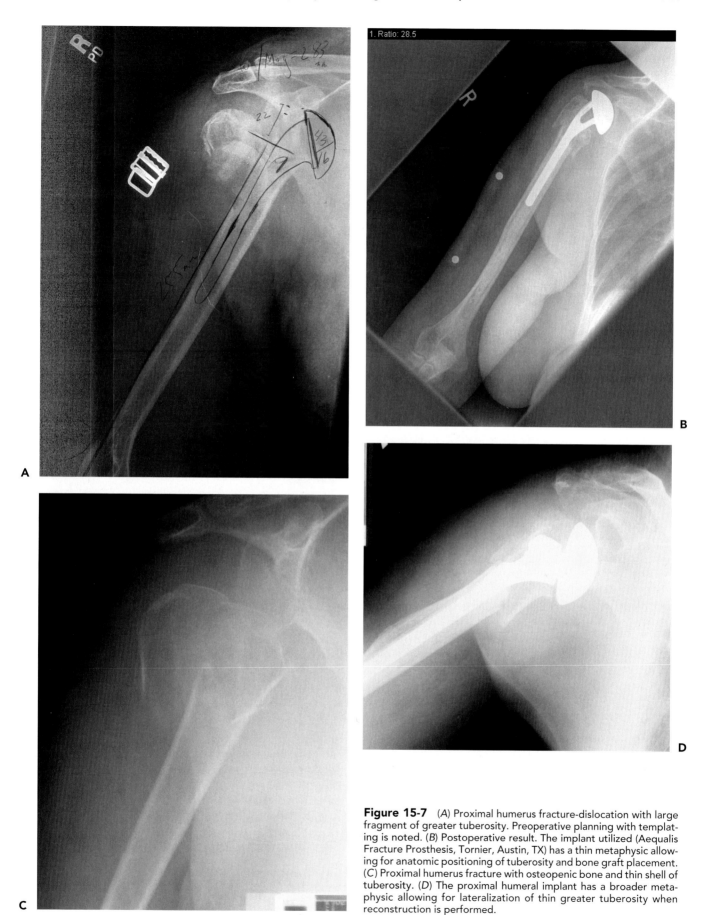

Figure 15-7 (*A*) Proximal humerus fracture-dislocation with large fragment of greater tuberosity. Preoperative planning with templating is noted. (*B*) Postoperative result. The implant utilized (Aequalis Fracture Prosthesis, Tornier, Austin, TX) has a thin metaphysic allowing for anatomic positioning of tuberosity and bone graft placement. (*C*) Proximal humerus fracture with osteopenic bone and thin shell of tuberosity. (*D*) The proximal humeral implant has a broader metaphysic allowing for lateralization of thin greater tuberosity when reconstruction is performed.

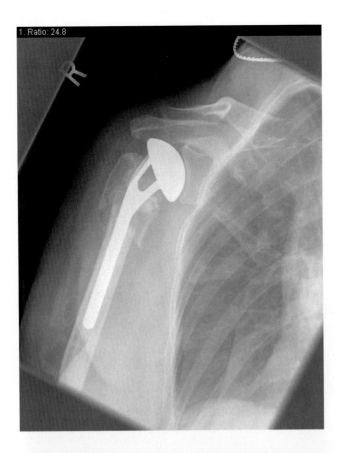

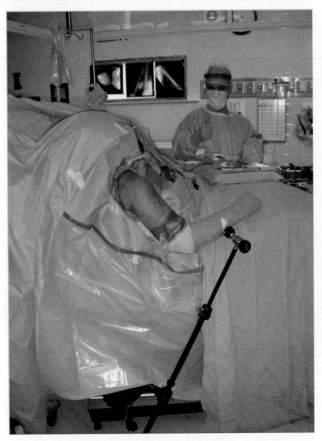

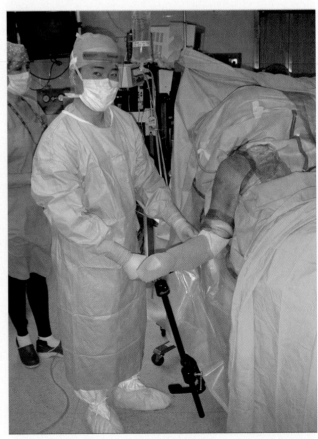

Figure 15-8 A fracture stem with low profile at the metaphysis leaves room for proper positioning of greater tuberosity.

A

B

Figure 15-9 (*A*) Patient positioning on a special beach chair (Tenet T-Max, Tenet Medical Engineering, Calgary, CANADA) and (*B*) using an articulated arm holder (McConnell Shoulder Holder, McConnell Co., Greenville, TX).

crest should be elevated with a roll so that access is available during the surgery.

SURGICAL APPROACH: HEMIARTHROPLASTY REPLACEMENT

Surgical Dissection

A straight incision is made, starting at the lateral aspect of the coracoid process and reaching the anterior aspect of the biceps muscle at the level of the deltoid insertion. The cephalic vein is identified and usually retracted laterally to preserve the venous outflow of the deltoid. This interval can be identified either proximally at the level of the coracoid process or in the distal portion of the incision where the tendon of the pectoralis major disappears under the tendon of the deltoid. A blunt Hohman retractor can be placed under the deltoid insertion around the humeral shaft by following the pectoralis major tendon. Abduction and forward flexion of the arm releases tension on the deltoid and facilitates exposure. The deltopectoral interval is developed, releasing all adhesions until the clavicle is exposed. A second blunt Hohman retractor is placed over the coracoacromial ligament. The fracture hematoma is removed and subdeltoid bursa is resected to expose the fracture. At this stage, the Browne deltoid retractor (George Innomed, Savannah, GA) can be placed easily under the deltoid to expose the anterior part of the fractured proximal humerus.

The first step of the procedure is to identify the fracture fragments. In most fractures requiring replacement arthroplasty, the fracture is a four-part fracture according to Neer, where the greater and the lesser tuberosities are detached from the humeral head and from the humeral shaft. The biceps course will help define the position of the tuberosity fragments (Fig. 15-10). The humeral head lies between the fragments free from any soft-tissue attachments. Once we identify the tuberosity fragments, the long head of the biceps is tenotomized and tenodesed at the completion of the procedure. We believe it may become entrapped in the fracture fragments, if not tenotomized, and it may be a source of motion loss and pain. The tuberosities are mobilized, and it is helpful to use a

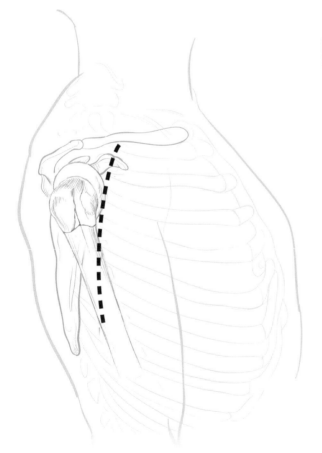

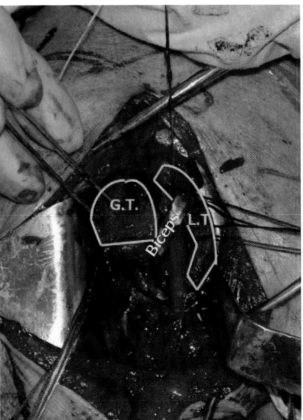

A   B

Figure 15-10   (*A,B*) Biceps defines greater (GT) and lesser (LT) tuberosities.

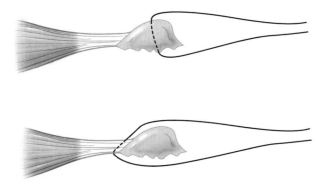

Figure 15-11 Placement of the suture around, rather than through, the tuberosity is stronger as the tendon is more secure than the osteopanic tuberosity.

large needle and strong braided nonabsorbable suture material placed through the tendons. Our preference is the use of No. 5 Fiberwire (Arthrex, Naples, FL). Usually, three to four sutures are placed through each tendon around the greater and lesser tuberosities (Fig. 15-11). Even in osteoporotic bone this gives excellent hold of the sutures and allows for manipulation of the tuberosity during surgery. During this step the axillary nerve is always visualized, and, in some cases, a vessel loupe is placed around it so that it can be protected with manipulation of the humeral shaft and rotator cuff.

After mobilization of the tuberosities, the head fragment can be extracted from the joint, which allows for exposure of the humeral shaft. This is then checked against the preoperative template of the normal side.

Determining Humeral Head Size

To determine humeral head size, the extracted original head is used and compared to trial heads available in the system (Fig. 15-12). If the head is comminuted, the fragments are put together like a puzzle to define head dimensions. This is then checked against the preoperative templating of the normal side.

Determining Humeral Head Height

Some surgeons suggest visual inspection or tension in the biceps tendon as a method to determine proper length.

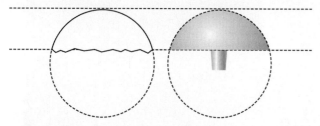

Figure 15-12 The size of the humeral head fragment approximates a portion of a circle and should be exactly replaced with the prosthetic head.

Others suggest assessment of soft-tissue tension. We have observed that all of these approaches are inaccurate. Our approach is based on our preoperative templating, as described previously, as well as an internal reference point, which we have defined.[8] This reference point is based on the upper border of the pectoralis major (Fig. 15-13). This is a constant reference point, which, in most cases of fracture, remains intact. The distance between this point and the top of the humeral head is 5.5 cm ± 0.5 cm. This is used as an internal check for our preoperative templating. The advantage of this method is that it does not require intraoperative jigs. We have determined that accuracy of this method is to within + 5 mm compared to the contralateral side when postoperative radiographs are obtained (Figs. 15-3 and 15-13).

Defining Head Retroversion

Reproducing the individual retroversion without metaphyseal reference is technically not possible. A mean 20 degrees to 30 degrees of retroversion has been recommended in fracture arthroplasty. The transepicondylar line is used as reference axis to determine retroversion. Retroversion is already fixed between head and shaft in some systems, allowing direct alignment of the stem of the prosthesis with the forearm (Fig. 15-14). A test reduction with a trial implant is recommended and may help depict mistakes in positioning. The shoulder is reduced into the glenoid and then the prosthesis is rotated so that the humeral head points directly at the glenoid with the forearm in neutral rotation. This position of the stem is then marked with electrocautery or a rongeur on the humeral shaft so it can be duplicated when the stem is definitively fixed (Fig. 15-14C).

FIXATION OF THE TUBEROSITIES AND STEM

Fixation of the tuberosities is of critical importance. Even with sutures and fixation to the shaft of the humerus, malpositioning of the humeral head will result in displacement of the tuberosities. Given this, we placed sutures through the shaft of the humerus so that the tuberosities can be fixed not only to the stem of the prosthesis and also to themselves, but also to the humeral shaft (Fig. 15-15). Usually, four sutures (Fiberwire No. 5) are placed. Additional sutures may also be placed through medial and lateral holes in the stem. A cement restrictor is placed to the proper depth, and the shaft is then irrigated and dried. Methacrylate cement is then inserted down the shaft, and the component is placed so that it is held in a position of height and retroversion, as determined by the methods noted previously (Figs. 15-14 and 15-16). When the cement is hardenend, the sutures through the medial hole in

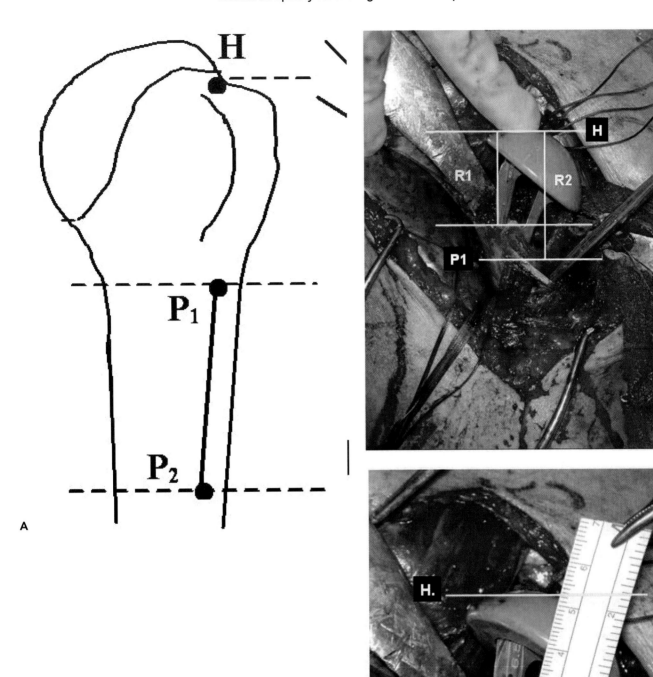

Figure 15-13 Determination of humeral head height is based on preoperative templating measurements and magnification adjusted long arm films. (*A*) The upper border of the pectoralis major is a useful reference point (see text for explanation). P1, upper border of pectoralis major tendon insertion; P2, lower border of pectoralis major tendon insertion; H, highest point of humeral head. (*B, C*) Intraoperative check of proper humeral head height. H, highest point of humeral head; P1, upper border of pectoralis major tendon; R1, reference line 1 (height of humeral head above diaphyseal edge of fracture); R2, reference line 2 (height of humeral head above upper border of pectoralis major tendon, P1; the length of this should be 5.5 cm ± 0.5 cm).

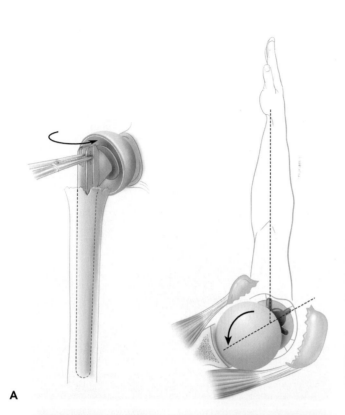

A

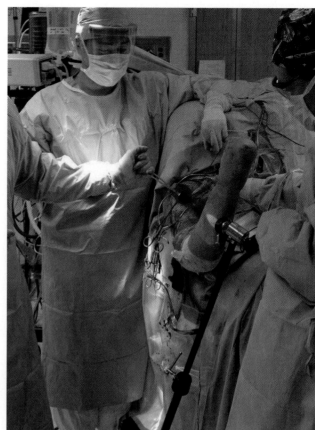

B

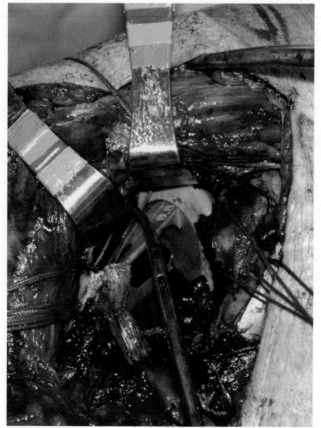

C

Figure 15-14   Determination of retroversion. (*A*) Proper version is determined by orienting the humeral prosthesis so that the head faces the glenoid with the arm in neutral rotation. (*B*) Intraoperative demonstration of determination of correct version with arm in neutral rotation. (*C*) The stem is rotated so that the humeral head points at the glenoid.

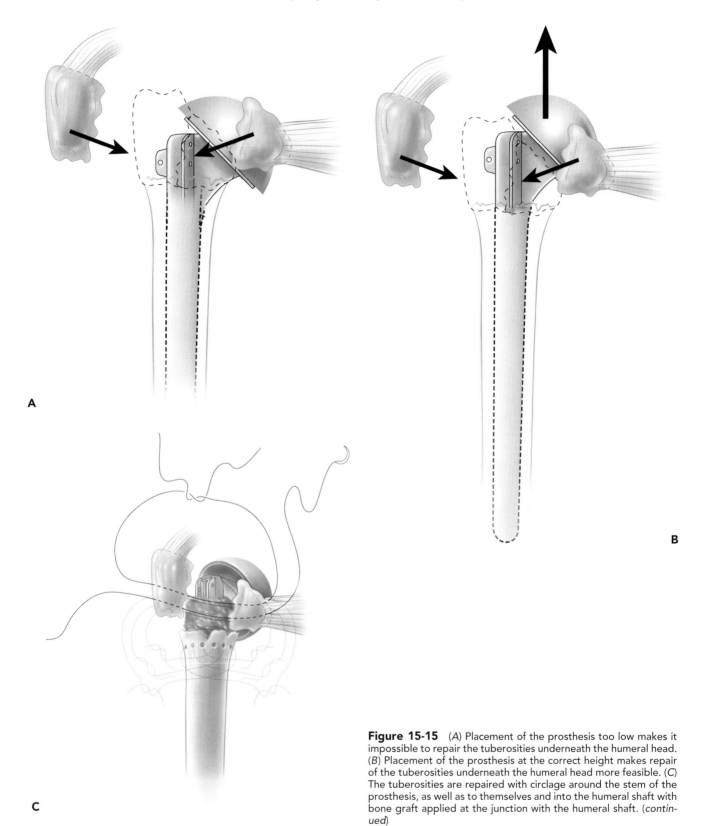

Figure 15-15 (*A*) Placement of the prosthesis too low makes it impossible to repair the tuberosities underneath the humeral head. (*B*) Placement of the prosthesis at the correct height makes repair of the tuberosities underneath the humeral head more feasible. (*C*) The tuberosities are repaired with circlage around the stem of the prosthesis, as well as to themselves and into the humeral shaft with bone graft applied at the junction with the humeral shaft. (*continued*)

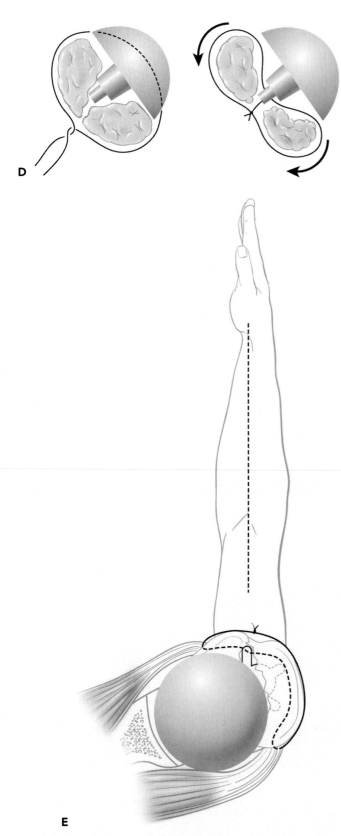

Figure 15-15 *(continued)* *(D)* Circlage of tuberosities around stem of prosthesis ensures secure fixation. If tuberosities are just fixed to the prosthesis, they will loosen with rotation of the humerus. *(E)* Correct version ensures secure tuberosity fixation around the humerus and underneath the humeral head.

the stem are placed in a circlage fashion through the subscapularis and infraspinatus so that these sutures will come over the tuberosities, locking them underneath the head of the prosthesis. The remaining sutures are then placed through the tuberosities so that they will be fixed directly to the shaft and to each other (Fig. 15-15).

Bone graft is utilized underneath the tuberosities and against the proximal humerus and stem as needed, depending on comminution. This can be obtained from the removed humeral head, and, if necessary, additional allograft bone (Fig. 15-15).

The tuberosities must be secured in a manner, which not only allows for secure attachment that prevents motion between the humeral shaft and prosthesis, but also so as not to overtension the rotator cuff. So as not to lose internal and external rotation, we fix the lesser tuberosity with the arm held in some external rotation and the greater tuberosity with the arm held in some external rotation. This will ensure an arc of tension-free rotation. Only the lateral part of the rotator interval is then closed (Figs. 15-16 and 15-17).

After the reconstruction is completed we assess the "safe zone" for passive range of motion to be performed by the therapist and communicate these limits to the therapist. The arm is rotated into internal and external rotation as well as taken into flexion to determine the point at which the repair comes under tension. This is then the limit for the first phase of postoperative rehabilitation, which is passive motion only.

POSTOPERATIVE REHABILITATION

Phase I (first 4 to 6 weeks): The goal of this initial phase is to avoid stiffness but maintain tuberosity security so that healing can occur. Passive range of motion is begun immediately after surgery, with a physical therapist bringing the shoulder to the limits of the "safe zone," which was defined during surgery. The patient is permitted to perform pendulum exercises. If available to the patient, we utilize an aquatherapy program. This seems to greatly enhance restoration of supple shoulder motion.

Phase II (6 to 12 weeks): Advancing to this phase requires reduced pain and radiographic confirmation of tuberosity healing. Passive motion and water therapy are advanced to include active-assisted motion so that the patient becomes more active in his or her program, using a home pulley as well as self-assisted exercises in the home.

Phase III (12 to 16 weeks): Active stretching continues and the patient now begins a strengthening program, initially using elastic bands and then advancing to light weights.

Phase IV (16 weeks): Return to all activities, including swimming, tennis, golf, and other overhead sports.

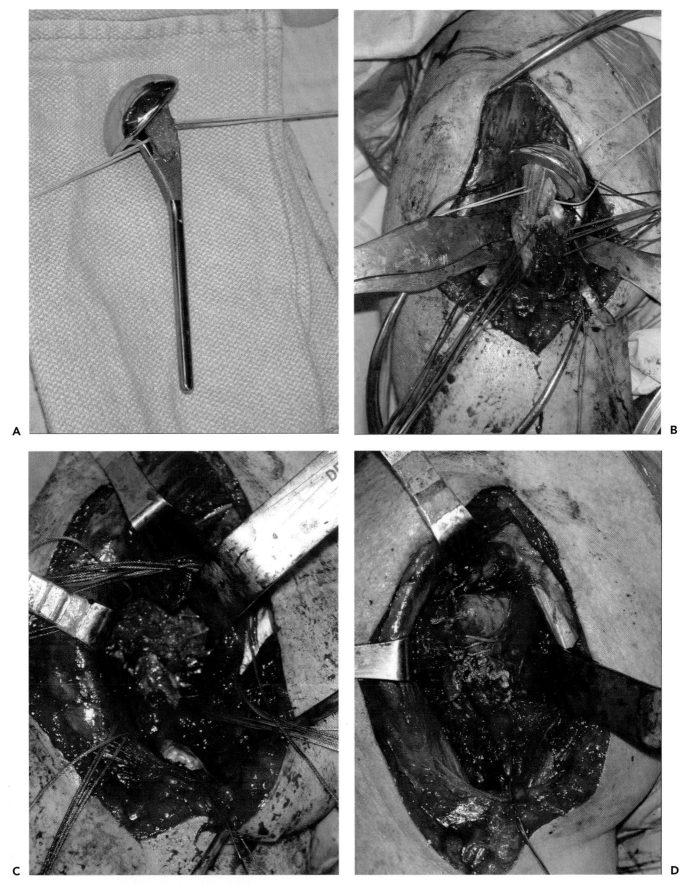

Figure 15-16 (*A*) Prosthesis with low profile of metaphysic with bone graft placed into it to promote tuberosity healing. Heavy braided sutures have been placed through medial hole and lateral hole of prosthesis for tuberosity fixation. (*B*) Prosthesis placed at proper height and version, as described in previous illustrations. Note medial and lateral sutures for tuberosity fixation as well as sutures in shaft of humerus. (*C*) Bone graft taken from humeral head is placed around proximal stem to promote tuberosity healing. (*D*) Tuberosity fixation over bone graft.

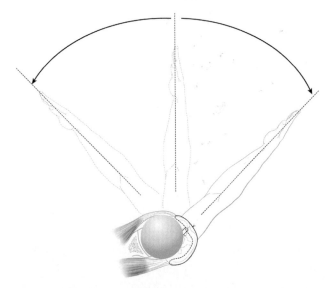

Figure 15-17 Determination of tuberosity fixation security and safe zone for passive motion after surgery.

Management of Severe Metaphyseal-Diaphyseal Comminution

Rare and challenging proximal humeral fractures can extend into the diaphysis with disruption of all landmarks. In such cases, preoperative radiographs of the contralateral shoulder provide the only frame of reference. It is also important to plan for the need of structural bone graft to bridge the proximal humeral deficiency and allow for tuberosity reconstruction at the proper height. A long stem prosthesis should be available as well (Fig. 15-18).

Results

Neer first popularized the treatment of irreparable complex proximal fractures with hemiarthroplasty.[16] Only few studies were able to reproduce the satisfactory results reported by Neer. For most authors, the overall results after hemiarthroplasty for proximal humeral fractures remain unpredictable and inferior to those obtained with hemiarthroplasty for osteoarthritis or avascular necrosis. This may be due, in part, to the fact that reconstructing individual anatomy is not possible in the fracture setting. A recent study[20] has shown that good functional outcome is most likely to happen in a younger individual who has no preoperative neurologic deficit, no postoperative complications, and a satisfactory radiographic appearance of the shoulder at 6 weeks. Functional outcome was poor in the elderly patients of the series, especially if they have a neurologic deficit, a postoperative complication requiring a reoperation, or an eccentrically located prosthesis with retracted tuberosities. Furthermore, hemiarthroplasty performed as a primary procedure leads to superior results when compared to hemiarthroplasty performed after a failed osteosynthesis.[17]

In our experiences, using the techniques of preoperative planning and anatomic surgical reconstruction, as described previously, we have observed accurate restoration of head height and tuberosity healing with near anatomical tuberosity offset restored. Many patients obtain overhead motion with good strength, though stiffness remains a major problem and is probably mainly due to the severe soft-tissue trauma sustained with these fractures (Fig. 15-19).

Complications

Secondary dislocation of the tuberosities is the most frequent complication after fracture arthroplasty, even in experienced hands.[20] Implant malpositioning, biologic factors involving blood supply of the tuberosities, and

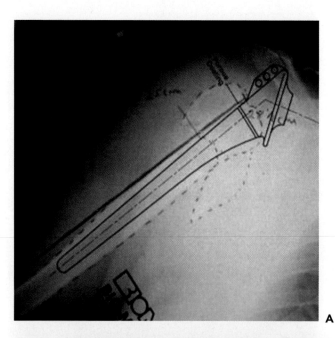

A

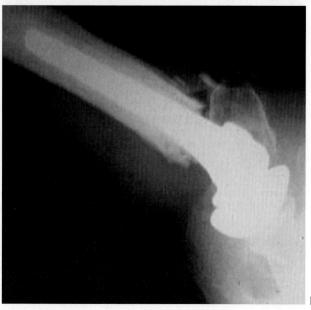

B

Figure 15-18 (A) Comminution of proximal humerus. (B) Restoration of length with tuberosity placement and bone grafting.

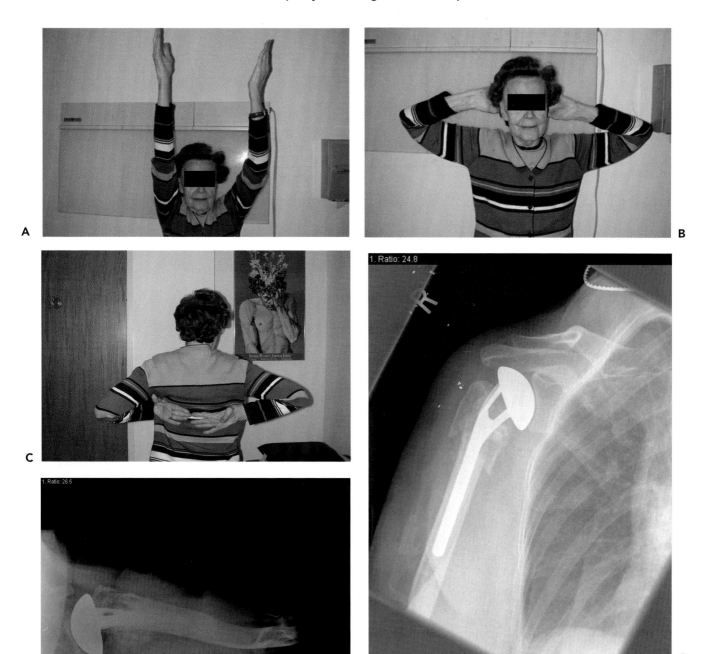

Figure 15-19 One year after hemiarthroplasty for proximal humerus fracture. (*A*) Forward flexion. (*B*) External rotation. (*C*) Internal rotation. (*D*) Tuberosity union on A-P view. (*E*) Tuberosity union on axillary view.

aggressive postoperative rehabilitation may explain failure. Secondary dislocation of the tuberosities, especially the greater tuberosity, is always associated with poor function (Fig. 15-20). Loss of rotator cuff function leads to superior and/or anterior subluxation of the prosthesis and to asymmetric load and wear of the glenoid (Fig. 15-21).

Implant malpositioning involves improper rotation, height, and/or head size. Precise implantation of the prosthesis in regard to retroversion is difficult due to the large variation among individuals. Free access to the the elbow

facilitated palpation of the epicondyles and definition of the transepicondylar line. Prostheses implanted too high or too low are a sign of poor preoperative planning. Correct selection of head size is almost always possible with the available modern implants.

Axillary nerve palsy and denervation of the anterior deltoid can be avoided when the approach is performed carefully. Infection may occur, especially if hemiarthroplasty is perfomed after failed osteosynthesis of the fracture. Loosening of the shaft occurs rarely in cemented prosthesis.

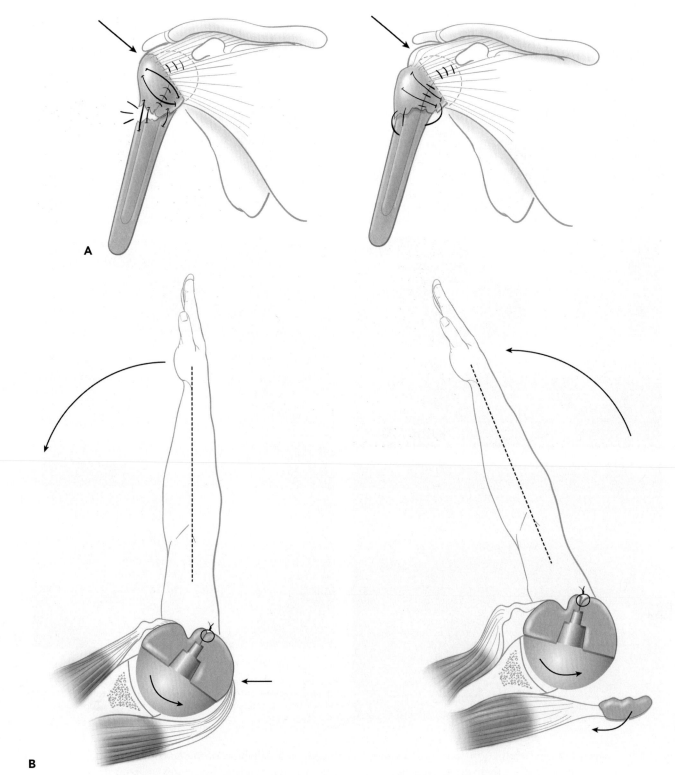

Figure 15-20 (*A*) Consequences of over-lengthening humerus. The greater tuberosity, fixation will fail. (*B*) Consequences of excessive retroversion. The greater tuberosity will fail.

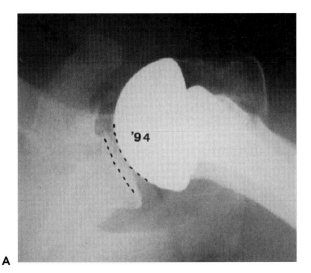

A

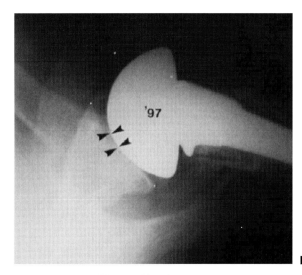

B

Figure 15-21 Glenoid erosion with malpositioned and incorrectly sized humeral head. (*A*) One month after hemiarthroplasty. (*B*) Three years after hemiarthroplasty.

Glenoid erosion occurs in unstable humeral components and nonanatomical head size.

CONCLUSIONS

The keys to successful outcome of proximal humeral reconstruction with hemiarthroplasty is proper patient selection, preoperative planning to establish anatomical guidelines for surgery, meticulous surgical technique, and a commitment to postoperative therapy through all four phases of the program.

REFERENCES

1. Boileau P, Coste JS, Ahrens PM, et al. Prosthetic shoulder replacement for fracture: results of the multicenter study. In: Walch G, Boileau P, Mole D, eds. 2000 Shoulder prosthesis: two to ten year follow-up, Montpelier, Sauramps Medical, 2002:561.
2. Boileau P, Krishnan SG, Tinsi L, et al. Tuberosity malposition and migration: reasons for poor outcomes after hemiarthroplasty for displaced fractures of the proximal humerus. J Shoulder Elbow Surg 2002;11(5):401.
3. Boileau P, Tinsi P, Le Huec J, et al. Results of shoulder arthroplasty in acute fractures of the proximal humerus. In: Walch G, Boileau P, eds. Shoulder arthroplasty. Berlin, Heidelberg, New York, Springer, 1999:331.
4. Boileau P, Walch G. Hemiprosthetic replacement in fractures of the proximal humerus. Semin Arthroplasty 2000;11(1):54.
5. Boileau P, Walch G. The three-dimensional geometry of the proximal humerus. Implications for surgical technique and prosthetic design. J Bone Joint Surg Br 1997;79(5):857.
6. Boileau P, Walch G, Krishnan SG. Tuberosity osteosynthesis and hemiarthroplasty for four-part fractures of the proximal humerus. Tech Shoulder Elbow 2000;1(2):96.
7. Frankle MA, Mighell MA. Techniques and principles of tuberosity fixation for proximal humeral fractures treated with hemiarthroplasty. J Shoulder Elbow Surg 2004;13:239.
8. Gerber A, Apreleva M, Harrold F, et al. Hemiarthroplasty for proximal humerus fracture: a new method to obtain correct length. Presented at the 10th International Congress of Surgery of the Shoulder. Washington, DC, June 4–8, 2004.
9. Gerber C, Hersche O, Berberat C. The clinical relevance of posttraumatic avascular necrosis of the humeral head. J Shoulder Elbow Surg 1998;7(6):586.
10. Gerber C, Warner J. Alternatives to hemiarthroplasty for complex proximal-humeral fractures. In: Warner J, Iannotti J, Gerber C, eds. Complex and revision problems in shoulder surgery, vol 1. Philadelphia, New York, Lippincott-Raven, 1997:215.
11. Hammon JW, Queale WS, Kim TK, et al. Surgeon experience and clinical and economic outcomes of shoulder arthroplasty. J Bone Joint Surg 2003;85A12:2318.
12. Hasan SS, Leith JM, Smith KL, et al. The distribution of shoulder replacement among surgeons and hospitals is significantly different than that of hip or knee replacement. J Shoulder Elbow Surg 2003;12:164.
13. Kralinger F, Schwaiger R, Wambacher M, et al. Outcome after primary hemiarthroplasty for fracture of the humeral head of the humerus. A retrospective multicenter study of 167 patients. J Bone Joint Surg 2004;86B:217.
14. Iannotti JP, Gabriel JP, Schneck SL, et al. The normal glenohumeral relationships. An anatomical study of one hundred and forty shoulders. J Bone Joint Surg Am 1992;74(4):491.
15. Le Huec JC, Boileau P, Sinnerton R, et al. Tuberosity osteosynthesis in shoulder arthroplasty. In: Walch G, Boileau P, eds. Shoulder arthroplasty. Berlin, Springer, 1999:323.
16. Neer C. Displaced proximal humeral fractures. II. Treatment of three-part and four-part displacement. J Bone Joint Surg Am 1970;52(6):1090.
17. Norris TR, Green A, McGuigan FX. Late prosthetic shoulder arthroplasty for displaced proximal humerus fractures. J Shoulder Elbow Surg 1995;4(4):271.
18. Parsons IM, Millett PJ, Warner JJP. Glenoid erosion after hemiarthroplasty. Clin Orthop 2004;421:120.
19. Robertson D, Yuan J, Bigliani L, et al. Three-dimensional analysis of the proximal part of the humerus: relevance to arthroplasty. J Bone Joint Surg 2000;82A:1594.
20. Robinson CM, Page RS, Hill RMF, et al. Primary hemiarthroplasty for treatment of proximal humeral fractures. J Bone Joint Surg Am 2003;85(7):1215.
21. Tanner RW, Cofield RH. Prosthetic arthroplasty for fracture and fracture-dislocation of the proximal humerus. Clin Orthop 1983; 179:116.

Nonunion of Proximal Humerus Fractures

16

Julie Y. Bishop   *Evan L. Flatow*

INTRODUCTION

Fractures of the proximal humerus are nondisplaced in the majority of cases and usually heal uneventfully with non-operative treatment.[15,27,29,41] Nonunions of the proximal humerus are uncommon and pose a very difficult problem to both the patient and the surgeon. For the patient, an established nonunion can be painful and functionally disabling. For the surgeon, treatment of these cases is extremely challenging, because various technical factors, such as soft bone, extensive scarring, and prior hardware, can limit the success of surgical treatment. However, successful treatment of a proximal humeral nonunion can be very rewarding when pain is abolished and functional use is restored to the patient.

PATHOETIOLOGY

Proximal humerus fractures are common, especially in elderly women.[2,7,14,16,21,35] Nonunions, although rare, are more commonly seen after displaced two-part fractures or after cases in which open reduction and internal fixation is the initial treatment.[6] Patients primarily present with a considerable amount of pain and varying degrees of functional loss. Patients are rarely able to perform their normal activities of daily living, and pain, which is often present at

rest, is generally exacerbated by any attempt to use the extremity. The causes of nonunion can be divided into factors that are unique to the fracture site, factors associated with the first method of treatment, and systemic and medical factors.

The weight of the arm causes a distraction force across the fracture site, which is compounded by the more cortical distal fragment that has poorer healing qualities compared to the more cancellous proximal fragment. A soft and cavitated head further decreases the healing potential of the bone in this area (Fig. 16-1). Soft-tissue interposition, such as the biceps tendon, can prevent fracture healing as well. Synovial fluid from the adjacent joint can communicate with the fracture site and limit the formation of hematoma and subsequent healing.

If the shaft is not properly reduced, the pectoralis major can continue to pull the shaft anteriorly, and the head can be further displaced through the pull of the rotator cuff. Improper immobilization can also create traction across the fracture site, also impeding bony apposition and healing. The arm must be immobilized across the front of the body, with the elbow anterior to the midline of the body in the coronal plane. This will neutralize the muscular forces across the fracture site (Fig. 16-2). Range-of-motion exercises, which are started before healing has begun, can also lead to nonunion of the fracture site. The upper extremity must move as a unit before any therapy is begun.

Finally, systemic disease and polytrauma are factors that may compromise a patient's ability to heal a fracture. Elderly patients can have severe osteopenia, complicated by nutritional deficiency and/or metabolic bone diseases, again hindering the ability to heal fractures. These medical

J. Y. Bishop: Mount Sinai School of Medicine, Department of Orthopaedic Surgery, New York, New York.
E. L. Flatow: Department of Orthopaedic Surgery, Mount Sinai Medical Center, New York, New York.

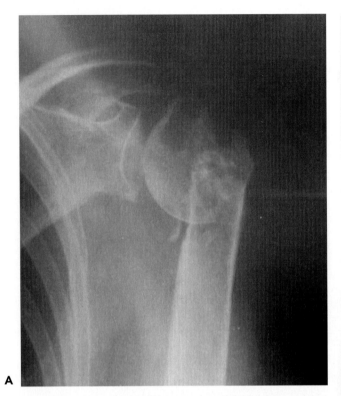

A

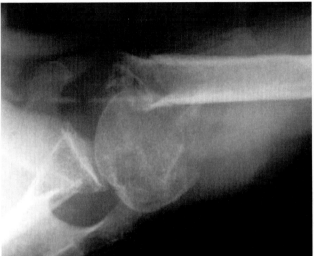

B

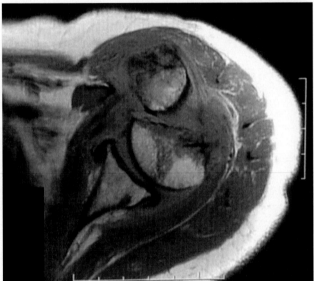

C

Figure 16-1 A surgical neck nonunion is shown demonstrating destruction of the medial calcar on both the (A) anteroposterior (AP) and (B) axillary views. The small amount of remaining head is further demonstrated on (C) the MRI scan, axial view.

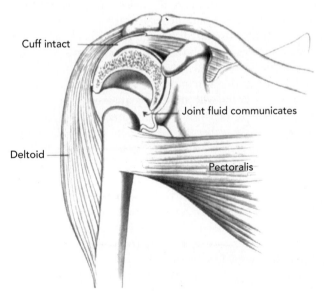

Cuff intact

Joint fluid communicates

Deltoid

Pectoralis

Figure 16-2 Diagram demonstrating muscular forces across the fracture site. The pectoralis can pull the muscle anterior and medial while the rotator cuff can further elevate and externally rotate the head. Synovial fluid from the adjacent joint can communicate with the fracture site and limit the formation of hematoma and subsequent healing. (Reprinted with permission from Neer CS. Glenohumeral arthroplasty. In: Shoulder reconstruction. Philadelphia, WB Saunders, 1990: 143, Fig. 3-65.)

issues should be recognized and addressed prior to subsequent surgery and a referral made to an internist, if necessary. In the series by Healy et al., 16 of the 25 patients had significant medical illnesses, and the results of treatment in this group were unsatisfactory overall.[14]

CLINICAL EVALUATION

The amount of pain and functional losses that a patient has must be carefully assessed. Because of the potential for increased morbidity associated with attempted treatment of this problem, conservative management may be indicated for the minimally symptomatic patient. A complete review of all prior records, especially any operative reports, is essential.

On physical examination, false motion may occur through the nonunion site, and thus passive "shoulder" motion may seem excellent, whereas active motion is generally poor due to a flail arm. In fibrous nonunions, there may be some stability, and motion may be limited by shoulder stiffness. A careful neurovascular examination must be performed, especially if operative intervention is being considered. Neurologic damage may have occurred at the time of the original injury, or at the initial surgery, if one was performed. Special attention should be directed to the axillary nerve and the status of the deltoid.

The status of the rotator cuff is often difficult to assess, because pain and weakness due to the original injury and subsequent nonunion may be significant. Overall disuse of the extremity may contribute to deltoid and periscapular muscular atrophy.

If the patient had prior surgical intervention, the possibility of sepsis must always be ruled out (Fig. 16-3). The skin should be carefully examined for any draining sinuses or other evidence of infection. When in doubt, appropriate lab work should be ordered and an aspiration performed with or without appropriate nuclear medicine imaging studies.

Finally, it is also very important to take into account the physiologic state of each patient and that patient's ability to heal a fracture in light of his or her medical conditions.

RADIOGRAPHIC EVALUATION

Adequate radiographic evaluation is a necessity, and the standard views are always obtained: anteroposterior in the plane of the scapula, a scapular lateral or "Y" view, and an axillary view. This should be sufficient to judge the position of the fracture fragments, the extent of bone loss, and the quality of the bone present. Computed tomography (CT) scanning may be helpful, if radiographs are inconclusive. This is more common when there is malunion of the greater tuberosity and nonunion of the surgical neck in a three-part proximal humerus fracture. Magnetic resonance imaging (MRI) is useful to demonstrate any soft-tissue abnormalities associated with the biceps tendon, rotator cuff, deltoid, or labrum.

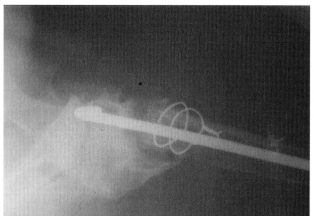

A   B

Figure 16-3 Infected nonunion after prior Ender's rod fixation of the surgical neck fracture. (*A*) Anteroposterior (AP) and (*B*) axillary views. *(continued)*

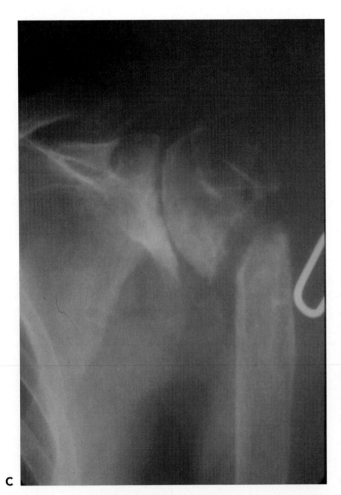

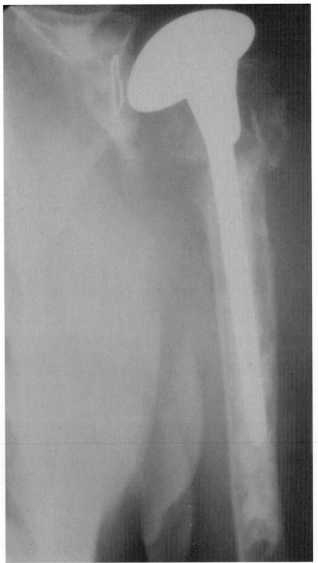

C   D

Figure 16-3 *(continued)* (*C*) Hardware removal and irrigation and debridement are performed in anticipation of a staged humeral head replacement. (*D*) AP radiograph after implantation of the humeral head prosthesis.

TUBEROSITY FRACTURE NONUNION

Tuberosity nonunions are rare unless markedly displaced; they usually heal to something and are more likely to develop a malunion. Gartsman and Taverna reported on a greater tuberosity nonunion, which was repaired arthroscopically, along with a concurrent rotator cuff tear.[13] If necessary, greater and lesser tuberosity nonunions can be repaired with the same techniques utilized for acute fractures (Fig. 16-4). However, a long-standing nonunion of a tuberosity may be quite retracted and adhesed to the soft tissues, necessitating an extensive release for mobilization of the fragment. Surgical indications are similar to those for malunions and include significant displacement

of the tuberosity and concurrent functional deficit caused by pain or significant limitation of range of motion.

SURGICAL NECK NONUNION

Surgical neck nonunions are more common than tuberosity nonunions and occur with or without tuberosity malunion, avascular necrosis of the humeral head, or posttraumatic glenohumeral arthritis[41] (Fig. 16-5). Indeed, surgical neck nonunion is more likely, if there is glenohumeral stiffness, because motion is shifted to the fracture site. Operative treatment of a surgical neck nonunion is a challenging undertaking, because there can be extensive bone resorp-

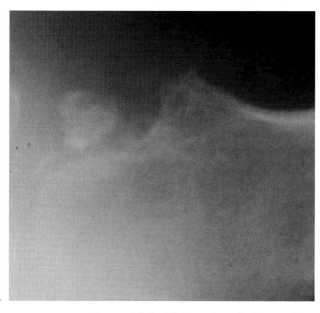
A

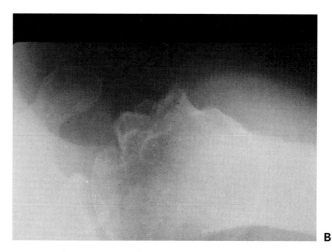
B

Figure 16-4   (*A*) Nonunion of a lesser tuberosity fracture, which was treated nonoperatively. (*B*) Axillary view after open reduction and suture fixation of the lesser tuberosity fragment.

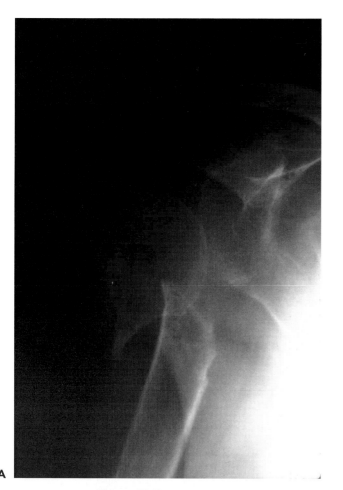
A

B

Figure 16-5   (*A*) Preoperative anteroposterior (AP) radiograph of a surgical neck nonunion. (*B*) Intraoperative picture demonstrating biceps tendon interposition at the fracture site, preventing reduction and fracture healing. *(continued)*

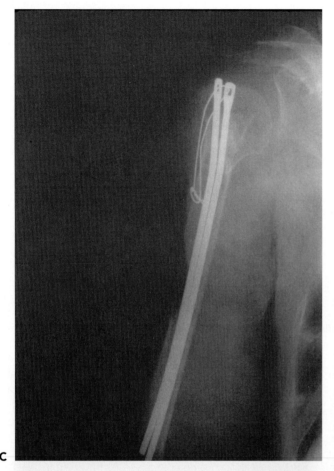

C

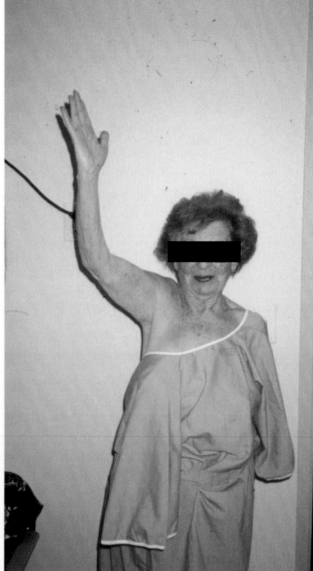

E

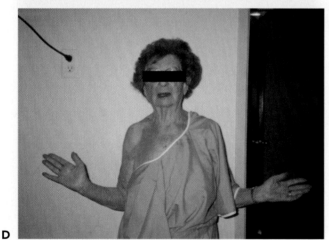

D

Figure 16-5 *(continued)* (C) Postoperative radiograph after fixation with Ender's rods and tension band suture fixation. (D,E) Clinical pictures taken 18 months after surgery; patient has symmetric motion and is pain-free.

tion, including a portion of the head by the pseudoarthrosis. In addition, the remaining bone is often osteoporotic and holds fixation poorly. Neer[25] noted in 1983 that there were only 29 reported cases in the literature, and then his paper added an additional 50 cases. Overall, the reported treatment results from the studies, subsequently in the literature, have been very mixed. Many types of treatment methods have been described[6,14,18,24,31,33,36,37] that consist pri-

marily of intramedullary fixation, open reduction and internal fixation, hemiarthroplasty, and "skillful neglect" or nonoperative treatment. Although some authors report reasonable results with humeral head replacement,[1,4,9,30,38] others have noted more reliable functional results following open reduction and internal fixation (ORIF).[3,4,8,30,31,33,36] In fact, one recent study recommends that replacement arthroplasty for surgical neck nonunions requiring greater tuberosity osteotomy be abandoned as a treatment option due to poor outcome.[4] Each method will be reviewed, followed by the senior author's treatment of choice.

NONOPERATIVE TREATMENT

A surgical neck fracture can be declared a nonunion at approximately 6 months after fracture. However, if there is no evidence of healing callus by 3 months, there should be suspicion that a delayed union or nonunion is developing. Given the potential for significant morbidity associated with surgical management of this problem, nonoperative treatment is an option, especially if it is the nondominant arm in an elderly person, and pain is not too severe. Healy et al.[14] reported poor results in patients treated nonoperatively at their institution; however, results of surgical treatment have been mixed, with several studies showing approximately 50% unsatisfactory results. Thus, nonoperative treatment is a viable option when pain is not severe.

Conservative treatment focuses on functional use. Range-of-motion exercises for the hand and elbow are used to prevent secondary stiffness. If the nonunion is flail, no shoulder motion exercises are used; they will generally only increase false motion at the nonunion. However, if there is a fibrous nonunion that moves as a unit, gentle exercises within the limits of comfort may be used to maintain motion at the shoulder. Some patients benefit from a humeral fracture brace to support the arm; in many it is a cumbersome nuisance.

OPERATIVE TREATMENT

Intramedullary Fixation

Reported results after intramedullary fixation for surgical neck nonunion have often been less than satisfactory, frequently due to mechanical impingement of the rods on the rotator cuff and the subacromial space. Often, the nonunions did heal; however, a secondary operation was necessary to remove the hardware, primarily Rush rods. One series[24] included 10 patients who were treated with Rush rods and a tension band and seven by humeral head replacement. All patients developed a clinical union; however, there were several complications, and eight required hardware removal. The tension bands were not incorporated into the rod fixation, which may be an important factor leading to impingement and failure. Another series of five patients showed failure to heal in four, and all showed symptoms of impingement and had unsatisfactory function. This was part of a larger series by Jupiter et al., in which 5 of 25 of their patients received nonreamed

intramedullary rods. These were the worst results of the series, and the authors did not recommend the technique.[14] There have been successful results reported, however, and they have been primarily with Ender's rods and suture fixation. Reliable pain relief was achieved, but functional results were modest.[9,31] Custom Ender's rods modified with a hole through the proximal aspect of the rod to allow incorporation of tension band sutures or wires may limit subsequent rod migration[9] (Fig. 16-6). However, impingement was still a problem in four of seven patients in one study, requiring hardware removal.[9] Humeral head comminution can lead to failure of fixation with rods and is a relative contraindication to this technique. Overall, intramedullary nails have not proven to have consistently good results, with impingement being a significant problem.

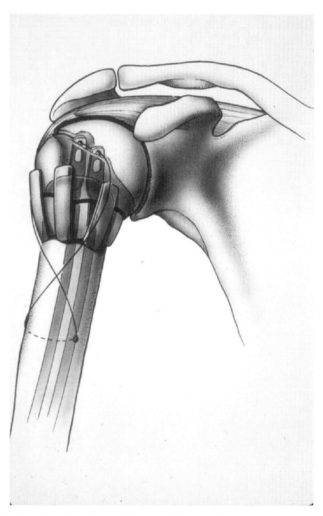

Figure 16-6 Diagram demonstrating calcar bone graft incorporation with the use of Ender's rod fixation and figure-of-eight suture. (Reprinted with permission from Duralde XA, Flatow EL, Pollock RG, et al. Operative treatment of non-unions of the surgical neck of the humerus. J Shoulder Elbow Surg 1996;5(3):169, Fig. 3.)

Plate Fixation

Open reduction and internal fixation has been a reliable treatment option for surgical neck nonunions, especially when there is sufficient bone stock within the humeral head. Several studies have shown good results.[14,36,37] Most commonly, T-plates or blade plates have been used, although blade plates do require less stripping of the lateral aspect of the proximal humerus and, subsequently, reduce avascular necrosis rates (Fig. 16-7). More recently, locking plates have been available, but no results are available.

Internal fixation can be difficult to achieve due to the poor fixation of screws within the humeral head. This is due to osteopenia within the head as well as the pull of the rotator cuff on the proximal humerus. Early papers did warn of this possibility,[6] and different methods have been used to avoid this.[19,39,40] Specialized plates were used, as well as a tension band, which was woven into the RTC and secured to the T-plate, which was used for shaft fixation. The tension band counteracted the pull of the humeral head away from the proximal humeral screws.

Walch et al. emphasized the importance of bone grafting and treating these kinds of fractures.[39] They had a 96%

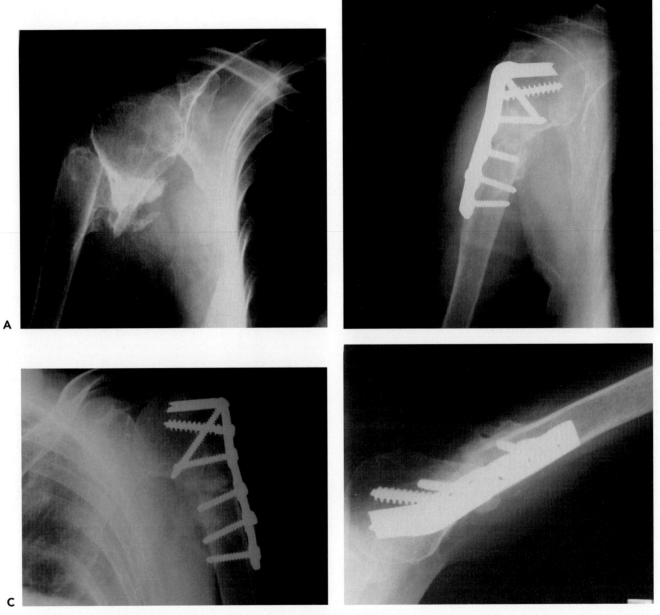

Figure 16-7 (*A*) Surgical neck nonunion visualized on an anteroposterior (AP) radiograph. (*B*) Patient was pain-free one year after open reduction and blade plate fixation of the nonunion. (*C*) AP and (*D*) axillary radiographs are shown.

union rate and an 85% satisfaction rate when intramedullary and cancellous bone grafting were used along with plate osteosynthesis. Healy et al. utilized T-plate fixation in 13 patients, in 12 of whom the fracture united; overall there were 9 good results.[14] They felt that the addition of bone graft was very important, as was a Krackow ligament stitch, placed through the rotator cuff to the plate. Sonnabend modified an AO semitubular plate into a blade-type plate and created two sharp spikes on the proximal end.[37] Combining this technique with bone graft led to union in five of six surgical neck nonunions. It was thought that this construct would decrease the incidence of screw cut-out. Also, a more inferior position on the humeral head may be possible with a blade plate than a T-plate and reduce the incidence of impingement.

Proximal humeral blade plates offer advantages over standard plate and screw fixation with potentially improved proximal fixation in the humeral head while serving as a tension band to counteract the pull of the rotator cuff. The broad fixed blade acts to maintain fracture alignment even when the bone quality is poor and does not depend on the engagement of threads within the bone to ensure the strength of fixation.[34] Blade plates require minimal dissection and therefore better preserve the blood supply to the humeral head, and unlike intramedullary nails, do not violate the rotator cuff. Jupiter and Mullaji reported on the early use of the blade plate for nine painful nonunions of the proximal humerus.[17] Only one patient did not achieve union and went on to a poor result. They followed up with a subsequent study of 25 nonunions in 2001.[34] Blade plate fixation and autogenous bone graft was used to repair all 25 nonunions. Healing was documented in 23 of the patients, and results were graded as good or excellent in 20. They felt that the blade plate provided a reliable, stable form of fixation for nonunions of the proximal humerus.

SURGICAL TECHNIQUES

Prosthetic Replacement

The biggest challenge in achieving internal fixation is the bone quality of the individual patient. Often the degree of osteopenia is substantial and can decrease the security of screw fixation. When the proximal fragment is too small or osteoporotic to gain stability with internal fixation, prosthetic replacement is a favorable option. Patients with poor bone quality and subsequent shaft resorption and head cavitation are poor candidates for internal fixation, but these factors may also limit the success of hemiarthroplasty. Neer reported early on on the technical difficulties, high complication rate, and overall poor and inconsistent results when shoulder arthroplasty is performed in the setting of old trauma.[25,26,28] Prosthetic replacement has been elected in cases with very poor bone quality, avascular

necrosis, significant glenohumeral arthritis, and fixed dislocation of the head.[32] However, there are very few papers in the literature on this subject, all with a small number of cases. Although there are definite times when a hemiarthroplasty is appropriate, the indications have not been firmly established; there is still no consensus on the best surgical technique, and no outcomes from the different studies showed uniform results.

Boileau et al. reported on hemiarthroplasty performed for six nonunions of the surgical neck.[4] These occurred in the setting of nonoperative three-part fractures (in which the head fragment rotated, the tuberosity healed in a malunited position, and the neck did not unite) or two- and four-part fractures that had undergone primary surgery. All cases required a greater tuberosity osteotomy, and two needed a lesser tuberosity osteotomy as well. They felt that greater tuberosity osteotomies led to a significant decrease in functional outcomes. The osteotomy devascularizes the greater tuberosity, leading to tuberosity nonunion, migration, and resorption. They felt that this was very likely responsible for the poor results.[5,8,10,26] Another contributing factor was believed to be the prosthesis preventing union of the tuberosities to the humeral shaft. The primary goal should be to obtain union of the tuberosities to the shaft. Given their results, especially in comparison to their prior published results on internal fixation with intramedullary bone grafting,[39] they believe that replacement arthroplasty should be abandoned in the treatment of surgical neck nonunions, except in the case of a long-standing nonunion in which the humeral head has collapsed.

Antuna et al. reported on 25 arthroplasties performed for pain and functional impairment due to proximal humerus nonunion.[4] They had one excellent, 11 satisfactory, and 13 unsatisfactory results; although, overall, 20 of the shoulders were either much better or better.[4] Fourteen of the shoulders underwent greater tuberosity osteotomy. In 12 shoulders, either the greater tuberosity was not healed, was malunited, or was resorbed at follow-up. Lack of tuberosity healing may account for the limited range of motion of these patients due to subsequent supraspinatus weakness. Tuberosity healing problems were the most common complication in their series. Unsatisfactory results were primarily due to poor motion and thus poor functional use. They concluded that although function was not completely restored in most of their patients, arthroplasty does allow most patients to obtain a high level of satisfaction and pain relief.

The preference of the senior author has been for blade-plate fixation when there has been preservation of the head, but in cases where the head is soft, cavitated, or eroded, a humeral head replacement utilizing the head for a cresenteric calcar bone graft has been the treatment of choice (Fig. 16-8). Recently, the author's experience with nine patients with surgical neck nonunions complicated by severe humeral head destruction and inadequate bone

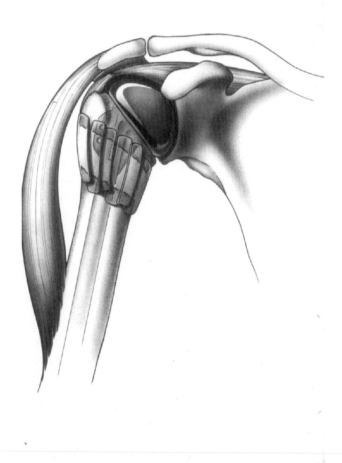

However, in a surgical neck malunion, the tuberosity is not healed to the shaft and therefore not in any constant relation to it. It may be malunited with respect to the head, but when replacement is elected, this relationship, too, no longer retains.

In a true surgical neck nonunion, the proximal fragment consists of the head, the greater tuberosity, and the lesser tuberosity. Once the head is osteotomized at the

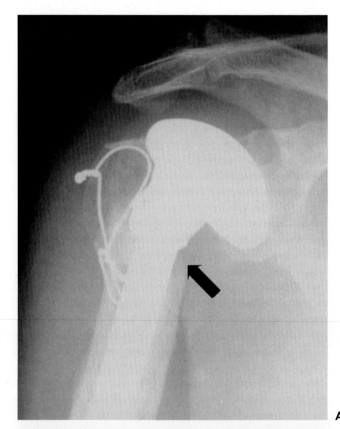

A

Figure 16-8   Diagram of a humeral head replacement for a surgical neck nonunion. Structural bone graft is placed around the calcar to improve stability and healing. (Reprinted with permission from Duralde XA, Flatow EL, Pollock RG, et al. Operative treatment of non-unions of the surgical neck of the humerus. J Shoulder Elbow Surg 1996;5(3):169, Fig. 4.)

stock was presented at the February 2003 annual meeting of the American Academy of Orthopaedic Surgeons.[23] All patients received humeral head replacement with calcar grafting, none required a greater tuberosity osteotomy, and all tuberosities healed (Fig. 16-9). Most patients achieved a dramatic improvement in range of motion as well as a dramatic decrease in pain. Complications were minimal with calcar graft resorption occurring in two cases.

There is perhaps some lack of clarity in the literature about exactly what constitutes an osteostomy of the greater tuberosity. With a malunited proximal humeral fracture, the healed greater tuberosity bears a fixed relation to the shaft, and, if there is a large degree of malunion, this can complicate treatment. When performing humeral head replacement in such cases, Neer argued that setting the prosthesis to the malunited tuberosity may be preferable to putting the prosthesis in the "correct" position and osteotomizing the tuberosity, if the deformity was not too severe.

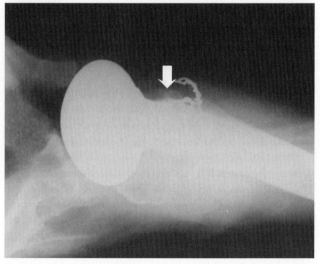

B

Figure 16-9   Radiographs showing a healed greater tuberosity with medial calcar graft resorption on the (A) anteroposterior (AP) and (B) axial views.

anatomical neck, only the two tuberosities remain, with or without a small calcar remnant. Even if the greater tuberosity has malunited, at this stage it is only with respect to the lesser tuberosity; a further osteotomy has never been necessary in our experience, because the ring of tuberosities and calcar may be rotated or tilted by the surgeons. When there has been calcar resorption, the greater and lesser tuberosities float freely as a single C-shaped fragment after the head is removed. This may be considered the functional equivalent of a tuberosity osteotomy with a known risk of poor healing. It is for this purpose that we employ a structural calcar graft, to complete the ring and improve stability and healing. With nonunions below the surgical neck, a tuberosity malunion presents a greater challenge, but the head and calcar are rarely eroded in such cases, and we generally prefer open reduction internal fixation and bone grafting.

The senior author feels that his results are satisfactory and comparable to at least three other studies.[4,16,17] Factors that contribute to the improved outcomes are (a) autologous bone grafting, (b) extensive surgical releases, (c) anatomic restoration of the humeral component, and (d) avoidance of greater tuberosity osteotomy.[31] The low complication rate and need for revision surgery is consistent with other studies that have reported more postoperative complications and a greater need for additional operations for patients who underwent ORIF when compared to those who underwent hemiarthroplasty.[9,12,24,30,41] This is a significant advantage because these procedures are often performed in the elderly population, who are particularly at risk for developing perioperative complications.[9,17,24] Thus, replacement arthroplasty with calcar grafting and an extensive surgical release is a good treatment option for symptomatic surgical neck nonunions of the humerus, especially when humeral head resorption and softening make internal fixation problematic.

It is interesting that Boileau concluded that his poor results may have been due to use of a "conventional" replacement, with too much proximal metal to allow bone grafting. He noted that early results with a lower profile prosthesis developed for fractures were encouraging. This may account for some of the variation in reported results, because available implants have a large range of geometrics. The good results reported by the senior author were with low-profile implants combined, as noted, with extensive proximal bone grafting.

SURGICAL PROCEDURE

An extended deltopectoral approach is utilized. The cephalic vein can be retracted medially with the pectoralis for protection from instrumentation during the procedure. The clavipectoral fascia is incised exposing the conjoined tendon, which is retracted medially to visualize the sub-

scapularis. The axillary nerve is palpated anterior to the subscapularis and protected for the remainder of the case. If the medial calcar is eroded from the nonunion, it is sometimes possible to avoid a subscapularis takedown. In such cases, the head may be removed through the rotator interval and "from below" (via the nonunion). If this is not possible, then the subscapularis is incised 1 cm medial to its insertion on the lesser tuberosity after ligating the circumflex vessels. Four No. 2, nonabsorbable sutures are placed through bone tunnels along the insertion site of the subscapularis for later repair. An extensive capsulectomy is performed to remove the anterior, inferior, and superior portions of the glenohumeral capsule.

The nonunion site can then be identified. Using periosteal elevators, osteotomes, and rongeurs, the nonunion site is debrided, removing any fibrous tissue or interposed soft tissue. Sagittal saws and osteotomes are then used to remove the humeral head along its anatomical neck. If the medial calcar is eroded from the nonunion, the greater and lesser tuberosities remained as a C-shaped fragment with an opening medially. If the calcar is preserved, a ring-shaped piece remains, which consists of the greater and lesser tuberosities and the calcar remnant. Sutures are placed around the tuberosities for later repair to the shaft after placing the prosthesis. The glenoid is then evaluated for evidence of articular damage. If significant full thickness diffuse chondral damage is present, then the glenoid is replaced.

The canal is prepared using progressively increased size reamers until cortical contact is achieved. An appropriately sized humeral trial is placed through the remaining humeral neck and into the humeral shaft and assessed for height and version. Stem height is determined using the medial cortex of the retained humerus as a guideline, and an attempt is made to restore the contour of the cortex (Fig. 16-10). Version is determined by using the epicondylar axis of the distal humerus. The canal is then debrided using pulsatile lavage, and any remaining blood is removed using thrombin and hydrogen peroxide-soaked gauzes. Cement is placed distally in the canal taking care to keep the proximal shaft free of cement to improve bone healing. The final prosthesis position is determined from the previously placed trial component making an attempt to restore anatomic height and version. If a ring-shaped piece remained, the stem of the final prosthesis skewers the remaining humeral neck and is placed into the canal. Cancellous bone from the osteotomized head is packed between the calcar and the shaft. If the medial calcar is resorbed leaving a C-shape, a large corticocancellous bone graft from the humeral head is wedged beneath the prosthesis head and the shaft to replace the medial calcar (Fig. 16-11).

The proximal fragment is repaired to the shaft with large nonabsorbable sutures incorporating the cuff tendon insertion. When bone quality allows, the fixation is augmented with a tension-band cable. The subscapularis is repaired to the lesser tuberosity and shaft using the previously placed sutures, which further secures the medial bone graft. A large hemovac drain is placed. The deltopectoral interval is loosely reapproximated, and the skin is closed with absorbable suture.

POSTOPERATIVE REHABILITATION

Patients begin full passive forward elevation and external rotation (to 40 degrees) on postoprative day one. Active-assisted exercises, including pulleys and external rotation with a stick, are incorporated into the rehabilitation program.

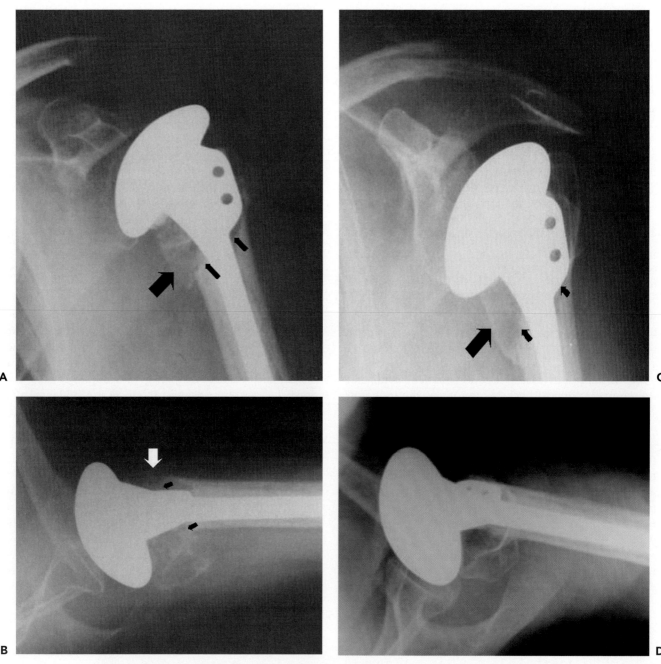

Figure 16-10   Humeral head replacement demonstrating restoration of humeral contour on both the (A) anteroposterior (AP) and (B) axillary views. The surgical neck non-union site (*small arrows*) and the bone graft (*large arrows*) are easily visualized at 6 weeks postop, whereas, at 2 years postop, the (C) AP and (D) axillary views show healing with obliteration of the radiolucent lines at the non-union site. Clinical pictures taken 4 years postop. *(continued)*

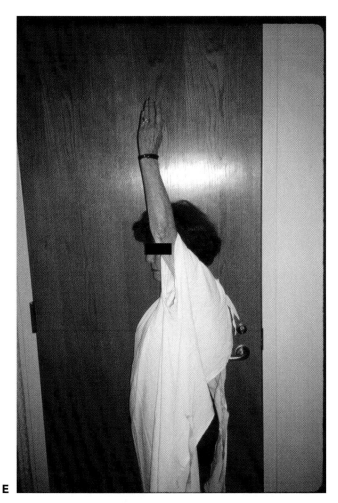

E

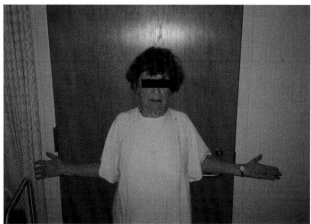

F

Figure 16-10 *(continued)*   Patient has regained (*E*) full elevation and (*F*) external rotation.

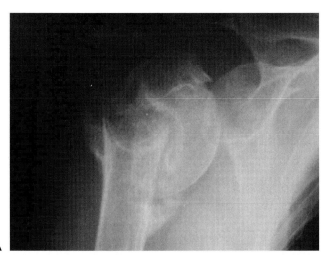

A

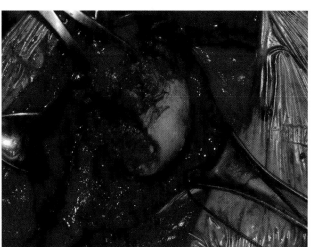

B

Figure 16-11   (*A*) A surgical neck nonunion demonstrating significant bone loss and calcar destruction on the anteroposterior (AP) radiograph. (*B*) Intraoperative picture showing the extreme cavitation of the humeral head. *(continued)*

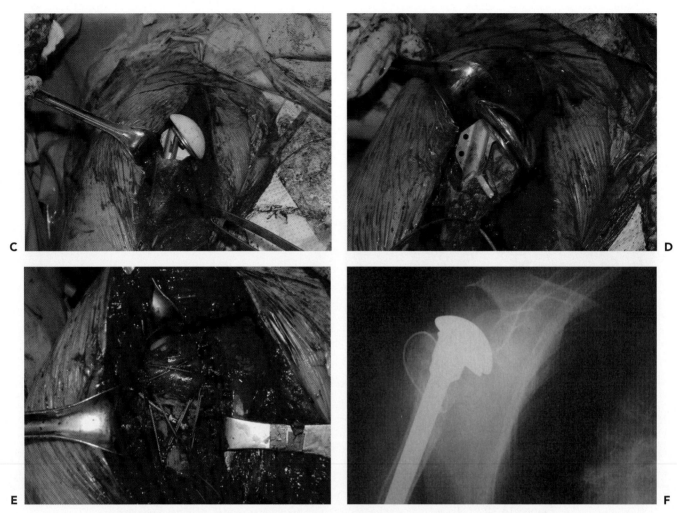

Figure 16-11 *(continued)*   *(C)* Trial prosthesis is evaluated for proper height and version. *(D)* Destruction of the medial cortex is visualized, demonstrating the need for bone graft, which is placed after the prosthesis has been cemented into the canal. *(E)* The graft is secured with a cable, and figure-of-eight suture fixation of the tuberosities further secures the medial bone graft. *(F)* Postoperative AP radiograph.

With the exception of physical therapy, the patient remains in the sling at all times for 6 weeks. Patients begin terminal stretches at 6 weeks to further maximize their range of motion. In addition, at 6 weeks the patient begins active motion with a gentle, progressive strengthening program.

THREE- AND FOUR-PART MALUNIONS AND NONUNIONS

Overall, three- and four-part proximal humerus fracture nonunions are not very common. Malunion of the tuberosities more commonly occur with surgical neck malunions. If nonunions do occur, prosthetic replacement is typically indicated. However, the results do not approach those obtained with prosthetic treatment of acute three- and four-part fractures.[11,22] In one study, Healy et al.[14] reported four good results and two fair re-

sults in a series of six three-part nonunions. Frich et al.[11] found that infection after primary open reduction and internal fixation often compromised the results of revision. Overall, failed primary surgical management of these fractures reduced the likelihood of a good result with revision arthroplasty.

SUMMARY

Nonunions of the proximal humerus are particularly debilitating to patients and pose a considerable technical challenge to the orthopedic surgeon. Successful treatment is possible, although pain relief has been more reliable than restoration of function. Several different treatment options are available, as each has different indications. If there is decent bone stock and the head is relatively well preserved, blade-plate fixation with bone grafting is a relatively good option. The recent introduction of locking plates may also be of help. However, in cases where there is erosion and cavitation of the head and medial bone loss, the senior author has found that symptomatic nonunions are best treated with extensive surgical releases, soft-tissue balancing, and hemiarthroplasty with calcar bone grafting utilizing a low-profile implant.

REFERENCES

1. Antuna SA, Sperling JW, Sanchez-Sotelo J, et al. Shoulder arthroplasty for proximal humeral non-unions. J Shoulder Elbow Surg 2002;11(2):114.
2. Bengner U, Johnell O, Redlun-Johnell I. Changes in the incidence of fracture of the upper end of the humerus during a 30-year period. Clin Orthop 1988;231:179.
3. Boileau P, et al. Sequelae of fractures of the proximal humerus: surgical classification and limits of shoulder arthroplasty. In: Walsh G, Boileau P, eds. Shoulder arthroplasty. Berlin, Springer-Verlag, 1999:349.
4. Boileau P, Trojani C, Walch G, et al. Shoulder arthroplasty for the treatment of the sequelae of fractures of the proximal humerus. J Shoulder Elbow Surg 200l;10(4):299.
5. Compito CA, Self EB, Bigliani LU. Arthroplasty and acute shoulder trauma: reasons for success and failure. Clin Orthop 1994; 307:27.
6. Coventry MB, Laurnen El. Ununited fractures of the middle and upper humerus. Clin Orthop 1970;69:192.
7. Depalma AF, Cautilli RA. Fractures of the upper end of the humerus. Clin Orthop 1961;20:73.
8. Dines DM, Klaarren RF, Altcheck DW, et al. Posttraumatic changes of the proximal humerus: mal-union, nonunion, and osteonecrosis. Treatment with modular hemiarthroplasty or total shoulder arthroplasty. J Shoulder Elbow Surg 1993;2:11.
9. Duralde XA, Flatow EL, Pollock RG, et al. Operative treatment of non-unions of the surgical neck of the humerus. J Shoulder Elbow Surg 1996;5(3):169.
10. Flatow EL, Neer CS II. Chronic anterior dislocation of the shoulder. J Shoulder Elbow Surg 1993;2:2.
11. Frich LH, Sojbjerg JO, Sneppen O. Shoulder arthroplasty in complex acute and chronic proximal humeral fractures. Orthopedics 1991;14:949.
12. Galatz L, Iannotti J. Management of surgical neck non-unions. Orthop Clin North Am 2001;31(1):51.
13. Gartsman GM, Taverna ET. Arthroscopic treatment of rotator cuff tear and greater tuberosity fracture nonunion. Arthroscopy 1996;12(2):242.
14. Healy WL, Jupiter J, Kristiansen T, et al. Nonunion of the proximal humerus: a review of 25 cases. J Orthop Trauma 1990;4(4): 424.
15. Heppenstall RB. Fractures of the proximal humerus. Orthop Clin North Am 1975;6(2):467.
16. Horak J, Nilsson BE. Epidemiology of fracture of the upper end of the humerus. Clin Orthop 197;112:250.
17. Jupiter JB, Mullaji AB. Blade plate fixation of proximal humeral non-unions. Injury 1994;25(5):301.
18. Leach R, Premer R. Nonunion of the surgical neck of the humerus: method of internal fixation. Minn Med 1965;45:318.
19. Leach RE, Premer RF. Nonunion of the surgical neck of the humerus: method of internal fixation. Minn Med 1965;48:318.
20. McCreoth SW. Delayed union and nonunion in fractures of the humeral shaft. J Bone Joint Surg 1975;578:393.
21. McGuigan FX, Norris TR, Sharkey PF. Delayed shoulder arthroplasty for cases of failed outcome in complex fractures of the proximal humerus. Orthop Trans 1992–1993;16:823.
22. Miller S, Lin JS, Klepps S. Effectiveness of replacement arthroplasty with calcar grafting for the treatment of surgical neck nonunions of the humerus. Presented at American Academy of Orthopaedic Surgeons annual meeting, New Orleans, LA, February 2003.
23. Nayak NK, Schickendantz MS, Regan WD, et al. Operative treatment of nonunion of surgical neck fractures of the humerus. Clin Orthop 1995;313:200.
24. Neer C. Nonunion of the surgical neck of the humerus. Orthop Trans 1983;3:389.
25. Neer CS. Old trauma in glenohumeral arthroplasty. In: Shoulder reconstruction. Philadelphia, WB Saunders, 1990:222.
26. Neer CS II. Displaced proximal humeral fractures I. J Bone Joint Surg 1970;52A(61):1077.
27. Neer CS II, Watson KC, Stanton FJ. Recent experience in total shoulder replacement. J Bone Joint Surg Am 1982;64:319.
28. Neviaser JS. Complicated fractures and dislocations about the shoulder joint. J Bone Joint Surg 1962;44A(5):984.
29. Nicholson GP, Flatow EL, Bigliani LU. Shoulder arthroplasty for proximal humerus fractures. In Friedman R, ed. Arthroplasty of the shoulder. New York, Thieme, 1994:183.
30. Norris T, Turner J, Bovill D. Nonunion of the upper humerus: an analysis of the etiology and treatment in 28 cases. In Post M, Morrey B, eds. Surgery of the shoulder. St. Louis, Mosby, 1990:63.
31. Norris TR. Prosthetic arthroplasty in nonunions and malunions of the proximal humerus. Semin Arthroplasty 1997;8:304.
32. Norris TR, Green A, McGuigan FX. Late prosthetic shoulder arthroplasty for displaced proximal humerus fractures. J Shoulder Elbow Surg 1995;4(4):271.
33. Ring D, McKee MD, Perey B. The use of a blade plate and autogenous cancellous bone graft in the treatment of ununited fractures of the proximal humerus. J Shoulder Elbow Surg 2001;10:501.
34. Rockwood CA, Pearce JC. Management of proximal humerus nonunions. Orthop Trans 1989;13:644.
35. Scheck M. Surgical treatment of non-unions of the surgical neck of the humerus. Clin Orthop 1982;167:255.
36. Sonnabend DH. Blade plate fixation of humeral neck fractures and nonunions in osteoporotic bone. J Shoulder Elbow Surg 1993;2(suppl):49.
37. Tanner MW, Cofield RH. Prosthetic arthroplasty for fractures and fracture-dislocations of the proximal humerus. Clin Orthop 1983;179:116.
38. Walch G, Badet R, Nove-Josserand L, et al. Nonunions of the surgical neck of the humerus: surgical treatment with an intramedullary bone peg, internal fixation, and cancellous bone grafting. J Shoulder Elbow Surg 1995;5:161.
39. Wang GJ, Reger SI, Stamp WG. Nonunion of fractures of the proximal humerus: a method of treatment using a modified Moe plate. South Med J 1977;70:818.
40. Young TB, Wallace WA. Conservative treatment of fractures and fracture dislocations of the upper end of the humerus. J Bone Joint Surg 1985;67B(3):373.
41. Duralde XA, Flatow EL, Pollock RG, et al. Operative treatment of nonunions of the surgical neck of the humerus. J Shoulder Elbow Surg 1996;5:169–180.

Malunions of the Proximal Humerus

17

Todd F. Ritzman   Joseph P. Iannotti

INTRODUCTION

Fractures of the proximal humerus are relatively common, accounting for approximately 5% of all fractures,[22] and their prevalence can be expected to increase as life expectancy and associated osteoporosis increase. Most proximal humerus fractures can be treated nonoperatively with expected good outcomes; initial surgical intervention is required in only 20% of acute fractures. Unfortunately, a small but not insignificant subset of those patients whose initial treatment was either surgical or conservative fail treatment and proceed to develop proximal humerus malunions. These patients often have debilitating pain, limitation of range of motion, and loss of function of the shoulder, leading to significant disability.

For symptomatic patients, realistic nonsurgical options to reduce pain and improve function do not exist, and surgical reconstruction is often necessary. Surgical treatment of proximal humerus malunions proves especially challenging due to associated disruption of normal anatomic relationships, soft-tissue scarring and contracture, rotator cuff pathology, postsurgical changes, neurologic impairment, and osteoporosis. This array of concomitant pathology renders the achievement of the operative goals of restoring premorbid functional status and relieving pain exceptionally challenging. The treatment of these complex problems requires thorough preoperative evaluation to determine the causative factors for the malunion and sound understanding and skilled

T. F. Ritzman: Department of Orthopaedic Surgery, Clinic Lerner School of Medicine, Cleveland, Ohio.
J. P. Iannotti: Department of Orthopaedic Surgery, Cleveland Clinic Foundation, Cleveland, Ohio.

application of the surgical techniques available to treat the entire spectrum of osseous and soft-tissue pathology.

ETIOLOGY

Proximal humerus malunion results from either inadequate reduction of the displaced fragments or loss of fixation following closed reduction, closed reduction and percutaneous pinning, or open reduction and internal fixation (ORIF). Although malunions sometimes occur following ORIF, they occur more commonly after nonoperative treatment. The higher incidence of malunion with nonoperative treatment may be secondary to the acceptance of a displaced fracture and unsatisfactory fracture configuration. Nonsurgical treatment of a displaced proximal humeral fracture may be a selected option in patients who are poor candidates for surgery or are severely injured. Occasionally, a malunion occurs because the treating physician failed to appreciate the extent of displacement either due to lack of experience or inadequate radiographs. The malunion seen after internal fixation is usually secondary to inadequate fragment fixation obtained in the cancellous bone of the proximal humerus.

Other contributing factors in proximal humerus malunions include inadequate immobilization, inadequate length of immobilization, or soft-tissue interposition at the fracture site. Excessively aggressive rehabilitation can result in loss of fracture reduction or fixation.

CLINICAL EVALUATION

Eliciting a careful history is essential in the evaluation of a patient with proximal humerus fracture malunion. The history should determine the mechanism of injury and subsequent treatment, with the goal of determining the cause of the malunion. Errors in diagnosis, such as a missed injury, may have occurred. Conditions that contribute to malunion include osteoporotic bone, premature or aggressive rehabilitation, high-energy multitrauma, and inadequate stability of operative fixation. Alcohol or steroid use may contribute to the development of humeral head avascular necrosis, which may provide additive joint incongruity to that attributable to the malunion.

The pain or disability associated with a proximal humerus fracture malunion varies considerably and must be addressed in terms of the patient's goals. This assessment is critical. A relatively painless malunion with adequate passive range of motion and strength may not require surgical management, especially in a sedentary patient with limited expectations for upper extremity function.

Essential to the clinical evaluation of the patient with a malunion is a complete neurovascular examination of the involved upper extremity. From the initial trauma, there may have occurred associated permanent axillary nerve or brachial plexus injuries, especially if fracture fragments were initially displaced medially to the coracoid process. Axillary nerve injury is often associated with inferior sub-

luxation of the proximal humerus (Fig. 17-1). Possible neurologic injury from previous surgery must also be ascertained. If prior nerve injury is suspected, electromyelographic examination can be helpful in determining the extent of injury and the prognosis for neurologic recovery.

The long head of the biceps tendon interposition can contribute to a malunion of the proximal humerus. Rotator cuff injury may have occurred during the initial trauma and must be addressed at the time of surgery. Iatrogenic injury from previous surgery can include detachment of the origin of the anterior deltoid or deltoid denervation,[16] transection of the long head of the biceps, or subscapularis tendon detachment.

Loss of motion is one of the primary management problems associated with proximal humeral malunion. Assessment of the degree of loss of passive versus active arcs of motion is necessary and should be considered in terms of the patient's current disability and treatment goals (Fig. 17-2). The progression or improvement of the patient's pain, weakness, and loss of motion must be considered as it relates to the rehabilitation program. If the passive motion is maintained, the rotator cuff is intact, and the surface of the joint is congruent, good function can be achieved (Fig. 17-3).

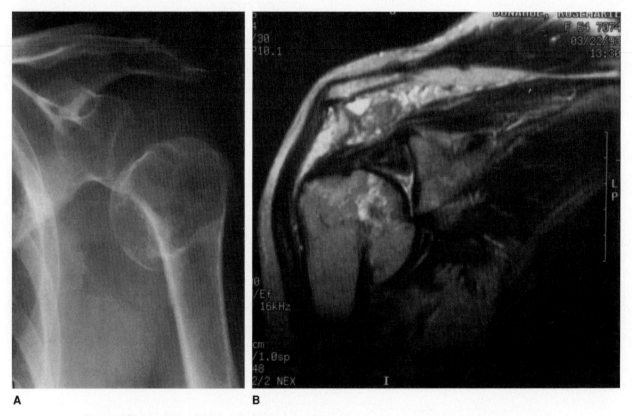

A   **B**

Figure 17-1   (A) Anatomic neck malunion in a 64-year-old woman with an associated axillary nerve injury and deltoid paralysis. (B) Magnetic resonance (MR) scan demonstrates a posttraumatic arthritis defect in the humeral head, early avascular necrosis, and marked deltoid and supraspinatus atrophy. In this case, the MR scan is helpful in diagnosing the avascular necrosis, determining the degree of atrophy and detecting posttraumatic arthritis.

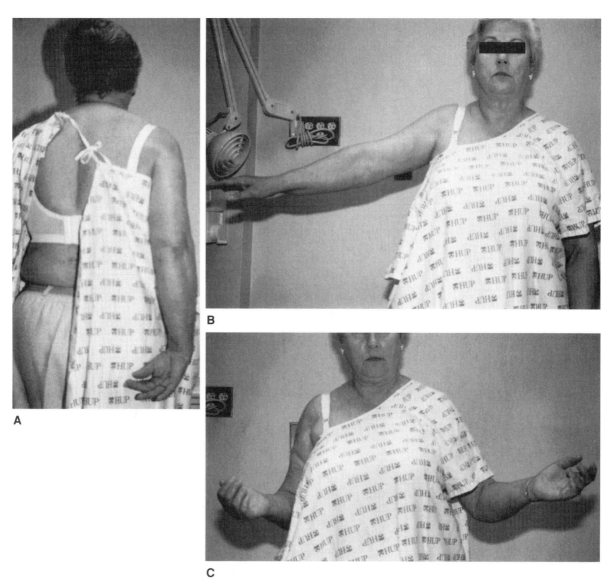

Figure 17-2 (A) The patient's functional disability from the marked loss of internal rotation, (B) abduction, and (C) external rotation, primarily resulting from capsular contracture, necessitating open capsular release.

The surgeon should keep in mind the possibility of shoulder sepsis complicating any malunion resulting from prior surgery. If infection is suspected, appropriate hematologic studies are required and aspiration arthrogram is warranted.[10]

RADIOGRAPHIC EVALUATION

Plain Radiographs

The most important aspect in the injury evaluation is to determine the position of the fracture fragments. Bone quality and the likelihood of healing must also be assessed. An adequate radiographic evaluation is required and includes an anteroposterior view in the plane of the scapula, axillary lateral, and transscapular lateral views[29] (Fig. 17-4). This series usually provides sufficient information to determine a treatment plan for most patients. Additional radiographic views, such as apical oblique view, which demonstrates posterolateral humeral head compression fractures, and the transscapular lateral view, which may be helpful in the evaluation of superiorly displaced greater tuberosity malunion, can be obtained.

Computed Tomography Scans

Computed tomography (CT) scans of proximal humerus malunions are needed when the plain radiographs are indeterminate. Computed tomography scans have been rec-

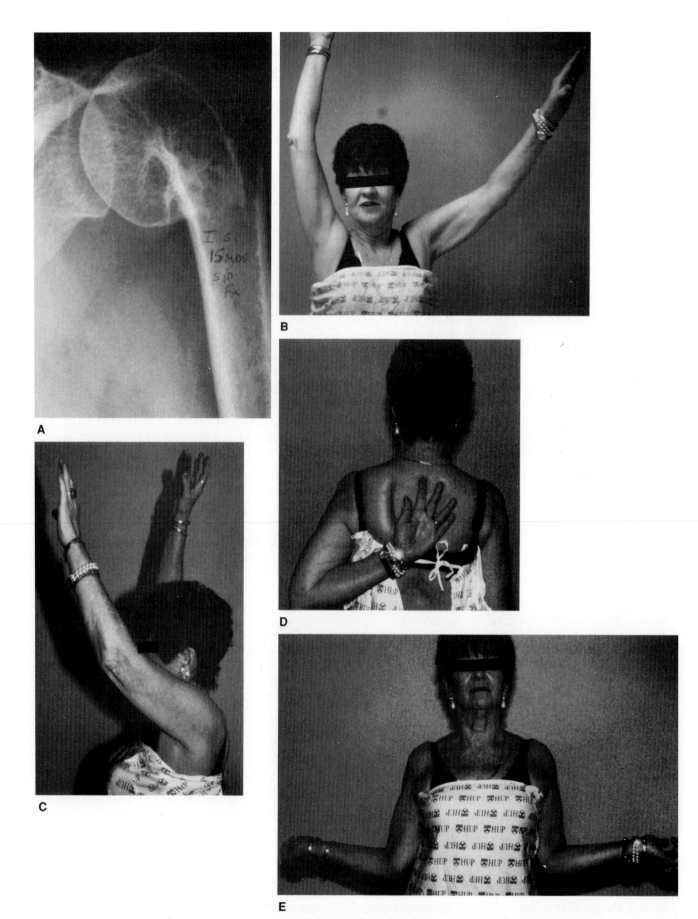

Figure 17-3 (*A*) A 60-year-old woman had a humeral neck malunion after prior surgery. The patient had excellent function in (*B*) abduction, (*C*) forward flexion, (*D*) internal rotation, and (*E*) external rotation.

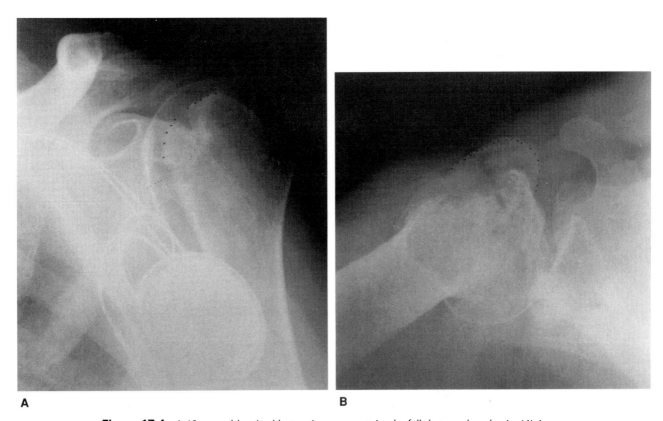

A   B

Figure 17-4   A 60-year-old retired but active man sustained a fall that produced pain. (*A*) An anteroposterior and inadequate scapular Y-view did not demonstrate the posterior humeral head dislocation. Malunion of a lesser tuberosity fracture with a posterior dislocation was initially unrecognized because of the lack of an axillary view at the time of the initial injury. (*B*) The axillary view obtained 6 months after injury clearly demonstrates posterior subluxation, malunited tuberosities, and posttraumatic arthritis. The dotted line represents the greater tuberosity.

ommended to evaluate the degree of tuberosity displacement and for clearly imaging articular impression fractures, head-splitting fractures, and chronic fracture dislocations (Fig. 17-5).[4,18,24] Morris et al. reported that CT identified axial malposition of the greater and lesser tuberosity that was not appreciated on plain radiographs in 10 and 18 out of 18 patients, respectively.[24] Additionally, several authors have recommended the utilization of three-dimensional CT reconstructions of the proximal humerus to better comprehend the position of malunited tuberosities (Fig. 17-6).[10,20]

Other Radiographic Modalities

Magnetic resonance imaging (MRI) can demonstrate associated soft-tissue problems of the deltoid, rotator cuff, biceps tendon, and glenoid labrum, which can be helpful in the management of patients who may have concomitant osseous and soft-tissue pathology (Fig. 17-1*B*). Avascular necrosis can be detected earlier with MRI than plain films, knowledge of which may affect treatment plans. It should be noted that patients with hardware from prior operative intervention may have signal artifact that can diminish the quality and utility of the MRIs.

CLASSIFICATION OF PROXIMAL HUMERUS MALUNIONS

There is presently no universally accepted classification system for proximal humerus malunions that provides a basis for comparing various subsets of malunions and different treatment outcomes. The absence of such a system lends to some difficulty in interpreting the relevant literature and comparing different treatments for specific subsets of malunions or posttraumatic sequelae across all reported cases. A few authors have recognized this shortcoming and have proposed classification systems useful in determining the treatment approach for proximal humerus malunions and evaluating outcomes.

Beredjiklian et al.[2] attempted to provide a method for systematic evaluation of both osseous and soft-tissue abnormalities. Osseous abnormalities were categorized as malposition of the greater or lesser tuberosity of greater than 1 cm (type-I malunion), incongruity or step-off of the articular surface of more than 5 mm (type-II malunion), and malalignment of the articular segment by more than 45 degrees of rotation in any plane (type-III malunion). Soft-tissue abnormalities were classified as soft-tissue

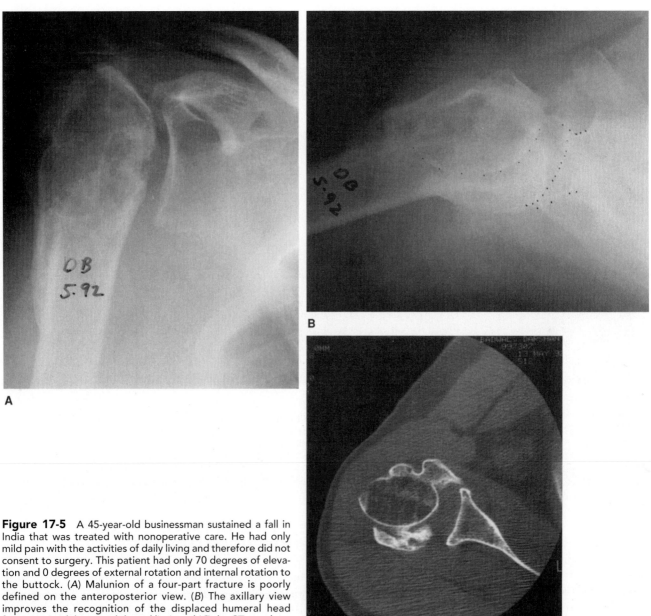

Figure 17-5 A 45-year-old businessman sustained a fall in India that was treated with nonoperative care. He had only mild pain with the activities of daily living and therefore did not consent to surgery. This patient had only 70 degrees of elevation and 0 degrees of external rotation and internal rotation to the buttock. (*A*) Malunion of a four-part fracture is poorly defined on the anteroposterior view. (*B*) The axillary view improves the recognition of the displaced humeral head fragment (*widely spaced dotted line*), and (*C*) the CT scan best defines the united tuberosities.

contracture, rotator cuff tear, and subacromial impingement. Any given patient often has multiple osseous and soft-tissue sequelae of their posttraumatic deformity, and this classification system is useful in enabling a holistic awareness of all involved pathology with the aim of treating each component.

In an attempt to simplify the surgical treatment and prognosis in treating the posttraumatic sequelae of the proximal humerus, Boileau et al.[5] proposed a general classification system for proximal humerus fracture sequelae that was not specific for but did include proximal humerus malunions. Intracapsular/impacted fracture sequelae (Category 1)

included both cephalic collapse and necrosis (type I) and chronic dislocation or fracture-dislocation (type II), in which a proximal humerus arthroplasty could be performed without a greater tuberosity osteotomy. Extracapsular/disimpacted fracture sequelae (Category 2) included both surgical neck nonunions (type III) and severe tuberosity malunions (type IV), in which the proximal humerus could not be reconstructed without a greater tuberosity osteotomy. This classification system enabled the prediction of posttraumatic deformities, which could be reconstructed with an arthroplasty with a predictably good outcome (Category 1) versus those which would yield an

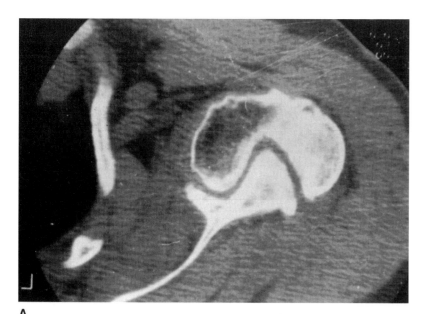

A

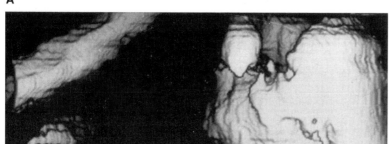

B

Figure 17-6 A 40-year-old laborer sustained a four-part fracture dislocation that was treated by attempted open reduction and internal fixation 15 years before referral to our center. (*A*) A computed tomography (CT) scan and (*B*) three-dimensional reconstruction of this malunited four-part fracture dislocation demonstrate the humeral head in a subcoracoid location and the humeral shaft articulating with the glenoid. This patient performed heavy labor for 15 years with what was essentially a fused "glenohumeral" joint, but pain increased over the years, and he was eventually treated with excision of the malunited head fragment and fusion of the proximal humerus to the glenoid. Successful fusion allowed him to return to heavy labor.

unpredictable and likely poor result with arthroplasty (Category 2) predicated on the need for greater tuberosity osteotomy and the associated possibility of postoperative displacement, malunion, or nonunion. This series excluded cases in which malunions could be treated with osteotomy and internal fixation without the use of shoulder arthroplasty in treating posttraumatic sequelae.

The most commonly utilized classification of proximal humerus malunions has been a simple modification of Neer's classification of acute proximal humerus fractures.[25] Several authors have utilized this classification and applied it to describe their series of malunions.[1,6,13,26,32] Because this is a commonly understood classification system, it will be utilized to structure the following discussion of specific subtypes of proximal humerus malunions.

SPECIFIC FRACTURE MALUNIONS

Two-Part Anatomic Neck Malunion

Isolated anatomic neck fractures are extremely rare, and malunions of this type have not been reported. Subse-

quent avascular necrosis of the articular surface is a common posttraumatic sequelae of this type of fracture. A prosthetic hemiarthroplasty would be selected as the treatment, if there is avascular necrosis with head collapse. Theoretically, an anatomic neck malunion could be treated by osteotomy and internal fixation, although risk of subsequent avascular necrosis would be of significant concern.

Two-Part Greater Tuberosity Malunion

Malunion of the greater tuberosity fracture is probably the most common proximal humeral malunion. Greater tuberosity fractures are often retracted superiorly and posteriorly by the deforming forces of the attached supraspinatus, infraspinatus, and teres minor muscles. The articular surface is unaffected by this fracture type and maintains its appropriate relationship with the humeral shaft. Posterior displacement of the greater tuberosity can lead to a rigid, bony block to external rotation, which can be evident on physical examination. In extreme cases, anterior glenohumeral instability can result as the posteriorly displaced greater tuberosity impinges on the posterior glenoid in external rotation.[9] Similarly, superior displacement of the greater tuberosity can block abduction and forward elevation and lead to subacromial impingement as the malunited tuberosity encroaches on the subacromial space.[9,17] Tuberosity malposition can result in rotator cuff weakness secondary to the shortened musculotendinous length of the external rotators.[30] Additionally, severe subacromial impingement can lead to rotator cuff attrition or tears. Thus, it is critical to examine the integrity of the rotator cuff on physical examination and intraoperative evaluation.

Greater tuberosity malunions that heal to the humeral shaft result in less deformity and soft-tissue contracture. These malunions are easier to mobilize and reduce to their anatomic site. On the other hand, greater tuberosity malunions that heal to the posterior part of the humeral head or glenoid result in severe shortening of the capsule and attached rotator cuff and can rarely be brought to their anatomic site and still achieve internal rotation to the abdomen.

Satisfactory closed reduction of chronically displaced, isolated greater tuberosity fracture is impossible, and malunion of this fracture is best treated by prevention through primary surgical management of the acute fracture. Conversely, fractures associated with an anterior glenohumeral dislocation are often successfully reduced with reduction of the dislocation.[19] Healing of these fractures must be monitored closely when they are treated by closed means because of the tendency for later displacement.[23]

Radiographic Evaluation

Careful radiographic evaluation of the suspected greater tuberosity is required; three high-quality orthogonal views of the shoulder should be obtained.[28] Small fragments isolated to the superior facet of the greater tuberosity often displace superiorly and are more commonly diagnosed on anteroposterior (AP) radiographs. Larger fragments containing the superior and posterior portion of the rotator cuff often displace posteriorly behind the humeral head and are more difficult to appreciate on AP radiographs. The scapular lateral view may be particularly useful in delineating posterior and superior displacement of the greater tuberosity, and the axillary view is particularly useful in determining posterior displacement. Malunion of the greater tuberosity is a result of not obtaining the correct views, obtaining poor-quality views, or not obtaining follow-up x-ray films. In any case, malunion of the greater tuberosity is preventable.

A CT scan of the proximal humerus can be particularly useful in evaluating the greater tuberosity malunion. As stated previously, Morris et al.[7] evidenced that CT scanning enabled accurate evaluation of tuberosity displacement, which was inaccurately identified with plain radiographs.

Surgical Indications

The Neer classification of proximal humerus fractures defines 1 cm as the criterion for significant displacement. In the case of greater tuberosity malunion, we think that for most patients the same criterion should be applied to correct the pathologic limitation in motion, rotator cuff weakness, and impingement. In an active patient with malunion of greater than 5 mm in the superior direction symptoms of subacromial impingement can occur and can warrant surgical intervention.

Surgical Technique

In patients with acceptable passive arcs of shoulder motion, greater tuberosity malunions can be surgically managed with the same techniques used for the acute fracture.[24] For small fragments, up to 3 cm in size, with superior displacement, satisfactory exposure can be achieved with a superior incision within the Langer lines centered on the anterolateral corner of the acromion. The deltoid is removed from the anterior acromion and split a distance of 4 cm from the acromion. Subacromial scar tissue is excised when present. For larger fragments or malunions with posterior displacement, a wider and more extensile exposure is required. In these cases an extended deltopectoral approach is performed.

The greater tuberosity fragment is mobilized by sharp dissection of a fibrous union or by osteotomy of a bony union. The greater tuberosity osteotomy is frequently biplanar,[10] beginning at the anterior callous. Craig describes the use of several drill holes prior to osteotomizing the tuberosity to mark the site and minimize fracture and fragmentation.[9] He emphasizes that care must be taken during the osteotomy to protect the axillary nerve posteriorly as it emerges from the quadrilateral space. When discrimination between tuberosity and fracture callous is difficult, good quality radiographs and a CT scan can assist in making this assessment. The donor defect from which the greater tuberosity has been displaced is adjacent to the bicipital groove. It is often filled with fibrous tissue or sclerotic bone and requires debridement and light decortication down to a bed of bleeding bone in preparation for the reduced greater tuberosity. Care should be taken to avoid removing all of the dense, cortical bone so as to preserve adequate bone stock for fixation. With severely posteriorly displaced fragments excision of the posterior capsule is required to mobilize the greater tuberosity and its attached rotator cuff to allow the greater tuberosity to reach its site of reattachment. The rotator interval is usually torn, and dissection of the scar in this area is necessary to mobilize the greater tuberosity fracture fragment. The rotator cuff must be brought to length, and any coexistent cuff tear should be first repaired. Temporary traction sutures placed in the rotator cuff insertion allow control of the greater tuberosity fragment to assist in lateral advancement during lysis of adhesions and contracture release. Prior to definitive repair of the rotator interval and fixation of the tuberosity fragment, it is important to inspect the anterior glenoid and labrum through the rotator interval to rule out associated pathology. This is especially true in cases in which the greater tuberosity fracture occurred in the setting of a traumatic anterior glenohumeral dislocation. If a Bankart lesion is identified, some authors advocate repair through the rotator interval prior to the bony repair.[9,30] In some cases, partial takedown of the subscapularis may be necessary to achieve exposure of the anterior inferior glenoid. Bankart repair would be recommended in the young, active patient and is usually not required in the older and more sedentary patient. In the senior author's experience only lesions that include a significant bony component and demonstrate instability prior to surgery are repaired. The vast majority of patients with greater tuberosity fracture associated with an anterior dislocation either do not have a Bankart lesion or the lesion does not require repair.

The greater tuberosity fragment can usually be anatomically reduced. In those cases where it cannot be anatomically reduced, the greater tuberosity is returned anteriorly as far as possible and below the top of the humeral head. It is necessary that the patient's arm can be brought passively to the abdomen prior to wound closure. The surgeon may use the supraspinatus, infraspinatus, and teres minor facets of the greater tuberosity as anatomic landmarks for anatomic reduction.

Two to four heavy, nonabsorbable sutures (No. 5 or No. 2 Fiberwire, Arthrex, Naples, FL) are placed vertically in a figure-of-eight configuration through the greater tuberosity and then through drill holes in the humeral shaft. Horizontal fixation can be achieved by placing intraosseous sutures to the lesser tuberosity area (Fig. 17-7).[27] Incorporation of the sutures in the rotator cuff tendon adjacent to the greater tuberosity fragment is important because the tendon substance is often stronger than that of the osteopenic bone of the tuberosities.

Alternatively, internal fixation of the greater tuberosity with screws and washers could be used in normal bone, if the tuberosity fragment is large. In such cases where there is a large fragment of bone with good bone quality, one or two interfragmentary bone screws can be used but should not be used without the additional use of the suture fixation described previously. Hardware loosening may require later removal.[33] The head of the screws should be placed lateral or distal to the greater tuberosity to avoid subacromial impingement. This method of fixation should be avoided in osteopenic bone. There is no place for a plate fixation in the management of an isolated greater tuberosity malunion because of the space constraints of the subacromial area. Wire fixation does not seem to offer any distinct advan-

tage over heavy nonabsorbable suture but does have the disadvantage of material failure and subsequent migration, requiring removal.

After reconstruction, the subacromial space is examined with the surgeon's index finger. If it is tight or if a rotator cuff repair was performed, a subacromial decompression is performed to protect the bony and soft-tissue repairs.

Passive and active-assisted range of motion is begun on the day of surgery, but internal rotation behind the back is avoided for 6 weeks. Active motion is begun at 6 weeks, followed soon by resistance exercises. For cases with severe posterior displacement and difficult mobilization of the fragment, we utilize an abduction orthosis to hold the arm in 0 degrees of rotation, and internal rotation to the abdomen is avoided for the first 4 weeks.

In patients with greater tuberosity malunions and loss of passive arcs of glenohumeral motion, an arthroscopic capsular release without correction of the malunion is usually unsuccessful in achieving acceptable passive arcs of motion with a minimum of 120 degrees of forward elevation. In cases of malunion, there is a significant extracapsular scarring; therefore, we prefer extended deltopectoral approach with open capsular release at the time that the malunion is corrected. Additionally, for large greater tuberosity fragments with metaphyseal-diaphyseal extension, the axillary nerve limits the extent of a deltoid split, further necessitating the use of a deltopectoral exposure. In cases with internal rotation contracture of greater than 20 degrees, subscapularis coronal plane Z-lengthening is performed. Cases with mild malunion and less severe internal rotation contracture require separation of the subscapularis from the underlying capsule, excision of the capsule and surrounding scar from the subscapularis tendon and muscle.

Results

Morris et al.[24] reported three greater tuberosity malunions that underwent osteotomy and repositioning. Shoulder elevation and external rotation motion arcs were both improved by 60 degrees. If significant shoulder stiffness and weakness have not yet occurred, the surgeon might expect the good healing rate and functional results that Flatow et al.[12] found in their series of acute, displaced greater tuberosity fractures treated by internal fixation using the nonabsorbable suture method.

Eleven of the 39 cases reported by Beredjiklian et al.[2] involved an isolated malunion of the tuberosity (type I malunion). Eight of these patients were treated definitively with an osteotomy of the tuberosity and soft-tissue reconstruction, and seven of these reconstructions corrected the bony deformity to within 5 mm of anatomical reduction. Pain relief was significant in all cases and rated as minimal or none in 88%. Functional capacity improved in 75% of patients, and, overall, six of eight patients had a satisfactory

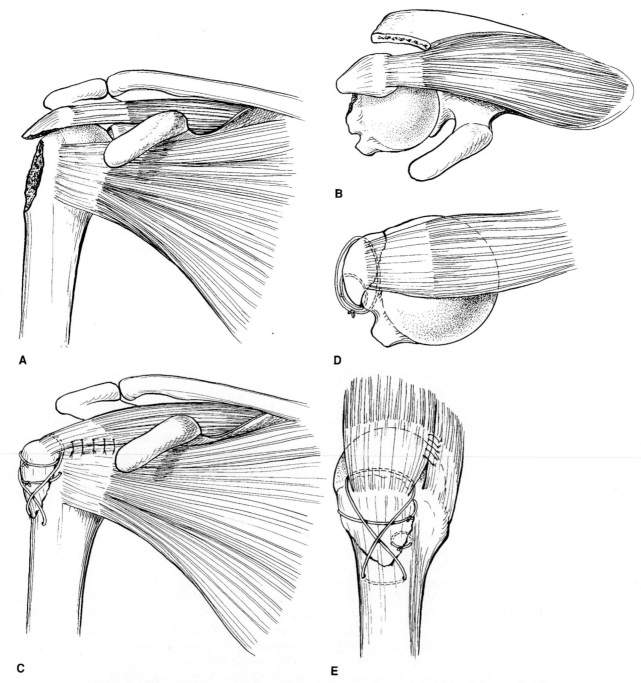

A

B

C

D

E

Figure 17-7 (*A,B*) Isolated greater tuberosity fracture with superoposterior displacement. (*C–E*) Reduction of the greater tuberosity and internal fixation using transosseous horizontal sutures and vertical figure-of-eight sutures. The horizontal sutures between the tuberosities are placed between the bone fragments, which helps to reduce the fragments, and in the rotator cuff tendon insertion sites, which provides the best tissue for maintaining the reduction during the postoperative evaluation. The vertical figure-of-eight suture also passes through the tendon insertion and then passes through a drill hole 2 cm distal to the metaphyseal fracture line. The vertical suture prevents superior displacement. The rotator interval between the subscapularis and supraspinatus is repaired, significantly improving stability.

result. The best outcomes among their 39 cases were seen in the group who had isolated malposition of the greater or lesser tuberosity and had all osseous and soft-tissue abnormalities corrected.

Two-Part Lesser Tuberosity Malunion

Two-part lesser tuberosity fractures are rare but often associated with posterior shoulder dislocations (Fig. 17-3, *A* and *B*). If a malunion fragment is large, it may act as an obstacle to internal rotation and may also involve the articular surface of the humeral head. Associated subscapularis weakness may be seen with significant medial displacement due to altered musculotendinous length.

Radiographic Evaluation

Trauma series radiographs or CT scans can assist in determining size and displacement of the lesser tuberosity fragment. Morris and associates[24] reported that plain radiographs were inadequate in determining lesser tuberosity position when compared with surgical findings and that CT evaluation improved accuracy.

Surgical Technique

A deltopectoral approach can provide access to the lesser tuberosity fragment. Open reduction and internal fixation with anatomic reduction of associated articular involvement can be performed with heavy nonabsorbable sutures. The smaller-sized lesser tuberosity fragment can be excised,[21] and the subscapularis tendon repaired directly to the proximal humerus with intraosseous sutures.[4] A chronically retracted fragment may require capsular release to mobilize the fragment. When necessary, we perform this from the inner aspect of the joint in the midcapsule. This approach avoids detaching the subscapularis.

Surgical Neck Malunion

Isolated surgical neck malunions usually involve anterior angulation and varus deformity secondary to anterior displacement of the shaft by the pectoralis major[11] and abduction of the head by the rotator cuff.[25] This deformity, if severe, can cause limited forward flexion and abduction with associated impingement.[8] However, in many cases, varus malunion does not result in significant loss in internal rotation and external rotation (Fig. 17-3).

Radiographic Evaluation

Plain radiographic views of the proximal humerus in various degrees of rotation are required to accurately assess angulation. Comparison radiographs of the contralateral shoulder can assist in estimating the degree of deformity and in planning the required osteotomy. Beredjiklian et al.[2] provided an excellent description of the method for determining the magnitude of this deformity radiographically.

Surgical Indications

If the surgical neck malunion reveals an increased anterior angulation greater than 45 to 55 degrees, forward elevation will be limited.[4,17] Varus deformity of similar magnitude can cause decreased abduction and forward elevation. These indications were supported by Beredjiklian et al.,[2,3] who classified malalignment of the articular segment of more than 45 degrees with the humeral shaft in any plane as a subtype of proximal humerus malunions requiring intervention.

Surgical Technique

If clinically indicated, osteotomy and internal plate fixation are performed at the malunion site. We prefer using a blade plate or a locking proximal humerus plate (Synthes, Paoli, PA). Open capsular release is usually necessary to restore satisfactory passive arcs of motion and is performed before osteotomy. Bone from the osteotomy can be used for the graft or harvested from the iliac crest. For patients with intra-articular fracture or posttraumatic arthritis/avascular necrosis, hemiarthroplasty is our preferred method of surgical management (Fig. 17-8A).

Results

Solonen and Vastamaki[31] described a valgus wedge derotational osteotomy with T-formed AO plate fixation through a deltopectoral approach in seven young patients with preoperative varus angulation ranging from 40 to 60 degrees. Five of the seven patients achieved normal or near normal results with significantly improved range of motion. Their two poor results were secondary to soft-tissue pathology rather than failures in fixation or union of the osteotomy.

Three- and Four-Part Malunions

Three- and four-part malunions are complex problems that can result in severe deformities and significant complications. These posttraumatic sequelae usually require prosthetic replacement. In selected three-part injuries, osteotomy of the fracture fragments, followed by internal fixation, may be attempted if there is no humeral head avascular necrosis or joint incongruity and the bone quality is good.

In three-part malunions, either the greater or lesser tuberosity is displaced along with the surgical neck. If the

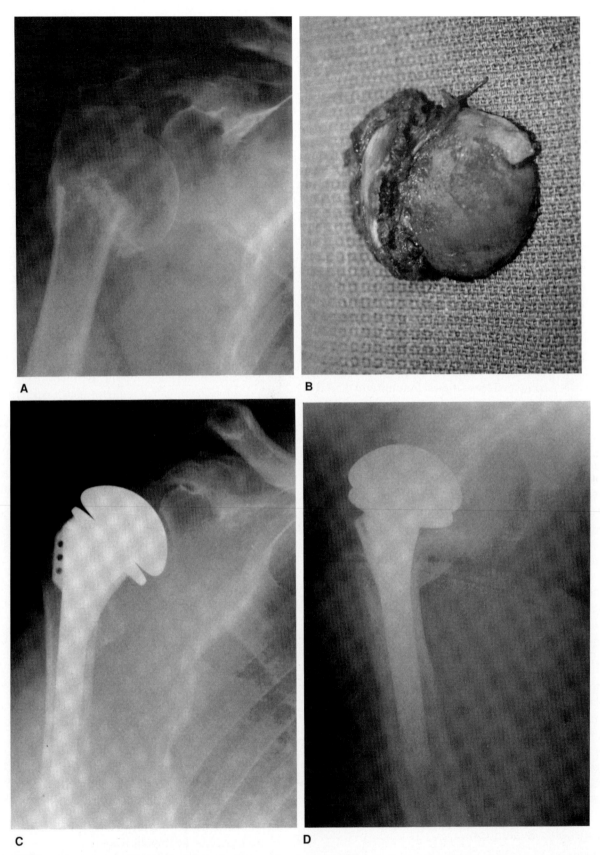

A

B

C

D

Figure 17-8 (A,B) A 60-year-old woman sustained a humeral head-splitting fracture that was initially treated with sling immobilization. (C,D) The humeral head-splitting, three-part fracture and malunion were treated with hemiarthroplasty without tuberosity osteotomy. After a trial insertion of the humeral component, the tuberosity did not impinge on the posterior glenoid with external rotation of the arm and did not impinge on the acromion with elevation of the arm. Based on these observations, a tuberosity osteotomy was not performed. Avoiding a tuberosity osteotomy obviates the possibility of tuberosity nonunion and the postoperative loss of fixation. These postoperative radiographs show both tuberosities below the collar of the prosthesis. At the 12-month follow-up examination, the patient had no pain, but active elevation was only 60 degrees because of deltoid weakness as a result of axillary nerve neuropraxia.

greater tuberosity is left intact, the head will be externally rotated and abducted secondary to the intact superior and posterior portion of the rotator cuff. The shaft will be pulled anteromedially by the pectoralis, and the lesser tuberosity will retract medially. Fractures in which the greater tuberosity is displaced will result in the articular surface being internally rotated by the pull of the subscapularis. The greater tuberosity is posterosuperiorly displaced by the intact cuff, and the humeral shaft is again retracted anteromedially. Malunions of this magnitude often lead to severe loss of function, decreased range of motion, and disabling pain. An increased incidence of posttraumatic degenerative arthritis and avascular necrosis of the humeral head is also prevalent.[14]

Four-part malunions are challenging to treat as both tuberosities and the surgical neck are significantly displaced leading to extreme humeral head distortion. These malunions are associated with significant soft-tissue injuries and adhesions, joint incongruity, and an increased incidence of osteonecrosis.[14] Patients with four-part malunions typically have severe pain and disability secondary to restricted range of motion, avascular necrosis, soft-tissue injuries, and contractures.

Radiographic Evaluation

Thorough preoperative radiographic studies are required in the treatment of three- and four-part malunions because tuberosity malunion is commonly present. We recommend CT scanning with three-dimensional reconstructions to determine tuberosity position, articular surface congruity, and bone integrity.

Surgical Technique

Most of these types of deformities occur in the elderly, and prosthetic replacement is usually required. The integrity of the glenoid articular surface determines whether humeral hemiarthroplasty or total shoulder arthroplasty is performed, and this determination can be made intraoperatively if preoperative radiographs are indeterminate (see Fig. 17-3, *A* and *B*).

An extensive deltopectoral approach preserving the deltoid origin is our preferred technique. Dissecting subacromial and intra-articular scarring is required to mobilize the rotator cuff and tuberosities and avoid neurovascular injury. Capsular contracture always exists, and an extensive capsular excision is required. Rotator cuff mobilization is enhanced by global excision of the capsule. The rotator cuff should be carefully inspected for tears, and these should be repaired.

Tuberosity position must be assessed before surgery and intraoperatively. A general guideline indicating the need for surgical correction of a tuberosity fracture is 1 cm of displacement. Greater tuberosity malunion with posterior displacement often blocks external rotation or forward elevation and results in postoperative anterior dislocation. Lesser tuberosity malunion may permit excessive posterior subluxation or block internal rotation because of coracoid impingement.

In some cases of tuberosity malposition, avoiding an osteotomy can be achieved with the use of a small stem, which is shifted in the medullary canal to accommodate for tuberosity malposition, and an eccentric humeral head, which is helpful to adapt the prosthesis to the malposition (Fig. 17-9). When these measures cannot restore a near normal relationship between the tuberosities and the humeral head, a tuberosity osteotomy should be performed. Tuberosity reconstruction requires osteotomy with an oscillating saw or osteotome. Large degrees of tuberosity displacement require osteotomy before osteotomy of the humeral head segment. Small displacements can be assessed after osteotomy of the humeral head, and, in some cases, tuberosity osteotomy is unnecessary (Fig. 17-9). The bicipital groove is a helpful landmark for tuberosity osteotomy. The osteotomy should produce a tuberosity fragment long enough to ensure contact with the bony humeral shaft on repositioning and large enough so that adequate rotator cuff is attached. The attached rotator cuff may need to be mobilized so as to achieve needed length as described earlier.

Tuberosity fixation is achieved by using several heavy nonabsorbable sutures (Fig. 17-10). Two sutures are passed through the middle portion of the tuberosities and the anterior flange of the prosthesis. Two more sutures are passed through both tuberosities, one each at the superior and inferior ends. Holes are drilled through the lateral and anterior aspect of the proximal humeral shaft. Two sutures are passed through these holes and, in figure-of-eight fashion, passed through the superior aspect of the tuberosities at the cuff insertion. These two sutures assist in bringing the tuberosities inferior to ensure contact of the tuberosities and the humeral shaft and placement below the top of the prosthetic humeral head. Local bone graft is usually available from the discarded head fragment and is used to increase tuberosity healing. Impingement can be avoided by making certain that the tuberosities are below the superior level of the humeral head.

A modular shoulder arthroplasty system, with a number of head component size options, allows better soft-tissue tensioning. Intraoperative prosthetic changes can be made to improve glenohumeral stability and tuberosity position.[10] Humeral shaft bone quality and humeral component stability determine whether a cemented or noncemented humeral prosthesis is used.

Postoperative immobilization in a Don Joy brace (Southern California Orthopedic Institute [SCOI], Van Nuys, CA) with slight abduction and neutral rotation for 4 weeks helps protect the tuberosity repair and allows for balanced scarring in both the anterior and posterior aspects of

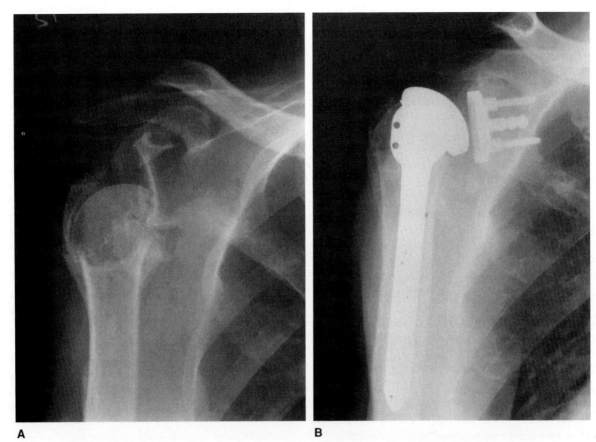

A   **B**

Figure 17-9 A 70-year-old retiree had an acute four-part, valgus-impacted fracture and complete axillary nerve paralysis that resulted in the initial decision for nonoperative treatment. (*A*) The axillary nerve neuropraxia recovered, but the fracture malunited and remained in a locked inferior subluxation. The patient had posttraumatic glenoid arthritis and a marked loss of passive range of motion because of capsular contracture. (*B*) The patient was treated with total shoulder arthroplasty without tuberosity osteotomy. Humeral height was restored using the humeral prosthetic, and the impacted humeral head was left in place and used as an in situ bone graft. At the 4-year follow-up examination, the patient continued to have minimal pain, but active elevation was only 80 degrees, and active external rotation was 20 degrees. He can function well for all waist-level activities but is not able to use his arm for chest-level or higher activities.

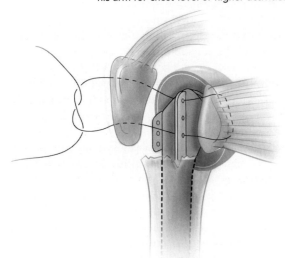

Figure 17-10 Suture fixation of tuberosities through holes in the anterior fin of the prosthesis and directly to the humeral shaft. (Printed with permission from Dines DM, Warren RF. Posttraumatic changes of the proximal humerus: malunion, nonunion, and osteonecrosis. Treatment with modular hemiarthroplasty or total shoulder arthroplasty. J Shoulder Elbow Surg 1993;2:20.)

the shoulder. The brace is removed several times a day for pendulum, active-assisted and passive range-of-motion exercises, and activities of daily living.

Results

There is a relative paucity of literature regarding the surgical treatment of three- and four-part fracture malunions. The majority of series addresses the entire spectrum of posttraumatic sequelae of proximal humerus fractures in whole without focusing particular attention on malunions. This leads to a rather confusing body of literature in which comparisons between series are difficult.

In general, the results of prosthetic arthroplasty of three- and four-part malunions are inferior to those of prosthetic treatment of similar acute fractures.[34] While pain relief is usually achieved, shoulder range of motion and strength are often limited. Patients with these malunions should be prepared for "limited goals" outcomes following prosthetic replacement.

Tanner and Cofield[32] reported their experience in performing proximal humeral arthroplasty in 49 shoulders with acute or chronic fractures of the proximal humerus. The chronic fracture group was composed of 27 shoulders with a mean time of 20 months from initial injury to arthroplasty. Sixteen of these 27 shoulders were documented as having malunion with incongruity of the articular surface. All of the patients in the acute fracture group and 25 of 28 shoulders in the chronic fracture group had satisfactory pain relief. Active abduction in the acute and chronic fracture group were 101 degrees and 112 degrees, respectively. Complications were noted to be more frequent in the chronic fracture group and were related to surgical difficulty, extensive tissue scarring, and anatomic distortion. Patients with the best function and motion also incurred less surgical insult to the cuff and tuberosity mechanism and did not require a tuberosity osteotomy. Cofield warned that late reconstruction of malunited proximal humerus fractures is "exceedingly complex" and that the results in terms of motion and strength are limited; thus, these procedures should be classified as "salvage procedures."[7]

Frich et al.[13] found better pain relief in four-part fractures treated with acute arthroplasty than in those treated after a surgical delay, which in their series was of at least 4 months duration. Of 11 patients in the chronic four-part fracture group treated with prosthetic replacement, only 1 had a good result, compared with 3 excellent results and 6 good results in the 15 patients treated with immediate replacement. There were no good or excellent results for the 9 patients with chronic three-part fractures. There was a high incidence of instability for the group with delayed surgery attributed to increased difficulty in soft-tissue tensioning, including rotator cuff reconstruction. The authors noted a remarkably limited range of motion in their series of chronic fractures and concluded that "treatment of chronic proximal humerus fractures to a large extent is a soft tissue problem and that the preoperative condition of the soft tissue around the shoulder determines the end result."[13]

Dines et al.[10] reported on a series of 20 shoulder arthroplasties performed for chronic posttraumatic changes of the proximal humerus, including malunion, nonunion, impression fractures, and osteonecrosis. Preoperative malunion of the tuberosities or humeral head was noted in 8 of 20 patients, and 12 patients required tuberosity osteotomy at the time of arthroplasty for malunited tuberosities. Fair, good, or excellent results were achieved in 90% of patients. Ninety percent and seventy-five percent of patients had pain relief at rest and with activity, respectively. Average postoperative motions were forward elevation of 111 degrees, external rotation of 30 degrees, and internal rotation to L2. However, patients requiring tuberosity osteotomy had resultant motion of 15 degrees less forward elevation and 9 degrees less external rotation

than those not requiring an osteotomy. Additionally, patients having undergone a tuberosity osteotomy had less improvement in the Hospital for Special Surgery (HSS) shoulder scoring system than those not requiring an osteotomy (73.6 vs. 82.3, respectively). Thus, avoiding tuberosity osteotomy is advised whenever feasible. The authors recommend the use of a modular-designed prosthesis to facilitate soft-tissue tensioning and tuberosity repair.

In a study of 39 consecutive patients with three- and four-part fractures treated with hemiarthroplasty, Bosch et al.[6] noted that the outcome of primary or secondary hemiarthroplasty was inversely proportional to the time between the injury and the prosthetic replacement. Their series included 17 patients with secondary humeral head replacements greater than 4 weeks post injury. Limited description of the presence or types of malunions was provided. All patients had satisfactory pain relief, and the only factor found to negatively influence outcome was the length of time from injury to operation.

Seventeen of 23 shoulders with failed treatment of three- and four-part proximal humerus fractures subsequently treated with arthroplasty reviewed by Norris et al.[15] were classified as malunions. All of the shoulders were initially treated nonoperatively, and 54% of those initially treated surgically had malunion as a complication. Tuberosity osteotomy was required in 57% of cases, and the authors warned that tuberosity osteotomy is a "formidable procedure" with technical difficulty and potential for complications. Pain was satisfactorily relieved in 95% of patients, average forward elevation increased from 68 to 92 degrees, and average external rotation increased from 6 to 27 degrees postoperatively. They concluded that late glenohumeral arthroplasty, albeit technically difficult, is a satisfactory reconstructive procedure when primary treatment of complex proximal humerus fractures is unsuccessful. It was also noted by these authors that results are inferior to those for acute humeral head replacement.

Beredjiklian et al.[2,3] retrospectively reviewed their experience in treating 39 patients with proximal humerus malunions categorized by the presence of osseous and soft-tissue abnormalities, as described previously. Overall, the result was satisfactory for 69% and unsatisfactory for 31% of patients at an average of 44 months postoperatively. It is notable that 96% of patients with a satisfactory result had operative correction of all osseous and soft-tissue abnormalities, whereas 66% of patients with an unsatisfactory result had incomplete operative correction of these abnormalities. Thus, the authors concluded that operative management of these patients is successful only if all osseous and soft-tissue abnormalities are corrected at the time of surgery. Additionally, 74% of patients with malunions and joint incongruity treated with prosthetic arthroplasty had a satisfactory result. The rate of complications in their study approached 30% and attests to the technical difficulty in treating proximal humerus malunions.

Sixteen of the 71 shoulders treated with arthroplasty for the posttraumatic sequelae of proximal humerus fractures in the series by Boileau et al.[5] were characterized as having severe malunions of the tuberosities. Overall, the results of arthroplasty for this heterogeneous group, including cephalic collapse, locked dislocations, surgical neck nonunions, or severe tuberosity malunions, were encouraging, with a significant reduction in pain and improvement in anterior elevation (74 to 102 degrees) and external rotation (0 to 34 degrees). However, the isolated results for those patients requiring tuberosity osteotomy for prosthesis implantation (16 patients with severe malunions of the tuberosity and 6 patients with surgical neck nonunions) were less favorable. All of the patients in this group had either fair or poor results and did not regain active elevation above 90 degrees (mean active elevation of 82 degrees vs. mean of 123 degrees in patients not requiring osteotomy). The authors concluded that greater tuberosity osteotomy is the most likely reason for poor and unpredictable results after shoulder arthroplasty for the sequelae of proximal humerus fractures and recommended avoiding an osteotomy whenever possible, even if that entails accepting distorted proximal humerus anatomy. Complications occurred in 27% of the cases in this series.

Antuna et al.[12] evaluated the long-term outcome of 50 patients who underwent shoulder arthroplasty as treatment for proximal humeral malunions with a mean of 9 years follow-up. Shoulder arthroplasty resulted in statistically significant pain relief with significant improvements in postoperative motion; active elevation improved from 65 to 102 degrees and external rotation improved from 12 to 32 degrees on average. Despite these promising results, 50% of patients in the series had an unsatisfactory result, as determined by the Neer result-rating system, with a 20% overall complication rate. Of note, there was statistically significant less postoperative motion in those patients who had undergone previous operative treatment of their initial fracture or who required a tuberosity osteotomy at the time of arthroplasty. Ten of the 24 shoulders that required tuberosity osteotomy had complications, including tuberosity nonunion,[29] tuberosity malunion,[10] and tuberosity resorption.[10] These results further attest to the technical difficulty in treating this complex group of patients.

GLENOHUMERAL SURGICAL FUSION

Glenohumeral fusion of a proximal humerus malunion is indicated in select cases only. A fusion may be required in the individual with concomitant rotator cuff and deltoid dysfunction.[27] A shoulder infection that cannot be eradicated with hardware removal, irrigation with debridement, and intravenous antibiotics may ultimately require fusion.[15]

CONCLUSION

Fortunately, proximal humerus malunions are relatively uncommon injuries. However, when present, they are painful and severely debilitating with little response to conservative, nonsurgical measures. As evidenced by the significant rate of complications experienced even in the clinical series of accomplished, respected shoulder specialists, these posttraumatic sequelae are among the most challenging and technically difficult disorders that a shoulder surgeon will encounter. Certainly, the best treatment for any proximal humerus malunion is prevention by adequately treating acute fractures. Several authors, citing the increase in complications and worse functional outcomes following late arthroplasty for proximal humerus malunions, warn against making the mistake of assuming that failed primary treatment can simply be corrected with late prosthetic arthroplasty.[6,13,26,27,30,32] Thus, they advocate prompt and proper acute treatment of proximal humerus fractures to avoid the later challenge of treating a malunion.

When faced with a proximal humerus malunion, it is critical to obtain an accurate history and perform a thorough physical exam. Workup should include adequate plain radiographs supplemented with CT scans, three-dimensional CT reconstructions, and MRI scans, when uncertainty remains after reviewing the plain films. The ultimate goal of every preoperative evaluation should be maximal understanding of all involved pathology, including osseous and soft-tissue deformities, so that an appropriate surgical plan, whose aim is treating all components of the posttraumatic pathology, can be formulated. The results for surgical correction of isolated tuberosity malunions are promising, and favorable outcomes can be expected. Although results of prosthetic arthroplasty for complex proximal humerus malunions are inferior to acute arthroplasty, results in the literature evidence are good potential for pain relief and some improvement in function with the likelihood for limited-goals function. It is essential to counsel patients preoperatively so as to equate postoperative expectations with attainable goals.

When it comes to the surgical treatment of proximal humerus malunions, we recommend an approach that addresses all osseous and soft-tissue abnormalities present in each posttraumatic shoulder. The treatment algorithm recommended by Beredjiklian et al.[2,3] provides a comprehensive, systematic method of evaluating and treating these complex cases in such a manner (Fig. 17-11). It is obvious from the literature that the necessity for a greater tuberosity osteotomy automatically increases the likelihood for complications and decreases the likelihood for favorable, predictable outcomes. Therefore, we recommend avoiding tuberosity osteotomy during arthroplasty by utilizing a modular prosthetic system and approximating the tuberosity to humeral head relationship. Thus, avoid tuberosity osteotomy unless absolutely necessary for

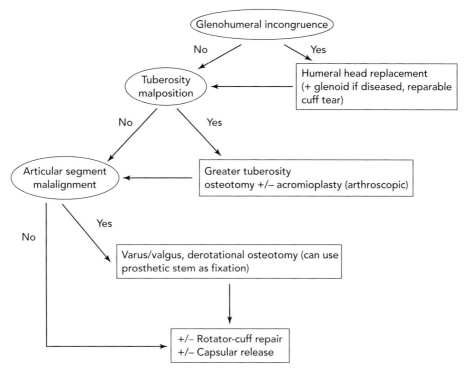

Figure 17-11   Algorithm for the categorization and operative treatment of malunions of the proximal aspect of the humerus. (Modified from Beredjiklian P, Iannotti JP, Norris TR, et al. Operative treatment of malunion of a fracture of the proximal aspect of the humerus. J Bone Joint Surg Am 1998;80:1484.)

prosthetic implantation. When all osseous and soft-tissue abnormalities are addressed surgically using appropriate technique and postoperative rehabilitation is monitored carefully, the outcome is satisfactory in most cases.

REFERENCES

1. Antuna S, Sperling JW, Sanchez-Sotelo J, et al. Shoulder arthroplasty for proximal humeral malunions: long-term results. J Shoulder Elbow Surg 2002;11:122.
2. Beredjiklian P, Iannotti JP, Norris R, et al. Operative treatment of malunion of a fracture of the proximal aspect of the humerus. J Bone Joint Surg 1998;80A(10):1484.
3. Beredjiklian P, Iannotti J. Treatment of proximal humerus fracture malunion with prosthetic arthroplasty. Instr Course Lect 1998;47:135.
4. Bigliani L. Fractures of the shoulder. Part I: fractures of the proximal humerus. In: Rockwood C, Green D, Bucholz R, eds. Fractures in adults. Philadelphia, JB Lippincott, 1991:884.
5. Boileau P, Trojani C, Walch G, et al. Shoulder arthroplasty for the treatment of the sequelae of fractures of the proximal humerus. J Shoulder Elbow Surg 2001;10:299.
6. Bosch U, Skuteck M, Fremery RW, et al. Outcome after primary and secondary hemiarthroplasty in elderly patients with fractures of the proximal humerus. J Shoulder Elbow Surg 1998;4:479.
7. Cofield R. Comminuted fractures of the proximal humerus. Clin Orthop 1988;230:49.
8. Connor P, Flatow E. Complications of internal fixation of proximal humeral fractures. Instr Course Lect 1997;46:25.
9. Craig E. Open reduction and internal fixation of greater tuberosity fractures, malunions and nonunions. In: Craig E, ed. Master techniques in orthopaedic surgery: the shoulder. New York, Raven Press, 1995.
10. Dines D, Warren RF, Altchek, DW, et al. Posttraumatic changes of the proximal humerus: malunion, nonunion, and osteonecrosis. Treatment with modular hemiarthroplasty or total shoulder arthroplasty. J Shoulder Elbow Surg 1993;2:11.
11. Duralde X, Flatow EL, Pollock RG, et al. Operative treatment of nonunions of the surgical neck of the humerus. J Shoulder Elbow Surg 1996;5:169.
12. Flatow E, Cuomo F, Maday MG, et al. Open reduction and internal fixation of two-part displaced fractures of the greater tuberosity of the proximal part of the humerus. J Bone Joint Surg 1991;73A:1213.
13. Frich L, Sojbjerg J, Sneppen O. Shoulder arthroplasty in complex acute and chronic proximal humeral fractures. Orthopedics 1991;14(9):949.
14. Gerber C, Hersche O, Berberat C. The clinical relevance of posttraumatic avascular necrosis of the humeral head. J Shoulder Elbow Surg 1998;7:586.
15. Goss T. Shoulder infections. In: Bigliani L, ed. Complications of shoulder surgery. Baltimore, Williams & Wilkins, 1993:202.
16. Groh GI, Simoni M, Rolla P. Loss of the deltoid after shoulder operations: an operative disaster. J Shoulder Elbow Surg 1994;3:243.
17. Keene JS, Huzienga RE, Engher WD, et al. Proximal humeral fractures: a correlation of residual deformity with long term function. Orthopedics 1983;6:173.
18. Kilcoyne R, Shuman W, FM III. The Neer classification of displaced proximal humerus fractures: spectrum on findings on plain radiographs and CT scans. Am J Radiol 1990;154:1029.
19. Kristiansen B, Christensen S. Proximal humeral fractures: late results in relation to classification and treatment. Acta Orthop Scand 1987;58:124.
20. Kuhlman J, Fishman EK, Ney DR, et al. Complex shoulder trauma: three-dimensional CT imaging. Orthopedics 1988;11:1561.
21. LaBriola J, Mohaghesh H. Isolated avulsion fracture of the lesser tuberosity of the humerus. J Bone Joint Surg 1975;57A:1011.
22. Lind T, Kroner T, Jensen J. The epidemiology of fractures of the proximal humerus. Arch Orthop Trauma Surg 1989;108:285.

23. McLaughlin H. Dislocation of the shoulder with tuberosity fracture. Surg Clin North Am 1963;43:1615.
24. Morris M, Kilcoyne R, Shuman W. Humeral tuberosity fractures: evaluation by CT scan and management of malunion. Orthop Trans 1987;11:242.
25. Neer C. Displaced proximal humerus fractures. Part I. Classification and evaluation. J Bone Joint Surg 1970;52A:1077.
26. Norris T, Green A, McGuigan F. Late prosthetic shoulder arthroplasty for displaced proximal humerus fractures. J Shoulder Elbow Surg 1995;4:271.
27. Norris T, Turner J, Bovill D. Nonunion of the upper humerus: an analysis of the etiology and treatment in 28 cases. In: Morrey B, Hawkins R, eds. Surgery of the shoulder. St. Louis, Mosby-Year Book, 1990:63.
28. Sidor ML, Zuckerman JD, Lyon T, et al. Classification of proximal humerus fractures: the contribution of the scapular lateral and axillary radiographs. J Shoulder Elbow Surg 1994;3:24.
29. Sidor M, Zuckerman J, Lyon T. The Neer classification system for proximal humeral fractures: an assessment of interobserver reliability and intraobserver reproducibility. J Bone Joint Surg 1993;75A:1745.
30. Siegel J, Dines D. Proximal humerus malunions. Orthop Clin North Am 2000;31(1):35.
31. Solonen K, Vastamaki M. Osteotomy of the neck of the humerus for traumatic varus deformity. Acta Orthop Scand 1985;56:79.
32. Tanner M, Cofield R. Prosthetic arthroplasty for fracrues and fracture-dislocations of the proximal humerus. Clin Orthop 1983;179:117.
33. Watson K. Complications of internal fixation of proximal humeral fractures. In: Bigliani L, ed. Complications of shoulder surgery. Baltimore, Williams & Wilkins, 1993:190.
34. Wiater J, Flatow E. Posttraumatic arthritis. Orthop Clin North Am 2000;31(1):63.

Scapular and Glenoid Fractures

18

Charles Getz   Allen Deutsch   Gerald R. Williams, Jr.

INTRODUCTION

The scapula is intimately linked to shoulder function and mobility. Through the clavicle, acromioclavicular, sternoclavicular, and glenohumeral joints, the shoulder connects the axial and appendicular skeletons and presents a stable platform for the upper extremity. Injury to the scapula may disrupt normal shoulder function. The incidence of scapular fracture has been reported to be 3% to 5% of shoulder girdle injuries[40,90] and 0.4% to 1% of all fractures.[75] The low incidence of scapula fracture is because of its protected position along the rib cage, the enveloping musculature, and its relative mobility, which permits dissipation of forces. Scapular fractures most commonly involve the scapular body (49%–89%), the glenoid neck (10%–60%), and the glenoid cavity (10%) (Fig. 18-1).[1,2,18,49,69,106]

Scapular fractures usually are sustained as the result of severe trauma. Most series report motor vehicle or motorcycle accidents as the cause of injury in more than 50% of the cases.[1,2,49,69,106] Associated injuries are common, including rib fracture, pneumothorax, and head injury. Rowe[90,91] reported that 71% of the patients in his series of scapular fractures had other associated injuries; 45% had fracture of other bones, including the ribs, sternum, and spine; 3% sustained a pneumothorax; 4% sustained brachial plexus injuries; and 19% sustained other shoulder girdle disloca-

tions. Since the earliest modern series of scapula fractures, emphasis has been placed on the high association of other serious injuries.[24,56,77,110] Table 18-1 summarizes the associated injuries with scapula fractures from several series.

ANATOMY AND BIOMECHANICS

Anatomy

The scapula is enveloped by multiple layers of muscles. The anterior surface provides attachment for the subscapularis, serratus anterior, omohyoid, pectoralis minor, conjoined tendon of the coracobrachialis and short head of the biceps, long head of the biceps, and long head of the triceps (Fig. 18-2).[37] The posterior surface of the scapula provides muscular attachment sites for the levator scapulae, the rhomboid major, the rhomboid minor, the latissimus dorsi, the teres major, the teres minor, a portion of the long head of the triceps, the deltoid, the trapezius, the supraspinatus, the infraspinatus, and a portion of the omohyoid (Fig. 18-2).[37] The intramuscular position of the scapula provides it with great mobility and a protective cushion that are no doubt responsible for the low incidence of scapular injury.

The close proximity of neurovascular structures to the scapula places them at risk for injury. The pectoralis minor tendon inserts at the base of the coracoid process and the lateral border of the suprascapular notch. The brachial plexus and axillary artery travel posterior to the pectoralis minor tendon. The suprascapular nerve traverses through the suprascapular notch to innervate the supraspinatus muscle, whereas the suprascapular artery passes over it. The suprascapular nerve continues through the spinoglenoid

C. Getz: Fellow, Shoulder and Elbow Service, Department of Orthopaedic Surgery, University of Pennsylvania, Philadelphia, Pennsylvania.

A. Deutsch: Department of Orthopaedic Surgery, Kelsey-Seybold Clinic, Houston, Texas.

G. R. Williams, Jr.: Chief, Shoulder and Elbow Service, Department of Orthopaedic Surgery, University of Pennsylvania, Philadelphia, Pennsylvania.

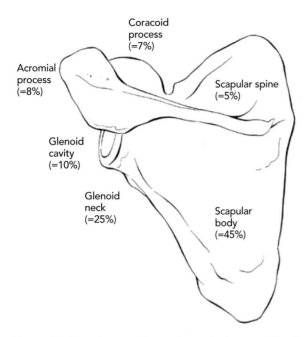

Coracoid
process
(=7%)

Acromial
process
(=8%)

Scapular spine
(=5%)

Glenoid
cavity
(=10%)

Glenoid
neck
(=25%)

Scapular
body
(=45%)

Figure 18-1 Relative incidence of scapular fractures. (Reprinted with permission from McGahan JP, Rab GT, Dublin A. Fractures of the scapula. J Trauma 1980;20(10):880.)

notch to innervate the infraspinatus muscle. At the medial border of the scapula, the dorsal scapular and spinal accessory nerves descend along the thorax, along with branches of the transverse cervical artery.

The osseous components of the scapula, which consist of the body and spine, coracoid process, acromion process, glenoid, and inferior angle, arise from several ossification centers.[67] At birth, the body and spine form one ossified

mass. However, the coracoid process, acromion process, glenoid, and inferior angle are all cartilaginous. The coracoid process is a coalescence of four or five centers of ossification. The center of ossification for the midportion of the coracoid appears at age 3 to 18 months and may be bipolar. The ossification center for the base of the coracoid, which includes the upper third of the glenoid, appears at 7 to 10 years. Two ossification centers appear at age 14 to 16 years: a center for the tip and a shell-like center at the medial apex of the coracoid process. The ossification centers for the base and the midportion of the coracoid coalesce during adolescence at age 14 to 16 years. The other ossification centers fuse at the age of 18 to 25 years.

The acromion is a coalescence of two or three centers of ossification that appear between the ages of 14 and 16 years, coalesce at the age of 19 years, and fuse to the spine at the age of 20 to 25 years. Failure of the anterior acromion ossification center to fuse to the spine gives rise to the os acromiale. This unfused apophysis is present in 2.7% of random patients and is bilateral in 60% of cases.[57] The size of the os acromiale depends on which of the four ossification centers of the acromion have failed to fuse (Fig. 18-3). The most common site of nonunion is between the meso-acromion and the meta-acromion, which corresponds to the midacromioclavicular joint level. An axillary lateral radiograph clearly demonstrates the lesion. Norris has reported that the os acromiale has been mistaken for fracture and that there is an association between the os acromiale and a rotator cuff tear.[78]

The inferior angle of the scapula arises from an ossification center that appears at age 15 years and fuses with the remainder of the scapula at age 20 years. The vertebral bor-

TABLE 18-1
ASSOCIATED INJURIES WITH SCAPULA FRACTURE

Study	Leung and Lam	Wilbur and Evans	Findlay	Ada and Miller	Nordqvist and Petersson	Zdravkovic and Damholt
Patients	15	40	37	113	129	40
Rib fracture	4 (27%)	17 (42.5%)	20 (54%)	NR*	28 (22%)	NR
Hemothorax/pneumothorax	2 (13%)	NR	NR	42 (37%)	7 (5%)	NR
Head injury	6 (40%)	2 (5%)	NR	38 (34%)	22 (17%)	NR
Pulmonary contusion	2 (13%)	NR	NR	8%	NR	NR
Long bone fracture	2 (13%)	7 (17.5%)	NR	NR	13 (10%)	NR
Spine fracture	1 (7%)	NR	NR	4 (3.5%)	8 (6%)	NR
Death	NR	NR	4 (11%)	NR	NR	4 (10%)
Ipsilateral clavicle fracture	15 (100%)	7 (17.5%)	NR	28 (25%)	18 (14%)	NR
Brachial plexus injury	NR	NR	NR	4 (3.5%)	NR	4 (10%)
Subclavian artery injury	NR	NR	NR	1 (<1%))	NR	1 (2.5%)
Ipsilateral acromioclavicular separation	NR	NR	NR	6 (5%)	NR	NR
Aorta injury	NR	NR	NR	NR	1 (<1%)	NR
Suprascapular nerve injury	NR	NR	NR	NR	1 (<1%)	NR

*No percentage reported but referred to as the most common associated injury.

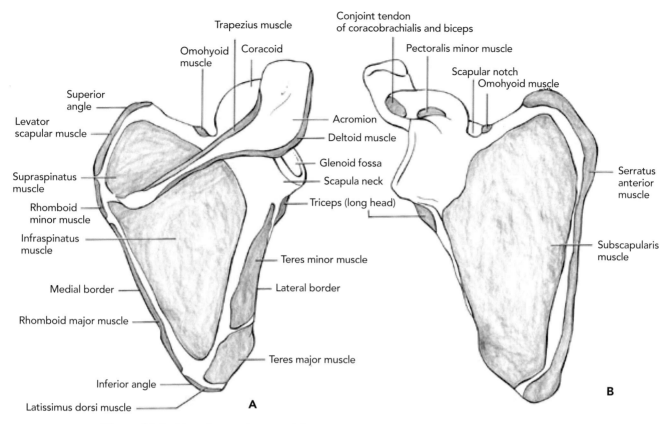

Figure 18-2 Muscular attachments of the posterior (A) and anterior (B) aspects of the scapula. (Reprinted with permission from Goss TP. Fractures of the scapula: diagnosis and treatment. In: Williams GR Jr., ed. Disorders of the shoulder: diagnosis and management. Philadelphia, PA, Lippincott Williams & Wilkins, 1999:597.)

der arises from an ossification center that appears at age 16 to 18 years and fuses by the age of 25 years.

The glenoid fossa ossifies from four sources: (a) the coracoid base (including the upper third of the glenoid), (b) the deep portion of the coracoid process, (c) the body, and (d) the lower pole, which joins with the remainder of the body of the scapula at age 20 to 25 years.

Caution must be exercised when interpreting radiographs of the scapula in adolescents and young adults. The os acromiale is the most frequently quoted unfused apophysis and can be confused with fracture.[57,78] In addition, the physes at the base of the coracoid and the tip of the coracoid process can be difficult to distinguish from fracture. In the appropriate setting, a radiograph of the contralateral scapula is useful in determining whether a radiographic "line" is truly a fracture or an unfused apophysis. Furthermore, the junction between the upper and lower glenoid in adults represents the coalescence of the previous ossification centers and is the site of origin of many glenoid fossa fractures with a transverse component.

Biomechanics

The scapula is suspended from the clavicle through the acromial clavicular joint and coracoclavicular ligament.

The clavicle, in turn, joins the trunk at the sternoclavicular joint. The sternoclavicular joint is the only true joint attaching the upper extremity to the body. However, the scapula articulates with the posterior chest wall and spine through numerous muscular attachments. Although not a

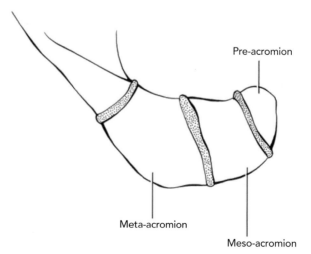

Figure 18-3 The types of os acromiale, depending on which ossification fails to fuse. (Reprinted with permission from Liberson F. Os acromiale—a contested anomaly. J Bone Joint Surg Am 1937;19:683.)

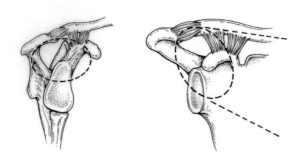

Figure 18-4 The superior shoulder suspensory complex (SSSC) described by Goss consists of a bone-soft-tissue ring supported by two bone struts.

synovial joint, the scapulothoracic articulation is a stable construct that is rarely disrupted.[16,17,45,83]

The reliance of overhead activity on the relationships among the clavicle, coracoclavicular ligaments, acromio-clavicular joint, acromion, and glenoid neck has led to the development of the concept of the superior shoulder suspensory complex (SSSC) by Goss.[32–34] He likened the SSSC to a ring with two links. The ring is composed of the clavicle lateral to the coracoclavicular ligament, the coracoclavicular ligament itself, the glenoid, the coracoid process, and the acromion. The links are composed of the clavicle and the lateral scapular body and scapular spine (Fig. 18-4). The SSSC is thought to provide stability for the shoulder complex. Moreover, disruption of two or more components of the SSSC may result in enough loss of stability of the shoulder complex to require operative fixation.[26,32–34, 40–42,60,99]

Williams and colleagues[107] investigated the biomechan-ics of the SSSC in a cadaveric model, with particular refer-ence to one specific type of double disruption of the SSSC—the "floating shoulder" (fracture of the glenoid neck and clavicular shaft). In their model, the coracoacro-mial ligament, which was not included in Goss's original description of the SSSC, provided significant stability to the shoulder girdle. Complete lack of suspensory support

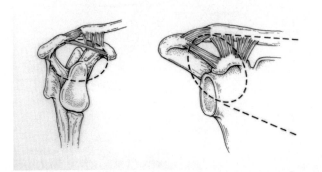

Figure 18-5 The coracoacromial ligament was not included in Goss's original description, but should be included.

of the shoulder did not occur as a result of ipsilateral clav-icle and glenoid neck fractures without additional injuries to the coracoacromial and acromioclavicular ligaments. Williams et al. suggested that the coracoacromial ligament should be added to the SSSC (Fig. 18-5).

MECHANISM OF INJURY

The body of the scapula is flat and encompassed within thick layers of muscle that allow movement in numerous directions. It has three projections, two synovial joints, and one articulation. In addition to its varied bony anatomy, the scapula serves as an attachment for 17 muscles. The body, a projection, an articulation, or a muscular attachment can be the site of a scapular frac-ture.[1,23,24,56,77,106,110] Fracture may occur through direct or indirect trauma.

Direct Trauma

Fractures of the scapula are the result of energy transmitted in one of several means. A direct blow to the body or any of the projections can result in a fracture. The scapula is well protected; therefore, the body, spine, glenoid neck, and coracoid fractures that occur by this mechanism are commonly secondary to high-energy injuries. Numerous reports cite motor vehicle accidents, falls, pedestrian-vehicle accidents, and motorcycle accidents as the most common precipitating events.

Indirect Trauma

Indirect Injury from the Humeral Head

Trauma that loads the arm and subsequently impacts the humerus into the glenoid may result in glenoid fracture. The direction of loading and position of the humeral head on the glenoid face at the time of loading determine the fracture pattern. If the humeral head is positioned anterior on the face when the energy is delivered, the resulting frac-ture will be an anterior rim fracture. Similarly, if the head is posterior on the face when impact occurs, a posterior glenoid rim fracture will occur. Medial impaction of the humeral head when it is centered on the glenoid fossa often produces a transverse glenoid fracture that may exit the superior, medial, or lateral borders of the scapula. The humerus has also been implicated in coracoid and acro-mial process fractures.[6,14,27,108,109]

Avulsion Fractures

Indirect trauma through forceful contraction of any of the scapular muscle attachments may cause an avulsion-type scapular fracture. Goss has proposed three mechanisms of injury: (a) severe contraction from seizure, electric shock, or electroconvulsive therapy; (b) overloading the strength of the bone by a forceful contraction; and (c) repetitive loading (stress or fatigue fractures).[35,43,50,53,93,97]

CLASSIFICATION

Several classification systems for scapular fractures have been reported in the literature. Classification systems that involve a specific anatomic location, such as the coracoid, acromion, or glenoid processes, will be discussed in the individual sections pertaining to those injuries. However, Zdravkovic and Damholt[110] divided scapular fractures into three general types: type I fractures, or fractures of the body; type II fractures, or fractures of the apophyses (including the coracoid and acromion); and type III fractures, or fractures of the superior lateral angle (i.e., scapular neck and glenoid). Zdravkovic and Damholt considered the type III fracture to be the most difficult to treat; these represented only 6% of their series.

Thompson and coworkers[98] presented a classification system that divided scapular fractures according to the likelihood that associated injuries would be present. Their cases all resulted from blunt trauma. Class I fractures included fractures of the coracoid and acromion process and small fractures of the body. Class II fractures comprised glenoid and scapular neck fractures. Class III fractures included major scapular body fractures. Thompson and colleagues reported that class II and III fractures were much more likely to have associated injuries.[98]

Wilbur and Evans[106] described 40 patients with 52 scapular fractures. The patients were divided into two groups based on fracture location: group I, which included patients with fractures of the scapular body, neck, and spine; and group II, which included patients with fractures of the acromion process, coracoid process, or glenoid. They reported unsatisfactory results of treatment in patients in group II because of residual pain and loss of glenohumeral motion.

CLINICAL EVALUATION

History and Physical Examination

It is important to reemphasize that scapular fracture is often associated with other injuries that require more urgent treatment. In these patients, the standard trauma protocol of stabilizing airway, breathing, and circulation must be performed before definitive evaluation. Once the patient has been stabilized, physical examination should be directed toward identifying any of the concomitant injuries previously described. McLennan and Ungersma[70] highlighted the importance of follow-up examination in

patients with scapular fracture, because the development of pneumothorax may be delayed 1 to 3 days.

Scapular fracture typically presents with the arm adducted and protected from all movements. Abduction is especially painful. Although ecchymosis is less than expected from the degree of bony injury present, severe local tenderness is a reliable finding.[10] Patients with scapular body fractures or coracoid process fractures frequently experience increasing pain with deep inspiration secondary to the pull of the pectoralis minor or serratus anterior muscles. Frequently, rotator cuff function is extremely painful and weak secondary to inhibition from intramuscular hemorrhage. This has been described as a "pseudo-rupture" of the rotator cuff and frequently resolves within a few weeks.[74] If this weakness does not resolve, concomitant rotator cuff or nerve injury should be suspected.

Radiographic Evaluation

Most scapular fractures can be adequately visualized with routine radiographic views. A true anteroposterior view of the scapula combined with an axillary or true scapular lateral view will demonstrate most scapular body or spine fractures, glenoid neck fractures, and acromion fractures. "Special" views may be required in selected circumstances. The Stryker notch view is useful for coracoid fractures (Fig. 18-6).[10] The apical oblique view, described by Garth et al.,[28] and the West Point lateral view are useful views for evaluating anterior glenoid rim fractures.[88]

The majority of scapula fractures can be diagnosed and classified properly by plain radiographs. Computed tomography (CT) is not necessary in most scapular fractures.[66] However, the evaluation of intra-articular glenoid fractures is facilitated by CT scanning. The contralateral normal shoulder may be scanned as well as the involved shoulder to provide a means for comparison of the pathologic findings noted in the involved shoulder, especially in adolescents.[10] CT scanning also allows for confirmation of the size, location, and degree of displacement of fracture fragments, and may detect the presence of instability. With the appropriate software, three-dimensional images can be generated and the humeral head can be subtracted from the image so that an unobstructed view of the scapula and glenoid can be obtained (Fig. 18-7). These three-dimensional CT reconstructions can be extremely useful in surgical planning.

TREATMENT

The recommended treatment for specific types of scapular fractures varies depending on the fracture's location (intra- or extra-articular), displacement, and effect on shoulder stability. The great majority of extra-articular fractures

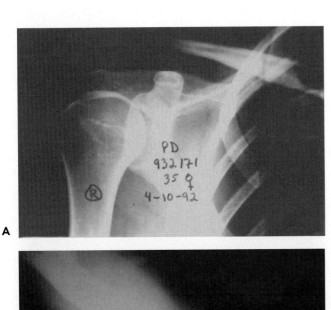

A

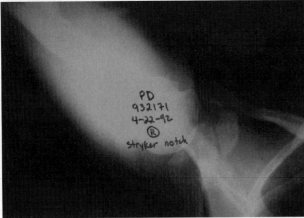

C

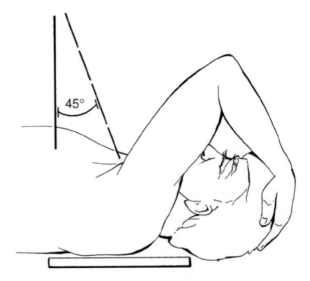

B

Figure 18-6 Fracture of the coracoid base is often not visualized well on routine anteroposterior radiographs (A), but are seen well on a Stryker Notch view (B and C).

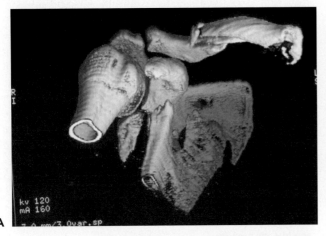

A

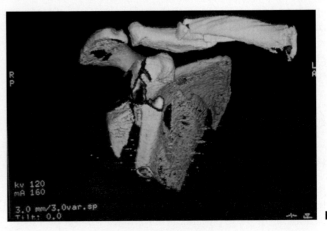

B

Figure 18-7 Computed tomography (CT) scans are not necessary in all scapular fractures but can aid in quantifying the amount of intra-articular displacement. Three-dimensional reconstruction allows visualization of the glenoid fossa with (A) and without (B) the humeral image.

(i.e., glenoid neck, scapular body, or spine, acromion, and coracoid fractures) are managed nonoperatively.[10,15,59] Intra-articular fractures, particularly those associated with glenohumeral instability or substantial displacement, are most often managed operatively.[15,34,46,73]

Extra-articular Fractures

Scapular Body Fracture

Fracture of the scapula's body is the most common type of scapular fracture and is correlated with the highest incidence of associated injury.[10] The musculature surrounding the scapula makes nonunion a rare occurrence. Scapular malunion is uncommonly associated with clinical symptoms.[15,90,91] Consequently, most authors favor a sling, ice, and supportive measures until the initial pain subsides, followed by early motion.[15,90,91] Several large series of scapular body fractures treated nonoperatively have been reported, with union generally being the rule.[23,24,77,110] Shoulder function scores are rarely reported, but function is generally referred to as good. Nordqvist and Petersson,[77] however, found poor long-term results in some patients with greater than 10 mm of displacement.

When scapular body malunion is associated with painful crepitus that interferes with range of motion, excision of the bony prominence is usually curative.[62] Nonunions of the scapular body often involve the inferior angle and its serratus anterior insertion. Therefore, weakness, pain, and limited motion are the common complaints. Fortunately, symptomatic nonunion routinely responds well to open reduction, internal fixation, and bone grafting (Fig. 18-8).[22,38] Although excision of small fragments may be successful,[51] caution should be exercised when considering excision of large inferior angle fragments because of the potential for serratus anterior insufficiency.

Author's Preferred Treatment

With the assumption that serious associated injuries have been ruled out, symptomatic treatment is indicated for almost all patients with scapular body fracture. Displacement is often well tolerated, except when the fracture traverses the inferior angle and the inferior fragment is displaced anteriorly, deep to the superior fragment. Under these rare circumstances, particularly when the inferior fragment is large and involves a large portion of the serratus insertion, primary open reduction and plate fixation are indicated. Stable fixation usually requires two plates—one along the lateral border and one along the medial border of the scapula. These can be placed through a single skin incision, paralleling the lateral border, midway between the medial and lateral margins of the scapula. The lateral border is exposed by anterior retraction of the posterior border of the latissimus dorsi and elevation of the dorsal origin of the teres minor and major. The medial border is exposed by superomedial retraction of the lateral border of the lower and middle trapezius. Rarely will detaching a small portion of the trapezius insertion on the base of the scapular spine be required (Fig. 18-9).

Nonoperative treatment for the majority of scapular body fractures consists of ice and sling immobilization, initially. Within 1 to 2 weeks, passive range of motion can be instituted. An overhead pulley is added at 3 to 4 weeks postinjury; active range of motion and progressive-resistance exercises can usually be instituted at 6 weeks postinjury. Recovery from fracture usually requires 6 to 12 months. This rehabilitation protocol is also followed postoperatively for stably fixed fractures.

Glenoid Neck

Fracture of the neck of the scapula is the second most common scapular fracture.[10] By definition, glenoid neck fractures are extra-articular. Three common fracture patterns have been described, depending on the point of exit of the superior extent of the fracture. These fracture patterns include one that exits the superior border of the scapula medial to the coracoid base, one that exits lateral to the coracoid base (anatomic neck), and one that exits the medial border of the scapula, inferior to the scapular spine, without traversing the glenoid neck (Fig. 18-10).[1,33,77,110] The most common fracture, by far, is the first pattern, whereby the fracture line exits the superior scapular border, medial to the base of the coracoid. Glenoid neck fractures have been classified as type I (nondisplaced) and type II (displaced), in which displacement is defined as 1 cm of translation or 40 degrees of angulation (Fig. 18-11).[1,33,77,110]

Recommended methods of closed treatment for glenoid neck fractures include closed reduction and olecranon pin traction for 3 weeks followed by a sling, closed reduction, and a shoulder spica cast for 6 to 8 weeks, and brief sling immobilization followed by progressive mobilization.[2,11,15,44,59,110] Regardless of the method of closed treatment, permanent reduction of glenoid neck displacement is unlikely.[15,59] Therefore, when nonoperative treatment is indicated, a brief period of sling immobilization followed by progressive mobilization seems most reasonable. Most series report good functional results in patients with glenoid neck fractures regardless of the treatment method.[2,44,110]

When the results of nonoperative management are stratified according to the degree of residual displacement, a relationship between displacement and end result is identified.[1,25,40] Gagey and colleagues[25] reported only one good result among 12 displaced glenoid neck fractures that were treated closed. They theorized that the glenoid neck, healing in the displaced position, would "disorganize the coracoacromial arch." Therefore, they recommended open reduction and internal fixation.

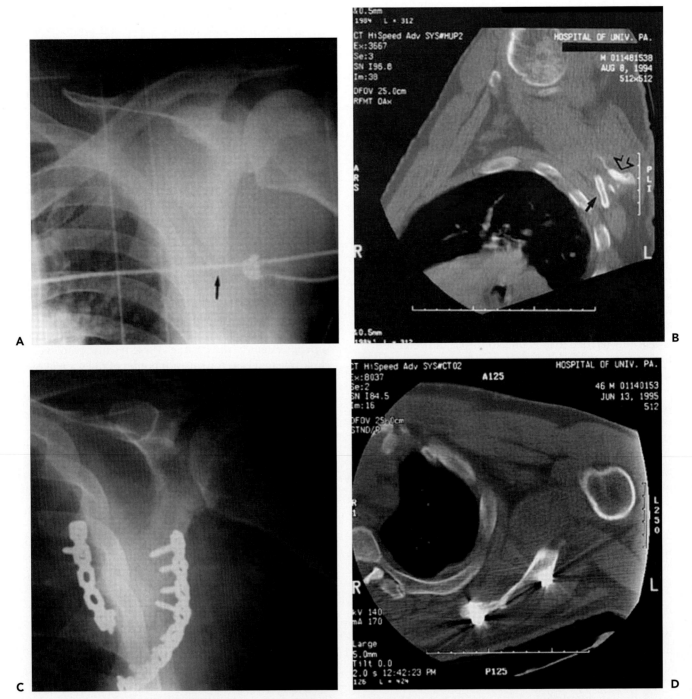

Figure 18-8   Anteroposterior radiograph *(A)* of initial scapular body fracture *(arrow)* and CT scan *(B)* of nonunion with inferior fragment *(smaller arrow)* incarcerated between the superior fragment *(larger arrow)* and the rib cage. Postoperative anteroposterior radiograph *(C)* and CT scan *(D)* after open reduction and internal fixation with two plates. (Reprinted with permission from Gupta R, Sher J, Williams GR, et al. Non-union of the scapular body. A case report. J Bone Joint Surg Am 1998;80(3):428.)

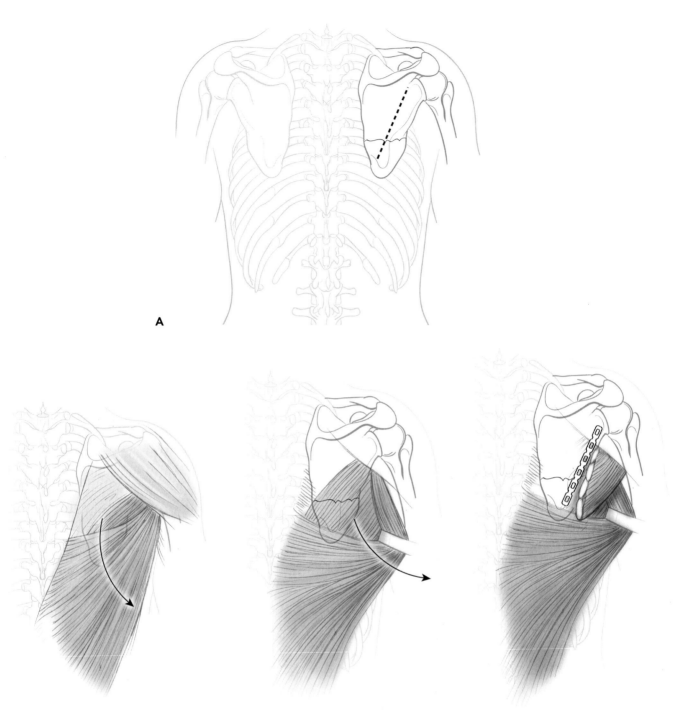

Figure 18-9 The skin incision (A) for open reduction and internal fixation of transverse scapular body fractures parallels the lateral border of the scapula, midway between the medial and lateral borders. A lateral plate can be placed (B) after exposure of the lateral border by retracting the latissimus dorsi anteriorly and releasing the dorsal portion of the teres minor and major origins. (continued)

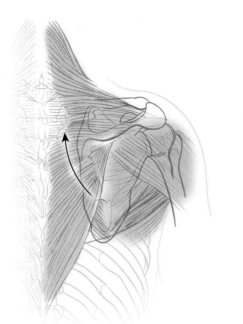
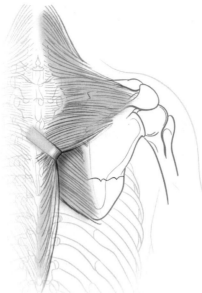
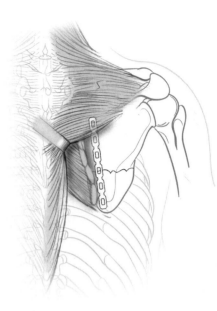

C

Figure 18-9 *(continued)* A medial plate can be placed *(C)* after exposure of the medial border by retracting the middle and inferior trapezius medially and releasing the dorsal portion of the rhomboid minor and major.

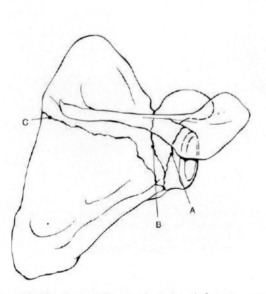

Figure 18-10 Three different glenoid neck fracture patterns have been recognized, with the most superior extent of the fracture exiting the scapula at the superior scapular border lateral to the base of the coracoid process *(A)*, medial to the base of the coracoid process *(B)*, and at the medial scapular border, inferior to the scapular spine *(C)*. (Reprinted with permission from Goss TP. Fractures of the scapula: diagnosis and treatment. In: Williams GR Jr., ed. Disorders of the shoulder: diagnosis and management. Philadelphia, PA, Lippincott Williams & Wilkins, 1999:597.)

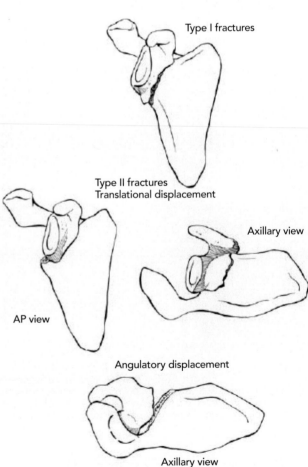

Type I fractures

Type II fractures
Translational displacement

AP view

Axillary view

Angulatory displacement

Axillary view

Figure 18-11 Glenoid neck fractures have been classified as nondisplaced (type I) and displaced (type II), for which displacement is defined as 1 cm of translation or 40 degrees of angulation. (Reprinted with permission from Goss TP. Fractures of the scapula: diagnosis and treatment. In: Williams GR Jr., ed. Disorders of the shoulder: diagnosis and management. Philadelphia, PA, Lippincott Williams & Wilkins, 1999:597.)

Ada and Miller[1] reported on 24 patients with displaced scapular neck fractures. Of the 16 patients treated conservatively, 50% complained of night pain, 40% had weakness of abduction, and 20% had decreased range of motion. Open reduction and internal fixation were used to treat eight patients with scapular neck fractures having greater than 40-degree angulation or more than 1 cm of medial displacement of the glenoid surface. None of these patients experienced night pain, and all regained at least 85% of abduction.

Suprascapular nerve paralysis may result from extension of the glenoid neck fracture into the suprascapular notch. This concomitant nerve injury has been reported to be an indication for early exploration, open reduction, and internal fixation.[18,95] However, this recommendation is made on few cases and with no control group.

The glenoid neck is one component of the SSSC and, as such, contributes substantially to the suspensory support of the entire shoulder girdle. When the most common fracture pattern occurs (i.e., the fracture line exits medial to the coracoid process), translatory displacement of the distal fragment is resisted by its attachment to the proximal fragment (coracoacromial ligament) and axial skeleton (clavicle, coracoclavicular ligament, and acromioclavicular capsule). The distal fragment becomes completely unstable (i.e., "floating shoulder") when it has lost all attachments to the proximal fragment and axial skeleton (Fig. 18-12). This situation can occur through concomitant fractures, ligamentous injuries, or combinations of the two.

Concomitant fractures that may result in a "floating shoulder" after glenoid neck fracture include fracture of the

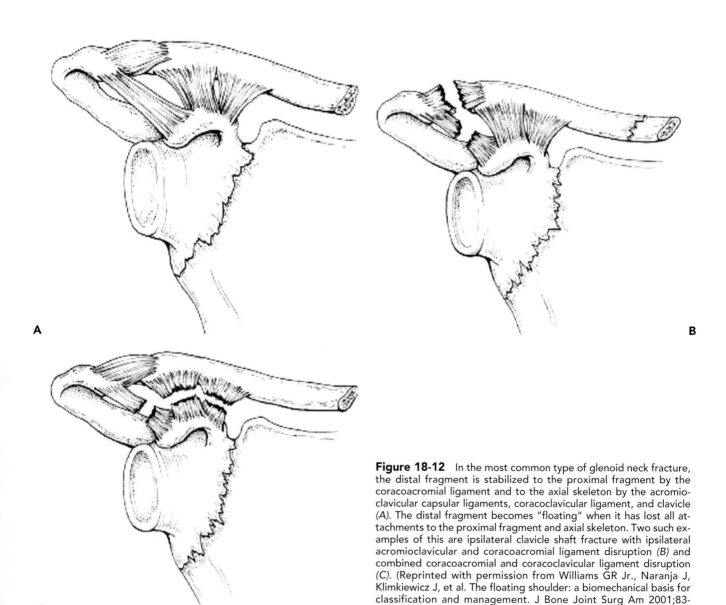

Figure 18-12 In the most common type of glenoid neck fracture, the distal fragment is stabilized to the proximal fragment by the coracoacromial ligament and to the axial skeleton by the acromioclavicular capsular ligaments, coracoclavicular ligament, and clavicle (A). The distal fragment becomes "floating" when it has lost all attachments to the proximal fragment and axial skeleton. Two such examples of this are ipsilateral clavicle shaft fracture with ipsilateral acromioclavicular and coracoacromial ligament disruption (B) and combined coracoacromial and coracoclavicular ligament disruption (C). (Reprinted with permission from Williams GR Jr., Naranja J, Klimkiewicz J, et al. The floating shoulder: a biomechanical basis for classification and management. J Bone Joint Surg Am 2001;83-A(8):1182.)

coracoid base and combined clavicle shaft and acromion/scapular spine fracture. Purely ligamentous injuries that result in complete instability of the distal fragment include combined disruption of the coracoacromial and coracoclavicular ligaments. Combined bone-ligament injuries that result in complete instability comprise clavicle shaft fracture with coracoacromial and acromioclavicular capsular ligament injury and acromion/scapular spine fracture with coracoclavicular and acromioclavicular capsular disruption.[107]

Rotational displacement is also likely to be resisted by the ligamentous attachments to the distal fragment. However, the amount of rotation allowed by intact stabilizers of the distal fragment is not known. The conjoined tendon of the coracobrachialis and short head of the biceps is potentially a significant deforming force and theoretically could cause inferior and medial rotation of the glenoid fragment.

Traditionally, floating shoulders (i.e., ipsilateral clavicle and glenoid neck fractures) were treated nonoperatively. However, more recently, there has been increased interest in open reduction and internal fixation of these fractures.[32–34,40–42,56] The importance of a concurrent ipsilateral clavicle fracture was first noted by Herscovici et al.,[41] who advocated open reduction and internal fixation of at least the clavicle fracture. No mention was made of the angulation of the glenoid or the amount of displacement of the clavicle before surgery. All seven of the seven patients who underwent open reduction and internal fixation had an excellent result. The two nonoperative patients had one excellent and one poor result. Both nonoperative patients were noted to have ptosis of the shoulder. Again, there was no mention of the displacement of the nonoperatively treated fractures.

Routine operative treatment of floating shoulder without regard to displacement has recently been questioned.[19,20,85–87,89,101] Ramos et al.[85] showed good or excellent results in 9 of 13 patients treated nonoperatively. Edwards found that shoulder function in 20 patients with floating shoulder who were treated nonoperatively had outcome comparable to previously published results of operative treatment.[19] They recommended nonoperative treatment, especially in patients with glenoid neck displacement of 5 mm or less.

Egol et al.[20] retrospectively compared outcomes in operatively and nonoperatively treated glenoid neck fractures associated with either acromioclavicular joint injury or clavicle fracture. The operatively treated group had greater shoulder elevation, but the functional results were not significantly different between groups. The authors concluded that routine operative management of floating shoulders could not be supported by their data.

Ramsey et al.[86] reported the results of nine patients who were managed nonoperatively with a floating shoulder. Six patients were graded with good or excellent results, and three were graded with fair results. Of those patients with fair results, one had a closed head injury, and one had a brachial plexus injury and heterotopic ossification. It is in-

teresting that five of the six excellent results were in patients whose initial medial displacement was less then 2 cm. The other patient with an excellent result had an initial displacement of 2.2 cm. Two of three of the fair results were in patients with greater than 3 cm of medial displacement. Other authors with larger numbers of patients have also correlated decreasing results with increasing glenoid neck angulation or displacement.[89,101]

Author's Preferred Treatment

Several factors contribute to the decision to treat a given glenoid neck fracture surgically. These factors include glenoid neck displacement, patient age and activity level, bone quality, comminution, and associated injuries. Operative treatment is reserved for displaced fractures in young, active patients with good bone quality and manageable comminution. Displacement is defined as translation greater than 2 cm medially or angulation greater than 40 degrees. These displacement criteria for operative management are followed for all glenoid neck fractures, even those associated with other disruptions of the SSSC (i.e., floating shoulders). Nonoperative management is undertaken in all fractures that do not meet these criteria. Surgery may not be indicated in older, more sedentary patients, in patients who have other more life-threatening injuries, and in patients with extensive medical comorbidities, even if the previously mentioned displacement criteria have been met.

When nonoperative treatment is indicated, a sling is used for comfort for the first 7 to 10 days postinjury. As pain subsides, pendulum exercises are instituted within 2 weeks postinjury. Supine passive elevation and passive external rotation exercises are instituted at 2 to 3 weeks. At 4 to 5 weeks, an overhead pulley program is added. Active range of motion, passive stretching in all planes, and strengthening exercises for the rotator cuff, deltoid, and scapular stabilizers are begun at 6 to 8 weeks after the fracture. Although the fracture will heal in the majority of cases during the first 6 to 8 weeks, full recovery will take 6 to 12 months.

Open reduction and internal fixation of displaced glenoid neck fractures are performed through a posterior approach with the patient in the lateral decubitus position. The weight of the involved arm results in a medially directed deforming force that can complicate the achievement and maintenance of an adequate reduction. Therefore, a traction setup, such as the one used for shoulder arthroscopy in the lateral decubitus position or a fracture distraction device that has one pin in the scapular spine (or clavicle if the scapular spine is fractured) and the other in the humeral head, may be useful.

The scapular neck is approached through a posterior axillary incision that begins at the scapular spine. approximately 3 to 4 cm medial to the posterolateral acromial corner, and extends inferiorly to the posterior axillary fold. If additional exposure of the superior portion of the lateral scapular border is needed, the incision is extended inferiorly and medially. Full-thickness skin flaps are created to allow exposure of the superior half of the lateral scapular border and the posterior deltoid margin. The posterior border of the deltoid is identified, and its overlying fascia is incised proximally, all the way to the scapular spine, and inferiorly into the axilla. The posterior deltoid is then retracted anterosuperiorly. The arm should be abducted to at least 90 degrees to relax the deltoid and facilitate retraction. This is easily accomplished if one is using an arthroscopy traction setup. Alternatively, if a fracture distractor is going to be used, a mechanical arm holder can be used to position the arm in abduction (Fig. 18-13).

The internervous plane between the infraspinatus and teres minor is identified. This interval is dissected laterally

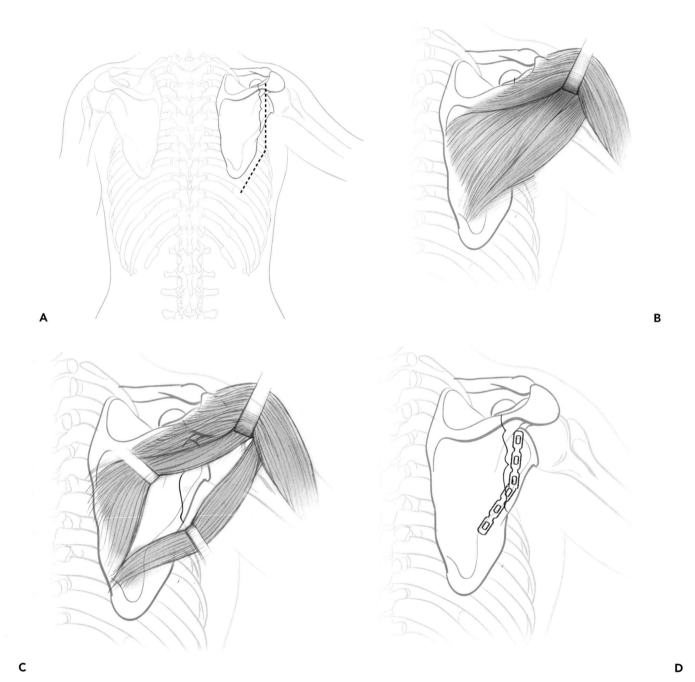

A   B

C   D

Figure 18-13 Scapular neck fractures are fixed through a posterior axillary incision (A) that can be extended inferomedially to aid in exposure of the upper portion of the lateral scapular border. Deep dissection (B) includes superior retraction of the posterior deltoid, dissection of the infraspinatus/teres minor interval, superior retraction of the infraspinatus and inferior retraction of the teres minor, and posterior capsulotomy to visualize the glenoid surface during screw placement. A contoured small pelvic reconstruction plate is placed (C) along the upper portion of the lateral scapular border and posterior glenoid.

to the humeral attachment site of the rotator cuff and medially onto the infraspinatus fossa. An elevator and a scalpel are used to release the infraspinatus muscle and tendon from the underlying posterior capsule. This allows greater superior retraction of the infraspinatus. The dorsal origins of the teres minor and major are partially detached from the lateral scapular border to expose the glenoid neck fracture. With the infraspinatus retracted superiorly and the teres minor and major retracted inferiorly, the fracture, lateral scapular border, and posterior glenoid are visualized. A medial-lateral incision is made in the posterior capsule, and enlarged superiorly and inferiorly if needed, to allow visualization of the joint during drilling and screw placement in the posterior glenoid.

The fracture is reduced and stabilized with a 3.5-mm dynamic compression or some other similarly sized plate. A minimum of two screws, preferably three, in each fragment should be used. The third screw in the lateral fragment may require bending of the plate superiorly or a curved pelvic reconstruction plate. Care should be taken to avoid injuring the suprascapular nerve with the edge of the plate or penetrating the articular surface of the glenoid with the most lateral screw(s) (Fig. 18-14). The capsule is closed, and the infraspinatus, teres minor, teres major, and posterior deltoid are allowed to fall back to their anatomic locations, and the skin is closed in standard fashion. The postoperative rehabilitation protocol is identical to the one described for nonoperative management in this chapter, assuming adequate fixation was attained.

If concomitant fractures of the clavicle and/or scapular spine/acromion also exist, it may be possible to reduce the glenoid neck fracture sufficiently by reducing the other fracture(s). In the acute setting (less than 7 days), this is the treatment of choice. In the subacute setting, it may be necessary to approach both (all) fractures to allow adequate reduction of the glenoid neck. Under these circumstances, both (all) fractures are also fixed. Because of the potential need for exposure of the glenoid neck, the lateral decubitus position is still used.

Coracoid process fractures that accompany glenoid neck fractures are not specifically reduced and stabilized unless the fracture involves the anterosuperior glenoid articular surface and is displaced. Adequate exposure of these fractures typically requires a more extensile posterior exposure, as described in the section on glenoid fossa fractures, or combined anterior and posterior exposures.

Acromion Fracture

Although fracture of the acromion is rare, when it does occur it is usually the result of one of two mechanisms. First, an acromion fracture can result from a downward blow directly applied to the superior aspect of the acromion. Second, acromion fracture can result from superior displacement or dislocation of the humeral head. When the

injury is a result of a downward blow to the acromion, acromioclavicular dislocation is much more common than acromion fracture. However, when a fracture does occur, it is usually minimally displaced. Caution should be used in distinguishing this minimally displaced fracture from an os acromiale. In questionable cases, a radiograph of the contralateral side may be helpful because the os acromiale is bilateral in 60% of the cases.[57] The supraspinatus outlet view may be useful in estimating the amount of displacement.[72] Significant displacement of an acromion fracture resulting from a downward blow to the acromion should alert the clinician to possible associated brachial plexus avulsions.[10,71] Significant superior displacement of the acromion associated with superior displacement or dislocation of the humeral head should alert the clinician to possible injury to the rotator cuff.[71]

Stress fractures of the acromion may occur in athletes. Ward et al.[103] reported that a professional football player with a stress fracture at the base of the acromion was a result of repeated microstresses secondary to weight lifting and blocking assignments. Veluvolu et al.[102] reported a case of an acromial stress fracture in a jogger using arm weights while running. Hall and Calvert[39] described a female golfer who sustained a stress fracture at the base of the acromion as a result of repetitive stress by repeated shots and contraction of the posterior deltoid as the club struck the golf ball. Stress fractures have also been reported after subacromial decompression secondary to thinning of the acromion.[61,64,104]

The majority of acromion fractures, because they are minimally displaced, are treated closed.[71,90,106] Neer[71] recommended symptomatic treatment only, except in the case of significant displacement. Wilbur and Evans,[106] on the other hand, recommended cast immobilization in 60 degrees of abduction, 25 degrees of flexion, and 25 degrees of external rotation for 6 weeks. Open reduction and internal fixation have only been reported for markedly displaced fractures to reduce the acromioclavicular joint and prevent nonunion, malunion, and secondary impingement.[30,35,54,58,68,71,79]

Kuhn and associates[54] recommended a classification system to help determine the need for operative intervention. Type I fractures with minimal displacement and type II displaced fractures without a decrease in the subacromial space warrant nonoperative treatment. In type II displaced fractures in which the subacromial space is diminished by the inferior pull of the deltoid on the acromial fragment, open reduction and internal fixation are required to prevent secondary impingement.

Author's Preferred Treatment

No criteria for displacement of acromial fractures have been established. Therefore, treatment decision making is imprecise and subject to individual surgeon variation.

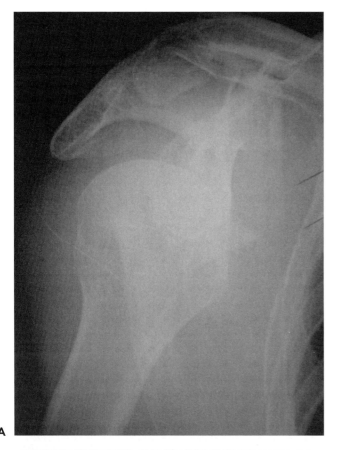

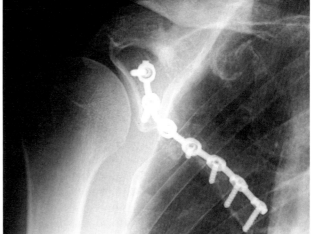

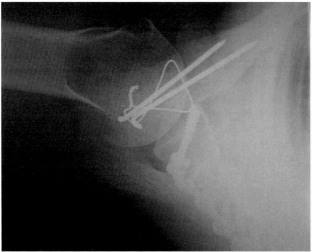

Figure 18-14   Anteroposterior radiograph (A) demonstrating a displaced scapular neck fracture in association with a displaced distal clavicle fracture. Fixation devices such as plates and screws should be placed lateral enough from the spinoglenoid notch to avoid the suprascapular nerve (B) and far enough away from the glenoid rim to avoid the articular surface (C).

Important factors include patient age and activity level, fragment apposition, and the presence of concomitant injuries, such as rotator cuff tears or nerve injuries. Nonoperative management is chosen 90% of the time. Operative intervention is reserved for young, active patients with less than 50% apposition of the fracture fragments and/or associated rotator cuff tear with retraction. This is suspected on the basis of lag signs and weakness in external rotation (posterior cuff) or internal rotation (anterior cuff).

When nonoperative treatment is chosen, a sling is used for comfort for 7 to 10 days. Pendulum exercises are begun within the first 2 weeks. Supine passive flexion and external rotation exercises are added at 3 to 4 weeks. An overhead pulley and active range of motion are added at 5 to 6 weeks postinjury. Stretching and strengthening exercises for the rotator cuff, deltoid, and scapular stabilizers are instituted at 6 to 8 weeks. Full recovery takes 6 to 9 months.

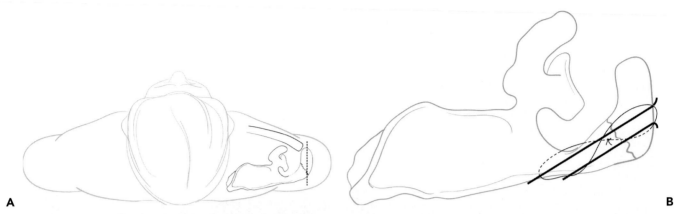

A

B

Figure 18-15 Most often, acromial fractures start at the posterior border of the acromioclavicular joint and extend posterolaterally toward the posterolateral corner. The skin incision *(A)* is in Langer's skin lines midway between the lateral acromial border and the acromioclavicular joint. The fracture can be fixed with a tension band wire construct *(B)*.

If anterior shoulder pain develops after fracture healing, it may be the result of subacromial impingement. Radiographs may reveal narrowing of the supraspinatus outlet. If the pain is temporarily relieved with subacromial local anesthetic, an arthroscopic acromioplasty is likely to result in substantial and long-term improvement of pain.

When open reduction and internal fixation are chosen because of inadequate fragment apposition or narrowing of the subacromial space, they are performed through a superior approach with the patient in the beach-chair position. The skin incision parallels Langer's skin lines, approximately midway between the acromioclavicular joint and the lateral acromial margin. It begins slightly anterior to the anterior acromial margin and extends slightly posterior to the posterior acromial margin. The fracture line typically traverses from the posterior corner of the acromioclavicular joint laterally and posteriorly, toward the posterolateral corner (Fig. 18-15). Occasionally, it is more medial than this, near the base of the scapular spine. In the former case, the fracture can be fixed with a tension band wiring technique. In the more medial fractures, a plate can be placed across the base of the scapular spine (Fig. 18-16). Take care to prevent excessive inferior protrusion of the lateral screws into the subacromial space. Postoperative rehabilitation is as described previously for nonoperative treatment.

Coracoid Process Fracture

Coracoid process fracture may occur in isolation or in combination with other injuries.[6,14,21,29,36,43,58,63,80,81,108,109] Commonly associated injuries include acromioclavicular dislocation, glenohumeral dislocation, and clavicle fracture. Stress fracture of the coracoid from repetitive athletic activity has also been reported.[8,93] Both operative and nonoperative treatments have been recommended. In general, surgical treatment has been recommended for patients with intra-articular extension and involvement of the suprascapular nerve.[21,29,36,63,80,81]

Ogawa et al.[80] proposed a simple classification system for coracoid fractures. The type I fracture occurs between the body of the scapula and the coracoclavicular ligaments. These fractures are frequently associated with additional shoulder injuries such as clavicle fracture, acromial fracture, acromioclavicular dislocation, or associated glenoid fracture. The type II fracture occurs distal to the coracoclavicular ligaments. This may be secondary to humeral head impaction or avulsion by the conjoined tendon. Ogawa et al. recommended surgical treatment for type I fractures and nonsurgical management for type II fractures.

Coracoid process fractures are uncommon, and reported results of both surgical and nonsurgical treatment are sparse. Eyres et al.[21] reported the results of coracoid fractures treated nonoperatively. Of nine patients, eight had excellent function, whereas one patient developed stiffness secondary to immobilization. Ogawa et al.[81] reviewed the outcome of 67 patients with coracoid process fractures.

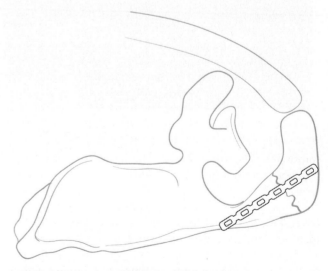

Figure 18-16 More medial acromial fractures can be treated with a plate and screws.

Operative treatment was reserved for patients with type I fractures mentioned previously. The results of the nonoperative patients were not significantly different than the results of those treated operatively. However, the selection criteria for nonoperative treatment called for treating the less severe injuries nonoperatively and may have selected the more favorable patients for nonoperative treatment.

Martin-Herrero et al.[63] presented the results of seven patients with nonoperative treatment of coracoid fractures. In six of the seven cases, there was an ipsilateral clavicle fracture, acromioclavicular dislocation, or extension into the glenoid cavity. All seven patients were considered to have satisfactory shoulder function after treatment.

Author's Preferred Treatment

Isolated fractures of the tip of the coracoid process are treated nonoperatively, almost without regard to displacement. The majority of fractures are minimally displaced. Moreover, even if the fracture heals with a fibrous union, symptoms severe enough to warrant treatment are uncommon. In the occasional circumstance that a symptomatic nonunion exists, it can be managed successfully with excision or open reduction, internal fixation, and bone grafting. In situations in which associated injuries exist (i.e., glenohumeral dislocation or brachial plexus injury), it is important to realize that the prognosis for recovery likely depends more on the associated injuries than on the coracoid fracture (Fig. 18-17).

Fractures of the base of the coracoid (i.e., type I fractures) are managed nonoperatively if there is no glenoid involvement or the associated glenoid fracture is displaced less than 5 mm. Nonoperative treatment may also be indicated in older, sedentary patients, particularly if extensive medical comorbidities exist, regardless of displacement.

Nonoperative treatment consists of a sling for comfort for 7 to 10 days. Pendulum exercises are instituted within the first 2 weeks. Passive elevation and external rotation exercises are added at approximately 3 to 4 weeks. An overhead pulley program is begun at 4 to 6 weeks postinjury. Formal stretching exercises, active range of motion, and strengthening for the rotator cuff, deltoid, and scapular stabilizers are added at the 6- to 8-week mark and progressed over the ensuing 2 to 3 months. Although most fractures are healed within 8 weeks, full recovery requires 6 to 9 months.

Operative stabilization is performed when the fracture involves the glenoid fossa and is displaced 5 mm or more. In addition, if the coracoid is angulated such that the coracohumeral distance is less than 5 mm, surgical reduction and stabilization are considered to prevent coracoid impingement. Coracoid fracture-associated acromioclavicular dislocation is not an indication for surgical management unless the fracture extends into the glenoid fossa. An acute coracoid fracture (i.e., less than 7 days) associated with acromioclavicular dislocation and intra-articular extension is one of the few indications for acromioclavicular fixation.

Under these circumstances, reduction of the acromioclavicular joint reduces the glenoid articular surface. Terminally threaded pins of at least 2 mm in size are passed from the acromion, through the acromioclavicular joint, and into the reduced clavicle. This is performed through an open, superior approach similar to the approach used for acromioclavicular reconstruction. If there is any question of adequate glenoid reduction, a C-arm or diagnostic arthroscopy can be used to confirm this. The pins are removed in 6 to 8 weeks. Restriction from overhead use of the arm is necessary until the pins are removed.

In the absence of other injuries, fractures of the base of the coracoid are fixed through a deltopectoral approach. The deltopectoral interval must be dissected superiorly to the clavicle. In most cases, the fracture can be visualized and the reduction can be attained by incising the rotator interval capsule and retracting the intact subscapularis inferiorly. If greater visualization is required, the subscapularis is detached and reflected medially. Fixation is accomplished using a cannulated, partially threaded screw (Fig. 18-18). Postoperative management is identical to the protocol outlined previously for nonoperative management.

Intra-articular (Glenoid Fossa) Fractures

Ideberg et al.[46,48] devised a classification system that divided scapula fractures with an associated intra-articular glenoid component into five types. This system was modified by Goss with inclusion of six types.[31,32,34] Type I fractures involve the glenoid rim and are subdivided into Ia, (anterior rim) and Ib (posterior rim). Types II to V fractures extend from the glenoid fossa to various exit points along the scapula. Type II fractures exit the lateral border of the scapula, below the infraglenoid tubercle. Type III fractures exit the superior border and typically extend medial to the base of the coracoid. Type IV fractures extend directly across the scapula to the medial border and usually exit superior to the scapular spine. Type V fractures are combinations of types II to IV. Type VI fractures encompass stellate glenoid fractures with extensive intra-articular comminution (Fig. 18-19).[31,32,34,46,48]

Historically, intra-articular glenoid fractures, in the absence of associated glenohumeral instability, have been managed nonoperatively.[10,106] Intact glenohumeral ligaments may act to prevent gross displacement of the fracture. Many authors have reported good early functional results in patients treated nonoperatively with intra-articular glenoid fractures without associated instability.[10,46,90] Surgical intervention was initiated only for glenoid fractures associated with glenohumeral instability.[3,15] These reports were limited because standardized outcome measures were lacking and the incidence of late glenohumeral arthritis was unknown. Surgical treatment of glenoid fractures has received greater attention recently.[4,5,12,31,34,52,55,56,65,73,76,94] Indications for open reduction and internal fixation of intra-

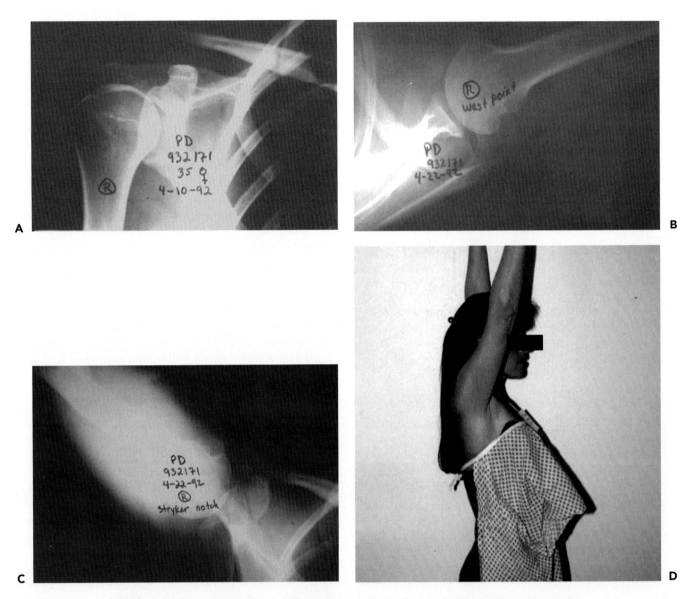

Figure 18-17 Anteroposterior radiograph *(A)* of a 32-year-old skier who fell and sustained an anterior glenohumeral dislocation, suprascapular nerve palsy, acromioclavicular dislocation, and fractures of the base and tip of the coracoid process. The tip of the coracoid process fracture and the Hill-Sachs defect are seen on the West Point lateral view *(B)*. The base of the coracoid process fracture is seen on the Stryker Notch view *(C)*. The patient was treated nonoperatively and achieved a good result *(D)*.

articular glenoid fractures depend on the fragment size, fracture displacement, and stability of glenohumeral joint.[4,5,12,13,15,31,34,46,47,52,55,56,65,73,76,90,92,94]

Type I Fractures

Glenoid rim fractures (type I) are usually sustained during traumatic glenohumeral subluxation or dislocation. In the setting of recurrent anterior instability, Rowe and coworkers[92] recommended excision of an anterior rim fragment of up to 25% of the articular surface with repair of the labrum

and capsule back to the remainder of the glenoid. DePalma[15] believed that glenohumeral instability would result if the fragment is greater than 25% of the anterior rim, greater than 33% of the posterior rim, or displaced more than 10 mm. He recommended immediate open reduction for these situations.[15] More recently, Weishaupt and colleagues[105] advocated craniocaudal length of glenoid rim fragments to predict instability. Specifically, fragments with a craniocaudal length of 1.2 cm or greater were predictive of instability. In addition, Burkhart and colleagues[9] quantitated the amount of glenoid bone loss arthroscopically by

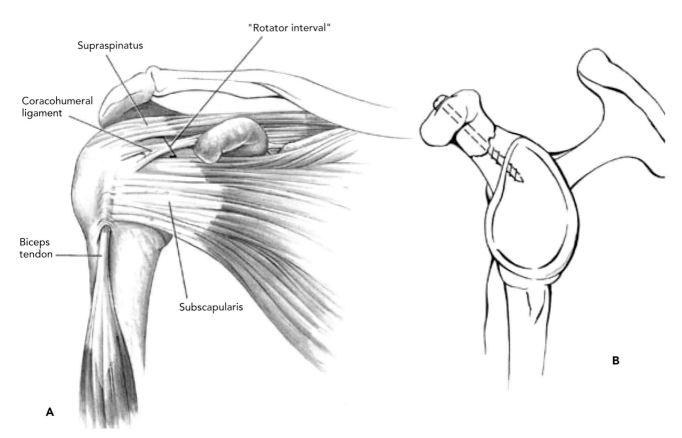

Figure 18-18 When fractures of the base of the coracoid are angulated enough to cause coracoid impingement, they are reduced through a deltopectoral approach by incising the rotator interval and retracting the subscapularis inferiorly (A). Fixation may be obtained with an interfragmentary screw (B). (Reprinted with permission from Goss TP. Fractures of the scapula: diagnosis and treatment. In: Williams GR Jr., ed. Disorders of the shoulder: diagnosis and management. Philadelphia, PA, Lippincott Williams & Wilkins, 1999:597.)

measuring the distance from the glenoid bare spot to the remaining glenoid edge. Although debate exists regarding the amount of displacement and fragment size that are acceptable, the concept of open reduction and internal fixation of glenoid rim fractures associated with persistent or recurrent instability is established.[3,10,15,40,47,76,94]

Fixation methods for glenoid rim fractures depend on the size of the fragment and degree of comminution. Screw fixation can be used for large, minimally comminuted fragments. Glenoid rim fragments that are too small or too comminuted to accommodate a screw can be reduced and stabilized with suture anchors in the glenoid and sutures passed through the fragment. Alternatively, if the rim fracture is so comminuted that it cannot be repaired, the fragment can be excised and reconstructed with a tricortical graft from the iliac crest.[31] Arthroscopic-assisted reduction and percutaneous fixation of a displaced intra-articular glenoid fracture have also been reported.[12,13] Careful monitoring of fluid extravasation is recommended. The results of operative fixation of glenoid rim fractures, regardless of fixation method, have been good.[3,4,7,10,12,13,76,94]

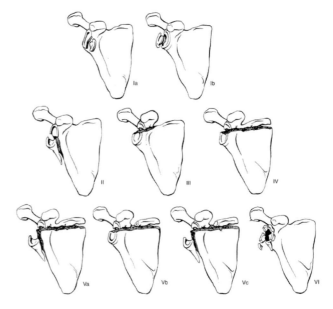

Figure 18-19 Classification of glenoid fossa fractures. (Reprinted with permission from Goss TP. Fractures of the scapula: diagnosis and treatment. In: Williams GR Jr., ed. Disorders of the shoulder: diagnosis and management. Philadelphia, PA, Lippincott Williams & Wilkins, 1999:597.)

Author's Preferred Treatment

Anterior glenoid fractures (type IA) associated with significant displacement (5 mm) or static subluxation are best treated acutely with surgical repair. This is true regardless of fragment size. However, small fragments (less than 5 mm) are not likely to be displaced or associated with static subluxation. If the fragment is of good quality and large enough to accept a small fragment screw, open reduction and internal fixation through an anterior deltopectoral approach are performed. The upper two-thirds of the subscapularis tendon is divided and reflected medially. The joint is entered through a laterally based capsulotomy. The fragment is reduced and held provisionally with a temporary wire, and a standard 3.5-mm cortical or partly threaded cancellous screw is used for definitive fixation. If a cortical screw is used, the anterior rim fragment should be "overdrilled" to allow compression. Alternatively, a cannulated screw can be used. Smaller or comminuted fractures may be fixed with suture anchors placed in the glenoid and sutures passed through the fragment (Fig. 18-20). Rarely is the fragment excised. Even very small fragments are left within the capsulolabral sleeve when it is reattached. The same is true of larger, comminuted fragments.

Pendulum exercises are begun immediately postoperatively. At 2 to 3 weeks postoperatively, the patient is encouraged to use the arm for everyday living activities, and gentle passive flexion and external rotation exercises are begun. At 6 to 8 weeks, stretching and strengthening exercises for the deltoid, rotator cuff, and scapular stabilizers are instituted. The fracture is usually healed by 10 weeks, but full recovery may require 6 to 9 months.

Posterior glenoid fractures (type IB) with significant displacement (5 mm) or posterior glenohumeral instability require acute operative intervention through a posterior approach with the patient in the lateral decubitus position. As in type IA fractures, this is true regardless of fragment size, with the proviso that small fragments (5 mm or less) are not likely to be displaced or associated with static subluxation. A deltoid-splitting approach is usually adequate. If the fragment is not too large, this may be combined with a muscle-splitting, internervous approach between the infraspinatus and teres minor or an infraspinatus-splitting approach. The more distal interval (i.e., between infraspinatus and teres minor) is preferred because it is extensile, allowing reflection of the infraspinatus and elevation of the dorsal portion of the teres minor origin, if necessary for adequate exposure. If the fragment comprises 25% or more of the articular surface, it is reduced and stabilized with a screw (Fig. 18-21). Smaller fragments or comminuted fragments are fixed by placing suture anchors within the remaining glenoid and passing the sutures through the fragment.

Postoperatively, an orthosis is used to maintain the arm in neutral or external rotation for 6 weeks. The brace is removed for pendulum exercises beginning 2 to 3 weeks postoperatively. Passive elevation is added at 4 to 6 weeks, depending on the degree of stiffness observed on examination. An overhead pulley program as well as stretching and strengthening exercises for the rotator cuff, deltoid, and scapular stabilizers are added at 6 weeks and progressed according to the patient's symptoms. Full recovery requires 6 to 9 months.

Types II to V Fractures

For types II to V glenoid fossa fractures, the amount of articular displacement and the degree of comminution determine the need for open reduction and internal fixation. Goss[34] recommended open reduction and internal fixation for an articular step-off of 5 mm or more. Kavanagh et al.[52] described successful surgical treatment of displaced (4–8 mm) intra-articular fractures of the glenoid fossa. They emphasized that uncertainty still remained with regard to the amount of glenoid articular incongruity that could be accepted without risking long-term pain, stiffness, and post-traumatic degenerative arthritis. Poppen and Walker[84] demonstrated that transarticular forces of 0.9 times body weight can be generated at the glenohumeral joint by lifting a 5-kg mass to shoulder height with the elbow extended. This suggests that disruption of articular congruence probably leads to unacceptable joint contact stress. Soslowsky and coauthors[100] demonstrated that the maximum thickness of glenoid articular cartilage is 5 mm. On the basis of this information, articular displacement of 5 mm or more has been adopted by many surgeons as the indication for reduction and stabilization.[3,5,52,56]

The results of operative fixation of displaced glenoid fossa fractures have been less predictable than those of extra-articular fractures. Bauer et al.[5] reported greater than 70% good or very good functional results for patients treated surgically for grossly displaced fractures of the glenoid rim, neck, fossa, and acromion. Leung and Lam[56] reported 9 excellent and 5 good results in 14 patients treated surgically for displaced intra-articular glenoid fractures. Mayo et al.[65] reviewed 27 displaced glenoid fossa fractures treated with open reduction and internal fixation at 43 months follow-up and found that 82% of patients had good or excellent results. Three patients had articular incongruities measuring 2 mm or less. Despite these variable results, it is likely that an anatomically reduced glenoid articular surface is preferable to residual displacement. Therefore, operative treatment of displaced glenoid fossa fractures will probably continue to gain in popularity.

Author's Preferred Treatment

Glenoid fossa fractures with less than 5 mm of displacement that are not associated with static subluxation or

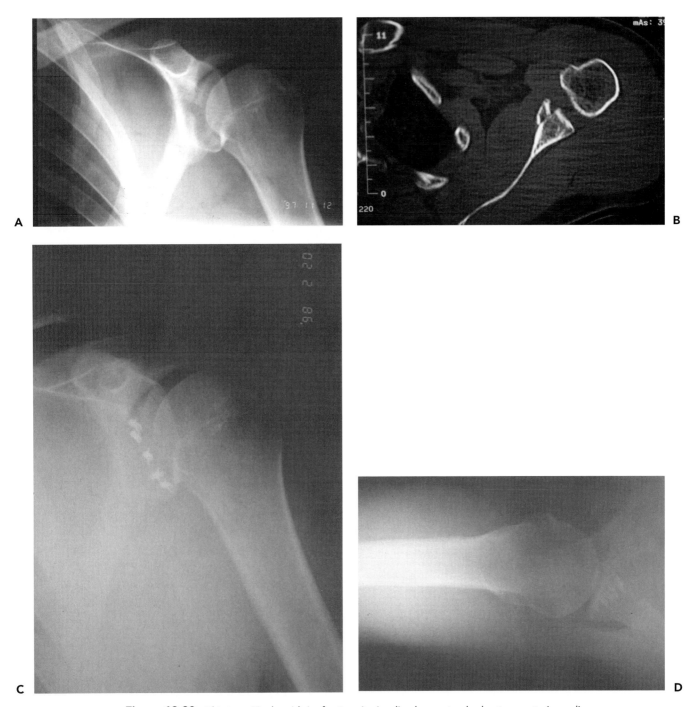

Figure 18-20 This type IA glenoid rim fracture is visualized on a standard anteroposterior radiograph *(A)*. Fragment size and displacement are accurately quantified on an axial CT image *(B)*. The fracture was fixed through an anterior deltopectoral approach with suture anchors *(C and D)*.

dislocation are treated symptomatically, with a sling for comfort, until pain permits range of motion exercises (7–10 days). Pendulum exercises are instituted within the first 2 postinjury weeks. Passive flexion and external rotation with the arm at the side are added at 2 to 3 weeks postinjury. An overhead pulley program is begun at 4 to 6 weeks. Passive stretching, active range of motion, and strengthening exercises for the deltoid, rotator cuff, and

scapular stabilizers are added at 6 to 8 weeks. The fracture is typically healed in 6 to 8 weeks, but complete rehabilitation often requires 9 to 12 months. This treatment may also be used for older, sedentary patients, even if the displacement criteria for open reduction and internal fixation are met.

Types II to V glenoid fossa fractures with 5 mm or greater of displacement are treated surgically. The approach de-

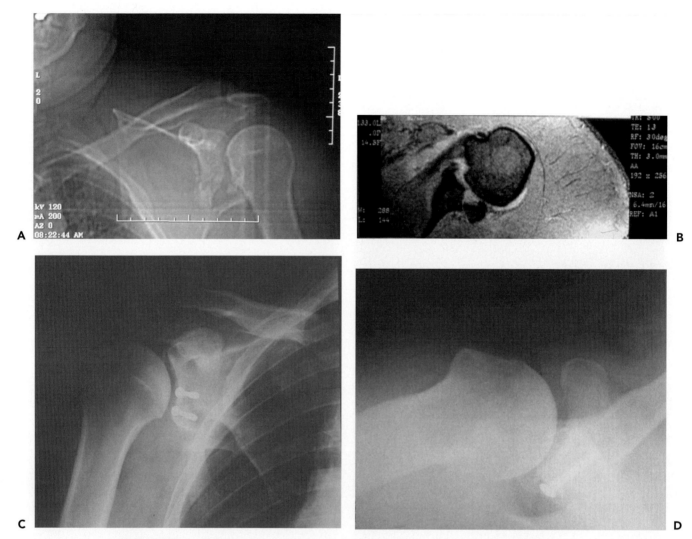

Figure 18-21 Comminuted fracture of the posterior glenoid rim (type IB) that extends into the lateral margin of the scapula (A). It is associated with posterior glenohumeral subluxation (B). The fragment was fixed through a posterior approach that preserved the deltoid origin, exploited the internervous plane between infraspinatus and teres minor, and preserved the infraspinatus insertion (C and D).

pends on whether extensile exposure of the lateral angle of the scapula is required. Extensile exposure of the anterior aspect of the lateral scapular border is limited because of the axillary nerve. The posterior approach is the most utilitarian approach and is used for most type II, IV, and V fractures. An extensile exposure may be obtained by reflecting the posterior deltoid origin from its attachment on the scapular spine. Displaced type III glenoid fossa fractures usually do not require exposure of the lateral scapular border and can frequently be stabilized through an anterior deltopectoral approach. If the posterior cortex is comminuted, a posterior deltoid-splitting approach may be used instead of or in addition to an anterior approach.

Glenoid fossa fractures that exit inferior to the glenoid, along the lateral scapular border (type II fractures), are usually most easily approached through a posterior axillary in-

cision with the patient in the lateral decubitus position. This is because the fracture line is usually slightly oblique from anterior-inferior to posterior-superior, creating a fragment that has a large posterior surface. The incision begins approximately 5 to 6 cm medial to the posterolateral acromial corner and extends laterally along the scapular spine for a short distance (2–3 cm) before curving inferiorly to the posterior axillary border. This incision and approach are similar to the upper two-thirds of the incision and approach used for complex glenoid fractures described in Figure 18-22. If additional exposure of the lateral scapular margin is required, the inferior extent of the incision can be extended inferiorly and medially, as described in Figure 18-22. The posterior border of the deltoid is identified, and its fascia is incised proximally to the scapular spine and distally toward the deltoid insertion. The deltoid is then re-

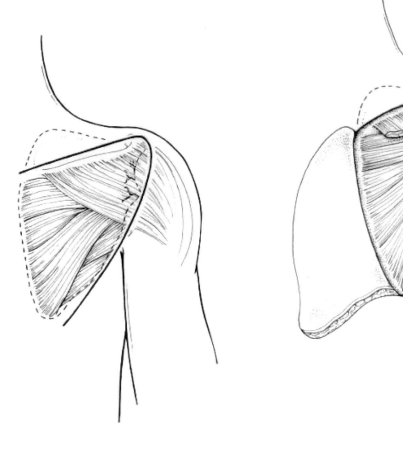

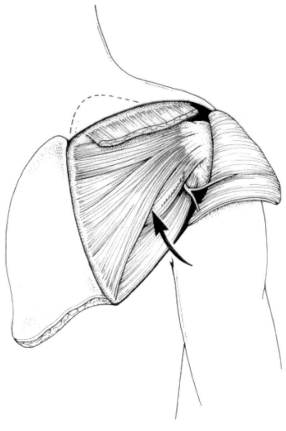

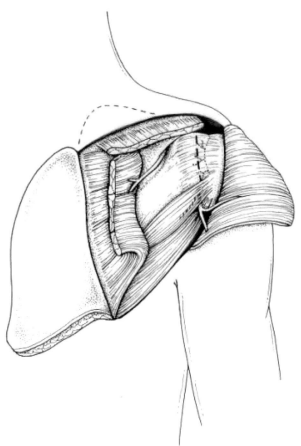

A

B

C

Figure 18-22 An extensile posterior exposure is used for type V glenoid fossa fractures. The skin incision starts at the base of the scapular spine and extends laterally. It then curves inferiorly and me-dially to follow the lateral scapular border *(A)*. The deltoid is released for its origin and retracted laterally to expose the posterior aspect of the scapula. The internervous plane between infraspinatus and teres minor is identified and dissected *(B)*. The infraspinatus is reflected medially, taking care to protect the suprascapular nerve, and the joint is opened to expose the articular surface *(C)*. *(continued)*

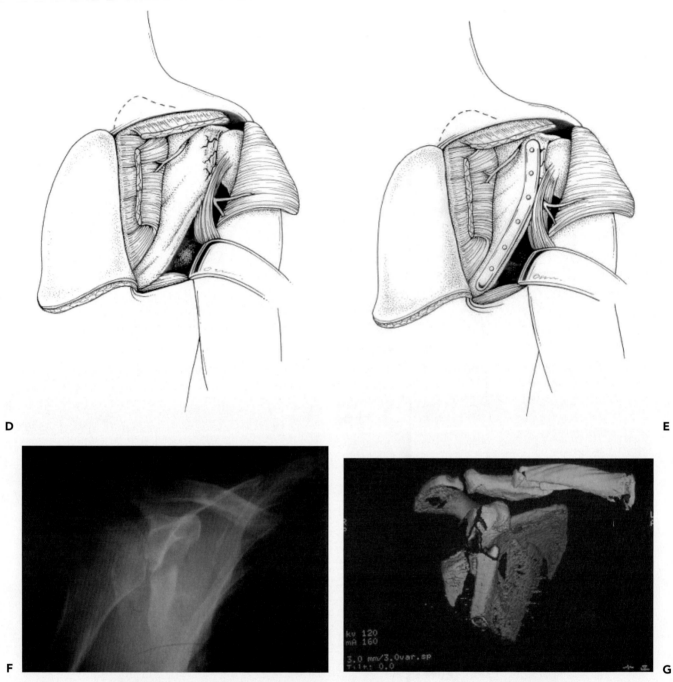

Figure 18-22 *(continued)* The dorsal origins of the teres minor and major are reflected off the lateral scapular border *(D)*. A contoured plate is applied to the reduced fracture *(E)*. Preoperative anteroposterior radiograph and three-dimensional reconstructed CT scan of a type V glenoid fossa fracture with ipsilateral clavicle fracture *(F and G)*. *(continued)*

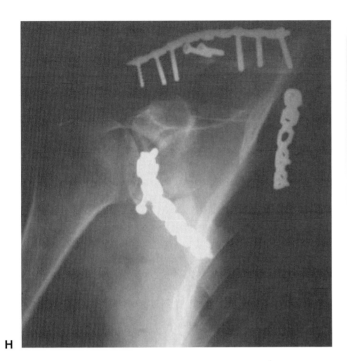

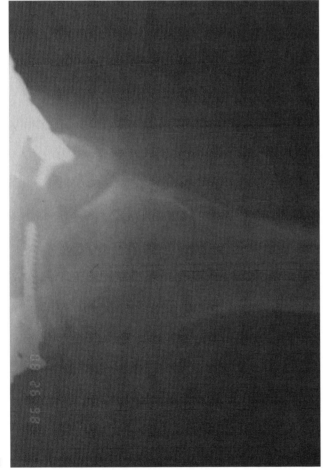

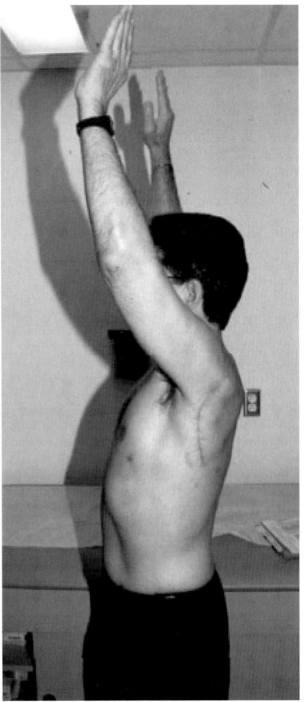

Figure 18-22 *(continued)* Postoperative anteroposterior and axillary lateral radiographs revealing anatomic reduction and medial and lateral plate fixation. The clavicle has also been fixed *(H* and *I)*. The clinical result is good *(J)*.

tracted superolaterally. If this does not provide adequate exposure, a portion of the posterior deltoid can be released from the scapular spine.

The internervous plane between the infraspinatus and teres minor muscles is identified and incised distally to the humerus. The procedure can often be performed without detaching the infraspinatus from the humerus. This requires that any capsular attachments to the teres minor and infraspinatus be released and that the dorsal portions of the teres minor and teres major origins be released from the lateral scapular margin. The joint is entered through a longitudinal capsulotomy, similar to the method described in Figures 18-13 and 18-22, except that it is made in line with and continuous with the posterior glenoid fracture. This requires that the incision go through the labrum. The fracture can then be displaced inferiorly and laterally to expose the joint and fracture surfaces.

The fracture is then reduced and fixed provisionally using two guide wires for partially threaded, cancellous cannulated screws. Using traction can aid reduction and visualization of the articular surface. Traction can be accomplished by using an arthroscopy traction setup or a fracture traction device, as discussed previously in the section on surgical neck fractures. The long head of the triceps forms a very broad attachment on the inferior glenoid fragment. The most dorsal attachment of this tendon is released from the fragment to create a surface for hardware placement. Paralysis is required to minimize the effect of the triceps on the inferior glenoid fragment during reduction. The course of the axillary nerve and posterior humeral circumflex vessels lateral and the circumflex scapular artery medial to the triceps origin should be remembered when placing the guide wires and screws. It is also important to realize that the screws must travel in a posteroinferior to an anterosuperior direction to cross the fracture site. An intraoperative c-arm may be used to confirm the reduction and screw placement. If fixation is inadequate, a plate can be placed along the lateral scapular border onto the inferior glenoid fragment. The capsulotomy is repaired; the infraspinatus, teres minor, teres major, and deltoid muscles are allowed to fall back to their normal anatomic positions; and the skin is closed routinely.

Postoperatively, an orthosis that maintains the arm in approximately 20 to 30 degrees of abduction and 0 to 20 degrees of external rotation is worn to protect the posterior deltoid origin (if it was detached and repaired), the infraspinatus insertion (if it was detached and repaired), and the teres minor and major origins. The brace is worn for 3 to 6 weeks and, within the first two postoperative weeks, is only removed to perform pendulum exercises. Passive flexion and external rotation exercises with the arm at the side are begun 3 to 4 weeks postoperatively. An overhead pulley program is instituted at 4 to 5 weeks postoperatively. Passive stretches, active range of motion, and strengthening ex-

ercises for the deltoid, rotator cuff, and scapular stabilizers are added at 6 to 8 weeks postoperatively. Full recovery requires 9 to 12 months.

Type III fractures often exhibit severe intra-articular displacement. This is likely to be secondary to the pull of the conjoined tendon of the short head of the biceps and coracobrachialis. Operative reduction is reserved for fractures in which the intra-articular displacement is 5 mm or more. Although the posterior approach is the "workhorse" for most glenoid fossa fractures that do not involve the anterior glenoid rim, the scapular spine impedes access to type III fractures, which usually do not extend below the equator of the glenoid. Therefore, the preferred approach is an anterior, deltopectoral approach. The upper two-thirds of the subscapularis tendon is incised, and the muscle is reflected medially. The joint is opened through a laterally based capsulotomy. Complete paralysis is helpful in negating the influence of the conjoined tendon on fracture reduction. A guide wire for a cannulated screw is passed percutaneously through the interval between the posterior border of the acromioclavicular joint and the anterior border of the scapular spine (i.e., Neviaser's portal) and into the superior fragment. The fragment is then reduced under direct visualization, and the guide wire is passed into the intact inferior glenoid. The guide wire can be used to help manipulate the superior fragment. A c-arm is recommended to help estimate appropriate position of the guide wire in the inferior glenoid and subsequent cannulated screw length. If additional rotational control is required, a plate can be placed on the anterior glenoid (Fig. 18-23). Postoperative rehabilitation follows the protocol outlined previously for type 2 fractures.

Type IV fractures are often not significantly displaced and are amenable to nonoperative management. However, when they are displaced (5 mm), a posterior approach with the patient in the lateral decubitus position is indicated. The skin incision is as described previously for type II fractures. Most often, a portion of the posterior deltoid is released, and the infraspinatus is reflected to gain adequate exposure. Once the fracture is reduced, a guide wire placed percutaneously through the region of Neviaser's portal can be passed through the superior fragment, across the fracture, and into the inferior fragment. Additional rotational control can be obtained through the use of a plate along the medial border of the scapula. This can be exposed adequately through the same skin incision by retracting the lateral border of the middle and inferior trapezius superomedially. A small portion of the trapezial attachment at the base of the scapular spine may need to be released. The medial scapular border is then exposed by elevating the dorsal insertions of the rhomboid major and minor. Postoperative management is as described previously for type II injuries.

Type V fractures are treated operatively if the degree of comminution is minor and will allow stable fixation. The

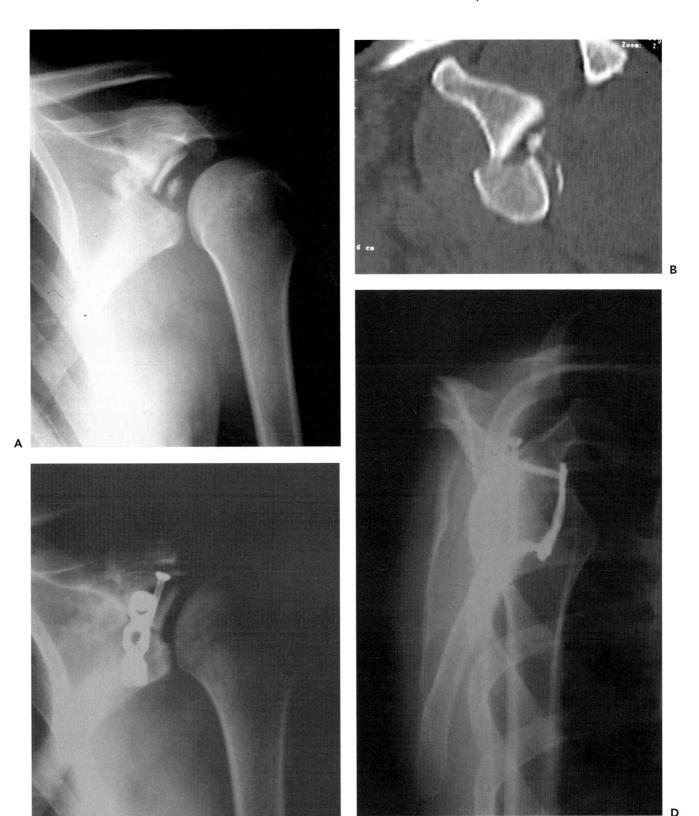

Figure 18-23 Anteroposterior radiograph (A) and CT scan (B) of a displaced type III glenoid fossa fracture. Note the small free fragment. This fracture was fixed through an anterior deltopectoral approach with an interfragmentary screw and anterior plate (C and D). (continued)

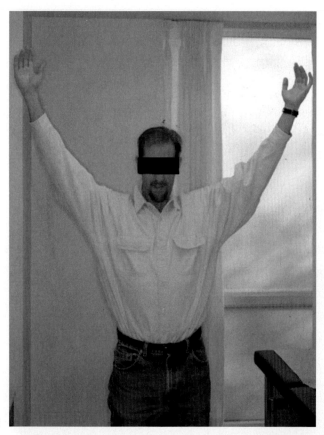

E

Figure 18-23 *(continued)* The clinical result was good *(E)*.

approach is an extensile posterior exposure in the lateral decubitus position, with reflection of the posterior deltoid origin, infraspinatus insertion, and dorsal teres minor and major origins, as described previously. Fixation is obtained through a combination of interfragmentary screws and plates (Fig. 18-22). If comminution is too severe to permit fixation of all fragments, then limited reduction and stabilization of the articular segment are performed if possible. If fracture comminution prevents even limited fixation, nonoperative management is used.

For type VI fractures, the degree of comminution dictates the method of treatment. Typically, the comminution associated with type VI fractures is too severe to allow internal fixation except in rare instances when limited fixation of larger fragments can be accomplished. To maximize functional results after operative intervention, fixation must be rigid enough to allow for early passive mobilization. Severe comminution that prevents stable fixation is best managed nonoperatively with early motion. Type VI fractures, in which the humeral head is well centered, are managed nonoperatively.

CONCLUSION

Scapular fractures often occur as the result of severe trauma and have a high incidence of associated injuries. Extra-artic-ular fractures involving the scapular body, coracoid process, acromion process, and glenoid or scapular neck are often managed nonoperatively. Operative treatment is reserved for glenoid neck fractures with displacement greater than 2 cm, coracoid fractures with intra-articular extension and displacement greater than 5 mm, acromion fractures with poor fragment apposition and subacromial space encroachment, and glenoid fossa fractures associated with instability or residual displacement of 5 mm or greater. Nonoperative treatment may be indicated in patients with enough displacement to justify operative treatment if those patients are older and sedentary, their fractures are excessively comminuted, or they have extensive medical comorbidities.

REFERENCES

1. Ada JR, Miller ME. Scapular fractures. Analysis of 113 cases. Clin Orthop 1991(269):174.
2. Armstrong C, Spuy JVD. The fractured scapula: importance and management based on a series of 62 patients. Injury 1984;15:324.
3. Aston JWJ, Gregory CF. Dislocation of the shoulder with significant fracture of the glenoid. J Bone Joint Surg 1973;55A:1531.
4. Aulicino PL, Reinert C, Kornberg M, et al. Displaced intra-articular glenoid fractures treated by open reduction and internal fixation. J Trauma 1986;26(12):1137.
5. Bauer G, Fleischmann W, Dussler E. Displaced scapular fractures: indication and long-term results of open reduction and internal fixation. Arch Orthop Trauma Surg 1995;114(4):215.
6. Benchetrit E, Friedman B. Fracture of the coracoid process associated with subglenoid dislocation of the shoulder. A case report. J Bone Joint Surg Am 1979;61(2):295.
7. Bigliani LU, Newton PM, Steinmann SP, et al. Glenoid rim lesions associated with recurrent anterior dislocation of the shoulder. Am J Sports Med 1998;26(1):41.
8. Boyer DW Jr. Trapshooter's shoulder: stress fracture of the coracoid process. Case report. J Bone Joint Surg Am 1975;57(6):862.
9. Burkhart SS, DeBeer JF, Tehrany AM, et al. Quantifying glenoid bone loss arthroscopically in shoulder instability. Arthroscopy 2002;18(5):488.
10. Butters KP. The scapula. In: Matsen FA, ed. The shoulder. Philadelphia, PA, WB Saunders Company, 1990:335.
11. Cain TE, Hamilton WP. Scapular fractures in professional football players. Am J Sports Med 1992;20(3):363.
12. Cameron SE. Arthroscopic reduction and internal fixation of an anterior glenoid fracture. Arthroscopy 1998;14(7):743.
13. Carro LP, Nunez MP, Llata JI. Arthroscopic-assisted reduction and percutaneous external fixation of a displaced intra-articular glenoid fracture. Arthroscopy 1999;15(2):211.
14. Cottias P, le Bellec Y, Jeanrot C, et al. Fractured coracoid with anterior shoulder dislocation and greater tuberosity fracture—report of a bilateral case. Acta Orthop Scand 2000;71(1):95.
15. DePalma AF. Surgery of the shoulder. 3rd ed. In: J. Lippincott, ed. Surgery of the shoulder. Philadelphia, PA, Lippincott Williams & Wilkins, 1983:366.
16. Ebraheim NA, An HS, Jackson WT, et al. Scapulothoracic dissociation. J Bone Joint Surg Am 1988;70(3):428.
17. Ebraheim NA, Pearlstein SR, Savolaine ER, et al. Scapulothoracic dissociation (closed avulsion of the scapula, subclavian artery, and brachial plexus): a newly recognized variant, a new classification, and a review of the literature and treatment options. J Orthop Trauma 1987;1(1):18.
18. Edeland HG, Zachrisson BE. Fracture of the scapular notch associated with lesion of the suprascapular nerve. Acta Orthop Scand 1975;46(5):758.
19. Edwards SG, Whittle AP, Wood GW 2nd. Nonoperative treatment of ipsilateral fractures of the scapula and clavicle. J Bone Joint Surg Am 2000;82(6):774.

20. Egol KA, Connor PM, Karunakar MA, et al. The floating shoulder: clinical and functional results. J Bone Joint Surg Am 2001;83-A(8):1188.
21. Eyres KS, Brooks A, Stanley D. Fractures of the coracoid process. J Bone Joint Surg Br 1995;77(3):425.
22. Ferraz IC, Papadimitriou NG, Sotereanos DG. Scapular body nonunion: a case report. J Shoulder Elbow Surg 2002;11(1):98.
23. Findlay R. Fractures of the scapula. Ann Surg 1931;93:1001.
24. Findlay R. Fractures of the scapula and ribs. Am J Surg 1937;38:489.
25. Gagey O, Curey JP, Mazas F. [Recent fractures of the scapula. Apropos of 43 cases]. Rev Chir Orthop Reparatrice Appar Mot 1984;70(6):443.
26. Ganz R, Noesberger B. [Treatment of scapular fractures]. Hefte Unfallheilkd 1975;(126):59.
27. Garcia-Elias M, Salo JM. Non-union of a fractured coracoid process after dislocation of the shoulder. A case report. J Bone Joint Surg Br 1985;67(5):722.
28. Garth WP, Slappey CE, Ochs CW. Roentgenographic demonstration of instability of the shoulder: the apical oblique projection. J Bone Joint Surg 1984;66A(9):1450.
29. Gil JF, Haydar A. Isolated injury of the coracoid process: case report. J Trauma 1991;31(12):1696.
30. Gorczyca JT, Davis RT, Hartford JM, et al. Open reduction internal fixation after displacement of a previously nondisplaced acromial fracture in a multiply injured patient: case report and review of literature. J Orthop Trauma 2001;15(5):369.
31. Goss TP. Fractures of the glenoid cavity. J Bone Joint Surg 1992;74A:299.
32. Goss TP. Double disruptions of the superior shoulder suspensory complex. J Orthop Trauma 1993;7:99.
33. Goss TP. Fractures of the glenoid neck. J Shoulder Elbow Surg 1994;3:42.
34. Goss TP. Scapular fractures and dislocations: diagnosis and treatment. J Am Acad Orthop Surg 1995;3(1):22.
35. Goss TP. The scapula: coracoid, acromial, and avulsion fractures. Am J Orthop 1996;25(2):106.
36. Goss TP. Fractures of the coracoid process. J Bone Joint Surg Br 1997;79(4):694.
37. Goss TP. Fractures of the scapula: diagnosis and treatment. In: Williams GR Jr., ed. Disorders of the shoulder: diagnosis and management. Philadelphia, PA, Lippincott Williams & Wilkins, 1999:597.
38. Gupta R, Sher J, Williams GR, et al. Non-union of the scapular body. A case report. J Bone Joint Surg Am 1998;80(3):428.
39. Hall RJ, Calvert PT. Stress fracture of the acromion: an unusual mechanism and review of the literature. J Bone Joint Surg Br 1995;77(1):153.
40. Hardegger FH, Simpson LA, and Weber BG. The operative treatment of scapular fractures. J Bone Joint Surg Br 1984;66(5):725.
41. Herscovici D Jr., Fiennes AG, Allgower M, et al. Ipsilateral clavicle and scapular neck fractures. J Bone Joint Surg Br 1992;6:499.
42. Herscovici D Jr., Fiennes AG, Allgower M, et al. The floating shoulder: ipsilateral clavicle and scapular neck fractures. J Bone Joint Surg Br 1992;74(3):362.
43. Heyse-Moore GH, Stoker DJ. Avulsion fractures of the scapula. Skeletal Radiol 1982;9(1):27.
44. Hitzrot J, Bolling R. Fractures of the neck of the scapula. Ann Surg 1916;63:215.
45. Hollinshead R, James KW. Scapulothoracic dislocation (locked scapula). A case report. J Bone Joint Surg Am 1979;61(7):1102.
46. Ideberg R. Fractures of the scapula involving the glenoid fossa. In: Welsh R, ed. Surgery of the shoulder. Philadelphia, PA, B.C. Decker, 1984:63.
47. Ideberg R. Unusual glenoid fractures: a report on 92 cases. Acta Orthop Scand 1987;58:191.
48. Ideberg R, Grevsten S, Larsson S. Epidemiology of scapular fractures. Incidence and classification of 338 fractures. Acta Orthop Scand 1995;66(5):395.
49. Imatani RJ. Fractures of the scapula: a review of 53 fractures. J Trauma 1975;15(6):473.
50. Ishizuki M, Yamaura I, Isobe Y, et al. Avulsion fracture of the superior border of the scapula. Report of five cases. J Bone Joint Surg Am 1981;63(5):820.
51. Kaminsky SB, Pierce VD. Nonunion of a scapula body fracture in a high school football player. Am J Orthop 2002;31(8):456.
52. Kavanagh BF, Bradway JK, Cofield RF. Open reduction and internal fixation of displaced intra-articular fractures of the glenoid fossa. J Bone Joint Surg 1993;75A:479.
53. Kelly J. Fractures complicating electroconvulsive therapy in chronic epilepsy. J Bone Joint Surg 1954;36B:70.
54. Kuhn JE, Blasier RB, Carpenter JE. Fractures of the acromion process: a proposed classification system. J Orthop Trauma 1994;8(1):6.
55. Lee SJ, Meinhard BP, Schultz E, et al. Open reduction and internal fixation of a glenoid fossa fracture in a child: a case report and review of the literature. J Orthop Trauma 1997;11(6):452.
56. Leung KS, Lam TP. Open reduction and internal fixation of ipsilateral fractures of the scapular neck and clavicle. J Bone Joint Surg Am 1993;75(7):1015.
57. Liberson F. Os acromiale—a contested anomaly. J Bone Joint Surg Am 1937;19:683.
58. Lim KE, Wang CR, Chin KC, et al. Concomitant fracture of the coracoid and acromion after direct shoulder trauma. J Orthop Trauma 1996;10(6):437.
59. Lindholm A, Leven H. Prognosis in fractures of the body and neck of the scapula. A follow-up study. Acta Chir Scand 1974;140(1):33.
60. Magerl F. [Osteosyntheses in the shoulder region. Pretubercular humeral fractures, scapular neck fractures]. Helv Chir Acta 1974;41(1-2):225.
61. Marr DC, Misamore GW. Acromion nonunion after anterior acromioplasty: a case report. J Shoulder Elbow Surg 1992;1:317.
62. Martin SD, Weiland AJ. Missed scapular fracture after trauma. A case report and a 23-year follow-up report. Clin Orthop 1994;(299):259.
63. Martin-Herrero T, Rodriguez-Merchan C, Munuera-Martinez L. Fractures of the coracoid process: presentation of seven cases and review of the literature. J Trauma 1990;30(12):1597.
64. Mathews RE, Cocke TB, D'Ambrosia RD. Scapular fractures secondary to seizures in patients with osteodystrophy. Report of two cases and review of the literature. J Bone Joint Surg Am 1983;65(6):850.
65. Mayo KA, Benirschke SK, Mast JW. Displaced fractures of the glenoid fossa. Results of open reduction and internal fixation. Clin Orthop 1998;(347):122.
66. McAdams TR, Blevins FT, Martin TP, et al. The role of plain films and computed tomography in the evaluation of scapular neck fractures. J Orthop Trauma 2002;16(1):7.
67. McClure JG, Raney RB. Anomalies of the scapula. Clin Orthop 1975;(110):22.
68. McGahan JP, Rab GT. Fracture of the acromion associated with an axillary nerve deficit: a case report and review of the literature. Clin Orthop 1980;(147):216.
69. McGahan JP, Rab GT, Dublin A. Fractures of the scapula. J Trauma 1980;20(10):880.
70. McLennan JG, Ungersma J. Pneumothorax complicating fracture of the scapula. J Bone Joint Surg Am 1982;64(4):598.
71. Neer CS II. Shoulder reconstruction. Philadelphia, PA, WB Saunders Company, 1990:416.
72. Neer CS II, Poppen NK. Supraspinatus outlet. Orthop Trans 1987;11:234.
73. Neviaser J. Traumatic lesions: injuries in and about the shoulder joint. Instru Course Lect 1956;13:187.
74. Neviaser R. Long-term follow-up of operatively treated intra-articular glenoid fractures. Presented at the 7th ICSS. Sydney, Australia, 1998.
75. Newell E. Review of over two thousand fractures in the past seven years. South Med J 1927;20:644.
76. Niggebrugge AH, van Heusden HA, Bode PJ, et al. Dislocated intra-articular fracture of anterior rim of glenoid treated by open reduction and internal fixation. Injury 1993;24(2):130.
77. Nordqvist A, Petersson C. Fracture of the body, neck, or spine of the scapula: a long-term follow-up study. Clin Orthop 1992;283:139.
78. Norris T. Unfused epiphysis mistaken for acromion fracture. Orthop Today 1983;3(10):12.
79. Ogawa K, Naniwa T. Fractures of the acromion and the lateral scapular spine. J Shoulder Elbow Surg 1997;6(6):544.

80. Ogawa K, Toyama Y, Ishige S, et al. [Fracture of the coracoid process: its classification and pathomechanism]. Nippon Seikeigeka Gakkai Zasshi 1990;64(10):909.

81. Ogawa K, Yoshida A, Takahashi M, et al. Fractures of the coracoid process. J Bone Joint Surg Br 1997;79(1):17.

82. Ogden JA, Phillips SB. Radiology of postnatal skeletal development. VII. The scapula. Skeletal Radiol 1983;9(3):157.

83. Oreck SL, Burgess A, Levine AM. Traumatic lateral displacement of the scapula: a radiographic sign of neurovascular disruption. J Bone Joint Surg 1984;66A(5):758.

84. Poppen NK, Walker PS. Forces at the glenohumeral joint in abduction. Clin Orthop 1978;135:165.

85. Ramos L, Mencia R, Alonso A, et al. Conservative treatment of ipsilateral fractures of the scapula and clavicle. J Trauma 1997;42(2):239.

86. Ramsey M, Williams G, Iannotti JP, et al. Ipsilateral glenoid neck and clavicle fracture, a clinical investigation. Presented at the American Academy of Orthopaedic Surgeons Annual Meeting. Anaheim, CA, 1999.

87. Rikli D, Regazzoni P, Renner N. The unstable shoulder girdle: early functional treatment utilizing open reduction and internal fixation. J Orthop Trauma 1995;9(2):93.

88. Rokous JR, Feagin JA, Abbott HG. Modified axillary roentgenogram. A useful adjunct in the diagnosis of recurrent instability of the shoulder. Clin Orthop 1972;82:84.

89. Romero J, Schai P, Imhoff AB. Scapular neck fracture—the influence of permanent malalignment of the glenoid neck on clinical outcome. Arch Orthop Trauma Surg 2001;121(6):313.

90. Rowe C. Fractures of the scapula. Surg Clin North Am 1963;43:1565.

91. Rowe CR. The shoulder. New York, NY, Churchill Livingstone, 1987;73.

92. Rowe CR, Patel D, Southmayd WW. The Bankart procedure: a long-term end-result study. J Bone Joint Surg Am 1978;60A(1):1.

93. Sandrock AR. Another sports fatigue fracture. Stress fracture of the coracoid process of the scapula. Radiology 1975;117(2):274.

94. Sinha J, Miller AJ. Fixation of fractures of the glenoid rim. Injury 1992;23(6):418.

95. Solheim LF, Roaas A. Compression of the suprascapular nerve after fracture of the scapular notch. Acta Orthop Scand 1978; 49(4):338.

96. Tachdjian M. Pediatric orthopaedics. Philadelphia, PA, WB Saunders, 1972:1553.

97. Tarquinio T, Weinstein ME, Virgilio RW. Bilateral scapular fractures from accidental electric shock. J Trauma 1979;19(2):132.

98. Thompson DA, Flynn TC, Miller PW, et al. The significance of scapular fractures. J Trauma 1985;25(10):974.

99. Tscherne H, Christ M. [Conservative and surgical therapy of shoulderblade fractures]. Hefte Unfallheilkd 1975;(126):52.

100. Soslowsky LJ, Flatow EL, Bigliani LU, et al. Articular geometry of the glenohumeral joint. Clin Orthop 1992;285:181.

101. van Noort A, te Slaa RL, Manti RK, et al. The floating shoulder. A multicentre study. J Bone Joint Surg Br 2001;83(6):795.

102. Veluvolu P, Kohn HS, Guten GN, et al. Unusual stress fracture of the scapula in a jogger. Clin Nucl Med 1988;13(7):531.

103. Ward WG, Bergfeld JA, Carson WG Jr., Stress fracture of the base of the acromial process. Am J Sports Med 1994;22(1):146.

104. Warner JP, Port J. Stress fracture of the acromion. J Shoulder Elbow Surg 1994;3:262.

105. Weishaupt D, Zanetti M, Nyffeler RW, et al. Posterior glenoid rim deficiency in recurrent (atraumatic) posterior shoulder instability. Skeletal Radiol 2000;29(4):204.

106. Wilbur M, Evans E. Fractures of the scapula: an analysis of forty cases and a review of the literature. J Bone Joint Surg 1977; 59A:358.

107. Williams GR Jr., Naranja J, Klimkiewicz J, et al. The floating shoulder: a biomechanical basis for classification and management. J Bone Joint Surg Am 2001;83-A(8):1182.

108. Wolf AW, Shoji H, Chuinard RG. Unusual fracture of the coracoid process. A case report and review of the literature. J Bone Joint Surg Am 1976;58(3):423.

109. Wong-Pack WK, Bobechko PE, Becker EJ. Fractured coracoid with anterior shoulder dislocation. J Can Assoc Radiol 1980; 31(4):278.

110. Zdravkovic D, Damholt VV. Comminuted and severely displaced fractures of the scapula. Acta Orthop Scand 1974;45:60.

Acute Fractures, Malunions, and Nonunions of the Clavicle

David Ring   *Jesse B. Jupiter*

INTRODUCTION

Recent observations emphasize that nonunion of the clavicle is more common than previously recognized[79,175,208,209] and that malunion with shortening can be associated with shoulder dysfunction.[15,28,55,56,122,161,209] As a result, primary operative treatment is becoming more commonplace. The indications and techniques of operative treatment are evolving. The operative treatment of nonunion and malunion can also be effective.

PATHOLOGY

Anatomy

The clavicle and scapula link the upper limb with the axial skeleton. The clavicle is linked to the scapula through the strong coracoclavicular and acromioclavicular ligaments.

D. Ring: Department of Orthopaedic Surgery, Massachusetts General Hospital, Cambridge, Massachusetts.

J. B. Jupiter: Department of Orthopaedic Surgery, Massachusetts General Hospital, Cambridge, Massachusetts.

Although it was once believed that the clavicle rotated with respect to the scapula,[81,82] experiments involving the insertion of Kirschner wires into awake volunteers have demonstrated that these two bones are tightly linked.[61,178] Elevation-depression, protraction-retraction, and rotation of the clavicle through the sternoclavicular articulation are associated with corresponding movements of the scapula with respect to the thorax.

Animals that bear weight on their forelimbs do not have clavicles.[10,30,44,110,155,156] The absence of a clavicle improves running and agility on four limbs. In such animals, the scapula is stabilized to the thorax by numerous powerful muscles. Clavicles are present in brachiating animals and apparently serve to help hold the upper limb away from the trunk to enhance more global positioning and use of the limb.

The clavicle has been considered by some to be an expendable bone.[73] Although children with congenital absence of the clavicle adapt suprisingly well,[58,116] and patients with tumors or infections treated with clavicular resections sometimes function adequately,[34,52,72,73,193,212] both have difficulty with overhead activities requiring strength or dexterity. Patients with clavicular resection may also have brachial plexus irritation related to instability of the clavicular fragments. Patients with a trapezius palsy do particularly poorly without a clavicle.[212] The authors believe that the evolutionary process has determined an important function for the clavicle and therefore always strive to preserve its length and alignment.

The clavicle is named for its S-shaped curvature with an apex anterior medially and an apex posterior laterally, resembling the musical symbol clavicula[127] (Fig. 19-1). The larger medial curvature widens the space for passage of neurovascular structures from the neck into the upper extremity through the costoclavicular interval. The transition from medial to lateral curvature occurs at approximately two-thirds the length of the bone as measured from its sternal end, a site that corresponds approximately to both the medial limit of attachment of the coracoclavicular ligaments and the entrance point of the main nutrient artery of the clavicle.[151]

The clavicle is made up of very dense trabecular bone lacking a well-defined medullary canal. In cross-section, the clavicle changes gradually between a flat lateral aspect, a tubular midportion, and an expanded prismatic medial end.[6]

The clavicle is subcutaneous throughout its length and makes a prominent aesthetic contribution to the contour of the neck and upper chest. The supraclavicular nerves run obliquely across the clavicle just superior to the platysma muscle, and the authors suggest identifying and protecting them during operative exposure to offset the development of hyperesthesia or dysesthesia over the chest wall (Fig. 19-2).

It is not surprising that the middle third is the most common site of clavicular fracture considering that the midportion (1) is the thinnest and narrowest portion of the bone, (2) represents a transitional region of the bone, both in curvature and in cross-sectional anatomy, making it a mechanically weak area, and (3) is the only area of the clavicle that is not supported by ligamentous or muscular attachments. It is possible that this circumstance was

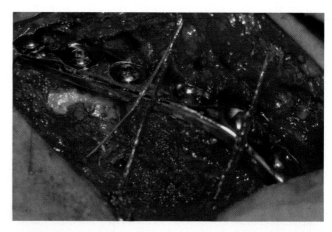

Figure 19-2   The supraclavicular nerves cross the clavicle and are at risk with incisions made either parallel or perpendicular to the clavicle. We attempt to protect these because injuring them can cause a painful neuroma or hypersensitive scar.

selected during evolution because clavicular fracture protects the brachial plexus during difficult births (shoulder dystocia).[153]

The intimate relation of the clavicle to the brachial plexus, to the subclavian artery and vein, and to the apex of the lung, belies the fact that injury to these structures in association with fracture of the clavicle is so uncommon. Brachial plexus palsy may develop weeks or years after injury as a result of hypertrophic callus with or without malalignment of the fracture fragments, leading to compromise of the costoclavicular space.[53,80,88,93,119,124,170,182,204,214] Narrowing of the costoclavicular space as a result of malunion or nonunion can also lead to a dynamic narrowing of the thoracic outlet.[5,9,20,31,59,11,126,162,195]

Shoulder Suspensory Complex

Although the effective treatment of most isolated fractures of the clavicle and scapula is relatively straightforward, combined injuries are regarded as more troublesome and are more readily considered for operative treatment.[68,76,108] An anatomic concept that facilitates understanding of these issues is the superior shoulder suspensory complex.[68] The complex consists of two struts (the clavicle and the lateral portion of the scapular body) linked by a combined bony and soft tissue ring (Fig. 19-3). The ring is composed of the coracoid process, coracoclavicular ligaments, distal clavicle, acromioclavicular ligaments, acromion, and glenoid process. Disruption of this complex at two sites can be far more problematic than disruption at one site. Common examples of double disruptions include complete acromioclavicular dislocation (e.g., disruption of the coracoclavicular and acromioclavicular ligaments), displaced fracture of the lateral clavicle (i.e., coraclavicular ligament injury and fracture of the distal clavicle), and fracture of the clavicle associated with fracture of the glenoid neck or scapulothoracic

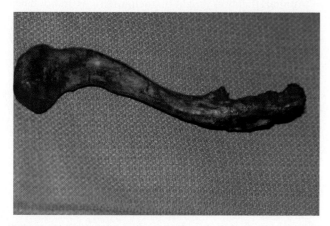

Figure 19-1   The clavicle is named for its resemblance to the musical symbol, clavicula. This S-curvature and change from flat lateral to round medial shape make internal fixation more difficult.

Classification and Epidemiology

The traditional division of the clavicle into thirds[1,136,137,180] seems arbitrary given that most fractures occur near the junction of the middle and distal thirds.[198] Other authors have suggested division of the clavicle into fifths with the middle three-fifths representing midclavicular fractures and the lateral one-fifth representing distal clavicular fractures.[175] The use of fractional divisions may not adequately distinguish fractures from injury to the coracoclavicular ligaments.

Neer[136] defined fractures of the lateral clavicle as lateral to the medial limit of the trapezoid ligament. He distinguished fractures of the distal clavicle with intact coracoclavicular ligaments (type 1) from those associated with tearing of these ligaments with wide displacement of the fracture fragments (type 2).[136] The wide displacement and instability of type 2 fractures place them at greater risk of nonunion. Intra-articular fractures (type 3) are rarely diagnosed acutely and were introduced into the classification in an attempt to explain later arthrosis or osteolysis.[36,135–137]

Rockwood's[176,177] distinction of distal third fractures with intact (type IIA) or disrupted (type IIB) coracoclavicular ligaments is confusing because there is no clear distinction between type IIA fractures and more distal midclavicle fractures.

It may be most useful to restrict the term "lateral clavicle fracture" to very far lateral fractures. These are essentially an alternative to an acromioclavicular dislocation in which the coracoclavicular ligaments tear but the acromioclavicular ligaments remain intact, the failure occurring through the distal clavicle instead (Fig. 19-4).

In unusual instances, fractures of the distal clavicle may be unstable in the absence of ligamentous injury. This occurs when both of the coracoclavicular ligaments remain attached to an inferior fracture fragment that lacks attachment to either of the primary medial or lateral fragments.[158]

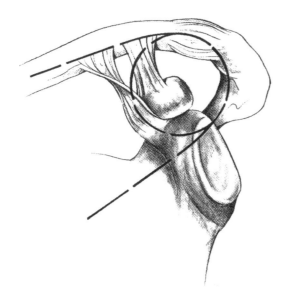

Figure 19-3 The combination of bone and ligament attachments that connect the trunk to the upper limb through the clavicle and shoulder girdle has been termed the "shoulder suspensory complex." This area is remarkably resilient in response to injury, but some have speculated that if the ring of structures is disrupted in two places, the chances of problems are higher and there may be a greater role for operative treatment.

dislocation. Although the role of operative treatment for these injuries is debated, each poses a more substantial risk to shoulder function than injuries that only disrupt one aspect of the shoulder suspensory complex.

Consequences of Fracture Malalignment

Some studies suggest a relationship between shortening of the clavicle and shoulder dysfunction.[55,56,122,152] Eskola and associates[55] evaluated 89 patients 2 years after clavicle fracture injury. Twenty-four (27%) had either slight pain on exercise or restricted shoulder movement, and four had major functional problems. Both primary fracture displacement of more than 15 mm and shortening greater than 15 mm at final follow-up were significantly associated with pain on exercise. It is possible that the shoulder dysfunction is related to the higher energy of the injury rather than the residual malalignment.

In contrast, Nordqvist and colleagues[147] evaluated 16 patients with 15 mm or greater shortening of the clavicle and found no measurable effect on mobility, strength, or Constant score. Oroko and colleagues[154a] found 3 of 13 adults with healed clavicle fractures with 15 mm or greater shortening had diminished Constant scores, but in each case the disability was explained by factors other than the shortening.

The authors believe that shortening of the clavicle may affect shoulder function in ways that are difficult to quantify and is probably only important in patients who place substantial demands on their shoulders.

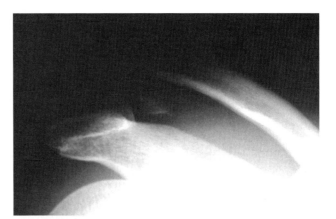

Figure 19-4 The classification of lateral clavicle fractures has been varied and inconsistent. Displaced lateral clavicle fractures may be best considered as an alternative injury pattern of complete acromioclavicular separations—instead of tearing the acromioclavicular ligaments, the distal clavicle fails.

Fractures of the medial end of the clavicle are uncommon and almost without exception are treated symptomatically. Craig[36] subdivided these as minimally displaced (type I), displaced (type II), intra-articular (type III), physeal separation (type IV), and comminuted (type V) fractures. Fractures in this region of the clavicle are so uncommon that the patterns of medial clavicular injury have rarely been described and studied, and it remains unclear how different fracture patterns influence treatment and prognosis.

Robinson[175] reviewed 1,000 fractures of the clavicle treated at the Royal Infirmary of Edinburgh over a 6-year period. He divided the clavicle into fifths, labeling the medial one-fifth as type I or medial clavicle fractures, the lateral one-fifth as type 3 or lateral clavicle fractures, and the middle three-fifths as midclavicular fractures (type 2). For midclavicular fractures he applied subclassifications that distinguished displacement greater than the width of the bone and segmental comminution of the fracture fragments. For medial and lateral clavicle fractures he distinguished displacement and articular involvement. He reported the following interesting facts: the incidence of medial clavicle fractures was 1 per 100,000 per year compared with 20 for midclavicular and 8 for lateral clavicular fractures; the midclavicular fractures were more often displaced than not by a ratio of 2.7 to 1; and the lateral clavicle fractures were more often nondisplaced by a ratio of approximately 2 to 1. Ten percent of displaced midclavicular fractures had delayed or arrested healing, and 6% were treated operatively. None of the nondisplaced fractures had healing problems. Segmental comminution of the fracture was also a risk factor for nonunion with 5% of noncomminuted fractures failing to heal, compared with 11.5% of comminuted fractures. Forty-four percent of displaced lateral clavicle fractures had healing problems, and 14% were treated operatively.

Other recent studies of the epidemiology of clavicle fractures found an incidence closer to 50 per 100,000 per year and suggest that lateral clavicle fractures are increasingly common among the elderly who have a simple fall from a standing height.[143,149,175] In another study, two-thirds of patients with a lateral clavicle fracture were alcoholics.[144]

Mechanism

In adolescents and adults, clavicle fractures in all regions typically result from moderate or high-energy traumatic impacts, such as those caused by a fall from a height, a motor vehicle accident, a sports injury, a blow to the point of the shoulder, or, rarely, a direct injury to the clavicle.[143,149,175] In elderly persons, clavicle fractures usually result from low-energy trauma such as a simple fall.

It has become clear that the clavicle fails most commonly in compression.[11,63,186,194] Failure in compression is seen after falls onto the shoulder and direct blows to the point of the shoulder. A direct blow to the clavicle, which can occur in sports in which sticks are wielded (e.g., lacrosse[191]), may also fracture the clavicle. Although a fall onto the outstretched hand has traditionally been considered a common mechanism of midclavicular fracture,[1] recent observations question this assumption.[194]

Stanley and colleagues[194] studied 122 of 150 consecutive patients with fractured clavicles who presented to two hospitals in Sheffield and provided detailed accounts of their injury. Eighty-seven percent resulted from a fall onto the shoulder, 7% resulted from a direct blow to the point of the shoulder, and 6% resulted from a fall onto an outstretched hand. A fall on the outstretched hand was the apparent mechanism of 5 (6.3%) of 79 midclavicular fractures and 2 (5.9%) of 34 distal clavicular fractures, suggesting that a direct injury to the shoulder is the most common mechanism of clavicular fracture at all sites. These authors hypothesized that even those patients who recall their injury as a fall onto the outstretched hand may have fallen secondarily onto the shoulder. This second impact may have been the injuring force, and an isolated fall onto the outstretched hand may actually be an unusual mechanism of injury.[194]

EVALUATION

Clinical Evaluation

Diagnosis is usually straightforward based on the mechanism of injury, the location of swelling and ecchymosis, and the examination for deformity, tenderness, and crepitation. Open clavicle fractures are uncommon, even after high-energy traumatic injury, and usually the result of a direct blow to the clavicle. Tenting of the skin by one of the major fracture fragments or by an intervening fragment of comminuted bone is not uncommon, but a true threat to the integrity of the skin is unusual.[169,175]

Neurovascular injury,[80] pneumothorax,[42,112,123,214] and hemothorax[180] have been reported in association with fracture of the clavicle but are uncommon. In contrast with late dysfunction of the brachial plexus after clavicular fracture, in which medial cord structures are typically involved, acute injury to the brachial plexus at the time of clavicular fracture usually takes the form of a traction injury to the upper cervical roots. Such root traction injuries usually occur in the setting of high-energy trauma and have a relatively poor prognosis.[8,106,189]

The prevalence of pneumothorax in association with fracture of the clavicle is 3%, based on Rowe's study of more than 600 fractures at Massachusetts General Hospital.[180] In that study, Rowe did not distinguish between moderate and high-energy injuries, nor did he distinguish isolated fractures from those injuries associated with ipsilateral scapular fracture or dissociation from the thorax or with ipsilateral upper rib injuries. The presence of these associated injuries indicates an injury mechanism of extremely high energy.[45,47,76,102,108,172,207] Pneumothorax and hemothorax are more common in this situation and more likely to result from a generalized chest wall injury than from a direct injury to the apical pleura by the fractured clavicle.[42,112,123,214] Nonetheless, evaluation for possible pneumothorax by physical examination and close inspection of an upright film that includes the ipsilateral upper lung field is important.

When a clavicle fracture occurs because of a high-energy traumatic injury (e.g., motor vehicle accident or fall from a height), then the evaluation of life-threatening lesions takes precedence. Major vascular disruption can occur in association with fracture of the clavicle, but it is extremely rare.[35,40,41,43,71,80,84,118,120,133,148,159,196] Injury to the thoracic duct has also been reported. Death after a tear of the subclavian vein with resultant pseudoaneurysm was recorded in the famous case of the death of Sir Robert Peel.[41,101] Arterial thrombosis may occur after intimal injury.[83,105,202] Most vascular injuries associated with clavicle fractures occur in combination with a scapulothoracic dissociation, which has been compared with a closed forequarter amputation.[45,47,102,154,181]

Evaluation of the vascular status of the upper extremity should include an assessment of relative temperature and color compared with the uninvolved extremity. Because of the extensive collateral blood supply to the upper extremity, these factors may appear normal despite the presence of a major vascular injury. A difference in peripheral pulses or blood pressure between injured and uninjured upper extremities may be the only clue that a vascular injury is present. If the limb is threatened or there is persistent unexplained hemorrhage, angiography can help to detect and localize any vascular injury and thereby assist with definitive management.

Radiographic Evaluation

An anteroposterior (AP) view of the clavicle identifies and localizes most clavicular fractures, and it should differentiate displaced from nondisplaced or minimally displaced fractures. The radiographic film should be large enough to evaluate both the acromioclavicular and the sternoclavicular joints as well as the remainder of the shoulder girdle and upper lung fields.[180] Oblique views can be used to further gauge the degree and direction of displacement.[180,167] Quesada recommended 45-degree caudad and cephalad views, which he believed would facilitate evaluation by providing orthogonal projection.[167] In practice, a single 20- to 60-degree cephalad-tilted view provides an adequate second view, because interference with thoracic structures is minimized. Medial clavicular fractures may be difficult to characterize on this view, and computed tomography is often necessary.

Evaluation of distal clavicular fracture displacement in the AP plane requires a different set of radiographs, because cephalad-tilted and caudad-tilted views are hindered by overlap of the bones of the shoulder and overexposure of the distal clavicle and often fail to accurately depict the degree of displacement. Neer[135] suggested a stress view (with 10 lb of weight in each hand) to evaluate the integrity of the coracoclavicular ligaments and 45-degree anterior and posterior oblique views to gauge displacement.

A combination of both AP and cephalad-caudad obliquity has been advocated in the evaluation of midclavicular fractures.[171,206] The so-called apical oblique view (tilted 45 degrees anterior and 20 degrees cephalad) may facilitate the diagnosis of minimally displaced fractures (e.g., birth fractures and fractures in children).[206] Ultrasound is also a sensitive diagnostic tool in the evaluation of birth fractures.[91]

The abduction lordotic view, taken with the shoulder abducted above 135 degrees and the central ray angled 25 degrees cephalad, is useful in evaluating the clavicle after internal fixation.[171] The abduction of the shoulder results in rotation of the clavicle on its longitudinal axis, which causes the plate to rotate superiorly and thereby expose the shaft of the clavicle and the fracture site under the plate.

ACUTE FRACTURES

Nonoperative Treatment

Closed reduction of clavicle fractures is rarely attempted because the reduction is usually unstable and there are no reliable means for providing external support. The reduction maneuvers described resemble those used for sternoclavicular joint dislocations.[21,33,157,168,201]

Of the many appliances that have been devised in an attempt to effect or maintain closed reduction and thereby minimize the deformity associated with fracture of the clavicle, most have proved to be cumbersome, painful, and even dangerous.[142] Dupuytren in 1831[43] and Malgaigne in 1859[113] argued that deformity of the clavicle was inevitable and emphasized the use of the simplest and most comfortable method of treatment; for Dupuytren, this consisted of placing the arm on a pillow until healing occurred.[43]

Nonetheless, devices intended for the maintenance of reduction and immobilization of clavicle fractures have remained popular and commonly take the form of either a figure-of-eight bandage, with or without a sling and, on rare occasions, a figure-of-eight plaster (Billington yoke[13]) or a shoulder spica cast.[1,157,168,180] Those who agree with Dupuytren and Malgaigne, that accurate reduction and immobilization of clavicular fractures is, as stated by Mullick, "neither essential nor possible,"[63,64,103,107,130,187] advocate the use of a simple sling for comfort, forgoing any attempts at reduction.

The advantage of the figure-of-eight bandage is that the arm remains free and can be used to a limited degree.

Disadvantages include the following: increased discomfort[2,63,64]; the need for frequent readjustment and repeat office visits[2,121]; the potential for complications, including axillary pressure sores[121,163] and other skin problems[2]; upper extremity edema and venous congestion[2,121,130]; brachial plexus palsy[186]; worsening of deformity[63,121,130]; and perhaps an increased risk of nonunion.[210]

A few investigations have compared treatment with a figure-of-eight or reducing bandage with the use of a simple sling or supporting bandage.[2,107,121,194] Although the details of patient selection and evaluation in these investigations remain unclear based on the meager data published, the authors claim to have found no difference with regard to shoulder function,[2,107,121] residual deformity,[2,121] or time to return to full range of motion and full activity.[194]

In the authors' opinion, the only way to address deformity is with operative treatment. This is equally true for midclavicle and lateral clavicle fractures. Because nonoperative treatment has little influence on alignment or healing, the authors prefer to use a simple sling for support and pain relief. The clavicle typically heals sufficiently to discontinue protection within 3 to 4 weeks in young children, 4 to 6 weeks in older children, and 6 to 8 weeks in adults.[180] Limitation of activity is usually encouraged for a minimum of 8 weeks after clinical and radiographic union to reduce the risk of refracture.

Operative Treatment

Until recently, the rate of nonunion of nonoperatively treated fractures of the clavicle was consistently reported as less than 3%.[57,99,107,134,180,186] Recent studies suggest that the rate of delayed and nonunion may approach 10% to 20% among widely displaced, comminuted fractures in adults.[79,146,175,208] Furthermore, although malunion has traditionally been considered a cosmetic concern,[142] some

reports exist of difficulties in shoulder function among patients with overriding clavicular fragments.[55,56] For these reasons, acute clavicle fractures are now considered for operative treatment in selected cases.

The indications for operative fixation of clavicular fractures remain uncertain. Absolute indications are rare, including open fracture, scapulothoracic dissociation,[45,47,102] and associated major vascular injury for which an open approach will be necessary for vascular repair.

The need for operative treatment of the so-called floating shoulder injury (displaced fractures of the clavicle and glenoid neck)[68,76,108,172] has been questioned recently,[50,51,203,211] but should be considered for patients who place substantial demands on their shoulders. For patients with multiple injuries, the rehabilitation of associated ipsilateral upper extremity lesions may be facilitated by operative fixation of the clavicle.

It is often stated that operative fixation should be considered if the skin is threatened by pressure from a prominent clavicular fracture fragment, and excision of a prominent spike is an occasional treatment recommendation[114]; however, it is rare for the skin to be perforated from within.[169] When a malaligned fracture causes brachial plexus compression,[53,119,124,170,182,204] realignment and stable fixation can help resolve the neurological dysfunction.

Widely displaced and comminuted fractures are associated with a higher risk of nonunion, and fractures with substantial shortening are associated with symptomatic malunion. These fractures are often considered for operative treatment. Patients and surgeons should be aware of the following: that the fracture will heal in most patients with these fracture patterns, and they will have good function; that operative treatment has risks; and that nonunion and malunion can be salvaged with secondary procedures if necessary. Nonetheless, very active and motivated patients often choose operative treatment (Fig. 19-5).

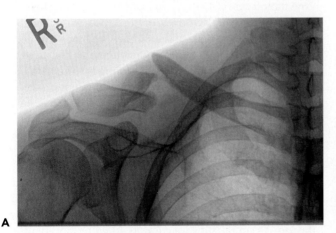
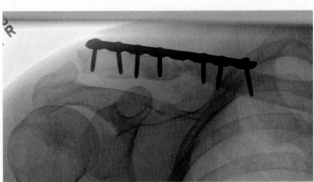

Figure 19-5 An active 43-year-old man had a widely displaced comminuted fracture of the diaphyseal clavicle after a fall from his bicycle. (*A*) Six weeks later there were no signs of healing, and the fracture remained unstable. (*B*) The patient elected to proceed with operative treatment, and union was achieved after reduction and plate and screw fixation.

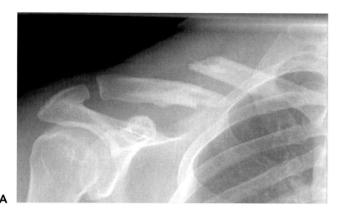

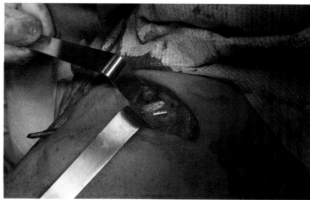

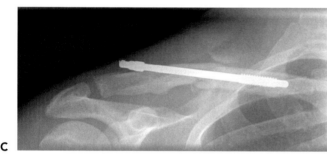

Figure 19-6 Intramedullary rod fixation is an alternative to plate fixation. *(A)* A 25-year-old man with a clavicle fracture after a motorcycle accident had a widely displaced diaphyseal fracture. After discussion of the risks and benefits of operative and nonoperative treatment, the patient elected to proceed with operative treatment. *(B)* The reduction and rod placement are achieved through an incision perpendicular to the clavicle at the fracture site. A second lateral incision is also required for rod placement and extraction. *(C)* The lateral portion of the rod is prominent and must be removed at a second operation.

The results of one recent study place this issue in perspective. A group of surgeons compared operative treatment with a 2.5-mm pin and nonoperative treatment with a figure-of-eight bandage in two comparable groups of 40 patients. They found similar Constant scores and satisfaction rates in both groups, with substantial complications in the patients who underwent operation, including the following: eight superficial infections, three refractures, two delayed unions with pin breakage, and two nonunions.[69] These results may not reflect optimum technique or implants, but they do reflect the occasionally meddlesome nature of operative intervention.

Intramedullary Fixation

Before the advent of modern techniques of plate fixation, the small, thin plates that were used for operative treatment of clavicle fractures gave poor results,[180] leading many to prefer intramedullary fixation with wires or screws.[22,100,104,126,131,141,160,180,183] The theoretical difficulties of intramedullary fixation of the clavicle, because of the curvature, the high density, and the poorly defined intramedullary canal of the bone,[180] have not been described in practice.[14,26,87,217] Intramedullary devices have been altered in attempts to prevent the complications associated with pin migration; threaded pins, pins with heads, and pins bent at the ends have been used. However, even threaded and bent pins can migrate, particularly if they break.[14,26,29,132,148,217]

The potential advantage of intramedullary fixation (i.e., a smaller, more cosmetic scar) is disputable considering that the incision required for open reduction is not a great deal smaller than that required for plate fixation, and a second, more lateral scar is necessary for implant removal (Fig. 19-6). The incision for intramedullary fixation is perpendicular to the clavicle and is claimed to produce a more aesthetic scar. The authors have used incisions both perpendicular and parallel to the clavicle for both plate and screw as well as intramedullary fixation and have found that the scars are not appreciably different in appearance, although a perpendicular scar may be easier to hide. The supraclavicular nerves cross both the perpendicular and the parallel incisions, and an attempt should be made to protect them.

The technique for intramedullary fixation is described in detail elsewhere in this text.

Plate and Screw Fixation

Plate and screw fixation can provide rigid fixation allowing immediate functional use of the limb. When the plate is placed on the superior portion of the bone, the plate can be prominent and symptomatic, but most patients do not request plate removal. Alternatively, the plate can be placed on the anterior surface of the clavicle where it is sometimes less prominent[95] (Fig. 19-7).

The authors use a supine, semi-sitting (beachchair) position. The iliac crest is prepared and draped when there is a chance that bone graft will be needed.

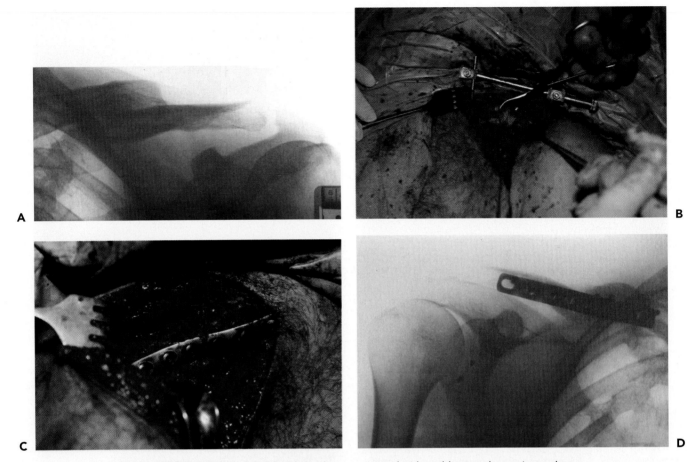

Figure 19-7 Malunion of the clavicle has been associated with problems such as pain, weakness, and neurovascular symptoms. *(A)* Substantial shortening (>2.5 cm) is particularly problematic. *(B)* In this case an oblique osteotomy was created at the old fracture site, and a small skeletal distractor was used to lengthen the clavicle and hold the provisional reduction. *(C)* Plate and screws were placed on the anterior surface of the clavicle after elevation of a part of the pectoralis major origin from the clavicle. *(D)* This anterior plate placement can be less prominent, and the drill for the screws is directed in a less dangerous direction.

The authors usually use an incision parallel and just inferior to the long axis of the clavicle, although an incision perpendicular to the clavicle can also be used. The crossing supraclavicular nerves are identified under loupe magnification and preserved to limit chest wall numbness and a potentially painful neuroma.

Reduction can be achieved by stripping the clavicle subperiosteally and manipulating the fragments with bone clamps, but this compromises the vascularity of the clavicle. We prefer to use a temporary external fixator or small skeletal distractor to facilitate gradual restoration of alignment (Fig. 19-8). This can be challenging if there is substantial shortening and overlap and partial healing of the fracture. Periosteal and muscle attachments are elevated only as needed to visualize the fracture site and gradually restore alignment.

The authors usually apply a 3.5-mm limited contact dynamic compression plate (LCDC Plate, Synthes, Paoli,

PA) to the superior or anterosuperior aspect of the clavicle. A minimum of three screws should be placed in each major fragment. If the fracture pattern allows it, placement of an interfragmentary screw greatly enhances the stability of the construct (Fig. 19-9).

Locking compression plates can be particularly useful for poor-quality bone. When a plate with locked screws is placed superiorly, it occasionally fails by axial pullout of the screws from the bone. This may represent a different mode of failure with delayed healing rather than a greater risk of failure with this type of plate.

When the vascularity to the fragments has been preserved, no bone graft is needed. When there is extensive stripping or gaps in the cortex opposite the plate, consider the addition of a small amount of autogenous iliac crest cancellous bone graft. A subcuticular suture is used to improve the appearance of the scar.

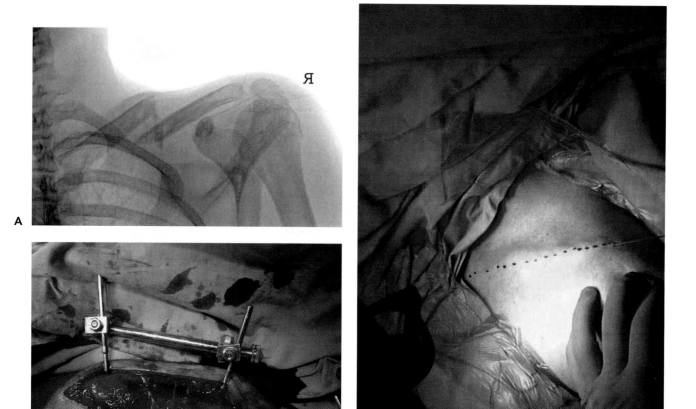

Figure 19-8   *(A)* A 34-year-old woman with a widely displaced, comminuted, and shortened clavicle fracture elected operative treatment. *(B)* An incision parallel to the clavicle was planned and infiltrated with dilute epinephrine. *(C)* A small skeletal distractor was used to realign the clavicle. The muscular and periosteal attachments were preserved, and the supraclavicular nerves were identified and protected. *(continued)*

The authors' current practice, provided there is confidence in the security of fixation, is to use a sling for patient comfort during the initial 7 to 10 postoperative days. Thereafter, the arm can be used for functional activities with the arm at the side and the sling used only as needed. Passive shoulder pendulum exercises are sometimes used. Active forward flexion and abduction are initiated between 2 and 6 weeks after injury depending on the fracture pattern and security of fixation. Once healing is demonstrated, progressive strengthening exercises are permitted. A return to all occupational duties and recreational pursuits is usually possible by 4 months after operative treatment.

In most cases, plate removal is unnecessary. When patients request plate removal for cosmetic or comfort reasons, we advise waiting at least 12 and preferably 18

months from the time of injury and verifying reconstitution of the cortex under the plate by using the abduction lordotic radiographic view.

Distal Clavicle Fractures

Fractures of the distal clavicle with little or no displacement are treated symptomatically with a sling. Although some cases of nonunion after such fractures have been reported,[145] the chance of nonunion is extremely low, and symptoms are variable.

Displaced distal clavicular fractures, on the other hand, are recognized as the only general type of clavicle fracture for which routine primary operative treatment should be considered. This is based on the work of Neer[135–137,145] and others[49,145] who found that 22% to 33% of these fractures

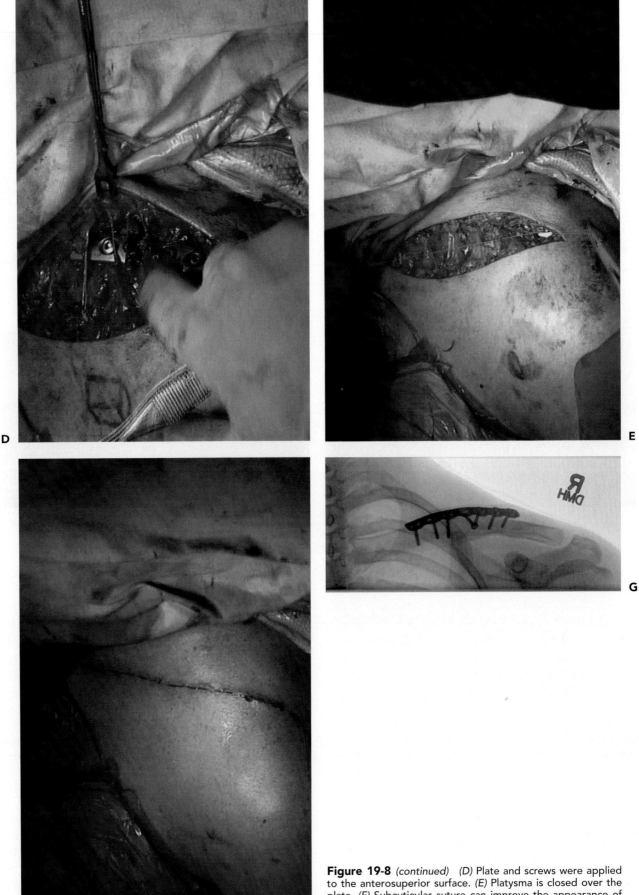

D

E

F

G

Figure 19-8 *(continued)* *(D)* Plate and screws were applied to the anterosuperior surface. *(E)* Platysma is closed over the plate. *(F)* Subcuticular suture can improve the appearance of the scar. *(G)* Fracture healed with good alignment and function.

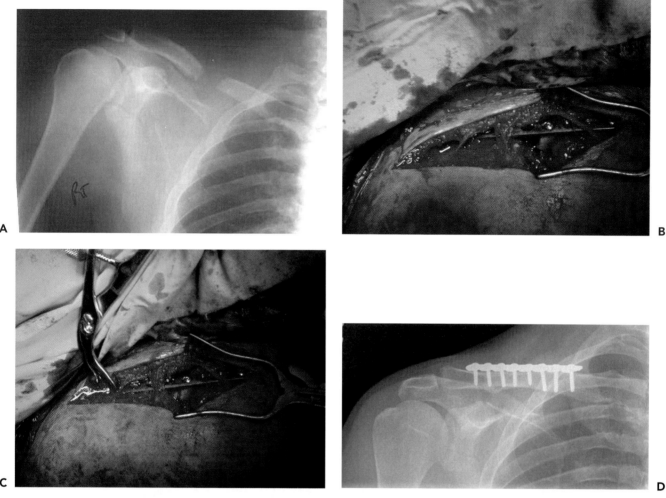

Figure 19-9 A 33-year-old man had multiple injuries in a motor vehicle accident. (A) The clavicle fracture was distracted. There was also a scapula fracture and likely a scapulothoracic dissociation. (B) The plate was applied first to the medial fragment through an incision parallel to the clavicle. (C) A push-pull screw and clamp were then used to reduce and compress the fracture. (D) The fracture healed in good alignment.

fail to unite after nonoperative treatment. An additional 45% to 67% require more than 3 months for the fracture to heal.[49,136] Good results have been reported with the operative treatment of type 2 fractures using a variety of techniques.[49,57,67,78,136,204]

A few authors report acceptable results with nonoperative treatment,[125,145,179] stating that those few nonunions that become symptomatic can be treated with a reconstructive procedure at a time remote from the injury, if necessary. Given that most complete acromioclavicular dislocations have acceptable results with nonoperative treatment, the addition of a small distal clavicle fracture to this type of injury may not appreciably alter the results.[179] There may be good reason to carefully consider the classification of these injuries and then reconsider the need for routine operative treatment. On the other hand, because these frac-

tures are so uncommon, they will be difficult to study. For now, the preference remains operative treatment.

Neer recommended stabilization of displaced distal clavicular fractures with two Kirschner wires inserted retrograde into the distal fragment through the fracture site.[125] Two wires are used to control rotation. The wires are passed through the acromioclavicular joint, through the acromion, and out the skin on the lateral aspect of the shoulder, and then passed into the medial fragment, bent to decrease the risk of migration, and cut beneath the skin. Shoulder motion must be restricted to prevent pin breakage and migration. Some surgeons have used a single wire,[75,158,180] threaded wires,[75] or screws,[75,138–141] and some have made a point of avoiding the acromioclavicular joint.[158] Kona and colleagues urge caution,[97] noting high rates of both nonunion and infection with transacromial wire techniques.

Alternative techniques for operative fixation of distal clavicular fractures include coracoclavicular screw fixation,[3,17,49] transfer of the coracoid to the clavicle,[27,60,92] and other coracoclavicular fixation.[67,78,205] The AO/ASIF group recommended use of a tension band wire construct in which two Kirschner wires enter on the superior aspect of the clavicle, avoiding the acromioclavicular joint.[74] In addition, they suggested consideration of a small plate, particularly a small T-shaped plate, with one of the screws directed into the coracoid.[74] A specially designed plate that is contoured so that its distal limit curves under the acromion, either through or posterior to the acromioclavicular joint, has also been used—the acromial hook plate[62,74] (Fig. 19-10).

Although the hook plate technique is appealing, a suitable plate is not yet widely available, and the authors' current preference is a tension band wire technique (Fig. 19-11). The distal clavicle and acromion are exposed through an incision parallel to the clavicle with the development of skin flaps. Provisional fracture reduction can be held with a transacromial Kirschner wire. Definitive fixation consists of two stout, smooth Kirschner wires passed through the posterolateral corner of the acromion and angled obliquely across the acromioclavicular joint and fracture to purchase in the solid cortex of the dorsal clavicle medial to the fracture. An 18-gauge wire is then looped through a drill hole medial to the fracture and around the tips of the wires, which are bent 180 degrees, turned downward, and impacted into the acromion. If either the trapezoid or the conoid ligament are torn and identified, an attempt is made to perform a suture repair. The wound is closed over a suction drain. The postoperative management differs

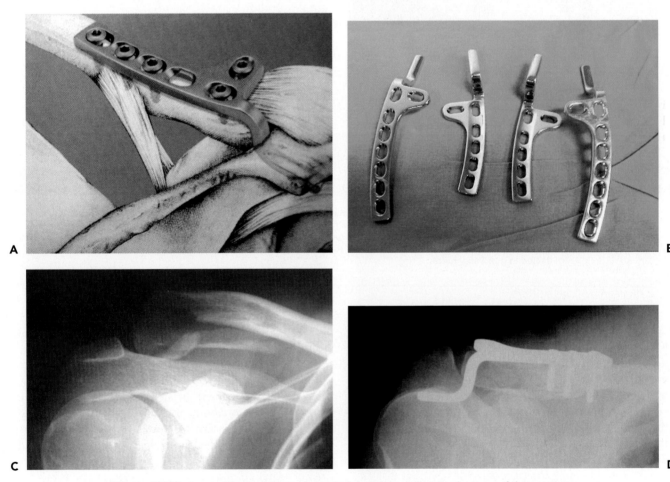

Figure 19-10 Internal fixation of lateral clavicle fractures is challenging because of the proximity to the acromioclavicular joint, the small distal clavicle fragment, and the poor hold of implants in the acromion. *(A)* Plate with an extension that hooks under the acromion has been used in several different designs. *(B)* In this design the plate extension goes under the posterior acromion without passing through the acromioclavicular joint. *(C)* Displaced lateral clavicle fracture with a bony fragment still attached to the conoid and trapezoid ligaments (type V lateral clavicle fracture). *(D)* Fixation with a clavicular hook plate achieved healing and good function. (Courtesy of Dr. A. D. Barrow, Witts University Orthopaedic Department, South Africa.)

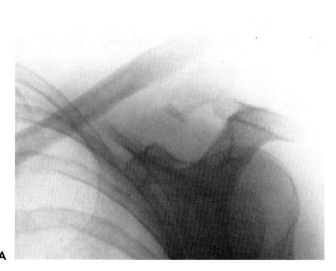

A

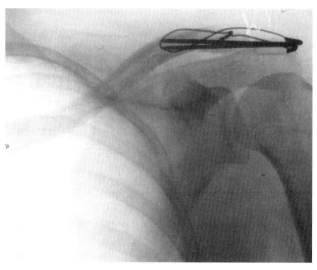

B

Figure 19-11 Tension band wiring of lateral clavicle fractures can also be effective. *(A)* Again, the true lateral clavicle fracture is characterized as an injury that is trying to be an acromioclavicular dislocation, but fails through bone rather than ligament at the acromioclavicular joint. *(B)* We place the Kirschner wires across the acromioclavicular joint and add a figure-of-eight tension band wire superiorly.

from that for the midclavicular fracture in that the patient is maintained in a sling for a minimum of 4 to 6 weeks. The hardware rarely migrates but is usually prominent and requires removal. The authors try to wait at least 6 months before removing the wires.

Medial Clavicle Fractures

Medial clavicle fractures are uncommon, and most practitioners have limited experience treating them. The literature offers little more than case reports, most describing medial physeal separation injuries.[24,65,89,109,165,216] Although some authors recommend open reduction internal fixation,[24,165] most advocate nonoperative treatment initially, with resection of the medial clavicle if symptoms persist.[1,24,32,36,55,77,107,109,137,180,216] Considering the risks attendant with insertion and migration of implants in this region, the authors rarely consider operative treatment. Displaced fractures must be evaluated with computed tomography scanning to be certain that posterior displacement of the fragments does not present a threat to neurovascular structures at the base of the neck.

NONUNION

Patients presenting with an ununited clavicle are likely to have specific complaints related to deformity (typically adduction, shortening, and internal rotation of the shoulder); altered shoulder function as a result of deformity or pain; or local compression of the underlying brachial plexus or vas-

cular structures.[88,185] Occasionally, patients present decades after the original injury to request treatment,[85,88,174,210] perhaps in part because they were advised previously that nothing operative could or should be done.

The neurovascular problems that may accompany a clavicular nonunion include thoracic outlet syndrome,[5,9,20,31,59,111,128,162,195] subclavian artery or vein compression[38,98] or thrombosis,[38,70,215] and brachial plexus palsy.[25,80,88,93] The prevalence of neurovascular dysfunction in patients presenting with clavicular nonunion has varied widely in reported series, from 6% to 52% of patients.[85,88,96,210]

In the treatment of clavicular nonunions, the authors prefer to distinguish between reconstructive procedures and salvage procedures. Reconstructive procedures seek relief from pain and neurovascular compression and seek enhanced function through the restoration of the alignment and the continuity of the clavicle. Salvage procedures, in which the clavicle is resected, contoured,[150] or avoided altogether (e.g., first rib resection[37]), seek the limited goal of relief of symptoms. Although treatment of clavicular nonunion with electrical stimulation has been attempted,[23,38] there are few indications for its use. Symptomatic clavicular nonunion typically has elements of both deformity and dysfunction, as well as neurovascular compromise, which are not addressed by electrical treatment.[132]

Improved techniques of stable fixation have improved the results of reconstructive procedures to the point that salvage operations are now largely of historical interest.[192] The only situation in which the authors would consider partial resection of the clavicle is in a chronically infected clavicle in a medically compromised patient or very distal clavicular nonunion. A small distal clavicular fragment can be resected, and the coracoclavicular ligaments can be securely attached to the outer end of the medial fragment.[192]

The treatment of clavicular nonunion has evolved from screw fixation of tibial or iliac crest bone grafts,[7,12,66,185] to intramedullary fixation,[85,117,134,197] which still has many advocates,[14,26,54,213] to the preferred method of rigid plate and screw fixation.[4,18,19,39,46,48,58,86,88,90,96,115,129,152,166,173,174,184,192,199,200,210]

In hypertrophic nonunions, the exuberant callus can be resected and saved for use as bone graft, making harvest of an iliac crest graft unnecessary in some cases. The nonunion site does not require debridement because the fibrocartilage progresses to union after stable internal fixation. If the fracture line is oblique, it is sometimes possible to secure the fragments with the use of an interfragmentary screw in addition to the plate. If lengthening is desired, the oblique fracture can be mobilized before placing the lag screw.[18]

Atrophic nonunions present sclerotic ends with interposed fibrous tissue, whereas pseudoarthroses have a false synovial joint. Resection of the ends of the fracture fragments and the intervening tissue is required in both situations. A small distractor often proves invaluable to help control the fragments and to attain the desired length and alignment. A sculptured tricortical iliac crest bone graft is useful to ensure restoration of length and alignment and to promote healing when there is an absolute bone defect (Figs. 19-12 and 19-13).

The authors harvest the iliac graft from the crest through an oblique incision along the midpoint of the ilium. The crest is exposed subperiosteally, and a tricortical section, measuring 1.5 times the anticipated size of the final graft, is

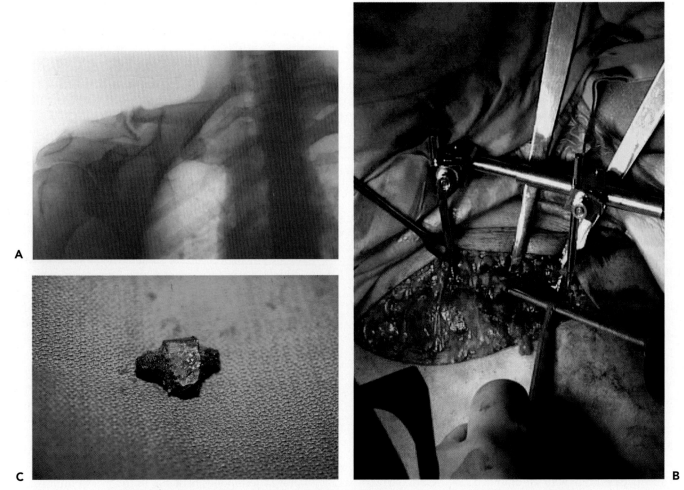

Figure 19-12   Plate fixation and structural bone graft for nonunion of the clavicle. *(A)* This long-standing nonunion was a synovial pseudoarthrosis. *(B)* After debridement of sclerotic bone and realignment, there was a bony defect. *(C)* Corticocancellous bone graft from the iliac crest was contoured to have cancellous pegs for interdigitation with the intramedullary spaces of the proximal and distal clavicle fragments. *(continued)*

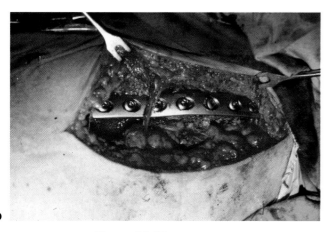

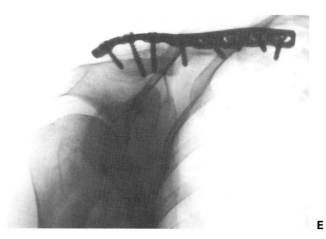

D

E

Figure 19-12 *(continued)* *(D)* Plate and screws are used for fixation. *(E)* Healing and improved function were achieved.

removed with either osteotomes or a small oscillating saw. The graft is then sculptured to create large cancellous pegs at each end, which plug into the medullary canals of the clavicular fragments. This interdigitation increases the stability of the construct and facilitates plate fixation. The graft is positioned so that the dorsal cortical margin of the iliac crest lies on the inferior surface of the clavicle, affording better purchase for a screw and more resistance to bend-

ing forces at the nonunion site. Additional cancellous graft from the iliac crest is compacted into the medullary canals of each fragment before the final impaction of the cortico-cancellous segmental graft.

A 3.5-mm LCDC plate is then applied with a minimum of three screws in each major fragment and a single screw transfixing the graft. Compression is applied to both surfaces of the graft to enhance early stability and healing with

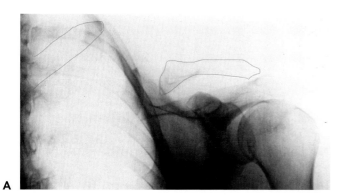

A

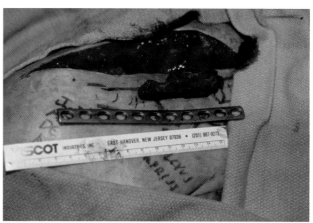

B

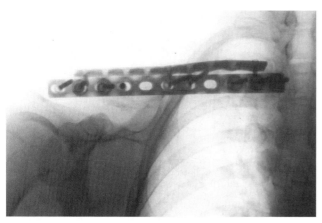

C

Figure 19-13 Even very large defects can be reconstructed. *(A)* Patient with a 5-cm defect in the clavicle after multiple procedures had an unstable medial fragment and symptoms consistent with brachial plexus dysfunction. *(B)* A large corticocancellous iliac crest craft was obtained. *(C)* Fracture and bone graft were secured with two orthogonal plates—one superior and one anterior. Healing was achieved, and the function improved.

little callus. The wound is closed with a subcuticular suture over suction drainage.

MALUNION

Malunion of the clavicle has been associated with exercise-related pain and other symptoms of shoulder dysfunction.[55,56,122,209] In addition, compression of underlying neurovascular structures has been reported in association with malaligned clavicle fractures as a result of narrowing of the costoclavicular space[5,9,20,31,53,59,111,119,124,128,162,182,195,204] and compression of the brachial plexus or the subclavian artery or vein.[25,38,70,80,88,93,98,214] Weeks or months after the injury, malunited fractures typically may give rise to neurological symptoms caused by proliferative callus.[5,31,53,59,170,182,204]

Osteotomy for symptomatic malunion of the clavicle is becoming more commonplace.[15,28,122,161] The malunion is osteotomized through the plane of deformity, realigned with the use of a small distractor, and secured with a plate and screws (Figs. 19-7 and 19-14).

COMPLICATIONS

Refracture

Repeat fracture of the clavicle usually occurs on premature resumption of full activity, in particular, contact sports activity. Because the typically vigorous healing response of the clavicle results in rapid decrease in pain and return of shoulder function, overenthusiastic patients often ignore their physicians' admonitions to avoid contact sports for at least 2 to 3 months after healing of the fracture. Refracture after plate removal is unusual if the plate remains in place at least 12 to 18 months after healing of the fracture.[164,192]

Nonunion After Operative Treatment

Traditional teaching held that the best way to get a nonunion of a clavicle fracture was to operate. According to Neer,[134] only 3 (0.1%) of 2,235 patients with midclavicular fractures treated by closed methods failed to heal, whereas 2 (4.6%) of 45 treated with immediate open reduction and fixation developed nonunion. Rowe[180] found 0.8% nonunion after closed treatment, compared with 3.7% after initial open treatment. The interpretation of these numbers should be tempered by the likelihood of a selection bias with more complex fractures being treated operatively.

Improvements in the techniques and implants for internal fixation of the clavicle have reduced but not eliminated nonunion after operative treatment. Failures are often related to technical shortcomings.

Khan and Lucas[94] noted no nonunions among 19 patients treated with primary plate fixation. Schwarz and Hocker[188] used 2.7-mm plates and reported nonunion in 3 of 36 patients, which they attributed to use of a plate of inadequate length. Poigenfurst et al.[164] reported nonunion in 5 (4.1%) of 122 patients treated operatively. They also re-

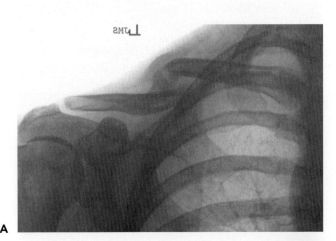
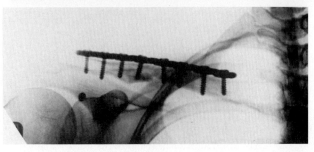
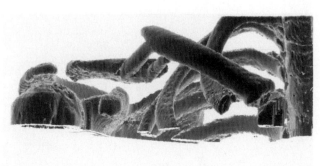

Figure 19-14 Malunion can cause a thoracic outlet syndrome. *(A)* Narrowing of the thoracic outlet because of fracture malalignment can be exacerbated by hypertrophic callus formation. *(B)* This three-dimensional computed tomography images shows the narrowing of the thoracic outlet well. *(C)* Plate and screw fixation of the realigned clavicle results in healing with less callus and can usually resolve the neurologic symptoms.

lated the failures to technical errors, including use of a plate of inadequate length or strength and devitalization of fracture fragments during operative exposure. Shen and colleagues[190] reported nonunion in 7 (3%) of 232 patients treated with plate fixation. All of the nonunions occurred in displaced fractures with segmental comminution (Robinson type 2B2). One was related to infection, and the other 6 were related to technical errors. Bostman and colleagues[16] reported 5 deep infections, 6 hardware failures, and 3 nonunions among 103 patients treated with plate fixation. The use of a plate of inadequate strength and size were responsible for the majority of the plate-related complications.

Injury to Adjacent Structures

Despite the proximity of important anatomic structures beneath the clavicle, intraoperative complications are rare. Eskola and coworkers[56] reported tearing of the subclavian vein, pneumothorax, air embolism, and brachial plexus palsy all in a single patient during dissection of a clavicular nonunion.

CONCLUSIONS

Operative treatment of a fracture of the clavicle can be accomplished with either intramedullary or plate and screw fixation and with a high success rate and acceptable complications. Given that most fractures will do well with nonoperative treatment, that only high-demand individuals are likely to have shoulder dysfunction from malunion, and that nonunion and malunion are responsive to reconstructive treatment, only a very motivated patient will select operative treatment for an acute fracture.

REFERENCES

1. Allman FL. Fractures and ligamentous injuries of the clavicle and its articulation. J Bone Joint Surg 1967;49A:774.
2. Andersen KJ, Jensen PO, Lauritzen J. Treatment of clavicular fractures. Acta Orthop Scand 1987;58:71.
3. Ballmer FT, Gerber C. Coracoclavicular screw fixation for unstable fractures of the distal clavicle. J Bone Joint Surg Br 1991;73:291.
4. Balmer FT, Lambert SM, Hertel R. Decortication and plate osteosynthesis for nonunion of the clavicle. J Shoulder Elbow Surg 1998;7:581.
5. Bargar WL, Marcus RE, Ittleman FP. Late thoracic outlet syndrome secondary to pseudarthrosis of the clavicle. J Trauma 1984;24:857.
6. Basmajian JV. The surgical anatomy and function of the arm trunk mechanism. Surg Clin North Am 1963;43:1471.
7. Basom WC, Breck LW, Herz JR. Dual grafts for non-union of the clavicle. South Med J 1947;40:898.
8. Bateman JE. Nerve injuries about the shoulder in sports. J Bone Joint Surg 1967;49A:785.
9. Bateman JE. Neurovascular syndromes related to the clavicle. Clin Orthop 1967;58:75.
10. Bechtol CO. Biomechanics of the shoulder. Clin Orthop 1980;146:37.
11. Bennett EH. The mechanism of fractures of clavicle. Ann Surg 1885;1:293.
12. Berkheiser EJ. Old ununited clavicular fractures in the adult. Surg Gynecol Obstet 1937;64:1064.
13. Billington RW. A new (plaster yoke) dressing for fracture of the clavicle. South Med J 1931;24:667.
14. Boehme D, Curtis RJ Jr, DeHann JT, et al. Non-union of fractures of the mid-shaft of the clavicle. J Bone Joint Surg Am 1991;73:1219.
15. Bosch U, Skutek M, Peters G, et al. Extension osteotomy in malunited clavicular fractures. J Shoulder Elbow Surg 1998;7:402.
16. Bostman O, Manninen M, Pihlajamaki H. Complications of plate fixation in fresh displaced midclavicular fractures. J Trauma 1997;43:778.
17. Bosworth BM. Acromioclavicular separation: a new method of repair. Surg Gynecol Obstet 1941;73:866.
18. Boyer MI, Axelrod TS. Atrophic nonunion of the clavicle. Treatment by compression plate, lag-screw fixation and bone graft. J Bone Joint Surg 1997;79B:301.
19. Bradbury N, Hutchinson J, Hahn D, et al. Clavicular nonunion. 31/32 healed after plate fixation and bone grafting. Acta Orthop Scand 1996;67:367.
20. Braun RM. Iatrogenic compression of the thoracic outlet. Johns Hopkins Med J 1979;145:94.
21. Breasthead JH. The Edwin Smith Surgical Papyrus: published in facsimile and hieroglyphic transliteration and commentary in two volumes, vol. 1. Chicago, IL, University of Chicago Press, 1930.
22. Breck LW. Partially threaded round pins with oversized threads for intramedullary fixation of the clavicle and the forearm bones. Clin Orthop 1958;11:227.
23. Brighton CT, Pollack SR. Treatment of recalcitrant non-union with a capacitively coupled electrical field. A preliminary report. J Bone Joint Surg Am 1985;67:577.
24. Brooks AL, Henning GD. Injury to the proximal clavicular epiphysis. J Bone Joint Surg Am 1972;54A:1347.
25. Campbell EH, Howard WP, Burkland CW. Clinical notes, suggestions and new instruments. JAMA 1949;139:91.
26. Capicotto PN, Heiple KG, Wilber JH. Midshaft clavicle nonunions treated with intramedullary Steinmann pin fixation and onlay bone graft. J Orthop Trauma 1994;8:88.
27. Caspi I, Ezra E, Oliver S, et al. Treatment of avulsed clavicle and recurrent subluxations of the ipsilateral shoulder by dynamic fixation. J Trauma 1987;27:94.
28. Chan KY, Jupiter JB, Leffert RD, et al. Clavicle malunion. J Shoulder Elbow Surg 1999;8:287.
29. Chu CM, Wang SJ, Lin LC. Fixation of mid-third clavicular fractures with Knowles pins: 78 patients followed for 2–7 years. Acta Orthop Scand 2002;73:134.
30. Codman EA. The shoulder: rupture of the supraspinatus tendon and other lesions in or about the subacromial bursa. Boston, MA, Thomas Todd, 1989.
31. Connolly JF, Dehne R. Nonunion of the clavicle and thoracic outlet syndrome. J Trauma 1989;29:1127.
32. Conwell HE. Fractures of the clavicle: a simple fixation dressing with a summary of the treatment and results attained in ninety-two cases. JAMA 1928;90:838.
33. Cook TW. Reduction and external fixation of fracture of the clavicle in recumbency. J Bone Joint Surg 1954;36A:878.
34. Copeland SM. Total resection of the clavicle. Am J Surg 1946;72:280.
35. Costa MC, Robbs JV. Nonpenetrating subclavian artery trauma. J Vasc Surg 1988;8:72.
36. Craig EV. Fractures of the clavicle. In: Rockwood CA Jr., Matsen FA III, eds. The shoulder. Philadelphia, PA, WB Saunders, 1990:367.
37. Dash UN, Handler D. A case of compression of subclavian vessels by a fractured clavicle treated by excision of the first rib. Am J Orthop 1960;42A:798.
38. Daskalakis E, Bouhoutsos J. Subclavian and axillary vein compression of musculoskeletal origin. Br J Surg 1980;67:573.
39. Davids PHP, Luitse JSK, Strating P, et al. Operative treatment for delayed union and nonunion of midshaft clavicular fractures: AO reconstruction plate fixation and early mobilization. J Trauma 1996;40:985.

40. DeBakey ME, Beall AC Jr, Wukasch DC. Recent developments in vascular surgery with particular reference to orthopedics. Am J Surg 1965;109:134.
41. Dickson JW. Death following fractured clavicle. Br Med J 1952;2:266.
42. Dugdale TW, Fulkerson JP. Pneumothorax complicating a closed fracture of the clavicle: a case report. Clin Orthop 1987;221:212.
43. Dupuytren G. Fracture de la clavicule en plusieurs fragments par cause indirecte. Gaz des hopitaux 1831;4:315.
44. Dvir Z Berme N. The shoulder complex in elevation of the arm: a mechanism approach. J Biomech 1978;11:219.
45. Ebraheim NA, An HS, Jackson WT, et al. Scapulothoracic dissociation. J Bone Joint Surg 1988;70A:428.
46. Ebraheim NA, Mekhail AO, Darwich M. Open reduction and internal fixation with bone grafting of clavicular nonunion. J Trauma 1997;42:701.
47. Ebraheim NA, Pearlstein SR, Savolaine ER, et al. Scapulothoracic dissociation (closed avulsion of the scapula, subclavian artery, and brachial plexus?: a newly recognized variant, a new classification, and a review of the literature and treatment options. J Orthop Trauma 1987;1:18.
48. Edvardsen P, Odegard O. Treatment of posttraumatic clavicular pseudoarthrosis. Acta Orthop Scand 1977;48:456.
49. Edwards DJ, Kavanaugh TG, Flannery MC. Fractures of the distal clavicle: a case for fixation. Injury 1992;23:44.
50. Edwards SG, Whittle AP, Wook GW. Nonoperative treatment of ipsilateral fractures of the scapula and clavicle. J Bone Joint Surg Am 2000;82A:774.
51. Egol KA, Connor PM, Karunakar MA, et al. The floating shoulder: clinical and functional results. J Bone Joint Surg Am 2001;83A:1188.
52. Elkin DC, Cooper FW Jr. Resection of the clavicle in vascular surgery. J Bone Joint Surg 1946;28A:117.
53. Enker SH, Murthy KK. Brachial plexus compression by excessive callus formation secondary to a fractured clavicle: a case report. Mt Sinai J Med 1970;37:678.
54. Enneking TJMQ, Hartlief MT, Fontijne WPJ. Rushpin fixation for midshaft clavicular nonunions. Good results in 13/14 cases. Acta Orthop Scand 1999;70:514.
55. Eskola A, Vainionpaa S, Myllynen P, et al. Outcome of clavicular fracture in 89 patients. Arch Orthop Trauma Surg 1986;105:337.
56. Eskola A, Vainionpaa S, Myllynen P, et al. Surgery for ununited clavicular fracture. Acta Orthop Scand 1986;57:366.
57. Eskola A, Vainionpaa S, Patiala H, et al. Outcome of operative treatment in fresh lateral clavicular fracture. Ann Chir Gynaecol 1987;76:167.
58. Fairbank HA. Cranio-cleido-dysostosis. J Bone Joint Surg 1949;31B:608.
59. Falconer MA, Weddell G. Costoclavicular compression of the subclavian artery and vein: relation to the scalenus anticus syndrome. Lancet 1943;2:539.
60. Falstie-Jensen S, Mikkelsen P. Psuedodislocation of the acromioclavicular joint. J Bone Joint Surg Br 1982;64:368.
61. Flatow EL. The biomechanics of the acromioclavicular, sternoclavicular and scapulothoracic joints. Instr Course Lect 1993;42:237.
62. Flinkkila T, Ristiniemi J, Hyvonen P, et al. Surgical treatment of unstable fractures of the distal clavicle: a comparative study of Kirschner wire and clavicular hook plate fixation. Acta Orthop Scand 2002;73:50.
63. Fowler AW. Fracture of the clavicle. J Bone Joint Surg 1962;44B:440.
64. Fowler AW. Treatment of the fractured clavicle. Lancet 1968;1:46.
65. Gearen PF, Petty W. Panclavicular dislocation. J Bone Joint Surg Am 1982;64:454.
66. Ghormley RK, Black JR, Cherry JH. Ununited fractures of the clavicle. Am J Surg 1941;51:343.
67. Goldberg J, Bruce WJM, Sonnabend DH, et al. Type 2 fractures of the distal clavicle: a new surgical approach. J Shoulder Elbow Surg 1997;6:380.
68. Goss TP. Double disruptions of the superior shoulder suspensory complex. J Orthop Trauma 1993;7:99.
69. Grassi FA, Tajana MS, D'Angelo F. Management of midclavicular fractures: comparison between nonoperative treatment and open intramedullary fixation in 80 patients. J Trauma 2001;50:1096.
70. Guilfoil PH, Christiansen T. An unusual vascular complication of a fractured clavicle. JAMA 1967;200:72.
71. Guillemin A. Dechirure de la veine sous-claviere par fracture fermee de la clavicule. Bull et Mem Soc Nat Chir 1930;56:302.
72. Gurd FB. The treatment of complete dislocation of the outer end of the clavicle: a hitherto undescribed operation. Ann Surg 1941;113:1094.
73. Gurd FB. Surplus parts of the skeleton: a recommendation for the excision of certain portions as a means of shortening the period of disability following trauma. Am J Surg 1947;74:705.
74. Heim U, Pfeiffer KM. Internal fixation of small fractures: technique recommended by the AO-ASIF Group, 3rd ed. New York, NY, Springer-Verlag, 1987.
75. Heppenstall RB. Fractures and dislocations of the distal clavicle. Orthop Clin North Am 1975;6:477.
76. Herscovici D Jr., Fiennes AG, Allgower M, et al. The floating shoulder: ipsilateral clavicle and scapular neck fractures. J Bone Joint Surg Br 1992;74:362.
77. Herscovici D Jr., Sanders R, Dipasquale T, et al. Injuries of the shoulder girdle. Clin Orthop 1995;318:54.
78. Hessman M, Kirschner R, Baumgaertel F, et al. Treatment of unstable distal clavicular fractures with and without lesions of the acromioclavicular joint. Injury 1996;27:47.
79. Hill JM, McGuire MH, Crosby LA. Closed treatment of displaced middle-third fractures of the clavicle gives poor results. J Bone Joint Surg Br 1997;79:537.
80. Howard FM, Shafer SJ. Injuries to the clavicle with neurovascular complications: a study of 14 cases. J Bone Joint Surg Am 1965;47:1335.
81. Inman VT, Saunders JB. Observations on the function of the clavicle. Calif Med 1946;65:158.
82. Inman VT, Saunders JB, Abbott LC. Observations of the function of the shoulder joint. J Bone Joint Surg 1944;26A:1.
83. Iqbal O. Axillary artery thrombosis associated with fracture of the clavicle. Med J Malaya 1971;26:68.
84. Javid H. Vascular injuries of the neck. Clin Orthop 1963;28:70.
85. Johnson EW Jr, Collins HR. Nonunion of the clavicle. Arch Surg 1963;87:963.
86. Joukainen J, Karaharju E. Pseudoarthrosis of the clavicle. Acta Orthop Scand 1977;48:550.
87. Jubel A, Andermahr J, Schiffer G, et al. Elastic stable intramedullary nailing of midclavicular fractures with a titanium nail. Clin Orthop 2003;408:279.
88. Jupiter JB, Leffert RD. Non-union of the clavicle. Associated complications and surgical management. J Bone Joint Surg Am 1987;69:753.
89. Kanoksikarin S, Wearne WM. Fracture and retrosternal dislocation of the clavicle. Aust N Z J Surg 1978;48:95.
90. Karaharju E, Joukainen J, Petonen J. Treatment of pseudoarthrosis of the clavicle. Injury 1981;13:400.
91. Katz R, Landman J, Dulitzky F, et al. Fracture of the clavicle in the newborn: an ultrasound diagnosis. J Ultrasound Med 1988;7:21.
92. Katznelson A, Nerubay J, Oliver S. Dynamic fixation of the avulsed clavicle. J Trauma 1976;16:841.
93. Kay SP, Eckardt JJ. Brachial plexus palsy secondary to clavicular nonunion: case report and literature survey. Clin Orthop 1986;206:219.
94. Khan MA, Lucas HK. Plating of fractures of the middle third of the clavicle. Injury 1977;9:263.
95. Kloen P, Sorkin AT, Rubel IF, et al. Anteroinferior plating of midshaft clavicular nonunions. J Orthop Trauma 2002;16:425.
96. Koelliker F. Behandlungsergebnisse der clavicula-pseudarthrose. Unfallchirurg 1989;92:164.
97. Kona J, Bosse MJ, Staeheli JW, et al. Type II clavicle fractures: a retrospective review of surgical treatment. J Orthop Trauma 1990;4:155.
98. Koss SD, Goitz HT, Redler MR, et al.. Nonunion of a midshaft clavicle fracture associated with subclavian vein compression: a case report. Orthop Rev 1989;28:431.

99. Kreisinger V. Sur le traitement des fractures de la clavicule. Rev Chir 1927;46:376.
100. Kuner EH, Schlickewei W, Mydla F. Operative therapie der claviculafrakturen, indikation, technik, ergebnisse. Hefte Unfallheilkunde 1982;160:76.
101. Sir Robert Peel's death (editorial). Lancet 1850;2:19.
102. Lange RH, Noel SH. Traumatic lateral scapular displacement: an expanded spectrum of associated neurovascular injury. J Orthop Trauma 1993;7:361.
103. Le Vay D. Treatment of midclavicular fractures. Lancet 1967; 1:723.
104. Lee HG. Treatment of fracture of the clavicle by internal nail fixation. N Engl J Med 1946;234:222.
105. Leese G, Belch JJ, Rickhos P, et al. Post-traumatic axillary artery thrombosis dissolution with low-dose intra-arterial streptokinase. Injury 1993;24:212.
106. Leffert RD, Seddon H. Infraclavicular brachial plexus injuries. J Bone Joint Surg Br 1965;47:9.
107. Lester CW. The treatment of fractures of the clavicle. Ann Surg 1929;89:600.
108. Leung KS, Lam TP. Open reduction and internal fixation of ipsilateral fractures of the scapular neck and clavicle. J Bone Joint Surg Am 1993;75:1015.
109. Lewonowski K, Bassett GS. Complete posterior sternoclavicular epiphysial separation: a case report and review of the literature. Clin Orthop 1992;281:84.
110. Ljunggren AE. Clavicular function. Acta Orthop Scand 1979; 50:261.
111. Lusskin R, Weiss CA, Winer J. The role of the subclavius muscle in the subclavian vein syndrome (costoclavicular syndrome) following fracture of the clavicle. Clin Orthop 1967;54:75.
112. Malcolm BW, Ameli FM, Simmons EH. Pneumothorax complicating a fracture of the clavicle. Can J Surg 1979;22:89.
113. Malgaigne JF. A treatise of fractures. Philadelphia, PA, J.B. Lippincott, 1859.
114. Mandalia V, Shivshanker V, Foy MA. Excision of a bony spike without fixation of the fractured clavicle in a jockey. Clin Orthop 2003;409:275.
115. Manske DJ, Szabo RM. The operative treatment of mid-shaft clavicular non-unions. J Bone Joint Surg Am 1985;67:1367.
116. Marie P, Sainton P. The classic: on hereditary cleido-cranial dysostosis. Clin Orthop 1968;58:5.
117. Marsh HO, Hazarian E. Pseudarthrosis of the clavicle. J Bone Joint Surg 1970;52B:793.
118. Matry C. Fracture de la clavicule gauche au tiers interne: blessure de la veine sous-claviere. Osteosynthese. Bull et Mem Soc Nat Chir 1932;58:75.
119. Matz SO, Welliver PS, Welliver DI. Brachial plexus neuropraxia complicating a comminuted clavicle fracture in a college football player: case report and review of the literature. Am J Sports Med 1989;17:581.
120. Maunoury G. Fracture de la clavicule compliquee de dechireure de la veine sous-claviere: operation. Mort par hemorrhagie et entree de l'air dans les veines. Progres Med (Paris) 1881;10:302.
121. McCandless DN, Mowbray MA. Treatment of displaced fractures of the clavicle: sling versus figure-of-eight bandage. Practitioner 1979;223:266.
122. McKee MD, Wild LM, Schemitsch EH. Midshaft malunions of the clavicle. J Bone Joint Surg 2003;85A:790.
123. Meeks RJ, Riebel GD. Isolated clavicle fracture with associated pneumothorax: a case report. Am J Emerg Med 1991;9:555.
124. Miller DS, Boswick JA Jr. Lesions of the brachial plexus associated with fractures of the clavicle. Clin Orthop 1969;64:144.
125. Miller MR, Ada JR. Injuries to the shoulder girdle. In: Browner BD, Jupiter JB, Levine AM, et al., eds. Skeletal trauma, 1st edition. Philadelphia, PA, E.B. Saunders, 1991:1291.
126. Moore TO. Internal pin fixation for fracture of the clavicle. Am Surg 1951;17:580.
127. Moseley HF. The clavicle: its anatomy and function. Clin Orthop 1968;58:17.
128. Mulder DS, Greenwood FA, Brooks CE. Posttraumatic thoracic outlet syndrome. J Trauma 1973;13:706.
129. Muller ME, Thomas RJ. Treatment of non-union in fractures of long bones. Clin Orthop 1979;138:141.
130. Mullick S. Treatment of mid-clavicular fractures. Lancet 1967; 1:499.
131. Murray G. A method of fixation for fracture of the clavicle. J Bone Joint Surg 1940;22A:616.
132. Naidoo P. Migration of a Kirschner wire from the clavicle into the abdominal aorta. Arch Emerg Med 1991;8:292.
133. Natali J, Maraval M, Kieffer E, et al. Fractures of the clavicle and injuries of the subclavian artery: report of 10 cases. J Cardiovasc Surg (Torino) 1975;16:541.
134. Neer CS. Nonunion of the clavicle. JAMA 1960;172:1006.
135. Neer CS. Fracture of the distal clavicle with detachment of the coracoclavicular ligaments in adults. J Trauma 1963;3:99.
136. Neer CS. Fractures of the distal third of the clavicle. Clin Orthop 1968;58:43.
137. Neer CS. Fractures about the shoulder. In: Rockwood CA Jr., Green DP, eds. Fractures. Philadelphia, PA, J.B. Lippincott Co., 1984:707.
138. Neviaser JS. The treatment of fractures of the clavicle. Surg Clin North Am 1963;43:1555.
139. Neviaser JS. Injuries of the clavicle and its articulations. Orthop Clin North Am 1980;11:233.
140. Neviaser RJ. Injuries to the clavicle and acromioclavicular joint. Orthop Clin North Am 1987;18:433.
141. Neviaser RJ, Neviaser JS, Neviaser TJ. A simple technique for internal fixation of the clavicle: a long-term evaluation. Clin Orthop 1975;109:103.
142. Nicoll EA. Miners and mannequins. J Bone Joint Surg 1954; 36B:171.
143. Nordqvist A, Petersson C. The incidence of fractures of the clavicle. Clin Orthop 1994;300:127.
144. Nordqvist A, Petersson CJ. Shoulder injuries common in alcoholics. An analysis of 413 injuries. Acta Orthop Scand 1996; 67:364.
145. Nordqvist A, Petersson C, Redlund-Johnell I. The natural course of lateral clavicle fracture: 15 (11–21) year follow-up of 110 cases. Acta Orthop Scand 1993;64:87.
146. Nordqvist A, Petersson CJ, Redlund-Johnell I. Mid-clavicle fractures in adults: end result study after conservative treatment. J Orthop Trauma 1998;12:572.
147. Nordqvist A, Redlund-Johnell I, vonScheele A, et al. Shortening of clavicle after fracture. Incidence and clinical significance, a 5-year follow-up of 85 patients. Acta Orthop Scand 1997;68:349.
148. Norrell H Jr, Llewellyn RC. Migration of a threaded Steinmann pin from an acromioclavicular joint into the spinal canal. J Bone Joint Surg 1965;47A:1024.
149. Nowak J, Mallmin H, Larsson S. The aetiology and epidemiology of clavicular fractures. A prospective study during a two-year period in Uppsala, Sweden. Injury 2000;31:353.
150. Nowak J, Stalberg E, Larsson S. Good reduction of paresthesia and pain after excision of excessive callus formation in patients with malunited clavicular fractures. Scand J Surg 2002;91:369.
151. Ogden JA, Conlogue GJ, Bronson ML. Radiology of postnatal skeletal development III. The clavicle. Skeletal Radiol 1979; 4:196.
152. Olsen BO, Vaesel MT, Sojbjerg JO. Treatment of midshaft clavicular nonunion with plate fixation and autologous bone grafting. J Shoulder Elbow Surg 1995;4:337.
153. Oppenheim WL, Davis A, Growdon WA, et al. Clavicle fractures in the newborn. Clin Orthop 1990;250:176.
154. Oreck SLB, Burgess A, Levine A. Traumatic lateral displacement of the scapula: a radiographic sign of neurovascular disruption. J Bone Joint Surg 1984;66A:758.
154a. Oroko PK, Buchan M, Winkler A, et al. Does shortening matter after clavicular fractures? Bull Hosp Jt Dis 1999;58(1):6–8.
155. Oxnard CE. The functional morphology of the primate shoulder as revealed by comparative anatomical, osteometric, and discrimination function techniques. Am J Phys Anthropol 1967; 26:219.
156. Oxnard CE. The architecture of the shoulder in some mammals. J Morphol 1968;126:249.

157. Packer BD. Conservative treatment of fracture of the clavicle. J Bone Joint Surg 1944;26B:770.

158. Parkes JC, Deland JT. A three-part distal clavicle fracture. J Trauma 1983;23:437.

159. Penn I. The vascular complications of fractures of the clavicle. J Trauma 1964;4:819.

160. Perry BF. An improved clavicle pin. Am J Surg 1966;112:143.

161. Peters G, Bosch U, Tscherne H. Die verlangerungsosteotomie bei fehlverheilter kalvikulafractur. Unfallchirurg 1997;100:270.

162. Pipkin G. Tardy shoulder hand syndrome following united fracture of the clavicle. Mo Med 1951;48:643.

163. Piterman L. The fractured clavicle. Aust Fam Physician 1982;11:614.

164. Poigenfurst J, Rappold G, Fischer W. Plating of fresh clavicular fractures: results of 122 operations. Injury 1992;23:237.

165. Prime HT, Doig SG, Hooper JC. Retrosternal dislocation of the clavicle: a case report. Am J Sports Med 1991;19:92.

166. Pyper JB. Non-union of fractures of the clavicle. Injury 1977;9:268.

167. Quesada F. Technique for the roentgen diagnosis of fractures of the clavicle. Surg Gynecol Obstet 1926;42:424.

168. Quigley TB. The management of simple fractures of the clavicle. N Engl J Med 1950;243:286.

169. Redmond AD. Letter to the editor. Injury 1982;13:352.

170. Reichenbacher D, Siebler G. Early post-traumatic plexus lesions: a rare complication after clavicle fractures. Unfallchirurg 1987;13:91.

171. Reimer BL, Butterfield SL, Daffner RH, et al. The abduction lordotic view of the clavicle: a new technique for radiographic visualization. J Orthop Trauma 1991;5:392.

172. Rikli DR, Regazzoni P, Renner N. The unstable shoulder girdle: early functional treatment utilizing open reduction and internal fixation. J Orthop Trauma 1995;9:93.

173. Ring D, Jupiter JB. Ununited fractures of the clavicle: treatment with a corticocancellous bone graft and plate fixation. Tech Hand Upper Extr Surg 1999;3(3):193–196.

174. Ring D, Barrick WT, Jupiter JB. Recalcitrant nonunion. Clin Orthop 1997;340:181.

175. Robinson CM. Fractures of the clavicle in the adult. J Bone Joint Surg 1998;80B:476.

176. Rockwood CA. Fractures and dislocations of the ends of the clavicle, scapula, and glenohumeral joint. In: Rockwood CA, Wilkins KE, King RE, eds. Fractures in children. Philadelphia, PA, J. B. Lippincott, 1984:624.

177. Rockwood CA Jr. Fractures of the outer clavicle in children and adults. J Bone Joint Surg 1982;64B:642.

178. Rockwood CA, Williams GR, Young DC. Disorders of the acromioclavicular joint. In: Rockwood CA, Matsen FA, eds. The shoulder. Second edition. Philadelphia, PA, WB Saunders, 1998:483.

179. Rokito AS, Zuckerman JD, Shaari JM, et al. A comparison of nonoperative and operative treatment of type II distal clavicle fractures. Bull Hosp Jt Dis 2002–2003;61:32.

180. Rowe CR. An atlas of anatomy and treatment of midclavicular fractures. Clin Orthop 1968;58:29.

181. Rubenstein JD, Ebraheim NA, Kellam JF. Traumatic scapulothoracic dissociation. Radiology 1985;157:297.

182. Rumball KM, Da Silva VF, Preston DN, et al. Brachial-plexus injury after clavicular fracture: a case report and literature review. Can J Surg 1991;34:264.

183. Rush LV, Rush HL. Technique of longitudinal pin fixation in fractures of the clavicle and jaw. Miss Doct 1949;27:332.

184. Sadiq S, Doyle J. Double plating technique for clavicle fractures, non-union/malunion. Injury 1999;30:559.

185. Sakellarides H. Pseudarthrosis of the clavicle: a report of twenty cases. J Bone Joint Surg 1961;43A:130.

186. Sankarankutty M, Turner BW. Fractures of the clavicle. Injury 1975;7:101.

187. Sayre LA. A simple dressing for fracture of the clavicle. Am Pract 1871;4:1.

188. Schwarz N, Hocker K. Osteosynthesis of irreducible fractures of the clavicle with 2.7 millimeter ASIF plates. J Trauma 1992; 33:179.

189. Seddon HJ. Nerve lesions complicating certain closed bone injuries. JAMA 1947;135:691.

190. Shen WJ, Liu TJ, Shen YS. Plate fixation of fresh displaced midshaft clavicle fractures. Injury 1999;30:497.

191. Silloway KA, McLaughlin RE, Edlich RF. Clavicular fractures and acromioclavicular joint injuries in lacrosse: preventable injuries. J Emerg Med 1985;3:117.

192. Simpson NS, Jupiter JB. Clavicular nonunion and malunion: evaluation and surgical management. J Am Acad Orthop Surg 1996;4:1.

193. Spar I. Total claviculectomy for pathological fractures. Clin Orthop 1977;129:236.

194. Stanley D, Norris SH. Recovery following fractures of the clavicle treated conservatively. Injury 1988;19:162.

195. Storen H. Old clavicular pseudarthrosis with late appearing neuralgias and vasomotoric disturbances cured by operation. Acta Chir Scand 1946;94:187.

196. Sturm JT, Strate RG, Mowlem A, et al. Blunt trauma to the subclavian artery. Surg Gynecol Obstet 1974;138:915.

197. Taylor AR. Some observations on fractures of the clavicle. Proc R Soc Med 1969;62:33.

198. Taylor AR. Non-union of fractures of the clavicle: a review of thirty-one cases. J Bone Joint Surg 1974;51B:568.

199. Thompson AG, Batten RL. The application of rigid internal fixation to the treatment of non-union and delayed union using the AO technique. Injury 1977;8:188.

200. Tregonning GM, McNab I. Post-traumatic pseudarthrosis of the clavicle. J Bone Joint Surg 1976;58B:264.

201. Trynin AH. The Bohler clavicular splint in the treatment of clavicular injuries. J Bone Joint Surg 1937;19:417.

202. Tse DH, Slabaugh PB, Carlson PA. Injury to the axillary artery by a closed fracture of the clavicle. J Bone Joint Surg Am 1980; 62:1372.

203. van Noort A, te Slaa RL, Marti RK, et al. The floating shoulder. A multicentre study. J Bone Joint Surg Br 2001;83B:795.

204. Van Vlack HG. Comminuted fracture of the clavicle with pressure on brachial plexus. J Bone Joint Surg 1940;22A:446.

205. Webber MCB, Haines JF. The treatment of lateral clavicle fractures. Injury 2000;31:175.

206. Weinberg B, Seife B, Alonso P. The apical oblique view of the clavicle: its usefulness in neonatal and childhood trauma. Skeletal Radiol 1991;20:201.

207. Weiner DS, O'Dell HW. Fractures of the first rib associated with injuries to the clavicle. J Trauma 1969;9:412.

208. White RR, Anson PS, Kristiansen T. Adult clavicle fractures: relationship between mechanism of injury and healing. Orthop Trans 1989;13:514.

209. Wick M, Muller EJ, Kollig E, et al. Midshaft fractures of the clavicle with a shortening of more than 2 cm predispose to nonunion. Arch Orthop Trauma Surg 2001;121:207.

210. Wilkins RM, Johnson RM. Ununited fractures of the clavicle. J Bone Joint Surg Am 1983;65:774.

211. Williams GR, Naranja J, Klimkiewicz J, et al. The floating shoulder: a biomechanical basis for classification and management. J Bone Joint Surg Am 2001;83A:1182.

212. Wood VE. The results of total claviculectomy. Clin Orthop 1986;207:186.

213. Wu CC, Shih CH, Chen WJ. Treatment of clavicular aseptic nonunion: comparison of plating and intramedullary nailing techniques. J Trauma 1998;45:512.

214. Yates AG. Complications of fractures of the clavicle. Injury 1976;7:189.

215. Yates AG, Guest D. Cerebral embolism due to an ununited fracture of the clavicle and subclavian thrombosis. Lancet 1928; 2:225.

216. Zaslav KR, Ray S, Neer CS 2nd. Conservative management of a displaced medial clavicular physeal injury in an adolescent male. Am J Sports Med 1989;17:833.

217. Zenni EJ Jr, Krieg JK, Rosen MJ. Open reduction and internal fixation of clavicular fractures. J Bone Joint Surg Am 1981; 63:147.

Acromioclavicular Joint: Difficult Problems and Revision Surgery

Young W. Kwon   *Joseph P. Iannotti*

INTRODUCTION

The acromioclavicular (AC) joint is one of the most commonly injured structures in the human body. Because of its subcutaneous location, the AC joint is highly susceptible to injury after direct trauma to the shoulder girdle. In addition, because of the repetitive nature of shoulder motion and the large amount of force that must transmit across a relatively small surface area, this structure is also prone to various degenerative conditions. The majority of AC joint pathology can be successfully treated without a surgical intervention. If, however, a surgical intervention is warranted, there are numerous procedures, both historic and contemporary, that can be used to treat pathologic conditions about the AC joint.

For patients with a difficult problem or condition that requires a revision surgery, understanding the nuances of a single pathology or a single procedure is of limited benefit. Rather, identifying the underlying pathology and restoring the physiologic biomechanical properties of the joint will be of greater value in successfully treating these patients. As such, instead of providing a detailed description of any single procedure, this chapter will focus on providing a general guideline in evaluating and treating patients with a complex AC joint pathology.

ANATOMY AND BIOMECHANICS

The AC joint is located between the lateral end of the clavicle and the medial aspect of the anterior acromion. Its articular surface is initially composed of hyaline cartilage, which subsequently changes to fibrocartilage during early adulthood.[88] The joint space is filled with fibrocartilaginous disks. These disks may be complete or meniscoid (i.e., partial). Overall size and dimensions of the meniscus can be quite variable.[30] Similar to the knee, this meniscus is generally believed to possess both a stabilizing and a protective role for the joint. However, for unknown reasons, the meniscus degenerates rapidly during early adulthood to become a nondistinct structure by the fourth decade.[30,70,73] As such, its exact role remains largely speculative.

Stability of the AC joint is provided by both dynamic and static restraints. Dynamic stabilization arises from

Y. W. Kwon: Assistant Professor, Department of Orthopedic Surgery, NYU-Hospital for Joint Disease, New York, New York.

J. P. Iannotti: Professor and Chairman, Department of Orthopedic Surgery, The Cleveland Clinic Foundation, Cleveland, Ohio.

various superficial muscles about the shoulder girdle. For example, the anterior deltoid muscle originates in part from the lateral end of the clavicle and inserts onto the deltoid tuberosity on the humerus. Thus, during its contraction, the generated force will tend to depress the clavicle against the acromion and provide a stabilizing effect on the AC joint. Similar stabilizing force is also generated from contractions of the middle deltoid and trapezius muscles.

Static stabilizers of the joint include the AC ligaments and coracoclavicular ligaments. The AC ligaments are confluent thickenings within the joint capsule and are named according to their location. These ligaments are thought to be the primary stabilizers along the anterior-posterior direction.[29,36,50] As such, significant amounts of translation may be observed in the anteroposterior direction even after isolated damage to the AC ligaments.[29] For small displacements, these ligaments can also provide significant stability in the superoinferior direction. For larger displacements in the superoinferior direction, however, the majority of the stability is provided by the coracoclavicular ligaments.[36] The coracoclavicular ligaments are composed of two primary structures. They are the conoid (medial) and trapezoid (lateral) ligaments, named after their approximate geometric shape. These ligaments arise from the coracoid process and attach onto the undersurface of the distal clavicle just medial to the joint. They span the coracoclavicular distance of approximately 13 mm.[11,18] Although the AC and coracoclavicular ligaments each possess a role as a primary stabilizer along a particular direction, in the absence of one, the other can compensate to act as the primary stabilizer for all directions.[36]

Both the scapulothoracic and the glenohumeral motion contribute to the overall movement of the upper extremity. Relative contributions of each can vary depending on the total arc of arm motion.[59] Primary motion of the clavicle during arm elevation is rotation around its long axis. Although overall rotation may reach up to 45 degrees, the majority of this motion appears to take place at the sternoclavicular joint rather than at the AC joint.[45] Physiologically, the clavicle and scapula move as a single unit. As such, rotation at the AC joint is typically limited to only 5 to 8 degrees.[26] Thus, full range of arm motion should be possible with minimal to no motion across the AC joint.[25,48,72]

PATHOLOGY

Acute Injuries of the Acromioclavicular Joint

Most acute injuries to the AC joint occur as a result of direct trauma. Because of the intrinsic stability of the sternoclavicular joint, most of the energy generated by an impact appears to be absorbed by the AC joint.[12] A common cause of AC joint injury is a fall onto the shoulder with the arm in an adducted position, because this force will displace the acromion inferiorly. In addition, because of its subcutaneous location, the AC joint is often a primary target of an external blow. As expected, the magnitude and location of the impact will determine the severity of the injury. Initially, the resulting force is absorbed by the AC ligaments. With additional force, the AC ligaments rupture and the coracoclavicular ligaments are damaged. If the force is severe enough, the deltotrapezial fascia and the coracoclavicular ligaments can also be ruptured. In such cases, the upper extremity will have lost its suspensory support from the clavicle and therefore sag inferiorly relative to the clavicle.

This sequence of injury progression has been summarized in an AC joint dislocation classification system. Originally proposed by Allman and Tossy et al., and subsequently modified by Rockwood et al., this system categorizes the severity of the injury on the basis of the damaged anatomic stabilizers and degree of overall joint displacement.[4,72,86] Type I injury describes a sprain of the AC ligaments with other intact stabilizers. Type II injury describes a rupture of the AC ligaments with a sprain of the coracoclavicular ligaments and intact deltotrapezial fascia. Type III injury signifies a rupture of both the AC and the coracoclavicular ligaments with an additional injury to the deltotrapezial fascia. As such, there is a complete dislocation of the AC joint with an inferior displacement of the acromion relative to the clavicle. In types IV, V, and VI injuries, all of the stabilizing structures about the AC joint are disrupted and there is a gross dislocation of the joint. Type IV injury is associated with a severe posterior displacement of the clavicle, often piercing into or through the trapezius muscle. In type V injury, there is a gross (i.e., more than 100% compared with the normal shoulder) inferior displacement of the acromion relative to the clavicle. In type VI injury, the clavicle is actually displaced inferiorly relative to the acromion and often locked under coracoid process. The overall classification system is summarized in Figure 20-1.

Degenerative Conditions of the Acromioclavicular Joint

Because of its small dimensions, the relative amount of force transmitted across the AC joint is quite large. As the intra-articular meniscus tends to become nondistinct by the fourth decade of life, its ability to provide protection for the articular surface is limited.[30,70,73] Thus, the AC joint is quite susceptible to degenerative changes. Systemic inflammatory diseases (e.g., rheumatoid arthritis, gout, or pseudogout), trauma, and previous operative procedures can also increase the likelihood of symptomatic AC joint degeneration. Although the true incidence of AC joint arthritis is unknown, it is generally believed to be the most common cause of AC joint pain.[43] According to

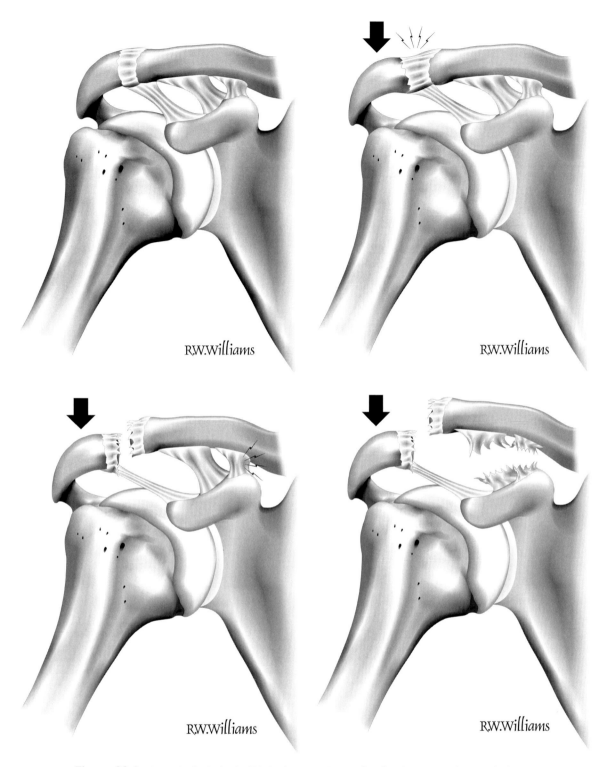

Figure 20-1   Acromioclavicular (AC) joint ligament injury classification system (see text). (Reproduced with permission from Rockwood CA, Williams GR, Young DC. Disorders of the acromioclavicular joint. In: Rockwood CA, Matsen FA, eds. The shoulder. Philadelphia: WB Saunders, 1998:445.) (*continued*)

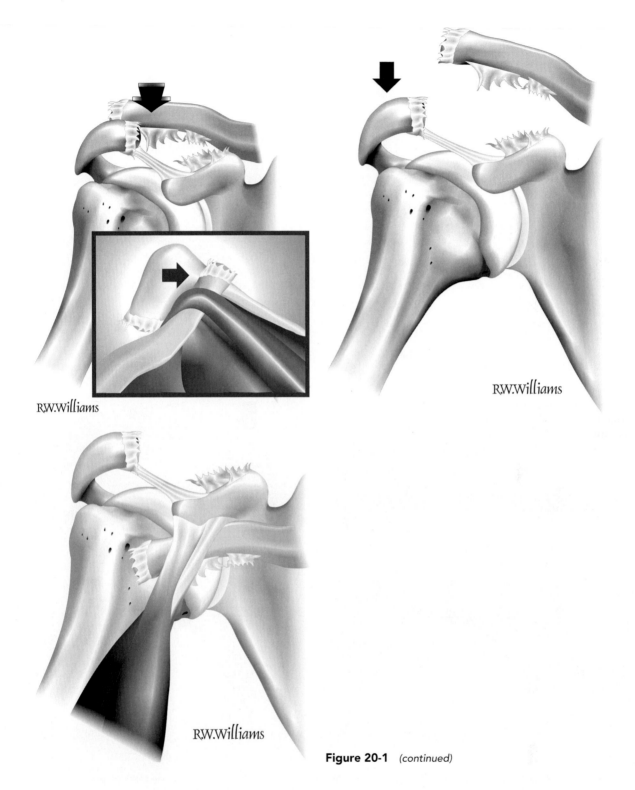

Figure 20-1 *(continued)*

one study, radiographic evidence of AC joint arthritis can be found in up to 57% of elderly patients, with 42% to 45% of these patients having associated joint tenderness.[44] In addition, up to 70% of patients with documented arthritis in other joints may also have tenderness in one or both AC joints.[92]

It is important to distinguish radiographic evidence of arthritis from the clinical symptomatic entity, because many patients with significant radiographic AC joint changes may be asymptomatic.[63,77] In one study, for example, up to 93% of patients with no shoulder symptoms had magnetic resonance imaging (MRI) findings consistent with AC joint osteoarthritis.[77] In addition, other pathologic changes about the shoulder girdle may coexist with symptomatic AC joint arthritis. In one series of patients, for example, more than 97% of patients with symptomatic AC joint degeneration had other coexisting shoulder pathology.[24]

An infrequent, but increasingly recognized, degenerative clinical entity of the AC joint is distal clavicle osteolysis. This condition is believed to be increasing in frequency because of the increasing emphasis by professional and recreational athletes on weight training. Histologic features of the condition include subchondral cysts, demineralization, and microscopic fractures.[62] These observations have led to the hypothesis that distal clavicle osteolysis is a result of repetitive microtrauma to the AC joint leading to fatigue failure and bone resorption.[23,24,62]

EVALUATION—GENERAL GUIDELINES

Clinical Evaluation

Acromioclavicular joint symptoms may present as an isolated pathology or in conjunction with other conditions about the shoulder girdle. Therefore, a thorough history and examination are necessary to identify the exact cause(s) of symptoms. For acute injuries, the history may be clear and simple to elucidate. For chronic cases or degenerative conditions, the history may be more subtle. In these patients, the duration and nature of the symptoms should be addressed. Notable activities that can initiate or exacerbate the symptoms as well as any recent change in the level or type of activities should be elicited. Prior trauma and prior treatments, including surgical interventions, should also be discussed, and the appropriate documents must be reviewed.

A careful evaluation of the cervical spine should accompany the physical examination, because radicular symptoms may mimic vague AC joint pathology.[38] Inspection may demonstrate prominence, and palpation may elicit crepitus or tenderness. Reproduction of the patient's usual symptoms with AC joint palpation is the most important finding on physical examination. Isolated pathology of the AC joint should not typically inhibit shoulder motion. Therefore, a restricted motion in a setting other than recent trauma may suggest other pathology about the shoulder girdle. Provocative maneuvers such as cross-body adduction with the arm elevated at 90 degrees or internal rotation of the arm reaching to the lumbar spine may elicit significant pain in the AC joint. The specificity of these maneuvers for AC joint pathology has not been validated in the literature. Thus, positive findings on these maneuvers suggest, but do not confirm AC joint pathology. Instability of the AC joint is difficult to elicit. Manual manipulation can be performed to trans-late the distal clavicle away from the acromion. A positive finding would reproduce the abnormal translation, in either superoinferior or anteroposterior direction, with characteristic pain. Unfortunately, correlation of this maneuver to the actual pathology has not been validated in the literature.

For patients with an unclear source of pathology, a diagnostic injection with a short-acting anesthetic agent can be very useful. Elimination of symptoms with an accurately placed injection can confirm the source of pain.[15,34] In addition to its diagnostic utility, an injection can also provide information regarding the potential benefit of a surgical intervention. For example, in patients with a degenerative joint, pain relief after an injection is typically considered to be the best prognostic factor for success after a distal clavicle excision.[99] For an injection to be informative, however, a patient must be able to consistently reproduce the symptoms. Furthermore, the injection must be placed accurately within the joint. According to a cadaveric study, AC joint injection by an orthopedic surgeon was successful in only 67% of the cases.[68] Inaccurate placement of the anesthetic agent into the subacromial space can actually lead to a false-positive diagnosis.

Radiographic Studies

Routine radiographs of the shoulder are inadequate for the examination of the AC joint. Because of its small size, these radiographs will typically "overpenetrate" the AC joint and fail to reveal any details. For most patients, approximately 50% of the voltage used for shoulder radiographs should be used when examining the AC joint. In addition, routine shoulder radiographs show an overlap of the AC joint against the scapula, which can prohibit detailed examination of the joint. For an acceptable evaluation, approximately 10 to 15 degrees of cephalic tilt should be used to project the x-ray beam.[100] This tilt will allow isolated visualization of the AC joint without a bony background. To evaluate subtle changes, a similar tilt can be used to project an x-ray beam across both AC joints onto a single wide cassette.[72] This view can allow comparison of the affected joint against the contralateral AC joint. In addition to these anteroposterior views, a lateral view of the AC joint should also be obtained and evaluated.[91]

Stress views of the AC joint can be helpful for a certain population of patients whose history and examination suggest instability. Routine use of stress views, however, is not recommended.[17] For examination of instability in the superior inferior direction, an anteroposterior radiograph with a cephalic tilted beam is obtained with approximately 10 to 15 pounds of weight that is either held by or tied to the wrist of the patient.[78] When examining instability in the anteroposterior direction, an axillary lateral view can be obtained with either a posteriorly directed force to the

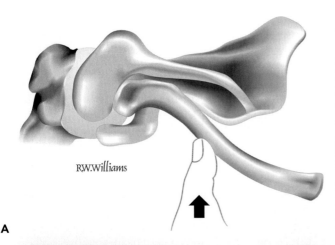

A

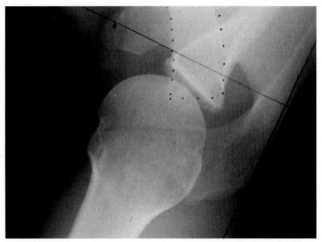

B

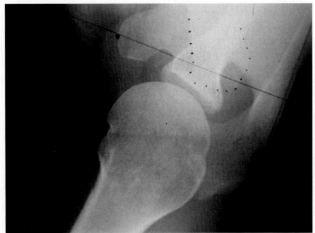

C

Figure 20-2   Stress radiographs for examination of the anterior-posterior instability. As illustrated in the schematic drawing (A), axillary lateral radiographs are obtained before (B) and after (C) a posteriorly directed force is applied to the midshaft of the clavicle. Alternatively, the radiographs may be obtained before and after an anteriorly directed force is applied to the acromion.

clavicle or an anteriorly directed force on the acromion.[16] This view is illustrated in Figure 20-2. An alternative is a scapula lateral view with the patient voluntarily protracting the affected shoulder forward, as this maneuver may displace the scapula anteriorly relative to the clavicle.[1,2,98] Typically, stress views are also obtained on the contralateral shoulder for comparison.

Other Studies

Routine use of other modalities for the evaluation of the AC joint is usually not necessary. In certain select cases, however, other studies can provide significant additional information. Computed tomography images can reveal a more detailed anatomy of the joint and exhibit subtle changes in the bony architecture. MRI can provide information regarding the soft tissues about the joint. Interpretation of the MRI should be performed with caution, however, because 75% to 93% of asymptomatic patients can exhibit signal changes consistent with arthritis.[63,77] For symptomatic patients whose radiographs are unremarkable, a technetium bone scan can reveal changes in the AC joint.[23] This can be especially useful in cases where distal

clavicle osteolysis is suspected in its early phase but the radiographs are inconclusive. Finally, various authors have shown the utility of ultrasonography in the evaluation of AC joint instability.[23,74,79] The dynamic nature of this study provides a unique perspective in assessing instability. However, because of its inherent limitations, such as user dependency, a routine use of ultrasonography to assess the AC joint has not gained wide popularity.

CONTROVERSIAL ACROMIOCLAVICULAR JOINT TREATMENT ISSUES

Surgical Versus Nonsurgical Treatment for Acute Dislocations

A general consensus seems to exist among orthopedic surgeons in treating acute type I and II AC joint dislocations. Typically, nonsurgical treatment is favored for acute cases, while surgical intervention is reserved for chronic, symptomatic patients.[4,28,72,90] General consensus also exists for the treatment of acute AC joint dislocation types

IV, V, and VI. For these patients, elective surgical treatments are typically recommended.[28,37,42,65,69,72] Open reduction and stabilization of the joint, with the repair of delto-trapezial fascia as needed, are associated with an improved clinical outcome for such cases.

For treatment of acute type III AC joint dislocations, however, much controversy still exists. As opposed to types IV, V, or VI, the AC joint in type III dislocation can, in theory, be anatomically reduced without an open reduction. Therefore, it has the potential for satisfactory healing without surgical intervention. Studies have supported this hypothesis, because patients treated without surgery have reported satisfactory outcomes.[5,8,39,82,84,97] Successful nonoperative methods of treatment for acute AC joint dislocations include adhesive strapping, sling and bandage, harness, figure-of-eight bandage, and casts. Still, the key issue remains: do patients with a surgical intervention have improved outcomes that would warrant the risks of an operative intervention?

Many recent studies seem to suggest that patients treated nonoperatively for type III AC joint separations have equivalent clinical outcome when compared with those treated surgically. In a prospective randomized study, patients treated for symptomatic relief had similar outcomes as those treated with an open reduction and internal fixation with a coracoclavicular screw.[8] In another prospective randomized study, patients treated without an operation reported similar outcome as those treated with an open reduction, repair of the ligaments, and fixation of the joint with Kirschner wires.[52] These authors found an increased rate of minor complications in patients who were treated operatively and thus recommended nonoperative treatment for most patients with acute type III AC joint dislocations. Recent surveys of orthopedic surgeons support this finding, as surgeons who participated in the survey overwhelmingly preferred nonoperative treatment.[28,67] Therefore, the current trend seems to favor nonoperative treatment for the type III acute AC joint separations in most patients.

For a certain select subset of the population, however, this general trend may not be applicable. For younger patients who participate in heavy labor or overhead athletic activities (i.e., baseball pitchers), many surgeons still consider open reduction and internal fixation as the primary mode of treatment.[8,28,67,72] It is possible that patients who participate in such activities endure increased forces across the AC joint and, thus, are more likely to have a poor outcome without surgical stabilization. In addition, in one series of patients, those who received early surgical repair (less than 3 months) fared better than those who received late surgical intervention.[94] Therefore, these patients may not benefit from a "wait-and-see" approach, where an operative intervention is recommended only to those patients whose symptoms persist. At this time, there is not enough scientific evidence to guide the treating surgeon, and the treatment of acute type III AC joint dislocations for this subset of patients still remains controversial.

Role of Acromioclavicular Joint "Co-planing"

Acromioclavicular joint arthrosis can lead to the formation of circumferential bony overgrowth on the distal clavicle. Bony spurs on the inferior surface of the distal clavicle as well as on the anterior medial aspect of the acromion may, in turn, be partially or predominantly responsible for the impingement on the rotator cuff tendons.[49,71] For symptomatic patients who are not responsive to nonoperative therapy, the impinging structures should be excised. This typically includes the anterior undersurface of the acromion as well as the inferior aspect of the distal clavicle (co-planing). Co-planing the distal clavicle can be performed as an open procedure or under arthroscopic visualization. Typically, bone from the undersurface of the distal clavicle is resected until it is co-planar or "flush" with the undersurface of the anterior acromion.

There is no clear evidence to support the hypothesis that the patients who undergo co-planing of the distal clavicle have superior results when compared with those patients who undergo isolated acromioplasty. However, in a minimum of 25 months follow-up, patients who underwent co-planing of the distal clavicle or partial resection of the AC joint did not exhibit increased AC joint symptoms.[9] Similar results were also reported in another series of patients who underwent distal clavicle co-planing; and show no increased rate of AC joint instability or pain at an average follow-up of four years.[21] Thus, appropriately performed co-planing of the distal clavicle does not seem to cause subsequent AC joint symptoms. Co-planing of the distal clavicle seems to be a safe procedure that can potentially benefit a certain population of patients.

Rather than co-planing, the decision may also be made to perform distal clavicle excision. For patients who experience impingement symptoms in addition to AC joint arthrosis, partial acromioplasty and distal clavicle excision performed in a single operative setting seem to be an excellent treatment option.[53,57] In fact, some have advocated that acromioplasty should be performed with routine excision of the distal clavicle for the treatment of rotator cuff impingement syndrome.[64] At this time, however, this recommendation has not gained wide popularity, because patients may be experiencing pain from impingement of the soft tissues or from arthritic changes within the AC joint. Accurate preoperative examination, including an injection test to determine the source of the pain, should guide the decision to perform excision or co-planing of the distal clavicle.

Ideal Amount of Bone Removal for Distal Clavicle Resection

It is generally believed that the distal clavicle resection should be performed until the bone can no longer contact the medial aspect of the acromion during a cross-body adduction maneuver. Various authors have suggested that this objective can be achieved after resection of only 5 to 6 mm

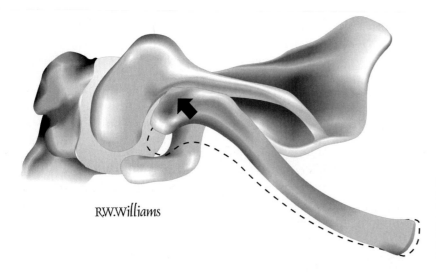

R.W.Williams

Figure 20-3 Possible mechanism of persistent shoulder pain after excessive distal clavicle resection. Significant AC joint instability in the anterior-posterior direction allows the posterior lateral aspect of the distal clavicle to abut against the scapular spine or posterior medial aspect of the acromion.

of bone from the distal clavicle.[19,35] Intraoperatively, the cross-body adduction maneuver can be performed passively by the surgeon or actively by the patient if local anesthesia is used.[10] On the other hand, excessive resection of the distal clavicle may lead to permanent joint instability. Instability in the anterior posterior direction can lead to excessive posterior translation of the distal clavicle to the point of allowing the bone to abut against the medial acromion or the scapular spine (Fig. 20-3). As such, the degree of instability seems to be directly correlated to the severity of the pain experienced by the patient.[16] Several studies have shown that the primary restraint against posterior displacement of the distal clavicle is provided by the posterior and superior AC ligaments.[36,50] Therefore, regardless of the amount of bony resection, preservation of these ligaments will likely decrease the likelihood of persistent and symptomatic joint instability.

As summarized by Shaffer,[76] the amount of resected bone has ranged between 4 to 25 mm among various reports. Despite this variability in the amount of resected bone, most studies report a successful clinical outcome. In addition, a clinical correlation between the amount of resected bone and the eventual outcome has not been clearly documented. Most surgeons seem to use 10 mm as a reasonable goal, because patients who underwent resection of distal clavicle in excess of 10 mm may be more likely to experience persistent shoulder pain.[31,76]

REVISION AND DIFFICULT ACROMIOCLAVICULAR JOINT SURGERY

Soft Tissue Coverage

Because of the shoulder's excellent blood supply, wound healing is generally not a significant problem after shoulder surgery. As such, available literature on this topic is limited. For patients with multiple prior surgeries, the loss of soft tissue may present a significant concern for wound coverage. In a small series of patients, Tarar and Quaba[83] used a local adipofascial turnover flap to cover the soft tissue defect after an open reduction and internal fixation of the clavicle. Case reports describing the use of the clavicular head of the pectoralis major muscle for coverage of the AC joint are also available in the literature.[85,96] As shown in Figure 20-4, this rotational muscle flap's approximate size and consistent anatomy suggest that it may be well suited for soft tissue coverage of the distal clavicle and AC joint.[96] Nevertheless, specific indications for the use of any soft tissue flap around the shoulder girdle have yet to be formulated.

Acromioclavicular Joint Instability in the Superior Inferior Direction Without Bone Loss

Operative interventions for these injuries attempt to reproduce, either statically or dynamically, the anatomic restraints that stabilize the AC joint. As such, the AC joint can be reapproximated using one of three stabilization techniques: (a) primary fixation across the joint; (b) secondary stabilization of the joint by recreating the anatomic linkage between the distal clavicle and the coracoid process; or (c) dynamic stabilization of the joint by creating an inferiorly directed force on the distal clavicle. Specifics of these procedures have been summarized elsewhere.[51,67,72] These three methods are not mutually exclusive, as they may be combined in a single operative setting to produce a final construct with superior mechanical stability.

Our stabilization procedure of choice is a transfer of the coracoacromial ligament to the distal clavicle. This construct is then augmented with a suture band between the coracoid process and the distal clavicle. Currently we

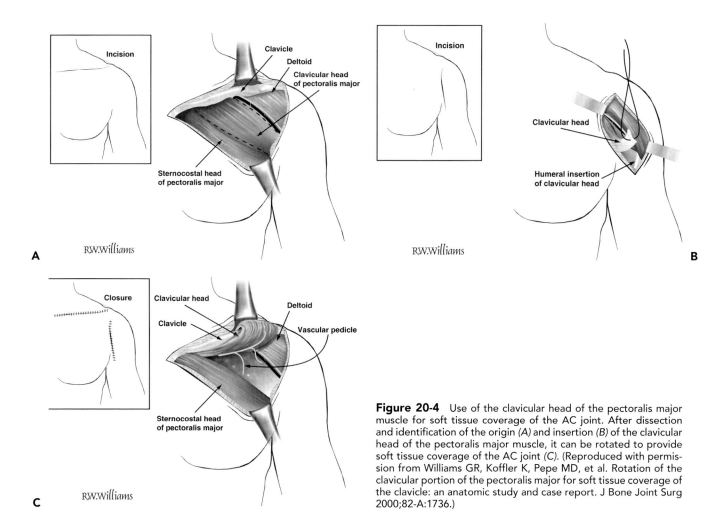

Figure 20-4 Use of the clavicular head of the pectoralis major muscle for soft tissue coverage of the AC joint. After dissection and identification of the origin (A) and insertion (B) of the clavicular head of the pectoralis major muscle, it can be rotated to provide soft tissue coverage of the AC joint (C). (Reproduced with permission from Williams GR, Koffler K, Pepe MD, et al. Rotation of the clavicular portion of the pectoralis major for soft tissue coverage of the clavicle: an anatomic study and case report. J Bone Joint Surg 2000;82-A:1736.)

prefer to use two strands of No. 2 fiberwire (Arthrex, Naples, FL). Typically, a wafer of bone from the acromion is transferred with the coracoacromial ligament to enhance subsequent healing. Care is taken to preserve and isolate the entire coracoacromial ligament. In patients with ligaments of insufficient length, however, releasing the anterolateral fasciculus of the ligament from the lateral waist of the coracoid process can provide additional length.[22,72] The released fasciculus is then sutured back onto the remaining ligament for additional strength. If the remaining coracoclavicular ligament is substantial and of adequate length, it can be repaired and used as a secondary stabilization construct in addition to the coracoclavicular suture band.

If the coracoacromial ligament is inadequate for a transfer, our procedure of choice is to fix the distal clavicle to the coracoid process with a screw.[18] This is then augmented with a semitendinosus autograft or allograft that is looped around the clavicle and the coracoid process.[46] The procedure is carried out after an open exploration and manual reduction, because percutaneous placement of this screw

has been associated with a high rate of technical failures.[87] In addition, soft tissues along the anticipated path of the screw are carefully dissected before its insertion. In this fashion, drilling, insertion of the depth gauge, and insertion of the screw can all be performed under direct visualization.

Postoperatively, patients are protected in a sling for 4 to 6 weeks. During this period, they are encouraged to perform gentle passive range-of-motion exercises and nonstrenuous activities at waist level. They are prohibited, however, from performing activities that stress the AC joint such as reaching, pushing, and pulling. Active range-of-motion exercises are then started with a progressive increase in their activity level. Strengthening exercises begin at approximately 8 weeks after the surgery, and contact sports are allowed between 16 and 20 weeks. Rehabilitation for patients with a revision surgery or a semitendinosus tendon loop is generally more protracted. As such, they may be placed in a more robust form of immobilization such as a Southern California Orthopaedic Institute brace (dj Orthopedics, LLC, Vista, CA) or a similar device.

The subsequent rehabilitation protocol sequence is similar to that described previously.

Acromioclavicular Joint Instability in the Anterior Posterior Direction Without Bone Loss

Acromioclavicular joint instability in the anteroposterior direction is often difficult to manage. Despite intact coracoclavicular ligaments and stability in the superior inferior direction, isolated damage to the AC ligaments may still lead to excessive distal clavicle motion in the anterior posterior direction.[29,50] This instability, in turn, can be associated with significant shoulder pain and disability.[16,33] Unfortunately, there are no clinical outcome studies addressing this specific pathology. The senior author has used various procedures to treat this condition and achieved mixed success. In general, procedures that eliminate, rather than stabilize, motion at the AC joint seem to be associated with improved outcomes. As such, our procedure of choice is coracoclavicular arthrodesis. Typically, the distal clavicle is rigidly fixed to the coracoid process with a screw.[18] This is followed by placing bone graft in the coracoclavicular interval. Postoperatively, the rehabilitation protocol for these patients is protracted with immobilization in a Southern California Orthopaedic Institute brace or a similar type of brace for 4 to 6 weeks. The remainder of the rehabilitation protocol is similar to that described previously.

Acromioclavicular Joint Instability with Bone Loss

Without sufficient bone, AC joint instability can be quite difficult to manage. In some cases, the treatment may involve replenishing the bone stock with bone grafts followed by a stabilization procedure at a later date. Either autografts or allografts can be fashioned and fixed to the remaining clavicle. In situations where the blood supply to the region is questionable, the senior author has used vascularized bone grafts, both fibula and iliac crest, with success (Fig. 20-5). After securely fixing the graft to the clavicle and/or scapular spine, it can then be stabilized to the coracoid process. Once again, for such situations, we prefer the using a coracoclavicular screw.[18] The construct can then be augmented with a semitendinosus autograft or allograft that is looped around the clavicle and the coracoid process.[46]

In situations where the bony deficit is so massive that bone grafting is precluded, a total claviculectomy can be considered. Total claviculectomy has been performed for various indications, including panclavicular instability, pathologic fractures, malignancy, thoracic outlet syndrome, infection, intractable pain, and severe cosmetic deformity.[7,55,80,81,98] Early experience suggested that, although total claviculectomy is generally associated with a good clinical outcome, these patients may demonstrate mild drooping of the shoulder and mild weakness.[7,80] Others, however, contest this view and suggest that there are minimal consequences after a total claviculectomy.[40,98] The only noted exceptions are patients with a dysfunctional trapezius, because total claviculectomy in these patients are associated with a poor functional result.[98] The senior author has also performed this operation and found the procedure to be associated with a generally good clinical outcome. Prognostic indicators for a favorable outcome were good preoperative periscapular musculature and the ability to participate in an aggressive postoperative strengthening rehabilitation. As reported in the early literature, a few of the patients exhibited mild shoulder drooping and weakness. However, most patients reported satisfactory function and were able to perform activities of daily living with minimal or no discomfort. Thus, this procedure may provide a viable treatment option in these difficult situations.

Acromioclavicular Joint Arthrosis

For symptomatic AC joint arthrosis, most patients are initially treated nonsurgically. An injection of steroids and a short-acting analgesic agent into the AC joint can provide lasting relief. In addition to its therapeutic value, this injection can also confirm the source of pain and provide predictive information regarding the potential benefit of a distal clavicle resection.

In patients with a history or symptoms consistent with joint instability in addition to arthrosis, isolated distal clavicle resection can be associated with a poor outcome.[15,34] Therefore, surgical treatment should include distal clavicle excision and stabilization of the joint. As mentioned previously, our procedure of choice for stabilization is a transfer of the coracoacromial ligament to the distal clavicle. This construct is then augmented with a suture band around the distal clavicle and the coracoid process. For patients with isolated joint arthrosis, our procedure of choice is distal clavicle resection. The procedure can be performed after an open exploration. For the majority of cases, however, it is performed arthroscopically with visualization of the joint from the subacromial space. Approximately 1 cm of the distal clavicle is resected. Damage to the superior or posterior AC ligaments may lead to subsequent joint instability.[50] Thus, care is taken to avoid violating the superior and posterior joint capsule to preclude damage to these ligaments. Under direct or arthroscopic visualization, a cross-body adduction maneuver is performed to ensure adequate resection of the bone. Postoperatively, patients are placed in a sling for a short period of time for comfort only.

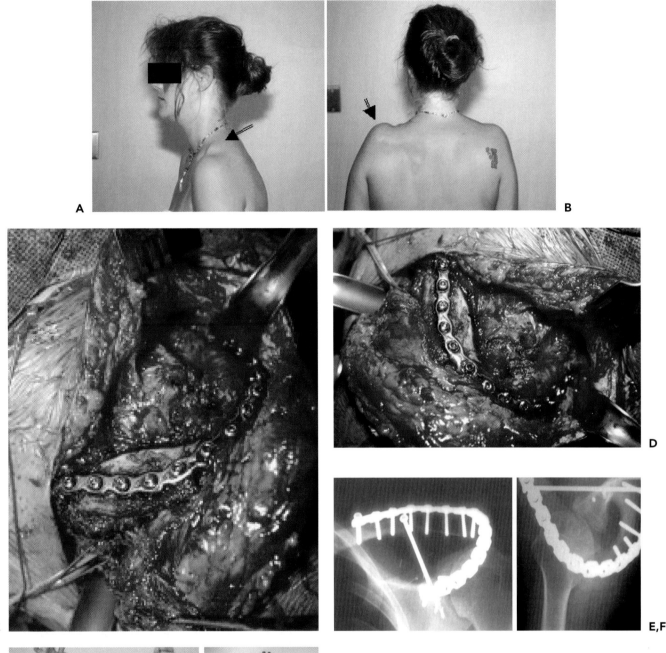

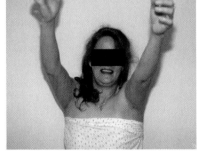
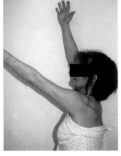

Figure 20-5 A patient who underwent AC joint stabilization with vascularized free iliac crest bone graft. After undergoing excessive distal clavicle resection, this patient complained of excessive pain with shoulder motion. Preoperative photographs *(A,B)* reveal the obvious deformity *(arrow)* associated with distal clavicle instability. Intraoperative photographs *(C,D)* and postoperative radiographs *(E,F)* reveal the final construct where the bone graft *(arrow)* has been fixed to the remaining clavicle and scapular spine. Postoperatively, the patient complained of minimal pain and functional range of motion *(G,H)*.

COMPLICATIONS

Complications after treatment of AC joint pathology include, but are not limited to, the following: erosion or fracture through the clavicle, hardware migration, heterotopic ossification, infection, joint arthritis, neurovascular injury, nonunion, poor cosmesis, recurrent deformity, and wound compromise.[41,72] Of these, some specific complications are noteworthy and deserve further discussion.

Hardware Migration

Multiple authors have reported their experience with the migration of implanted hardware from the shoulder girdle.[54,56,58,66,75] After its placement in the shoulder region, small hardware, such as pins and Kirschner wires, can migrate to distant structures including the eye, heart, abdomen, lung, spinal cord, liver, and aorta. Therefore, this complication can be associated with significant morbidity and possible mortality. To lessen the likelihood of this complication, some authors have recommended that the placed hardware be bent or have a restraining device that prevent migration.[56] In addition, most authors currently recommend hardware removal at the completion of the treatment. Alternatively, other authors have recently advocated the use of bioabsorbable fixation devices. Although clinical experiences with such devices are relatively limited, the use of bioabsorbable implants has been associated with good to excellent short-term clinical results.[47,61]

Heterotopic Ossification and Calcification

After an acute injury to the AC joint, soft tissues in the coracoclavicular interval may become ossified.[6,89,90] The incidence is variable, ranging from 57% to 83%, among different authors.[6] This finding can occur as early as 3 weeks after the injury and does not appear to depend on whether the patient was treated with or without an operation.[60] The bone also does not appear "de novo." Rather, it seems to result after ossification of native soft tissues.[6] Despite the formation of a possible bony bridge between the coracoid process and the clavicle, overall clinical outcome in most patients does not appear to be affected.[3,72,95] As such, other than patient reassurance, no treatment is usually necessary.

Unlike the coracoclavicular interval, heterotopic bone formation in the AC joint interval after distal clavicle resection can be associated with persistent symptoms.[13] Although rare in occurrence, symptoms from the newly formed bone are difficult to treat nonoperatively. For many of the patients, one or more surgical interventions are required to adequately treat this condition. As such, prophylactic therapy for heterotopic ossification should be considered for patients who are at high risk of developing this complication (e.g., patients with hypertrophic pulmonary osteoarthropathy or spondylitic arthropathy, or patients with a history of previous heterotopic ossification).[13]

Joint Arthritis

The relative risk of developing arthritis after an operative intervention to the AC joint is largely unknown. According to one article, degenerative changes after a surgical intervention can occur in as many as 24% of the patients.[27] In other studies, posttraumatic development of arthritic symptoms occurred in 42% of the patients.[14,82] However, it is unclear whether these degenerative changes were a direct result of the surgical trauma or from the normal aging process. Certainly, it can be inferred that any trauma to the joint, including the original injury and placement of the hardware, can increase the likelihood of subsequent joint arthritis. As such, some authors recommend a routine distal clavicle excision during an open treatment of the AC joint.[27,93] This protocol, however, has not been universally accepted. Without clinical or intraoperative evidence of articular damage, most authors do not routinely excise the distal clavicle.

REFERENCES

1. Alexander OM. Radiography of the acromioclavicular joint. Radiography 1948;14:139.
2. Alexander OM. Dislocation of the acromioclavicular joint. Radiography 1949;15:260.
3. Alldredge RH. Surgical treatment of acromioclavicular dislocation. Clin Orthop 1969;63:262.
4. Allman FL. Fractures and ligamentous injuries of the clavicle and its articulation. J Bone Joint Surg 1967;49-A:774.
5. Ansel SH, Streitz WL. Acute acromioclavicular injuries: a report of nineteen cases treated non-operatively employing dynamic splint immobilization. Clin Orthop 1974;103:143.
6. Arner O, Sandahl U, Ohrling H. Dislocation of the acromioclavicular joint: review of the literature and a report of 56 cases. Acta Chir Scand 1957;113:140.
7. Attarian DE. Atraumatic floating clavicle and total claviculectomy. J South Orthop Assoc 1999;8:293.
8. Bannister GC, Wallace WA, Stableforth PG, et al. The management of acute acromioclavicular dislocation: a randomized prospective controlled trial. J Bone Joint Surg 1989;71-B:848.
9. Barber FA. Coplaning of the acromioclavicular joint. Arthroscopy 2001;17:913.
10. Bassett FH. Distal clavicle resection under local anesthesia. Orthop Trans 1994;18:766.
11. Bearden JM, Hughston JC, Whatley GS. Acromioclavicular dislocation: method of treatment. J Sports Med 1973;1:5.
12. Bearn JG. Direct observations on the function of the capsule of the sternoclavicular joint in clavicular support. J Anat 1967;101:159.
13. Berg EE, Ciullo JV. Heterotopic ossification after acromioplasty and distal clavicle resection. J Shoulder Elbow Surg 1995;4:188.
14. Bergfeld JA, Andrish JT, Clancy WG. Evaluation of the acromioclavicular joint following first and second degree sprains. Am J Sports Med 1978;6:153.
15. Bigliani LU, Nicholson GP, Flatow EL. Arthroscopic resection of the distal clavicle. Orthop Clin North Am 1993;24:133.
16. Blazar PE, Iannotti JP, Williams GR. Anteroposterior instability of the clavicle after distal clavicle resection. Clin Orthop 1998; 348:114.
17. Bossart PJ, Joyce SM, Manaster BJ, et al. Lack of efficacy of "weighted" radiographs in diagnosing acute acromioclavicular separation. Ann Emerg Med 1988;17:47.

18. Bosworth BM. Complete acromioclavicular dislocation. N Engl J Med 1949;241:221.
19. Branch TP, Burdette HL, Shahriari AS, et al. The role of the acromioclavicular ligaments and the effect of distal clavicle resection. Am J Sports Med 1996;24:293.
20. Brown JN, Roberts SNJ, Hayes MG, et al. Shoulder pathology associated with symptomatic acromioclavicular joint degeneration. J Shoulder Elbow Surg 2000;9:173.
21. Buford D, Mologne T, McGrath S, et al. Midterm results of arthroscopic co-planing of the acromioclavicular joint. J Shoulder Elbow Surg 2000;9:498.
22. Cadenat FM. The treatment of dislocations and fractures of the outer end of the clavicle. Int Clin 1917; 1:145.
23. Cahill BR. Osteolysis of the distal part of the clavicle in male athletes. J Bone Joint Surg 1982;64-A:1053.
24. Cahill BR. Atraumatic osteolysis of the distal clavicle: a review. Sports Med 1992;13:214.
25. Caldwell GD. Treatment of complete permanent acromioclavicular dislocation by surgical arthrodesis. J Bone Joint Surg 1943; 25:368.
26. Codman EA. Rupture of the supraspinatus tendon and other lesions in or about the subacromial bursa. In: The shoulder. Boston, MA, Thomas Todd & Co., 1934.
27. Cook DA, Heiner JP. Acromioclavicular joint injuries. J Orthop Rev 1990;19:510.
28. Cox JS. Current method of treatment of acromioclavicular dislocations. Orthopedics 1992;15:1041.
29. Debski RE, Parsons IM, Woo SLY, et al. Effect of capsular injury on acromioclavicular joint mechanics. J Bone Joint Surg 2001;83A: 1344.
30. DePalma AF. The role of the disks of the sternoclavicular and acromioclavicular joints. Clin Orthop 1959;13:7.
31. Eskola A, Santavirta S, Viljakka HT, et al. The results of operative resection of the lateral end of the clavicle. J Bone Joint Surg 1996;78-A:584.
32. Fenkl R, Gotzen L. Sonographic diagnosis of the injured acromioclavicular joint: a standardized examination procedure. Unfallchirurgie 1992;95:393.
33. Flatow EL. The biomechanics of the acromioclavicular, sternoclavicular, and scapulothoracic joints. Instr Course Lect 1993; 42:237.
34. Flatow EL, Cordasco FA, Bigliani LU. Arthroscopic resection of the outer end of the clavicle from a superior approach: a critical, quantitative, radiographic assessment of bone removal. Arthroscopy 1992;8:55.
35. Flatow EL, Duralde XA, Nicholson GP, et al. Arthroscopic resection of the distal clavicle with a superior approach. J Shoulder Elbow Surg 1995;4:41.
36. Fukuda K, Craig EV, An K-N, et al. Biomechanical study of the ligamentous system of the acromioclavicular joint. J Bone Joint Surg 1986;68-A:434.
37. Gerber C, Rockwood CA. Subcoracoid dislocation of the lateral end of the clavicle: a report of three cases. J Bone Joint Surg 1987;69-A:924.
38. Gerber C, Galantay RV, Hersche O. The pattern of pain produced by irritation of the acromioclavicular joint and the subacromial space. J Shoulder Elbow Surg 1998;7:352.
39. Glick JM, Milburn LJ, Haggerty JF, et al. Dislocated acromioclavicular joint: follow-up study of 35 unreduced acromioclavicular dislocations. Am J Sports Med 1977;5:264.
40. Gurd FB. The treatment of complete dislocation of the outer end of the clavicle: a hitherto undescribed operation. Ann Surg 1941; 113:1094.
41. Guttmann D, Paksima NE, Zuckerman JD. Complications of treatment of complete acromioclavicular joint dislocations. Instr Course Lect 2000;49:407.
42. Hastings DE, Horne JG. Anterior dislocation of the acromioclavicular joint. Injury 1979;10:285.
43. Henry MH, Liu SH, Loffredo AJ. Arthroscopic management of the acromioclavicular joint disorder: a review. Clin Orthop 1995; 316:276.
44. Horvath F, Kery L. Degenerative deformations of the acromioclavicular joint in the elderly. Arch Gerontol Geriatr 1984; 3:259.
45. Inman VT, Saunders JB, Abbott LC. Observations on the function of the shoulder joint. J Bone Joint Surg 1944;26:1.
46. Jones HP, Lemos MJ, Schepsis AA. Salvage of failed acromioclavicular joint reconstruction using autogenous semitendinosis tendon from the knee. Am J Sports Med 2001;29:234.
47. Keller HW, Rehm KE. Treatment of acromioclavicular dislocations without metallic implants. Unfallchirurgie 1991;94:511.
48. Kennedy JC, Cameron H. Complete dislocation of the acromioclavicular joint. J Bone Joint Surg 1954;36-B:202.
49. Kessel L, Watson M. The painful arc syndrome. Clinical classification as a guide to management. J Bone Joint Surg 1977;59-B:166.
50. Klimkiewicz JJ, Williams GR, Sher JS, et al. The acromioclavicular capsule as a restraint to posterior translation of the clavicle: a biomechanical analysis. J Shoulder Elbow Surg 1999;8:119.
51. Kwon YW, Iannotti JP. Operative treatment of acromioclavicular joint injuries and results. Clin Sports Med 2003;22:291.
52. Larsen E, Bjerg-Nielsen A, Christensen P. Conservative or surgical treatment of acromioclavicular dislocation: a prospective, controlled, randomized study. J Bone Joint Surg 1986;68-A:552.
53. Levine WN, Barron OA, Yamaguchi K, et al. Arthroscopic distal clavicle resection from a bursal approach. Arthroscopy 1998; 14:52.
54. Lindsey RW, Gutowski WT. The migration of a broken pin following fixation of the acromioclavicular joint: a case report and review of the literature. Orthopedics 1986;9:413.
55. Lord JW, Wright IS. Total claviculectomy for neurovascular compression in the thoracic outlet. Surg Gynecol Obstet 1993; 176:609.
56. Lyons FA, Rockwood CA. Migration of pins used in operations on the shoulder. J Bone Joint Surg 1990;72-A:1262.
57. Martin SD, Baumgarten TE, Andrews JR. Arthroscopic resection of the distal clavicle with concomitant subacromial decompression. J Bone Joint Surg 2001;83-A:328.
58. Mazet RJ. Migration of a Kirschner wire from the shoulder region into the lung: report of two cases. J Bone Joint Surg 1943;25-A:477.
59. McClure PW, Michener LA, Sennett BJ, et al. Direct 3-dimensional measurement of scapular kinematics during dynamic movements in vivo. J Shoulder Elbow Surg 2001;10:269.
60. Millbourn E. On injuries to the acromioclavicular joint: treatment and results. Acta Orthop Scand 1950;19:349.
61. Monig SP, Burger C, Helling HJ, et al. Treatment of complete acromioclavicular dislocation: present indications and surgical technique with biodegradable cords. Int J Sports Med 1999; 20:560.
62. Murphy OB, Bellamy R, Wheeler W, et al. Post-traumatic osteolysis of the distal clavicle. Clin Orthop 1975;109:108.
63. Needell SD, Zlatkin MB, Sher JS, et al. MR imaging of the rotator cuff: peritendinous and bone abnormalities in an asymptomatic population. Am J Roentgenol 1996;166:863.
64. Neviaser TJ, Neviaser RJ, Neviaser JS, et al. The four-in-one arthroplasty for painful arc syndrome. Clin Orthop 1982;163:108.
65. Nieminen S, Aho AJ. Anterior dislocation of the acromioclavicular joint. Ann Chir Gynaecol 1984;73:21.
66. Norrell H, Llewellyn RC. Migration of a threaded Steinmann pin from an acromioclavicular joint into the spinal canal: a case report. J Bone Joint Surg 1965;47-A:1024.
67. Nuber GW, Bowen MK. Acromioclavicular joint injuries and distal clavicle fractures. J Am Acad Orthop Surg 1997;5:11.
68. Partington PF, Broome GH. Diagnostic injection around the shoulder: hit and miss? A cadaveric study of injection accuracy. J Shoulder Elbow Surg 1998;7:147.
69. Patterson WR. Inferior dislocation of the distal end of the clavicle. J Bone Joint Surg 1967;49-A:1184.
70. Petersson CJ. Degeneration of the acromioclavicular joint: a morphological study. Acta Orthop Scand 1983;54:434.
71. Petersson CJ, Gentz CF. Rupture of the supraspinatus tendon: the significance of distally pointing acromioclavicular osteophytes. Clin Orthop 1983;174:143.
72. Rockwood CA, Williams GR, Young DC. Disorders of the acromioclavicular joint. In: Rockwood CA, Matsen FA, eds. The shoulder. Philadelphia, PA, WB Saunders, 1998:483.
73. Salter EG, Nasca RJ, Shelley BS. Anatomical observations on the acromioclavicular joint and supporting ligaments. Am J Sports Med 1987;15:199.

74. Schmid A, Schmid F. Use of arthrosonography in diagnosis of Tossy III lesions of acromioclavicular joints. Aktuel Traumatol 1988;18:134.

75. Sethi GK, Scott SM. Subclavian artery laceration due to migration of a Hagie pin. Surgery 1976;80:644.

76. Shaffer BS. Painful conditions of the acromioclavicular joint. J Am Acad Orthop Surg 1999;7:176.

77. Shubin-Stein BE, Wiater JM, Pfaff HC, et al. Detection of acromioclavicular joint pathology in asymptomatic shoulders with magnetic resonance imaging. J Shoulder Elbow Surg 2001;10:204.

78. Sluming VA. A comparison of the methods of distraction for stress examination of the acromioclavicular joint. Br J Radiol 1995;68:1181.

79. Sluming VA. Technical note: measuring the coracoclavicular distance with ultrasound—a new technique. Br J Radiol 1995; 68:189.

80. Spar I. Total claviculectomy for pathological fractures. Clin Orthop 1977;129:236.

81. Srivastava KK, Garg LD, Kocklar VL. Osteomyelitis of the clavicle. Acta Orthop Scand 1974;45:662.

82. Taft TN, Wilson FC, Oglesby JW. Dislocation of the acromioclavicular joint: an end-result study. J Bone Joint Surg 1987;69-A:1045.

83. Tarar MN, Quaba AA. An adipofascial turnover flap for soft tissue cover around the clavicle. Br J Plast Surg 1995;48:161.

84. Tibone J, Sellers R, Tonino P. Strength testing after third degree acromioclavicular dislocations. Am J Sports Med 1992;20:328.

85. Tobin GR. Pectoralis major segmental anatomy and segmentally split pectoralis major flaps. Plast Reconst Surg 1985;75:814.

86. Tossy JD, Mead NC, Sigmond HM. Acromioclavicular separations: useful and practical classification for treatment. Clin Orthop 1963;28:111.

87. Tsou PM. Percutaneous cannulated screw coracoclavicular fixation for acute acromioclavicular dislocations. Clin Orthop 1989;243:112.

88. Tyurina TV. Age related characteristics of the human acromioclavicular joint. Arkh Anat Gistol Embriol 1985;89:75.

89. Urist MR. Complete dislocation of the acromioclavicular joint: the nature of the traumatic lesion and effective methods of treatment with an analysis of 41 cases. J Bone Joint Surg 1946; 28:813.

90. Urist MR. The treatment of dislocation of the acromioclavicular joint. Am J Surg 1959;98:423.

91. Waldrop JI, Norwood LA, Alvarez RG. Lateral roentgenographic projections of the acromioclavicular joint. Am J Sports Med 1981;9:337.

92. Waxman J. Acromioclavicular disease in rheumatologic practice—the forgotten joint. J La State Med Soc 1977;129:1.

93. Weaver JK, Dunn HK. Treatment of acromioclavicular injuries, especially complete acromioclavicular separation. J Bone Joint Surg 1972;54-A:1187.

94. Weinstein DM, McCann PD, McIlveen SJ, et al. Surgical treatment of complete acromioclavicular dislocations. Am J Sports Med 1995;23:324.

95. Weitzman G. Treatment of acute acromioclavicular joint dislocation by a modified Bosworth method: report on twenty four cases. J Bone Joint Surg 1967;49-A:1167.

96. Williams GR, Koffler K, Pepe MD, et al. Rotation of the clavicular portion of the pectoralis major for soft tissue coverage of the clavicle: an anatomic study and case report. J Bone Joint Surg 2000;82-A:1736.

97. Wojtys EM, Nelson G. Conservative treatment of grade III acromioclavicular dislocations. Clin Orthop 1991;268:112.

98. Wood VE. The results of total claviculectomy. Clin Orthop 1986; 207:186.

99. Worcester JN, Green DP. Osteoarthritis of the acromioclavicular joint. Clin Orthop 1968;58:69.

100. Zanca P. Shoulder pain: involvement of the acromioclavicular joint—analysis of 1,000 cases. Am J Roentegenol 1971;112: 493.

Sternoclavicular Joint: Primary and Revision Reconstruction

Michael A. Wirth   *Charles A. Rockwood*

PATHOLOGY AND EVALUATION

Biomechanics and Mechanisms of Injury

The sternoclavicular (SC) joint is freely moveable and functions almost like a ball-and-socket joint with motion in almost all planes, including rotation.[2,11] The clavicle, and therefore the SC joint, in normal shoulder motion is capable of 30 to 35 degrees of upward elevation, 35 degrees of combined forward and backward movement, and 45 to 50 degrees of rotation around its long axis (Fig. 21-1). It is most likely the most frequently moved joint of the long bones in the body, because almost any motion of the upper extremity is transferred proximally to the SC joint.

Either direct or indirect force can produce a dislocation of the SC joint. Because the SC joint is subject to practically every motion of the upper extremity and because the joint is small and incongruous, one would think that it would be the most commonly dislocated joint in the body. However, the ligamentous supporting structure is strong and so well designed that it is, in fact, one of the least commonly dislocated joints in the body. A traumatic dislocation of the SC joint usually occurs only after a tremendous force, either direct or indirect, has been applied to the shoulder.

M. A. Wirth: Department of Orthopaedics, University of Texas Health Science Center at San Antonio, San Antonio, Texas.
C. A. Rockwood: Department of Orthopaedics, University of Texas Health Science Center at San Antonio, San Antonio, Texas.

Direct Force

When a force is applied directly to the anteromedial aspect of the clavicle, the clavicle is pushed posteriorly behind the sternum and into the mediastinum. This can occur in a variety of ways: an athlete lying on his or her back on the ground is struck by the knee of a jumper landing directly on the medial end of the clavicle; a kick is delivered to the front of the medial clavicle; a person lying supine is run over by a vehicle; or a person is pinned between a vehicle and a wall (Fig. 21-2). Anatomically, it is essentially impossible for a direct force to produce an anterior SC dislocation.

Indirect Force

A force can be applied indirectly to the SC joint from the anterolateral or posterolateral aspects of the shoulder. This is the most common mechanism of injury to the SC joint. Mehta and coworkers[14] reported that three of four posterior SC dislocations were produced by indirect force, and Heinig[8] reported that indirect force was responsible for eight of nine cases of posterior SC dislocations. Indirect force was the most common mechanism of injury in the authors' 185 patients. If the shoulder is compressed and rolled forward, an ipsilateral posterior dislocation results; if the shoulder is compressed and rolled backward, an ipsilateral anterior dislocation results. One of the most common causes that the authors have seen is a pile-on in a football game. In this instance, a player falls on the ground,

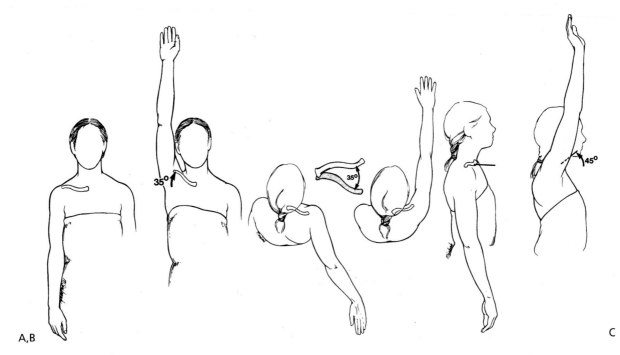

A,B   C

Figure 21-1 Motions of the clavicle and sternoclavicular (SC) joint. (*A*) With full overhead elevation, the clavicle elevates 35 degrees. (*B*) With adduction and extension, the clavicle displaces anteriorly and posteriorly 35 degrees. (*C*) The clavicle rotates on its long axis 45 degrees as the arm is elevated to the full overhead position. (Reprinted with permission from Rockwood CA, Green DP, Bucholz RW, et al., eds. Fractures in adults. 5th ed. Philadelphia, PA, Lippincott Williams & Wilkins, 2001.)

landing on the lateral shoulder; before he can get out of the way, several players pile on top of his opposite shoulder, which applies significant compressive force on the clavicle down toward the sternum. If, during the compression, the shoulder is rolled forward, the force directed down the clavicle produces a posterior dislocation of the SC joint. If the shoulder is compressed and rolled backward, the force directed down the clavicle produces an anterior dislocation

of the SC joint. Other types of indirect forces that can produce SC dislocation are a cave-in on a ditch digger, with lateral compression of the shoulders by the falling dirt; lateral compressive forces on the shoulder when a person is pinned between a vehicle and a wall; and a fall on the outstretched abducted arm, which drives the shoulder medially in the same manner as a lateral compression on the shoulder.

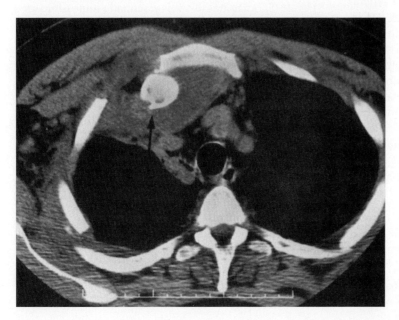

Figure 21-2 Computed axial tomogram of a posterior SC joint dislocation that occurred when the driver's chest impacted the steering wheel during a motor vehicle accident. The vehicle was totaled, and the steering wheel was fractured from the driving column. (Reprinted with permission from Rockwood CA, Green DP, Bucholz RW, et al., eds. Fractures in adults. 5th ed. Philadelphia, PA, Lippincott Williams & Wilkins, 2001.)

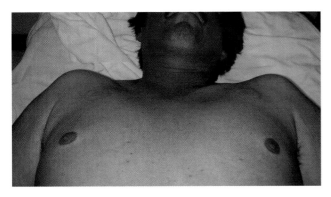

Figure 21-3 Patient with a traumatic right posterior dislocation (note the subtle asymmetry).

History and Physical Examination

It is very important to take a careful history and perform a thorough physical examination. The physician should obtain x-rays, tomograms, computed tomography (CT) scans, or angio-CT scans to document whether there is any compression of the great vessels in the neck or arm and to determine whether there is a structural cause for difficulty in swallowing or breathing. It is also important to determine whether the patient has any feeling of choking or hoarseness. If any of these symptoms are present, indicating pressure on the mediastinum, the appropriate cardiovascular or thoracic specialist should be consulted.

Although the diagnosis of anterior or posterior injury of the SC joint used to be made based on a physical examination, it is now known that anterior swelling and firmness are not diagnostic of an anterior injury. The authors have been fooled on several occasions when the patient appeared to have an anterior dislocation on physical examination, but x-rays documented a posterior problem (Fig. 21-3). Therefore, the authors recommend that the clinical impression *always* be documented with appropriate x-rays before making any decision to treat or not to treat.

Radiographs

The older literature reflects that routine x-rays of the SC joint, regardless of the special views, are difficult to interpret. Special oblique views of the chest have been recommended, but because of the distortion of one of the clavicles over the other, interpretation is difficult.

Heinig View

With the patient in a supine position, the x-ray tube is placed approximately 30 inches from the involved SC joint, and the central ray is directed tangential to the joint and parallel to the opposite clavicle. The cassette is placed against the opposite shoulder and centered on the manubrium (Fig. 21-4).

Hobbs View

In the Hobbs view, the patient is seated at the x-ray table, high enough to lean forward over the table. The cassette is on the table, and the lower anterior rib cage is against the cassette (Fig. 21-5). The patient leans forward so that the nape of his or her flexed neck is almost parallel to the table. The flexed elbows straddle the cassette and support the head and neck. The x-ray source is above the nape of the neck, and the beam passes through the cervical spine to project the SC joints onto the cassette.

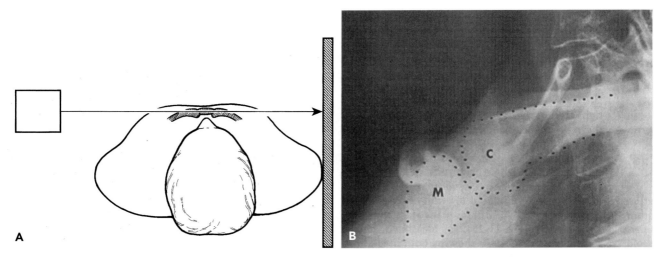

Figure 21-4 *(A)* Positioning of the patient for radiographic evaluation of the SC joint, as described by Heinig. *(B)* Heinig view demonstrating a normal relationship between the medial end of the clavicle (C) and manubrium (M). (Reprinted with permission from Rockwood CA, Green DP, Bucholz RW, et al., eds. Fractures in the adult. Philadelphia, PA, JB Lippincott, 1996.)

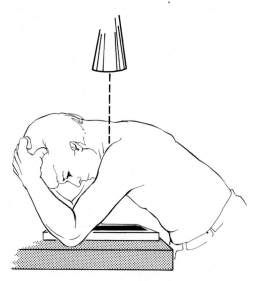

Figure 21-5 Hobbs view. Positioning of the patient for x-ray evaluation of the SC joint, as recommended by Hobbs. (Modified from Hobbs DW. SC joint; a new axial radiographic view. Radiology 1968;90:801.) (Reprinted with permission from Rockwood CA, Green DP, Bucholz RW, et al., eds. Fractures in the adult. Philadelphia, PA, JB Lippincott, 1996.)

Serendipity View

The "serendipity view" is aptly named because that is the way it was developed. The senior author accidentally noted the next best thing to having a true cephalocaudal lateral view of the SC joint is a 40-degree cephalic tilt view. The patient is positioned on his or her back squarely and in the center of the x-ray table. The tube is tilted at a 40-degree angle off the vertical and centered directly on the sternum (Fig. 21-6).

Computed Tomography, Magnetic Resonance Imaging, and Other Studies

Computed Tomography Scans

Without question, the CT scan is the best technique to study any or all problems of the SC joint. It clearly distinguishes injuries of the joint from fractures of the medial clavicle and defines minor subluxations of the joint. The orthopedist must ask for CT scans of both SC joints and the medial one-half of both clavicles so that the injured side can be compared with the uninjured side.

Magnetic Resonance Imaging Scans

When there are questions of diagnosis between dislocations of the SC joint or physeal injury in children and young adults, the MRI scan can be used to determine whether the epiphysis has been displaced with the clavicle or is still adjacent to the manubrium.

Tomograms

Tomograms can be very helpful in distinguishing between SC dislocation and medial clavicle fracture. They can also help distinguish fractures from dislocation and evaluate arthritis changes in questionable anterior and posterior dislocation of the SC joint.

Concomitant Injuries

Injuries that occur in association with trauma to the SC joint are primarily posterior dislocations. These injuries have been associated with significant morbidity and include the fol-

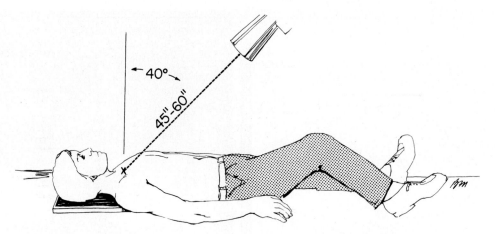

Figure 21-6 Positioning of the patient to take the "serendipity" view of the SC joints. The x-ray tube is tilted 40 degrees from the vertical position and aimed directly at the manubrium. The non-grid cassette should be large enough to receive the projected images of the medial halves of both clavicles. In children, the tube distance from the patient should be 45 inches; in thicker-chested adults, the distance should be 60 inches. (Reprinted with permission from Rockwood CA, Green DP, eds. Fractures (3 vols.), 2nd ed. Philadelphia, PA, JB Lippincott, 1984.)

lowing: pneumothorax and laceration of the superior vena cava[21]; respiratory distress, venous congestion in the neck, rupture of the esophagus with abscess and osteomyelitis of the clavicle[3]; pressure on the subclavian artery in an untreated patient[12]; occlusion of the subclavian artery late in a patient who was not treated[8]; compression of the right common carotid artery by a fracture-dislocation of the SC joint[12]; brachial plexus compression[17]; hoarseness of the voice, onset of snoring, and voice changes from falsetto with movement of the arm and a fatal tracheoesophageal fistulae.[27]

STERNOCLAVICULAR INSTABILITY: ANTERIOR

Acute Versus Chronic Subluxation

Patients who develop anterior SC instability may present acutely or several months after the development of this condition. In addition, anterior instability can develop in the absence of trauma. In a review by Rockwood and Odor[22] of 37 patients with spontaneous atraumatic subluxation, 29 were managed without surgery and 8 were treated with a surgical reconstruction elsewhere. With an average follow-up of more than 8 years, all 29 patients who did not undergo operation were doing well without limitations of activity or lifestyle. The 8 patients treated with surgery had increased pain, limitation of activity, alteration of lifestyle, persistent instability, and a significant scar. In many instances, the patient, before a previous reconstruction or resection, had minimal discomfort, had an excellent range of motion, and only complained of the "bump" that slipped in and out of place with certain motions. Postoperatively, the patient still had the bump, along with a scar and painful range of motion.

Nonoperative Management

For an acute subluxation of the SC joint, application of ice is recommended for the first 12 hours, followed by heat for the next 24 to 48 hours. The joint may be reduced by drawing the shoulders backward as if reducing and holding a fracture of the clavicle. A clavicle strap can be used to hold the reduction. A sling and swath should also be used to hold up the shoulder and prevent motion of the arm. The patient should be protected from further possible injury for 4 to 6 weeks. Plaster figure-of-eight dressing, a simple sling to support the arm, a soft figure-of-eight bandage with a sling, and, occasionally, adhesive strapping over the medial end of the clavicle have all been recommended.

Is There Ever a Role for Operative Treatment?

Occasionally, after conservative treatment of an anterior SC subluxation, the pain lingers and the symptoms of popping and grating persist. This may require joint exploration. On several occasions the authors have noted a degenerative tear of the intra-articular disc ligament. Analogous to a torn meniscus in the knee, the symptomatic SC joint demonstrated mechanical symptoms of popping, catching, and even locking when the arm was put in various positions or when the shoulders were repeatedly protracted and retracted. After excision of the intra-articular disc and repair of the capsule, the symptoms were eliminated.

Technique for Removal of the Intra-articular Disc and Repair of the Anterior Capsular Ligament

This approach is a modified approach to the one described previously in this chapter. The patient is supine on the table

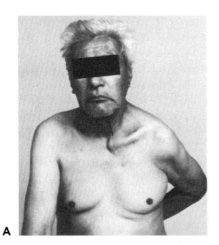
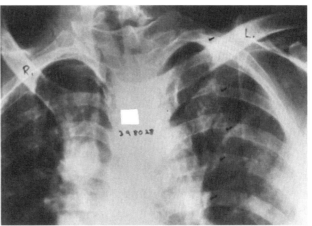

Figure 21-7 Unreduced anterior traumatic dislocations of the SC joint. *(A)* This patient has an anterior unreduced dislocation of the left SC joint. He works as a laborer and has few if any complaints. *(B)* The injury occurred 5 years before the photograph when he had a dislocation and multiple fractures of the ribs. (Reprinted with permission from Rockwood CA, Green DP, eds. Fractures (3 vols.), 2nd ed. Philadelphia, PA, JB Lippincott, 1984.)

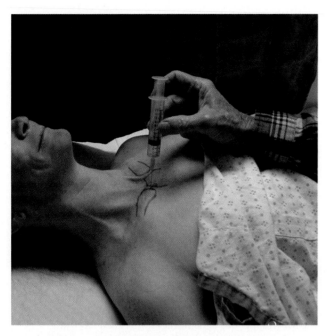

Figure 21-8 Diagnostic injection of the SC joint.

with two or three folded towels in between the scapulae. The anterior incision parallels the superior border of the medial 2 inches of the clavicle and then extends downward over the manubrium. The anterior SC ligament is divided, taking care to not divide the superior portion of the transverse ligament running across to the opposite medial clavicle. With the joint open, the intra-articular ligament is easily removed. Occasionally, it will have an inferior attachment that will need to be sharply divided. Loose fragments of ligament are removed. The bolster between the shoulders is then removed from between the scapulae, which allows the SC joint to close and makes it easier to repair the anterior capsular ligament. Because the costoclavicular ligament and the posterior ligament are still intact, the joint will remain stable. After surgery the patient's shoulder is held in a sling for 2 weeks to allow healing of the soft tissues.

As previously described, most patients with an unreduced and permanent anterior dislocation of the SC joint are not very symptomatic, have almost a complete range of motion, and can work and even perform manual labor with few problems (Fig. 21-7). Because the joint is so small and incongruous and because the results seen in patients who have had attempted reconstructions are so miserable, the authors usually recommend a nonoperative, skillful neglect type of treatment.

If the patient has persistent symptoms of traumatic arthritis for 6 to 12 months after a dislocation, and if the symptoms can be completely relieved by injection of local anesthesia into the SC joint region, we would perform an arthroplasty of the SC joint (Fig. 21-8). This would include a resection of the medial 1 inch of the clavicle with a beveling of the superoanterior corner for cosmetic purposes, a

debridement of the intra-articular disc ligament, and stabilization of the remaining clavicle to the first rib with either 1-mm or 3-mm cottony Dacron tape. If the costoclavicular ligaments are incompetent, it is important to ensure some stabilization between the medial clavicle and the first rib. Usually, stabilization is completed by passing several 1-mm cottony Dacron sutures around the medial end of the clavicle securing the periosteal tube of the clavicle down to the periosteal tissue and the remnants of the costoclavicular ligament. The technique is described in more detail later in the chapter.

STERNOCLAVICULAR INSTABILITY: POSTERIOR

Nonoperative Management

If children and adults younger than 22 to 23 years of age have no symptoms from the pressure of the posteriorly displaced clavicle into the mediastinum, the physician can wait and watch to see whether the physeal plate remodeling process removes the posteriorly displaced bone.[22]

Indeed, as with other childhood fractures, the potential for remodeling is significant and may extend until the 24th or 25th year. Several reports have noted successful treatment of posteriorly displaced medial clavicle physeal injuries in young patients with CT documentation of remodeling, most probably within an intact periosteal tube.[14,15]

Closed Reduction

The patient is placed in the supine position with a 3- to 4-inch–thick sandbag or three to four folded towels between the scapulae to retract the shoulders. The dislocated shoulder should be over toward the edge of the table so that the arm and shoulder can be abducted and extended. If the patient is having extreme pain and muscle spasm and is quite anxious, the authors use general anesthesia; otherwise, narcotics, muscle relaxants, or tranquilizers are given through an established intravenous route in the normal arm. First, gentle traction is applied on the abducted arm in line with the clavicle while countertraction is applied by an assistant who steadies the patient on the table. The traction on the abducted arm is gradually increased while the arm is brought into extension.

Reduction of an acute injury usually occurs with an audible pop or snap, and the relocation can be noted visibly. If closed reduction is not successful, the skin should be surgically prepared and a sterile towel clip used to gain purchase on the medial clavicle (Fig. 21-9). The towel clip is used to grasp completely around the shaft of the clavicle, and the reduction maneuver is repeated while applying anteriorly directed force on the clavicle. After the reduction, a padded figure-of-eight clavicle strap is ap-

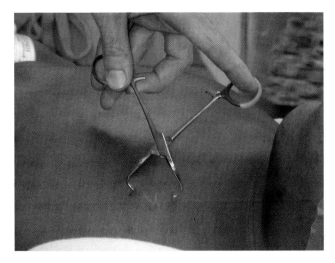

Figure 21-9 Application of a sterile towel clip to assist in closed reduction of a posterior SC dislocation.

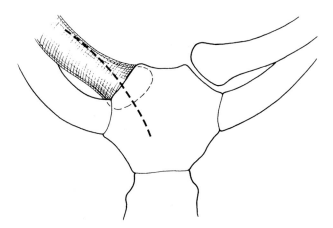

Figure 21-10 Proposed skin incision for open reduction of a posterior SC dislocation. (Reprinted with permission from Rockwood CA, Green DP, eds. Fractures (3 vols.), 2nd ed. Philadelphia, PA, JB Lippincott, 1984.)

Operative Treatment: Indications, Techniques, and Aftercare

Potential complications of an unreduced posterior SC dislocation in adults are numerous; thoracic outlet syndrome,[9] vascular compromise,[3] and erosion of the medial clavicle into any one of the many vital structures that lie posterior to the SC joint have all been reported. Therefore, in adults, if closed reduction fails to reduce the dislocation, an open procedure should be performed.

The patient is supine on the table with three to four towels or a small sandbag placed between the scapulae. The upper extremity should be draped out free so that lateral traction can be applied during the open reduction. In addition, a folded sheet around the patient's thorax should be left in place so that it can be used for countertraction if necessary. An anterior incision is used that parallels the superior border of the medial 3 to 4 inches of the clavicle and then extends downward over the sternum just medial to the involved SC joint (Fig. 21-10). The trick is to remove sufficient soft tissues to expose the joint but to leave the anterior capsular ligament intact. The reduction can usually be accomplished with traction and countertraction while lifting up anteriorly with a clamp around the medial clavicle, but it may be necessary to use an elevator to lever the clavicle back to its articulation with the sternum. When the reduction has been obtained, and with the shoulders held back, the reduction is usually stable. If the anterior capsule is damaged or is insufficient to prevent anterior displacement of the medial end of the clavicle, the authors recommend excising the medial 1 to 1 1/2 inches of the clavicle and securing the residual clavicle to the first rib with 1-mm Dacron tape. The medial clavicle is exposed by careful subperiosteal dis-

section (Fig. 21-11). When possible, any remnant of the capsular or intra-articular disk ligaments should be identified and preserved because these structures can be used to stabilize the medial clavicle (Fig. 21-12). The capsular ligament covers the anterosuperior and posterior aspects of the joint and represents thickenings of the joint capsule. This ligament is primarily attached to the epiphysis of the medial clavicle and is usually avulsed from this structure with posterior SC dislocations. Similarly, the intra-articular disc ligament is usually intact where it arises from the synchondral junction of the first rib and sternum and is avulsed from its attachment site on the medial clavicle.

If the sternal attachment site of these structures is intact, a nonabsorbable No. 1 cottony Dacron suture is woven back and forth through one or both ligaments so that the ends of the suture exit through the avulsed free end of the tissue. The medial end of the clavicle is resected, being careful to protect the underlying structures (Fig. 21-13). The medullary canal of the medial clavicle is drilled and curetted to receive the transferred capsular or intra-articular disc ligament. Two small drill holes are then placed in the superior cortex of the medial clavicle, approximately 1 cm lateral to the site of resection (Fig. 21-14). These holes communicate with the medullary canal and will be used to secure the suture in the transferred ligament. The free ends of the suture are passed into the medullary canal of the medial clavicle and out the two small drill holes in the superior cortex of the clavicle (Fig. 21-15). While the clavicle is held in a reduced and anteroposterior position in relationship to the first rib and sternum, the sutures are used to pull the ligament tightly into the medullary canal of the clavicle. The suture is tied, thus securing the transferred ligament into the clavicle. The stabilization procedure is completed by passing several 1-mm cottony Dacron sutures around the medial end of the remaining clavicle and securing the periosteal sleeve of the clavicle to the costoclavicular ligament (Fig. 21-16). Postop-

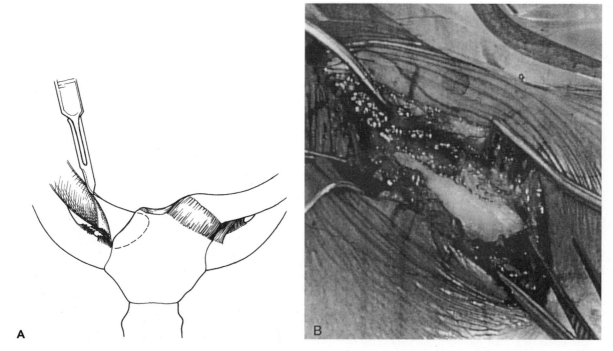

Figure 21-11 (*A,B*) Subperiosteal exposure of the medial clavicle. Note the posteriorly displaced medial end of the clavicle. (Reprinted with permission from Rockwood CA, Green DP, Bucholz RW, et al., eds. Fractures in the adult. Philadelphia, PA, JB Lippincott, 1996.)

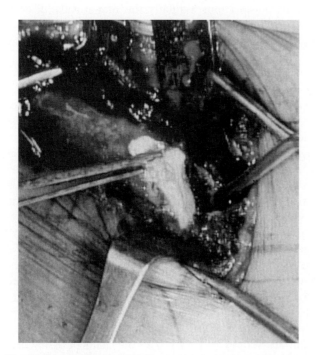

Figure 21-12 Forceps holding the anterior portion of the SC ligament, which was avulsed from its attachment on the medial clavicle. The sternal attachment site of this ligament was intact. (Reprinted with permission from Rockwood CA, Green DP, Bucholz RW, et al., eds. Fractures in the adult. Philadelphia, PA, JB Lippincott, 1996.)

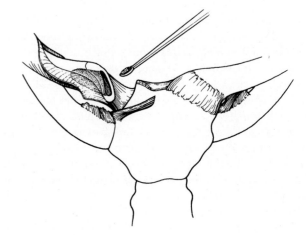

Figure 21-13 Medullary canal of the medial clavicle is curetted in preparation for receiving the transferred SC capsular ligament. (Reprinted with permission from Rockwood CA, Green DP, Bucholz RW, et al., eds. Fractures in the adult. Philadelphia, PA, JB Lippincott, 1996.)

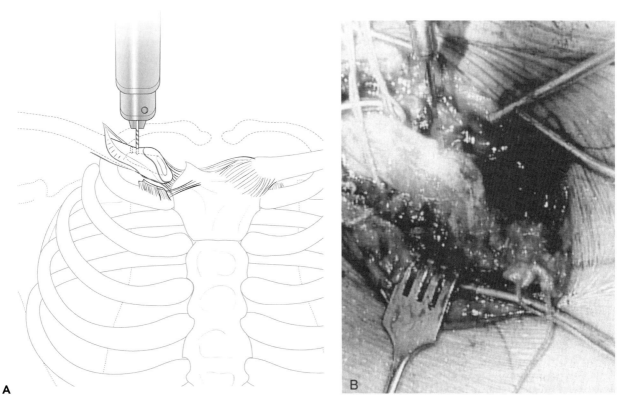

Figure 21-14 *(A,B)* Drill holes are placed in the superior cortex of the clavicle, approximately 1 cm lateral to the osteotomy site. *(A* Reprinted with permission from Rockwood CA, Green DP, Bucholz RW, et al., eds. Fractures in the adult. Philadelphia, PA, JB Lippincott, 1996.)

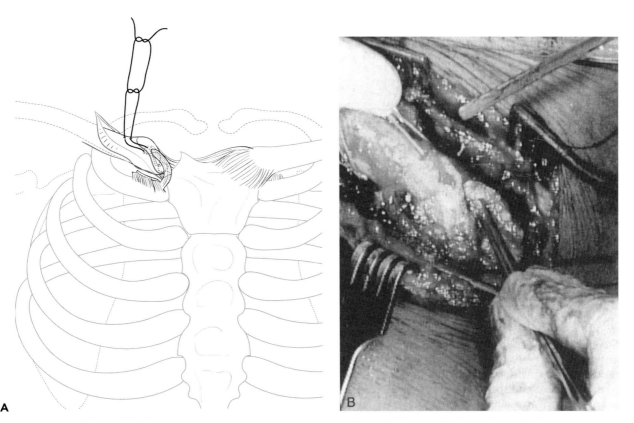

Figure 21-15 Free ends of the suture are passed into the medullary canal and out the two holes in the superior cortex. (Reprinted with permission from Rockwood CA, Green DP, Bucholz RW, et al., eds. Fractures in the adult. Philadelphia, PA, JB Lippincott, 1996.)

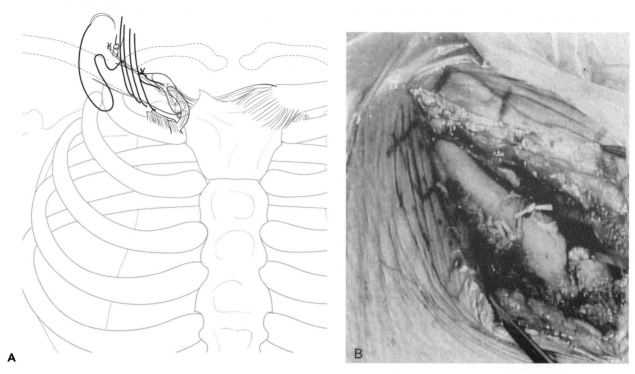

Figure 21-16 Transferred capsular ligament is secured into the medial clavicle by tying the sutures exiting from the superior cortex of the clavicle. (Reprinted with permission from Rockwood CA, Green DP, Bucholz RW, et al., eds. Fractures in the adult. Philadelphia, PA, JB Lippincott, 1996.)

TABLE 21-1
RESULTS

Authors	No. Patients	Procedure	Mean Follow-up (yr)	Results
Rockwood et al. 1997[23]	15	Resectional arthroplasty	7.7 (range, 2.0–14.5)	Uniformly excellent in patients who had an intact costo-clavicular ligament
Acus et al. 1995[1]	15	Resectional arthroplasty	4.6 (range, 1–14)	13 excellent (relief of pain) 2 poor results (because of regeneration of the clavicle)
Rockwood et al. 1989[22]	29 nonoperative 8 operative	Resectional arthroplasty (3) Reconstruction with autogenous tissue (4) Osteotomy with open reduction internal fixation (1)	8.4 (range, 1–24)	Nonoperative patients improved over time; poor results with operative treatment
Nettles and Linscheid 1968[18]	14	Capsulorrhaphy/fascial sling (1) Wire loop or transfixing pins (3) Resectional arthroplasty (2)	7.2 (range, 1–29)	8 good or excellent 4 fair or poor 2 inadequate follow-up

eratively, the patient should be held with his shoulders comfortably retracted in a figure-of-eight dressing for 4 to 6 weeks to allow for healing of the soft tissues (Table 21-1).

MEDIAL CLAVICLE FRACTURES AND FRACTURE DISLOCATIONS

Anterior Physeal Injuries of the Medial Clavicle

If the anterior physeal injury is recognized or if the patient is younger than 25 years, closed reduction, as described for anterior dislocation of the SC joint, should be performed. The shoulders should be held back in a clavicular strap or figure-of-eight dressing for 3 to 4 weeks, even if the reduction is stable. Healing is prompt, and remodeling will occur at the site of the deformity.

Posterior Physeal Injuries of the Medial Clavicle

Closed reduction of a posterior displacement of the medial clavicle should be performed in the manner described for posterior dislocation of the SC joint. The reduction is usually stable with the shoulders held back in a figure-of-eight dressing or strap. Immobilization should continue for 3 to 4 weeks. If the posterior physeal injury cannot be reduced, the patient is not having symptoms, and the patient is younger than 23 years, the physician can wait to see whether remodeling eliminates the posterior displacement of the clavicle.

Open reduction of the physeal injury is seldom indicated, except for an irreducible posterior displacement in a patient with significant symptoms of compression of the vital structures in the mediastinum. After reduction, the shoulders are held back with a figure-of-eight strap or dressing for 3 to 4 weeks.

REVISION STERNOCLAVICULAR SURGERY

Figuring Out What Went Wrong and Is Reoperation Justified?

In our experience, the two most common problems leading to revision surgery of the SC joint involve either "too much" or "too little" medial clavicle resection. In the former case, resection of the medial portion of the clavicle can result in cephalad displacement and instability of the remaining portion of the clavicle if the resection includes attachment site of the costoclavicular ligament. This is especially symptomatic with cross-body adduction when the medial clavicle rides across the midline of the sternum. In

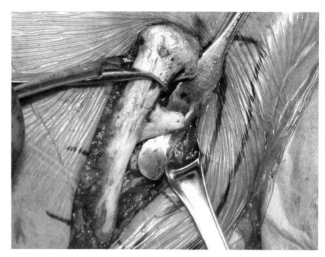

Figure 21-17 Chronic anterior SC dislocation. Note the ossified periosteum/rhomboid ligament that was projecting posteriorly into the mediastinal structures.

addition, the medial border of the clavicle will be displaced cephalad by the pull of the clavicular head of the sternocleidomastoid muscle in any attempt to elevate the arm or do any lifting. This produces a gross disfigurement of the front of the shoulder and is wholly unsatisfactory to the patient. There is a high rate of failure to restabilize the clavicle, which has led us to recommend subtotal claviculectomy as the salvage procedure (Fig. 21-17). Although some periscapular symptoms persist because the shoulder girdle is no longer supported by the axial skeleton, pain relief is usually satisfactory. In respect to inadequate resection, CT is most helpful in identifying structural impingement between the residual medial clavicle and the manubrium. In addition, a localized injection of lidocaine into this suspected area will confirm symptomatic impingement. Elimination of symptoms suggests that revision resection would be beneficial, bearing in mind that the costoclavicular ligament must be preserved to maintain stability of the medial portion of the clavicle.

Principles, Techniques, and Aftercare of Revision Surgery

The surgeon must be totally familiar with the anatomy immediately cephalad and posterior to the SC joint before the operation. In addition, we recommend that a thoracic surgeon be available as an integral part of the surgical team in the event of vascular complication. The risk of potentially fatal complications are particularly high with chronic unreduced posterior complication.

Procedure When the Costoclavicular Ligament Is Intact

After exposure of the medial portion of the clavicle, a curved 1- or 2-cm–wide retractor is passed posterior to the clavicle to isolate it and protect the vital posterior vascular structures during resection. The caudad aspect of the osteotomy must be medial to the costoclavicular ligament to avoid compromising the stabilizing role of the ligament. Excision of the medial portion of the clavicle is facilitated by drilling a series of holes through both cortices of the clavicle at the intended site of the osteotomy. An air-powered drill with a side-cutting bit is used to make the holes and to complete the osteotomy. The anterior and superior corners of the clavicle are beveled with an air burr. The periosteal tube is carefully repaired around the residual portion of the clavicle.

Procedure When the Costoclavicular Ligament Is Absent

When the costoclavicular ligament is absent, as is usually the case in chronic dislocation of the SC joint, it is necessary to reestablish the continuity of the remaining portion of the clavicle to the first rib. After any prominence of the remaining medial portion of the clavicle has been resected, two or three nonabsorbable sutures (1-mm Dacron tape) are passed around the remaining medial end of the clavicle and its periosteal tube and then through the residual scar of the costoclavicular ligament on the dorsal surface of the first rib. Closure of the periosteal tube stabilizes the medial portion of the clavicle to the first rib. The authors have not found it necessary to use fascial grafting to substitute for the costoclavicular ligaments. In some patients it may be necessary to pass additional sutures around or through holes in the first rib for stability. If the intra-articular disc ligament is preserved, it should be used as previously described.

Postoperative Management

All shoulders are immobilized in a sling for 6 weeks. On the second day, patients are allowed to perform gentle pendulum exercises but are cautioned against active flexion or abduction of the shoulder above 90 degrees. Forceful pushing, pulling, and lifting are avoided for 3 months. Beginning at 8 to 12 weeks, the patient can begin strengthening exercises. If the costoclavicular ligament is intact, the patient can be permitted to return to his or her usual activities, including manual labor, at 8 to 12 weeks. However, if the costoclavicular ligament is irreparable and Dacron tape was used to stabilize the clavicle down to the first rib as previously described, then the patient is restricted from returning to strenuous manual labor.

RESULTS AND COMPLICATIONS

Complications after operative treatment of the SC joint can be quite ominous because of the vital structuring in close proximity to the precarious joint. One of the easiest ways to avoid some of the more severe life-threatening complications is to avoid the use of pins that transfix the SC joint (Table 21-2).

Because of the degree of motion at the SC joint, tremendous leverage force is applied to pins that cross the SC joint resulting in hardware migration and fatigue breakage of the pins. Through 2000, eight deaths,[5,10,15,18,22,24,25] four near deaths,[4,6,20,25] and six additional cases of intrathoracic K-wire migration from complications of transfixing the SC joint with Kirschner wires of Steinman pins have been reported. The migration of the pins, either intact or broken,

TABLE 21-2
COMPLICATIONS

Authors	No. Patients	Procedure	Complications
Eskola et al. 1989[7]	12	Reconstruction with a tendon graft	4 poor (painful restriction of motion and weakness)
		Resection of sternal end of clavicle	1 loss of reduction (local tenderness, and pain radiating to the arm)
		Stabilization with fascial loop	
Lunseth et al. 1975[16]	4	Threaded Steinman transfixation pin	1 loss of reduction
Omer 1967[19]	4	Horizontal Z or step-cut transverse osteotomy	1 postoperative infection
			2 arthritic symptoms
Brown 1961[4]	10	K-wire transfixation pin	2 broken pins (required sternotomy for retrieval)
			1 pulmonary artery injury (required a thoracotomy secondary to pericardial tamponade)

into the heart, pulmonary artery, innominate artery, or aorta is common. *Consequently, the authors do not recommend any type of transfixing pins, large or small, across the SC joint.*

ACKNOWLEDGMENT

The authors express their appreciation to Debbie Mucha, R.N., C.R.R.N., for her assistance with the preparation of this chapter.

REFERENCES

1. Acus RA 3rd, Bell RH, Fisher DL. Proximal clavicle excision: an analysis of results. J Shoulder Elbow Surg 1995;4(3):182.
2. Bankart ASB. An operation for recurrent dislocation (subluxation) of the sternoclavicular joint. Br J Surg 1938;26:320.
3. Borrero E. Traumatic posterior displacement of the left clavicular head causing chronic extrinsic compression of the subclavian artery. Phys Sportsmed 1987;15:87.
4. Brown JE. Anterior sternoclavicular dislocation—a method of repair. Am J Orthop 1961;31:184.
5. Clark RL, Milgram JW, Yawn DH. Fatal aortic perforation and cardiac tamponade due to a Kirschner wire migrating from the right sternoclavicular joint. South Med J 1974;67:316.
6. DePalma AF. Surgical anatomy of acromioclavicular and sternoclavicular joints. Surg Clin North Am 1963;43:1541.
7. Eskola A, Vainiopaa S, Vastamaki M, et al. Operation for older sternoclavicular dislocation. Results in 12 cases. J Bone Joint Surg 1989;71-B(1):53.
8. Franquet T, Lecumberri F, Rivas A, et al. Condensing osteitis of the clavicle. Report of two new cases. Skeletal Radiol 1985;14:184.
9. Gangahar DM, Flogaites T. Retrosternal dislocation of the clavicle producing thoracic outlet syndrome. J Trauma 1978;18:369.
10. Gerlach D, Wemhoner SR, Ogbuihi S. [On two cases of fatal heart tamponade due to migration of fracture nails from the sternoclavicular joint.] Z Rechtsmed 1984;93:53.
11. Holmdahl HC. A case of posterior sternoclavicular dislocation. Acta Orthop Scand 1954;23:218.
12. Howard FM, Shafer SJ. Injuries to the clavicle with neurovascular complications. A study of fourteen cases. J Bone Joint Surg Am 1967;49A:755.
13. Hsu HC, Wu JJ, Lo WH, et al. Epiphyseal fracture-retrosternal dislocation of the medial end of the clavicle. A case report. Chinese Med J 1993;52:198.
14. Jelesijevic V, Knoll D, Klinke F, et al. Penetrating injuries of the heart and intrapericardial blood vessels caused by migration of a Kirschner pin after osteosynthesis. Acta Chir Iugosl 1982;29:274.
15. Leonard JW, Gifford RW. Migration of a Kirschner wire from the clavicle into pulmonary artery. Am J Cardiol 1965;16:598.
16. Lunseth PA, Chapman KW, Frankel VH. Surgical treatment of chronic dislocation of the sternoclavicular joint. J Bone Joint Surg 1975;57-B(2):193.
17. McKenzie JMM. Retrosternal dislocation of the clavicle. A report of two cases. J Bone Joint Surg 1963;45B:138.
18. Nettles JL, Linscheid R. Sternoclavicular dislocations. J Trauma 1968;8:158.
19. Omer GE. Osteotomy of the clavicle in surgical reduction of anterior sternoclavicular dislocation. J Trauma 1967;7:584.
20. Pate JW, Wilwhite J. Migration of a foreign body from the sternoclavicular joint to the heart. A case report. Am Surg 1969;35:448.
21. Paterson DC. Retrosternal dislocation of the clavicle. J Bone Joint Surg 1961;43B:90.
22. Rockwood CA, Odor JM. Spontaneous atraumatic anterior subluxations of the sternoclavicular joint in young adults. Report of 37 cases. Orthop Trans 1988;12:557.
23. Rockwood CA, Groh GI, Wirth MA, et al. Resection arthroplasty of the sternoclavicular joint. J Bone Joint Surg Am 1997;79:387.
24. Salavator JE. Sternoclavicular joint dislocation. Clin Orthop 1968;58:51.
25. Simurda MA. Retrosternal dislocation of the clavicle. A report of 4 cases and a method of repair. Can J Surg 1968;11:487.
26. Stankler L. Posterior dislocation of clavicle: a report of 2 cases. Br J Surg 1962;50:164.
27. Wayslenko MJ, Busse EF. Posterior dislocation of the clavicle causing fatal tracheoesophageal fistula. Can J Surg 1981;24:626.
28. Zaslav KR, Ray S, Neer CS. Conservative management of a displaced medial clavicular physeal injury in an adolescent athlete. Am J Sports Med 1989:17:833.

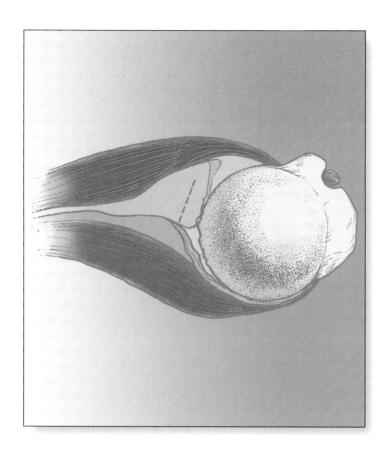

Alternatives to Total Shoulder Arthroplasty

22

Brian D. Cameron   Joseph P. Iannotti

INTRODUCTION

The primary goals in the management of the painful arthritic shoulder are pain relief and function restoration.[85] Total shoulder arthroplasty offers the most favorable functional results and successful pain relief among patients with rheumatoid arthritis and advanced osteoarthritis of the glenohumeral joint.[9,15,37,86,88] Favorable prognostic indicators include low-demand patients with moderate to severe disease, competent and intact or reparable rotator cuff, and minimal glenoid bone loss.[34,55] Variables occasionally exist that curb the surgeon's enthusiasm for total shoulder replacement. These include mild to moderate arthritic changes, young physiologic age, higher activity requirements, rotator cuff deficiency, severe glenoid bone loss, and brachial plexus injury.[2,35,68,108,114] Before recommending shoulder arthroplasty, the surgeon should weigh the risks associated with hemiarthroplasty or prosthetic glenoid resurfacing and consider all potential alternatives, including nonoperative management, arthroscopic debridement of loose cartilage and osteophytes, glenoidplasty, open or arthroscopic capsular release, synovectomy, periarticular osteotomy, corrective osteotomy, resection arthroplasty, soft tissue interpositional arthroplasty, and arthrodesis. Humeral prosthetic hemiarthroplasty with interpositional glenoid resurfacing represents an alternative to total shoulder arthroplasty in young active patients with advanced disease of both the humerus and glenoid.

B. D. Cameron: Stevens Orthopedic Group, Edmonds, Washington.
J. P. Iannotti: Chairman, Department of Orthopedics, Professor Cleveland Clinic Lerner School of Medicine, Cleveland Clinic Foundation, Cleveland, Ohio.

Short of total shoulder arthroplasty, complete amelioration of pain is not achieved with the same rate of success. However, improvement in the pain level is often acceptable and may delay the need for total shoulder replacement. Many symptomatic patients with early glenohumeral arthritis will benefit from nonsurgical management. When the disease has become recalcitrant to conservative measures, surgical intervention is considered.

CLASSIFICATION AND IMAGING

Natural History of Arthritis

Each of the glenohumeral arthritides is associated with particular patterns of osteoarticular damage. Although the causes are disparate, they share the common features of progressive, irreversible destruction. Articular destruction is accompanied by varying degrees of secondary involvement of the periarticular soft tissues, including the synovium, capsule, glenohumeral ligaments, and rotator cuff. Specific interventions may not be similarly effective for each condition. Therefore, successful diagnosis and treatment require an understanding of the glenohumeral arthritides. The main categories of glenohumeral arthritis include primary and secondary osteoarthritis, inflammatory arthritis, avascular necrosis, capsulorrhaphy arthropathy, and rotator cuff tear arthropathy.

Osteoarthritis

Primary osteoarthritis of the glenohumeral joint is uncommon relative to other major joints, has the highest average

age of onset, and presents more frequently in females.[23,84,98] When it occurs in men and younger individuals, it is often related to acute or repetitive trauma, and is often associated with a posterior glenoid bone loss and on occasion osteochondral fracture (Fig. 22-1).[56] Posttraumatic osteoarthritis and posterior subluxation of the humeral head may develop and is associated with posterior glenoid bone loss. Glenoid dysplasia, glenoid hypoplasia, and static subluxation of the humeral head may increase the risk of developing osteoarthritis.[115,120] Secondary osteoarthritis may be related to a previous fracture, chronic dislocation, or instability, or may be the result of failed surgical attempts to correct glenohumeral instability. Whether it is the result of an age-related inability to accommodate to normal forces or a failure to respond to excess loading, the process is an imbalance between reparative and degradative factors. The disorder is mechanically driven and biomechanically mediated.[29]

Articular changes are characterized by asymmetric joint space narrowing, subchondral sclerosis, cyst formation, and development of large osteophytes. Early articular thinning, surface fibrillation, and fissuring may remain subclinical for years.[13,28] These changes usually begin on the glenoid and then progress to the humeral head. Hypertrophic osteophyte formation occurs circumferentially around the neck of the humerus and glenoid rim. These osteophytes occupy intra-articular volume and restrict capsular excursion. Asymmetric contracture of the anterior capsule and subscapularis progressively limits external ro-

tation of the arm and causes obligate posterior translation of the humeral head relative to the glenoid. Preferential posterior glenoid erosion occurs, and a crista may develop between the intact anterior glenoid cartilage and the posteriorly eburnated bone. Osteochondral loose bodies may float within the recesses of the joint or may attach to adjacent bone or synovium.

Patients with primary osteoarthritis frequently present with complaints of shoulder pain and restricted motion. Although there exists a global loss of motion, the most profound losses usually develop in forward elevation and external rotation of the arm. Patients often complain of difficulty sleeping at night, especially on the affected side.[74] They may also describe a sense of weakness and atrophy. In contrast with rheumatoid arthritis, rotator cuff defects do not commonly occur in association with osteoarthritis.

Severe secondary or posttraumatic osteoarthritis may result from identifiable insults such as fracture, chronic dislocation, or surgery.[5,52,110] Alterations in the joint anatomy, biology, or mechanics will contribute to the development of arthritis or osteonecrosis. The reported rate of osteonecrosis associated with proximal humerus fractures varies according to the severity of injury, personality of the fracture, and method of treatment.[42,47,58,62,106] Traumatic and iatrogenic intra-articular fractures may result in some degree of arthropathy because of intra-articular incongruity or the development of osteonecrosis.[38,48] Chronic unreduced dislocations will develop softening and fragmentation of the cartilage and subchondral bone in the absence of normal physiologic joint forces. Large articular impression fractures will further contribute to the joint destruction. Osteoarthritis in the setting of fracture or chronic dislocation may result from a combination of intra-articular injury, malunion, instability, vascular disruption, and capsular contracture. Treatment of these problems can be very complex.

Iatrogenic causes of osteoarthritis may follow the treatment of instability. Periarticular implants that have been improperly placed or have dislodged may abrade the articular surfaces.[90,110,128] Intra-articular or extra-articular bone augmentation may lead to impingement, articular abrasion, and abnormal contact forces.[52] Procedures that are associated with excessive scarring (Bristow) may result in secondary osteoarthritis through pathologic compressive and shear forces across the articular surfaces.[70] Intra-articular fractures as a result of posterior glenoid osteotomy may result in a combination of osteonecrosis and osteoarthritis.[48]

Capsulorrhaphy arthropathy describes the arthritic condition that follows excessive surgical tightening of one side of the joint in the treatment of instability.[45] This complication occurs more commonly after nonanatomic repairs such as the Putti-Platt, Bristow, or Magnuson-Stack reconstruction.[40,46,53,70] However, it may also occur after a unidirectional repair in the treatment of multidirectional instability or excessive tightening of an "anatomic" repair.[71] Excessive anterior tightening after an anterior repair will restrict

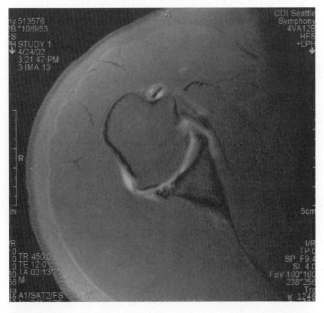

Figure 22-1 Axillary magnetic resonance imaging (MRI) of a young male with early glenohumeral osteoarthritis, posterior glenoid fracture, and posterior humeral subluxation. (Reprinted with permission from author.)

external rotation of the arm and push the humeral head posteriorly. Attempts to externally rotate the arm will lead to further obligate posterior translation of the humeral head relative to the glenoid. This constant eccentric loading of the glenoid results in posterior glenoid erosion and rapid destruction of the joint over a 10- to 15-year time period.

Rheumatoid Arthritis

Rheumatoid arthritis is the most common form of inflammatory arthritis and is representative of the pathologic and clinical manifestations seen in the glenohumeral joint. Shoulder pain develops in up to 90% of patients with rheumatoid arthritis, with 30% to 60% of patients experiencing significant pain or functional impairment.[99,112] Symptomatic shoulder involvement typically occurs in early middle-aged females who test positive for rheumatoid factor and variably involves the acromioclavicular joint, subacromial bursa, rotator cuff, and glenohumeral joint. Although the shoulder is commonly affected, rarely is it the primary manifestation of the disease or the only involved joint. The clinical course is one of insidious onset and gradual progression of pain and dysfunction.[22] Morning stiffness, weakness, and fatigue are common complaints. Shoulder pain, especially nocturnal pain, is the most common complaint of patients with glenohumeral rheumatoid arthritis. However, the actual source of pain in these patients may be difficult to locate. Cervical radiculopathy or myelopathy may produce shoulder pain and weakness. In addition, pain from the acromioclavicular joint, subacromial bursa, or rotator cuff may mimic or coexist with glenohumeral arthritis. A thorough history and physical examination, combined with radiographs and selective local anesthetic injections, will assist in accurately identifying the sources of pain and determining the appropriate treatment.

The destructive inflammatory process initially affects the periarticular soft tissues. Proliferation of the inflamed synovium and pannus, and the resulting reactive effusion, will distend the capsule and lead to an intensely painful joint that is exacerbated by motion. Clinically, the patient will try to limit this pain by avoiding the end ranges of motion. The proliferative pannus not only causes indirect damage through the release of destructive inflammatory mediators such as proteases and collagenase but also directly invades the adjacent cartilage, bone, tendon, and ligaments. The rotator cuff and biceps tendon are affected early in the disease process, leading to progressive attenuation and dysfunction. The incidence of rotator cuff defects and biceps tendon ruptures at the time of arthroplasty is approximately 40% and 60%, respectively.[8,9] Superior migration of the humeral head occurs in 20% of patients even in the presence of an intact rotator cuff. This is thought to occur through a muscular imbalance between a dysfunctional rotator cuff incapable of centering the head within the glenoid concavity in the presence of a properly functioning deltoid muscle. Degradative

enzymes from the inflammatory synovium, combined with direct invasion of pannus and altered cartilage nutrition from decreased joint motion, contribute to the destruction of the articular cartilage surfaces.[73,75] Synovial infiltration of the marginal bone characteristically begins along the superomedial aspect of the greater tuberosity, adjacent to the concomitant rotator cuff disease. Periarticular erosions and cysts become evident at the margins of the joint. Central and medial glenoid erosion progresses toward the base of the coracoid. The final result is severe glenohumeral incongruity and bone loss, symmetric capsular contracture, and an incompetent rotator cuff, which manifests as a very painful, poorly functioning shoulder.[101] Most shoulder surgeons advocate early intervention before the loss of bone stock and rotator cuff tissue.

Osteonecrosis

Osteonecrosis is often referred to as avascular necrosis, or aseptic necrosis. Occurring through a variety of traumatic or atraumatic means, osteonecrosis' common denominator is vascular embarrassment and bone death.[21] The ascending branch of the anterior humeral circumflex artery is the primary blood supply to the proximal humerus. Traumatic vascular disruption of the articular segment of the humeral head may occur after trauma or surgical intervention, variably resulting in osteonecrosis. Atraumatic osteonecrosis is associated with a variety of conditions such as steroid use, alcohol use, smoking, vascular disorders, coagulopathies, infiltrative marrow disorders, sickle cell disease, and Caisson's disease.[14,20,25,61,116] The disease process is believed to occur through a disturbance of the microcirculation, which results in ischemia and infarction of the marrow elements. The reparative response to remove and repair the necrotic bone leaves the subchondral bone weakened and vulnerable to compressive forces. Microfracturing and trabecular incompetence lead to collapse of the subchondral bone. Articular incongruity of the humeral head eventually leads to arthritic changes involving both the humeral head and glenoid.

Pain develops insidiously and is the primary complaint of patients with osteonecrosis. Pain may be related to bone infarction, elevated intraosseous pressure, or microfracturing of the subchondral cancellous trabeculae. Progressive subchondral collapse may produce painful mechanical symptoms such as catching or locking. Although the development of arthritis may be associated with weakness and atrophy, the rotator cuff and deltoid are generally intact.

Imaging

Plain Radiographs

Imaging studies are obtained to confirm the pathologic process and determine its extent. Plain radiographs are the initial studies of the shoulder and include three orthogonal views: an anteroposterior (AP) view in the scapular plane, a scapular lateral (Y) view, and an axillary view.[39] Except in the earliest stages, glenohumeral arthritis is usually easily detected on plain radiographs. External and internal rotation AP views of the humerus (35 degrees) or weight-bearing abduction views may facilitate the detection of early joint narrowing. Important radiographic features include joint space narrowing, proximal humeral migration, and amount and direction of bone loss. Other pathologic features may include postsurgical changes, periarticular erosions, hypertrophic marginal osteophytes, and the presence of calcifications or loose bodies.

Particular radiographic features are disease specific and offer important information regarding treatment options. Progressive osteoarthritic changes include joint space narrowing, subchondral sclerosis, subchondral cystic changes, and humeral head and glenoid flattening.[84] The classic inferomedial humeral osteophyte becomes prominent on the AP view. Although posterior subluxation of the humeral head and posterior erosion of the glenoid will be evident on the axillary view, it may not reveal the actual extent of osseous erosion.

Radiographic characteristics of rheumatoid arthritis are related to the duration and severity of the disease and include periarticular osteopenia, marginal erosions, joint space narrowing, and medial migration of the humeral head into the glenoid.[39,64] The axillary view reveals symmetric central erosion of the glenoid. End-stage disease is often accompanied by rotator cuff insufficiency and superior humeral head migration. Narrowing of the acromiohumeral interval and superior glenoid bone loss are seen on the AP view.[67] Resorption and collapse of the humeral head may allow the medial humeral metaphysis to articulate with the inferior aspect of the glenoid.

The radiographic features of osteonecrosis have been described by Cruess and are based on the Ficat staging system.[19–21] Focal sclerosis without collapse (stage II) may be apparent on the AP film with the humerus in external rotation. Stage III represents mild collapse of subchondral bone (1–2 mm) as depicted by a "crescent sign" on the AP view in external rotation. The articular cartilage is soft and bollotable but has not collapsed. Collapse of the humeral head articular surface and secondary degenerative changes of the glenoid (stages V and VI) may follow.

Computed Tomography Scanning and Magnetic Resonance Imaging

Advanced imaging studies should not replace a series of high-quality plain radiographs. When indicated, computed tomography (CT) scanning and magnetic resonance imaging (MRI) are useful adjunctive tests in determining the extent of the disease and in surgical planning. Computed tomography scanning allows an accurate assessment of bony architecture, whereas MRI offers exceptional noninvasive visualization of the articular cartilage and soft tissues.

Rarely, CT scanning may be performed as a primary study when it is not possible to obtain an adequate axillary view. Stiffness, severe pain, or obesity may prevent proper patient positioning for a quality study. In most cases, CT scanning is obtained to assess alterations in bony anatomy, especially in determining glenoid version and the extent and pattern of glenoid erosion.[7,36,83] Although the accuracy may vary slightly depending on scapular rotation, it is more accurate than plain radiographs, which will frequently underestimate the degree of osteoarticular destruction. Glenoid erosion is variable among the arthritides, occurring posteriorly in cases of osteoarthritis and capsulorrhaphy arthropathy, superior and central in patients with cuff-tear arthropathy or rheumatoid arthritis, and either anteriorly or posteriorly in association with a chronic dislocation of the shoulder. The degree of erosion will influence the available surgical options. Computed tomography scanning is also particularly useful in assessing proximal humeral bone stock, tuberosity malunion, and deformity of the proximal humerus and shaft, which occurs in cases of posttraumatic arthritis and in the revision setting.[31]

The role of MRI in the evaluation of the painful shoulder continues to expand.[50,87] Recent advances in magnetic resonance sequencing have improved the ability to detect early osteochondral abnormalities, which were previously underestimated by MRI and plain radiographs.[97,103] Currently, MRI is the best imaging study for detecting early osteoarthritis.[102] The loose bodies associated with synovial chondromatosis may only be evident by MRI. The ability to identify the presence of inflammatory synovitis and joint effusions may represent a clinical application in the early detection and treatment of patients with inflammatory arthropathies of the shoulder.[104,111,124] The high accuracy afforded by MRI provides valuable information regarding rotator cuff retraction and muscular atrophy.[57] In the setting of concomitant rotator cuff disease and glenohumeral arthritis, MRI is useful in assessing both the integrity of the rotator cuff and the degree of osteoarticular destruction.

Early osteonecrosis (stage I) is also often only detectable by MRI. This is superior to bone scanning, which has a poor sensitivity in diagnosing osteonecrosis.[81] Magnetic resonance imaging features are similar to those found in osteonecrosis of the femoral head.[79] The "double line sign" corresponds to the histologic changes that occur.[44] The hypointense line corresponds to the outer layer of osteoclastic proliferation and bone sclerosis, whereas the hyperintense line highlights an area of hypervascularity and granulation tissue.

Once the disease process has been defined, the clinician must determine the appropriate course of management for each patient. From the onset of the disease, the patient's function gradually deteriorates. Myotendinous shortening, muscular weakness, and capsular contracture (or attenuation) lead to functional impairment. Painful motion restriction may be related to articular destruction, soft tissue contracture, joint effusion, and synovial inflammation. With disease progression, the clinical manifestations resulting from articular erosion, ligamentous changes, and rotator cuff dysfunction may be profound. However, pain perception may be variable and may not directly correlate with radiographic disease stage. Patients with glenohumeral arthritis frequently have mechanical, inflammatory, and psychologic components to their pain.[26] It is not entirely clear whether psychologic distress or the effect of the joint condition is the cause of a heightened pain response. An appropriate treatment plan should take into account all of these variables.

Nonoperative Treatment

Patient satisfaction may suffer when the patient and physician are pursuing dissimilar goals. Education regarding the natural course of the disease and the patient's activity level and lifestyle requirements will help in making the patient's expectations commensurate with the prognosis.[105] Patients should be shown how to monitor clinical improvements as well as identify harmful symptoms to self-govern their therapy program.[113] Acute inflammatory episodes are best treated with a short period of rest, ice, analgesics, and an oral anti-inflammatory medication. Prolonged periods of rest may result in joint stiffness and muscle atrophy. Chronic inflammatory pain may be managed by the application of heat in the form of hot packs, hydrotherapy, and therapeutic ultrasound. These interventions seem to alleviate pain and enhance joint mobility by improving blood flow and increasing tissue elasticity.[65,66] They are also a useful adjuvant to physical therapy in restoring motion to the stiff shoulder.

The mainstay of physical therapy is to improve motion and strength.[27,54,72] Motion provides nutrition to the articular cartilage and minimizes the severity of capsular contracture that normally accompanies the disease process. Clinically, range of motion seems to be inversely related to pain levels. Active-assisted stretching exercises should be performed through an arc of motion that minimizes pain. Isometric and isotonic strengthening exercises, using light weights or elastic bands, are then added. The therapy program should avoid exacerbating the underlying condition and should be individualized to the specific needs and expectations of each patient. Methods to decrease exercise-induced inflammation include using ice, cortisone phonophoresis, and anti-inflammatory medications. Nonsteroidal anti-inflammatory drugs are clearly more effective than other oral analgesics (salicylates, acetaminophen, and codeine) when treating symptomatic inflammatory arthritides.[60] In patients with osteoarthritis, nonsteroidal anti-inflammatory drugs are as effective as simple analgesics.[30] Oral glucosamine may mitigate the pain associated with osteoarthritis.[10] However, it is unclear whether there exists a chondroprotective effect.

Selective local anesthetic injections, with or without a corticosteroid, may be both diagnostic and therapeutic. Pain relief after a glenohumeral injection will confirm an intra-articular cause and allow the patient to comfortably participate in the physical therapy program. Persistent pain immediately after an intra-articular injection suggests an alternative or concomitant source of pain, or an improperly placed injection. Intra-articular steroids provide longer lasting pain relief in patients with rheumatoid arthritis compared to those with osteoarthritis. Among patients with painful, stiff, rheumatoid shoulders, local injections and physical therapy seem to be equally effective.[24] Intra-articular viscosupplementation has been approved as a treatment for knee osteoarthritis.[121] To date there are no published reports supporting its use in the treatment of glenohumeral osteoarthritis.

Operative Treatment

Arthroscopic Debridement

Early arthritis of the glenohumeral joint poses a diagnostic and therapeutic challenge. Managing arthritis at any stage in the young or active patient is even more challenging because joint replacement may not be desirable in these patients and nonoperative treatment may not provide sufficient improvement in their levels of pain. Early articular changes of the humeral head or glenoid, including Outerbridge grade IV lesions, may be occult to detection by contemporary imaging techniques or clinical examination.[13] Previously unrecognized grades II to IV lesions have been detected as incidental findings at the time of arthroscopy.[32,33] The clinical significance of these early lesions, as well as their propensity to progress, is not well defined. Equally unclear is the ability of arthroscopic surgery to either alter or improve the natural course of the disease.

The results of arthroscopic debridement of knee osteoarthritis may be influenced by a strong placebo effect.[82] To date, there does not exist a similar randomized study of the effects of arthroscopic debridement in the management of glenohumeral osteoarthritis. Several studies have indicated that the results are related to the severity of the osteochondral lesions. Improvements in postoperative function and pain levels have been shown to reliably improve in 66% to 80% of patients with mild (grades I–III) changes and in 75% of patients with moderate (grade IV) lesions.[91,93,122] The surgical technique includes a complete inspection of the glenohumeral joint and subacromial space. Loose osteochondral fragments are extricated from the joint. A motorized shaver is used to debride degenerative labral tissue and to bring unstable chondral flaps back to a stable base. Grade III articular cartilage is debrided, and the margins are tapered. Microfracturing or drilling of the intact subchondral bone is performed with the intent that it will create bleeding of the bone to bring cells that differentiate into new cartilage-like tissue. Degenerative tissue on either side of the rotator cuff is debrided, and all reactive synovium and bursal tissue are removed. A capsular release should be performed in patients who exhibit a 20-degree[13] capsular contracture in any plane (compared with the unaffected side) or have posterior humeral head subluxation. The shoulder is injected with a long-acting local anesthetic combined with a corticosteroid, and motion exercises are started in the recovery room. The ideal candidate for arthroscopic debridement is the patient with a congruent, well-centered joint, little or no osteophyte formation, mild or no subchondral sclerosis or cyst formation, and an osteochondral defect that does not exceed 2 cm².[13] Lesions larger than this are at risk for return of pain and clinical failure.

Arthroscopic debridement is not often performed as an isolated procedure. Concomitant osteochondral lesions frequently coexist with other lesions such as impingement syndrome, partial thickness rotator cuff tears, acromioclavicular arthropathy, and capsular contracture. It is incumbent on the surgeon to define these abnormalities through preoperative clinical evaluation, selective injections, and appropriate imaging studies. Several studies demonstrate that the presence of early osteoarthritis is not a contraindication to concomitant surgical procedures when the surgeon is confident about the diagnosis.[13,33,41] Favorable results have been achieved when arthroscopic debridement is combined with arthroscopic bursectomy, subacromial decompression, distal clavicle excision, labral debridement, or debridement of partial thickness rotator cuff tears. The surgeon should not abandon an original diagnosis that is based on a thorough preoperative evaluation merely on encountering unsuspected grade IV osteochondral lesions. In many cases, there are several causes of shoulder pain, and the preoperative diagnosis based on examination, injection tests, and preoperative imaging will often remain an accurate method of identifying these other causes of shoulder pain. In many cases, these causes of shoulder pain should be addressed at the time of surgery despite identifying previously unsuspected arthritis.

Several authors have reported successful results after arthroscopic debridement of the glenohumeral joint among patients with synovial chondromatosis and early associated arthritic changes.[18,107,127] Surgery includes debridement of the reactive synovium and degenerative cartilage in addition to removal of the loose bodies. Arthroscopic debridement of early avascular necrosis of the humeral head may produce favorable results when the lesion is small and localized.[43,49,81] This includes debridement of the articular lesion and removal of loose osteochondral fragments (Fig. 22-2). Very little data exist regarding the value of arthroscopic debridement among patients with rheumatoid arthritis of the glenohumeral joint.[127] Rotator cuff disease is inevitably present, and the addition of a subacromial decompression to include only minimal smoothing and

bursectomy seems to improve functional and pain levels in up to 80% of patients.[112] A conservative decompression should not diminish the anterior to posterior dimension of the acromion or compromise the structural integrity of the coracoacromial arch.

The early results of arthroscopic debridement for early glenohumeral arthritis are encouraging, whereas long-term results have yet to be established. Whether it slows the progression of cartilage degeneration is not known. Despite radiographic progression, well-selected patients show a significant clinical benefit from arthroscopic debridement. For others it may represent only a palliative procedure, delaying prosthetic replacement.

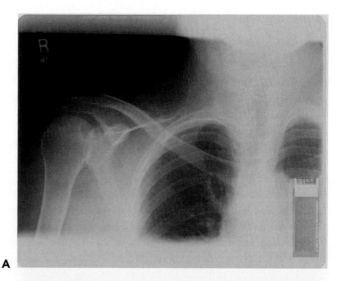

A

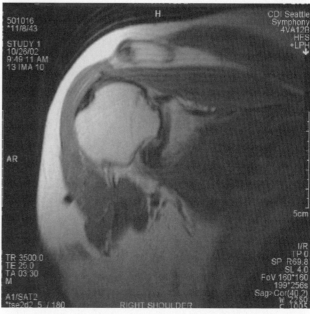

B

Figure 22-2 *(A)* Plain film reveals stage III osteonecrosis of the superior humeral head in a steroid-dependent woman. (Reprinted with permission from author.) *(B)* Coronal and axial MRI reveal significant osteochondral destruction of the humeral head.

Capsular Release

Loss of shoulder motion is a frequent clinical manifestation of glenohumeral osteoarthritis. Anterior capsular contracture results in a loss of external rotation of the arm at the side. Obligate posterior translation of the humeral head occurs as a secondary phenomenon, resulting in asymmetric posterior glenoid erosion. In addition, mechanical irritation of the joint may produce a more globally frozen shoulder. Capsular contractures exist in up to 30% of patients undergoing arthroscopic debridement of glenohumeral osteoarthritis.[13,93] Regaining and retaining full arcs of motion are crucial in obtaining a favorable result. Arthroscopic debridement alone will not restore normal motion in patients with capsular contractures. Capsular release is recommended when the patient has lost 20 degrees of motion in any plane compared with the unaffected side.

We perform the capsular release with either a radiofrequency probe or an arthroscopic Bovie cautery. The rotator interval capsule and coracohumeral ligament are incised in the midsubstance. The anterior capsule is incised 1 cm lateral to the glenoid rim. The middle glenohumeral ligament is released, and the thick capsule covering the subscapularis is divided to the anterior inferior capsular pouch. The subscapularis tendon should not be disrupted. Its tendon fibers are oriented transversely compared with the amorphous appearance of the capsule. The inferior capsule is then scored with the electrocautery, and the shoulder is manipulated after removing the arthroscopic equipment. An inferior posterior portal is useful for surgical release of the inferior capsular pouch. If necessary, a posterior capsular release is performed using the posterior portal, incising the capsule midway between the humeral and glenoid attachments.

Capsulorrhaphy arthropathy is a well-recognized complication after excessive imbrication of the anterior capsule and subscapularis for the treatment of glenohumeral instability.[46] Patients with persistent pain, mild to moderate arthritic changes, and limited external rotation are candidates for open capsular release. Capsular release is ideally performed before there is radiographic evidence of arthritis. If the subscapularis tendon was shortened at the time of the initial surgery, then subscapularis lengthening is added to capsular release. Although instability does not appear to recur after the procedure, no long-term follow-up data are available regarding the progression of arthrosis.

Inflammatory arthropathy of the glenohumeral joint will clinically manifest in a progressive, symmetric loss of shoulder motion. Manipulation under anesthesia should be avoided in the rheumatoid patient with a stiff shoulder because of the risk of fracture or rotator cuff tear. Arthroscopic capsular release is preferred.

Synovectomy

The treatment of early rheumatoid glenohumeral arthritis is directed at eliminating the offending synovial tissue, before destruction of the soft tissues and articular surfaces. The orthopedic surgeon should become involved in the early stages of the disease when systemic therapy has failed, before destructive changes have become apparent. Synoviorthosis, or synovectomy, may be obtained by either medical or surgical means. Medical synovectomy is achieved through the intra-articular placement of chemical or radioactive agents that are designed to eradicate the pathologic synovium.[76,77] Success rates of approximately 50% have been reported, with pain relief and functional improvements lasting 3 to 5 years. Pathologic synovial tissue usually regenerates, requiring multiple treatments. Potential complications associated with these chemical agents include infection, skin necrosis, allergic reaction, and neoplastic changes.

Surgical synovectomy may be achieved by open or arthroscopic techniques.[96,123] Surgery is indicated in a narrow spectrum of patients who present in the early stages of the disease, exhibiting little or no radiographic evidence of articular destruction.[94,95,100] Arthroscopic synovectomy is particularly attractive because it facilitates early active motion, which is essential for a favorable result.[59,92] It is appropriately performed when the rotator cuff is intact, providing reliable pain relief in 80% of patients and significantly improved motion in nearly all patients. In the presence of a repairable full-thickness rotator cuff tear, synovectomy and bursectomy should be combined with a conservative subacromial decompression and open rotator cuff repair. Regeneration of the pathologic synovium may warrant repeat synovectomies. Open synovectomy performed in later stages of the disease (extensive soft-tissue damage, articular destruction) has been shown to provide pain relief in 50% of patients and improved motion in 70% of patients through a 6-year follow-up period.[118] The poorest outcomes are associated with extensive rotator cuff and subacromial bursal disease.

Glenoidplasty

Arthroscopic glenoidplasty with osteocapsular arthroplasty is a novel application of arthroscopic technique for advanced glenohumeral osteoarthritis in patients in whom shoulder replacement is either unsuitable or undesirable.[89] It is essentially an effort to sculpt the incongruous glenohumeral joint. Glenoidplasty is directed at correcting the combination of eccentric posterior glenoid erosion and fixed posterior subluxation of the humeral head. This is achieved by converting a biconcave glenoid into a single concave surface. Arthroscopic contouring of the anterior glenoid cartilage and vertical central crista is performed with an arthroscopic burr and rasp, creating a concentric glenohumeral articulation. Restoring the position of the humeral head may increase the joint contact surface area, improve stability, and relax the anterior soft tissues. Glenoidplasty is not necessary if the joint is already concentric.

Osteocapsular arthroplasty is directed at relieving pain and improving motion in patients with advanced glenohumeral osteoarthritis. It is indicated in patients with large humeral osteophytes and capsular contracture when there is a relative contraindication to total shoulder arthroplasty because of young age or high activity level. Marginal osteophytes and loose bodies are removed to alleviate impingement pain. An arthroscopic synovectomy is performed to improve pain at rest and at the end range of motion. Finally, contracted capsular structures are arthroscopically released. Multiple portals may be needed to access the large osteophytes, and multiple outflow sites may be needed to prevent fluid extravasation.

Early results of these procedures seem encouraging, with consistent relief of impingement and rest pain.[89] Pain relief in the mid arc of motion is less predictable. Functional improvements appear to be directly correlated to postoperative pain levels, whereas postoperative improvements in range of motion appear to slowly decline. Favorable prognostic indicators include impingement pain at the end range of motion, association with large humeral osteophytes, posterior glenoid erosion, humeral head subluxation, and large loose bodies. Negative predictive variables include pain in the mid range of motion, painful crepitus, pain with glenohumeral compression during humeral rotation, and a concentric glenohumeral articulation. Little is known regarding progressive glenoid erosion.

Corrective Osteotomy

In cases of early eccentric glenohumeral osteoarthritis with posterior glenoid erosion, an attempt may be made to correct the acquired retroversion of the posterior glenoid,[56] which is achieved by performing a posterior opening wedge osteotomy of the glenoid (Fig. 22-3). The osteotomy is combined with intra-articular interposition of the posterior capsule to resurface the eburnated posterior glenoid surface. The posterior capsule can be used in this manner when it is of sufficient length such that suturing it to the glenoid surface will not result in excessive tightening of the posterior capsule or excessive loss of internal rotation. The objective is to reduce the posterior humeral subluxation and create a concentric glenohumeral joint. The anticipated effect is a decrease in shear forces and a more even distribution of joint contact forces. Improvements in pain and function have been reported. The procedure is considered for young or active symptomatic individuals with significant glenoid retroversion, fixed subluxation, or early eccentric glenohumeral osteoarthritis. Complications include infection, nonunion, secondary arthritis, and osteonecrosis.

Glenoid hypoplasia or dysplasia may be associated with excessive glenoid retroversion.[54,126] Some of these patients may develop glenohumeral instability or degenerative glenohumeral arthritis. It is not known whether these patients will benefit from a posterior opening wedge osteotomy.

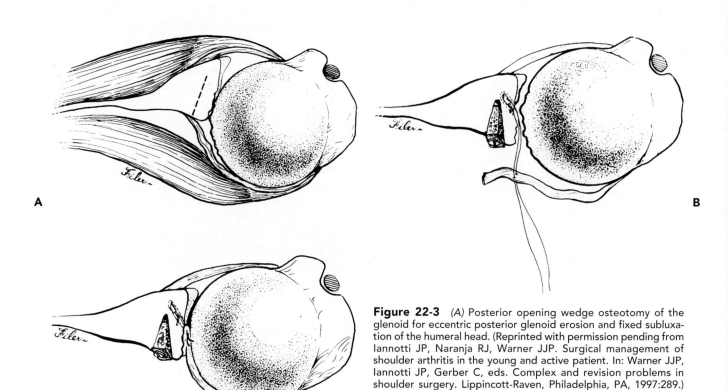

Figure 22-3 (A) Posterior opening wedge osteotomy of the glenoid for eccentric posterior glenoid erosion and fixed subluxation of the humeral head. (Reprinted with permission pending from Iannotti JP, Naranja RJ, Warner JJP. Surgical management of shoulder arthritis in the young and active patient. In: Warner JJP, Iannotti JP, Gerber C, eds. Complex and revision problems in shoulder surgery. Lippincott-Raven, Philadelphia, PA, 1997:289.) (B) Placement of a posterior bone graft. (C) Posterior capsule is used to cover the eburnated bone on the posterior glenoid.

Humeral derotational osteotomy has been advocated as a method to correct malunited fractures and to address glenohumeral instability. It may also provide reasonable pain relief among patients with rheumatoid arthritis who have a severe limitation of external rotation.[1]

Interpositional Arthroplasty

Recontouring the arthritic glenohumeral joint and biologic interpositional arthroplasty is generating considerable interest as an alternative to total joint arthroplasty in the young or active patient. First described by Baer in 1918, interpositional arthroplasty has been performed as a treatment for both osteoarthritis and rheumatoid arthritis, using tissues ranging from pig's bladder to lyophilized dura mater.[3,78,117] The humeral head is debrided of osteophytes and is reshaped to decrease the diameter of the humeral head and increase humeral retroversion. This debulking may facilitate rotator cuff repair if a tear is present. The glenoid is then reamed to create a single concave surface and is covered with a biologic membrane, such as the anterior capsule, Achilles tendon allograft, or fascia lata (Fig. 22-4).[4] Several authors have reported favorable results in up to 85% of patients, with significant improvements in pain and functional levels.

A hybrid prosthetic alternative combines biologic resurfacing of the glenoid with hemiarthroplasty (Fig. 22-5) for the treatment of osteoarthritis in the young, active patient.[11,12] Originally described by Burkhead,[11] this hybrid approach addresses several important issues. First, humeral loosening is exceedingly rare in the absence of a prosthetic glenoid component.[16,125] Second, hemiarthroplasty alone for the treatment of osteoarthritis provides inferior pain relief compared with total shoulder arthroplasty, especially in the presence of asymmetric glenoid erosion.[17,68,114] Finally, prosthetic glenoid resurfacing in the young or active patient confers a higher risk of mechanical glenoid loosening, as well as polyethylene wear-related aseptic loosening of the components. The goal of hemiarthroplasty with interpositional glenoid arthroplasty is to provide pain relief that approaches that of total shoulder arthroplasty, while mitigating the risks of wear and mechanical loosening that are associated with a polyethylene glenoid component. Surface humeral prosthetic arthroplasty with soft tissue interposition glenoplasty may provide a more conservative bone-sparing approach than using a standard stemmed humeral prosthetic. When one uses a surface humeral hemiarthroplasty, glenoid exposure is more difficult and will require complete anterior inferior capsular release to optimize glenoid exposure.

Appropriate preoperative imaging studies should reveal the degree of posterior glenoid erosion. Neutral glenoid version may be restored by preferentially reaming the high side of the glenoid. The humeral prosthesis may be

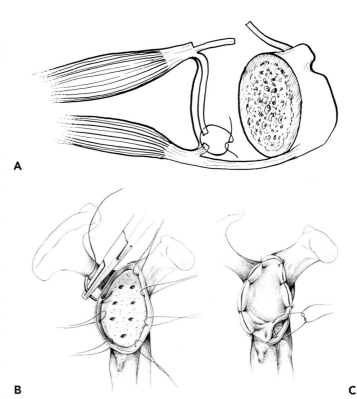

Figure 22-4 *(A)* Interposition arthroplasty using the anterior capsule as a biologic covering for the glenoid. (Reprinted with permission pending from Iannotti JP, Naranja RJ, Warner JJP. Surgical management of shoulder arthritis in the young and active patient. In: Warner JJP, Iannotti JP, Gerber C, eds. Complex and revision problems in shoulder surgery. Lippincott-Raven, Philadelphia, PA, 1997:289.) *(B,C)* Interposition arthroplasty using fascia lata autograft as a biologic covering for the glenoid. (Reprinted with permission from Hauzeur J, Sintzoff S, Appelboom T, et al. Relationship between magnetic resonance imaging and histologic findings by bone biopsy in nontraumatic osteonecrosis of the femoral head. J Rheumatol 1992; 19(3):385.)

placed in slightly less retroversion if neutral glenoid version cannot be obtained. The entire glenoid surface should be denuded of articular cartilage and concentrically reamed. The graft is then sutured to the glenoid using drill holes, suture anchors, or a combination of both. If possible, the anterior capsule is dissected free from the subscapularis tendon and sutured over the face of the glenoid. If this is not adequate, then autogenous fascia lata, Achilles tendon allograft, or fascia lata allograft may be used. Lateral meniscal allograft has recently been introduced as an alternative to the currently used interposition materials.[5] The wedge shape of the meniscus seems to assist in restoring glenoid contour and improving version. The relative size match of the meniscus and glenoid usually allows adequate coverage (Fig. 22-6). Overall, the early results of hemiarthroplasty with biologic glenoid resurfacing are satisfactory to excellent in 90% of patients.

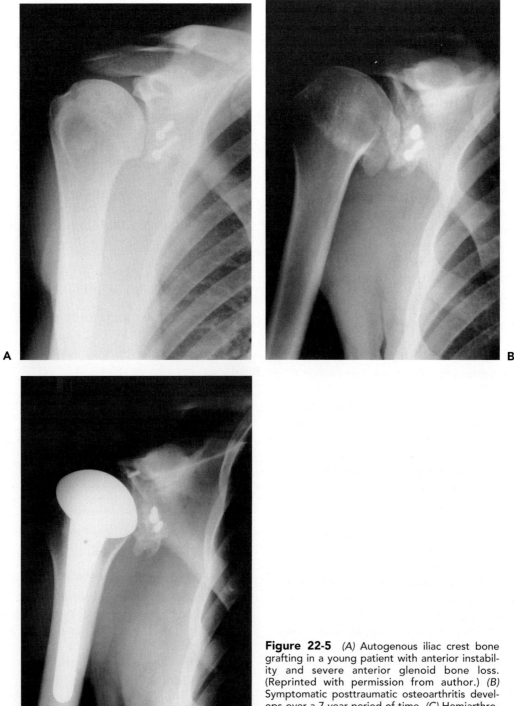

Figure 22-5 (A) Autogenous iliac crest bone grafting in a young patient with anterior instability and severe anterior glenoid bone loss. (Reprinted with permission from author.) (B) Symptomatic posttraumatic osteoarthritis develops over a 7-year period of time. (C) Hemiarthroplasty with glenoid interpositional arthroplasty using the anterior capsular tissue.

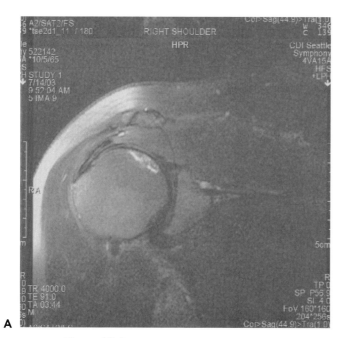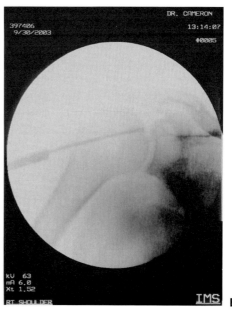

Figure 22-6 *(A,B)* Interpositional arthroplasty using lateral meniscal allograft as a biologic covering for the glenoid. (*A* reprinted with permission from Burkhead WZ Jr., Hutton KS. Biologic resurfacing of the glenoid with hemiarthroplasty of the shoulder. J Shoulder Elbow Surg 1995;4(4):263. *B* reprinted with permission from Skedros JG, O'Rourke PJ, Zimmerman JM, et al. Alternatives to replacement arthroplasty for glenohumeral arthritis. In: Iannotti JP, Williams GR, eds. Disorders of the shoulder: diagnosis and management. Philadelphia, PA, Lippincott Williams & Wilkins, 1999:485.)

Core Decompression

The use of core decompression in the treatment of early osteonecrosis has been advocated by several authors.[63,80,81,109,119] Ten-year follow-up studies have shown successful resolution of symptomatic precollapse and early collapse lesions (90% good or excellent results for stages I and II, 70% good or excellent results for stage III lesions). Although most of these patients experience immediate pain relief and improvement in function, it is unclear whether core decompression is superior to nonoperative treatment in preventing progressive radiographic changes. The beneficial effect of core decompression for stage III lesions is controversial, although it may delay the need for hemiarthroplasty.[69] Core decompression does not appear to alter the progression of stage IV or V disease, for which prosthetic arthroplasty is recommended.

The patient is placed in the supine or semirecumbent position with a wedge or saline bag placed under the affected scapula. Biplane fluoroscopy is used to localize the lesion. A small anterior axillary incision is made in the deltopectoral interval. The insertion site for the drill or cannula should be made lateral to the bicipital groove to avoid injury to the arterial blood supply, and two to four tunnels are created depending on the size of the lesion. We currently prefer to evaluate the glenohumeral joint arthroscopically, before core decompression, to evaluate the integrity of the articular cartilage and perform any necessary joint debridement. Currently, no studies are available evaluating the combined use of core decompression and arthroscopic debridement in the treatment of osteonecrosis.

SUMMARY

Total shoulder replacement represents the best treatment option for many older patients with advanced arthritis of the glenohumeral joint. Among patients with mild articular changes, and in the young, active patient, joint-sparing alternatives should be considered. On the basis of the current literature and our clinical experience, we generally avoid placing a glenoid component in these patients. We do not advocate periarticular osteotomy or humeral derotation osteotomy for the treatment of glenohumeral osteoarthritis. We will perform arthroscopic debridement of the joint in cases of mild to moderate glenohumeral osteoarthritis. Concomitant surgical procedures are conducted according to a thorough preoperative clinical evaluation. Intraoperative motion restoration is imperative, and is accomplished through appropriate capsular releases. When eccentric posterior glenoid wear and posterior subluxation of the humeral head are encountered, a posterior opening wedge osteotomy of the glenoid may be performed.

We will perform arthroscopic synovectomy of the rheumatoid shoulder when there is evidence of minimal joint destruction. When clinically apparent, defects of the rotator cuff are repaired and a capsular release is performed.

We have been performing hemiarthroplasty with biologic glenoid interposition in young, active patients with primary glenohumeral osteoarthritis, as well as in the revision setting. We have also performed isolated glenoid biologic resurfacing in cases of severe glenoid erosion in association with mild changes of the humeral articular surface. Our early results have been encouraging with regard to pain relief and restoration of function, and we believe that this represents an excellent alternative to total shoulder arthroplasty in well-selected patients. It is not a substitute prosthetic arthroplasty in older patients with advanced glenohumeral osteoarthritis. We have not had clinical experience with this technique in patients with rheumatoid arthritis.

REFERENCES

1. Allieu Y, Lussiez B, Desbonnet P, et al. External deterioration osteotomy of the humerus in rheumatoid arthritis. Rheumatology 1989;12:60.
2. Arntz CT, Jackins S, Matsen FA III. Prosthetic replacement of the shoulder for the treatment of defects in the rotator cuff and the surface of the glenohumeral joint. J Bone Joint Surg 1993;75A(4):485.
3. Baer WS. Arthroplasty with the help of animal membrane. Am J Orthop Surg 1918;16.
4. Baghian S, Font-Rodriguez D, Williams GR. Soft-tissue interposition without hemiarthroplasty for treatment of degenerative glenohumeral arthritis in young patients. Presented at the American Academy of Orthopaedic Surgeons 70th Annual Meeting. New Orleans, LA, February 8, 2003.
5. Ball CM, Galatz LM, Yamaguchi K. Meniscal allograft interposition arthroplasty for the arthritic shoulder: description of a new surgical technique. Tech Shoulder Elbow Surg 2001;2(4):247.
6. Barrett WP, Thornhill TS, Thomas WH, et al. Nonconstrained total shoulder arthroplasty in patients with polyarticular rheumatoid arthritis. J Arthroplasty 1989;4(1):91.
7. Bokor DJ, O'Sullivan MD, Hazan GJ. Variability of measurement of glenoid version on computed tomography scan. J Shoulder Elbow Surg 1999;8(6):595.
8. Boyd AD, Aliabadi P, Thornhill TS. Postoperative proximal migration in total shoulder arthroplasty. J Arthroplasty 1991;6(1):31.
9. Boyd AD, Thomas WH, Scott RD, et al. Total shoulder arthroplasty versus hemiarthroplasty. J Arthroplasty 1990;5:329.
10. Brief AA, Maurer SG, Di Cesare PE. Use of glucosamine and chondroitin sulfate in the management of osteoarthritis. J Am Acad Orthop Surg 2001;9(2):71.
11. Burkhead WZ Jr. Hemiarthroplasty with biologic resurfacing of the glenoid for glenohumeral arthritis. J Shoulder Elbow Surg 1993;2(1):29.
12. Burkhead WZ Jr., Hutton KS. Biologic resurfacing of the glenoid with hemiarthroplasty of the shoulder. J Shoulder Elbow Surg 1995;4(4):263.
13. Cameron BD, Galatz LM, Ramsey ML, et al. Non-prosthetic management of grade IV osteochondral lesions of the glenohumeral joint. J Shoulder Elbow Surg 2002;11(1):25.
14. Chung SM, Ralston EL. Necrosis of the humeral head associated with sickle cell anemia and its genetic variants. Clin Orthop 1972;80:105.
15. Cofield RH. Total shoulder arthroplasty with the Neer prosthesis. J Bone Joint Surg 1984;66A:899.
16. Cofield RH. Uncemented total shoulder arthroplasty. A review. Clin Orthop 1994;(307):86.
17. Cofield RH, Frankle MA, Zuckerman JD. Humeral head replacement for glenohumeral arthritis. Semin Arthroplasty 1995;6(4):214.
18. Covall DJ, Fowble CD. Arthroscopic treatment of synovial chondromatosis of the shoulder and biceps tendon sheath. Arthroscopy 1993;9(5):602.
19. Cruess RL. Steroid-induced avascular necrosis of the head of the humerus. J Bone Joint Surg 1976;53B(3):313.
20. Cruess RL. Experience with steroid-induced avascular necrosis of the shoulder and etiologic considerations regarding osteonecrosis of the hip. Clin Orthop 1978;130:86.
21. Cruess RL. Osteonecrosis of bone. Clin Orthop 1986;208:30.
22. Curran JF, Ellman MH, Brown NL. Rheumatologic aspects of painful conditions affecting the shoulder. Clin Orthop 1983;173:27.
23. Cushnaghan J, Dieppe PA. Study of 500 patients with limb osteoarthritis. 1. Analysis by age, sex and distribution of symptomatic joint sites. Ann Rheum Dis 1991;50:8.
24. Dacre JE, Beeney N, Scott DL. Injections and physiotherapy for the painful stiff shoulder. Ann Rheum Dis 1989;48:322.
25. David HG, Bridgman SA, Davies SC, et al. The shoulder in sickle-cell disease. J Bone Joint Surg 1993;75-B(4):538.
26. Davis MA, Ettinger WH, Neuhaus JM, et al. Correlates of knee pain among US adults with and without radiographic knee osteoarthritis. J Rheumatol 1992;19(12):1943.
27. Dean MT, Burkhead WZ. Nonoperative treatment of anterior shoulder instability. Sports Med Arthrosc Rev 1993;1:202.
28. DePalma AF, White JB, Gallery G. Degenerative lesions of the shoulder joint at various age groups which are compatible with good function. In: Blount W, Edwards JW, eds. American Academy of Orthopaedic Surgeons Instructional Course Lectures. Vol. VII. Ann Arbor, MI, J. W. Edwards, 1950:168.
29. Dequeker J, Dieppe P. Osteoarthritis and related disorders. In: Klippel JH, Dieppe PA, eds. Rheumatology. Philadelphia, PA, Mosby, 1999:2.
30. Dieppe P. Drug treatment of osteoarthritis. J Bone Joint Surg Br 1993;75:673.
31. Dines DM, Warren RF, Altchek DW, et al. Posttraumatic changes of the proximal humerus: malunion, nonunion and osteonecrosis. treatment with modular hemiarthroplasty or total shoulder arthroplasty. J Shoulder Elbow Surg 1993;2:11.
32. Ellman H, Harris E, Kay S. Early degenerative joint disease simulating impingement syndrome: arthroscopic findings. Arthroscopy 1992;8(4):482.
33. Ellowitz AS, Rosas R, Rodosky MW, et al. The benefit of arthroscopic decompression for impingement in patients found to have unsuspected glenohumeral osteoarthritis. Presented at the Annual Meeting of American Academy of Orthopaedic Surgeons, San Francisco, CA, February 15, 1997.
34. Figgie HE, Inglis AE, Goldberg VM, et al. An analysis of factors affecting the long-term results of total shoulder arthroplasty in inflammatory arthritis. J Arthroplasty 1988;3(2):123.
35. Franklin JL, Barrett WP, Jackins SE, et al. Glenoid loosening in total shoulder arthroplasty. J Arthroplasty 1988;3(1):39.
36. Friedman RJ, Hawthorne KB, Genez BM. The use of computerized tomography in the measurement of glenoid version. J Bone Joint Surg 1992;74A:1032.
37. Gartsman GM, Roddey TS, Hammerman SM. Shoulder arthroplasty with or without resurfacing of the glenoid in patients who have osteoarthritis. J Bone Joint Surg 2000;82-A(1):26.
38. Gerber C, Hersche O, Berberat C. The clinical relevance of posttraumatic avascular necrosis of the humeral head. J Shoulder Elbow Surg 1998;7:586.
39. Green A, Norris TR. Imaging techniques for glenohumeral arthritis and glenohumeral arthroplasty. Clin Orthop 1994;307:7.
40. Green A, Norris TR. Shoulder arthroplasty for advanced glenohumeral arthritis after anterior instability repairs. J Shoulder Elbow Surg 2001;10(6):539.
41. Guyette TM, Bae H, Warren RF, et al. Results of arthroscopic subacromial decompression in patients with subacromial impingement and glenohumeral degenerative joint disease. J Shoulder Elbow Surg 2002;11(4):299.
42. Haag O, Lundberg B. Aspects of prognostic factors in comminuted and dislocated proximal humerus fractures. In: Bateman J, Welsh R, eds. Surgery of the shoulder. Philadelphia, PA, Decker, 1984:51.
43. Hardy P, Decrette E, Jeanrot C, et al. Arthroscopic treatment of bilateral humeral head osteonecrosis. Arthroscopy 2000; 16(3):332.
44. Hauzeur J, Sintzoff S, Appelboom T, et al. Relationship between magnetic resonance imaging and histologic findings by bone biopsy in nontraumatic osteonecrosis of the femoral head. J Rheumatol 1992;19(3):385.

45. Hawkins RH, Hawkins RJ. Failed anterior reconstruction for shoulder instability. J Bone Joint Surg 1985;67B(5):709.
46. Hawkins RJ, Angelo RL. Glenohumeral osteoarthrosis. A late complication of the Putti-Platt repair. J Bone Joint Surg 1990; 72A(8):1193.
47. Hawkins RJ, Bell RH, Gurr K. The three-part fracture of the proximal part of the humerus. J Bone Joint Surg 1986;68A(9):1410.
48. Hawkins RJ, Koppert G, Johnston G. Recurrent posterior instability (subluxation) of the shoulder. J Bone Joint Surg 1984; 66A(2):169.
49. Hayes JM. Arthroscopic treatment of steroid-induced osteonecrosis of the humeral head: a case report. Arthroscopy 1989;5(3):218.
50. Herzog RJ. Magnetic resonance of the shoulder. J Bone Joint Surg 1997;79-A(6):934.
51. Hovelius L, Augustini BG, Fredin H, et al. Primary anterior dislocation of the shoulder in young patients. J Bone Joint Surg 1996;78-A(11):1677.
52. Hovelius LK, Sandstrom BC, Rosmark DL, et al. Long-term results with the Bankhart and Bristow-Laterjet procedures: recurrent shoulder instability and arthropathy. J Shoulder Elbow Surg 2001;10(5):445.
53. Hovelius L, Thorling J, Fredin H. Recurrent anterior dislocation of the shoulder. J Bone Joint Surg 1979;61-A(4):566.
54. Hurley JA, Anderson TE, Dear W, et al. Posterior shoulder instability. Surgical versus conservative results with evaluation of glenoid version. Am J Sports Med 1992;20(4):396.
55. Iannotti JP, Norris TR. Influence of preoperative factors on outcome of shoulder arthroplasty for glenohumeral osteoarthritis. J Bone Joint Surg 2003;85-A(2):251.
56. Iannotti JP, Naranja RJ, Warner JJP. Surgical management of shoulder arthritis in the young and active patient. In: Warner JJP, Iannotti JP, Gerber C, eds. Complex and revision problems in shoulder surgery. Philadelphia, PA, Lippincott-Raven, 1997:289.
57. Iannotti JP, Zlatkin MB, Esterhai JL, et al. Magnetic resonance imaging of the shoulder: sensitivity, specificity and predictive value. J Bone Joint Surg 1991;73A:17.
58. Jakob RP, Miniaci A, Anson PS, et al. Four-part valgus impacted fractures of the proximal humerus. J Bone Joint Surg Br 1991; 73(2):295.
59. Johnson LL. The shoulder joint. Clin Orthop 1987;223:113.
60. Kaplan SR, Lally EV. Part I. Steroids, NSAIDS, gold and D-penicillamine, and antimalarials. Decision points in the management of rheumatoid arthritis. J Musculoskelet Med 1986;46.
61. Kenzora JE, Glimcher MJ. Accumulative cell stress: the multifactorial etiology of idiopathic osteonecrosis. Orthop Clin North Am 1985;16:669.
62. Kristiansen B, Christiansen S. Plate fixation of proximal humerus fractures. Acta Orthop Scand 1986;57:320.
63. LaPorte D, Mont M, Mohan V, et al. Osteonecrosis of the humeral head treated by core decompression. Clin Orthop 1998;335:254.
64. Larsen A, Dale K, Eek M. Radiographic evaluation of rheumatoid arthritis and related conditions by standard reference films. Acta Radiol Diagn 1977;18:481.
65. Lehmann JF, DeLateur BJ. Application of heat and cold in the clinical setting. In: Lehmann JF, ed. Therapeutic heat and cold. Baltimore, MD, Williams and Wilkins, 1990:633.
66. Lehmann JF, DeLateur BJ. Therapeutic heat. In: Lehmann JF, ed. Therapeutic heat and cold. Baltimore, MD, Williams and Wilkins, 1990:417.
67. Lehtinen JT, Belt EA, Lyback CO, et al. Subacromial space in the rheumatoid shoulder: a radiographic 15-year follow-up study of 148 shoulders. J Shoulder Elbow Surg 2000;9(3):183.
68. Levine WN, Djurasovic M, Glasson J, et al. Hemiarthroplasty for glenohumeral osteoarthritis: results correlated to degree of glenoid wear. J Shoulder Elbow Surg 1997;6(5):449.
69. L'Insalata J, Pagnini M, Warren R, et al. Humeral head osteonecrosis: clinical course and radiographic predictors of outcome. J Shoulder Elbow 1996;5:355.
70. Lombardo SJ, Kerlan RK, Jobe FW, et al. The modified Bristow procedure for recurrent dislocation of the shoulder. J Bone Joint Surg 1976;58A(2):256.
71. Lusardi DA, Wirth MA, Wurtz D, et al. Loss of external rotation following anterior capsulorrhaphy of the shoulder. J Bone Joint Surg Am 1993;75(8):1185.
72. Mahowald ML, Krug H, Steveken MN, et al. Exercises and other physical therapies of rheumatoid arthritis. J Musculoskeletal Med 1990;7(6):52.
73. Maini R, Zvaifler NJ. Rheumatoid arthritis and other synovial disorders. In: Klippel JH, Dieppe PA, eds. Rheumatology. Philadelphia, PA, Mosby, 1999:2.
74. Matsen FA, Ziegler DW, DeBartolo SE. Patient self-assessment of health status and function in glenohumeral degenerative joint disease. J Shoulder Elbow Surg 1995;4:345.
75. Matteson EL, Goronzy JJ, Weyland CM, et al. Rheumatoid arthritis. In: Klippel JH, ed. Primer on the rheumatic diseases. Atlanta, GA, Arthritis Foundation, 2001:209.
76. Menkes CJ. Is there a place for chemical and radiation synovectomy in rheumatic diseases? Rheumatol Rehabil 1979;28(2):65.
77. Menkes CJ, Millet B. Synoviorthosis of the shoulder joint in rheumatoid arthritis. Rheumatology 1989;12:46.
78. Miehlke RK, Thabe H. Resection interposition arthroplasty of the rheumatoid shoulder. Rheumatology 1989;12:73.
79. Mitchell D, Rao V, Dalinka M. Femoral head avascular necrosis: correlation of MR imaging, radiographic staging, radionuclide imaging, and clinical findings. Radiology 1987;162:709.
80. Mont MA, Maar DC, Urquhart MW, et al. Avascular necrosis of the humeral head treated by core decompression. J Bone Joint Surg 1993;75-B(5):785.
81. Mont M, Payman R, Laporte D, et al. Atraumatic osteonecrosis of the humeral head. J Rheumatol 2000;27(7):1766.
82. Moseley JB, O'Malley K, Peterson NJ, et al. A controlled trial of arthroscopic surgery for osteoarthritis of the knee. New Engl J Med 2002;347(2):81.
83. Mullaji AB, Beddow FH, Lamb GH. CT measurement of glenoid erosion in arthritis. J Bone Joint Surg 1994;76B:384.
84. Nakagawa Y, Hyakuna K, Otani S, et al. Epidemiologic study of glenohumeral osteoarthritis with plain radiography. J Shoulder Elbow Surg 1999;8(6):580.
85. Neer CSII. Replacement arthroplasty for glenohumeral osteoarthritis. J Bone Joint Surg 1974;56A(1):1.
86. Neer CSII, Watson KC, Stanton FJ. Recent experience in total shoulder replacement. J Bone Joint Surg 1982;64A(3):319.
87. Nelson MC, Leather GP, Nirschl RP, et al. Evaluation of the painful shoulder. J Bone Joint Surg 1991;73A(5):707.
88. Norris TR, Iannotti JP. Functional outcome after shoulder arthroplasty for primary osteoarthritis: a multicenter study. J Shoulder Elbow Surg 2002;11(2):130.
89. O'Driscoll SW. Arthroscopic glenoidplasty and osteocapsular arthroplasty for advanced glenohumeral osteoarthritis. Presented at the American Academy of Orthopaedic Surgeons 67th Annual Meeting. Orlando, FL, March 18, 2000.
90. O'Driscoll SW, Evans DC. Long term results of staple capsulorrhaphy for anterior instability of the shoulder. J Bone Joint Surg 1993;75A:249.
91. Ogilvie-Harris DJ. Arthroscopy and arthroscopic surgery of the shoulder. Semin Orthop 1987;2(4):246.
92. Ogilvie-Harris DJ, D'Angelo G. Arthroscopic surgery of the shoulder. Sports Med 1990;9(2):120.
93. Ogilvie-Harris DJ, Wiley AM. Arthroscopic surgery of the shoulder. A general appraisal. J Bone Joint Surg 1986;68-B(2):201.
94. Pahle JA. The shoulder joint in rheumatoid arthritis: synovectomy. Reconstr Surg Traumatol 1981;18:33.
95. Pahle JA. Experiences with synovectomy of the shoulder. Rheumatology 1989;12:31.
96. Patzakis MJ, Mills DM, Bartholomew BA, et al. A visual, histological, and enzymatic study of regenerating rheumatoid synovium in the synovectomized knee. J Bone Joint Surg 1973; 55:287.
97. Peterfy CG, Majumdar S, Lang P, et al. MR imaging of the arthritic knee: improved discrimination of cartilage, synovium, and effusion with pulsed saturation transfer and fat-suppressed T1-weighted sequences. Radiology 1994;191(2):413.
98. Petersson CJ. Degeneration of the glenohumeral joint. An anatomical study. Acta Orthop Scand 1983;54:277.
99. Petersson CJ. Painful shoulders in patients with rheumatoid arthritis: prevalence, clinical and radiological features. Scand J Rheumatol 1986;15:275.

100. Petersson CJ. Shoulder surgery in rheumatoid arthritis. Acta Orthop Scand 1986;57:222.
101. Pollock RG, Deliz ED, McIlveen SJ, et al. Prosthetic replacement in rotator cuff-deficient shoulders. J Shoulder Elbow Surg 1992;1(4):173.
102. Recht MP. Practical options for MR imaging of articular cartilage. In: De Smet AA, ed. Musculoskeletal MRI: normal anatomy and key pathology. Seattle, WA, American Roentgen Ray Society, 2001:129.
103. Recht MP, Kramer J, Marcelis S, et al. Abnormalities of articular cartilage in the knee: analysis of available MR techniques. Radiology 1993;187(2):473.
104. Recht MP, Kramer J, Petersilge CA, et al. Distribution of normal and abnormal fluid collections in the glenohumeral joint: implications for MR arthrography. J Magn Reson Imaging 1994; 4(2):173.
105. Recommendations for the medical management of osteoarthritis of the hip and knee: 2000 update. American College of Rheumatology Subcommittee on Osteoarthritis Guidelines. Arthritis Rheum 2000;43(9):1905.
106. Resch H, Beck E, Bayley I. Reconstruction of the valgus-impacted humeral head fracture. J Shoulder Elbow Surg 1995;4(2):73.
107. Richman JD, Rose DJ. The role of arthroscopy in the management of synovial chondromatosis of the shoulder. A case report. Clin Orthop 1990;257:91.
108. Rodosky MW, Bigliani LU. Indications for glenoid resurfacing in shoulder arthroplasty. J Shoulder Elbow Surg 1996;5(3):231.
109. Rutherford C, Cofield R. Osteonecrosis of the shoulder. Orthop Trans 1987;11:239.
110. Samilson RL, Prieto V. Dislocation arthropathy of the shoulder. J Bone Joint Surg 1983;65A(4):456.
111. Schweitzer ME, Magbalon MJ, Fenlin JM, et al. Effusion criteria and clinical importance of glenohumeral joint fluid: MR imaging evaluation. Radiology 1995;194(3):821.
112. Simpson NS, Kelley IG. Extra-glenohumeral joint shoulder surgery in rheumatoid arthritis: the role of bursectomy, acromioplasty, and distal clavicle excision. J Shoulder Elbow Surg 1994;3:66.
113. Skedros JG, O'Rourke PJ, Zimmerman JM, et al. Alternatives to replacement arthroplasty for glenohumeral arthritis. In: Iannotti JP, Williams GR, eds. Disorders of the shoulder: diagnosis and management. Philadelphia, PA, Lippincott Williams & Wilkins, 1999:485.
114. Sperling JW, Cofield RH, Rowland CM. Neer hemiarthroplasty and Neer total shoulder arthroplasty in patients fifty years old or less. J Bone Joint Surg 1998;80-A(4):464.
115. Sperling JW, Cofield RH, Steinmann SP. Shoulder arthroplasty for osteoarthritis secondary to glenoid dysplasia. J Bone Joint Surg 2002;84-A(4):541.
116. Taylor LJ. Multifocal avascular necrosis after short-term high-dose steroid therapy. J Bone Joint Surg 1984;66-B(3):431.
117. Tillmann K, Braatz D. Resection interposition arthroplasty of the shoulder in rheumatoid arthritis. Rheumatology 1989; 12:68.
118. Tressel W, Köhler G, Mohing W. Synovectomy of the shoulder joint in rheumatoid arthritis. Rheumatology 1989;12:40.
119. Urquhart M, Mont M, Maar D, et al. Results of core decompression for avascular necrosis of the humeral head. Orthop Trans 1992;16:780.
120. Walch G, Ascani C, Boulahia A, et al. Static posterior subluxation of the humeral head: an unrecognized entity responsible for glenohumeral osteoarthritis in the young adult. J Shoulder Elbow Surg 2002;11(4):309.
121. Watterson JR, Esdaile JM. Viscosupplementation: therapeutic mechanisms and clinical potential in osteoarthritis of the knee. J Am Acad Orthop Surg 2000;8(5):277.
122. Weinstein D, Bucchieri J, Pollock R. Arthroscopic debridement of the shoulder for osteoarthritis. Arthroscopy 1993;9:366.
123. Wilkinson MC, Lowry JH. Synovectomy for rheumatoid arthritis. J Bone Joint Surg 1965;47B(3):482.
124. Winalski CS, Aliabadi P, Wright RJ, et al. Enhancement of joint fluid with intravenously administered gadopentate dimeglumine: technique, rationale, and implications. Radiology 1993; 187(1):179.
125. Wirth MA, Rockwood CA Jr. Complications of total shoulder-replacement arthroplasty. J Bone Joint Surg Am 1996;78(4):603.
126. Wirth MA, Lyons FR, Rockwood CA Jr. Hypoplasia of the glenoid. A review of sixteen patients. J Bone Joint Surg Am 1993;75(8):1175.
127. Witwity T, Uhlmann R, Nagy MH, et al. Shoulder rheumatoid arthritis associated with chondromatosis, treated by arthroscopy. Arthroscopy 1991;7(2):233.
128. Zuckerman JD, Matsen FA. Complications about the glenohumeral joint related to the use of screws and staples. J Bone Joint Surg 1984;66A:175.

Shoulder Arthroplasty in the Young, Active Patient

Edward W. Lee   *Evan L. Flatow*   *Jon J. P. Warner*

INTRODUCTION

As success with shoulder arthroplasty has grown, and orthopedists have become more familiar and adept with the technique, the indications for shoulder arthroplasty have expanded. Those patients refractory to an extensive trial of nonoperative treatment and unsuitable for, or having failed, arthroscopic treatment may be considered for prosthetic replacement. In young patients with severe proximal humerus fractures; avascular necrosis (AVN); and posttraumatic, postsurgical, inflammatory, and degenerative arthritides, humeral head replacement (HHR) and total shoulder arthroplasty (TSA) remain viable options.[20,31,32,34] It is critical, however, to remember the limits of the technique; to remain clear on the indications and contraindications; and to accurately educate patients on the risks, benefits, alternatives, and expected outcomes of shoulder arthroplasty. This is especially the case in a young, active patient who may have expectations for active participation in sports and work for many years.

E. W. Lee: Clinical Shoulder Fellow, Department of Orthopaedic Surgery, Mount Sinai Medical Center, New York, New York.

E. L. Flatow: Lasker Professor of Orthopaedic Surgery, Chief of Shoulder Surgery, Department of Orthopaedic Surgery, Mount Sinai Medical Center, New York, New York.

J. J. P. Warner: Professor of Orthopaedic Surgery, Chief, The Harvard Shoulder Service, Harvard Medical School, Massachusetts General Hospital, Boston, Massachusetts.

CAUSE

Cause plays an important part in the natural history and prognosis after arthroplasty. The shoulder joint is an uncommon site of primary osteoarthritis (OA). Osteoarthritis in the shoulder presents with large inferior osteophytes, sclerosis, subchondral cysts, and posterior erosion of the glenoid (Fig. 23-1). In young patients, glenohumeral OA is less common than arthritis secondary to trauma[38] or prior instability repair. Humeral trauma or surgery that alters the biomechanics and results in humeral roughness or eccentric loading of the glenoid can eventually progress to glenoid arthrosis.[31,34,40] Furthermore, associated soft-tissue insufficiency or contractures may be relevant to the overall pathology that will require treatment. Roentgenographic findings do not necessarily correlate with symptoms.

In rheumatoid arthritis (RA), the glenohumeral joint is commonly involved and usually part of a polyarthropathy[3] (Fig. 23-2). Symptomatic RA of the shoulder typically occurs in women between 35 and 55 years-old who test positive for rheumatoid factor, with rotator cuff tears occurring in approximately 25% of these patients.[38]

Avascular necrosis can occur in patients with trauma, steroid use, alcoholism, sickle cell disease, hemophilia, history of decompression sickness, lipid storage diseases, or lupus.[18,24,34] Often the cause is unknown. Disease progression was staged by Cruess as follows: preradiographic stage (I), humeral head involvement (II), subchondral humeral head fracture (crescent sign, III), humeral head collapse

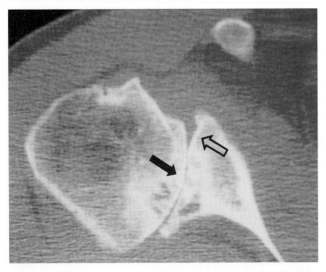

Figure 23-1 Computed tomography scan showing eccentric posterior glenoid wear in patient with osteoarthritis (OA). Native glenoid contour *(hollow arrow)*. Posterior eroded contour *(solid arrow)*.

(IV), and glenoid involvement (V) (Fig. 23-3). The later stages of AVN are typically more symptomatic, are more likely to progress, and most often require prosthetic replacement.[24]

Degenerative glenohumeral arthritis can result from glenohumeral instability and is the most common cause of arthritis in patients less than 40 years-old.[6,11] This may result from postsurgical, iatrogenic subluxations; persistent multidirectional instability; inadequate or inappropriate surgery; or a hardware complication. The cause is often multifactorial in nature[11] (Fig. 23-4). In a series by Bigliani et al.,[6] symptomatic arthrosis required pros-

thetic replacement at an average of 16 years after the initial stabilization.

EVOLUTION OF GLENOHUMERAL PROSTHETIC REPLACEMENT FOR ARTHRITIS

A number of changes have occurred in prosthetic design and technology as well as surgical technique in shoulder arthroplasty. First-generation arthroplasty for the shoulder used a "monoblock" design with few options to accommodate the variable anatomy between different patients (Fig. 23-5). Despite this lack of prosthetic variability, the "old design" performed well with Torchia et al.[42] providing relief of moderate to severe pain in 83% of patients' shoulders in their study.

Second-generation shoulder arthroplasty introduced humeral head modularity and more stem sizes, which theoretically allowed for better soft-tissue tensioning. A number of various pegged and keeled glenoid designs were also introduced in an attempt to optimize fixation of the polyethylene component. Several problems with second-generation components became apparent, including nonanatomic head sizing, which prevented the restoration of proper offset and resulted in suboptimal cuff tension, overstuffing the joint, and eccentric glenoid loading. Survival problems became evident with early glenoid osteolysis and may have been multifactorial (overstuffing the joint, head/glenoid curvature mismatch, and material failure [i.e., Hylamer, DePuy, Warsaw, IN]) (Fig. 23-6).[43] Humeral-sided complications arose as well, with stress-shielding and proximal bone loss from large and stiff stems.

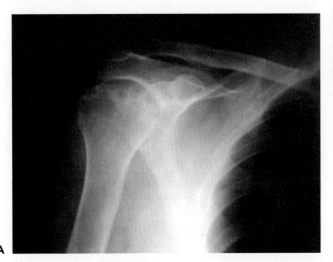

A

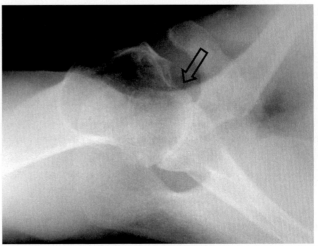

B

Figure 23-2 *(A)* Anteroposterior (AP) view of patient with glenohumeral rheumatoid arthritis (RA). Note the subchondral erosions, relative osteopenia, and absence of osteophytes. *(B)* Axillary view of same patient. Note central glenoid erosion, relative osteopenia, periarticular erosions, and lack of osteophytes. Anterior periarticular erosion *(hollow arrow)*.

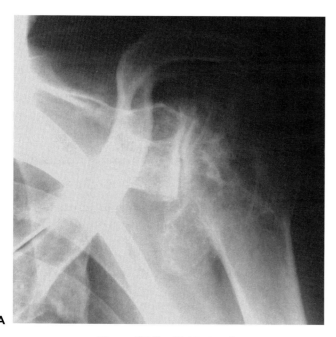

A

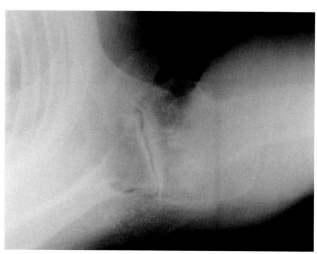

B

Figure 23-3 *(A)* AP view demonstrating Cruess stage V idiopathic avascular necrosis (AVN). Note joint space narrowing, large inferior humeral osteophyte, and humeral head collapse. *(B)* Axillary view of same patient. Flattened humeral head caused reciprocal damage to the glenoid.

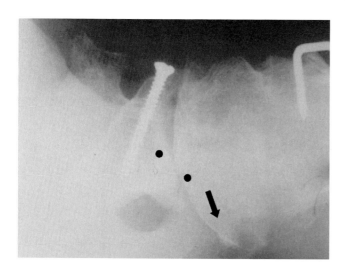

Figure 23-4 Axillary view of 32 year-old with painful arthritis of the glenohumeral joint after multiple procedures for instability, including a coracoid transfer and Putti-Platt procedure. Center of the glenoid and humerus *(dots)*. Fixed posterior subluxation *(arrow)*.

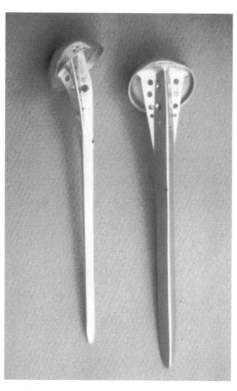

Figure 23-5 First-generation Neer shoulder prosthesis.

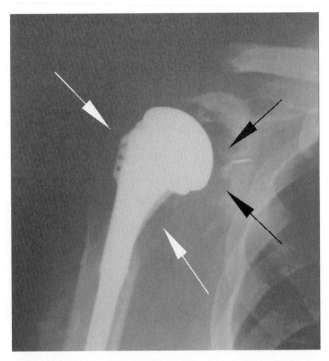

Figure 23-6 *Second-generation shoulder prosthesis. Note severe osteolysis of the proximal humerus (white arrows) and glenoid (black arrows).*

Third-generation, or "anatomic," systems have more prosthetic adaptability with offset heads and variable neck angles, better glenoid surface designs, and newer instrumentation to minimize bone loss and improve cement integration (Fig. 23-7, *A* and *B*). Better restoration of

anatomy may minimize or avoid eccentric loading of the glenoid component or reduce glenoid wear after an HHR (Fig. 23-8, *A* and *B*).

HUMERAL HEAD REPLACEMENT VERSUS TOTAL SHOULDER ARTHROPLASTY WITH CONSIDERATIONS IN THE YOUNG, ACTIVE PATIENT

Currently, some confusion still exists in defining the indications for resurfacing the glenoid in glenohumeral arthritis. Advantages of hemiarthroplasty include a relatively easier procedure, a shorter operating time with less blood loss, less risk of instability, and the ability to convert to a TSA in the future. However, the disadvantages include less consistent pain relief and progressive erosion of the glenoid leading to deteriorating functional results over time (Figs. 23-9 and 23-10).

In contrast, TSA provides more consistent pain relief and restores the glenohumeral fulcrum, providing better active motion. Arguments against resurfacing the glenoid include a more difficult procedure with longer operative time and greater blood loss and glenoid wear resulting in bone loss and loosening of both components. The surgical technique has been well described in the literature.[26]

A number of current studies examining the clinical results of HHR versus TSA have favored glenoid resurfacing. In their short-term follow-up of 600 TSAs and 89 HHRs for primary OA, Edwards et al.[19] found superior results with

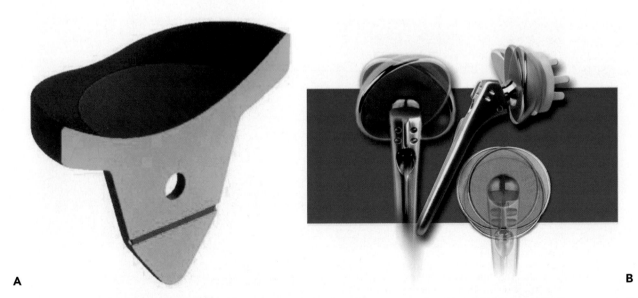

A   **B**

Figure 23-7 *(A)* Third-generation glenoid surface design with central "conforming zone" and peripheral "translational" zone. (Courtesy of Zimmer, Warsaw, IN.) *(B)* Third-generation humeral design (Anatomical Shoulder, Sulzer Orthopedics Inc., Austin, TX), which allows for variable placement of head to accommodate three-dimensional anatomy of proximal humerus: humeral head offset, neck-shaft angle, and humeral version. (Courtesy of Zimmer, Warsaw, IN.)

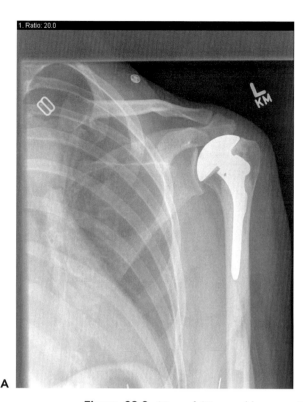
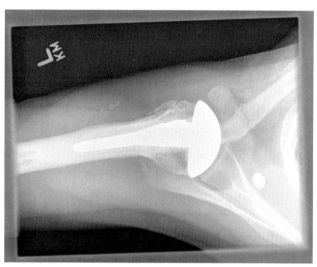

Figure 23-8 View of 35-year-old woman 3 years after hemiarthroplasty for avascular necrosis (AVN) with anatomic restoration of articular humeral anatomy. There is no joint space narrowing in anteroposterior (AP) view *(A)* or axillary view *(B)*, and the patient has motion symmetric with contralateral normal side.

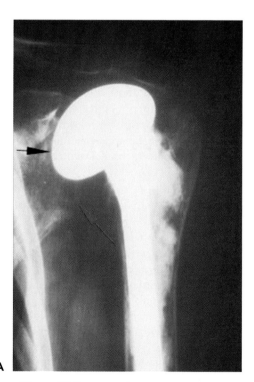
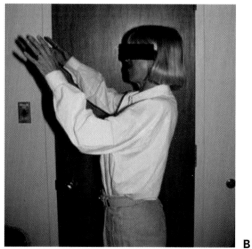

Figure 23-9 Hemiarthroplasty in patient with rheumatoid arthritis (RA) 5 years postoperatively. *(A)* Anteroposterior (AP) view demonstrating glenoid wear. Level of native glenoid *(red arrow)*; level of medial wear and bone loss *(black arrow)*. *(B)* Clinical photograph demonstrating difficulty with forward elevation.

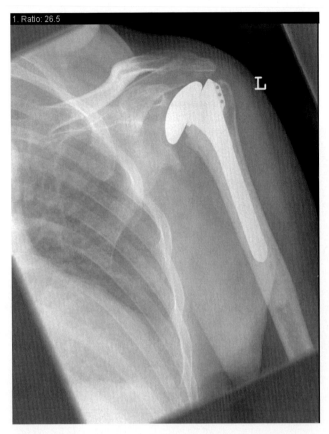

Figure 23-10   Hemiarthroplasty with nonanatomic (inferior) placement of humeral head associated with glenoid erosion and pain.

TSA compared with HHR with statistically significant differences with respect to pain, mobility, and activity. Similarly, Bell and Gschwend[5] found better average elevation and pain relief with glenoid resurfacing in their study of 11 TSAs and 17 HHRs. In their randomized clinical series, Gartsman et al.,[21] Sandow et al.,[37] and Kirkley et al.[27] found better pain relief with TSA but no significant differences in functional outcome with HHR at short-term follow-up.

A number of investigators have also considered the glenoid to prognosticate of the results with hemiarthroplasty. Levine et al.[29] retrospectively reviewed 30 patients and 31 shoulders after hemiarthroplasty, classifying glenoid surface wear as either concentric or nonconcentric. Although pain relief was similar in both groups, overall satisfaction was higher in the concentric group and was attributed to better motion in this subset. Rockwood et al.[35] also concluded that hemiarthroplasty is successful in OA with concentric wear but fails with a flat, eroded glenoid and associated posterior head subluxation. Warner and Parsons,[43] however, found that, although progressive glenoid wear was observed in all patients undergoing HHR, there was no statistically significant correlation between glenoid erosion and poor functional outcome or the need to convert to TSA. Kirkley et

al.[27] found no correlation with glenoid wear pattern and conversion to TSA in "cross-over" patients (those requiring subsequent TSA after hemiarthroplasty).

The few studies examining the results of arthroplasty in the young patient caution against the high rates of unsatisfactory results and revision surgery. Sperling et al.[39] examined 33 patients (average age 46 years-old) with glenohumeral arthritis after instability surgery. Despite significant improvement in pain relief and function, there was a high rate of revision surgery (3/10 HHRs and 8/21 TSRs) and unsatisfactory results because of component failure, instability, and pain. In a separate study, Sperling et al.[41] retrospectively reviewed their long-term experience with 62 HHRs and 29 TSRs in patients 50 years-old or less. Their results demonstrated significant long-term pain relief and improvement in function with no significant difference between the two procedures with respect to these outcomes. However, they noted that 38% of the glenoid resurfacing group and 45% of the hemiarthroplasty group had unsatisfactory results.

Hardware-related complications, specifically glenoid fixation, remain an unsolved problem. The incidence of glenoid-cement interface radiolucency is high with reports in the literature ranging from 30% to 96%.[2,12,14,25,33] Although the association of radiolucency with component loosening and declining patient satisfaction is not fully understood, Torchia et al.[42] reported the presence of radiolucent lines at the bone-cement interface of glenoid components in 84% of their patients followed for an average of 12 years. By radiographic signs, 44% were "definitely loose," and loosening was associated with pain. In our experience, however, the ache associated with loosening is often not enough in the patient's opinion to warrant a revision operation (Fig. 23-11). Nevertheless, glenoid loosening remains the most common prosthesis-related cause of revision surgery, with rates ranging from 0% to 12.5%.[10,36,45] Accelerated loosening and premature wear become even greater concerns in the younger, more active patient compared with the typically older osteoarthritic population.

In an attempt to reduce the incidence of glenoid component lucency and loosening, uncemented porous-coated or tissue-ingrowth components have been developed. A finite element analysis study of cemented and uncemented, metal-backed glenoid designs demonstrated stress-shielding and separation between the metal/polyethylene bond; however, the implant-bone interface seemed less likely to fail compared with the cemented designs.[23] Despite these findings, several studies have reported on accelerated polyethylene wear and poor clinical results of metal-backed designs (Fig. 23-12).[9,14–17] More recent efforts in uncemented glenoid designs have shown more promising early results. Wirth et al.[44] compared fixation of a conventional cemented keeled glenoid component with an uncemented flanged pegged implant ("Magic Peg," Depuy,

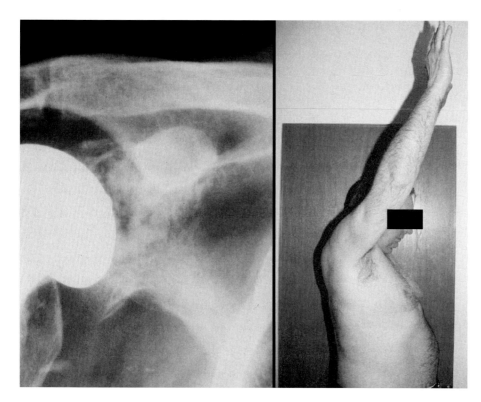

Figure 23-11 Glenoid loosening in a patient with 19-year follow-up. He has good function and only mild ache, and does not desire revision for current level of symptoms.

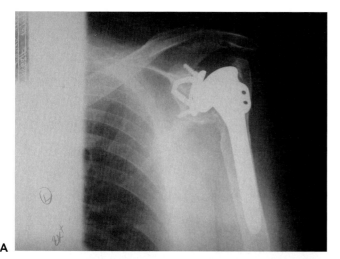

A

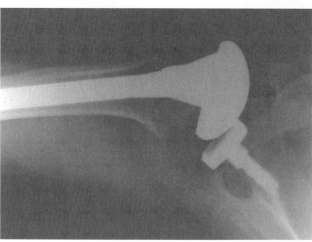

C

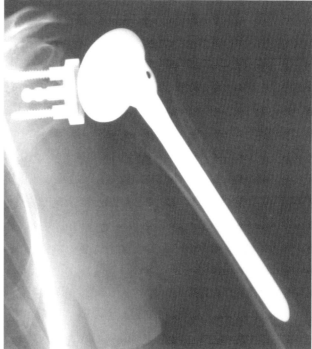

B

Figure 23-12 (*A*) Metal-backed glenoid in which wear has produced polyethylene debris. The particles can travel through the screw holes, accelerating osteolysis. (*B,C*) View of 28-year-old woman 2 years after total shoulder replacement for avascular necrosis (AVN). Note anterior subluxation on axillary view. This was associated with polyethylene fracture and metallosis.

Warsaw, IN) in a weight-bearing canine model. Results demonstrated that mean fixation strength of the fluted peg component increased significantly between 0 and 3 months after surgery, and remained strong through 6 months. In contrast, the conventional cemented keeled implant had partial or complete lucent lines around the keel, and mechanical testing demonstrated weakened mean fixation strength between 0 and 3 months after surgery, which remained weak through 6 months (Fig. 23-13).

The clinical experience with Trabecular Metal (Zimmer, Warsaw, IN) technology in the shoulder has been, thus far, limited, but has also shown encouraging early results. Trabecular Metal implants are constructed from elemental tantalum metal and vapor deposition techniques that create a metallic strut configuration similar to trabecular bone. Trabecular Metal consists of interconnecting pores resulting in a structural biomaterial that is 80% porous, reportedly allowing approximately 2 to 3 times greater bone ingrowth compared with conventional porous coatings and double the interface shear strength,[8] as well as low stiffness to minimize stress shielding. A transcortical implant animal study demonstrated that new bone infiltrated the Trabecular Metal 8 weeks after surgery. At 4 weeks, the bone interface shear strength of Trabecular Metal was double that of sintered beads[7,8] (Fig. 23-14).

Newer surgical techniques have also attempted to solve the problem of postoperative radiolucency around conventional cemented glenoid components. Gross et al.[22] reported on a "weep-hole" technique that involves transcoracoid suction through an osseous channel to improve cement penetration in the glenoid vault. After using this technique, 27 of 29 consecutive patients' shoulders had no evidence of radiolucent lines.

Another study by Klepps et al.[28] used specialized cement pressurization instrumentation and compared the incidence of radiolucent lines with glenoid components implanted with traditional manually packed cementing techniques. The newer instrumented pressurization group had a significantly lower incidence of radiolucent lines than the manually packed group ($P < .002$) (Fig. 23-15). Furthermore, pegged components had a lower incidence of radiolucent lines than keeled components in this study ($P < .05$).

OTHER ARTHROPLASTY OPTIONS

Most surgeons are reluctant to offer prosthetic replacement to young, active, high-demand patients for fear of loosening and eventual failure. Several alternatives to traditional arthroplasty have been proposed and reported throughout the literature.

Biologic resurfacing arthroplasty has been advocated to improve the results of hemiarthroplasty and as a primary procedure for young patients with end-stage glenohumeral arthritis. Burkhead and Hutton[13] reported on their early results of biologic resurfacing the glenoid with autogenous fascia lata or anterior shoulder capsule with a porous-coated HHR in the young patient with glenohumeral arthritis. The capsule is harvested from the undersurface of the subscapularis to create a medially based flap (Fig. 23-16). Care is taken to preserve the length of the capsular flap so that it can reach the posterior and superior edges of the glenoid. The glenoid is then reamed to a bleeding surface. Finally, the capsular flap is then sewn to the glenoid peripherally through the labrum and anchored centrally with suture anchors. Excellent results were

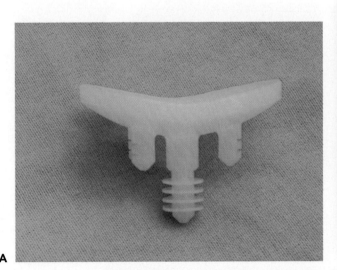

A

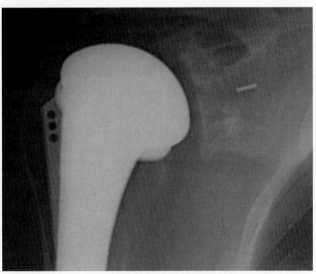

B

Figure 23-13 *(A)* "Magic Peg" glenoid (DePuy, Warsaw, IN). *(B)* Anteroposterior (AP) view at 12-month follow up. (Case courtesy of M. Wirth, M.D., San Antonio, TX.)

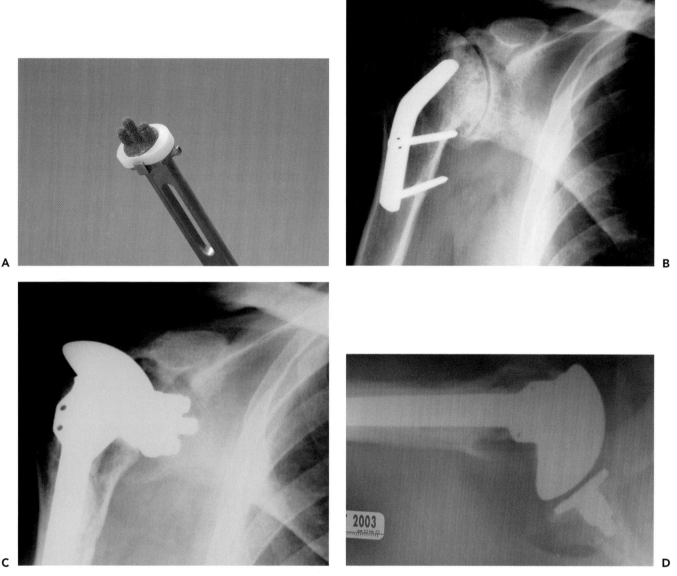

Figure 23-14   (A) Trabecular metal glenoid component (Zimmer, Warsaw, IN). The patient is a 56 year-old who underwent (B) open reduction internal fixation for a proximal humerus fracture at age 16 years and developed posttraumatic arthritis. (C) Anteroposterior (AP) and (D) axillary views after total shoulder arthroplasty (TSA) with a trabecular metal glenoid implant.

obtained in five of six patients at a minimum of two years follow-up, with excellent pain relief and significant gains made in motion.

Ball et al.[1] and Baumgarten et al.[4] recently described meniscal allograft interposition arthroplasty as another variation on the resurfacing concept. Prosthetic replacement combined with use of a meniscal allograft secured to the glenoid has been used in an attempt to improve functional results and pain relief in young, active patients with asymmetric wear or structural damage to the glenoid. Absolute contraindications include skeletal immaturity, ac-

tive septic arthritis, or osteomyelitis. After performing humeral preparation and exposing the glenoid, recontouring the articular surface can be undertaken, being careful to preserve remaining bone stock. A lateral meniscus graft is preferred because of its smaller size and more circular shape to allow a better fit with the glenoid surface. The graft is secured to the glenoid rim with transosseous sutures or suture anchors, adjusting the rotation of the meniscus to enhance stability, depending on glenoid version and amount of wear. In their preliminary study, six consecutive patients underwent the procedure. All patients

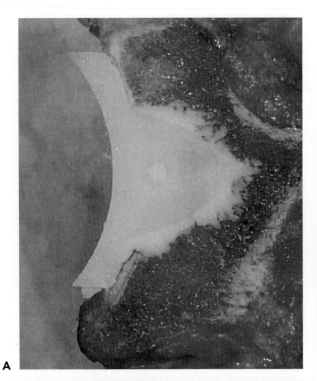
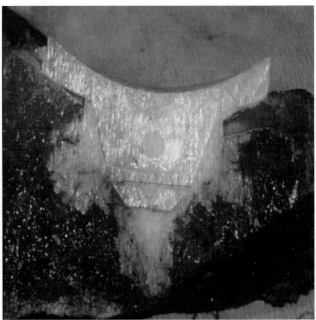

Figure 23-15 *(A)* Cadaveric specimen cut in coronal plane after cementing the glenoid with standard "finger packing" technique. *(B)* Cadaveric specimen cut in coronal plane after cementing the glenoid with third-generation technique: serial pressurization of "wet" cement with special pressurization tools and sponges.

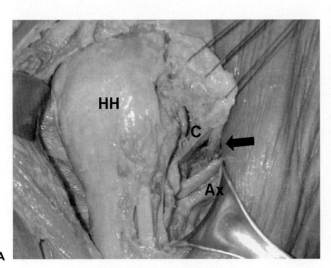
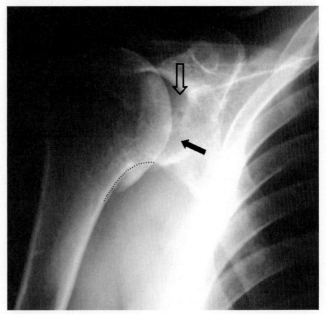

Figure 23-16 *(A)* Cadaveric dissection after subscapularis release before dividing the capsule off the posterior aspect of the subscapularis. The anterior labrum can be left to deepen the socket in hemiarthroplasty cases. The capsule can be harvested off the subscapularis and reflected over the freshened glenoid surface for biologic resurfacing. In total shoulder arthroscopy (TSA), the anterior capsule and labrum are excised. HH, humeral head; C, capsule; Ax, axillary nerve. Subscapularis anterior to the capsule *(solid arrow)*. Thirty-five year-old with painful glenohumeral arthritis and stiffness after multiple prior instability procedures. *(B)* Anteroposterior (AP) view with inferior osteophyte noted below the *dotted line* outlining native cortex. Change in contour of humeral head from flattening *(solid arrow)*. Nonmetallic anchor hole from prior instability repair *(hollow arrow)*. *(continued)*

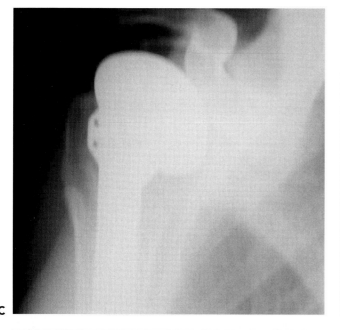

C

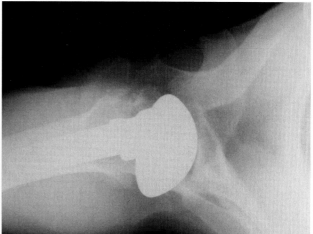

D

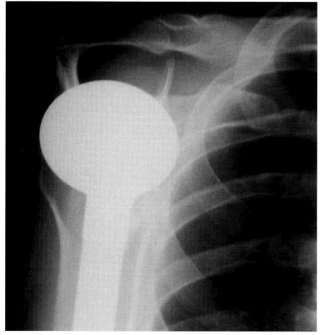

E

Figure 23-16 *(continued)* *(C)* Anteroposterior, *(D)* axillary, and *(E)* scapular lateral views after hemiarthroplasty and biologic resurfacing with anterior capsule.

demonstrated satisfactory outcomes postoperatively after a mean follow-up of 24 months (Fig. 23-17).

Humeral-sided resurfacing implants attempt to preserve bone stock and humeral length. Levy and Copeland[30] have had the most extensive experience with this technology with up to 13 years of experience with Copeland's prosthesis, the Copeland Cementless Surface Replacement Arthroplasty (CSRA) (Biomet, Warsaw, IN). The CSRA uses a press-fit pegged cobalt-chrome cap implanted through a standard deltopectoral or anterosuperior approach. The

theoretic advantages include avoidance of periprosthetic fractures and maintenance of bone stock and humeral length should revision surgery or arthrodesis become necessary in the future. In a retrospective study of 39 total shoulder arthroplasties and 30 hemiarthroplasties (minimum follow-up 2 years, mean 7.6 years) using this implant, age-adjusted Constant scores improved from 33.8% to 94% for total shoulder replacement and from 40% to 91% for hemiarthroplasty. Active elevation improved from a mean of 59.9 degrees to 128 degrees for total shoulder

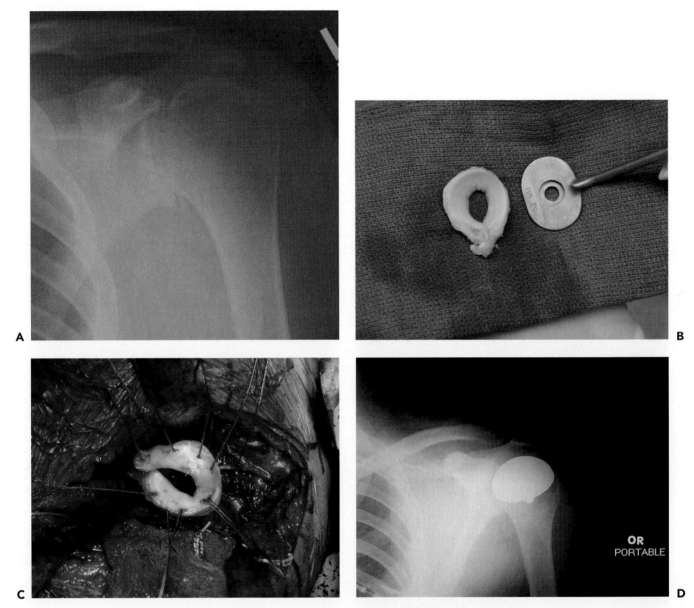

Figure 23-17 Meniscal allograft interposition arthroplasty. (A) Anteroposterior (AP) view of 19 year-old with chondrolysis after thermal capsulorraphy. The patient had virtually no glenohumeral motion and severe pain. (B) Meniscal allograft beside glenoid sizing tool. (C) Suture fixation of allograft. (D) Anteroposterior view after interposition arthroplasty and humeral resurfacing. The patient is now free of pain with 160 degrees of forward elevation. (Case courtesy of K. Yamaguchi, M.D., St. Louis, MO.)

replacement and to a mean of 124 degrees for hemiarthroplasty. Patient satisfaction was high, with 89.9% considering the shoulder to be better or much better as a result of the surgery[30] (Fig. 23-17D).

More recently, the HemiCAP (Arthrosurface, Franklin, MA) was developed and can be used to treat contained humeral articular surface defects. Similar to the Copeland prosthesis, the HemiCAP is a rounded, caplike implant made from a cobalt chrome alloy with a central post on the implanted side. The implant comes in a variety of sizes and curvature profiles designed for different surface anatomies.

Experience is currently limited with the HemiCAP, but it is a promising surgical option for isolated articular surface defects in which traditional prosthetic replacement would not be indicated (Fig. 23-18).

DISCUSSION

In the young patient with glenohumeral arthritis, shoulder arthroplasty can result in excellent pain relief and significant gains in active motion. Care must be taken to exhaust

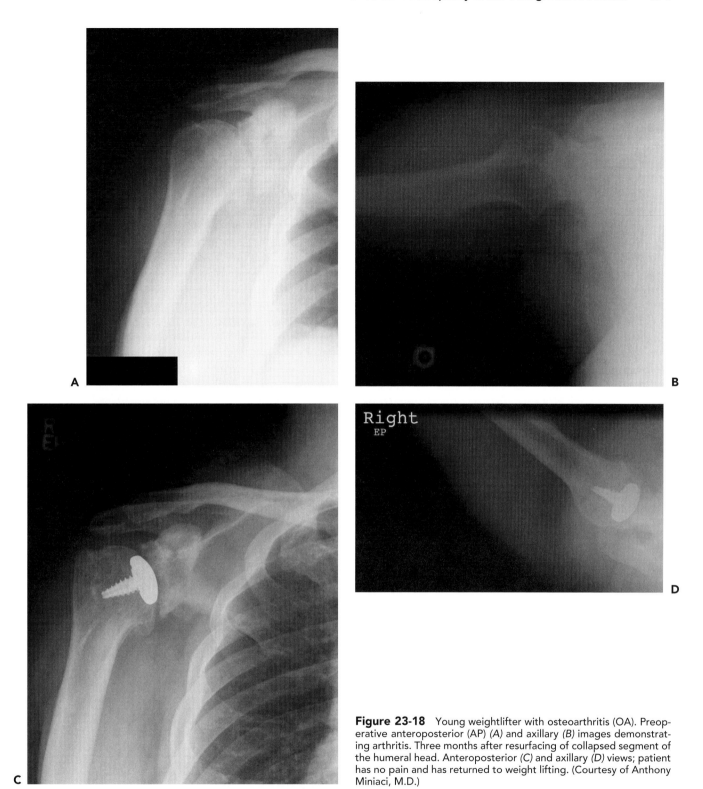

Figure 23-18   Young weightlifter with osteoarthritis (OA). Preoperative anteroposterior (AP) (A) and axillary (B) images demonstrating arthritis. Three months after resurfacing of collapsed segment of the humeral head. Anteroposterior (C) and axillary (D) views; patient has no pain and has returned to weight lifting. (Courtesy of Anthony Miniaci, M.D.)

nonoperative and joint-sparing surgical options in the young, active patient.

Careful preoperative studies help select and plan the appropriate procedure. History, physical examination, radiographic studies, and diagnostic injections can isolate the pain generators about the shoulder, including or excluding the acromioclavicular joint, subacromial bursa, glenohumeral joint, and sites outside the shoulder including the cervical spine.

Nonoperative means must be fully used to restore comfort and function, including activity modification; stretching and strengthening; ice, heat, and other physical modalities; pharmaceuticals; and judicious use of steroid injections. Other procedures, such as debridement arthroscopy, subacromial decompression, distal clavicle resection, rotator cuff repair, and capsular releases, may play a role depending on the clinical setting.

Knowledge of cuff and deltoid integrity and neurovascular status about the shoulder is vital in planning shoulder arthroplasty. If any doubt exists, preoperative studies such as magnetic resonance imaging or electromyograms should be considered.

The results of shoulder arthroplasty are significantly influenced by the underlying pathogenesis, degree of arthrosis, and any concomitant soft-tissue and bony pathology around the shoulder. Patients with OA typically fare very well with respect to pain relief and function restoration, although pure OA requiring shoulder arthroplasty in patients less than 40 years-old is rare. Arthroplasty after fractures reliably relieves pain and results in significant gains of motion, but restoration of function and full active motion is less predictable. In AVN, results are typically excellent in steroid-induced and other nontraumatic causes of osteonecrosis. Prosthetic replacement of traumatic AVN can be technically more difficult, and results are inferior compared with the atraumatic setting. In RA, prosthesis survival is statistically better than in the posttraumatic setting. Pain relief is excellent, but restoration of function depends to a large degree on the condition of the rotator cuff.

Subtle, unique nuances in pathogenesis (arthritis of dislocation) and unique clinical considerations (return to the work force and patient longevity) are encountered in the young patient. Furthermore, prosthetic survivorship is much more pertinent in the young patient. Current consensus is that hemiarthroplasty should be considered in the younger, active patient with concentric glenoid wear after all other, less invasive, options have been exhausted and in the patient in whom it is not possible to implant a glenoid component. Furthermore, glenoid replacement is not performed in the setting of unresolved infections, for nonfunctioning deltoid or rotator cuff, for a tight shoulder despite releases, or in patients who will be noncompliant with postoperative restrictions. Additional procedures (meniscal allograft or capsular/fascial interposition) have not yet undergone vigorous randomized clinical trials to prove their efficacy, but serve as promising adjuncts to existing technology. Understanding the unique pathogenesis, surgical alternatives, technical considerations, and clinical results with arthroplasty in the young patient can help the shoulder surgeon choose wisely when offering surgical solutions to young patients with glenohumeral arthritis. Ultimately, young and active patients will grade their outcome according to the active lifestyle they can maintain as well as durable pain relief (Fig. 23-19).

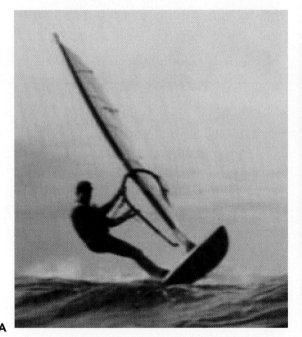
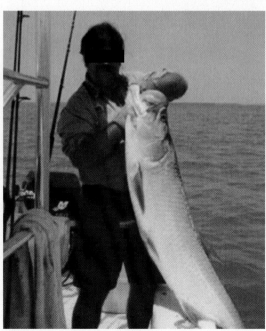

A

B

Figure 23-19 *(A)* View of 38-year-old man 2 years after total shoulder replacement; he has no pain and desires to ocean wind surf. *(B)* View of 39-year-old electrician 3 years after bilateral total shoulder replacement; patient desires to deep sea fish.

REFERENCES

1. Ball CM, Galatz LM, Yamaguchi K. Meniscal allograft interposition arthroplasty for the arthritic shoulder: description of a new surgical technique. Tech Shoulder Elbow Surg 2001;2(4):247.
2. Barrett WP, Franklin JL, Jackins SE, et al. Total shoulder arthroplasty. J Bone Joint Surg 1987;69:865.
3. Barrett WP, Thornhill TS, Thomas WH, et al. Nonconstrained total shoulder arthroplasty in patients with polyarticular rheumatoid arthritis. J Arthroplasty 1989;4(1):91.
4. Baumgarten KM, Lashgari CJ, Yamaguchi K. Glenoid resurfacing in shoulder arthroplasty: indications and contraindications. Instr Course Lect 2004;53:3.
5. Bell SN, Gschwend N. Clinical experience with total shoulder arthroplasty and hemiarthroplasty of the shoulder using the Neer prosthesis. Int Orthop 1986;10(4):217.
6. Bigliani LU, Weinstein DM, Glasgow MT, et al. Glenohumeral arthroplasty for arthritis after instability surgery. J Shoulder Elbow Surg 1995;4(2):87.
7. Bobyn JD, Hacking SA, Chan SP, et al. Characterization of a new porous tantalum biomaterial for reconstructive orthopaedics. Presented at the Scientific Exhibit, Proc. of American Academy of Orthopaedic Surgeons, Anaheim, CA, February 4–8, 1999.
8. Bobyn JD, Stackpool G, Toh K-K, et al. Bone ingrowth characteristics and interface mechanics of a new porous tantalum biomaterial. J Bone Joint Surg 1999;81:907.
9. Boileau P, Avidor C, Krishnan SG, et al. Cemented polyethylene versus uncemented metal-backed glenoid components in total shoulder arthroplasty: a prospective, double-blind, randomized study. J Shoulder Elbow Surg 2002;11(4):351.
10. Brems J. The glenoid component in total shoulder arthroplasty. J Shoulder Elbow Surg 1993;2:47.
11. Brems JJ. Arthritis of dislocation. Orthop Clin North Am 1998;29(3):453.
12. Brenner BC, Ferlic DC, Clayton ML, et al. Survivorship of unconstrained total shoulder arthroplasty. J Bone Joint Surg 1989;71:1289.
13. Burkhead WZ, Hutton KS. Biologic resurfacing of the glenoid with hemiarthroplasty of the shoulder. J Shoulder Elbow Surg 1995;4(4):263.
14. Cofield RH. Total shoulder arthroplasty with the Neer prosthesis. J Bone Joint Surg 1984;64:319.
15. Cofield RH. Uncemented total shoulder arthroplasty: a review. Clin Orthop 1994;307:86.
16. Cofield RH, Daly PJ. Total shoulder arthroplasty with a tissue-ingrowth glenoid component. J Shoulder Elbow Surg 1992;1:77.
17. Cofield RH, Sperling JW. Radiographic assessment of ingrowth total shoulder arthroplasty. Abstract 236. Presented at the Congress of the European Society for Surgery of the Shoulder and Elbow Convention (ESSE-SECEC) Meeting. La Hague, Netherlands, September 8–11, 1999.
18. Cruess RL. Experience with steroid-induced avascular necrosis of the shoulder and etiologic considerations regarding osteonecrosis of the hip. Clin Orthop 1978;130:86.
19. Edwards TB, Kadakia NR, Boulahia A, et al. A comparison of hemiarthroplasty and total shoulder arthroplasty in the treatment of primary glenohumeral osteoarthritis: results of a multicenter study. J Shoulder Elbow Surg 2003;12(3):207.
20. Friedman R, ed. Total shoulder arthroplasty. Orthop Clin North Am. Vol. 29. Philadelphia, PA, WB Saunders Company, 1998.
21. Gartsman GM, Roddey TS, Hammerman SM. Shoulder arthroplasty with or without resurfacing of the glenoid in patients who have osteoarthritis. J Bone Joint Surg 2000;82(1):26.
22. Gross RM, McCarthy JA, Skowron Lomneth C, et al. Cemented glenoid fixation with the 'weep-hole' technique. Presented at the 2nd Annual Douglas T. Harryman II Shoulder and Elbow Society Meeting, Seattle, Washington, July 22–24, 2002.
23. Gupta S, van der Helm FC, van Keulen F. The possibilities of uncemented glenoid component—a finite element study. Clin Biomech (Bristol, Avon) 2004;19(3):292.
24. Hattrup S. Osteonecrosis of the humeral head: relationship of disease stage, extent, and cause to natural history. J Shoulder Elbow Surg 1999;8(6):559.
25. Hawkins RJ, Bell RH, Jallay B. Total shoulder arthroplasty. Clin Orthop 1989;242:188.
26. Hayes PR, Flatow EL. Total shoulder arthroplasty in the young patient. Instr Course Lect 2001;50:73.
27. Kirkley A, Lo IKY, Griffin S, et al. Hemiarthroplasty versus total shoulder arthroplasty in the treatment of osteoarthritis of the shoulder: a prospective randomized trial. American Shoulder and Elbow Meeting, Miami Beach, FL, 2000:115.
28. Klepps S, Miller S, Chiang AS, et al. Incidence of early radiolucent glenoid lines in patients undergoing total shoulder replacement. Presented at the American Academy of Orthopaedic Surgeons 70th Annual Meeting, New Orleans, LA, February 5–9, 2003.
29. Levine WN, Djurasovic M, Glasson JM, et al. Hemiarthroplasty for glenohumeral osteoarthritis: results correlated to degree of glenoid wear. J Shoulder Elbow Surg 1997;6(5):449.
30. Levy O, Copeland SA. Cementless surface replacement arthroplasty (Copeland CRSA) for osteoarthritis of the shoulder. J Shoulder Elbow Surg 2004;13(3):266.
31. Matsen F, Rockwood CA, Wirth MA, et al. Glenohumeral arthritis and its management. In: Rockwood CA, Matsen FA, eds. Philadelphia, PA, WB Saunders, 1998:840.
32. Neer CS. Shoulder reconstruction. Philadelphia, PA, WB Saunders, 1990.
33. Neer CSII, Watson KC, Stanton FJ. Recent experience in total shoulder replacement. J Bone Joint Surg 1982;64:319.
34. Post M. Operative treatment of degenerative and arthritic diseases of the glenohumeral joint. In: Cooke D, ed. The shoulder: operative technique. Baltimore, MD, Williams and Wilkins, 1998:73.
35. Rockwood CA Jr, Jensen KL, Wirth MA. Hemiarthroplasty vs. total shoulder arthroplasty in patients with osteoarthritis. International Congress on Surgery of the Shoulder, Sydney, Australia, October 5–8, 1998:99.
36. Rodosky MW, Bigliani LU. Indication for glenoid resurfacing in shoulder arthroplasty. J Shoulder Elbow Surg 1996;5:231.
37. Sandow MJ, David HG, Bentall SJ. Hemi-arthroplasty or total replacement for shoulder osteoarthritis preliminary results of a PRCT with intra-operative randomization. International Congress on Surgery of the Shoulder, Sydney, Australia, October 5–8, 1998: 100.
38. Skedros J, O'Rourke PJ, Zimmerman JM, et al. Alternatives to replacement arthroplasty for glenohumeral arthritis. In: Iannotti J, Williams GR, eds. Disorders of the shoulder: diagnosis and management. Philadelphia, PA, Lippincott, Williams & Wilkins, 1999:485.
39. Sperling JW, Antuna SA, Sanchez-Sotelo J, et al. Shoulder arthroplasty for arthritis after instability surgery. J Bone Joint Surg 2002;84(10):1775.
40. Sperling JW, Cofield RH. Revision total shoulder arthroplasty for the treatment of glenoid arthrosis. J Bone Joint Surg 1998;80(6):860.
41. Sperling JW, Cofield RH, Rowland C. Minimum 15 year follow-up of Neer hemiarthroplasty and total shoulder arthroplasty in patients 50 years old or less. Presented at the American Academy of Orthopaedic Surgeons 70th Annual Meeting, New Orleans, LA, February 5–9, 2003.
42. Torchia ME, Cofield RH, Settergren CR. Total shoulder arthroplasty with the Neer prosthesis: long-term results. J Shoulder Elbow Surg 1997;6(6):495.
43. Warner JP, Parsons IM. Quantification of radiographic glenoid wear after shoulder hemiarthroplasty. American Shoulder and Elbow Surgeons 15th Open Meeting, Anaheim, CA, February 4–8, 1999:29.
44. Wirth MA, Korvick DL, Basamania CJ, et al. Radiologic, mechanical, and histologic evaluation of 2 glenoid prosthesis designs in a canine model. J Shoulder Elbow Surg 2001;10(2):140.
45. Wirth MA, Rockwood CA Jr. Complications in shoulder arthroplasty. Clin Orthop 1994;307:47.

Special Issues in Inflammatory Arthritis

24

Ian G. Kelly

INTRODUCTION

The inflammatory conditions affecting the shoulder include rheumatoid arthritis (RA) and the seronegative spondyloarthropathies such as psoriatic arthritis, Reiter's syndrome, and ankylosing spondylitis. Shoulder involvement in the seronegative spondyloarthropathies is uncommon, with the acromioclavicular joint being most commonly affected. This chapter will discuss the management of shoulder problems in the patient with RA. Emery et al.[9] have presented an excellent account of shoulder problems encountered in patients with ankylosing spondylitis.

Rheumatoid arthritis is the most common inflammatory joint disease and is a prominent and often dominant part of rheumatoid disease, a systemic illness. The arthritis is polyarticular and can thus involve one or more parts of the complex of joints that comprise the shoulder.

PATHOLOGY AND DIAGNOSIS

Although the cause of rheumatoid disease remains unknown, the disease process involves a synovitis, a vasculitis, and secondary changes, such as anemia.

The initial changes are confined to the soft tissues, and it has been suggested that it is the synovial sheath of the intra-articular portion of the tendon of the long head of biceps that is first involved. It appears that the process commences with vascularization followed by hyperplasia of the

synovium and the formation of pannus. Pannus is abnormal synovium that secretes hyaluronate, collagenase, proteolytic enzymes, and proteoglycan proteases, and thus contributes to joint destruction.

When the inflammatory process involves tendon sheaths, it is in a confined area and may infiltrate the tendon to a variable degree. The rotator cuff tendons do not have a synovial sheath, but the subacromial bursa is intimately connected to the superior surface of the supraspinatus tendon, which is always involved when there is a bursitis.

In addition to producing bony erosions, the rheumatoid process stimulates osteoclast activity through the secretion of prostaglandins and cytokines. This contributes to the osteopenia seen in these patients.

The wide variety of pathologic processes involved in rheumatoid disease are reflected in the diverse clinical presentations with different aspects dominating in different patients.

THE SHOULDER COMPLEX IN RHEUMATOID ARTHRITIS

Involvement of the subacromial "joint" occurs in 10% to 15% of patients and is often seen in the absence of radiologic evidence of disease in other parts of the shoulder. In some patients, the bursa is very large (Fig. 24-1) and will contain multiple "melon seed" bodies, but in most it is not palpable. Because of the intimate relationship of the bursa to the rotator cuff, large bursae are usually associated with cuff deficiency or tears.

The acromioclavicular joint is said to be involved in up to 55% of symptomatic shoulders.[10,39] Dijkstra et al.,[8] in a

I. G. Kelly: Consultant Orthopaedic Surgeon, Glasgow Royal Infirmary, Glasgow, Scotland.

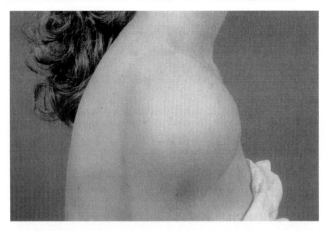

Figure 24-1 Very large subacromial bursa. It contained numerous "melon seed" bodies, and the rotator cuff was thinned with a number of small perforations.

radiologic study, indicated that acromioclavicular (AC) joint involvement was independent of the extent of glenohumeral disease. Local tenderness is usually present, and, rarely, synovitis will be palpable, although this may be a herniation from the subacromial bursa. At the AC joint, there is a widening of the joint space with increasing severity of rheumatoid involvement (Fig. 24-2). However, it should be noted that typical degenerative changes with narrowing of the joint space can be seen, especially in patients who develop RA in later life.

The glenohumeral joint is not involved clinically as often as the subacromial or acromioclavicular joints,[21] but radiologic involvement is common. Ennevara[10] found changes in 67.5% of his patients.

The most widely used grading system is that of Larsen et al.[27] It has stages for both the acromioclavicular joint and the glenohumeral joint (Fig. 24-3). The system was not constructed as a clinical classification, although there is a tendency for the radiologic changes to pass through these stages as the severity increases. Lehtinen et al.[28] demonstrated that the subacromial space decreases significantly between Larsen grades III and IV, indicating that substantial rotator cuff pathology had developed.

In a recent study, Olofsson et al.[36] found shoulder involvement in 50% of 80 patients who had RA for a median period of 8 months; 30 patients had evidence of reduced shoulder function in at least one shoulder. Decreased function was associated with higher disease activity. Thus, the shoulder complex is not only frequently involved in RA but also involved from an early stage. However, not all affected shoulders progress.

From a surgical point of view it is important to be able to identify the shoulder that will progress. Hirooka and colleagues[18] contributed to our understanding of this when they reported five radiologic patterns of disease in the rheumatoid shoulder in a group of 83 patients (133 shoulders) followed for 5 to 23 years (mean 14 years) (Fig. 24-4). Significantly, the largest group was the nonprogressive type (74 shoulders), in which there was only osteopenia or minor erosions at 15 to 20 years. The

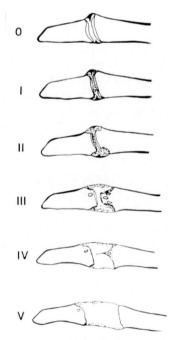

Figure 24-2 Larsen classification for the acromioclavicular joint.[27] Note the widening of the joint space with increasing severity of disease.

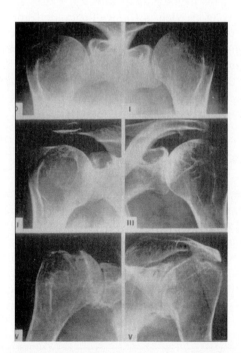

Figure 24-3 Standard reference films for the Larsen classification[27] of the glenohumeral joint.

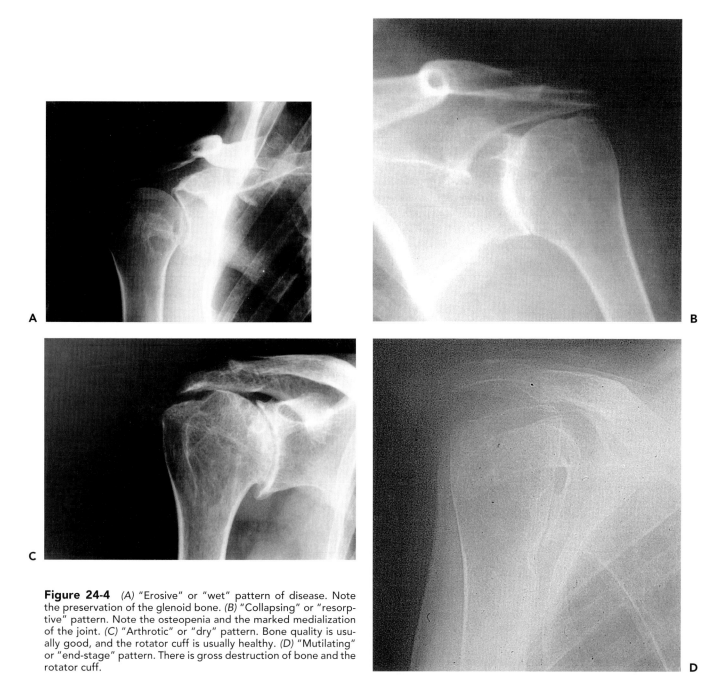

Figure 24-4 *(A)* "Erosive" or "wet" pattern of disease. Note the preservation of the glenoid bone. *(B)* "Collapsing" or "resorptive" pattern. Note the osteopenia and the marked medialization of the joint. *(C)* "Arthrotic" or "dry" pattern. Bone quality is usually good, and the rotator cuff is usually healthy. *(D)* "Mutilating" or "end-stage" pattern. There is gross destruction of bone and the rotator cuff.

second type was "erosive" (22 shoulders), in which there were marginal erosions but the articular surface was well preserved until 10 years after the onset of the disease, after which joint destruction progressed slowly. The "collapse" pattern was the most commonly seen (34 shoulders), and these shoulders developed osteopenia rapidly with associated subchondral cysts. This progressed to collapse of the subchondral bone and advanced joint destruction after 5 to 10 years. The "arthrosis" group (12 shoulders) showed osteophytes and subchondral sclerosis with joint structure

being well preserved for a long time. Finally, the mutilans group (14 shoulders) showed extensive and rapid bone resorption.

Neer[33] described four patterns of the rheumatoid shoulder. These were wet, dry, resorptive, and end stage. The terms were purely descriptive and not related to presentation. Hirooka et al.[18] compared their patterns with those described by Neer and believed that there was some overlap of their patterns with his. My experience suggests that the patterns of Hirooka et al. match those of Neer very closely with the "wet" corresponding to the "erosive," the "resorptive" corresponding to the "collapsing," and the "dry" corresponding to the "arthrotic."

Applying these terms to the preoperative radiographs of 104 shoulders undergoing arthroplasty, we found 30 "wet" shoulders, 10 "dry" shoulders, 56 "resorptive" shoulders, and 8 end-stage shoulders. The operative findings were correlated with the patterns. Of the 30 wet shoulders, 15 were found to have normal glenoid bone stock; they were the only shoulders in the group to have this. Further, 21 of the 30 wet shoulders had ruptured rotator cuffs, with the remainder all being described as "thin." Four cuff tears were found in the 56 resorptive shoulders, 2 in the 10 dry shoulders, and 4 in the 8 end-stage shoulders. All of the shoulders in the resorptive group had thin rotator cuffs.

Our own study relates the soft tissue changes to the observed patterns, and, together with the data from Hirooka et al.,[18] provides some indication of the likely rate and type of progression of glenohumeral disease in the rheumatoid shoulder. Thus, the wet shoulder is a shoulder "at risk" with a high incidence of cuff rupture, which often occurs before there is a significant amount of bony damage. Crossan and Vallance[7] drew attention to this subgroup in their classification, emphasizing that cuff failure could occur acutely and before significant bony damage was evident. In contrast, the "dry" pattern appears to be protective. Although a consecutive group of 53 rheumatoid patients with shoulder pain contained 16 "dry" shoulders, the group of 104 shoulders undergoing shoulder arthroplasty contained only 10 with the "dry" pattern.

ASSESSMENT OF THE EXTENT OF SHOULDER DISEASE

The frequent radiographic appearance of superior subluxation of the humeral head (Fig. 24-5) resulted in the belief that rotator cuff rupture was common in RA. However, studies by Neer et al.,[34] Cofield,[6] Kelly et al.,[23] Sledge et al.,[45] Sneppen et al.,[46] and Stewart and Kelly[49] demonstrated that between 70% and 80% of these shoulders have intact rotator cuffs, although the majority will be abnormally thin. This thinning, together with the cephalic destruction of the glenoid, contributes to the radiographic superior subluxation. Ultrasound can be valuable for studying the state of the rotator cuff or for assessing the state and extent of the subacromial bursa.[19] In advanced disease, the bony deformity and limitation of motion can make this technique difficult to use and interpret.

Computed tomography (CT) can be very useful in assessing the bone stock available for arthroplasty[1,32] both in the humeral head and the glenoid. Plain radiographs are

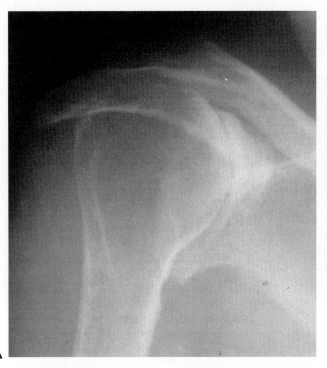
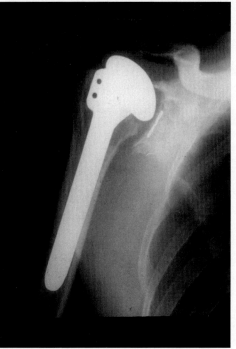

Figure 24-5 (A) Superior subluxation of the humeral head as a consequence of cephalic erosion of the glenoid. The shoulder is medialized, and the cuff is usually intact although thin. (B) If an arthroplasty is inserted without correction of the deformity, the humeral component will ride high and eccentrically load the glenoid component.

usually sufficient to assess the humeral head, but if a cup arthroplasty is to be used, CT scanning will sometimes demonstrate the presence of large cysts within the head that cannot otherwise be seen. Glenoid erosion is usually central in RA, but significant glenoid bone loss in a cephalic direction is occasionally encountered. Again, plain radiographs usually suffice, but CT scanning should be performed if there is any doubt about bone stock.

Magnetic resonance imaging (MRI) of the rheumatoid shoulder has been widely reported. Kieft et al.[25] demonstrated the range of pathology in the glenohumeral joint but found that the acromioclavicular joint was difficult to image. They also commented that damage to the soft tissues was present even when radiographs showed normal results. I have not found MRI to be particularly useful in the surgical management of patients with rheumatoid shoulders.

THE PATIENT

Matsen et al.[30] demonstrated that patients with RA presenting for shoulder arthroplasty had significantly more health impairment than patients with osteoarthritis presenting for the same procedure. In patients with RA, shoulder surgery should never be performed without considering the state of other joints and the overall health and function of the patient. If the shoulder problem is part of a generalized flare of the disease, assessment is difficult and may not be reliable. Appropriate medical measures should be instituted, and the patient should be reviewed at a later date. I prefer not to operate on patients who are having a flare of disease. Although some flares will settle after surgery, some will not, and this is likely to adversely affect their rehabilitation.

Cervical spine disease may be present in up to 80% of patients with RA with severe disease.[20] This is usually at the atlanto-axial joint, but subaxial problems and vertical subluxation or cranial settling will also be seen. Because a high proportion of patients with significant subluxation will be asymptomatic, it is important to assess the cervical spine in all rheumatoid patients undergoing surgery to avoid problems during intubation or positioning. Flexion and extension lateral projections suffice in most patients, but if there is a suspicion of a myelopathy, MRI should be used.

There is little point in operating on the shoulder if problems with the ipsilateral elbow, wrist, and hand will not permit the limb to function. In such an instance, hand surgery should take precedence. Whether to operate on the elbow or shoulder first may be a difficult decision. If one is more painful than the other it would seem reasonable to deal with that joint first. However, a painful and unstable elbow can interfere with shoulder rehabilitation. Simultaneous ipsilateral shoulder and elbow arthroplasty has been reported[26] with good results, matching those reported for separate surgery, and a recent long-term follow-up of a large

series from the same unit has revealed durable results (Neumann, personal communication). In a study of 31 patients who had undergone ipsilateral shoulder and elbow arthroplasty at separate operations, Friedman and Ewald[12] found that the results were as good as if either joint had been operated on alone. However, if the elbow was operated on first, there was a longer interval until the second operation, suggesting that this should be performed first. Gill et al.[14] concluded that shoulder and elbow arthroplasty in RA were independent events and that the sequence and interval between them should be guided by clinical need alone.

The shoulder becomes a major load-bearing joint when the patient has to use walking aids, especially after lower limb surgery, which must be considered when planning the order of surgery in a polyarthritic patient.

The general functional status of the patient can be classified according to the American Rheumatology Association criteria reported by Steinbrocker et al.[48]

Grade I: Capable of all activities
Grade II: moderate restrictions—adequate for normal activities
Grade III: marked restrictions—self-care only
Grade IV: bed and/or chair—little or no self-care

Although this classification system gives a guide to the functional status of the entire patient, very few reports of shoulder surgery in the rheumatoid patient refer to it.[13]

WHERE IS THE PAIN FROM?

The location of the pain in the shoulder can provide a useful guide to the site of the pathology in some patients.[24] However, the majority of rheumatoid patients present with pain felt over the point of the shoulder that radiates toward the area of the deltoid insertion and/or to the root of the neck.[21] Local tenderness is a poor guide to the site of the problem, and radiographs and other imaging modalities correlate poorly with the clinical presentation.

In many patients, it is difficult to be certain of the site of the pain. In this situation, I use small injections of local anesthetic to locate the painful site(s).[21] First, 1 mL of 1% lignocaine is injected into the joint most likely to be involved on the basis of clinical assessment. I then wait 2 to 3 minutes for the anesthetic to act before asking the patient to carry out previously painful movements. If the pain has been completely abolished, the test is complete. If the anesthetic has had no effect or has been only partially successful, I try another site, usually the acromioclavicular joint. The test is complete when total pain relief has been achieved or the glenohumeral joint has been injected. Failure to achieve relief from any of these sites should give cause to reconsider the source of the pain.

In our series of 75 shoulders assessed by using injection testing, the acromioclavicular joint was involved alone in

24, the subacromial joint was involved alone in 14, both joints were involved in combination in 21, and a glenohumeral joint injection was required in 16. Thus, despite 62 shoulders having Larsen III, IV, or V changes at the glenohumeral joint, 60% of this group experienced pain in a location other than the glenohumeral joint.

COORDINATING WITH THE RHEUMATOLOGIST

Patients with inflammatory joint disease typically run a variable course with intermittent flares of disease activity and polyarthritic involvement. Although there are still some centers where rheumatoid surgeons manage the patient's entire case, the tendency, even in Europe, has been toward regional subspecialization among orthopaedic surgeons. Therefore, it is only the rheumatologist who sees the whole picture and is in the position to coordinate the medical and surgical treatment of these patients. However, this demands that the rheumatologist know the surgical procedures that are available and their indications. Close collaboration between surgeon and rheumatologist is essential.

The surgeon must also understand the medical therapy of the arthritis and the implications of this therapy for surgery. The adverse effects of the corticosteroids on wound healing and their undesirable masking of infections are well recognized, but the need to stop agents such as methotrexate is more controversial. There have been a number of reports concerning the need to stop methotrexate before surgery, but most have failed to provide a clear answer. In a prospective randomized trial of 388 patients with RA undergoing orthopaedic procedures, Grennan et al.[16] found that continuing methotrexate treatment did not increase the risk of either infection or surgical complications during the first postoperative year. However, they also demonstrated that other drugs used to treat RA, such as penicillamine, cyclosporine, hydroxychloroquine, and prednisolone, all increased the risk of problems. The newer anti-tumor necrosis factor-α agents may also have implications for surgery, but, currently, experience with these drugs is limited in surgical patients. In those few patients presenting for shoulder arthroplasty, we have stopped the drug several weeks before the procedure.

INJECTIONS

Intra-articular steroid injections are very valuable in the management of these patients both from a diagnostic (discussed previously) and therapeutic standpoint. However, the proper use of injections demands one understand the shoulder's complex anatomy and the nature of this anatomy's involvement in the specific disease. Unfortunately, rheumatologists, and even orthopaedic surgeons,

do not always possess such understanding, and, unless the site of previous failed injections is known, the shoulder surgeon should always consider repeating at least the diagnostic injection.

In my practice, injections are always used diagnostically initially, as outlined previously, but, once the site of pain is identified, the therapeutic steroid is administered, often to more than one of the joints in the shoulder complex.

I consider using injections:

- When the site of pain is unclear.
- When there is pain but no bone or joint changes.
- When there is glenohumeral joint involvement but the status of the acromioclavicular joint is unclear.

By using this approach, I will only repeat the injection if there has been a response lasting 2 or more months. Failure to produce a lasting response is an indication for surgery.

Encouraging results have been reported when using suprascapular nerve blocks to manage glenohumeral pain in rheumatoid patients. Brown et al.[4] obtained particularly good and lasting results by using a radiofrequency heat probe located under image intensification. They emphasized that this approach only relieved superior and posterosuperior pain and that the best results were obtained when there was some passive motion demonstrable in the joint before the injection. Good results were reported by Shanahan et al.[43] in a randomized double-blind placebo study for bupivacaine and methylprednisolone acetate suprascapular injections over a 12-week period.

NONARTHROPLASTY SURGERY

We have obtained good results from operating on the acromioclavicular joint and/or the subacromial region, according to the results of the injection studies.[44] Nineteen shoulders underwent excision of the outer clavicle and anterior acromioplasty, with two further shoulders undergoing removal of much enlarged subacromial bursae and one shoulder undergoing an anterior acromioplasty and rotator cuff repair. At a follow-up between 18 and 50 months, most patients had no or minimal pain, and there was good recovery in range of motion and function. One patient progressed to require glenohumeral arthroplasty. It is of particular note that 17 of these shoulders had radiographic evidence of advanced glenohumeral disease (Larsen grade IV or V) but that this joint was not the source of pain in the injection studies.

Petersson[39] reported good results from combining excision of the acromioclavicular joint with synovectomy of the glenohumeral joint and subacromial bursectomy. Weber and Bell[52] reported good results using arthroscopic subacromial surgery in 12 patients with RA, 5 of whom had glenohumeral chondral damage. Selection was reported to be on the basis of severe subacromial symptoms and unresponsiveness to conservative treatment. Poor results correlated with advanced glenohumeral chondral damage.

Synovectomy of the glenohumeral joint has received scant attention in recent literature. This is probably the result of the relative success of shoulder arthroplasty, but it may also be because many patients with rheumatoid shoulder problems present late and because synovectomy has been shown to be most effective in glenohumeral joints at Larsen grades I and II.[38] Of the 54 shoulders reported by Pahle and Kvarnes,[38] only 10 still had pain or had undergone arthroplasty at a mean follow-up of 5.3 years. However, all of the patients studied had shoulder disease in Larsen grades I, II, or III, and all of those with shoulder disease in grade III also underwent debridement of any bony abnormalities. In a further study, Pahle[37] demonstrated that, despite a successful clinical outcome, all shoulders advanced by at least one Larsen grade at the time of follow-up. Although good results can be obtained, it is doubtful whether this procedure provides protection for the joint.

Arthroscopic synovectomy avoids the need to interfere with deltoid or subscapularis and is popular in many European centers. However, there have been few reports of its use. Ogilvie-Harris[35] reported significant improvement in 12 of 15 patients with early disease who were followed between 1 and 2 years.

SPECIAL ISSUES FOR JOINT REPLACEMENT

Indications for and Timing of Arthroplasty

Much has been made of the timing of shoulder arthroplasty in the patient with RA. Authors have stated that if they had been able to operate earlier before there was significant cuff disease or loss of glenoid bone stock they would have achieved better results, and rheumatologists have been criticized for not referring patients earlier. Although it is intuitive that performing an arthroplasty before there is bone and soft tissue destruction will give better results, there is no good evidence to support that view. Many patients with RA with significant shoulder pathology do not present to any doctor until they have reached an advanced stage of disease. It appears that shoulder pain is often intermittent, undergoing exacerbations with flares of disease after each of which there may be a small loss of motion, especially external rotation. It is only when this loss of motion impinges on the patient's function or the pain becomes more persistent that the patient presents. Further, our own work has shown that a significant number of patients with advanced radiologic changes at the glenohumeral joint can do well with surgery to other joints in the shoulder complex.

In my practice, patients with RA presenting with significant pain and limitation of function are assessed clinically, radiologically, and, in most cases, diagnostically, using injections of local anesthetic. If radiographs demonstrate that glenohumeral disease is establish and external rotation is restricted, arthroplasty is likely to be indicated. If the sphericity of the humeral head is preserved, I will usually perform local anesthetic injection studies to exclude the subacromial region and acromioclavicular joint as the site of pain. When humeral head sphericity is preserved, the external rotation range can often be restored by subacromial injection.

The radiologic pattern of the glenohumeral joint also has to be considered. The "wet" shoulder may not develop radiologic changes in the glenohumeral joint until later, but it may have cuff failure and pain early. When glenohumeral joint space loss is present and associated with pain in this group, I proceed to surgery swiftly. This is a situation in which I will consider synovectomy, but, if arthroscopy reveals significant chondral damage and erosions, I will proceed to arthroplasty. The "resorptive" shoulder progresses slowly and relentlessly with loss of mainly glenoid bone stock, thinning of the rotator cuff, and marked osteoporosis. Glenohumeral joint space may be lost early, but humeral head sphericity is often preserved until late in the disease, and this group of patients often present with extensive bone loss. It is this group who might benefit from earlier arthroplasty, but it is difficult to persuade patients of this if they do not have much pain and are managing their usually limited activities of daily living. Further, our own work has shown that a significant number of patients with advanced radiologic changes at the glenohumeral joint can do well with surgery to other joints in the shoulder complex. The "dry" pattern is uncommon, and these patients do not often come to arthroplasty. However, these patients' shoulders behave very much like osteoarthritic shoulders, and bone stock and the rotator cuff are usually well preserved.

Finally, mention has already been made of the need to consider the general health of these patients, and factors such as disease control and the state of the cervical spine must always be taken into account.

SURGICAL TECHNIQUE

The technique of unconstrained arthroplasty in the rheumatoid shoulder differs little from that in other pathologies. However, there are some areas in which the rheumatoid disease process necessitates adaptations.

I use the beach-chair position for surgery, as these patients frequently have thin skin and great care must be taken to *protect pressure areas*. The position of the head and neck, especially when using a head rest, should be monitored.

Many rheumatoid shoulders are markedly medialized, and the deltoid muscle is nearly always thinned. I have found that using a more laterally positioned *skin incision* commencing in front of the acromioclavicular joint and extending distally parallel to the chest wall results in the need for less retraction of the deltoid muscle and the frequently thin skin. The deltoid is further protected by ensuring that the deltopectoral interval is opened up to the clavicle and the muscle is elevated from the underlying clavipectoral fascia and humeral insertion by using blunt finger dissection.

The management of the *cephalic vein* varies greatly between surgeons. My preferred method in the rheumatoid patient is to tie the vein in continuity, ensuring that the proximal ligature is positioned at the point where the cephalic vein dips through the clavipectoral fascia. This ensures that the thin-walled vein is controlled if it is damaged by the deltoid retractor, a not uncommon event.

Most rheumatoid patients presenting for shoulder arthroplasty have greatly *reduced external rotation*, or even internal rotation deformities. Z-lengthening of the subscapularis tendon is not appropriate in RA because the subscapularis tendon is usually too thin to permit its use. In most patients, it is possible to section the tendon of subscapularis 5 mm lateral to its humeral insertion and gain sufficient length by releasing the muscle and its tendon from the scapular neck and underside of the coracoid process. Effective lengthening is, of course, also gained by attending to glenoid rim osteophytes when present. If the tendinous portion cannot be reached and/or the tendon is thin, access should be gained by osteotomizing the lesser tuberosity and elevating this along with the tendon. Avoid elevating the tendon by sharp dissection from the lesser tuberosity when the tendon is thin, because the tendon tends to fray when unsupported by bone.

The risk of failure of the *subscapularis repair* must also be recognized.[31] My preferred method of subscapularis reattachment over the past 20 years has been direct suture of the tendon to its stump using long-term absorbable sutures (PDS, Ethicon, Sommerville, NJ). If a good hold on the tendon or its stump is not possible (an unusual situation), I have added transosseous sutures. Using the belly-press test to assess subscapularis function in recent years has suggested that failure of the repair is a rare event. Nevertheless, the surgeon must be sure that the repair is sound and advise the therapist about postoperative management.

The *coracoacromial ligament* is usually intact, and an attempt should be made to preserve it because it may act as a superior restraint when there is a thin or absent rotator cuff.

Because all of these shoulders have medialized to some extent, *soft tissue releases* are required. I divide the inferior capsule under direct vision while protecting the axillary nerve, which also facilitates dislocation of the humeral head. The anterior capsule is usually very thin and rarely produces the restriction seen in osteoarthritic shoulders. However, I will excise it if it is tethering the subscapularis tendon. The posterior capsule may need to be levered off the back of the glenoid rim, but more formal releases are not usually required.

In rheumatoid patients, the supraspinatus is frequently thin and *cuff tears* are difficult to repair. Rozing and Brand[41] have reported on the difficulty of such repairs but have also indicated that, where they are possible, the result is superior to arthroplasty with a torn cuff. In shoulders with the resorptive pattern, the cuff is usually thin and the joint is much medialized. Although the tendon may be intact when first inspected, lateralizing the joint may well result in loss of integrity. The quality of the tendon usually means that repair is not possible. In this situation, the surgeon should be aware of the vulnerability of the cuff and be prepared to limit the releases and use a short neck length.

The glenoid is usually eroded centrally with no excessive anterior or posterior erosion, although in some wet shoulders it may be completely preserved. The erosion usually progresses in a cephalad direction with the superior glenoid being eroded toward the base of the coracoid process, but the inferior pole being preserved. If this position is accepted, any implanted glenoid component will also face cephalad, which will result in a reduced range of elevation and eccentric loading of the glenoid (Fig. 24-5). It is my preference to remove the inferior pole using a burr whether I am implanting a glenoid component or not. This further reduces the amount of glenoid bone and, in theory, may weaken the glenoid,[11] but the resulting arthroplasty is better balanced, and I have not experienced any glenoid fractures or early glenoid loosening.

The *osteopenia* present in all of these patients puts them at risk of intraoperative fracture. Displacement of the humerus to allow access to the glenoid may result in a fracture of the greater tuberosity unless adequate releases have been performed. Bringing the humerus back into joint after preparing the glenoid also risks fracturing the tuberosity or humeral shaft if the shaft catches on the posterior glenoid rim.

Because of the osteoporotic nature of rheumatoid bone, the humeral medullary cavity is usually capacious. Some press-fit humeral components are, therefore, unreliable, which has been confirmed in a long-term follow-up in this unit,[49] as well as in a study from Denmark.[46] Whereas cemented stems gave virtually no problems for 8 years, a significant proportion of noncemented stems subsided and loosened. More recently, Trail and Nuttall[51] have reported the use of the Global Shoulder Arthroplasty (DePut Orthopaedics, Warsaw, IN) in rheumatoid patients and have not seen any subsidence of uncemented humeral components. This is probably because the broader proximal body of that prosthesis was designed for noncemented use. The surgeon should be aware of the characteristics of the prosthesis being used, assess the quality of the proximal humeral bone, and use these factors to make the decision about the use of cement. If there is any doubt, cement should be used.

When there is painful disease of the *acromioclavicular joint*, diagnosed clinically or with injection tests, the outer end of the clavicle should be excised at the same time as glenohumeral arthroplasty. Failure to do so will likely

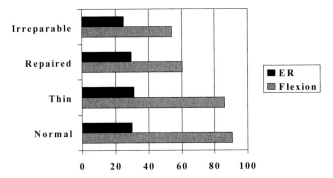

Figure 24-6 Outcome of shoulder arthroplasty in rheumatoid arthritis (RA) according to the status of the rotator cuff. A thin but intact rotator cuff tendon allows almost as good elevation as a healthy cuff.

compromise the result. Subacromial disease rarely requires attention because the bursa is decompressed by exposure of the shoulder and the positioning of the humeral component prevents impingement of the greater tuberosity.

The elbow is frequently affected in patients presenting for shoulder arthroplasty, and any instability will cause problems if the forearm is used to judge retroversion. Care should be taken in this situation to use landmarks such as the bicipital groove and the rotator cuff insertion when deciding on cut placement. If there has been a previous ipsilateral elbow replacement, care must be taken to choose a humeral prosthesis of appropriate size. It may be necessary

to consider a short-stemmed component or a resurfacing prosthesis. An attempt should be made to reduce the stress riser effect by filling the gap between the stems with cement.

CUFF DEFICIENCY

Some surgeons classify all rheumatoid shoulders as being cuff deficient. While it is true that 80% of patients presenting for shoulder arthroplasty have abnormal cuffs, only 20% to 30% have tears. We have shown that the results for patients with normal cuffs is only slightly better than for those patients with thin but intact cuffs, whereas the outcome for torn cuffs is significantly worse than for thin cuffs (Fig. 24-6). Rheumatoid arthritis is part of a systemic disease in which primary muscle disease is frequently present. Thus, many rheumatoid patients have poor muscle function, which is reflected in the poor elevation often seen after arthroplasty. This situation must be distinguished from that in which there is loss of infraspinatus and/or subscapularis as well as supraspinatus.

When supraspinatus alone is absent, acceptable results in terms of pain relief and activities of daily living can be achieved by using a humeral head replacement with the usual attention to soft tissue balancing. I have found that the use of an oversized cup arthroplasty placed in a valgus orientation, resurfacing both the humeral head and greater tuberosity, can be particularly effective in this situation (Fig. 24-7).

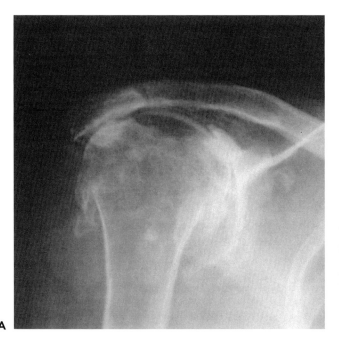
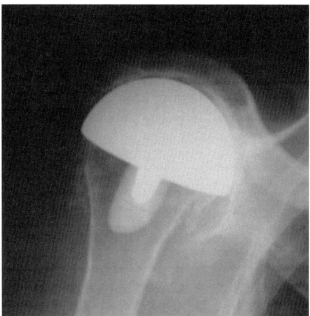

A   B

Figure 24-7 *(A)* Cuff-deficient rheumatoid shoulder with an absent supraspinatus but remnants of functional infraspinatus and subscapularis and major loss of glenoid bone stock. *(B)* Copeland cup arthroplasty placed in a valgus orientation, resurfacing both the humeral head and greater tuberosity.

With more extensive cuff deficiency (an unusual situation in the rheumatoid patient), it may be necessary to consider the use of a constrained arthroplasty.

The reversed geometry prosthesis described by Grammont and Baulot[15] has gained considerable popularity in recent years, and there have been two reports of its use in the rheumatoid shoulder. Unfortunately, the pathology of RA means that there is frequently very poor glenoid bone stock. This will either preclude the use of this device or increase the risk of loosening of the glenoid component. Rittmeister and Kerschbaumer[40] reported that, on eight Larsen grade V shoulders followed for 48 to 73 months, the Constant score improved from a mean of 17 to a mean of 63, but there were three glenoid loosenings, one of which was septic. The authors also drew attention to the fact that deltoid strength was crucial for adequate function. Woodruff et al.[53] reported on the use of the Delta III prosthesis in 17 rheumatoid patients, seven of whom had Larsen grade III shoulders, five Larsen IV grade shoulders, and only one Larsen V grade shoulder. All had massive tearing or "gross attenuation" of the cuff at surgery. Of the 13 shoulders followed for more than 5 years, pain relief was good and the mean Constant score was 59, but glenoid radiolucencies were present in five cases, with this equating to loosening in two. All shoulders demonstrated proximal stress shielding around the humeral component. The high proportion of Larsen grade III shoulders in this series suggests that glenoid bone stock was probably well preserved. The high rate of glenoid radiolucencies is, therefore, of serious concern.

If it is not possible to use a constrained prosthesis, and the cuff deficiency is causing painful instability, arthrodesis will have to be considered. Useful results have been achieved in patients with RA when careful attention has been paid to the position selected and the preservation of elbow motion.[42]

TOTAL REPLACEMENT OR HUMERAL HEAD REPLACEMENT?

Many surgeons find inserting the glenoid component to be difficult. In my experience, this is usually because of inadequate exposure secondary to inadequate soft tissue release. However, even if good exposure is obtained, correct preparation of the glenoid bone can be demanding. Does humeral head replacement give inferior results compared with total joint replacement? Unfortunately, there have been no prospective randomized trials in rheumatoid patients to provide an answer to this question.

Gschwend and Bischof[17] found that there was no difference in the results for total or hemiarthroplasty in the rheumatoid shoulder in terms of pain relief, motion, or function. However, when patients were asked whether they were "improved" or "much improved," a much higher proportion of those receiving a total replacement regarded themselves as "much improved." Clayton et al.[5] found no difference between total and hemiarthroplasty in their consecutive series. Boyd et al.[2] found no difference between the two forms of treatment in osteoarthritic patients, but recommended total arthroplasty in rheumatoid patients because overall pain relief, range of movement, and patient satisfaction were better with total replacement.

There are few long-term studies of the outcome of hemiarthroplasty in the rheumatoid shoulder. In our unit, we reviewed 43 shoulders in 41 patients managed with humeral head replacement.[23] Follow-up ranged from 1 to 9 years. Although 39 shoulders experienced good or excellent pain relief and 40 patients believed they were improved or much improved, 17 shoulders showed increased glenoid erosion, some as early as 1 year postoperatively. All 17 of these patients had torn or deficient rotator cuffs, and 15 were of the "wet" pattern. Sperling et al.[47] recently compared the results of Neer II hemiarthroplasty and total shoulder arthroplasty in a nonrandomized study at a mean follow-up of approximately 12 years. They concluded that there was no significant difference between the procedures with respect to pain relief and movement improvement.

My indications for the use of a humeral head replacement depend on the available shoulder space to accommodate the prosthetic components. Thus, I perform an extensive soft tissue release, remove any osteophytes, and trim the inferior pole of the glenoid if there has been cephalic erosion. If I can insert both a humeral component and a glenoid component into the resulting space while permitting 30 degrees of external rotation after closure of subscapularis, 30% to 50% anteroposterior translation and 90 degrees of internal rotation with the arm at 90 degrees of abduction, I will proceed to total replacement. Otherwise, I will insert only a humeral component with a head size that will fulfill these criteria. However, if there is a "wet" pattern of disease, I prefer to use a total replacement, and I will sometimes ream the glenoid more medially, sometimes accepting less motion to do so.

AFTERCARE

Unless there is the need to protect a tuberosity fracture or a repaired rotator cuff, rehabilitation should commence on the first postoperative day. We follow the regimen as outlined by Neer,[33] commencing with passive motion of the shoulder but progressing to assisted-active and then active movements as the patient is able. We have found that the patient is unwilling to externally rotate up to the range achieved at surgery in the early stages, but we do not allow extension for the first 3 weeks to protect the repair of the subscapularis tendon.

Isometric strengthening is introduced between 4 and 6 weeks, and dynamic strengthening is carried out thereafter.

Patients usually interact with their physiotherapists for approximately 12 weeks.

Hydrotherapy is particularly beneficial for patients with multiple joint problems. It can be used in place of the stated regimen or to complement it.

RESULTS

The results of shoulder arthroplasty in RA are generally inferior to those obtained in osteoarthritis in terms of range of movement (Table 24-1). This reflects the inferior quality of the rotator cuff and bone in these patients. It is very difficult to compare the results of the many series of shoulder arthroplasty reported in the literature, due to the variability of the information provided and the differences in methods of assessment. Thus, some articles do not give information about the radiologic stage of disease or the preoperative status of the patient, some record gains in motion and do not provide absolute values, and all use varying functional assessments. Few long-term follow-up studies have been reported. On occasion, even when a series contains long-term results, those for the short-term follow-up patients are included, so the average presented obscures important detail.

COMPLICATIONS

Few complications have been reported after shoulder arthroplasty in rheumatoid patients. Despite the known increased susceptibility to infection occasioned by the disease and the use of cytotoxic drugs, infection has been rarely encountered. Glenoid and humeral shaft fractures have occurred, and anterior instability has been reported. However, these problems do not seem to be any more frequent in this group. Late failure of the rotator cuff has been seen, and while it impairs the ability to use the arm against gravity, it appears to have very little effect on the patient's capacity to perform activities of daily life.

In a study from the Mayo Clinic, Lynch et al.[29] found neurologic problems in 4% of their patients who were in several different diagnostic groups. They also found that rheumatoid patients receiving methotrexate were at higher risk of developing neurologic problems. Half of the patients receiving this drug, not known to be neurotoxic, developed a neurologic complication. However, nearly all neurologic complications resolved fully and did not interfere with the long-term outcome of the arthroplasty. Of the three patients who have developed neurologic complications in my practice, all were receiving methotrexate and all recovered fully within 8 weeks.

Brenner et al.[3] found that there was 73% survivorship at 11 years when considering all diagnoses together, but, for rheumatoid patients, the survival rate was 92%. Torchia et

TABLE 24-1
CLINICAL AND RADIOLOGIC RESULTS OF SHOULDER ARTHROPLASTY IN RHEUMATOID ARTHRITIS

Author	No. Shoulders	Follow-up (yr)	Prosthesis Type*	Pain Relief	Active elevation° (gain)	External Rotation° (gain)	Internal Rotation Range**	Glenoid Loosening (%)	Humeral Loosening (%)
Cofield[6]	24	3 (1–6)	T	92	NR	35 (14)	PI/T8	4	0
Boyd et al.[2]	27	3.6 (2–12)	H	92	72 (14)	32 (22)	100 (24)	—	NR
Freidman et al.[13]	24	4.5 (2–10)	T	92	81 (40)	51 (11)	35 (22)	8	0
Trail and Nuttall[51]	40	5.1 (2–9)	T	88	78 (17)	36 (20)	4.6 (2.2)	53	0
	65	5.1 (2–9)	H	88	78 (17)	36 (20)	4.6 (2.2)*	—	0
Sneppen et al.[46]	62	7.7 (4–12)	T	89	75 (31)	28 (22)	S/L5	40	8
Stewart and Kelly[49]	37	9.5 (7–13)	T	88	75 (22)	38 (33)	B/T5	25	25
Torchia et al.[50]	42	12 (5–17)	T	82	103 (43)	47 (10)	Abd/T8	36	38

*Constant score values.
T, total arthroplasty; H, humeral head replacement; PI, posterior ilium; B, buttock; S, sacrum; Abd, abdomen; NR, not recorded.

al.[50] found that the survival rate for all diagnostic groups was 88% at 15 years.

PRACTICAL ADVICE ON DEALING WITH RHEUMATOID PATIENTS

Clinical Assessment

■ Site and severity of pain; functional analysis.
■ Is there a palpable or visible subacromial bursa?
■ Is external rotation reduced (suggests glenohumeral disease)?

Radiographs

■ Which joints are involved (if any)?
■ What is the (Larsen) grade of the involvement?
■ What is the pattern of disease?
■ How much glenoid bone remains?

Injection Tests: What Is the Site of the Pain?

■ Subacromial joint.
■ Acromioclavicular joint and subacromial joint.
■ Glenohumeral joint.

Subacromial Bursa

■ Inject steroid and review at 3 weeks.
■ If no resolution and bursa is palpable, proceed to surgery at an early date to decompress or remove bursa and repair cuff.
■ If no resolution and bursa is not palpable, consider subacromial decompression and bursal clearance. Arthroscopic techniques may be advantageous.
■ Division of the coracoacromial ligament does not adversely affect the results.

Subacromial and Acromioclavicular Joint Pain

■ If no or limited response to steroid, consider excising the outer end of clavicle and excising the bursa. Anterior acromioplasty may be needed if there is an acromial osteophyte. These measures are independent of the radiologic appearance of the glenohumeral joint.

Glenohumeral Pain

■ Usually responds to intra-articular steroid before radiologic changes are apparent.
■ If external rotation is preserved and joint is Larsen grade III or less, consider synovectomy.
■ With Larsen IV or V grade changes: Is the rotator cuff intact? Is the deltoid functioning?

1. With absent cuff and poor deltoid function consider arthrodesis.
2. With a functioning deltoid ± rotator cuff, consider arthroplasty. Small cuff tears may be repaired, but reversed geometry prostheses should be considered for massive cuff tears in older patients.

■ Arthroplasty: Insert total or humeral head replacement according to soft tissue tension unless there is an irreparable cuff tear when a humeral head replacement should be used. Attempt to use a total replacement in a "wet" shoulder.

REFERENCES

1. Albertsen M, Egund N, Jonsson E, et al. Assessment at CT of the rheumatoid shoulder with surgical correlation. Acta Radiologica 1994;35:164.
2. Boyd AD, Thomas WH, Scott RD, et al. Total shoulder arthroplasty versus hemiarthroplasty. Indications for glenoid resurfacing. J Arthroplasty 1990;5:329.
3. Brenner BC, Ferlic DC, Clayton ML, et al. Survivorship of total shoulder arthroplasty. J Bone Joint Surg 1989;71A:1289.
4. Brown DE, James DC, Roy S. Pain relief by suprascapular nerve block in glenohumeral arthritis. Scand J Rheumatol 1988;17:411.
5. Clayton ML, Ferlic DC, Jeffers PD. Prosthetic arthroplasties of the shoulder. Clin Orthop 1982;164:184.
6. Cofield RH. Total shoulder arthroplasty with the Neer prosthesis. J Bone Joint Surg 1984;66-A:899.
7. Crossan JF, Vallance R. The shoulder joint in rheumatoid arthritis. In: Bayley I, Kessel L, eds. Shoulder surgery. Berlin, Springer Verlag, 1982:131.
8. Dijkstra J, Dijkstra MD, Klundert WVD. Rheumatoid arthritis of the shoulder. Description and standard radiographs. Fortschrift Roentgenstr 1985;142:179.
9. Emery RJ, Ho EK, Leong JC. The shoulder girdle in ankylosing spondylitis. J Bone Joint Surg Am 1991;73:1526.
10. Ennevaara K. Painful shoulder joint in rheumatoid arthritis. Acta Rheumatol Scand 1967;(Suppl 11):108.
11. Frich LH, Jensen NC, Odgaard A, et al. Bone strength and material properties of the glenoid. J Shoulder Elbow Surg 1997;6:97.
12. Friedman RJ, Ewald FC. Arthroplasty of the ipsilateral shoulder and elbow in patients who have rheumatoid arthritis. J Bone Joint Surg 1987;69A:661.
13. Friedman RJ, Thornhill TS, Thomas WH, et al. Nonconstrained total shoulder replacement in patients who have rheumatoid arthritis and class IV function. J Bone Joint Surg 1989;71A:494.
14. Gill DRJ, Cofield RH, Morrey BF. Ipsilateral total shoulder and elbow arthroplasties in patients who have rheumatoid arthritis. J Bone Joint Surg 1999;81-A:1128.
15. Grammont PM, Baulot E. Delta shoulder prosthesis for rotator cuff rupture. Orthopedics 1993;16:65.
16. Grennan DM, Gray J, Loudon J, et al. Methotrexate and early postoperative complications in patients with rheumatoid arthritis undergoing elective orthopaedic surgery. Ann Rheum Dis 2001; 60(3):214.
17. Gschwend N, Bischof A. Clinical experiences in arthroplasty according to Neer. J Orthop Rheumatol 1991;4:135.
18. Hirooka A, Wakitani S, Yoneda M, et al. Shoulder destruction in rheumatoid arthritis. Acta Orthop Scand 1996;67:258.
19. Jantsch S, Zenz P, Schwagerl W. Radiologic and sonographic screening study of shoulder joints of patients with rheumatoid arthritis. Z Gesamte Inn Med 1991;46:512.
20. Johnston RA, Kelly IG. Surgery of the rheumatoid cervical spine. Ann Rheum Dis 1990;49(Suppl 2):845.
21. Kelly IG. The source of shoulder pain in rheumatoid arthritis: usefulness of local anaesthetic injections. J Shoulder Elbow Surg 1994;3:62.

22. Kelly IG. The place of hemiarthroplasty in the rheumatoid shoulder. In: Vastamaki M, Jalovaara P, eds. Surgery of the shoulder. Amsterdam, Elsevier, 1995.

23. Kelly IG, Foster RS, Fisher WD. Neer total shoulder replacement in rheumatoid arthritis. J Bone Joint Surg Br 1987;69-B:723.

24. Kessel L, Bayley I. Clinical disorders of the shoulder. 2nd ed. Edinburgh, Churchill Livingstone, 1986.

25. Kieft GJ, Dijkmans BAC, Bloem JL. Magnetic resonance imaging of the shoulder in patients with rheumatoid arthritis. Ann Rheum Dis 1990;49:7.

26. Kocialkowski A, Wallace WA. One stage arthroplasty of the ipsilateral shoulder and elbow. J Bone Joint Surg 1990;72B:520.

27. Larsen A, Dale K, Eek M. Radiographic evaluation of rheumatoid arthritis and related conditions by standard reference films. Acta Radiol Diagn 1977;18:481.

28. Lehtinen JT, Belt EA, Lyback CO, et al. Subacromial space in rheumatoid shoulder. A radiographic 15 year follow up study of 148 shoulders. J Shoulder Elbow Surg 2000;9:183.

29. Lynch NM, Cofield RH, Silbert PL, et al. Neurologic complications after total shoulder arthroplasty. J Shoulder Elbow Surg 1996;5:53.

30. Matsen FA, Smith KL, DeBartolo, SE, et al. A comparison of patients with late-stage rheumatoid arthritis and osteoarthritis of the shoulder using self-assessed shoulder function and health status. Arthritis Care Res 1997;10:43.

31. Miller SL, Hazrati Y, Klepps S, et al. Loss of subscapularis function after total shoulder replacement: a seldom recognised problem. J Shoulder Elbow Surg 2003;12;29.

32. Mullaji AB, Beddow FH, Lamb GHR. CT measurement of glenoid erosion in arthritis. J Bone Joint Surg 1994;76B:384.

33. Neer CS. Shoulder reconstruction. Philadelphia, PA, WB Saunders, 1990.

34. Neer CS, Watson KC, Stanton FC. Recent experience in total shoulder arthroplasty. J Bone Joint Surg 1982;64A:319.

35. Ogilvie-Harris D. Arthroscopy and arthroscopic surgery of the shoulder. Semin Orthop 1987;2:246.

36. Olofsson Y, Book C, Jacobsson LT. Shoulder involvement in patients with newly diagnosed rheumatoid arthritis. Prevalence and associations. Scand J Rheumatol 2003;32:25.

37. Pahle JA. Synovectomy of the shoulder. In: Friedman R, ed. Arthroplasty of the shoulder. New York, Thieme Medical Publishers Inc., 1994:113.

38. Pahle JA, Kvarnes L. Shoulder synovectomy. Ann Chir Gynaecol 1985;198(Suppl 74):37.

39. Petersson CJ. The acromioclavicular joint in rheumatoid arthritis. Clin Orthop 1987;223:86.

40. Rittmeister M, Kerschbaumer F. Grammont reverse total shoulder arthroplasty in patients with rheumatoid arthritis and nonreconstructible rotator cuff lesions. J Shoulder Elbow Surg 2001;10(1):17.

41. Rozing PM, Brand R. Rotator cuff repair during shoulder arthroplasty in rheumatoid arthritis. J Arthroplasty 1998;13(3):311.

42. Rybka V, Raunio P, Vainio K. Arthrodesis of the shoulder in rheumatoid arthritis. A review of 41 cases. J Bone Joint Surg 1979;61B:155.

43. Shanahan EM, Ahern M, Smith M, et al. Suprascapular nerve block (using bupivacaine and methylprednisolone acetate) in chronic shoulder pain. Ann Rheum Dis 2003;62:400.

44. Simpson NS, Kelly IG. Extra-glenohumeral joint shoulder surgery in rheumatoid arthritis: the role of bursectomy, acromioplasty and distal clavicle excision. J Shoulder Elbow Surg 1994;3:66.

45. Sledge CB, Kozinn SC, Thornhill TS, et al. Total shoulder arthroplasty in rheumatoid arthritis. In: Lettin AWF, Petersson C, eds. Rheumatoid arthritis surgery of the shoulder. Vol. 12. Basel, Switzerland, Karger, 1989.

46. Sneppen O, Fruensgaard S, Johannsen HV, et al. Total shoulder replacement in rheumatoid arthritis: proximal migration and loosening. J Shoulder Elbow Surg 1996;5:47.

47. Sperling JW, Cofield RH, Rowland CM. Neer hemiarthroplasty and Neer total shoulder arthroplasty in patients fifty years old or less. J Bone Joint Surg 1998;80-A:464.

48. Steinbrocker O, Traeger CH, Batterman RC. Therapeutic criteria in rheumatoid arthritis. JAMA 1949;140:659.

49. Stewart MPM, Kelly IG. Total shoulder replacement in rheumatoid arthritis. A seven to thirteen year follow up of 37 joints. J Bone Joint Surg 1997;79B:68.

50. Torchia ME, Cofield RH, Settergren CR. Total shoulder arthroplasty with the Neer prosthesis: long term results. J Shoulder Elbow Surg 1995;6:495.

51. Trail IA, Nuttall D. The results of shoulder arthroplasty in patients with rheumatoid arthritis. J Bone Joint Surg 2002;84B:1121.

52. Weber A, Bell S. Arthroscopic subacromial surgery in inflammatory arthritis of the shoulder. Rheumatology 2001;40:384.

53. Woodruff MJ, Cohen AP, Bradley JG. Arthroplasty of the shoulder in rheumatoid arthritis with rotator cuff dysfunction. Int Orthop 2003;27:7.

Rotator Cuff Arthropathy: The Unconstrained Arthroplasty

25

INTRODUCTION

The combination of an irreparable rotator cuff tendon tear and severely damaged glenohumeral joint is the common end-stage result of several disease processes such as rheumatoid arthritis (RA), rotator cuff tear arthropathy (RCTA), and Milwaukee shoulder syndrome. By creating a substantial defect in the rotator cuff tendons, these disease processes lead to destabilization of the glenohumeral joint with subsequent superior migration of the humeral head and secondary severe damage to both the intra-articular and extra-articular elements. The result is a painful, dysfunctional shoulder that necessitates, in many cases, a surgical solution to be carried out to decrease patients' morbidity. However, to date there has been no one surgical procedure to provide an optimal solution for this difficult problem. The aim of this chapter is to focus on the unconstrained arthroplastic solutions for the RCTA. We will begin by reviewing the pathomechanics, differential diagnosis, and some of the nonarthroplasty solutions available.

O. Safran: Fellow, Orthopedic Department, Cleveland Clinic Foundation, Cleveland, Ohio.

J. P. Iannotti: Chairman, Orthopedic Department, Cleveland Clinic Foundation, Cleveland, Ohio.

PATHOMECHANICS

The glenohumeral joint lacks significant intrinsic bony stability and thus relies largely on its soft tissue components. The rotator cuff tendons provide a major contribution to the dynamic stabilization of the glenohumeral joint by increasing the concavity-compression force in the joint.[5,19,22,25,45] By their synchronous action, the rotator cuff tendons oppose the displacing effect of the strong deltoid muscle, keeping the humeral head centered in the glenoid fossa throughout its movement.[37,46,47] The coupled work of the infraspinatus and subscapularis muscles has been shown to be a major factor in superior glenohumeral stability, whereas the contribution of the supraspinatus is less significant.[18,40] A massive tear, consisting of the supraspinatus and at least one of the other rotator cuff tendons[17] (in most cases the infraspinatus), may render the rotator cuff's anterior and posterior force couple ineffective in both the vertical and the transverse planes. The result is a diminution of joint reaction force and a change in the overall direction of the joint force that leads to the destabilization of the glenohumeral joint.[32] In cases in which the long head of biceps is still functional, it may oppose, to some extent, the superior migration of the humeral head.[23,24] Once the proximal pull of

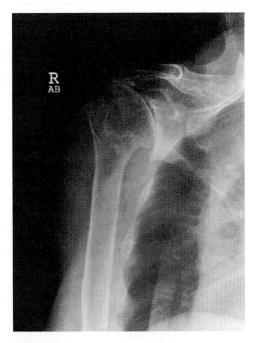

Figure 25-1 X-ray of shoulder joint with rotator cuff-deficient arthritis (RCDA). Notice the "acetabularization of the "socket."

the deltoid is left unopposed, the humeral head migrates superiorly toward the coracoacromial (CA) arch. The humeral head articulates with the CA arch superiorly and the superior glenoid rim inferiorly, leading to flattening of the superior part of the humeral head and tuberosities ("femoralization"), rounding and thinning of the CA arch ("acetabularization"), and destruction of the superior glenoid region (Fig. 25-1). The acromioclavicular joint is also frequently involved in the process, joining its cavity with that of the now joined synovial intra-articular and subacromial bursae spaces. The deltoid, which has lost its fulcrum, has a smaller mechanical advantage and. Therefore, must generate more force to perform its function.[40] The end result is an incongruous, unstable joint with a

Type Ia: Centered stable	Type I b: Centered – Medialized	Typ II a: Decentered – limited stable	Type II b: Dencenterd unstable	Relation- ship of the lever-arms of deltoid and of the upper limb
No superior migration		Superior Translation	Anterior-superior Dislokation	
Acetabularisation of c.a. arch; Femoralisation of humeral head	Medial erosion of the glenoid	Minimun stabilization by c.a. arch	No stabilization by c.a. arch	

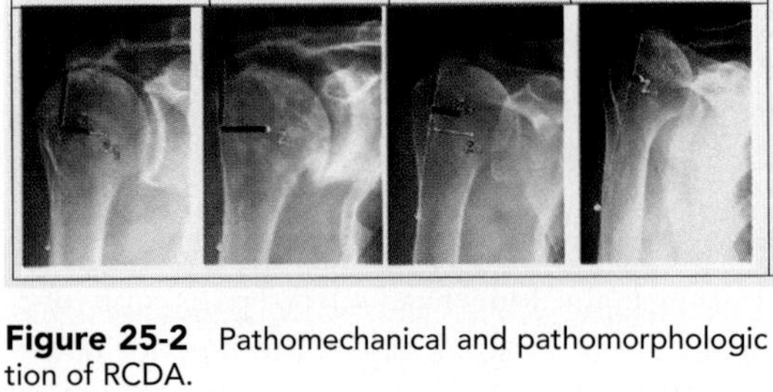

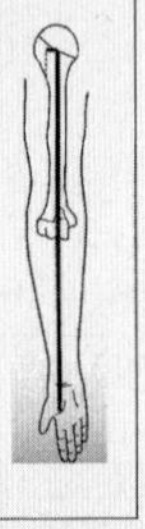

Figure 25-2 Pathomechanical and pathomorphologic classification of RCDA.

higher joint friction and superiorly malpositioned center of rotation.

A pathomechanistic and pathomorphologic classification of glenohumeral rotator cuff-deficient arthritis (RCDA), based on the position and stability of the humeral head, is presented in Figure 25-2. [36]

The classification is independent of the underlying pathologic conditions and is based on two critical issues for the function of the deltoid muscle: the glenohumeral center of rotation and the degree of anterior-superior instability.

DIFFERENTIAL DIAGNOSIS

Although the end result is similar, it is important to recognize the various disease processes leading to glenohumeral RCDA.

Rheumatoid arthritis is the most common cause of RCDA. Between 48% and 65% of patients with RA have significant glenohumeral joint involvement. Approximately 24% of those having glenohumeral arthritis will have a simultaneous rotator cuff tear.[26,38] Superimposed on the aforementioned changes are severe osteopenia, erosions of the entire glenoid without osteophyte formation, and medialization of the glenohumeral joint.

Rotator cuff tear arthritis is the extreme product of a massive rotator cuff tear. The term, coined by Neer et al. in 1983,[30] refers to a primary massive rotator cuff tear that by virtue of mechanical superior instability and nutritional effects leads to a secondary glenohumeral joint destruction.[21] It is believed that between 0% and 25% of massive rotator cuff tears will result in RCTA, but it is difficult, if not impossible, to predict which of the massive tears will result in RCTA.

The Milwaukee shoulder syndrome was originally described by McCarty et al. in 1981.[29] This is an uncommon entity affecting shoulders of elder people, predominantly women. It consists of a massive rotator cuff tear, joint instability, bony destruction, and large, bloodstained joint effusion containing basic calcium phosphate crystals, detectable protease activity, and minimal inflammatory elements. Its relation to RCTA is not clear, and it might represent one of the elements just described.[1] The role of the basic calcium phosphate crystals in creating this syndrome is still controversial. Whether it is the cause of the articular damage, through macrophage spillage of proteases, or just the result of the osteoarthritic process is still unknown.[21]

Primary glenohumeral osteoarthritis is the most common cause for shoulder joint replacement. Although recent data have shown an increase in glenohumeral cartilage damage in cadavers with concurrent rotator cuff tears,[13,20] cartilage damage did not correlate with the size of tear. Clinically, primary glenohumeral osteoarthritis is infrequently associated with irreparable rotator cuff tears.

CLINICAL PICTURE

Patients with an arthritic shoulder and irreparable massive cuff deficiency are primarily elderly people, with female gender predominance. Their main complaints are of severe shoulder pain, limited range of movement, and, in some cases, recurrent swelling of the shoulder. The pain is constant, aggravated by shoulder motion and at nighttime,[30] and felt at the periacromial region and glenohumeral joint line. On physical examination, atrophy of the infraspinatous and supraspinatus muscles, decrease in active and passive glenohumeral motion, and crepitus while moving the patient's shoulder is observed.[21] The x-ray image is typical and consists of a superiorly positioned humeral head, an "acetabularized" socket built up from thinned sclerotic acromion, and an eroded upper glenoid fossa (Fig. 25-1). Occasionally, the acromioclavicular joint and distal clavicle are also damaged and are thus included in the "socket." Cases of secondary stress fractures of the thinned acromion have also been published.[9]

The combination of the clinical and radiologic information is, in most cases, sufficient to make the proper diagnosis, although other modalities such as computed tomography and magnetic resonance imaging may be needed for treatment planning.

TREATMENT

Rotator cuff tear arthropathy combines severe articular damage, bone destruction, osteoporosis, and loss of stabilizing rotator cuff tendons. In contrast with the more common primary degenerative shoulder arthrosis, the inherent instability of the rotator cuff-deficient shoulder necessitates specific consideration. Severe pain and shoulder dysfunction lead many of these patients to seek medical advice. Treatment armamentarium available is variable and includes both conservative and nonsurgical treatment, as well as surgical procedures such as humeral head replacement, total shoulder arthroplasty, and even arthrodesis and resection arthroplasty.

The responsibility of the orthopedic surgeon is to tailor the best treatment option for the particular patient, taking into account the patient's symptoms, functional needs, and the bone and soft tissue conditions of the shoulder joint.

TREATMENT OPTIONS

Conservative Nonsurgical

Patients with mild symptoms and mild limitation in functional range of motion and activities of daily living should be treated nonsurgically. This includes the use of analgesics and physical therapy to maintain range of motion and strengthen the deltoid muscle. It has been shown that by strengthening the middle third of the deltoid, some improvement with superior stability control can be gained.[16] The use of repeated steroid injections is discouraged, but an occasional injection may be helpful in managing the most acute symptoms.

Surgical intervention should be considered in those patients with unremitting pain, significant motion-related pain, and limitation in range of motion and activities of daily living.

Glenohumeral Arthrodesis

The basic concept of fusion is to eradicate pain with elimination of motion. However, there are several drawbacks to its use in patients with glenohumeral arthrodesis.

1. Arthrodesis necessitates good function in the opposite shoulder. In as many as 40% of patients with RCTA, the opposite shoulder is involved in a similar process.
2. The involved shoulder is, in most cases, severely osteopenic and, thus, is more prone to fixation failure and nonunion.
3. Increased scapulothoracic motion needed after glenohumeral arthrodesis exposes the already damaged acromioclavicular joint to excessive motion and therefore pain.
4. Most of the patients involved are elderly. Elderly patients have difficulties submitting to the demanding postoperative rehabilitation process necessary after this procedure.[31]

Cofield and Briggs,[8] in 1979, reported on 12 patients, with an average age of 50 years, with rotator cuff tear who had their shoulders fused. Two of 12 patients developed nonunion, and 6 of 12 patients required a second operation for acromioclavicular pain, nonunion, or proximal migration.

It seems proper to apply the recommendations of Arntz et al.[2] and others[7] and to consider using arthrodesis in irreparable rotator cuff tears only in combination with irreparable deficiencies of the deltoid muscle or in the younger patient with demands for substantial strength at low angles of flexion.

Resection arthroplasty is a poor solution; it yields an unstable, nonfunctional, often painful shoulder, and, thus, should not be carried out as a primary surgical treatment in patients with glenohumeral arthrodesis.

Constrained Total Shoulder Arthroplasty

The lack of joint stability led surgeons to use constrained designs of total shoulder arthroplasty in cases of RCTA to create a steady fulcrum for deltoid function. Although initial reports showed good clinical results, longer-term follow-up showed a high percentage of glenoid component loosening and breakage of implants. Post and Jablon[34] reported that glenoid component radiolucent lines appeared in 30% of primary constrained arthroplasties used in shoulders with RCDA. Lettin and colleagues[27] reported on 10 of 49 shoulders that developed relatively early glenoid component loosening. It appeared that the inherent constraints in the prosthesis transferred strong shear forces to the glenoid component-bone interface, which, when coupled with the osteopenic nature of the bone and small surface area of the interface, led to the glenoid loosening. Given the unacceptable high failure rates, almost all surgeons abandoned the use of constrained, fixed fulcrum, total shoulder construct for RCTA.

More recently, the use of a constrained reverse ball in socket shoulder prosthesis (Delta III [Grammont] prosthesis; DePuy Johnson and Johnson, New Brunswick, NJ) has been used extensively in Europe for the cuff-deficient arthritic shoulder with good deltoid function. The European results with this prosthesis have been good and significantly better than the functional results obtained with unconstrained humeral hemiarthroplasty, particularly in patients with superior humeral head instability and CA arch deficiency.

Unconstrained Shoulder Arthroplasty

Two different types of unconstrained shoulder arthroplasty have been used for RCTA: (1) total shoulder arthroplasty using anatomic design with no additional built-in constraints and (2) humeral hemiarthroplasty.

Unconstrained Total Shoulder Arthroplasty

In 1982, Neer et al.[31] published their experience with prosthetic replacement of 273 shoulders, of which 16 were diagnosed with RCTA. Eight shoulders with RCTA received an unconstrained total shoulder prosthesis, whereas the rest were treated with a semiconstrained (hooded) implant. Eleven patients had a follow-up of more than 24 months. According to the "limited goals rehabilitation" criteria set by Neer et al.,[31] successful results were reported in 10 of 11 patients. Although 30% of shoulders and 33% of the shoulders with RCTA had glenoid lucent lines (less than 1 mm), clinically detected loosening was not found in any of these 273 shoulders. Lohr et al.[28] found unconstrained shoulder replacements to provide better pain relieve than hemiarthroplasty in 22 shoulders with RCDA. However, a high rate of radiologic and clinical loosening was noted in their patients. In a prospective study performed in 1987, Barrett et al.[4] reported on 44 patients who underwent total shoulder arthroplasty. Nine of the patients had a massive tear of the rotator cuff at the time of surgery. Glenoid loosening was found in four patients, all of whom had previous massive rotator cuff tear. Three of these patients required surgical revision. It was hypothesized that the unstable shoulder

joint causes repeated exaggerated translation of the humeral head on the glenoid component, allowing joint compression forces to be put on the superior glenoid margin rather than in the center of the glenoid, leading to loosening. Franklin et al.[15] tried to correlate different clinical and radiographic parameters with glenoid loosening in patients undergoing total shoulder replacement in the presence of massive rotator cuff tear. They found that the amount of superior migration of the humeral head was closely correlated with an increased glenoid loosening rate. They emphasized the eccentric forces applied by the unstable, translated humeral head on the glenoid component resembling the movement of a "rocking horse," leading to the loosening of the glenoid component. Because these high loosening rates are found relatively early in the postoperative course, unconstrained total shoulder implants have been disfavored.

HUMERAL HEAD REPLACEMENT

The relatively early loosening of the glenoid component has led surgeons to propose hemiarthroplasty with replacement of only the humeral head as a solution for shoulders with RCTA. With this approach, significant pain reduction in 47% to 86% of patients and significant, yet variable, gain in forward elevation have been reported on an average follow-up of 2 to 5 years.[14,33,35,44,48] According to Neer's limited-goal criteria,[31] successful results have been achieved in 63% to 83% of patients. Pollock and coworkers[33] found similar pain relief and better forward elevation gain in hemiarthroplasty versus total shoulder replacement in 30 shoulder with RCDA and arthritis.

The inherent instability of hemiarthroplasty in these patients, where no significant soft tissue support is available, has nourished several debates concerning the implant design and associated procedures needed to stabilize these shoulders.

Humeral Component Size

One of the first solutions to gain better stability was the use of a larger humeral head component. The rationale was that a large humeral component can articulate better with the large "acetabulum" (consisting of the superior glenoid and undersurface of CA arch), therefore creating a relatively stable and more congruent joint. However, potential disadvantages to the use of large humeral components included overstuffing of the joint, which led to increased joint reaction forces and accelerated bone resorption of both the glenoid and acromion, causing pain and instability.[35] In addition, with the use of a larger humeral head, any attempt to augment or partially repair the deficient rotator cuff became much more difficult. The disadvantages of a large-diameter humeral component and the need for additional joint contact area with the acromion and CA arch have led to the use of a specially designed humeral component, the cuff tear arthropathy head. This component is anatomic in size and has a smooth extension of the articular surface facing superiorly (Fig. 25-3). This design, at least theoretically, enlarges the joint contact area without overstuffing the joint.

Humeral Head Version

The most common problem with humeral hemiarthroplasty is the superior migration and superior instability of the prosthetic, with, in some cases, loss of contact of the CA arch. This problem can be decreased by properly sizing the humeral head, preserving the CA arch, and placing the humeral head in 15 degrees of further retroversion. The increased retroversion better positions the humeral head under the acromion for any degree of external rotation.

Reconstruction and Augmentation of the Rotator Cuff Elements

Pollock et al.,[33] Cantrell et al.,[6] and DiGiovanni et al.[10] have advocated attempts to repair or augment the torn rotator cuff tendons. One of the options suggested is to transfer the subscapularis tendon to a more superior position for superior humeral head stabilization.[10,43] This option is obviously limited to those patients with a functional, unshortened subscapularis tendon. However, others reported satisfactory results without any attempt to repair or augment the torn supraspinatus and infraspinatus tendons. Williams and Rockwood[44] published satisfactory results

with pain relief for 18 of 21 patients by using no cuff reconstruction and balancing the remaining cuff muscles by fine-tuning the humeral head component size. Zuckerman et al.,[48] who also did not try to repair or augment the torn supra and infraspinatus tendons, published similar results. Sanchez-Sotelo et al.[35] reported on 33 shoulders in 30 patients who received a hemiarthroplasty for the diagnosis of rotator cuff arthropathy. Medium-sized humeral head components were used in most shoulders. A statistically significant correlation was found between attempts to partially repair the rotator cuff tendons and postoperative, clinically significant anterior instability. The authors believe that their repair attempts created a muscle force imbalance.

Augmentation of Superior Bone Elements

The importance of maintaining the CA arch in RCTA cannot be overemphasized.[2,35,44,48] The deficiency in superior bony restraints, secondary in most cases to previous surgical decompression of the subacromial space, creates an extremely difficult scenario. Sanchez-Sotelo et al.[35] reported poorer results and increased susceptibility to anterosuperior instability in a subgroup of patients with RCTA who had undergone previous surgical CA arch decompression. Several solutions have been proposed for restoring these superior bony restraints. Wiley[43] described using autologous tricortical iliac bone graft that was fixed between the coracoid and acromion in cases in which the CA arch has been compromised by previous subacromial decompression. Engelbrecht and Heinert[12] introduced another technique in which augmentation of the glenoid rim was achieved by fixing an autologous bone graft to the superior

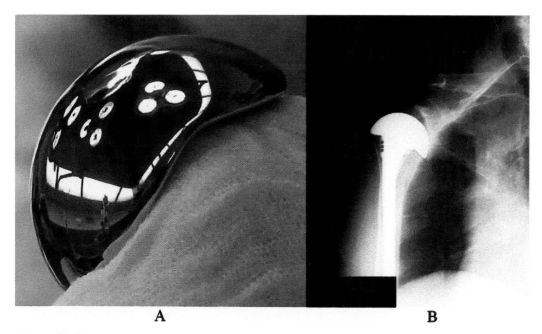

Figure 25-3 *(A)* Cuff tear arthropathy head prosthesis. *(B)* X-ray of cuff tear arthropathy hemiarthroplasty.

glenoid rim, thus deepening and widening the actual articulating surface of the glenoid and counteracting superior directed forces applied by the humeral head. These procedures have not been performed by many others, so their effectiveness cannot be verified.

Bipolar Humeral Prosthesis

The bipolar humeral component design was presented by Swanson et al.[39] in 1989 as a solution for patients with advanced glenohumeral arthritis and poor rotator cuff tissue as part of a total shoulder design. The rationale was to decrease prosthetic contact forces by a larger "articular" surface and by the secondary motion possible within the bipolar humeral prosthesis itself. At a follow-up of 5 years, pain relief was rated good to excellent in 31 of the 35 shoulders that underwent operation. Arredondo and Worland[6,45] reported their results using a newer, lower profile bipolar design that allows for less bony resection during insertion. At a mean follow-up of 3.1 years (range 2–6 years), satisfactory results were found in 92% of their patients by using the limited-goals criteria, including both pain relief and improved range of motion. The authors also reported prosthetic birotational motion (head-shell and shell-glenoid motion), which persisted in all shoulders. Vrettos

et al.,[45] using the same bipolar prosthesis, reported less favorable results. Six of the seven patients reported moderate to severe pain and were unhappy with the results. No glenohumeral or intrinsic bipolar motion was found in radiographs taken in different angles of abduction. A recent report by Duranthon et al.[11] on 13 shoulders with RCTA, with a mean follow-up of 28 months, revealed good pain relief with less than satisfactory range of motion improvement. Significant glenoid wear was found in three of the seven shoulders that were observed 2 years after surgery.

To date, bipolar hemiarthroplasty has not gained popularity. Concerns of "overstuffing" the shoulder and secondary glenoid wear, the rupture of the subscapularis tendon because of the vertical orientation of the component, the effect of polyethylene wear,[21] and the relatively short follow-up reported have prevented bipolar hemiarthroplasty from gaining more acceptance.

The inherent instability of hemiarthroplasty in shoulders with RCDA has been at least partially counteracted by using the aforementioned methods with relatively good clinical results. One of the still existing concerns is the durability achieved with the use of hemiarthroplasty in cuff-deficient shoulders. Sanchez-Sotelo et al.[35] reported on 33 shoulders in 30 patients who had a hemiarthroplasty for the diagnosis of rotator cuff arthropathy with an average

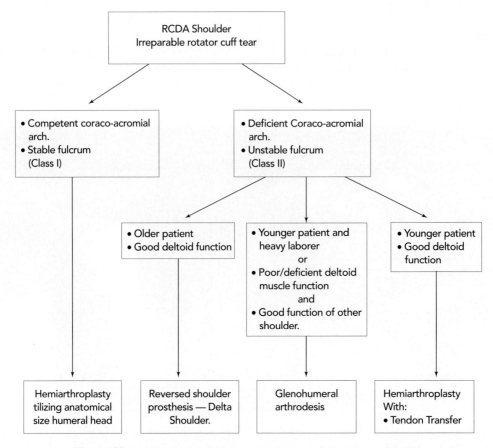

Figure 25-4 Algorithm for surgical management of shoulder with RCDA.

follow-up of 5 years (range 2–11 years). Most shoulders received medium-sized humeral heads. Progressive superior migration and progressive glenoid bone loss were reported in 8 of 33 shoulders, and acromial bone loss was reported in 16 of 33 shoulders, leading to acromion fracture in two patients. Poorer results and more severe anterosuperior instability were found in a subgroup of patients who had previous surgical CA arch decompression.

CONCLUSION

Hemiarthroplasty is a good surgical solution for a difficult clinical problem. Although not perfect, hemiarthroplasty provides good pain relief and moderate range-of-motion gain for most patients, which is relatively long lasting. Because of the high rates of glenoid component loosening, unconstrained total shoulder replacement should not be considered for joints with RCDA. No study has demonstrated an advantage of rotator cuff partial repair or augmentation in these circumstances over simple debridement. A competent CA arch is a keystone for successful result and therefore should not be damaged during the surgical procedure. In cases of preexistent CA deficiency, the use of an augmentation procedure for the CA arch, in addition to the hemiarthroplasty or the use of reversed shoulder prosthesis, should be considered. Progressive bone loss and progressive anterosuperior instability could lead to a growing number of unsatisfactory results in long-term follow-up periods (more than 5 years).

Figure 25-4 is an algorithm for the surgical management of RCDA.

REFERENCES

1. Antoniou J, Tsai A, Baker D, et al. Milwaukee shoulder: correlating possible etiologic variables. Clin Orthop 2003;(407):79.
2. Arntz CT, Matsen FA 3rd, Jackins S. Surgical management of complex irreparable rotator cuff deficiency. J Arthroplasty 1991;6(4):363.
3. Arredondo J, Worland RL. Bipolar shoulder arthroplasty in patients with osteoarthritis: short-term clinical results and evaluation of birotational head motion. J Shoulder Elbow Surg 1999;8(5):425.
4. Barrett WP, Franklin JL, Jackins SE, et al. Total shoulder arthroplasty. J Bone Joint Surg Am 1987;69(6):865.
5. Bassett RW, Browne AO, Morrey BF, et al. Glenohumeral muscle force and moment mechanics in a position of shoulder instability. J Biomech 1990;23:405.
6. Cantrell JS, Itamura JM, Burkhead WZ. Rotator cuff tear arthropathy. In: Warner JJ, Iannotti JP, Gerber C. Complex and revision problems in shoulder surgery. Philadelphia, PA, Lippincott-Raven Publishers, 1997.
7. Clare DJ, Wirth MA, Groh GI, et al. Shoulder arthrodesis. J Bone Joint Surg Am 2001;83-A(4):593.
8. Cofield RH, Briggs BT. Glenohumeral arthrodesis. Operative and long-term functional results. J Bone Joint Surg Am 1979; 61(5): 668.
9. Dennis DA, Ferlic DC, Clayton ML. Acromial stress fractures associated with cuff-tear arthropathy. A report of three cases. J Bone Joint Surg Am 1986;68(6):937.
10. DiGiovanni J, Marra G, Park JY, et al. Hemiarthroplasty for glenohumeral arthritis with massive rotator cuff tears. Orthop Clin North Am 1998;29(3):477.
11. Duranthon LD, Augereau B, Thomazeau H, et al. Bipolar arthroplasty in rotator cuff arthropathy: 13 cases. Rev Chir Orthop Reparatrice Appar Mot 2002;88(1):28.
12. Engelbrecht E, Heinert K. More than ten years experience with unconstrained shoulder replacement. In: Kolbel R, Helbig B, Blauth W, eds. Shoulder replacement. Berlin, Springer-Verlag, 1987:85.
13. Feeney MS, O'Dowd J, Kay EW, et al. Glenohumeral articular cartilage changes in rotator cuff disease. J Shoulder Elbow Surg 2003;12(1):20.
14. Field LD, Dines DM, Zabinski SJ, et al. Hemiarthroplasty of the shoulder for rotator cuff arthropathy. J Shoulder Elbow Surg 1997;6(1):18.
15. Franklin JL, Barrett WP, Jackins SE, et al. Glenoid loosening in total shoulder arthroplasty. Association with rotator cuff deficiency. J Arthroplasty 1988;3(1):39.
16. Gagey O, Hue E. Mechanics of the deltoid muscle. A new approach. Clin Orthop 2000;(375):250.
17. Gerber C, Fuchs B, Hodler J. The results of repair of massive tears of the rotator cuff. J Bone Joint Surg Am 2000;82(4):505.
18. Halder AM, Zhao KD, O'Driscoll SW, et al. Dynamic contributions to superior shoulder stability. J Orthop Res 2001;19(2):206.
19. Hsu HC, Boardman ND 3rd, Luo ZP, et al. Tendon-defect and muscle-unloaded models for relating a rotator cuff tear to glenohumeral stability. J Orthop Res 2000;18(6):952.
20. Hsu HC, Luo ZP, Stone JJ, et al. Correlation between rotator cuff tear and glenohumeral degeneration. Acta Orthop Scand 2003; 74(1):89.
21. Jensen KL, Williams GR Jr., Russell IJ, et al. Current concepts review—rotator cuff tear arthropathy. J Bone Joint Surg Am 1999; 81:1312.
22. Karduna AR. Kinematics of the glenohumeral joint: influences of muscle forces, ligamentous constraints, and articular geometry. J Orthop Res 1996;14(6):986.
23. Kido T, Itoi E, Konno N, et al. Electromyographic activities of the biceps during arm elevation in shoulders with rotator cuff. Acta Orthop Scand 1998;69(6):575.
24. Kido T, Itoi E, Konno N, et al. The depressor function of biceps on the head of the humerus in shoulders with tears of the rotator cuff. J Bone Joint Surg Br 2000;82(3):416.
25. Lee SB, Kim KJ, O'Driscoll SW, et al. Dynamic glenohumeral stability provided by the rotator cuff muscles in the mid-range and end-range of motion. A study in cadavera. J Bone Joint Surg Am 2000;82(6):849.
26. Lehtinen JT, Kaarela K, Belt EA, et al. Relation of glenohumeral and acromioclavicular joint destruction in rheumatoid shoulder. A 15 year follow up study. Ann Rheum Dis 2000;59(2):158.
27. Lettin AW, Copeland SA, Scales JT. The Stanmore total shoulder replacement. J Bone Joint Surg Br 1982;64(1):47.
28. Lohr JF, Cofield RH, Uhthoff HK. Glenoid component loosening in cuff tear arthropathy. J Bone Joint Surg 1991;73B(Suppl 2): 106.
29. McCarty DJ, Halverson PB, Carrera GF, et al. "Milwaukee shoulder"—association of microspheroids containing hydroxyapatite crystals, active collagenase, and neutral protease with rotator cuff defects. I. Clinical aspects. Arthritis Rheum 1981;24(3):464.
30. Neer CS 2nd, Craig EV, Fukuda H. Cuff-tear arthropathy. J Bone Joint Surg Am 1983;65(9):1232.
31. Neer CS 2nd, Watson KC, Stanton FJ. Recent experience in total shoulder replacement. J Bone Joint Surg Am 1982;64(3):319.
32. Parsons IM, Apreleva M, Fu FH, et al. The effect of rotator cuff tears on reaction forces at the glenohumeral joint. J Orthop Res 2002; 20(3):439.
33. Pollock, RG, Deliz ED, McIlveen SJ, et al. Prosthetic replacement in rotator cuff deficient shoulders. Orthop Trans 1993;16;774.
34. Post M, Jablon M. Constrained total shoulder arthroplasty. Long-term follow-up observations. Clin Orthop 1983;(173):109.
35. Sanchez-Sotelo J, Cofield RH, Rowland CM. Shoulder hemiarthroplasty for glenohumeral arthritis associated with severe rotator cuff deficiency. J Bone Joint Surg Am 2001;83-A(12): 1814.

36. Seebauer L. Optimierung der endoprothetischen versorgung der omarthritis und defektarthropathie-konventionelle, bipolare oder inverse prothese. Z Orthop 2002;140S:121.
37. Sharkey NA, Marder RA. The rotator cuff opposes superior translation of the humeral head. Am J Sports Med 1995;23(3):270.
38. Smith KL, Matsen FA. Total shoulder arthroplasty versus hemi-arthroplasty—current trends. Orthop Clin North Am 1998; 29(3):491.
39. Swanson AB, Swanson GG, Sattel AB, et al. Bipolar implant shoulder arthroplasty. Long-term results. Clin Orthop 1989;249: 227.
40. Thompson WO, Debski RE, Boardman ND 3rd, et al. A biome-chanical analysis of rotator cuff deficiency in a cadaveric model. Am J Sports Med 1996;24(3):286.
41. Vrettos BC, Wallace WA, Neumann L. Bipolar hemiarthroplasty of the shoulder for the elderly patient with rotator cuff arthropathy (abstract). In: Proceedings of the British Elbow and Shoulder Society. J Bone Joint Surg 1998;80B(Suppl I):106.
42. Warner JJP, Bowen MK, Deng XH, et al. Effect of joint compression of inferior stability of the glenohumeral joint. J Shoulder Elbow Surg 1999;8(1):31.
43. Wiley AM. Superior humeral dislocation. A complication following decompression and debridement for rotator cuff tears. Clin Orthop 1991;(263):135.
44. Williams GR Jr., Rockwood CA Jr. Hemiarthroplasty in rotator cuff-deficient shoulders. J Shoulder Elbow Surg 1996;5(5):362.
45. Worland RL, Arredondo J. Bipolar shoulder arthroplasty for painful conditions of the shoulder. J Arthroplasty 1998;13(6): 631.
46. Yamaguchi K, Sher JS, Andersen WK, et al. Glenohumeral motion in patients with rotator cuff tears: a comparison of asymptomatic and symptomatic shoulders. J Shoulder Elbow Surg 2000;9(1):6.
47. Zeman CA, Arcand MA, Cantrell JS, et al. The rotator cuff-deficient arthritic shoulder: diagnosis and surgical management. J Am Acad Orthop Surg 1998;6(6):337.
48. Zuckerman JD, Scott AJ, Gallagher MA. Hemiarthroplasty for cuff tear arthropathy. J Shoulder Elbow Surg 2000;9(3):169.

The Reversed Prosthesis

François Sirveaux   Daniel Molé   Pascal Boileau

INTRODUCTION

Although Grammont et al.[26] developed the reversed shoulder prosthesis nearly 20 years ago, it took two decades for this concept to be fully accepted in both Europe and North America. The reticence of many surgeons to accept this seemingly radical concept was because of the nonanatomic design and a long list of prior constrained prosthetic designs that led to dismal clinical failures. Currently, in Europe, the reversed shoulder prosthesis has become an important standard of care in the treatment of difficult reconstructive problems of the shoulder. Indeed, it has become one of the most commonly used prosthesis to treat rotator cuff tear arthroplasty and failed prior arthroplasty in the setting of soft-tissue loss. As such, it has greatly changed the habits of most surgeons who must confront these difficult problems. The reason for this great shift in clinical approach is the dramatic improvement of functional outcome because of the geometry of this prosthesis. In fact, the concept of "limited goal surgery," by Neer et al.,[38] in the case of rotator cuff tear arthropathy and revision surgery has become antiquated in many cases because of the reliability of the reverse prosthesis in compensating for loss of rotator cuff function.

It is widely accepted that the outcome of an anatomic prosthesis depends on the status of the rotator cuff. Rotator cuff insufficiency often results in anterosuperior subluxation of the humeral head, which hinders deltoid action. The loss of a fixed fulcrum for rotation thus leads to loss of active elevation of the arm. Many surgeons attempted to design a constrained or reversed prosthesis that compensated for this biomechanical deficiency, but virtually all

failed because of faulty biomechanical design. Grammont's[26] legacy of the reversed shoulder prosthesis was based on his belief in the concept of reestablishing a fixed fulcrum for rotation while respecting the forces across the glenoid. His design allowed for both of these goals to be achieved. This chapter will discuss the history and biomechanical aspects of the reversed prosthesis as well as the surgical technique, indications, and results.

HISTORY AND DESIGN RATIONALE

In the absence of an effective rotator cuff, active elevation is hindered because there is loss of the normal fulcrum for rotation that allows the deltoid to lift the arm. In fact, the orientation of the deltoid muscle fibers causes superior movement of the humeral head because the force coupled with the rotator cuff is now imbalanced. The coracoacromial arch forms the last barrier to this superior movement. The only way to restore shoulder motion in this situation is to restore a fixed fulcrum for rotation so the deltoid can have a sufficiently efficient lever arm to elevate the humerus. This can be achieved with the reversed shoulder prosthesis designed by Grammont.[26] Prior reversed shoulder designs have attempted to apply biomechanical principles normally appropriate for hip arthroplasty.[8,9,32,34,41] These designs failed as the result of a high rate of glenoid loosening because they all moved the fulcrum for rotation lateral to its normal position and thus created increased shearing forces across the glenoid during elevation.[41]

The principle of a reversed prosthesis was suggested in the 1970s by Neer.[36] The advantage of a reversed design was to alter the vector of forces starting from the center of rotation to create centripetal forces, which would maintain the compression of the humeral cup onto the sphere during the elevation. The use of a large-diameter sphere was theorized to increase the mobility and lever arm of the deltoid by lateralizing the greater tuberosity.[3,20,36] Neer ob-

F. **Sirveaux:** Clinique de Traumatologie et d'Orthopédie, Nancy, France.

D. **Molé:** Clinique de Traumatologie et d'Orthopédie, Nancy, France.

P. **Boileau:** Hôpital de l'Archet, Nice, France.

served, however, that this type of implant would not reestablish active external rotation when the infraspinatus was torn. Thus, he abandoned this line of implant design in 1974. Moreover, all prostheses using a fixed rotation center outside the scapula were given up for the same reasons (Reeves prosthesis,[42] Kolbel,[31] Kessel,[6,52] and Jefferson and Fenlin prostheses,[20] Gerard and Lannelongue prosthesis,[24] and Liverpool and Beddow prosthesis[2]). Three component prostheses suggested by Buechel et al.[7] and Gristina and Webb[27] remained at the experimental stage and never progressed further.

In 1987, Grammont et al.[26] (Dijon, France) developed an original reverse prosthesis design, based on experimental biomechanical studies. The aim of Grammont et al. was to design a stable prosthesis by improving deltoid efficiency while limiting risk of glenoid loosening. According to the work of Fischer and coworkers,[21] a prosthesis was conceived in which the center of rotation remained inside the glenoid. This geometry was achieved by fixing a hemisphere to a baseplate covering the glenoid to allow lateralization of the deltoid lever arm while at the same time reducing shearing forces across the glenoid and promoting compression forces across the joint during deltoid contraction and arm elevation (Figs. 26-1 to 26-3).

The increase of the deltoid lever arm (torque) is caused by the medial displacement of the center of rotation, and, thus, an increase in the force magnitude exerted by the muscle during elevation (Torque = force × distance) (Fig. 26-2). A study on an anatomic simulator showed that a 10-mm medialization of the center of rotation increased the deltoid torque by 20% to 60%.[26] Because of the orientation of the force vector produced by the deltoid, lowering the center of rotation also induces an increase of the lever arm (lowering of 10 mm increases the abduction torque by 30%–60%). The increase of the deltoid forces is related to the middle deltoid tensioning, which improves the efficiency of the contraction of the muscular fibers. Furthermore, the medialization of the center of rotation also increases the abduction component of the anterior and posterior part of the deltoid (Fig. 26-3).

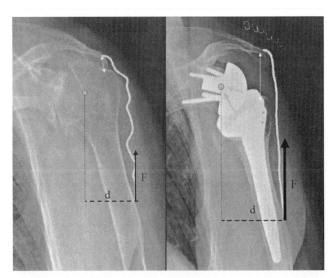

Figure 26-2   Middle deltoid torque is increased because of the medialization of the center of rotation, which increases the muscle lever arm and tension of the muscular fibers.

Using a large-diameter sphere allows an increase in the range of motion at the level of the prosthesis and increases the stability of a constrained design similar to the design of hip arthroplasty. The choice of a 36-mm or 42-mm sphere corresponds, according to the designer, to the average volume of the joint.[1] Beyond 45 degrees, the constraints applicable to the glenoid are centered on the bone/implant interface and participate in joint stability. The medialization and lowering of the rotation center tends to incline the diaphysis and open the angle between the humeral shaft and the scapula pilar. This tends to diminish the shearing constraints, which are persistent at the start of the elevation. For Grammont et al.[26] the existence of these constraints justifies the use of a noncemented glenoid implant with a central peg and a divergent fixation by screws fixed to the baseplate.

The initial prototype used by Grammont et al.[26] consisted of a cemented glenoidal implant corresponding to two-thirds of a sphere 42 mm in diameter, which would fit on a cylinder prepared with a crown saw. The humeral implant was polyethylene, forming a cup corresponding to one-third of a sphere (Fig. 26-4).

In 1987, Grammont et al.[26] reported their preliminary results on eight cases with an average follow-up of 8 years. There were three cases of postradiotherapy necrosis, four cases of revision prostheses, and one case of inflammatory arthritis. The approach included an osteotomy of the acromion. In three cases, patients recovered an active elevation of 100 to 130 degrees, and the author emphasized the swiftness of the functional recovery. From 1989 onward, Grammont conceived the Delta 3, in which the initial model consisted of a sphere screwed on the glenoid

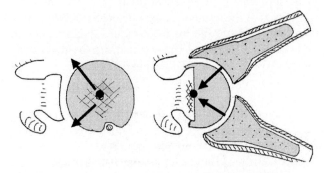

Figure 26-1   Reverse disposal of the prosthesis enables the forces to be focused on the center of the sphere and glenoid baseplate.

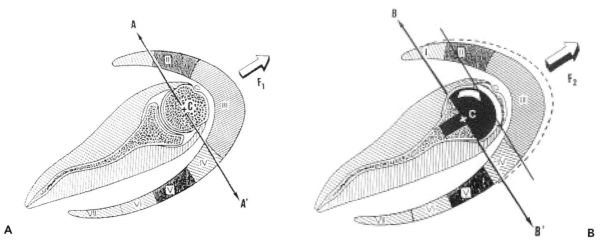

Figure 26-3   Medialization of the rotation center increases the abducting component of the anterior and posterior parts of the deltoid.

baseplate (Fig. 26-4). Because of the complication of unscrewing the sphere, the fixation of the sphere was modified in 1995 by a Morse taper locked by a central screw. The humeral stem was conical and available in its cemented or uncemented form, covered by hydroxyapatite, and in three different lengths (100, 150, or 180 mm). The proximal part was screwed on the stem and designed with an antirotation fin. The humeral cup was made available in two thicknesses (0 and 6 mm) with the possibility of adding a metallic extension of 9 mm or using deeper versions in case of instability. The Delta prostheses 1 and 2 correspond to an anatomic version of the prosthesis with a metallic head to be fixed on the humeral implant (Delta 1) and an anatomic glenoid implant (Fig. 26-5).

PLANNING AND SURGICAL TECHNIQUE

Patient Evaluation

In addition to the appreciation of pain, loss of active mobility (pseudo-paralytic), and the usual functional criteria (muscular strength, daily activity, and Constant score), the following points need to be assessed before implanting a reversed prosthesis:

- Surgical history: The status of the remaining acromial arch, rotator cuff tendons, and prior surgical approaches used are important to guide the subsequent prosthetic surgery.

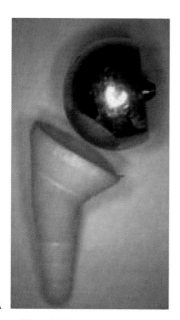
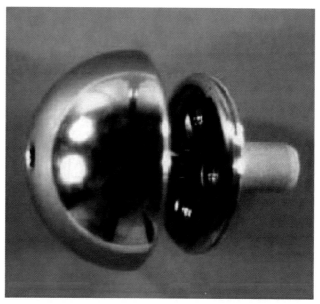

Figure 26-4   Initial prototype of Grammont's reverse prosthesis (A). Fixation system of the second version of the prosthesis with the sphere screwed on the baseplate (B).

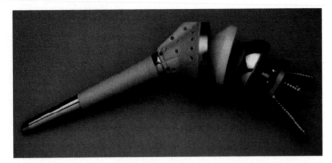

Figure 26-5 Delta prosthesis in its current configuration.

- External active rotation, elbow to the side (lag sign, belly press test) and in elevation: The patient should be asked about the functional consequences of the deficit, bearing in mind that it might increase if a reversed prosthesis is used.
- The passive mobility, especially in anterior elevation and external rotation: The presence of associated stiffness can influence the choice of the approach, because an inferior capsular release is more easily performed through an anterior deltopectoral approach than a superior approach.
- The essential integrity of the deltoid and the axillary nerve.

Preoperative imaging should consist of the following:

- X-ray: A true anterior-posterior image with the arm in neutral rotation will demonstrate glenoid wear that may have a bearing on implantation of the component. Superior displacement and disruption of the acromial arch may also be observed in cases of failed treatment of massive rotator cuff tears. An axillary view will demonstrate fixed displacement and glenoid erosion in that plain radiograph as well.
- Computed tomography (CT) scan or arthro-CT: These three-dimensional studies allow for assessment of the loss of bone stock, the glenoid orientation in the horizontal plane, and the degree of atrophy and fatty infiltration (Goutallier classification) of the cuff muscles (importance of the teres minor).
- Magnetic resonance imaging: Cuff lesions and degree of synovial inflammation can be seen on these images.

Preoperative Planning

Good preoperative anterior and posterior radiographs will allow for proper preoperative templating of the components needed for the surgical reconstruction.

- The diaphyseal axis and entry point of the humeral instruments (frequent variations).
- The sizes of the metaphysis and prosthetic sphere among the possible choices (diameter 36 or 42 mm). The choice is, in most cases, a 36-mm implant.
- The length and diameter of the humeral stem. Usually

the stem must be as short as possible (100 mm), and caution should be taken not to oversize its diameter to reduce the risk of fracture. The use of a cemented stem is generally advised.

- The level of the humeral cup, making sure to determine a reproducible landmark on the bone (lateral facet of the greater tuberosity).
- The glenoidal preparation: location of the entry point on the frontal plane and horizontal plane; orientation and amount of reaming relative to the loss of bone stock and to achieve optimal glenoid positioning; and orientation of the fixation screws of the baseplate.

Surgical Technique

Setup and Surgical Approach

The patient is positioned in a beach-chair position with the affected shoulder completely free from the table. The patient's head is carefully positioned rotated away from the operative shoulder to ensure good access to humeral preparation. The arm is left free so that manipulation is possible because this helps humeral component insertion. The following two approaches can be used (Fig. 26-6).

The **deltopectoral approach** allows for adequate inferior exposure to manage complex revision cases and significant contractures. However, a drawback is that it requires the section of the remaining subscapularis tendon and anterior capsule, and, in our experience, the risk of postoperative shoulder instability is greater than with the superior approach.

The **anterosuperior approach,** although having the disadvantage of compromising the deltoid origin, does allow preservation of remaining inferior soft tissue that may reduce the risk of instability. It is, however, difficult to perform revision cases with component removal from this approach.

- The deltopectoral approach presents an advantage because it respects the integrity and insertion of the del-

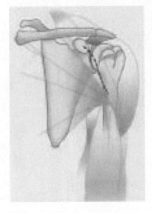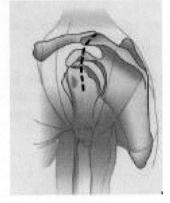

Figure 26-6 Deltopectoral approach and anterosuperior approach.

toid; it also enables an inferior capsular release in case of joint stiffness. Nevertheless, its drawback is that it requires the section of the remaining subscapularis tendon and anterior capsule, which carries a risk of postoperative dislocation.

■ The anterosuperior approach (along the anterior border of the acromion with division of the anterior deltoid) has the inconvenience of compromising the deltoid insertion; however, it has the double advantage of facilitating the exposure of the humeral head and glenoid in addition to enabling the respect of the anterior stabilizing structures (subscapularis tendon and capsule), decreasing the risk of postoperative instability.

Humeral Head Resection and Humeral Reaming (Author's Preferred Technique)

After resection of the remaining upper cuff, the humeral head is exposed by anterosuperior luxation (arm in extension, external rotation, pushing up on the elbow) when using the anterosuperior approach or by anterior dislocation (arm in extension, abduction and external rotation) when using the deltopectoral anterior approach.

The epiphysis entry hole is drilled at the top of the humeral head just medial to the bicipital groove at a location predetermined from preoperative templating (Fig. 26-7). The guide is introduced, and the humeral head is cut with an oscillating saw. The height of the cut should be consistent with preoperative planning. In the event of stiffness, resection should be slightly more aggressive with the humeral osteotomy somewhat lower than the guide. With the anterosuperior approach, the aim is that the medial edge of the humeral resection should align with the inferior pole of the glenoid.

The approach is one based on surgeon preference. In the case of a deltopectoral approach, the risk of dislocation is more of a concern; therefore it is preferable to position the

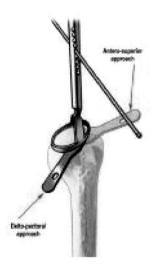

Figure 26-7 Humeral section.

humerus component in 20 degrees of retroversion. In the case of a superior approach, the risk of dislocation is decreased so the choice of the retroversion angle is less of a concern. In the case of a stiff shoulder, the risk of dislocation is less relevant, whereas the risk of inferior scapular notching is more of a concern; thus, a 0-degree retroversion angle seems preferable. If the shoulder is supple, a 20-degree retroversion angle is preferable to limit the risk of dislocation. Furthermore, if the shoulder is supple, then the glenoidal component can be fixed in such a way to decrease the risk of inferior impingement.

The metaphysis is then reamed to the appropriate diameter, as guided by preoperative templating, and the intraoperative fit is judged by achieving adequate depth. The diaphysis is prepared to the length and diameter planned preoperatively. After the diaphyseal and epiphyseal parts are assembled, the trial humeral prosthesis is inserted and covered by a cup protector.

The humeral section is performed with a retroversion angle between 0 and 20 degrees, depending on the anatomy of the proximal humerus and choice of the surgeon. A 0-degree retroversion enables us to avoid, in adduction, contact between the medial part of the epiphysis and the scapular pillar. Thus, the risk of scapular notching is decreased. However, the risk of anterior prosthetic dislocation is most likely to be increased. A 20-degree retroversion limits the risk of instability but increases the risk of an inferior glenoid notching.

Exposure and Preparation of the Glenoid

The glenoid surface is prepared with a surfacing rasp, corresponding to the diameter of the chosen implant (Fig. 26-8). Reaming may sometimes require withdrawing the retractors to fit the reamer in place on the glenoid. In case of fragile bone, it is preferable to perform this step manually using a hand reamer rather than reaming with a power drill. Reaming should be performed until a smooth area of the subchondral bone is created. At the completion of the reaming, it is necessary to reposition the retractors and check for any bony prominence that may remain outside the peripheral groove of the reamer. This can impede correct insertion of the glenoid baseplate.

The uncemented glenoid baseplate implant (the diameter having been chosen) is attached to the impactor and then inserted, checking the alignment of the inferior screwing hole with the scapular pillar. The inserter is withdrawn, and the contact between the baseplate and the osseous surface is checked.

The baseplate is then fixed; two threaded head screws are used for the superior and inferior holes, whereas two spherical head screws are used for the anterior and posterior holes. We recommend that initial fixation should be achieved with the two anterior and posterior screws with compression by using adequate drills and gauges perpen-

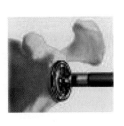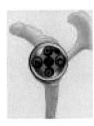

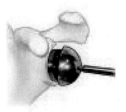

Figure 26-8 Glenoid is exposed by positioning the double point extractor under the axillary border, the points being located on both sides of the triceps tendon and scapular pillar. The retractor pushes down on the superior end of the humerus, which remains protected by the trial prosthesis. Other retractors are positioned anteriorly, posteriorly, and superiorly to the glenoid. Capsula release and its location are decided according to preoperative stiffness. Exposure is completed by resection of the remaining labrum, biceps tendon, and osteophytes, which could compromise the correct positioning of the implant. The central hole is created with the adequate cannulated drill. Its location and direction take into account the orientation of the joint area, analyzed beforehand by computed tomography (CT) scan, and the need for a portioning as low as possible, with a slight inferior tilt. The baseplate can be used as a guide if turned so that it is positioned backward on the glenoid. This tilt helps to limit the incidence of the inferior impingement and scapular notch. The use of a drilling guide can be useful to ensure that the positioning is compatible with inferior screwing. Use of a protected drill enables an adequate width.

dicular to the glenoidal axis. The inferior screw is then positioned and directed toward the axis of the scapular pillar with, ideally, an angle of 30 degrees inferiorly and 10 degrees posteriorly. The use of a gauge is essential so that this screw, normally long, can have an adequate length and stability. The same procedure is used for the superior screw, the purpose being to purchase the screw in the base of the coracoidal apophysis with an angle of 20 degrees superiorly and 20 degrees anteriorly.

Trial Reduction

The trial sphere with the adequate diameter (36 or 42 mm) is attached to the baseplate. The trial humeral insert is fixed on the humeral implant. The components are then reduced by traction and pushing posteriorly on the humeral epiphysis. Mobility and stability of the shoulder are then checked, as well as confirming the absence of humeroscapular contact with the inferior glenoid. The purpose of this trial is to decide the size of the humeral insert, available in several thicknesses, with the possible use of a metallic extension. The determination of proper soft-tissue tension and placement of a component of adequate thick-

ness are according to surgeon judgment, but the goal is to achieve stability throughout all ranges and maintain a mobile joint. Proper tension of the deltoid is the important criterion, although precise guidelines are not available.

Assembling and Installation of the Final Components

After removal of the trial implants, the sphere is attached to the baseplate by use of a double process of fixation with a central screw and impaction of the Morse taper. The security of this assembling may be checked with a hook.

The humeral component is assembled by attachment of the modular diaphyseal and epiphyseal parts. We recommend the use of a cemented humeral implant. The impactor is equipped with a retroversion control system. The prosthetic epiphysis should be cleaned and dried before fixation of the definitive polyethylene insert. In case of any doubt, trial inserts can still be used with the definitive stem.

The prosthesis is then reduced, and the wound is closed routinely. If an anterosuperior approach was used, then the anterior deltoid is reinserted to the acromion using transosseous nonabsorbable sutures. If the deltopectoral approach is used, it is recommended to suture, even partially, the remaining subscapularis to reduce the risk of instability.

Postoperative Care

The arm is placed in a sling in internal or neutral rotation. During the first week or two, use of a slight abduction splint may be useful, especially if pain is felt by the patient on the lateral side of the arm. This may be caused by excessive tension of the deltoid, and use of an abduction splint will allow the deltoid to gradually adapt by lengthening. Passive range of motion and aqua-therapy should start early. Movements of active rotation in abduction are restricted during the first 6 weeks after surgery. Afterward, active exercises can start with a muscular reinforcement of the deltoid and rotators. Functional motion is usually achieved for daily living activities after 6 weeks.

Technical Concerns Related to Cause

The type of arthropathy leading to the choice of a reversed prosthesis may influence the surgical approach.

■ Osteoarthritis (OA) with massive cuff tear and cuff tear arthropathy are the most frequent indications. The technical modalities described previously are applicable in most cases. Previous operations (cuff repair and subacromial decompression) can also influence the choice of the approach. There is not, however, any proof that a previous acromioplasty will compromise the healing of the anterior deltoid if the choice is an anterosuperior approach. Finally, any surgical precedent should motivate caution regarding the capsular resection (passive mobility and preoperative release) and the infection risk (preoperative biology and preoperative bacteriology).

- Prosthesis revision: The problem is different whether the revision concerns a hemiarthroplasty or total prosthesis. Of major importance regarding the approach (normally deltopectoral), the risk of infection (preoperative laboratory studies), or associated stiffness are relevant to anticipating the loss of bone stock during revision. In such cases, the reversed prosthesis is used as a revision salvage procedure.

- If the revised prosthesis is a hemiarthroplasty, the removal of the implant is the first step in the revision. A large soft tissue release may be required before the humeral component can be dislocated anteriorly. Adequate extractors are not always available. Difficulties are greater in case of uncemented humeral prosthesis because bony ingrowth of the humeral stem may make removal difficult. A longitudinal humeral osteotomy is sometimes necessary for the extraction, and restoring the humeral shaft may be necessary by using cerclage wiring. A long-stem cemented prosthetic stem may then be necessary to bypass the defect created by removal of the primary stem. Because there is usually a significant amount of capsular and tendinous soft tissue loss, we recommend implantation of the humeral component in 20 degrees of retroversion to reduce the risk of instability. Moreover, in these cases the glenoid is often fragile from erosion, so we prefer to perform reaming preparation manually rather than under power to avoid fracture.

- If the revised prosthesis is a total prosthesis, then one must anticipate loosening of the glenoid component and some loss of glenoid bone. Removal of the glenoid is thus not usually difficult. Three different situations can be schematically distinguished.

    - Simple loss of glenoid bone substance (grade 1): The glenoid rim is preserved, and the bone loss is central. This stable peripheral rim can be used as a guide for the glenoid reamer until a smooth area is obtained. The central defect can then be filled with bone graft, and the sclerotic peripheral rim can be used for fixation of screws from the base plate. Usually in this situation, fixation is secure because the remaining bone along the glenoid periphery as well as the inferior and superior glenoid is of good quality.

    - Intermediary loss of glenoid bone substance (grade 2): The loss of glenoid bone substance is more extensive and involves not only central bone loss but also disruption of the peripheral cortex. Even with reaming there is not sufficient bony contact to stabilize the glenoid baseplate. Usually, use of a bulk corticocancellous bone graft is necessary with fixation to the remaining scapula and then reaming for placement of the baseplate. This can be a challenging surgical problem.

    - Major loss of glenoid bone substance (grade 3): This situation may not be compatible with the implantation of the baseplate. An alternative to abandoning this approach is a two-stage surgery in which bulk bone grafting is first performed to reestablish a glenoid surface. Then after bony incorporation, the reverse prosthesis can be implanted in the second surgical stage.

- Rheumatoid arthropathy: In its advanced stages there is profound thinning of the rotator cuff or complete tearing of the cuff tendons with marked superior displacement of the humeral head. Hemiarthroplasty has been advocated, but results are unpredictable and often disappointing in terms of functional restoration. Even in the case of a reversed shoulder prosthesis, where one might imagine restoration of shoulder elevation, there is an increased risk of complications because of the poor-quality bone and soft tissues often inherent to rheumatoid disease of the shoulder. These include an increased risk of infection and more frequent fractures. For example, erosion of the humerus or glenoid may compromise component fixation, and erosion of the acromion may predispose to its fracture because of tension on the deltoid after reverse shoulder implantation. In these cases, we recommend the surgeon carefully use instruments with only manual reaming and avoidance of excessive tension on the deltoid by not overlengthening the humerus when the component is placed. The humeral component should be cemented, and use of an abduction splint may protect the acromion for a period of time after the surgery by reducing tension on the deltoid.

- Posttraumatic arthritis: The unique problems encountered are shoulder stiffness and the distortion of the proximal humerus anatomy. This requires detailed implant planning. Stiffness is best managed with an anterior deltopectoral approach, an extended capsular release, and, most of the time, the excision of the remaining superior rotator cuff. It is also necessary, sometimes, to excise the superior part of the tuberosities malunion that interferes with prosthesis placement. Preoperative planning, using bilateral long-arm radiographs with comparative measurement of both humeral lengths, will sometimes aid in determining the appropriate length for the prosthesis when no bony landmarks are available because of malunion or bone loss. The integrity of the deltoid and axillary nerve function should be evaluated preoperatively, especially in these conditions.

- Humeral head fractures: This is a rare condition, but in our experience, an anterosuperior approach is preferable. Implantation requires that the upper part of the lesser tuberosity is removed, taking with it the biceps and its groove. The upper part of the greater tuberosity is also sectioned, taking with it the supraspinatus tendon. The use of a trial prosthesis is important to assess the deltoid tension. Once the prosthesis is implanted, the low part of the tuberosities should be fixed to the prosthesis fin and bone section. Healing of the lesser tuberosity is an important element of the surgery to improve the functional outcome and reduce the risk of prosthetic instability.

INDICATIONS AND RESULTS

The reversed prosthesis has become an important alternative method for treatment of difficult reconstructive problems in Europe. The outcome over the short- and midterm has met expectations because it has demonstrated restoration of function that would otherwise be impossible when using conventional nonconstrained arthroplasty in difficult conditions.

Osteoarthritis and Massive Cuff Rupture

In 1991, Grammont[26] used the reversed prosthesis to treat a case of rotator cuff tear arthropathy. This situation corresponds to cuff tear arthropathy described by Neer et al. in 1983,[38] which is a condition of unchecked superior migration of the humeral head with associated articular necrosis and humeral head collapse. A similar condition was described by MacCarty et al.[36] in 1981 with the name of Milwaukee shoulder. De Seze et al.[11] in 1967 also reported on a similar condition, and Lequesne et al.[33] in 1982 identified a similar condition that they called "arthrite destructive rapide." In 1995, Baulot et al.[1] published their initial results of the reversed prosthesis in 16 cases with an average follow-up of 27 months (Table 26-1). They emphasized the complication associated with the use of the transacromial approach and the limitation of the internal rotation, which they attributed to placement of the prosthetic stem in retroversion. In 1997, De Buttet et al.[10] presented a poster reporting the result of a multicenter series of 70 cases. With an average Constant score of 59 points at 24

months follow-up, 80% of the patients subjectively judged their results as good or excellent. The authors described four cases of complications associated with component failure, and three of these were unscrewing of the glenoidosphere from the baseplate. (This early version of the reverse prosthesis was a screw-in linkage rather than a Morse taper and locking screw.)

Authors' Short-Term Results

In a multicenter study in 1998, we reviewed 42 cases of reversed prosthesis with an average follow-up of 25 months.[19] There were 36 cases of cuff tear arthropathy, 3 cases of centered OA with rotator cuff rupture, and 3 cases of rheumatoid arthritis. The mean age at the time of surgery was 71 years (43–86 years). The initial functional deficit was severe with an average Constant score of only 17 of a possible 100 points and an average active flexion of 60 degrees. After 25 months, the main complication found was the unscrewing of the sphere, which occurred in 9 of the 42 cases. This complication was attributable to the early design of this system that we used, in which the sphere screwed onto the baseplate. In 4 cases, this complication led to glenoid implant loosening, which required revision. The average Constant score at final follow-up was 55 points, with an average anterior active elevation of 120 degrees. The Constant score was not significantly influenced by the initial status of the rotator cuff, but the recovery of the internal rotation was significantly better when the subscapularis was intact and the active external rotation remained limited when the infraspinatus and teres minor were absent. Follow-up postoperative radiographs demonstrated a radiolucent line at the glenoid-bone interface in 21 cases, which seemed to progress in half of the cases. In 20 cases, we observed a notch that developed inferior to the glenoid adjacent to the scapula pillar. This was more frequent when a nonlateralized cup was used (Fig. 26-10).

From this experience we have concluded that the reversed prosthesis offers the opportunity to restore better function while achieving good pain relief when compared with conventional nonconstrained arthroplasty. However, complica-

TABLE 26-1

PUBLISHED SERIES OF DELTA REVERSED PROSTHESIS FOR CUFF TEAR ARTHROPATHY

Author, Year	Number/Average Age (yr)	Follow-up (mo)	Active Elevation pre/revision	Constant pre-/postoperative	Reoperation Rate
Baulot et al. 1995[1]	16/67	27	—	14/69	13%
De Buttet et al. 1997[10]	71/70	24	-/120°	19/59	4.2%
Favard et al. 1998[19]	36/72	25	60°	18/60	11%
Jacobs et al. 2001[30]	7/72	16	—	18/56	0
Valenti et al. 2001[48]	39/70	84	60°/120°	21/63	15%
Sirveaux et al. 2004[46]	80/72	44	73°/138°	22/65	5%

tions have been documented, and these remain a concern. The modification of the sphere and baseplate linkage into a Morse taper should eliminate unscrewing of the glenoidosphere. The significance of the inferior scapular notching that we observed is unclear because although it might be considered a risk to long-term component stability, thus far it has not been directly correlated to the outcome. Delloye et al.[15] believed that the notch was mainly caused by a mechanical conflict between the ridge of the prosthesis and the inferior scapula with the arm in an adducted position. During some cases of revision surgery we performed, we noticed, as did Delloye et al.,[15] that there was an erosion of the polyethylene on the medial side of the cup and an osteolysis of the medial part of the humerus leading to a polyethylene granuloma.

Classification of Osteoarthritis with Massive Cuff Tear

The occurrence of the scapula notch, described during the multicenter study, can have various origins. It can be linked to a granuloma caused by polyethylene particles or to a mechanical conflict between the medial part of the humeral implant and the glenoid implant, the position which is determined by the morphology of the glenoid shape. The assessment of the shape and wear of the glenoid must be done before placing a reversed prosthesis. Thus, it seemed to us essential to establish a classification of the different forms of osseous pathology of OA with massive cuff tear and to assess the results according to this classification.

In a multicenter European study, we evaluated a population of 1542 patients requiring a prosthesis for a chronic shoulder pathology, and we isolated 148 patients presenting with an OA with an associated massive rotator cuff rupture.[29] The preoperative status of the rotator cuff, initial Constant score, and mobility were analyzed. A precise study of the acromiohumeral distance and radiographic aspect of the humerus, acromion, and glenoid were performed for each case, and then a statistical analysis was performed.

In these 148 patients, the mean age was 72 years. The average preoperative Constant score was 23 points with an average active anterior elevation of 75 degrees. The loss of mobility in active external rotation (elbow to the side) was correlated to the extension of the rupture to the teres minor. Four types of acromion were identified: normal, slimmed, eroded, and hypertrophic. The anterior active elevation was significantly better when the acromion was normal or hypertrophic. The Constant score and active motion were correlated with wear of the humeral head and the existence of a subscapular rupture. Four types of glenoid wear were identified (Fig. 26-9). The E0 type corresponds to a normal glenoid, the E1 type corresponds to a concentric wear of the glenoid, the E2 type corresponds to a superior wear with an appearance of double concavity, and the E3 type corresponds to extension of superior wear into the bottom of the coracoid process.

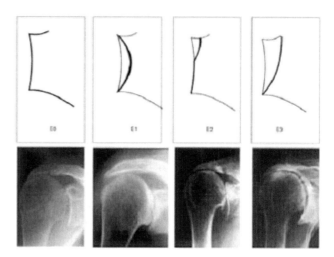

Figure 26-9 Classification of the glenoid erosion in shoulder arthropathy with a cuff tear.

This study allowed us to better understand the evolution of OA when associated with a massive rotator cuff tear. In some cases the humeral head remains centered on the glenoid with a normal or hypertrophic acromion, without wear of the superior glenoid. In these cases, an ossification of the coracoacromial ligament can lead to an acetabulum-like wear of the glenohumeral joint and an observable medialization of the humeral head. In another type, there is also an erosion of the acromion associated to asymmetric wear of the glenoid (type E2). These two different conditions allow for planning for glenoid component placement to avoid malpositioning, which might lead to inferior scapular notching or instability.

Midterm Results of a Multicenter Study

In a multicenter study in Europe with data collected from eight different centers, we collected information on 92 patients with OA associated with massive cuff tear who underwent operation between December 1991 and March 1999, with a minimum of 2 years of follow-up.[46] Six patients could not be located, and six of the patients were deceased at the time of the study; 80 prostheses in 77 patients were thus included in our study. The mean age at the time of the operation was 72 years (60–86 years). All patients were reexamined; clinical outcome and radiographic examination were also performed. A Kaplan-Meier survivorship curve was calculated, with a 95% confidence interval and three endpoints: surgical revision, surgical implant failure, or persistent pain (pain score less than 10 points).

With an average follow-up of 44 months (24–96), the average Constant score increased from 22 to 65 points (preoperative), with a significant improvement of all the parameters. The average active anterior elevation improved from 73 to 138 degrees. The clinical results were significantly worse when the teres minor tendon was initially torn with persistence of a "hornblower sign" (loss of external rotation

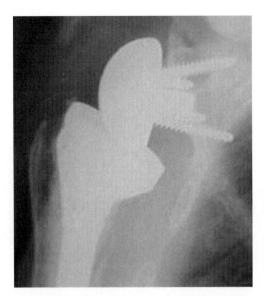 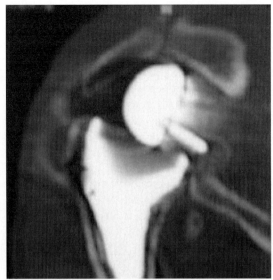

Figure 26-10 Scapula notch grade 3. Note on the CT scan the osteolysis around the inferior screw, which is compatible with a polyethylene granuloma.

with the shoulder abducted). Radiographic analysis demonstrated an obvious glenoid loosening in 6.5% of the cases and a stable radiolucent line in 30% of the cases. An unscrewing of the sphere on the baseplate occurred in 7 cases. An inferior scapula notch was observed in 63% of the cases. A classification of the notches was established. The presence of a notch affected the Constant score in a significant way, when it was voluminous (grade 3/4) (Fig. 26-10) but did not affect outcome when it was smaller. The occurrence of a notch was more frequent when the initial morphology of the glenoid was of type E2 or E3, because this resulted in the glenoidosphere being inclined superiorly on the scapula. The cumulative probability of the implant survivorship was 95% (92%–97%) after 8 years when the endpoint "revision" was considered. It was 91% (87%–95%) after 5 years and 30% (7%–52%) after 8 years when the endpoint was defined as "revision" or "implant failure."

This study confirmed that the midterm results were comparable to the short-term analysis and that the component was durable. It also validated the OA classification that we have proposed and allowed us to establish a scapula notch classification. The poor results in terms of implant survivorship after 7 years were linked to the inclusion, in some of the patient studies, of the initial design of the prosthesis, which was modified in 1995 because of the unscrewing of the glenoidosphere from the baseplate. A long-term follow-up seemed necessary to appreciate the consequences of the scapular notching on the stability of the implant.

Hemiarthroplasty Versus Reverse Prosthesis

The previous studies have shown the quality of the results obtained with a reversed prosthesis, but rigorous compari-

son with the results of unconstrained prosthesis was difficult because of the variability of assessment methodology used to determine outcome in the literature.[32,40,50,52] We have, however, been able to develop some insight by comparing results with our retrospective analysis of a population of similar patients who we treated with hemiarthroplasty and then evaluated with the same criteria used in our reverse prosthesis patient analysis.[18]

A nonparametric comparison was performed comparing the results of 80 reverse prostheses with 62 unconstrained prostheses. The preoperative parameters were similar in both groups in terms of age, Constant score, and mobility. The follow-up was 45 months in the reverse prosthesis group and 43 months in the "hemiarthroplasty" group. The comparison based on the parameters of the Constant score demonstrated a significantly better outcome in the reverse prosthesis group. This included parameters of pain, level of activity, mobility, and strength and mobility in active anterior elevation. However, the gain of mobility in external rotation with the elbow at the side was superior in the hemiarthroplasty group. The total Constant score was better in the reversed prosthesis group. The radiographic analysis demonstrated that there was, in both groups, an alteration in the bone structures, which concerned the acromion for the hemiarthroplasty group and the scapula for the reversed prosthesis group.

Both therapeutic options enabled patients to achieve better function of the shoulder while decreasing pain to a significant degree. At midterm follow-up, the comparison of both types of implants favored the reverse prosthesis. Clinically, the only element in favor of hemiarthroplasty was a better recovery of the active external rotation with the elbow at the side, whereas external rotation of the abducted shoulder was similar in both groups. The main advantage of hemiarthroplasty seems to be the reduced risk of loosening and lack of mechanical problems, which can be associated with the reversed shoulder prosthesis; however, anterosuperior instability is not corrected with this implant. Thus, we believe hemiarthroplasty should not be recommended in cases of a previous acromioplasty; it should remain a salvage procedure for young patients when the acromial arch is maintained and there is a concentric wear of the glenoid. The reversed prosthesis seems to have the advantage of enabling a quicker recovery of mobility, but the presence of the scapula notching remains a concern. On the basis of this study, we believe the indications for this prosthesis shoulder remain according to the previously described criteria but only in patients aged more than 70 years.

Long-Term Results

During the Nice symposium in 2001, Valenti et al.[48] reported the results of more than 5 years follow-up (an average of 7 years) of 39 reverse prostheses for OA with massive rotator cuff rupture. At final follow-up, the average Constant score had improved from 21 to 63 points with an average active anterior elevation of 120 degrees. The authors observed six complications: three unscrewings of the glenoidosphere from the baseplate, two infections, and one glenoid loosening. On final radiographic review, 11 patients on final radiographic review had a voluminous scapula notch without any significant consequence to the functional outcome or loosening of the component.

Recently, Guery et al.[28] established the survivorship curves from a multicenter study collecting patients with more than 5 years of follow-up. The initial cause was OA with massive cuff defect in 66 cases, rheumatoid arthritis in 8 cases, a recent fracture in 4 cases, and a prosthesis revision in 2 cases. The average follow-up was 69.6 months (60–121 months). Six patients underwent reoperation for prosthesis revision. All revision were performed in the first 3 years after implantation of the prosthesis.

The cumulative probability of not having a revision of the prosthesis was 91% after 120 months. It was 95% for OA with massive cuff defect, whereas it was only 77% for the other causes ($P = .015$). Seven cases of glenoid loosening were observed.

When failure was defined as revision or loosening, the survivorship was 91% after 96 months and 84% after 120 months for all patients studied. It was 96% after 96 months and 87% after 120 months for OA with massive cuff defect, whereas it was 77% after 120 months for the other causes. When failure was defined not only as revision or loosening but also significant pain, the survivorship of the prosthesis was 72% after 96 months and 61% after 120 months, without any significant difference according to the initial cause. Two breaks appear on the survivorship curve. The first break corresponds to mechanical complications that occurred after the first 2 years related to disassociation of the

sphere from the baseplate as the result of unscrewing (only seen with the first version of the prosthesis). The second break corresponds to pain and appearance of an inferior notching of the scapula.

This study confirmed that good functional results can be achieved and are relatively durable, although the survivorship analysis shows an increase in failure after the seventh year. This is the basis for our recommendation to proceed with caution in any patient aged less than 70 years. The weakest link in durability appears to be long-term fixation of the glenoid component.

On the basis of experience with the reversed prosthesis in cuff tear arthropathy, Gerber et al.[25] suggested that the indications for implantation of this device can be extended to massive rotator cuff tears that cause a painful pseudoparalysis even without arthritis change in individuals aged more than 70 years.

Rheumatoid Arthritis

In rheumatoid arthritis, the outcome of unconstrained prosthesis is dependent on the status of the rotator cuff.[45] In the advanced form of the disease, the rotator cuff can be ruptured and not functional, and this would justify the need for a reversed prosthesis. However, in three cases reviewed in the short term in our list,[19] we noticed osseous complications: a fracture of the acromion (Fig. 26-11), a nonunion of the acromion, and fracture of the external part of the clavicle. In Rittmeister and Kerschbaumer's series,[43]

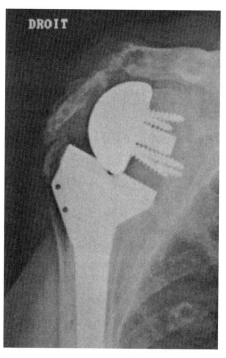

Figure 26-11 Secondary fracture of the acromion after implantation of a reverse prosthesis for rheumatoid arthritis with a voluminous scapula notch.

consisting of eight cases with an average follow-up of 54 months, six patients had complications: one had septic loosening, two had aseptic loosening, and three had a nonunion of the acromion when the transacromial approach was performed. In this disease condition, a transacromial approach should be avoided, and the precise quality of the osseous structures (acromion, glenoid) should be assessed.

Fractures in the Elderly

For the past 2 years we have been conducting a prospective randomized study comparing the reverse prosthesis with the hemiarthroplasty in the treatment of comminuted proximal humerus fracture in the elderly.[47] The main problem that we and others have encountered with an attempted anatomic reconstruction with a hemiarthroplasty prosthesis for fractures has been the fixation and healing of tuberosities. Several studies have shown that the clinical results for elderly patients are often poor in terms of function, and that this is attributable to poor-quality bone, postoperative immobilization (which is often required), and rehabilitation compliance.[4,44] Reversed prosthesis might thus be an alternative to hemiarthroplasty in fractures in elderly patients because tuberosity healing and postoperative rehabilitation would not be problematic.

The preliminary results of this study concern 13 cases in each group, reviewed with an average follow-up of 10 months (minimum 6 months). So far we have observed that the results of the reverse prosthesis for the treatment of proximal humerus fractures are not as good as in OA with massive cuff tear.[47] The analysis of the results showed that the patients treated with a reverse prosthesis achieved an average of 113 degrees of active elevation (range 80–140 degrees) compared with the hemiarthroplasty group, who achieved an average elevation of 88 degrees (range 20–140 degrees). With hemiarthroplasty, we observed better results when the tuberosities were observed to have healed on postoperative radiographs. When this did not occur, the result was marked weakness and patient inability to elevate the arm. For reversed prosthesis, the results were better when the lesser tuberosity was healed. Reversed prosthesis overall was observed to allow a faster recovery, without immobilization, and with a more predictable functional outcome. This study is ongoing, so no long-term conclusion can be made about the durability of results (Fig. 26-12).

Fracture Sequelae (Malunions and Nonunions)

Revision to a shoulder prosthesis for sequelae of fractures (malunion and nonunion) is especially difficult because of distorted bony and soft-tissue anatomy. We recommend preoperative CT scan to appreciate the displacement of the tuberosities and the fatty degeneration of the rotator cuff muscles. According to the experience of Boileau et al.,[5] the necessity of performing an osteotomy of the tuberosities to place a nonconstrained prosthesis increases the risk of complications and represents the major downside to use of hemiarthroplasty in these challenging reconstructions. In the case of severe posttraumatic deformity (major disimpacted fracture with severe tuberosity malunion), the reversed prosthesis is an alternative to hemiarthroplasty because the anticipated outcome with the latter is so poor (Fig. 26-13).[5]

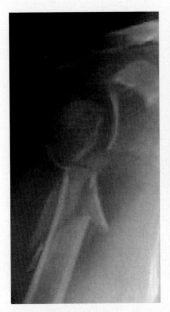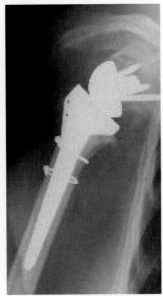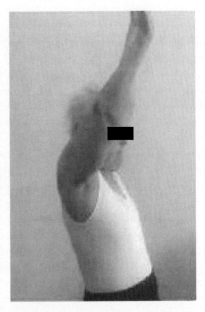

Figure 26-12 Complex fracture of the proximal right humerus in a 72-year-old patient treated with a reverse prosthesis. X-ray results and clinical results at 6 months follow-up.

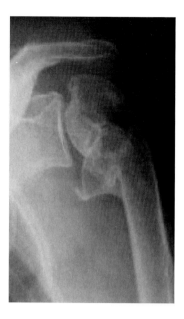
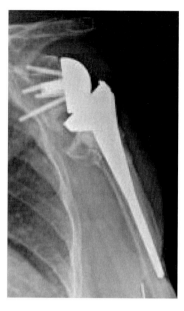

Figure 26-13 Severe fracture sequela with marked malunion of the proximal humerus in a 65 year-old. The patient underwent reconstruction with a reverse shoulder prosthesis on her left shoulder in 2002. X-ray at 2 years follow-up.

Reversed Prosthesis for Tumor

Wide resection of a tumor of the proximal humerus can require resection of the rotator cuff as well (Fig. 26-14). The reconstruction options can include a reverse prosthesis, as long as the axillary nerve, deltoid, and glenoid are preserved. These would be extra-articular tumors located in the S3 zone according to the Musculosketal Tumor Society Society classification.[17] According to De Wilde et al.,[13] the indication can be extended to the S4 zone as long as the deltoid is reinserted. According to the diaphysis resection level, the reconstruction of the proximal humerus may call for an autograft or allograft, or a reimplantation of the bone segment after irradiation.[14] The total resection of the rotator cuff can impose a significant risk of postoperative instability and leave a definitive external active rotation deficit. De Wilde et al. reported 4 cases of luxation in a group of 13 cases. In this study, the Constant score at final review was 72 points with an active elevation between 60 and 90 degrees. The instability risk leads us to set the humeral implant with 20 degrees of retroversion and to delay formal rehabilitation for 6 weeks after surgery.

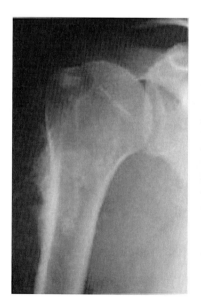
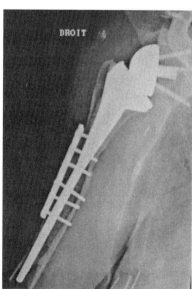
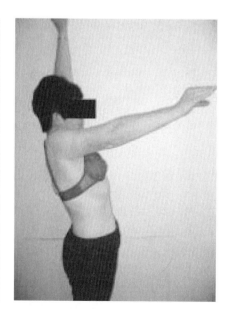

Figure 26-14 Chondrosarcoma of the proximal right humerus for a 42-year-old patient; reconstruction with a reverse prosthesis with massive allograft of the proximal humerus and functional result at 1 year follow-up.

Revision Arthroplasty

The revision of an unconstrained prosthesis may lead to marked bone loss and loss of the rotator cuff; thus the use of a reversed prosthesis makes sense (Fig. 26-15). When an hemiarthroplasty fails, the status of the glenoid bone is usually compatible with the fixation of a baseplate and sphere. Preoperative planning should concentrate on the conditions of removal of the implant to plan for the use of a longer stem component and bone graft if necessary. The approach should take into account the approach used beforehand and the need for a potential osteotomy for removal of the humeral stem whether cemented or uncemented.[49] The reversed prosthesis can also be indicated in cases of failed hemiarthroplasty for cuff tear arthropathy, necrosis or displacement of the tuberosities for a fracture hemiarthroplasty, or prosthetic instability.[12,16,22,23]

The revision of a total shoulder prosthesis requires a rigorous analysis of the glenoid bone stock. If the bone stock is sufficient, a reversed prosthesis can be set using a bone graft if necessary. In the study by Neyton et al.,[39] this technique was used in five cases with a bone graft in three cases. The average active anterior elevation was 118 degrees at revision (vs. 78 degrees preoperatively) with a functional gain of 23 points in the average Constant score. In case of a large bone defect, the authors performed a corticocancellous bone graft on the glenoid as a first stage in one case, and then after incorporation of the bone a second-stage surgery allowed the reversed prosthesis to be placed.

The results of the reversed prosthesis for revision are inferior to primary prosthesis results, but the analysis of the series shows a significant improvement of pain and mobility.[12,16] In Ekelund's[16] series (23 cases with a minimal follow-up of 2 years), the average Constant score went from 9 to 35 points, with an average anterior active elevation of 86 degrees. The recovery of active external rotation depends essentially on the status of the infraspinatus and teres minor, which can be appreciated on a preoperative CT scan. The main complications of revision surgery are infection and prosthetic instability. When determining the positioning height of the prosthesis, one should consider the proximal bone defect in the humerus and the tension of the deltoid during the operation because proper tension will reduce the risk of instability.

Contraindications

■ Deltoid dysfunction: In case of previous surgical treatment, it is essential to check the function of the deltoid before using a reverse prosthesis. The existence of weakness of the deltoid does not represent a strict contraindication, as long as the muscle remains contractile at clinical examination. A preoperative electromyograph is required in case of any doubt. The choice of the approach depends on the previous approach to preserve the deltoid in the best way.

■ Infection: Revision surgery is one of the most frequent indications for a reversed prosthesis. In all cases the patient must be evaluated to rule out infection. This should include aspiration arthrogram and hematologic analysis for markers of infection (erythrocyte sedimentation rate and C-reactive protein). In cases in which doubt about

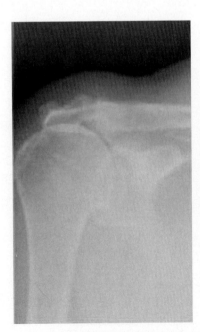 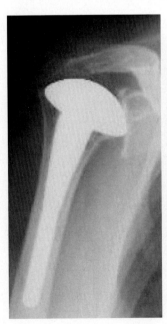 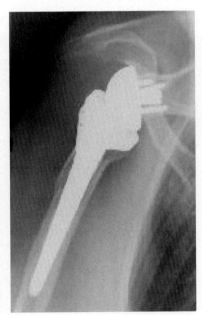

Figure 26-15 Cuff tear arthropathy for a 62-year-old patient who underwent operation in 1992 by hemiarthroplasty. Bad clinical results and rise of the head. Reoperation in 1994 to install a reverse prosthesis. X-ray result at 6 years follow-up.

infection may remain, a two-stage approach may be performed: The first stage is extraction of the prosthesis and quantitative tissue analysis for infection, and the second stage is implantation using cement impregnated with antibiotics.

- Bone loss: Because the reversed prosthesis is a constrained prosthesis, it is necessary to check the primary implant stability and have sufficient bone stock to have secondary fixation of the uncemented glenoid implant. A CT scan is part of the systematic preoperative planning. These precautions are recommended in case of cuff tear arthropathy in which the necrosis component could involve the glenoid. The existence of an asymmetric wear of E2 or E3 type can impose the addition of a bone graft. In case of revision surgery, bone stock should be reconstituted to ensure the solid fixation of the components.
- Anticipated activity level: The current data in the literature give concern regarding the durability of fixation of

the glenoid implant in the long term. The constraints on the glenoid implant remain important especially at the start of the elevation. Functional recovery can enable a quick return to activities. Nevertheless, it is preferable to advise the patient to avoid carrying weights, and it is not recommended to suggest this type of operation to manual workers requiring strength. Reversed prosthesis can be a salvage solution in exceptional situations for young patients, but the patients must be informed of the potential risk of failure of the glenoid implant over time.

CONCLUSION

The reversed prosthesis provides good results in patients in whom an anatomic prosthesis would give only limited results. The medialization and stability of the center of rotation allow for restoration of the deltoid lever arm and

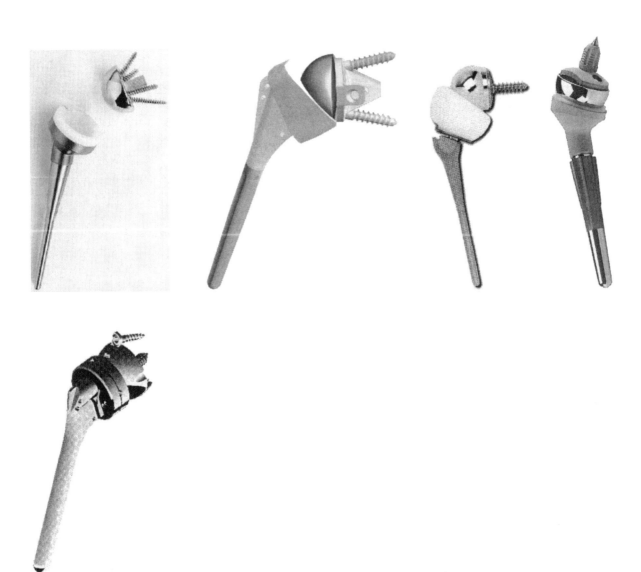

Figure 26-16 New type of reverse shoulder prosthesis.

enable active elevation greater than 90 degrees with reasonable strength return. Most patients are satisfied, even if they have a limited active external rotation. The design does not cause glenoid loosening in the short-term or even in the midterm follow-up. Thus, there is real cause for optimism for use of this technique of reconstruction.

Unfortunately there is a risk of excessive use because of failure of realization of limits to the technique. The early complications should not be ignored: Hematoma, acromial fracture, pain on the lateral side of the arm, prosthetic instability, and infection are problems that could vitiate the final results. In the longer term, we should remain watchful of the occurrence of inferior scapular notching. These notches can be explained by the mechanical impingement caused by the absence of a prosthetic neck. Their extensiveness is probably caused by the polyethylene wear and induced osteolysis. The frequency and size of the notches increase with time. To date, the results of the analysis do not show an accelerated rate of glenoid loosening with formation of this notching. Nevertheless, a comparison must be established between the occurrence and the evolution of these notches on the one hand and the survivorship curves on the other hand. Initial indications are that there is a deterioration of the functional result after 8 to 10 years.

Awareness of all these problems will allow the surgeon to adapt the surgical technique to avoid many problems. These include lower positioning of the glenoidosphere with inferior tilt (avoiding inferior notching). New designs may offer solutions to these problems as well (Fig. 26-16).

Reversed prosthesis has a bright future. Rigorous analysis of results and the description of salvage solutions in case of failure will enable modification of its use and precise definition of its indications.

ACKNOWLEDGMENT

We acknowledge Pierre Msika for translation.

REFERENCES

1. Baulot E, Chabernaud D, Grammont P. Résultats de la prothèse inversée de Grammont pour les omarthroses associées à de grandes destruction de la coiffe: à propos de 16 cas. Acta Orthop Belg 1995;61(Suppl I):112.
2. Beddow F, Elloy M. Clinical experience with the Liverpool shoulder replacement. In: Bayley I, Kessel L, eds. Shoulder surgery. New York, Springer-Verlag, 1982:164.
3. Bodey W, Yeoman P. Prosthetic arthroplasty of the shoulder. Acta Orthop Scand 1983;54:900.
4. Boileau P, Krishnan SG, Tinsi L, et al. Tuberosity malposition and migration: reasons for poor outcomes after hemiarthroplasty for displaced fractures of the proximal humerus. J Shoulder Elbow Surg 2002;11(5):401.
5. Boileau P, Trojani C, Walch G, et al. Shoulder arthroplasty for the treatment of the sequelae of fractures of the proximal humerus. J Shoulder Elbow Surg 2001;10(4):299.
6. Brostrom LA, Wallensten R, Olsson E, et al. The Kessel prosthesis in total shoulder arthroplasty. A five-year experience. Clin Orthop 1992;277:155.
7. Buechel F, Pappas M, De Palma A. Floating socket total shoulder replacement: anatomical, biomechanical, and surgical rationale. J Biomed Mater Res 1978;12:89.
8. Cofield R. Status of total shoulder arthroplasty. Arch Surg 1977;112:1088.
9. Coughlin M, Morris J, West W. The semiconstrained total shoulder arthroplasty. J Bone Joint Surg Am 1979;61-A(4):574.
10. De Buttet A, Bouchon Y, Capon D, et al. Grammont shoulder arthroplasty for osteoarthritis with massive rotator cuff tears. J Shoulder Elbow Surg 1997;6(2):197.
11. De Seze M, Hubault A, Rampon S. L'épaule sénile hémorragique, L'actualité rhumatologique. Paris, Expansion Scientifique Française, 1967:107.
12. De Wilde L, Mombert M, Van Petegem P, et al. Revision of shoulder replacement with a reversed shoulder prosthesis (Delta III): report of five cases. Acta Orthop Belg 2001;67(4):348.
13. De Wilde L, Sys G, Julien Y, et al. The reversed Delta shoulder prosthesis in reconstruction of the proximal humerus after tumour resection. Acta Orthop Belg 2003;69(6):495.
14. De Wilde L, Van Ovost E, Uyttendaele D, et al. Résultats d'une prothèse d'épaule inversée après résection pour tumeur de l'humérus proximal. Rev Chir Orthop 2002;88:373.
15. Delloye C, Joris D, Colette A, et al. [Mechanical complications of total shoulder inverted prosthesis]. Rev Chir Orthop Reparatrice Appar Mot 2002;88(4):410.
16. Ekelund A. Delta reversed shoulder arthroplasty for failed standard shoulder arthroplasties. Minimum 2 years follow-up. Presented at the 9th International Congress on Surgery of the Shoulder (ICSS), Washington DC, Poster Session N, No 12, 2004.
17. Enneking W, Dunham W, Gebhardt M, et al. A system for classification of skeletal resection. Chir Organi Mov 1990;75(Suppl 1):217.
18. Favard L, Lautman S, Sirveaux F, et al. Hemiarthroplasty versus reverse arthroplasty in the treatment of osteoarthritis with massive rotator cuff tear. In: Walch G, Boileau P, Molé D, eds. 2000 shoulder prosthesis. Two to ten year follow-up. Montpellier, Sauramps Medical, 2001:261.
19. Favard L, Sirveaux F, Mestdagh H, et al. La prothèse inversée de Grammont dans le traitement des arthropathies de l'épaule à coiffe détruite. Résultats d'une étude multicentrique de 42 cas. Rev Chir Orthop 1998;84(Suppl II):82.
20. Fenlin J. Total glenohumeral joint replacement. Orthop Clin North Am 1975;6(2):565.
21. Fischer J, Carret J, Gonon G, et al. Etude cinématique des mouvements de l'articulation scapulo-humérale. Rev Chir Orthop 1977;63(Suppl II):108.
22. Frankle M. Reverse shoulder prosthesis: a successful treatment after failed hemiarthroplasty for proximal humerus fracture. Presented at the 9th International Congress on Surgery of the Shoulder (ICSS), Washington DC, Poster Session 1, No, 23, 2004.
23. Frankle M. Reverse shoulder prosthesis can successfully treat patients that failed due to recurrent instability. Presented at the 9th International Congress on Surgery of the Shoulder (ICS), Washington DC, Poster Session 1, No, 24, 2004.
24. Gerard Y, Leblanc J, Rousseau B. Une prothèse totale d'épaule. Chirurgie 1973;99:655.
25. Gerber A, Roache P, Gerber C. The Delta III reversed prosthesis: weapon of the devil or acceptable salvage procedure? Presented at the 8th International Conference on Surgery of the Shoulder (ICSS), Cape Town (South Africa), April 25, 2001.
26. Grammont P, Trouilloud P, Laffay J, et al. Etude et réalisation d'une nouvelle prothèse d'épaule. Rhumatologie 1987;39(10):407.
27. Gristina A, Webb L. The trispherical total shoulder replacement. In: Bailey I, Kessel L, eds. Shoulder surgery. New York, Springer-Verlag, 1982:153–157.
28. Guery J, Favard L, Oudet D, et al. Prothèses d'épaule inversées de Grammont: courbes de survie à cinq ans. Presented at the 37 ème congrès annuel de la Société d'Orthopédie de l'ouest. Nantes, June 10, 2004.
29. Huguet D, Favard L, Lautman S, et al. Epidémiologie, imagerie, classification de l'omarthrose avec rupture massive et non répara-

ble de la coiffe. In: Walch G, Boileau P, Molé D, eds. 2000 shoulder prosthesis. Two to ten year follow-up. Montpellier, Sauramps Medical, 2001:233.

30. Jacobs R, Debeer P, De Smet L. Treatment of rotator cuff arthropathy with a reversed Delta shoulder prosthesis. Acta Orthop Belg 2001;67(4):344.

31. Kolbel R, Friedebold G. Moglichkeiten der alloarthroplastik an der schulter. Arch Orthop Unfallchir 1973;76:31.

32. Laurence M. Replacement arthroplasty of the rotator cuff deficient shoulder. J Bone Joint Surg Br 1991;73-B(6):916.

33. Lequesne M, Fallut M, Coulomb R, et al. L'arthropathie destructive rapide de l'épaule. Rev Rheumatol 1982;49:427.

34. Lettin A, Copeland S, Scales J. The Stanmore total shoulder replacement. J Bone Joint Surg Br 1982;64-B(1):47.

35. McCarty D, Halverson P, Carrera G, et al. "Milwaukee shoulder." Association of microspheroids containing hydroxyapatite crystals, active collagenase, and neutral protease with rotator cuff defects. Clinical aspect. Arthritis Rheum 1981;2(3):464.

36. Neer CS. Glenohumeral arthroplasty. In: Neer CS, ed. Shoulder reconstruction. Philadelphia, PA, WB Saunders Company, 1990: 143.

37. Neer C, Craig E, Fukuda H. Cuff tear arthropathy. J Bone Joint Surg Am 1983;65-A(9):1232.

38. Neer C, Watson K, Stanton F. Recent experience in total shoulder replacement. J Bone Joint Surg Am 1982;64-A(3):319.

39. Neyton L, Sirveaux F, Roche O, et al. Résultats des reprises pour descellment glenoïdien, a propos d'une série multicentrique de 37 prothèses d'épaule. Rev Chir Orthop 2004;90:111.

40. Pollock R, Deliz E, McIlveen S, et al. Prosthetic replacement in rotator cuff-deficient shoulders. J Shoulder Elbow Surg 1992;1:173.

41. Post M. Constrained arthroplasty of the shoulder. Orthop Clin North Am 1987;18(3):455.

42. Reeves B, Jobbins B, Flowers M. Biomechanical problems in the development of a total shoulder endoprosthesis. J Bone Joint Surg Br 1972;54-B:193.

43. Rittmeister M, Kerschbaumer F. Grammont total shoulder arthroplasty in rheumatoid patients with nonreconstructible rotator cuff lesions. J Shoulder Elbow Surg 2001;10(1):17.

44. Robinson CM, Page RS, Hill RM, et al. Primary hemiarthroplasty for treatment of proximal humeral fractures. J Bone Joint Surg Am 2003;85-A(7):1215.

45. Rozing PM, Brand R. Rotator cuff repair during shoulder arthroplasty in rheumatoid arthritis. J Arthroplasty 1998;13(3):311.

46. Sirveaux F, Favard L, Oudet D, et al. Grammont inverted total shoulder arthroplasty in the treatment of glenohumeral osteoarthritis with massive rupture of the cuff. Results of a multicentre study of 80 shoulders. J Bone Joint Surg Br 2004;86(3):388.

47. Sirveaux F, Roche O, Raphoz A, et al. Hemiarthroplasty versus inversed prosthesis in the treatment of proximal humerus fractures: a prospective randomised study in the elderly. Presented at the 17th Congress of the European Society for Surgery of the Shoulder and Elbow (ESSE-SECEC). Heidelberg, Germany, September 26, 2003.

48. Valenti P, Boutens D, Nerot C. Delta 3 reversed prosthesis for arthritis with massive rotator cuff tear: long term results. In: Walch G, Boileau P, Molé D, eds. 2000 shoulder prosthesis. Two to ten year follow-up. Montpellier, Sauramps Medical, 2001:253.

49. Walch G, Edwards TB, Boulahia A. Revision of the humeral stem, technical problems and complications. In: Walch G, Boileau P, Molé D, eds. 2000 shoulder prosthesis. Two to ten year follow-up. Montpellier, Sauramps Medical, 2001:443.

50. Williams G, Rockwood C. Hemiarthroplasty in rotator cuff-deficient shoulders. J Shoulder Elbow Surg 1996;5:362.

51. Wretenberg P, Wallensten R. The Kessel total shoulder arthroplasty: a 13 to 16 year retrospective follow-up. Clin Orthop 1999;365:100.

52. Zuckerman J, Scott A, Gallagher M. Hemiarthroplasty for cuff tear arthropathy. J Shoulder Elbow Surg 2000;9:169.

Management of Bony Insufficiency of the Glenoid and Humerus with Arthroplasty

27

Julie Y. Bishop   Evan L. Flatow

INTRODUCTION

Unconstrained shoulder arthroplasty has become a commonly performed procedure for many acute and chronic shoulder disease processes. Its success has been well established and largely depends on the status of the soft tissues, especially the rotator cuff and deltoid. However, the bone stock available for implant fixation is also of great importance. In the primary shoulder arthroplasty, glenoid bone loss is more often a problem than humeral loss. Patients with severe osteoarthritis may have significant posterior glenoid erosion, and the rheumatoid patient may have an eroded or medialized glenoid. Dramatic glenoid or humeral bone loss may be encountered during revision shoulder arthroplasty and with reconstruction after en bloc resection of bone for tumors of the shoulder girdle, especially in relation to the proximal humerus. In the revision situation, glenoid loosening is more common than humeral loosening and overall has been found to be the most common long-term complication of total shoulder replacement.[2,5,6,7,11,17,36,49,51]

Concern for glenoid component survival has prompted many to consider humeral replacement without glenoid resurfacing ("hemiarthroplasty") for glenohumeral arthritis, especially in cases in which poor glenoid bone stock would make glenoid resurfacing difficult. However, recent studies, including randomized prospective trials comparing humeral head replacement with the nonconstrained total shoulder replacement, have reported better pain control and function in patients undergoing total shoulder arthroplasty.[21,36,39] Thus, the reconstructive shoulder surgeon requires strategies to deal with the difficulties of bony deficiency in the primary arthroplasty setting, as well as in the revision situation.[18,48,50,51,53]

PATTERNS OF BONY LOSS

Preoperative evaluation for patients undergoing total shoulder arthroplasty consists of the standard medical history, preoperative examinations, and radiographic imaging. Although the radiographic and intraoperative evaluations are the key to assessing glenoid deficiency, certain clues as to glenoid bone stock may come from the history

J. Y. **Bishop:** Clinical Shoulder Fellow, Department of Orthopaedic Surgery, Mount Sinai Medical Center, New York, New York.
E. L. **Flatow:** Lasker Professor of Orthopaedic Surgery, Chief of Shoulder Surgery, Department of Orthopaedic Surgery, Mount Sinai Medical Center, New York, New York.

and examination. The patient's diagnosis, in particular, may provide the most insight into the type of potential bone loss that may be present.

Osteoarthritis

Some conditions are less likely to lead to glenoid bone erosion such as posttraumatic arthritis or avascular necrosis. In contrast, osteoarthritis or secondary arthritis resulting from previous instability repair are prone to posterior glenoid erosion (Fig. 27-1). In these patients, the case is often complicated with an instability pattern. This is classically described in patients undergoing previous stabilization procedures who have posterior subluxation because of an overly tightened anterior capsule and, thus, the subsequent posterior glenoid erosion (Fig. 27-2). In patients with primary osteoarthritis, the shoulder is usually stiff and not "unstable" in the sense of having uncontrolled translations, but they have stiff anterior tissues, a fixed posterior humeral subluxation, eccentric posterior glenoid wear, and a large posterior capsule. Therefore, in these patients, not only

must the bony loss be addressed, but, to avoid recurrent posterior subluxations and an overall failure, the soft tissues must be balanced[3,56] and the glenoid not implanted in retroversion.

Rheumatoid Arthritis

The pathology seen in shoulders with rheumatoid arthritis varies from mild to very severe.[65] Neer[47] classified the pattern of rheumatoid involvement in the shoulder as dry, wet, or resorptive, with the possibility of low-grade, intermediate, or severe changes within each group. With the dry form, there is a tendency for joint space loss, periarticular sclerosis, bone cysts, and stiffness. In the wet form, there is abundant synovial disease with marginal erosions and protrusion of the humeral head into the glenoid. The characteristic feature of the resorptive form is bony resorption. Thus, commonly, the patients with rheumatoid arthritis or other inflammatory arthritides often develop severe medialization of the glenoid with central erosions (Fig. 27-3). The bone quality is often osteopenic to vary-

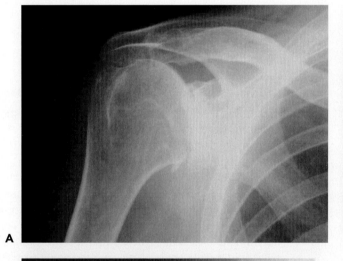

A

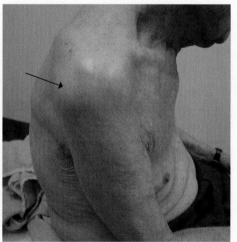

C

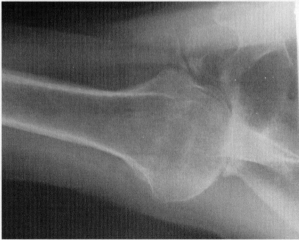

B

Figure 27-1 Severe primary osteoarthritis. *(A,B)* Significant arthritic changes with posterior subluxation caused by posterior glenoid bone wear, seen on anteroposterior (AP) and axillary views. *(C)* Posterior subluxation of the humeral head is evidenced by posterior fullness on physical examination.

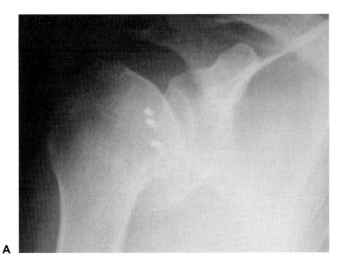

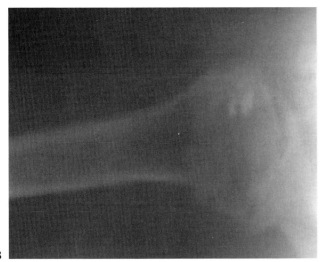

Figure 27-2 Secondary arthritis 15 years after Magnusson-Stack performed for instability. *(A,B)* Anteroposterior (AP) and axillary views.

within the glenoid vault, whereas noncontained defects involve some loss of cortical support usually along the posterior rim of the glenoid (i.e., posterior glenoid erosion). Glenoids with contained defects have historically been treated by filling the smaller defects with cement and larger

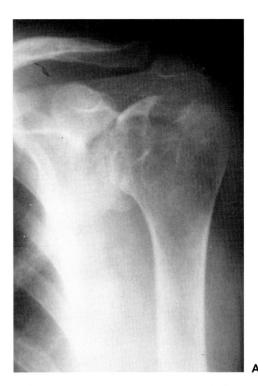

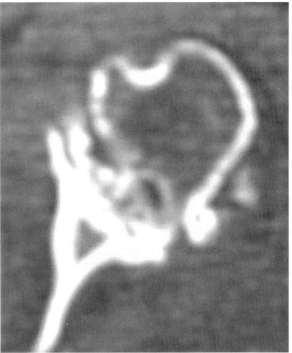

Figure 27-3 *(A)* Anteroposterior (AP) view demonstrating medialization and glenoid bone loss resulting from rheumatoid arthritis. *(B)* Computed tomography (CT) scan allows good visualization of significant medialization in this rheumatoid patient.

ing degrees, further complicating the bony loss. Many rheumatoid patients may have rotator cuff disease and cuff loss, which may contribute to the pattern of arthritis. They may present with a pattern more like a cuff-tear arthropathy, in which there is more superior bone loss as the head articulates with an "acetabularized" coracoacromial arch, coracoid bone, superior glenoid, and acromioclavicular joint. All of these factors make the management of bony loss in the patient with long-standing rheumatoid arthritis especially challenging.

Bone Loss in Revision Surgery

When undertaking a revision total shoulder arthroplasty, the surgeon will often encounter bony defects in either the humerus or glenoid. Bone lesions of the glenoid may simply be classified according to their composition (contained, uncontained, or combined) and location (peripheral or central). Contained defects involve the loss of cancellous bone defects with bone graft. Cancellous bone grafting has been recommended for focal bone loss more than 3 mm in size.[53] Overall, the contained defects are somewhat easier to address in the revision situation. Noncontained defects and huge cavitary lesions can be the most devastating to encounter in a revision. For a noncontained deficit, such as posterior wear, early attempts using an uneven cement mantle to correct glenoid version led to an increased rate of component breakage and loosening (Fig. 27-4).[12,51,59] More recent efforts have focused on eccentric reaming in an attempt to correct mild glenoid erosion; however, severe glenoid deficiency may require grafting (which will be discussed in detail later in the chapter). Finally, when the glenoid deficiency cannot be corrected with bone grafting, especially when there is medialization of the glenoid, resurfacing of the glenoid may need to be abandoned (Fig. 27-5).

Humeral defects encountered in the revision situation are typically found in either the proximal metaphyseal region or distally in the cortical region. Minimal to moderate metaphyseal deficiencies can be discrete bony defects, or at times large losses of metaphyseal bone can be present. The diaphysis can have large and sometimes isolated defects. Defects present after resection for neoplasm are mostly large, segmental losses of bone.

Bone Loss Encountered in Fracture/Tumor Surgery

A traumatic injury to the shoulder can result in certain fracture patterns that can lead to bone loss in either the glenoid or humerus. Severe glenoid crush fractures can lead to a special pattern of bone loss, specific to the type of fracture. Severely comminuted proximal humerus fractures may have significant bone loss at presentation. Hemiarthroplasty for these situations has achieved widespread acceptance.[14,46,48,50,52,63] Although there are many technical aspects to this treatment alternative, one of the most challenging is reestablishing the proper height of the prosthesis, especially when severe comminution or bone loss at the surgical neck exists. This problem is even more difficult in the revision setting, in which a prosthesis was placed too low, leading to poor function or instability.[8,50,69] Neer and Kirby[50] found this problem to be common after reconstruction for fractures in which there had been loss of humeral bone. Of 27 failed arthroplasties for fractures in their study, 18 had instability of the prosthesis and inadequate deltoid power because more than 2 cm of humeral length had been lost (58–book). If there is difficulty securing the tuberosities, either because of tuberosity bone loss or loss of bone at the shaft precluding adequate fixation, then tuberosity fixation should be supplemented with generous cancellous bone graft.

Tumors of the shoulder girdle can lead to significant glenoid or humeral loss after resection. The challenge of shoulder reconstruction after removal of a segmental portion of bone for neoplasm is immense. The proximal humerus is the second most common site of long bone primary tumors[9]; however, metastatic lesions of the shoulder girdle are common as well. After an appropriate amount of resection has been performed to maximize disease eradication, the generally accepted options for skeletal reconstruction of the proximal humerus include four techniques:

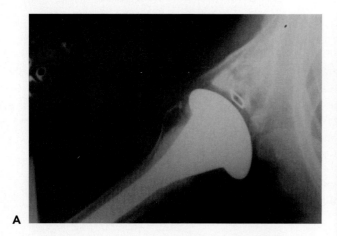

A

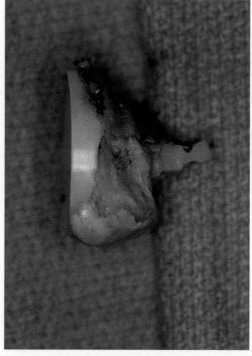

B

Figure 27-4 (A) Axillary radiograph of a total shoulder arthroplasty (TSA) demonstrating a glenoid component implanted in the correct version but supported posteriorly by a thick, asymmetric cement mantle. This method has a high risk of failure. (B) Intraoperative picture demonstrating cement buildup on the extracted glenoid component.

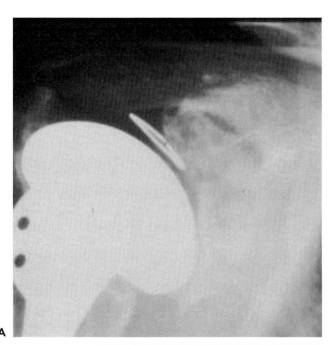

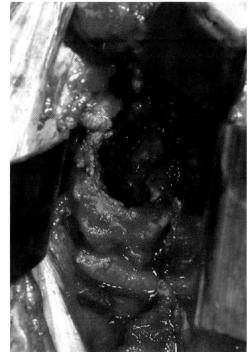

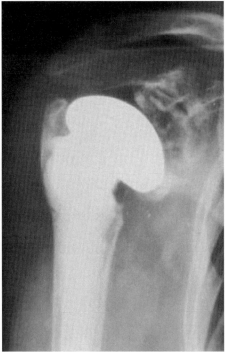

Figure 27-5 Uncontained defect in failed arthroplasty. *(A)* Preoperative anteroposterior (AP) radiograph shows loose glenoid component 16 years after total shoulder arthroplasty (TSA). *(B)* Intraoperative photograph shows large uncontained glenoid defect. *(C)* Glenoid reimplantation was not possible, and the TSA was converted to a humeral head replacement, as visualized on the AP radiograph.

arthrodesis, all-metal prosthesis, osteoarticular allograft, or allograft-composite.

IMAGING

The diagnosis of bony deficiency of the arthritic shoulder is made with a proper radiographic evaluation. Imaging techniques, including plain radiographs, computed tomography (CT) scans, and possibly magnetic resonance imaging (MRI), truly remain the cornerstone of preoperative planning, whether for the primary arthroplasty or revision situation. Proper evaluation and subsequent anticipation of the magnitude of bony loss will help prepare the surgeon to deal with any situation that arises at the time of reconstruction.

Radiographs

The radiographic series should consist of a true "scapular" anteroposterior (AP) view, a lateral "Y" scapular view, and an axillary view (Fig. 27-6, *A* and *B*). The axillary view is best for evaluating the amount of posterior wear, which is common in osteoarthritis or in patients who have undergone stabilization procedures. However, the axillary view can sometimes be inaccurate, and superimposition of the superior and inferior glenoid can make assessment of the glenoid vault difficult. If possible, serial radiographs including preoperative and postoperative x-rays (in the revision cases) should be assessed for radiolucent lines, osteolysis, prosthetic position, and prosthetic migration. If glenoid or humeral loosening is suspected, fluoroscopically guided radiographs may aid in demonstrating radiolucent lines at the bone-cement interface.[11,35] Fluoroscopy also has been recommended as useful in evaluation of glenoid wear, as opposed to CT, which more commonly is used to assess the extent of glenoid damage.[19,43,57]

Computed Tomography Scan

Although a CT scan is not an absolute necessity in every case, the narrow-cut (3-mm) cross-section imaging can provide important information about the implant positioning, humeral and glenoid bony loss, glenoid version, and posterior glenoid erosion (Fig. 27-6C).[20,25] Axillary radiographs can be inaccurate especially as to glenoid version, and CT is very useful in assessment of the available glenoid bone stock. It is important to fully examine the lower, middle, and upper glenoid cuts for a full understanding of the glenoid vault. The normal glenoid version has been shown by transverse CT studies to be approximately 6 degrees retroverted in relation to the angle between the glenoid fossa and the scapular blade.[43] This information can be useful in the preoperative assessment of glenoid deficiency and bone stock available for reconstruction, especially when there is difficulty in attaining a good axillary view. Magnetic resonance imaging is rarely necessary in the evaluation of bony deficiencies for a primary or revision

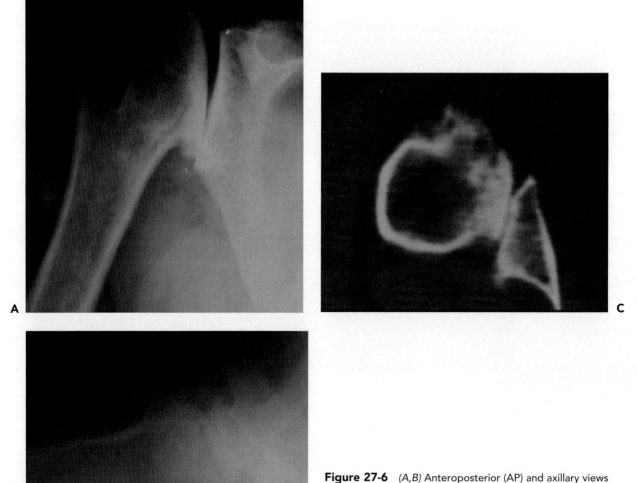

Figure 27-6   *(A,B)* Anteroposterior (AP) and axillary views of shoulder with osteoarthritis and posterior glenoid wear. Although posterior glenoid bone loss is clear, *(C)* Computed tomography (CT) scan is very helpful in delineating the true dimensions of the glenoid vault.

surgery. However, if the status of the rotator cuff is in question, MRI can be used; however, it will provide less detail about the condition of the bone. Good MRIs can be obtained in the face of a prosthesis, and good information can be obtained when special techniques to reduce metal artifact are used.[30]

GLENOID BONE LOSS: TECHNIQUES

Successful implantation of a glenoid component during a primary or revision total shoulder arthroplasty requires adequate exposure, appropriate soft-tissue balancing, careful glenoid preparation, and meticulous implant techniques. In the face of glenoid bone loss, an adequate assessment of the deficiency can only truly be performed if there is sufficient exposure of the glenoid. Although preoperative history and radiographic assessment are extremely important, the final evaluation of the extent of glenoid bony deficiency is achieved after direct inspection and palpation in the operating room. Of course, this will only be possible if the surgeon has performed the necessary releases and exposed the glenoid properly (Fig. 27-7).

Exposure and Releases

A standard deltopectoral approach is used extending proximally from the anterior edge of the clavicle just lateral to the coracoid and distal to the anterior deltoid insertion. Although it is technically possible to use a smaller incision, in this patient population scar length is usually not a concern and can limit the ease of exposure. Because resurfacing of the glenoid demands adequate exposure, especially when

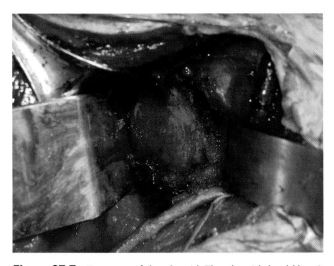

Figure 27-7 Exposure of the glenoid. The glenoid should be visualized *en face*, which requires extensive releases, especially in the revision situation. Although difficult, adequate evaluation of the extent of bony losses is only possible after full exposure. A Fukuda retractor is placed behind the posterior glenoid rim, and a spiked, curved retractor is used to expose the anterior glenoid margin.

bony deficiency is present, an extensile deltopectoral approach is warranted. Any previous incisions are incorporated if possible.

Generous skin flaps are raised, and the deltopectoral interval is developed. It is easiest to initially locate the deltopectoral interval proximally or distally. The cephalic vein is identified and retracted medially or laterally depending on the ease of dissection. We preferentially retract the cephalic vein medially with the pectoralis major, which prevents inadvertent damage during reaming of the humeral canal or during deltoid retraction. The anterior deltoid is then retracted laterally, and the conjoined tendon is gently retracted medially.

At this point, subdeltoid and subacromial adhesions are released and/or resected, and a small anterior portion of the coracoacromial ligament is excised (maintaining its integrity), easing exposure of the rotator interval. This is not performed in rheumatoid patients or in patients without a functioning rotator cuff. The subscapularis and biceps tendons are then identified, and the axillary nerve is palpated and identified at the lower border of the subscapularis tendon. The axillary nerve can usually be identified approximately 3 to 5 mm medial to the musculotendinous junction. After identification, the axillary nerve is protected and periodically reexamined throughout the procedure. The anterior humeral circumflex vessels are then ligated and divided.

If bone quality allows, an osteotomy of the lesser tuberosity, with the attached subscapularis tendon and underlying capsule, is then performed; this permits bone-to-bone healing after repair. Otherwise, the tendon is sharply released. The subscapularis tendon is then tagged, and a 360-degree release of the subscapularis is performed restoring the normal length-tension relationship of the muscle. This includes a rotator interval release to the base of the coracoid, complete mobilization of the strap muscles from the underlying subscapularis, and separation of the inferior surface of the subscapularis from the inferior capsule. In addition, the anterior capsule, located on the undersurface of the subscapularis, is resected, completing the mobilization (Fig. 27-8). Care is taken to avoid injury to nerves supplying the subscapularis medially.

Exposure of the glenohumeral joint, particularly in cases of severe arthrosis or revision arthroplasty, can be difficult and time-consuming. Inadequate release of soft tissue contractures is the most common reason preventing dislocation of the glenohumeral joint. One should resist the temptation of forcibly dislocating the glenohumeral joint, which risks fracturing the humerus or glenoid. Usually release of the soft tissue envelope from the humeral neck will permit atraumatic glenohumeral dislocation.

After joint dislocation, the humeral shaft is prepared, and a trial prosthesis is implanted. The humeral component (without the humeral head) is retained within the humeral shaft during glenoid resurfacing to decrease the risk of humeral fracture.

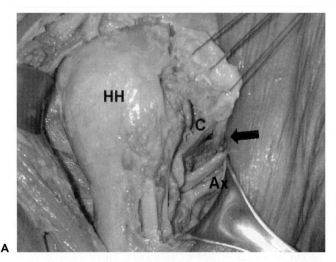
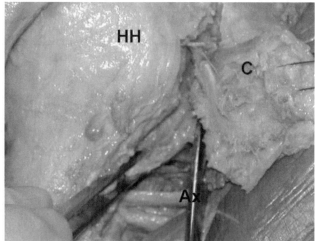

Figure 27-8 Capsular release of the subscapularis is performed to restore normal length-tension relationship of the muscle. *(A)* Subscapularis is tagged. Note the close proximity of the axillary nerve *(A)*. The anterior capsule (C) is adhered to the undersurface of the subscapularis and resected *(B)* to complete the mobilization

Glenoid Exposure

After humeral preparation, attention is turned toward the glenoid. A Fukuda ring retractor or bone hook is initially used to retract the humerus posteriorly and laterally away from the glenoid, and a spiked, curved retractor is used to expose the anterior glenoid margin. Further exposure is provided by an inferior Darrach retractor, which protects the axillary nerve.

To permit a complete, unobstructed view of the glenoid *en face*, the inferior capsule and superior capsule must be released. With the axillary nerve carefully protected, the inferior capsule is released with electrocautery. It is important during this procedure to place the arm in adduction and internal rotation, which allows the nerve to fall away from the glenoid rim. Furthermore, if the patient is not paralyzed, observing for deltoid muscle contraction during release is an indicator of nerve proximity. The superior capsule is released next by developing the interval between the superior capsule and the supraspinatus tendon. This interval is then sharply released. In most cases a posterior capsular release is not necessary, and in fact the posterior capsule will not be contracted but will be capacious secondary to posterior humeral subluxation. Inadvertently releasing the capsule in this situation can predispose to postoperative posterior instability. In rare cases with global tightness (e.g., avascular necrosis), a posterior capsular release may be necessary. After completion of these releases, the glenoid face is usually easily visualized and can be accessed by using straight instruments.

Eccentric Reaming

After exposure of the glenoid, all overlying soft tissues and osteophytes are removed from the glenoid rim. Care must

be taken when removing the osteophytes to avoid fracturing the glenoid or removing an excessive amount of bone, which could prohibit glenoid implantation. The glenoid can then be inspected for bony losses.

An estimation of glenoid version can be made by palpating the anterior glenoid neck and comparing intraoperative findings with preoperative imaging. In the cases of posterior glenoid erosion, there is often substantial retroversion of the glenoid. Although mild degrees of glenoid retroversion may be accepted, if one inserts a glenoid component in a retroverted position, this can commonly lead to penetration of the anterior glenoid neck by the glenoid component or to postoperative posterior instability. Furthermore, biomechanical studies suggest that even small version abnormalities can stress component fixation, possibly predisposing to long-term loosening. One most avoid the temptation of supporting a glenoid component with asymmetric buildup of cement beneath the glenoid component (Fig. 27-4). Over time this will lead to cement fragmentation and glenoid component loosening. Instead, glenoid version must be corrected by lowering the prominent side (usually the anterior rim) with eccentric reaming (Fig. 27-9). Eccentric reaming is performed by initially lowering the high side using a high speed burr and then drilling a provisional centering hole to accommodate the glenoid reamer. A deep drill hole is avoided because the final version of the glenoid component will be different after eccentric reaming. The final glenoid version is then adjusted by reaming the "high" side until a concentric glenoid is established in the appropriate version. As one reams eccentrically, the contact of the reamer to the glenoid will be observed to progress from anterior to posterior in a semicircular fashion. We prefer to have a minimum of 270 degrees of contact to ensure adequate support of the

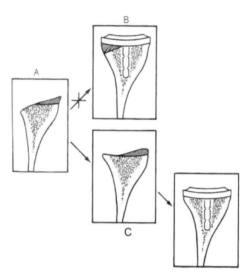

Figure 27-9 Eccentric reaming. *(A)* Wear of the posterior glenoid is apparent and must be corrected. *(B)* Posterior glenoid deficiency should not be corrected by asymmetric cement buildup because this has a high risk of cement fragmentation and component loosening. *(C)* Alternatively, the "high" side should be eccentrically reamed allowing implantation of a glenoid component in the appropriate version. (Reprinted with permission: Post M, Pollack PG. Operative treatment of degenerative and arthritis diseases of the glenohumeral joint. In: Post M, Flatow EL, Bigliani LU, et. al, eds. The Shoulder: Operative Techniques. Philadelphia:Lippincott Williams & Wilkins, 1998:73–131.)

glenoid component. Meticulous attention to glenoid preparation will allow intimate contact between the posterior surface of the glenoid component and native glenoid face, improving the stability of the glenoid component.[12]

Accepting Altered Version

The glenoid vault becomes shallow and narrow as one reams medially; therefore, high-side resection should be limited to less than 1 cm. If resection more than 1 cm is required, a small increase in retroversion (up to 5–10 degrees) may be accepted with a compensatory decrease in humeral component retroversion. The combined retroversion of the humeral and glenoid components should not exceed approximately 40 degrees.[48] Small amounts of residual retroversion may also be dealt with by using an augmented glenoid component. We have not found instability of the prosthetic components to be a problem when using these criteria. If there is less than 1 cm of glenoid bone stock available, bone grafting is considered, but usually glenoid resurfacing is just omitted.

Bone Grafts

When glenoid version is restored or corrected as best as possible given the remaining glenoid bone stock, the remaining bony deficiency can be reassessed. Glenoid deficiency can make proper seating of the glenoid component very difficult, and at this point, bone grafting may be con-

sidered. Several studies have been performed to evaluate the efficacy of bone grafting the glenoid. Neer and Morrison[51] reported that only 4% of 463 shoulders required a large, internally fixed bone graft for the treatment of glenoid deficiency at the time of total shoulder arthroplasty; 16 of the 19 patients they reported on had excellent results with no evidence of loosening or nonunion at an average of 4.4 years after grafting. Fixation screws broke in two of the patients, and there was wear of a fixation screw in a third patient. Cofield[10] reported on 28 patients who underwent bone grafting for glenoid deficiency, 23 (82%) of whom had excellent or good results. All grafts healed and appeared intact, whereas two had symptomatic loosening. Recently, Hill and Norris[29] reported on 17 glenoid bone grafts with less positive results. A satisfactory result was obtained in 9 of the 17 shoulders, and 5 were deemed failures, all of which were treated with component removal. All of their patients had some form of preoperative instability, and 12 of 17 had metal-backed components, both of which may have contributed to the higher failure rate. It should be impressed that even in the hands of a tertiary care shoulder surgeon, bone grafting of the glenoid is a very uncommon procedure (Fig. 27-10).

In the rare case of severe glenoid deficiency caused by posterior wear, glenoid bone grafting may be necessary. Although no set rules exist, guidelines and recommendations on when to consider bone grafting have been developed. These include (a) alignment that cannot be corrected to within 15 degrees of neutral by less than 1 cm of eccentric reaming[20,51,61] and (b) reaming that would leave less than 1 cm of glenoid remaining (thus increasing the risk of glenoid penetration).[29] In the primary arthroplasty situation, the resected humeral head usually provides an adequate amount of bone graft. In this case, a contoured graft is initially held in place by temporary K-wire fixation and then definitively fixed with two 3.5-mm cortical screws (Fig. 27-11).

Glenoid Bone Loss at Revision

Glenoid revision surgery for glenoid component loosening is commonly associated with osteolysis and significant bone loss.[37] Asymmetric wear, aseptic loosening with bone lysis associated with polyethylene debris, and bone loss associated with removal of a glenoid component all may contribute to the often severe bone loss. Again, these types of defects are either contained defects that involve a loss of cancellous bone within the glenoid vault or noncontained defects that involve some loss of cortical support usually along the posterior rim of the glenoid. These types of noncontained defects are often the result of a malpositioned glenoid in which the glenoid retroversion was not corrected at the primary arthroplasty.

Initially, glenoid bony loss encountered at revision surgery is handled in a similar fashion as just described.

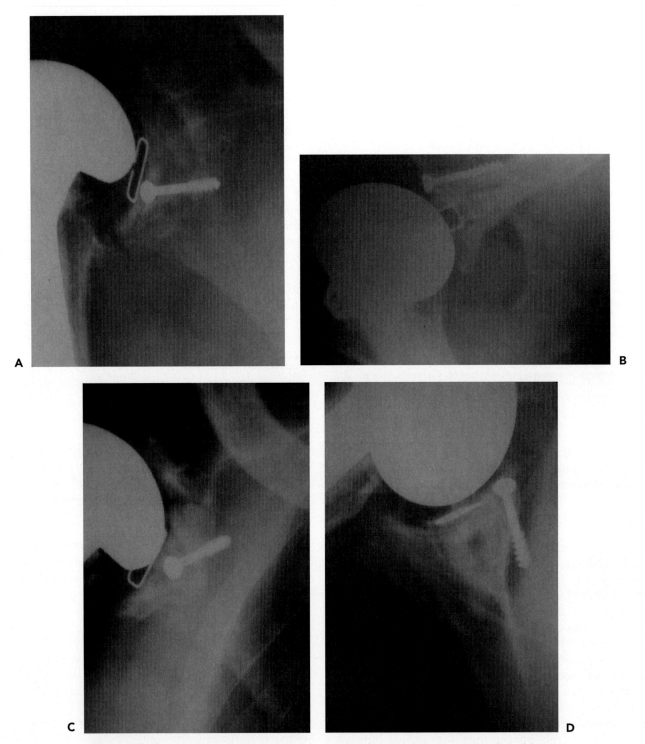

Figure 27-10 (A,B) Anteroposterior (AP) and axillary radiographs demonstrating glenoid bone grafting with cortical screw fixation after revision total shoulder arthroplasty (TSA). (C,D) AP and axillary views 12 years later demonstrate loosening and implant migration.

Version is addressed and can be corrected with eccentric reaming. Then, once again, bony deficiency can be reassessed. The small, contained defects may be filled with cement during glenoid component insertion. Larger central defects should be curetted and packed tightly with cancellous bone graft. If cortical penetration is present then the hole may be packed with cancellous bone graft to prevent cement extrusion during glenoid implantation. Significant retroversion remaining after eccentric reaming is addressed with a contoured bone graft as described previously for

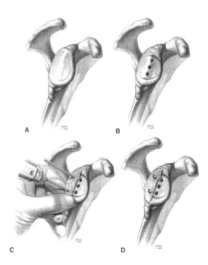

Figure 27-11 Technique of bone graft placement. *(A)* Segmental erosion of the posterior half of the bony glenoid. *(B)* Preparation of the anterior portion of the glenoid subchondral bone and placement of centering holes. *(C)* Placement of humeral head graft (or allograft) to the deficient area of the glenoid. The graft is temporarily held in place with drill bits or K-wires. *(D)* Replacement of temporary fixation with 3.5-mm cortical screws. The graft is then further contoured to match the slightly concave anterior surface. (Reprinted with permission: Steinman SP, Cofield RH. Bone grafting for glenoid deficiency in total shoulder replacement. J Shoulder Elbow Surg 2000;9:364.)

primary glenoid implantation (Fig. 27-11). However, in revision cases, an iliac crest or allograft is usually required. Once the version has been corrected and the bone grafting is complete, the glenoid component is cemented into position.

In revision total shoulder replacement, the glenoid deficiency is often too severe to be corrected by bone grafting (Fig. 27-5). In these circumstances, glenoid resurfacing is often abandoned and only a hemiarthroplasty is performed. Large, uncontained defects do not provide a stable enough base for component placement. Patients with large, contained defects may undergo cancellous bone grafting. In fact, simple removal of a loose component with cancellous bone grafting may result in satisfactory pain relief.[1,26,34,55] Grafting the defect not only reinforces the glenoid to articulate with the humeral component but also potentially recreates sufficient bone stock with graft incorporation for a possible later glenoid replacement.[1,20,56] If the decision has been made not to implant a glenoid because of severe bony loss, and a staged reconstruction is not planned, it is reasonable to treat the remaining glenoid conservatively. The surface can be sculpted to provide as congruous an articulating surface as possible for the humeral head. The remaining rim of peripheral cortical bone should be preserved as best as possible to articulate with the humeral component and enhance stability.

Technical Pitfalls

A major technical factor limiting glenoid component longevity is glenoid bone stock deficiency. Thus, lack of adequate bone stock is a leading contraindication to glenoid resurfacing. An inadequate preoperative and intraoperative assessment of glenoid bony detail could lead to glenoid penetration during reaming and subsequently early postoperative loosening. Similarly, failure to recognize and evaluate glenoid version can easily lead to several intraoperative and postoperative complications. If glenoid retroversion is not corrected, anterior perforation of the cortex can occur during glenoid preparation. Failure to recognize cortical perforation can lead to extrusion of cement behind the glenoid during implantation. Failure to correct version will thus also lead to component malposition and possible early loosening.

The condition of the soft tissues is often overlooked when performing glenoid resurfacing. Significant soft tissue deficits can preclude glenoid component placement or affect the decision to use bone graft. A strong contraindication for glenoid resurfacing is an irreparable rotator cuff tear or cuff tear arthropathy, because this can result in early loosening of the glenoid because of asymmetric motion between the humeral head and the glenoid.[6,19,45] Excessive posterior laxity is common in patients with primary osteoarthritis or who have undergone anterior stabilization procedures. These patients can have a combination of glenoid retroversion, bony loss, and posterior instability because of capsular laxity. Recurrent postoperative posterior instability is very possible if the soft-tissues are not balanced and, as stated previously, if the glenoid is also implanted in retroversion.

In the revision situation for a malpositioned glenoid, the component can often be solidly fixed. Great care must be taken when removing the glenoid component. First the glenoid face must be separated from the keel or pegs using a sharp osteotome, and then the keel or pegs can be removed with osteotomes or a high-speed burr. Hasty removal could lead to more extensive bony loss in the glenoid or, worse, cause fracture. Careless or aggressive retraction can also lead to glenoid fracture.

When bone grafting the glenoid, the surgeon must be cognizant of possibly lateralizing the glenoid. The humeral head will often need to be downsized to accommodate the increased thickness of the glenoid. Failure to do so can cause overstuffing of the glenohumeral joint and subsequent stiffness.

Humeral Bone Loss

Bony deficiency involving the humeral side of a shoulder arthroplasty is much less common than that of the glenoid. The most common scenarios in which this is a clinical problem include posttraumatic deformities of the proximal humerus, revision arthroplasty in which humeral bone loss has occurred after prosthetic removal, and proximal humeral deficits after resection for tumor or infection.

Humeral bone loss after prosthetic removal in the revision procedure is the most common and a challenge to manage. Although sometimes bone loss is unavoidable, it is very important to learn the appropriate techniques to avoid bony deficiencies and the errors that lead to problems in the revision situation.

Technique of Humeral Head Removal

The widespread usage of modular humeral head replacements helps to decrease the incidence of this complication by facilitating glenoid implantation or revision without removing the stem and by allowing minor adjustments in soft tissue balancing by exchanging only the modular component.[12,16,44] Unfortunately, significant errors in humeral position, prosthetic infection, or aseptic loosening often necessitate removal of the entire humeral prosthesis. The use of humeral hemiarthroplasty in the acute situation for severe proximal humerus fractures can be technically challenging. If the humeral height is not reestablished properly, patients may have poor function and instability.[8,40,69] Therefore, the reconstruction surgeon needs to be meticulous in his or her extraction techniques and be certain to have available all the appropriate instruments.

In the revision situation, once the joint has been dislocated, the humeral shaft and prosthesis are first evaluated for the necessity of component revision. Initially, all the fibrous soft tissues must be circumferentially removed from the proximal cement-bone or prosthesis-bone interface, and micromotion of the humeral implant is evaluated. Humeral component loosening is uncommon and should raise the suspicion of infection. Aseptic loose humeral components and well-fixed but grossly malpositioned humeral components may lead to instability.[23,28,32,44,66–68]

Removal of the well-fixed humeral prosthesis and surrounding polymethyl methacrylate usually requires the use of specialized equipment including prosthesis-specific extraction equipment, ultrasonic cement removal devices, high-speed low-torque drills, and cement removal instruments. We initially attempt to manually remove the prosthesis using osteotomes and chisels to circumferentially loosen the implant proximally. Usually the humeral component can then be manually extracted with osteotomes or by using a universal extractor that is applied under the collar of the prosthesis. If the prosthesis cannot be removed by using these techniques, then the shaft may need to be "windowed" to avoid destroying or fracturing the humerus with repeated attempts at removal.

To "window" the humerus, the anterior humeral shaft is first exposed subperiosteally between the deltoid and pectoralis major proximally and between the brachialis and triceps distally. With a sagittal saw, two parallel longitudinal cuts are created along the anterior cortex of the humerus approximately 1.5 to 2 cm apart, starting proximally at the osteotomized humeral neck and ending distally approximately 3 to 4 cm proximal to the tip of the cement mantle. A transverse cut is then made distally connecting the two longitudinal cuts, and the rectangular cortical section of bone is gently lifted away from the prosthesis/cement using wide, thin osteotomes. Alternatively, one longitudinal cut may be made and the window "trap-doored" by cracking the other side. Usually the prosthesis can now be easily removed by using the techniques just described. All intramedullary cement within the canal and on the undersurface of the cortical section is removed along with the pseudomembrane of the prosthesis/cement-bone interface. Image intensification can be very helpful during cement removal to verify that high-speed burrs are in the shaft, avoiding perforation.

Before reimplantation of a new humeral component, the cortical section is replaced and secured with multiple cerclage wires or cables. When an osteotomy has been performed, we prefer to implant a long-stem prosthesis 2 to 3 cortical diameters distal to the osteotomy site.

Small Humeral Defects

Even when all efforts are made to maintain bone stock of the humerus, it may often be unavoidable. Therefore, once the humeral component and all cement have been removed, an assessment of the amount of bone loss should be made. Proximal humeral bone loss is particularly prevalent in a prosthesis that uses a large wedge-shaped metaphyseal body designed for ingrowth (Fig. 27-12). In these cases, metaphyseal bone loss from stress-shielding can significantly compromise the fixation of the rotator cuff, and care must be taken to protect and potentially secure the tuberosities.

Usually, there is not adequate humeral bone stock present in this situation to allow press-fit, ingrowth fixation. The component is cemented in the appropriate version and height to reestablish the proper soft tissue tension. Humeral height is estimated by restoring the tension within the soft tissue envelope and by comparing radiographs or scanograms to the opposite humerus. If there is a significant bone gap between the prosthetic head and the shaft, autogenous iliac crest bone graft or allograft tibial or fibular struts may be used. If the security of the tuberosities is compromised, then additional fixation to the humeral shaft may be performed in a manner similar to tuberosity fixation during hemiarthroplasty for fracture. In both cases, tuberosity fixation should be supplemented with generous cancellous bone graft.

Large Humeral Defects

In patients with large metaphyseal and diaphyseal defects or large isolated diaphyseal defects, especially common in

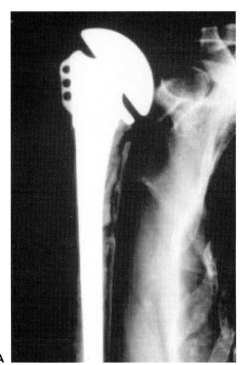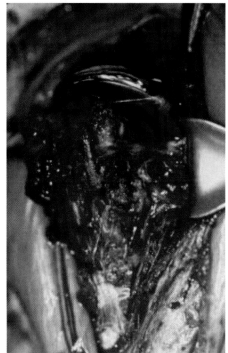

A   B

Figure 27-12 Proximal humeral bone loss is particularly prevalent in prostheses that use a large wedge-shaped body. *(A)* Anteroposterior (AP) radiograph of wedge-shaped implant with bone loss. *(B)* Intraoperative photograph of a patient with proximal bone loss.

the setting of a segmental resection performed for neoplasm, various reconstructive options exist. Some are aimed at preservation of shoulder mobility, whereas others are aimed at shoulder arthrodesis. Proximal humeral reconstructions that preserve shoulder mobility can be achieved using an endoprosthesis, osteoarticular humeral allograft, or allograft prosthetic composite arthroplasty.

Endoprosthesis

The use of a segmental, modular, all-metal proximal humerus prosthesis has been advocated by many.[15,40–42,60] The advantages of this technique include the maintenance of normal humeral length, preservation of elbow and hand function, and excellent cosmesis. Because there are no specific sites for attachment of the rotator cuff or deltoid, the success of this procedure depends on static and dynamic suspension with the use of Dacron tape and multiple muscle transfers about the prosthesis.[40,42] One study reported overall poor functional scores (66%), which were even worse if the shoulder abductors were not preserved (52%).[54] Many patients had unsatisfactory hand positioning, functional activity, and lifting ability. Complications were high and included subluxation, loosening, stress shielding, and infection. Several have reported a high incidence of loosening and instability when this prosthesis is used in young, active patients.[4,9,22]

Osteoarticular Allograft

The concept of osteoarticular allograft reconstruction of segmental defects of the proximal humerus was introduced as a treatment alternative in the younger patient after tumor excision. One of the bigger advantages is that the articular surface can be used to reconstruct the shoulder joint anatomically. However, the durability of the articular portion of the graft has not been reliable (Fig. 27-13). Osteoarticular allografts have been found to have a 20% incidence of subchondral fracture.[22] Recently Getty and Peabody[24] showed that although this procedure provides good pain relief and preserves manual dexterity, there was an extremely high complication rate, including joint instability, fracture of the allograft, and infection of the allograft. With time, they found a progressive decrease in function and an increased prevalence of complications related to the allograft. They have abandoned the technique.

Allograft Prosthetic Composite

Allograft prosthetic composite arthroplasty has been the more reproducible and reliable technique for reconstruction of the proximal humerus after segmental bone loss.[13,34] Allograft prosthetic composite arthroplasty has many advantages, including easy availability, restoration of bone stock, customization with conventional implant

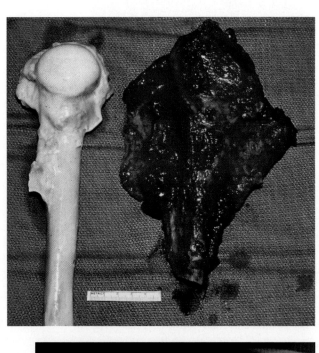

A

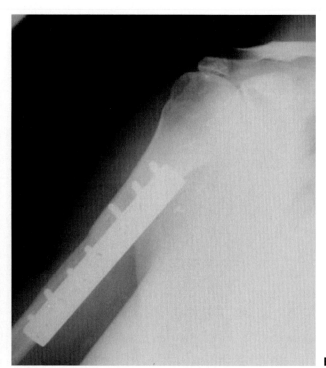

B

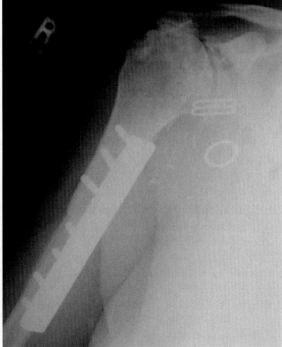

C

Figure 27-13 *(A)* Operative view of a frozen osteoarticular allo-graft with the remaining capsule and rotator cuff visualized around the articular surface. Resected specimen *(right)*. *(B)* Anteroposterior (AP) radiograph shows postoperative osteoarticular allograft re-construction and plate fixation. There is no evidence of a radiolu-cent line noted consistent with graft-host union. *(C)* AP radiograph taken 5 years after placement of the allograft shows significant ar-ticular degeneration.

components, soft tissue attachment of tendons and liga-ments, and preservation of the medullary canal of the host bone. Good functional results have been reported by many.[13,27,33,38,58,62] It is also a good alternative for a failed modular oncology prosthesis and failed osteoarticular allo-graft because it restores bone stock.[27] This technique evolved into use for shoulder arthroplasty in part because

of the need to salvage failed articular surfaces in patients with osteoarticular grafts and to provide a joint surface for those patients in whom osteoarticular grafts could not be used.[9,22]

The allograft proximal humerus can be prepared on the back table, placing the humeral cut in the anatomic amount of retroversion.[64] A long-stem prosthesis can be press-fit or

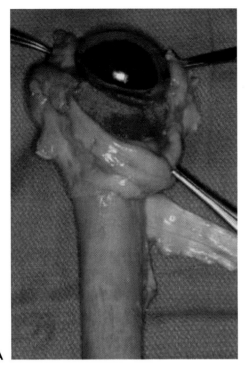
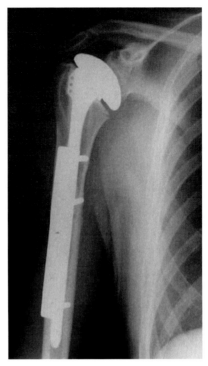

A

B

Figure 27-14 Allograft reconstruction of the proximal humerus. *(A)* Allograft-prosthetic composite is prepared on a back table. Note that the soft tissue attachment sites have been maintained. *(B)* Anteroposterior (AP) radiograph showing the reconstruction secured with plate fixation.

cemented into the allograft bone (Fig. 27-14). The allograft-host junction should be bone grafted. and the prosthetic stem should bypass this junction by at least 5 or 6 cm. The soft tissues can then be reattached at their anatomic sites.

CONCLUSION

Humeral bone deficiency is uncommonly of great significance during shoulder arthroplasty and usually is managed by a *larger* stem and bone grafting. Occasionally allograft reconstruction is added. Glenoid deficiency is most severe during revision surgery, when it may preclude glenoid resurfacing. In the more common setting of primary replacement for osteoarthritis, posterior glenoid erosion and increased retroversion are usually dealt with by eccentric reaming, although bone grafting occasionally may be used.

REFERENCES

1. Antuna SA, Sperling JW, Cofield RH, et al. Glenoid revision surgery after total shoulder arthroplasty. J Shoulder Elbow Surg 2001;10:217.
2. Barrett WP, Franklin JL, Jackins SE, et al. Total shoulder arthroplasty. J Bone Joint Surg Am 1987;69(6):865.
3. Bigliani LU, Weinstein DM, Glasgow MT, et al. Glenohumeral arthroplasty for arthritis after instability surgery. J Shoulder Elbow Surg 1995;4(2):87.
4. Bos G, Sim F, Pritchard D, et al. Prosthetic replacement of the proximal humerus. Clin Orthop 1987;224:178.
5. Boyd AD Jr., Aliabadi P, Thornhill TS. Postoperative proximal migration in total shoulder arthroplasty. Incidence and significance. J Arthroplasty 1991;6(1):31.
6. Boyd AD Jr., Thomas WH, Scott RD, et al. Total shoulder arthroplasty versus hemiarthroplasty. Indications for glenoid resurfacing. J Arthroplasty 1990;5(4):329.
7. Brenner BC, Ferlic DC, Clayton ML, et al. Survivorship of unconstrained total shoulder arthroplasty. J Bone Joint Surg Am 1989;71(9):1289.
8. Caldwell GL, Dines D, Warren R, et al. Revision shoulder arthroplasty. Abstract: Presented at the American Shoulder and Elbow Surgeons Annual Meeting, San Francisco, CA, February, 1993.
9. Cheng EY, Gebhardt MC. Allograft reconstructions of the shoulder after bone tumor resections. Orthop Clin North Am 1991;22:37.
10. Cofield RH. Total shoulder arthroplasty with the Neer prosthesis. J Bone Joint Surg Am 1984;66(6):899.
11. Cofield RH, Edgerton BC. Total shoulder arthroplasty: complications and revision surgery. Instr Course Lect 1990;39:449.
12. Collins D, Tencer A, Sidles J, et al. Edge displacement and deformation of glenoid components in response to eccentric loading. The effect of preparation of the glenoid bone. J Bone Joint Surg Am 1992;74(4):501.
13. Dick HM, Steinman SP, Cannot RM, et al. Limb salvage for malignant tumors of the shoulder girdle. Orthop Trans 1991;15:702.
14. Dines DM, Warren RF, Altchek DW, Moeckel B. Posttraumatic changes of the proximal humerus: malunion, nonunion, and osteonecrosis: treatment with modular hemiarthroplasty or total shoulder arthroplasty. J Shoulder Elbow Surg 1993;2:11.
15. Fabroni RH, Castagno A, Aguilera AL, et al. Long-term results of limb salvage with the Fabroni custom made endoprosthesis. Clin Orthop 1999;358:41.
16. Fenlin JM, Ramsey ML, Allardyce TJ, et al. Modular total shoulder replacement: design rationale, indications, and results. Clin Orthop 1994;307:37.

17. Fenlin JM Jr., Vaccaro A, Andreychik D, et al. Modular total shoulder: early experience and impressions. Semin Arthroplasty 1990;1(2):102.
18. Flatow EL. Unconstrained shoulder arthroplasty. In: Kohn D, Wirth CJ, eds. Die schulter: aktuelle operative therapie. Stuttgart, Thieme, 1992:216.
19. Franklin JL, Barrett WP, Jackins SE, et al. Glenoid loosening in total shoulder arthroplasty. Association with rotator cuff deficiency. J Arthroplasty 1988;3(1):39.
20. Friedman RJ, Hawthorne KB, Genez BM. The use of computerized tomography in the measurement of glenoid version. J Bone Joint Surg Am 1992;74:1032.
21. Gartsman GM, Roddey TS, Hammerman SM. Shoulder arthroplasty with or without resurfacing of the glenoid in patients who have osteoarthritis. J Bone Joint Surg 2000;82(1):26.
22. Gebhardt M, Roth Y, Mankin H. Osteoarticular allografts for reconstruction in the proximal part of the humerus after excision of a musculoskeletal tumor. J Bone Joint Surg 1990;72A:334.
23. Gerber A, Ghalambor N, Warner JJ. Instability of shoulder arthroplasty: balancing mobility and stability. Orthop Clin North Am 2001;32:661.
24. Getty PJ, Peabody TD. Complications and functional outcomes of reconstruction with an osteoarticular allograft after intra-articular resection of the proximal aspect of the humerus. J Bone Joint Surg 1999;81:1138.
25. Green A, Norris TR. Imaging techniques for glenohumeral arthritis and glenohumeral arthroplasty. Clin Orthop 1994;307:7.
26. Hawkins RJ, Greis PE, Bonutti PM. Treatment of symptomatic glenoid loosening following unconstrained shoulder arthroplasty. Orthopedics 1999;22:229.
27. Hejna MJ, Gitelis S. Allograft prosthetic composite replacement for bone tumors. Semin Surg Oncol 1997;13:18.
28. Hennigan SP, Iannotti JP. Instability after prosthetic arthroplasty of the shoulder. Orthop Clin North Am 2001;32:649.
29. Hill JM, Norris TR. Long-term results of total shoulder arthroplasty following bone grafting of the glenoid. J Bone Joint Surg Am 2001;83A(6):877.
30. Sperling JW, Potter HG, Craig EV, et al. Magnetic Resonance imaging of painful shoulder arthroplasty. J Shoulder Elbow Surg 2002;11(4):315–321.
31. Imbriglia JE, Neer CS, Dick HM. Resection of the proximal one half of the humerus in a child for chondrosarcoma. J Bone Joint Surg 1978;60A:262.
32. Jahnke AH Jr., Hawkins RJ. Instability after shoulder arthroplasty: causative factors and treatment options. Semin Arthroplasty 1995;6:289.
33. Jensen KL, Johnston JO. Proximal humeral reconstruction after excision of a primary sarcoma. Clin Orthop 1995;311:164.
34. Jensen KL, Toro P, Wirth MA, et al. Salvage of failed glenoid components: conversion to hemiarthroplasty. Proceedings of the 66th Annual Meeting of the American Academy of Orthopaedic Surgeons 39, 1999.
35. Kelleher I, Cofield RH, Becker DA, et al. Fluoroscopically positioned radiographs of total shoulder arthroplasty. J Shoulder Elbow Surg 1992;1:306.
36. Kirkley A, Jackowski D, Gartsman G, et al. A meta-analysis of hemi versus total shoulder arthroplasty for osteoarthritis of the shoulder. Presented at the 8th International Congress on Surgery of the Shoulder. Cape Town, South Africa, 2001.
37. Klepps S, Hazrati Y, Flatow E. The management of glenoid bone deficiency during shoulder replacement. Tech Shoulder Elbow Surg 2002;4(1):4–17.
38. Kneisl JS. Function after amputation, arthrodesis, or arthroplasty for tumors about the shoulder. J South Orthop Assoc 1995;14: 228.
39. Levine WN, Djurasovic M, Glasson JM, et al. Hemiarthroplasty for glenohumeral osteoarthritis: results correlated to degree of glenoid wear. J Shoulder Elbow Surg 1997;6(5):449.
40. Malawer M, Meller I, Dunham W. Shoulder girdle resections for bone and soft tissue tumors. In: Yamamuro T, ed. New developments for limb salvage in musculoskeletal tumors. Tokyo, Springer-Verlag, 1989:519.
41. Malawer MM, Chou LB. Prosthetic survival and clinical results with use of large-segment replacements in the treatment of high-grade bone sarcomas. J Bone Joint Surg 1995;77A:1154.
42. Malawer M, Pereless C. Limb-sparing surgery for bone and soft tissue tumors of the shoulder girdle: clinical experience of 50 patients and a proposed (modified) classification system. Presented at the Tenth Open Meeting of the American Shoulder and Elbow Surgeons, New Orleans, LA February, 1994.
43. Mallon WJ, Brown HR, Vogler JB III, et al. Radiographic and geometric anatomy of the scapula. Clin Orthop 1992;277:142.
44. Moeckel BH, Altchek DW, Warren RF, et al. Instability of the shoulder after arthroplasty. J Bone Joint Surg 1993;75A:492.
45. Mow VC, Flatow EL, Foster RJ. Biomechanics. In: Simon SR, ed. Orthopaedic basic science. Rosemont, IL, American Academy of Orthopaedic Surgeons, 1994:397.
46. Neer CS. Articular replacement of the humeral head. J Bone Joint Surg 1955;37A:215.
47. Neer CS. The rheumatoid shoulder. In: Cruess RR, Mitchell NS, eds. Surgery of rheumatoid arthritis. Philadelphia, PA, JB Lippincott, 1971:117.
48. Neer CS. Glenohumeral arthroplasty. In: Shoulder reconstruction. Philadelphia, PA, WB Saunders, 1990:143.
49. Neer CS 2nd. Replacement arthroplasty for glenohumeral osteoarthritis. J Bone Joint Surg Am 1974;56(1):1.
50. Neer CS, Kirby RM. Revision of humeral head and total shoulder arthroplasties. Clin Orthop 1982;170:189.
51. Neer CS, Morrison DS. Glenoid bone-grafting in total shoulder arthroplasty. J Bone Joint Surg Am 1988;70(8):1154.
52. Neer CS, Brown TH, McLaughlin HL. Fracture of the neck of the humerus with dislocation of the head fragment. Am J Surg 1953;85:252.
53. Neer CS, Watson KC, Stanton FJ. Recent experience in total shoulder replacement. J Bone Joint Surg 1982;64A:319.
54. O'Connor MI, Sim FH, Chao EY. Limb salvage for neoplasms of the shoulder girdle: intermediate reconstructive and functional results. J Bone Joint Surg 1996;78A:1872.
55. Petersen SA, Hawkins RJ. Revision of failed total shoulder arthroplasty. Orthop Clin North Am 1998;29:519.
56. Pritchett JW, Clark JM. Prosthetic replacement for chronic unreduced dislocations of the shoulder. Clin Orthop 1987;216:89.
57. Randelli M, Gambrioli PL. Glenohumeral osteometry by computed tomography in normal and unstable shoulders. Clin Orthop 1986;208:151.
58. Rock M. Intercalary allograft and custom Neer prosthesis after en bloc resection of the proximal humerus. In: Enneking WF, ed. Limb salvage in musculoskeletal oncology. New York, Churchill Livingstone, 1987:586.
59. Rodosky MW, Bigliani LU. Indications for glenoid resurfacing in shoulder arthroplasty. J Shoulder Elbow Surg 1996;5(3): 231.
60. Ross AC, Wilson JN, Scales JT. Endoprosthetic replacement of the proximal humerus. J Bone Joint Surg 1987;69B:656.
61. Steinmann SP, Cofield RH. Bone grafting for glenoid deficiency in total shoulder replacement. J Shoulder Elbow Surg 2000;9(5): 361.
62. Takagishi K, Shinohara N. Prosthetic replacement due to giant-cell tumor in the proximal humerus. A case report. Clin Orthop 1989;247:106.
63. Tanner MW, Cofield RH. Prosthetic arthroplasty for fractures and fracture-dislocations of the proximal humerus. Clin Orthop 1983;179:116.
64. Tillett E, Smith M, Fulcer M, et al. Anatomic determination of humeral head retroversion: the relationship of the central axis of the humeral head to the bicipital groove. J Shoulder Elbow Surg 1993;255:9.
65. Vainio K. Orthopaedic surgery in the treatment of rheumatoid arthritis. Ann Clin Res 1975;7:216.
66. Warren RF, Coleman SH, Dines JS. Instability after arthroplasty: the shoulder. J Arthroplasty 2002;17(Suppl):28.
67. Wirth MA, Rockwood CA Jr. Complications of shoulder arthroplasty. Clin Orthop 1994;307:47.
68. Wirth MA, Rockwood CA Jr. Complications of total shoulder-replacement arthroplasty. J Bone Joint Surg Am 1996;78:603.
69. Wirth MA, Seltzer DG, Senes HR, et al. An analysis of failed humeral head and total shoulder arthroplasties (abstract). Presented at the American Shoulder and Elbow Surgeons Tenth Annual Open Meeting. New Orleans, LA, 1994.

The Failed Arthroplasty: Options for Revision

28

Julie Y. Bishop   Evan L. Flatow

INTRODUCTION

Revision shoulder arthroplasty is a demanding procedure that usually involves not only component revision but also complex reconstruction of soft tissue contracture, muscle deficiency, and bone loss. It is undertaken only after careful evaluation of the causes of failure, especially ensuring that infection is not the underlying cause. Meticulous planning is also essential for a favorable outcome. Although clinical results of revision shoulder arthroplasty are generally inferior to primary shoulder arthroplasty, careful patient selection and adherence to surgical principles can lead to satisfactory results.

EVALUATION

Several factors must be evaluated when considering revision surgery, including the patient factors and expectations, cause of the implant and/or clinical failure, careful review of the operative reports for any clues as to the cause of failure, integrity of the soft tissue and bony envelope, and ability to satisfactorily improve the patient's condition. In many cases, the cause of primary arthroplasty failure is multifactorial, and thus several different reconstructive procedures may need to be performed during revision surgery. Thus, careful evaluation of the cause of failure, in

particular, ensuring that the cause is not infection, is mandatory before attempting revision arthroplasty.

Patient Goals

When a patient presents with complaints after shoulder arthroplasty, it is important to identify the chief complaint. Although most patients will present with the general complaint of pain and loss of function, these problems must be separated if possible. It is important to understand what bothers patients the most and what they hope to gain from revision surgery. Are they primarily seeking pain relief, or do they have tolerable pain but are dissatisfied with a poor functional outcome? This is especially important in cases in which severe structural loss make it unlikely that major functional gains can be expected. Sometimes it can be helpful to play a thought experiment: The patient is asked which of two procedures he or she would choose: one that would relieve all of the pain but not improve motion or strength or one that would increase function but leave pain unaltered.

History

Although it can be long and tedious, it is important to go carefully through the patient's history. The patient should always be asked about any history of infection or poor wound healing. The details of the postoperative rehabilitation may give clues as to any current stiffness. Understanding the onset of problems after the prior surgery may provide clues as to the cause of failure. Patients with an acute postoperative infection or instability commonly present with ongoing pain without improvement after surgery. Patients with delayed infection, glenoid arthrosis,

J. Y. Bishop: Clinical Shoulder Fellow, Department of Orthopaedic Surgery, Mount Sinai Medical Center, New York, New York.
E. L. Flatow: Lasker Professor of Orthopaedic Surgery, Chief of Shoulder Surgery, Department of Orthopaedic Surgery, Mount Sinai Medical Center, New York, New York.

or aseptic loosening more commonly present with a period of pain relief followed by a new onset of symptoms.

All prior operative reports must be obtained and reviewed. A surgeon should not make a final evaluation, and certainly not undertake revision surgery, without this important piece of information. When a primary arthroplasty fails, the evaluating surgeon should think of himself or herself as a detective. No stone should be left unturned, and every possible reason for failure should be examined. Thus, the prior operative report is an essential "clue" as to the cause of failure. It contains information that most patients may not know or understand and thus cannot articulate to the evaluating surgeon. Any complications, especially any neurovascular abnormalities or complications, should be noted. Most important, the type and size of the prosthetic implant should be noted in the report. In addition, every effort should be made to obtain the previous radiographs, office notes of clinical follow-up, and postoperative rehabilitation program. It can be very helpful, if the patient gives permission, to speak with the original surgeon. Much useful information, not in the written record, may be obtained, particularly about the patient's personality and adherence to postoperative instructions.

Physical Examination

The physical examination begins with inspection for surgical scars, abnormal posture, and muscular atrophy. Active and passive range of motion of the shoulder are assessed, and if any loss of motion is detected one should attempt to determine the cause of motion loss (i.e., whether by soft tissue contracture, bony impingement, or prosthetic impingement). The strength of the shoulder and upper extremity should be assessed with particular attention to rotator cuff and deltoid function. The stability of the joint is examined, documenting the degree and direction of any instability. A click or clunk during range of motion or instability examination may be indicative of a loose glenoid component. Careful attention should be paid to which movements and positions elicit pain as well. Finally, a neurologic examination of the upper extremity should be performed and investigated with electrodiagnostic studies if a deficit is suspected.

Imaging

A standard radiographic series should be performed in all patients to include anteroposterior views of the shoulder and glenohumeral joint, a lateral "Y" scapular view, and an axillary view. If possible, serial radiographs including preoperative and postoperative x-rays should be assessed for radiolucent lines, osteolysis, prosthetic position, and prosthetic migration (Fig. 28-1). If glenoid or humeral loosening is suspected, fluoroscopically guided radiographs may aid in demonstrating radiolucent lines at the bone-cement interface.[68]

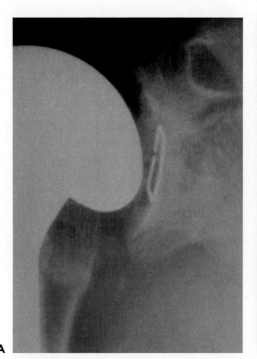
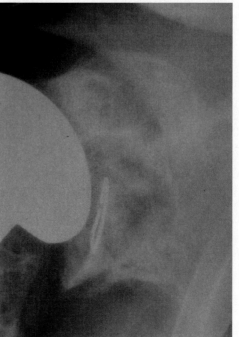

A   B

Figure 28-1 Anteroposterior (AP) serial radiographs revealing progression of radiolucent lines surrounding the glenoid component, indicative of loosening. *(A)* AP radiograph taken in the immediate postoperative period. Small circumferential radiolucent line is visualized. *(B)* AP radiograph taken 12 years later. There has been obvious progression of the radiolucency, bone loss, and shifting of the glenoid component.

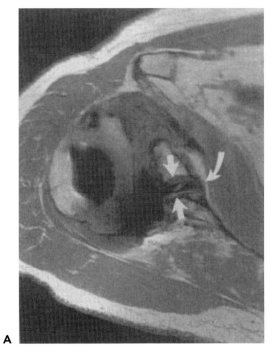

A

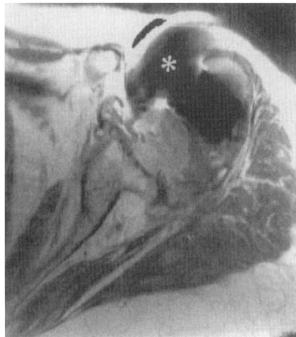

B

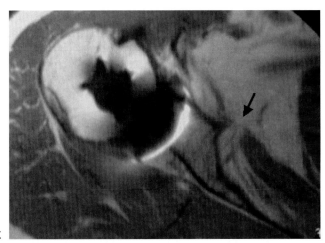

C

Figure 28-2   Axial fast spin-echo magnetic resonance imaging (MRI) of painful total shoulder replacements. *(A)* A 73-year-old patient with a loose glenoid component. Note the rind of intermediate signal intensity surrounding the keel of the glenoid component *(straight arrows)* and the cortical penetration of the tip of the keel toward the medial cortex of the scapula *(curved arrow)*. *(B)* A 76-year-old patient with pain and weakness after a hemiarthroplasty. The humeral component *(*)* is markedly anteverted relative to the glenoid, such that the articular surface of the humeral component faces the anterior subcutaneous soft tissues. The humeral anteversion was not prospectively detected on plain radiographs. (Reprinted with permission: Sperling JW, Potter HG, Craig EV, et al. Magnetic resonance imaging of painful shoulder arthroplasty. J Shoulder Elbow Surg 2002;11:315.) *(C)* Image of an unstable arthroplasty demonstrating a subscapularis tendon rupture retracted medial to the glenoid *(arrow)*.

Although not necessarily a prerequisite to surgery, cross-section imaging, that is, computed tomography and magnetic resonance imaging (MRI), may provide important information on implant positioning, humeral and glenoid bone loss, glenoid version, remaining glenoid bone stock, and posterior glenoid erosion[47,53] (Fig. 28-2, A and B). Determination of overall bony losses and bone stock should be done before surgery and should not be a surprise intraoperative finding for which one is unprepared to handle. Finally, limited pulse-sequence parameter modification makes it possible for MRI to provide information on the status of the rotator cuff and residual cartilage despite the presence of an implant[103] (Fig. 28-2C).

Infection

Infection should always be ruled out before embarking on revision surgery. This starts with a careful history, specifically asking about any postoperative wound complications, fever, chills, remote site of any infections, or any recent invasive procedures (e.g., colonoscopy and cystoscopy), all of which should raise suspicions of a prosthetic infection. Careful inspection of the wound and surrounding skin should be performed, looking in particular for any evidence of draining sinuses, persistent erythema, warmth, and lymphadenopathy.

One should routinely order a white blood cell count, erythrocyte sedimentation rate, and C-reactive protein as general measures of inflammation/infection. If infection is suspected, an indium-labeled white blood cell scan is ordered, the joint is aspirated, and cultures for gram-positive bacteria, gram-negative bacteria, acid fast bacilli and fungi are obtained.

INDICATIONS FOR REVISION

Patient Goals and Characteristics

Pain relief is the primary indication for revision shoulder arthroplasty. Although joint motion, strength, and function may also be achieved, the results after revision shoulder arthroplasty are more variable.[3,28,33,34,58,60,66,80,87,88,92,113,114] It is important during evaluation that patient disability and expectations are adequately assessed. In patients with minimal pain and disability despite a "failed" shoulder arthroplasty, nonoperative management may provide a satisfactory outcome. Similarly, elderly or medically compromised patients may have limited functional demands or be unfit for surgery. In these patients, nonoperative treatment including physical therapy, anti-inflammatory medications, and bracing (e.g., sling) may provide some benefit.

In patients with severe pain and disability who are good surgical candidates and have a complete understanding of the risks of surgical intervention, the prolonged rehabilitation program and the potential result of surgery, revision shoulder arthroplasty, should be considered. Specific indications for surgery include joint contractures and adhesions, joint instability, component malposition, component loosening, and/or wear, infection, and fracture.

Anatomic Factors

During revision shoulder arthroplasty, a number of anatomic lesions may coexist and contribute to the complexity of surgery. For example, prosthetic instability may be secondary to a combination of factors including contracture in the opposite direction of instability, soft tissue deficiency in the direction of instability, and component malposition. Further, component loosening and wear may contribute to osteolysis and bone loss. As already stated, the degree of bony loss should be predetermined, because this can affect the feasibility of implanting or revising a component, especially the glenoid. Knowing the degree of bony and/or soft tissue deficits preoperatively is essential to preoperative planning and certainly affects what can and cannot be done in the revision situation. Thus, before embarking on revision total shoulder arthroplasty it is important to construct a careful preoperative plan to ensure that the proper personnel and equipment are available. Intraoperatively, all pathologic findings including adhesions and contractures, soft tissue loss, bone loss, component malpositioning, component loosening/wear, and instability should be addressed to ensure a satisfactory outcome. Contraindications to revision shoulder arthroplasty are similar to contraindications to primary shoulder arthroplasty and include active infection, significant neurologic impairment, and inability to participate in a prolonged rehabilitation program, and patients whose medical or mental status precludes surgery.

PREPARATION FOR REVISION

Operative Planning

Careful and thorough preparation for the revision arthroplasty is essential because these cases can be long and arduous even for the most prepared of surgeons. The revision arthroplasty surgeon will be challenged enough by the complexity of the surgery itself, with no need to add the additional hardship of being unprepared. Before the case, all prior operative reports should be reread and any essential details about the anatomy, vascularity, and components noted. The current prosthesis should be exactly identified, and the proper personnel should be notified to bring any essential equipment. This includes proper extractors for the specific prosthesis and a universal extractor (Fig. 28-3). A long-stem prosthesis should be available in case of fracture, as well as cerclage wires or cables and other fixation equipment. If glenoid arthrosis is likely the problem and there is a chance that the humeral component will be retained, then the proper matching glenoid system should be available even if it is not the one routinely used by the operative surgeon. Different sizes of humeral heads should be available as well if only the humeral head, and not the entire prosthesis, needs to be changed. However, one should be prepared to remove the entire humeral prosthesis. Thus, in addition to the proper prosthesis-specific extractors, cement removal equipment must be available if the primary implant was cemented. This includes ultrasonic cement removal devices, high-speed low-torque drills, and cement removal instruments such as osteotomes and chisels.

Bony deficits are a common problem in the revision surgery and were explored in more detail in the previous chapter. However, in the planning stages, if one expects large humeral deficits or large segmental losses, bulk allograft should always be available. For glenoid bony losses, usually a small amount of allograft such as a femoral head allograft is typically enough, or if preferable, an iliac autograft may be planned.

Standard radiographs can be taken intraoperatively, but C-arm image intensification has proven to be very useful in evaluating component positioning, version, height, bone stock, and any possible fractures after component insertion or removal. Furthermore, image intensification can be used to verify the intrashaft position of high-speed tools used to

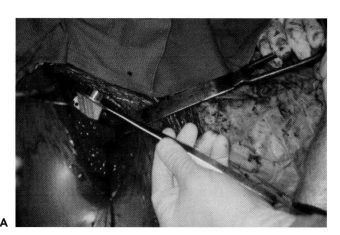 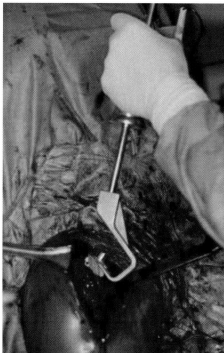

Figure 28-3 After the humeral prosthesis has been initially loosened proximally, the humeral component may be manually extracted with (A) osteotomes or (B) a universal extractor.

remove cement safely. In the revision situation, even the most prepared surgeon can run into difficulties with neurovascular structures, whether because of abnormalities, extensive scarring, or damage from the prior surgery, which cannot always be ascertained preoperatively. Therefore, it is wise to have a trained microvascular surgeon available during difficult cases.

THE STIFF ARTHROPLASTY

Postoperative stiffness can be a common cause of failure of the primary shoulder arthroplasty and is a difficult and complex problem. The stiffness can be caused by inadequate release of contracted tissues at the time of the primary arthroplasty, extensive postoperative scarring because of an intense inflammatory healing response, or slow rehabilitation. Extra-articular and intra-articular adhesions may contribute to the loss of motion.

When surgical release is used to treat the stiff arthroplasty, early range-of-motion exercises and physical therapy are crucial for maintaining the increased motion that was obtained intraoperatively.[57,77,79,85,111] Using a postoperative interscalene catheter for continuous regional block may be helpful in obtaining early postoperative pain-free range of motion.[30] When postoperative pain, which can be extensive, is managed with either intravenous or oral narcotics, doses are often high, and even if pain is controlled,

patients are typically too sleepy or nauseated to participate in physical therapy. When used in conjunction with interscalene regional anesthesia, the patient can avoid general anesthesia altogether, obtains excellent postoperative pain control, and subsequently is awake and alert and can start physical therapy the same day as surgery.[30] There are also psychologic benefits to using an interscalene catheter because the patient can immediately see the motion gains obtained during surgery. The patient can then see and believe that this motion is possible and can be achieved. Also, patients are more apt to participate willingly in physical therapy when the initial sessions are less painful.[9,22] The catheter provides excellent pain relief, is safe, and has been found to have a high rate of patient satisfaction as well.[30] However, an infusion rate that retains protective sensation is advisable, lest tendon repairs be compromised by a temporarily "insensate" joint.

Technique of Release

Although the senior author does not routinely perform shoulder arthroscopy before open revision shoulder arthroplasty, shoulder arthroscopy may be beneficial in patients with stiffness caused by capsular contracture (in which capsular release is performed).[58,108] However, when extra-articular scarring is present, between the subscapularis, strap muscles, deltoid, and pectoralis, arthroscopic release alone is inadequate and a formal open release is necessary.

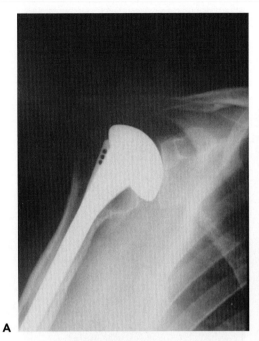

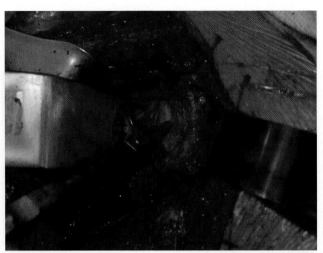

Figure 28-4 A 52-year-old woman with a painful, stiff shoulder 2 years after humeral head replacement (HHR). (A) Preoperative anteroposterior (AP) radiograph demonstrating loss of joint space. (B) Intraoperative view of exposed glenoid after extensive releases. No glenoid cartilage is left; the knife is directly on bone.

Arthroscopy also allows the identification and possible treatment of any associated pathology. It may also guide the surgeon toward an open approach if more significant problems, such as glenoid loosening, are found as well.

When an open revision arthroplasty for the stiff shoulder is carried out, extensive releases are performed (Fig. 28-4). After the standard deltopectoral exposure, which may be extended for the revision surgery, subdeltoid and subacromial adhesions are released and/or resected first. The coracohumeral ligament is released as well because it is often contracted in the revision cases. These structures must all be meticulously released to restore soft tissue mobility. The subscapularis and biceps tendons are then identified, and the axillary nerve is palpated and identified at the lower border of the subscapularis tendon. The axillary nerve can usually be identified approximately 3 to 5 mm medial to the musculotendinous junction.

In revision cases, this relationship may be distorted and the axillary nerve is often scarred and difficult to identify. The "tug test" has proved to be useful to confirm the identity of the axillary nerve. The "tug test" is performed by placing a finger under the deltoid on the anterior branch of the axillary nerve and another finger from the opposite hand on what one thinks is the axillary nerve as it passes inferior to the subscapularis tendon.[39] As one gently presses on the nerve with one finger, the force is transmitted through the axillary nerve and felt in the opposite finger, confirming the identity of the axillary nerve. After identification, the axillary nerve is protected and periodically reexamined throughout the procedure. When there is

a preoperative suspicion of nerve injury, or a high degree of scarring precluding simple identification of the nerve, the assistance of a microsurgeon to locate and free the nerve (and plexus as needed) may be helpful.

The subscapularis tendon is then thoroughly inspected for its continuity and quality. In revision cases, the subscapularis tendon is commonly scarred and contracted and limits external rotation of the shoulder. The subscapularis tendon, along with the underlying capsule, is then sharply released from its insertion on the lesser tuberosity. If bone quality allows, the insertion of the subscapularis is released with a thin wafer of bone using an osteotome (Fig. 28-5). This permits bone–bone healing after repair.

The subscapularis is then tagged, and a release of the subscapularis is performed by releasing the superior structures (i.e., rotator interval, coracohumeral ligament), anterior structures (i.e., adhesions between the subscapularis and subcoracoid space/strap muscles), inferior structures (i.e., adhesions between subscapularis and inferior capsule/axillary nerve), and posterior structures (i.e., anterior capsule) (Fig. 28-6).

To release the anterior capsule from the subscapularis tendon, a plane is initially bluntly developed between the anterior capsule and subscapularis. This is then sharply released, restoring the excursion of the subscapularis tendon. A complete capsular release is confirmed when the normal elastic feeling (or bounce) of the subscapularis tendon is restored when pulling on the traction sutures. Care is taken to avoid the subscapularis innervation medially.

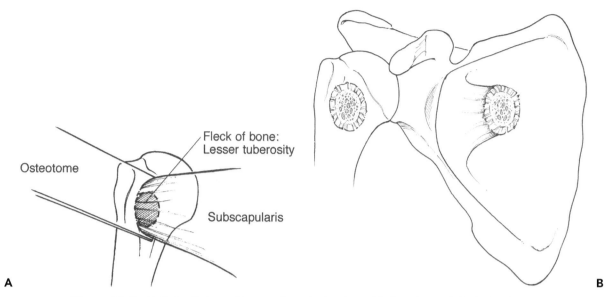

Figure 28-5   (A,B) Small piece of lesser tuberosity is taken with the subscapularis during the release from the humerus. This allows bone-to-bone healing.

A complete subscapularis release is usually all that is required to restore the normal soft-tissue tension of the anterior structures. If external rotation is still limited, then a medial transfer of the subscapularis insertion may be performed by repairing the subscapularis tendon to the humeral osteotomy at the completion of the procedure. This effectively further lengthens the subscapularis tendon. To further lengthen the subscapularis, a coronal Z-plasty lengthening has been described.[87,91] However, in revision cases the subscapularis is often atrophic and tissue quality is inadequate to permit a safe Z-plasty lengthening, unless the subscapularis was previously shortened (Putti-Platt).

After any necessary work is performed on the humerus, attention is turned toward the posterior inferior capsule. Exposure of the glenoid also provides access to this aspect of the capsule, which must be assessed and released in the stiff shoulder. A Fukuda ring retractor or bone hook is used to retract the humerus away from the glenoid, and a spiked, curved retractor is used to expose the anterior glenoid margin (Fig. 28-4B). With the inferior capsule exposed and

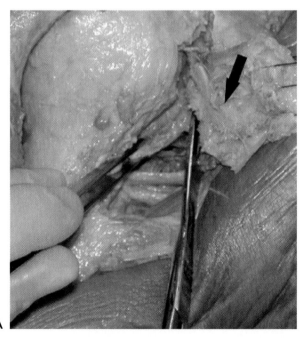
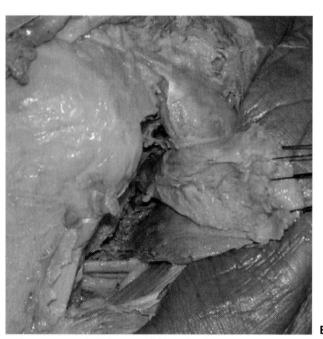

Figure 28-6   (A) Cadaveric example of technique for resection of the capsule from the undersurface of the subscapularis (black arrow). (B) Improved mobilization of the subscapularis noted.

axillary nerve protected, the inferior capsule is then incised with electrocautery. It is important during this procedure to place the arm in adduction and internal rotation, which allows the nerve to fall away from the glenoid rim. If the patient is not paralyzed, incising the capsule with electrocautery and observing for deltoid muscle contraction during release is also an indicator of nerve proximity. Similarly, the superior capsule is sharply dissected off the supraspinatus tendon, and the capsule is released.

With the humerus retracted posterior and lateral, the posterior capsule can now be evaluated. In most cases the posterior capsule will not be contracted but may be capacious secondary to posterior humeral subluxation. In this instance, inadvertently releasing the capsule can predispose to postoperative posterior instability. In general, posterior capsular redundancy is treated by releasing the tight anterior structures (i.e., 360-degree subscapularis release), effectively balancing the shoulder. However, in the stiff shoulder, posterior contracture may be present, and a final assessment can be made with the trial components in situ. At this point, any capsular contracture may be corrected with release, because severe stiffness may require global capsular release.

Rehabilitation

The postoperative management of patients after revision shoulder arthroplasty performed for stiffness is tailored specifically to the diagnosis and operative procedure. In this instance, immediate motion and stretching are instituted as the interscalene catheter allows pain-free motion. The only restriction is that external rotation is usually limited to 45 degrees for the first 6 weeks to protect the subscapularis repair. Patients remain in the hospital for 2 to 3 days for vigorous supervised physical therapy while the interscalene catheter provides pain relief. Patients must understand the importance of their postoperative rehabilitation program. Surgical release of the contracted tissues is only half of the battle, and all patients should be committed to their rehabilitation and understand their role in obtaining a successful outcome. After the patient is discharged from the hospital, he or she should have a supervised physical therapy session five times per week for the first 2 weeks, which is then reduced to three times per week. In addition, patients should perform the stretches they learn on their own four times per day. The therapy should be focused on vigorous stretches and range of motion in all planes, using pulleys, external rotation with a stick, and so forth. If patients are not diligent in their therapy, all the initial gains made in range of motion will be quickly lost.

THE UNSTABLE ARTHROPLASTY

Instability is one of the more common complications after shoulder arthroplasty with the reported prevalence ranging from 0% to 29%, with an overall average in the literature reported in one study at 2.8%.[37,38,50,75,90,106,112,115] Causes include bony insufficiency, malposition of components, and soft tissue deficiency. Once instability is addressed and corrected at surgery, a careful postoperative rehabilitation plan is critical to success.

Glenoid and Humeral Version

Excessive retroversion of the glenoid component with accompanying posterior instability is commonly a result of uncorrected posterior glenoid erosion. This is especially prevalent after arthroplasty for postcapsulorraphy arthritis, chronic posterior dislocations, or severe osteoarthritis. Humeral component malpositioning is less likely as a cause of instability, although it can occur[50,60,61,64,78,114] (Fig. 28-7). Anterior glenoid insufficiency is less common but may be seen in patients with chronic anterior dislocations or rheumatoid arthritis, or after glenoid fractures. Failure to correct this with placement of the glenoid in anteversion can lead to anterior instability.

Preoperative assessment of component position requires careful radiographs, although axillary radiographs may be misleading as to glenoid component version. Image intensification can be used to profile the humeral component, and simultaneous inspection of the forearm position allows estimation of humeral version. However, magnetic resonance scanning with special sequences is likely the most reliable imaging option for glenoid component version[102] (Fig. 28-8).

Intraoperative assessment at revision surgery of the glenoid component version requires adequate visualization. All overlying soft tissues and osteophytes are removed from the glenoid rim, allowing adequate exposure of the glenoid. By palpating the anterior glenoid neck and comparing intraoperative findings to preoperative imaging, one can estimate the version of the glenoid.

If there is substantial malposition of a well-fixed glenoid component, the component must be revised. Removing a solidly fixed glenoid component can be performed by first separating the glenoid face from the keel (or pegs) by using a sharp osteotome and then by removing the keel (or pegs) with osteotomes or a high-speed burr. If the native glenoid or remaining glenoid after component removal is maloriented (usually retroverted), then the prominent side (usually anterior rim) may be lowered with eccentric reaming. One must avoid the temptation of supporting a new glenoid component with asymmetric buildup of cement beneath the glenoid component. Over time, this will lead to cement fragmentation and glenoid component loosening. Eccentric reaming is performed by first initially lowering the high side using a high-speed burr and then drilling a centering hole to accommodate the glenoid reamer. The final glenoid version is then adjusted by reaming the "high" side until a concentric glenoid is established in the appropriate version (Fig. 28-9). Because the glenoid vault becomes shallow and narrow as one reams medially, high-side resection should be

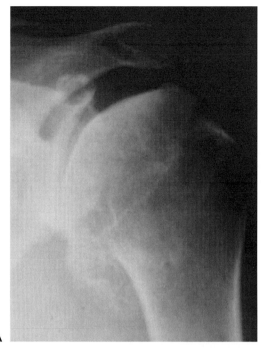

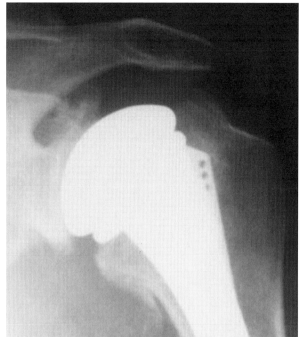

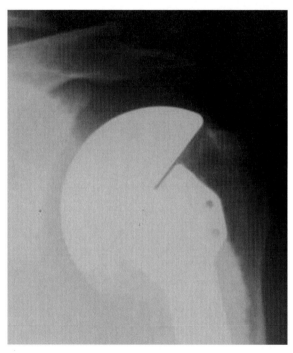

Figure 28-7 Serial radiographs demonstrating correction of malpositioning of the humeral component. *(A)* Initial AP radiograph demonstrating osteoarthritis. *(B)* Primary total shoulder arthroplasty (TSA) demonstrating a nonanatomic humeral component implanted in varus. *(C)* Revision shoulder arthroplasty demonstrating anatomic positioning of the humeral component. (Case courtesy of X. Duralde, M.D.).

limited to less than 1 cm. Also, at least some of the subchondral plate should be retained to support the component. If resection greater than 1 cm is required or cancellous bone starts to become exposed, mild retroversion (up to 10–15 degrees) may be accepted with a compensatory decrease in the retroversion of the humeral component. If there is less than 1 cm of glenoid bone stock available, the senior author does not resurface the glenoid.

In rare cases, the version cannot be corrected completely by eccentric reaming, and then bone grafting can be performed.[62,81,104] In revision cases, an iliac crest or allograft is usually required. In this situation, a contoured graft is ini-

tially held in place by temporary K-wire fixation and then definitively fixed with two 3.5-mm cortical screws. When placing the screws, one should take care to avoid interfering with the eventual position of the glenoid component. The finer details of bone grafting and assessing bony deficiency are covered in more depth in the chapter on bony deficits.

Soft Tissue Insufficiency and Difficulties

In some revision cases the subscapularis tendon may be absent or the tissue inadequate to permit a functional anterior soft tissue repair. These cases are commonly associated with

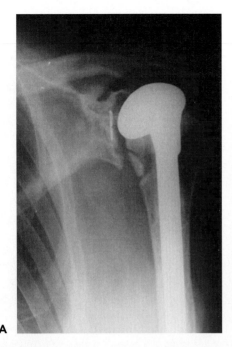

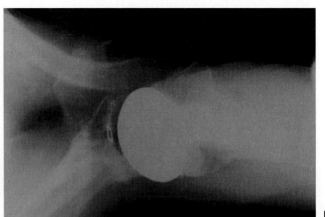

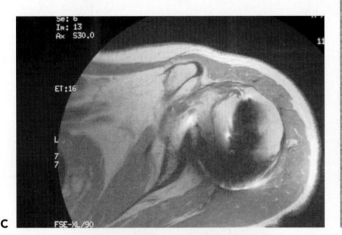

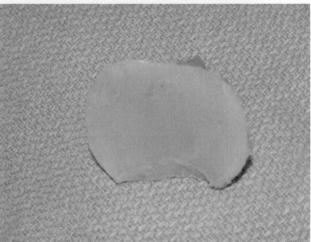

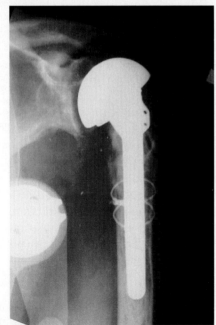

Figure 28-8 A 70-year-old man with pain 10 years after total shoulder arthroplasty (TSA). *(A,B)* Preoperative radiographs, anteroposterior (AP) and axillary views, show a well-fixed humeral component, but axillary suggests posterior subluxation of the humeral component. *(C)* Magnetic imaging resonance (MRI) shows more clearly the posterior subluxation. *(D)* Intraoperative picture of the glenoid component, showing significant posterior wear. *(E)* Postoperative AP radiograph. Cortical section of the humerus was removed to extract the humeral prosthesis and then replaced later with cerclage wires. Glenoid bone grafting was necessary to securely seat the glenoid component in the appropriate version.

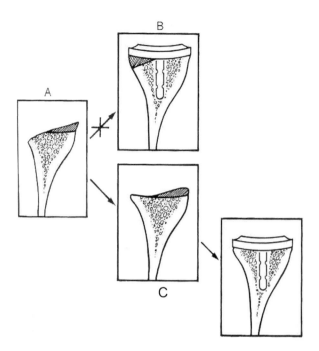

Figure 28-9 Diagrammatic representation of eccentric reaming. *(A)* Wear of the posterior glenoid is apparent and must be corrected. *(B)* Posterior glenoid deficiency should not be corrected by asymmetric cement buildup because this has a high risk of cement fragmentation and component loosening. *(C)* Alternatively, the "high" side should be eccentrically reamed allowing implantation of a glenoid component in the appropriate version. (Reprinted with permission: Shoulder and elbow arthroplasty. In: The shoulder. Lippincott, Williams & Wilkins.)

anterior instability.[50,61,64,78,112] Moeckel et al.[78] reported on the findings and results of reoperation in seven patients who developed anterior instability after arthroplasty. All seven were found to have a disruption of the sutured subscapularis tendon, which was then repaired. Three patients had a recurrence of the anterior instability, which was subsequently addressed with a bone-Achilles tendon allograft. In addition to allograft, for subscapularis tendon insufficiency, a pectoralis major transfer can also be performed to replace the function of the subscapularis tendon.[94,116] Although several variations are possible, the senior author prefers to transfer the sternocostal head of the pectoralis major tendon deep to the conjoined tendon, accurately reproducing the orientation of the subscapularis tendon.[71] In addition, transferring the sternocostal head superficial to the musculocutaneous nerve (but deep to the conjoint tendon) decreases the tension on the musculocutaneous nerve after transfer.[71] This minimizes the potential risk of nerve injury. During transfer it is important to carefully identify and visualize the musculocutaneous nerve to ensure that excessive tension is not created in the nerve. Occasionally, the proximal branches of the musculocutaneous nerve must be released to decrease the tension in the musculocutaneous nerve proper.[71] In some cases, altering of the humeral component version may also be necessary. A slight increase in the humeral component retroversion may help to prevent

anterior dislocation. Anterior placement of the humeral head on the shaft or an oversized component can further stress the anterior stability as well as the subscapularis repair. Rotating an offset humeral head to a more posterior position can help avoid anterior instability to some extent.

Large rotator cuff tears can lead to superior humeral head migration and instability. The rotator cuff functions as a humeral head stabilizer, and when it fails, the elevation of the extremity results in superior subluxation of the humeral component. If a tear is present, it should be mobilized and repaired using extracapsular and intracapsular releases as necessary. As a rule, the coracoacromial arch should be preserved because it provides the final restraint to anterior-superior migration of the humeral head in the rotator cuff-deficient shoulder.[40–44,89] The posterior capsule and posterior rotator cuff tendons provide the major restraints to posterior subluxation[84]; thus, a careful assessment should be made of the posterior aspect of the rotator cuff. If rotator cuff repair is not achievable, then consideration should be given at the time of revision surgery to concomitant latissimus dorsi and/or teres major transfer to recreate the abduction and external rotation moment of the posterior rotator cuff.[32,49,51,109,110] It is important to remember that in cases of unreconstructable rotator cuff deficiency, glenoid component implantation should be avoided because of the high risk of glenoid loosening.[2,13]

The surgeon and patient should always realize that when either a pectoralis major or latissimus dorsi transfer is performed, the goal of surgery is not strength, but stability of the prosthetic joint. In rare instances, despite tendon transfer and well-positioned prosthetic components, prosthetic instability may still persist. If there is still a significant soft tissue deficit, most commonly the anterior capsular tissues, consideration should be given to further reconstruction of the soft tissue envelope.[78] Reconstruction can be approached with a variety of methods, including autografts, allografts (e.g., Achilles tendon), and ligament xenografts (e.g., porcine submucosa). The use of an Achilles allograft has been reported for anterior or anterior-superior reconstructions in the case of a deficient coracoacromial ligament.[112] The coracoacromial arch can also be reconstructed by using a strip of the conjoined tendon. Wirth and Rockwood[114] reported using a 0.5 × 3 cm strip that was proximally based at its origin on the coracoid and mobilized in a proximal direction, securing the free distal end to the anterolateral aspect of the acromion.

In contrast with soft tissue deficiency, instability may also be the result of asymmetric soft tissue balancing. Most commonly this is seen in the patient with restricted external rotation and a tight, contracted anterior soft tissue envelope. The posterior capsule is stretched and has an increased volume leading to posterior instability. In this situation, the subscapularis and capsule are released as described in the section on capsular release for stiffness. The upper portion of the pectoralis major may also need to be released from its humeral insertion.[114] The final step is to assess the glenohumeral stability after trial component reduction and perform a posterior capsulorrhaphy if posterior instability still persists despite proper component positioning.

Inability to restore the resting tension in the deltoid will render it ineffective and can lead to weakness during elevation, inability to raise the arm above the horizontal level, and inferior instability. This most commonly occurs as a complication of treatment for proximal humerus fractures. Severe comminution can distort the proximal humeral anatomy, and subsequent determination of the true proximal humeral length becomes difficult. Achieving sufficient humeral component height is essential to restoring the proper resting tension of the deltoid.[82,114] If inferior instability becomes problematic, revision surgery should focus on restoration of the anatomic humeral length to restore the resting length of the deltoid and rotator cuff.

Postoperative Treatment

The final step in restoring stability is a carefully directed rehabilitative program. The choice of brace should be directed toward the direction of the preoperative instability because the brace will maintain the upper extremity in a "safe" position. The postoperative therapy should be adjusted as well in an effort to preserve stability, but also prevent stiffness. This requires close and frequent communication with the therapist and the commitment of the patient to cooperate with the postoperative bracing and therapy. An uncooperative patient or overzealous therapist may easily negate even the best surgical results.

THE LOOSE ARTHROPLASTY

Symptomatic loosening of the glenoid and humeral components after a total shoulder arthroplasty is common and has been reported to account for approximately one-third of all complications that are associated with total shoulder arthroplasty.[4,6,13,17,19,21,27,35,36,54,59,64,69,76,78,80,82,86,88,90,95,105,109] Glenoid component loosening after total shoulder arthroplasty occurs more frequently than aseptic humeral component loosening.[59] However, aseptic loosening of an uncemented humeral component has been reported.[70] Radiographic evidence of loosening often occurs in the absence of clinical symptoms; therefore, pain in association with radiographic evidence of loosening or migration of the component is the indication for revision.

Evaluation of Loosening

Evidence of radiographic loosening has been reported in 12% to 94% of glenoid components.[6,8,13,24,25,82] Early glenoid loosening can be caused by unequal stress distribution because of abnormal migration of the humeral

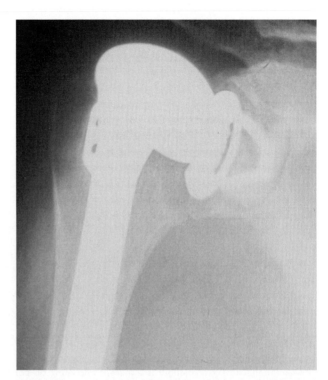

Figure 28-10 Anteroposterior (AP) radiograph demonstrating proud placement of the humeral component, which led to eccentric superior loading and loosening of the glenoid component.

component as occurs with rotator cuff deficiency[45] or shoulder instability[6,31,46,59,89,105] (Fig. 28-10). Other possible causes for early loosening include prosthetic design (i.e., metal backed),[11] infection, inadequate bone stock, or poor fixation to bone.[13]

Immediate postoperative radiolucent lines around the glenoid component (up to 94%) may indicate inadequate immediate fixation resulting from the surgical technique.[117] However, although several studies have a reported a high incidence of radiolucent lines, direct correlation to symptomatic loosening has not been found. Furthermore, the exact significance of the size and location of the radiolucent lines has not been found. A lucent line that is progressive in extent around the perimeter of the component or one that is seen to widen on serial radiographs should cause more concern for true loosening. Lucent lines that progress or exceed 1.5 to 2 mm in width appear to be of more significance for true, symptomatic loosening.[15,96] Of course, any translation of the glenoid component (i.e., shifting or tilting) or overall displacement of the component is a clear indication of component loosening. Recently the senior author has reported that new, instrumented cement pressurization techniques can reduce the incidence of immediate glenoid radiolucent line formation.[20]

Much less information is available on humeral radiolucent lines and overall radiographic assessment of the humeral component fixation. Even less information has been reported on the treatment of the loosened humeral component. This is primarily because mechanical failure of the humeral component after shoulder arthroplasty is uncommon.[70] Some reported values are as low as 0.3% to 0.6%.[29] When aseptic loosening occurs, it is primarily in humeral stems that have been press-fit, but it can also occur because of polyethylene debris-associated osteolysis or after a humeral shaft fracture.[29] However, radiographic changes at the implant-bone interface are occasionally noticed and do raise the concern for future implant failure.[25,107] Neer et al. and other investigators indicated that radiographic evaluations in the short- and intermediate-term follow-up studies have revealed a small but definite prevalence of implant subsidence or complete radiolucent lines.[6,13,25,28,82] Radiolucent lines have been reported more frequently around uncemented humeral components.[6,7,13,25,28,54,82] In a recent study, Sanchez-Sotelo et al.[96] defined the "at risk" humeral component to be a component in which two of three observers identified tilt or subsidence or a radiolucent line 2 mm or greater in width was present in three or more zones. In general, any component with subsidence or shift in position is typically deemed to be loose. Endosteal erosions, which are localized areas of bone resorption around the implant or bone-cement interface, are also evidence of component loosening. In their study they showed that cemented humeral components exhibited superior radiographic behavior in relation to component fixation, relative to ingrowth fixation and particularly press-fit fixation.[96,97,100] They also found a much higher rate of radiolucent lines around humeral components in the total shoulder arthroplasties versus the hemiarthroplasties, 13 of 20 versus 3 of 23, respectively. This was attributed to polyethylene particles that resulted from wear of the glenoid component; however, the exact role that glenoid wear debris plays in humeral periprosthetic changes is still unclear.[96] However, Matsen et al.[74] more recently reported on the outcomes of press-fit fixation of humeral components with a tapered metaphyseal segment. They found results comparable to cemented components, with no component showing shift or subsidence and only 11 of 127 had radiolucencies greater than or equal to 1 mm in width. The prevalence of radiolucencies did not differ between patients with hemiarthroplasty versus total shoulder arthroplasty.[74]

Component Removal

The final diagnosis of loosening is made intraoperatively. As stated earlier, the senior author does not routinely perform arthroscopy before revision shoulder arthroplasty, but it may be of significant help when performed to definitively diagnose glenoid loosening.[58,108] However, it is not particularly helpful in the evaluation of humeral stem loosening. After joint dislocation in the open cases, the humeral shaft and prosthesis are evaluated, and the necessity of component revision is assessed. Initially, the fibrous soft tissues must be circumferentially removed from the proximal cement-bone or prosthesis-bone interface, and micromotion around the

humeral implant is evaluated. Infection should be suspected preoperatively in the work-up for the failed arthroplasty, especially if component loosening is seen in the first 10 years after replacement. If the preoperative evaluation for infection was negative, intraoperative cultures, stat Gram stain, and frozen section should also be performed before continuing on with the revision arthroplasty. Removal of the loose humeral implant should not be difficult; however, if any resistance is met, similar techniques as described for removal of a well-fixed implant should be used.

In patients with suspected loose glenoid components, the soft tissues are first removed to allow evaluation of the cement-bone interface. In contrast with glenoid revision for arthrosis, glenoid revision surgery for glenoid component loosening is commonly associated with osteolysis and significant bone loss.[73] Thus, if there is any resistance at all to any aspect of glenoid removal, care should again be taken as if removing a solidly fixed glenoid implant. Cutting the component into pieces may allow safer removal with less damage to the glenoid vault. Speedy and careless removal of implants can lead to catastrophic bone loss, greater than what may already be present.

Total Shoulder Revision Versus Conversion to Hemiarthroplasty

Often, after component removal, there may be a rather sizable defect in the glenoid (Fig. 28-11). If glenoid bone loss is severe, especially when there is medialization of the glenoid, component implantation may be impossible. In general, placement of a new component is preferable and should be attempted if enough bone remains to support a glenoid component. However, simple removal of the loose implant with cancellous bone grafting of the defect may result in satisfactory pain relief.[58,66,87,110] Grafting the defect reinforces the glenoid to articulate with the humeral component, and with graft incorporation, a second-stage glenoid reconstruction may be performed.[2] Because every glenoid loosening pattern and bony loss pattern is different, there is no clear answer as to what approach is best. Cofield et al.[29] stated that approximately half of the cases that have been reported have had a new glenoid replaced and half have had the loosened glenoid component removed and left as is or restored with some bone grafting. Again, in cases of an unreconstructable rotator cuff deficiency, glenoid component implantation should be avoided, and the shoulder should be revised to a hemiarthroplasty.[13,40]

Particulate Debris

Polyethylene wear debris is a difficult problem that has been rarely reported on in association with total shoulder prostheses.[70,117] The capacity of wear debris to induce macrophage and giant cell-mediated osteolysis of periprosthetic bone has been well documented in association

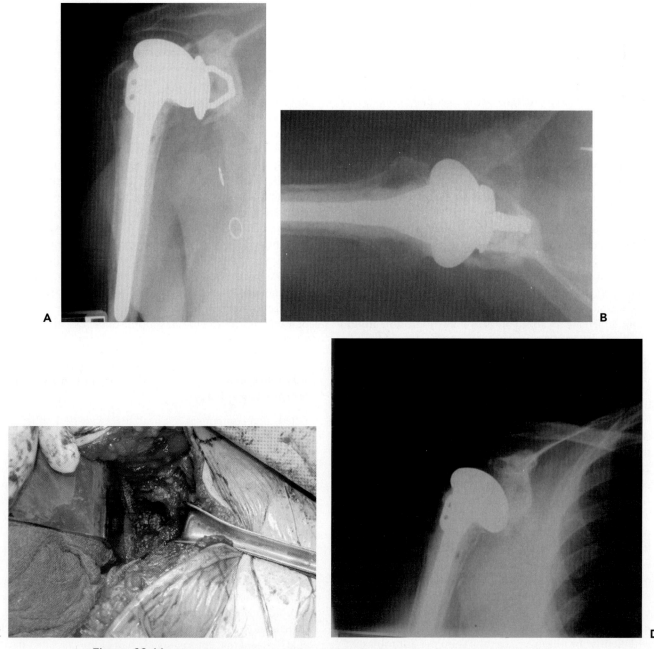

Figure 28-11 *(A,B)* Anteroposterior (AP) and axillary radiographs of a painful total shoulder arthroplasty (TSA) with a loose glenoid component. *(C)* Intraoperative picture of large glenoid defect after component removal. Defect was bone-grafted, but a new component was unable to be placed. *(D)* Postoperative AP radiograph after the TSA was converted to an HHR.

with aseptic loosening of total hip and knee prostheses.[56,63,65,67,82,98] A recent study by Wirth et al.[117] looked at the characterization of polyethylene wear debris associated with osteolysis after total shoulder arthroplasty. Specimens obtained from the vicinity of the osteolytic lesions demonstrated dense fibrous tissue with foci of intense histiocytic infiltration, foreign-body giant cells, and foamy macrophages. No acute inflammatory changes were seen. At the time of surgery, they found that the components were easy to remove and that fibrous membranes were found in the humeral canal, proximal humerus, and glenoid cavity.

These fibrous membranes are soft, but can be thick, and are less mechanically stable; thus loosening can occur. All the glenoid components had obvious signs of wear and delamination. On the glenoid component, the cement was mainly attached to the keel, although some cement remained in the glenoid trough. Overall, they found that the wear particles in the shoulder tended to be bigger and more fibrillar than those from hips, suggesting different wear mechanisms. They thought that the wear particles were indeed associated with the progressive periprosthetic osteolysis and subsequent aseptic loosening of the components.

INFECTION

Infection after shoulder arthroplasty remains one of the most devastating complications that necessitates revision surgery.[102] The prevalence of deep periprosthetic infection involving shoulder arthroplasty has been reported to be between 0% and 3.9% for unconstrained shoulder arthroplasties.[28] Unlike the hip and knee infection literature, which is more extensive with detailed algorithms, there are much less data to guide clinical decision making in the infected shoulder arthroplasty. Thus, successful management can be a challenge. Treatment possibilities include antibiotic suppression, debridement with prosthesis retention, direct exchange, delayed reimplantation, resection arthroplasty, arthrodesis, and amputation.[23,28,80,114]

Antibiotic Suppression

Glenohumeral infection has been found to be associated with rheumatoid arthritis, diabetes mellitus, advanced age, remote sites of infection, malnutrition, and immunosuppressive chemotherapy.[5,114] Infection after joint arthroplasty has been associated with diabetes and chronic disease.[48] Sperling et al.[102] recently reported on 33 patients with an infected glenohumeral arthroplasty, in which 20 of 33 patients were found to have at least one risk factor for infection including chronic disease. Therefore, this is often not a very healthy population, and unless the patient is septic, undergoing another large surgical procedure may not always be the best treatment. These situations are indeed rare, because there are few reports in the literature on the treatment of acute septic joint arthroplasties with intravenous antibiotics alone.[10] Suppression is an option when the patient is very sick, has minimal pain, or is not septic with a very localized infection.

Surgical Intervention

Surgery for infection requires special consideration. Intraoperatively, cultures should be repeated and tissue is sent to pathology for frozen sectioning before the administration of intravenous antibiotics. If there are a significant number of white blood cells on intraoperative frozen section, then infection should be strongly considered. Polymerase chain reaction may hold promise in occult detection of infectious organisms.[45] However, widespread use in the shoulder literature has yet to be reported.

Irrigation and Debridement

If the diagnosis is made early and the organism is highly sensitive to antibiotics, then debridement alone by arthroscopic or open means may be considered, particularly in an elderly patient. An infection is generally considered acute when it is discovered within 4 to 6 weeks after the surgical procedure. Thus, very acute infections may sometimes be eradicated with immediate and aggressive irrigation and debridement; however, some do believe that any evidence of chronicity necessitates component removal.[15] The more virulent gram-negative organisms may not become clinically apparent as rapidly as the more common gram-positive organisms, and these also need more than just irrigation and debridement. Sperling et al.[102] reported their experience with six infections in which debridement and prosthesis retainment were performed, and the results were poor. Three of the six patients had reinfection, requiring subsequent component removal. Sperling and colleagues believed that debridement with retainment of the prosthesis should be reserved for the patients with an acute infection within the first month after arthroplasty or in the patient with an acute hematogenous infection of an otherwise well-functioning and fixed prosthesis. Although debridement can be performed arthroscopically, there are little data evaluating the overall efficacy of this technique.

Immediate Exchange and Reimplantation

Immediate reimplantation may be considered after debridement and implant removal if the infection has been caused by a low-virulence organism.[23] Some surgeons do recommend this treatment in the acute phase for gram-positive infections; however, there are many who believe that a more conservative approach with a two-stage reimplantation after 6 weeks of intravenous antibiotics is more appropriate.[6,12,14,16] Sperling et al.[102] reported on two patients in whom immediate reimplantation was performed, and one subsequently required a resection arthroplasty at 9 months. Antibiotic impregnated cement used for prosthetic fixation has been shown to decrease the recurrence of deep infection[55]; however, further investigation is needed to determine the efficacy of this in preventing reinfection in shoulder arthroplasty.

Staged Implantation

In cases of acute infection secondary to high-virulence organisms, or in late infections, a two-stage reimplantation provides the most consistent results with long-term infection-free survival[93,99] (Fig. 28-12). It is generally agreed on that retainment of the prosthesis in these situations is not possible, and removal of both the prosthesis and cement mantle, combined with joint debridement, drainage, and intravenous antibiotics, is necessary.[6,14,93] This has become the accepted method of management for selected joints such as the hip and knee.[48,55] However, in this situation in the shoulder, the soft tissue sleeve can become very deficient and contracted over time. This can lead to poor functional recovery and a continued low level of pain, leading some to recommend resection arthroplasty instead.[15] Thus, at the time of debridement, an attempt should be made to reapproximate cuff tendons to their physiologic length.[15] In addition to the local delivery of antibiotics, placement of an antibiotic cement spacer will help to maintain a

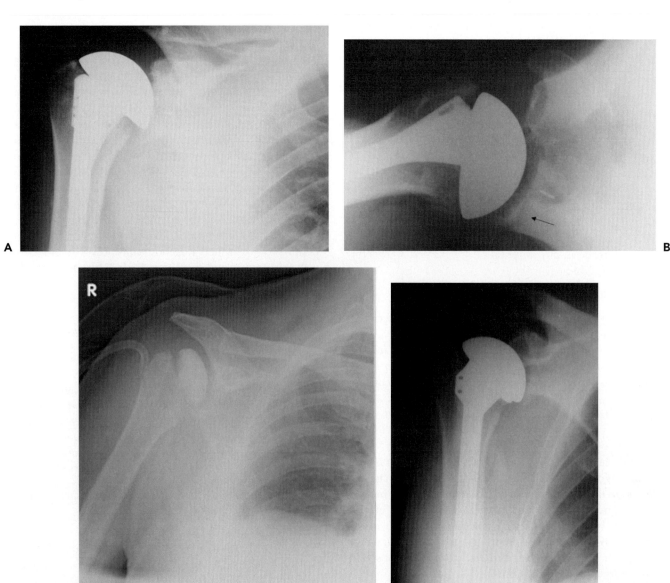

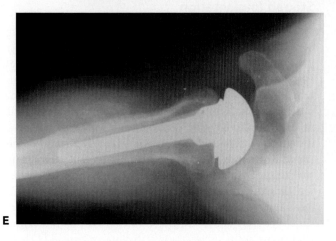

Figure 28-12 *(A,B)* A 62-year-old man with continued severe pain 6 months after total shoulder arthroplasty (TSA). Anteroposterior (AP) and axillary radiographs are shown. Note the radiolucency *(arrows)* around the glenoid component. However, the treating surgeon did not recognize that the glenoid loosening was the result of infection and reoperated only to remove the glenoid component. When pain continued, a second opinion was sought; indium white blood cell scans and laboratory work raised the strong suspicion for infection, and staged reimplantation was performed. Cultures were taken at the implant removal, which grew *Staphylococcus aureus*. *(C)* A cement spacer was placed, and intravenous antibiotics were administered for 6 weeks. *(D,E)* Patient returned for a humeral head reimplantation only, because the rotator cuff and glenoid bone stock were subsequently insufficient for glenoid replacement. AP and axillary views are shown.

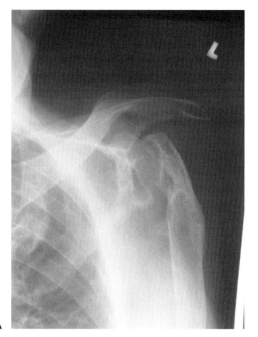

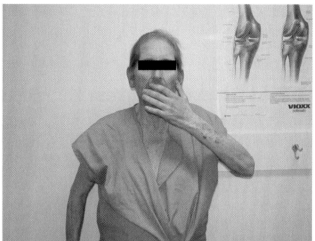

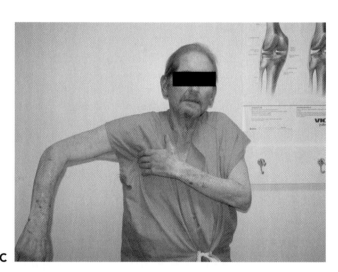

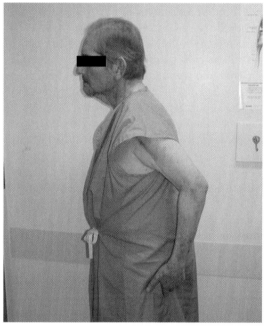

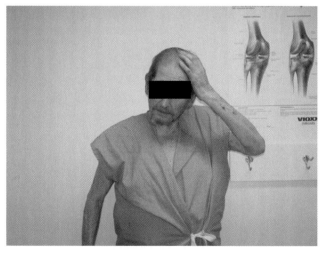

Figure 28-13 A 68-year-old man 1 year after resection arthroplasty for an infected total shoulder arthroplasty (TSA). The patient was not interested in undergoing reimplantation. Subsequently, he has good pain relief and is able to perform his basic activities of daily living. *(A)* AP radiograph after resection of components. Patient is able to reach his mouth *(B)*, opposite axilla *(C)*, back pocket *(D)*, and head *(E)*.

functional soft tissue envelope for later reconstruction and prevent soft tissue and capsular contraction.[93] Surgery should include aggressive debridement and removal of all infected tissues, extraction of all cement and particulate debris, removal of prosthetic components, and curettage and reaming of the intramedullary canal and glenoid. The antibiotic cement spacer (Palacos; Biomet, Warsaw, IN) is then fashioned in the shape of the humeral head, providing concentrated local antibiotics and maintaining the tension of the soft tissue envelope.[93,99] Patients are placed on a minimum of 6 weeks of antibiotic therapy adjusted according to the virulence of the organism. Postoperatively, in addition to clinical evaluation, the erythrocyte sedimentation rate, C-reactive protein, and white blood cell count are followed. At reimplantation, cultures of tissues should be repeated including an intraoperative frozen section to confirm resolution of infection. The standard techniques of revision are then undertaken if the infection appears to be eradicated.

There have been several authors reporting successful results and advocating a two-stage reimplantation,[1,7,14,18,28,52,101] and there are several who believe it offers better functional results than resection arthroplasty.[93,102] Codd et al.[23] reported on four staged reimplantations and believed that these patients had a better outcome and function than those who underwent resection arthroplasty. Sperling et al.[102] reported on three patients who underwent delayed implantation and had two good functional results and one fair result in a patient who underwent a custom prosthesis. However, there were no reinfections or reoperations in this group, and all had adequate pain relief. They believe that delayed reimplantation may offer the best hope for pain relief, eradication of infection, and maintenance of shoulder function. Seitz and Damacen[99] reported on eight patients who underwent staged implantation 6 months after debridement, cement spacer, and 3 months of antibiotics. All experienced pain relief and moderate functional improvement.

However, careful consideration must be given to the effect of the infection and subsequent resection on the soft tissue and bone stock present when determining the feasibility of performing a reimplantation. Persistent or refractory infections, serious medical conditions, significant bone stock deficiency, and inadequate soft tissue about the shoulder including the rotator cuff and deltoid may preclude reimplantation.[102]

Resection Arthroplasty

As stated previously, there are many situations in which resection arthroplasty should be considered, especially in the elderly, in low-demand patients with intractable infection, and in cases of significant rotator cuff loss.[15,80] In the literature, resection arthroplasty has been reported to have mixed results in regard to pain relief. Some have reported relief in only 50% to 66% of patients,[26] whereas others report relief in 80% to 100% of patients.[15] Some investigators believe

that even when infection is controlled, shoulder function is severely limited in addition to the variable pain relief.[74] However, Brems[15] reported that functional recovery is largely dependent on the patient, and that a well-structured, supine, eccentric deltoid muscle-strengthening program can give good functional results. Sperling et al.[102] reported on 11 resection arthroplasties, of which 7 received pain relief, 8 of 10 had fair/poor strength, and 8 of 11 overall had an unsuccessful clinical grade. They found a high reinfection rate and complication rate. Overall, they found that pain relief was satisfactory, but that function was quite limited. Attempting to perform revision surgery some months after resection arthroplasty can be very difficult and challenging, leading Sperling et al. to recommend delayed reimplantation as the initial treatment. Overall, it is the authors' view that there are certain scenarios in which patients will benefit from resection arthroplasty and achieve pain relief and the function that they need for their daily needs (Fig. 28-13).

CONCLUSION

Revision total shoulder arthroplasty performed for the failed primary arthroplasty remains a technically demanding procedure. Despite recent advances in component design, total shoulder arthroplasty will continue to have a finite life span necessitating revision procedures. It is a challenge to the orthopedic shoulder surgeon to adequately address all the components of revision surgery to optimize the potential for a satisfactory result. Although pain relief can be frequently achieved, range of motion, strength, and function are commonly compromised, emphasizing the importance of both patient education and patient selection.

REFERENCES

1. Amstutz HC, Thomas BJ, Kabo BJ, et al. The DANA total shoulder arthroplasty. J Bone Joint Surg Am 1988;70A:1174.
2. Antuna SA, Sperling JW, Cofield RH, et al. Glenoid revision surgery after total shoulder arthroplasty. J Shoulder Elbow Surg 2001;10:217.
3. Arroyo JS, Marra G, Pollock RG, et al. Revision of modular humeral components. J Shoulder Elbow Surg 1999;8:188.
4. Averill RM, Sledge CB, Thomas WH. Neer total shoulder arthroplasty. Orthop Trans 1980;4:287.
5. Bade HA, Warren RF, Ranawat CS, et al. Long term results of Neer total shoulder replacement. In: Bateman JE, ed. Surgery of the shoulder. St. Louis, MO, CV Mosby, 1984:294.
6. Barrett WP, Franklin JL, Jackens SE, et al. Total shoulder arthroplasty. J Bone Joint Surg 1987;69A:865.
7. Barrett WP, Thornhill TS, Thomas WH, et al. Nonconstrained total shoulder arthroplasty in patients with polyarticular rheumatoid arthritis. J Arthroplasty 1989;4:91.
8. Bell SN, Gschwend N. Clinical experience with total arthroplasty and hemiarthroplasty of the shoulder using the Neer prosthesis. Int Orthop 1986;10(4):217.
9. Bigliani LU, Codd TP, Duralde XA, et al. Intermittent interscalene catheter in resistant stiff or frozen shoulder as an adjunct for postoperative shoulder physical therapy with long term results. Orthop Trans 1994;18:659.
10. Bodey WN, Yeoman PM. Prosthetic arthroplasty of the shoulder. Acta Orthop Scand 1983;54:900.

11. Boileau P, et al. Polyethylene versus metal-backed glenoid components in total shoulder arthroplasty: a prospective randomized study. Presented at the American Academy of Orthopaedic Surgeons, Shoulder and Elbow Specialty Day. Dallas, TX, 2002.
12. Bonutti PM, Hawkins RJ. Component loosening following total shoulder arthroplasty. Orthop Trans 1990;14:254.
13. Boyd AD Jr, Thomas WH, Scott RD, et al. Total shoulder arthroplasty versus hemiarthroplasty. Indications for glenoid resurfacing. J Arthroplasty 1990;5:329.
14. Boyd AD, Thomas WH, Sledge CD, et al. Failed shoulder arthroplasty. Orthop Trans 1990;14:255.
15. Brems J. The glenoid component in total shoulder arthroplasty. J Shoulder Elbow Surg 1993;2:47.
16. Brems JJ, Wilde AH, Borden LS, et al. Glenoid lucent lines. Orthop Trans 1986;10:231.
17. Brostorm LA, Kronberg M, Wallensten R. Should the glenoid be replaced in shoulder arthroplasty with an unconstrained Dana or St. George prosthesis? Ann Chir Gynaecol 1992;81:54.
18. Brownlee RC, Cofield RH. Shoulder replacement in cuff tear arthropathy. Orthop Trans 1986;10:230.
19. Brumfield RH Jr., Schilz J, Flinders BW. Total shoulder replacement arthroplasty: a clinical review of 21 cases. Orthop Trans 1981;5:398.
20. Chiang AS, Klepps S, Miller S, et al. Incidence of immediate radiolucent glenoid lines in patients undergoing total shoulder replacement. Submitted 2002.
21. Clayton ML, Ferlic DC, Jeffers PD. Prosthetic arthroplasties of the shoulder. Clin Orthop 1982;164:184.
22. Codd TP, Duralde XA, Brown AR, et al. Indwelling interscalene catheter for post-arthroscopy shoulder physical therapy. Arthroscopy 1994;10:354.
23. Codd TP, Yamaguchi K, Flatow EL. Infected shoulder arthroplasties: treatment with staged reimplantation versus resection arthroplasty. Orthop Trans 1996/1997;20:59.
24. Cofield RH. Total joint arthroplasty. The shoulder. Mayo Clin Proc 1979;54(8): 500.
25. Cofield RH. Total shoulder arthroplasty with the Neer prosthesis. J Bone Joint Surg Am 1984;66(6):899.
26. Cofield RH. Shoulder arthrodesis and resection arthroplasty. Instr Course Lect 1985;34:268.
27. Cofield RH, Daly PJ. Total shoulder arthroplasty with a tissue-ingrowth glenoid component. J Shoulder Elbow Surg 1992;1:77.
28. Cofield RH, Edgerton BC. Total shoulder arthroplasty: complications and revision surgery. Instr Course Lect 1990;39:449.
29. Cofield RH, Chang W, Sperling JW. Complications of shoulder arthroplasty. In: Iannotti JP, Williams GR, eds. Disorders of the shoulder: diagnosis and management. Philadelphia, PA, Lippincott Williams & Wilkins, 1999.
30. Cohen NP, Levine WN, Marra G, et al. Indwelling interscalene catheter anesthesia in the surgical management of stiff shoulder: a report of 100 consecutive cases. J Shoulder Elbow Surg 2000;9:268.
31. Collins D, Tencer A, Sidles J, et al. Edge displacement and deformation of glenoid components in response to eccentric loading. J Bone Joint Surg 1992;74A:501.
32. Combes JM, Mansat M. Lambeau de muscle grand rond dans les ruptures massives de la coiffe des rotateurs. Etude experimente. In: Bonnel F, Blotman F, Mansat M, eds. L'epaule. L'epaule degenerative, L'epaule traumatique, L'epaule du sportif. Paris, Springer-Verlag, 1993:318.
33. Connor PM, Levine WN, Arroyo JS, et al. The surgical management of failed shoulder arthroplasty. Orthop Trans 1997;27:6.
34. Deutsch A, Kelly II J, Williams GR. Diagnosis and management of glenoid loosening after total shoulder arthroplasty: clinical results of 32 patients. Proceedings of the 68th Annual Meeting of the American Academy of Orthopaedic Surgeons. 2001;2:647.
35. Faludi DD, Weiland AJ. Cementless total shoulder arthroplasty: preliminary experience with thirteen cases. Orthopedics 1983; 6:428.
36. Fenlin JM Jr. Total glenohumeral joint replacement. Orthop Clin North Am 1975;67:565.
37. Field LD, Dines DM, Zabinski SJ, et al. Hemiarthroplasty of the shoulder for rotator cuff arthropathy. J Shoulder Elbow Surg 1997;6:18.
38. Figgie MP, Inglis AE, Figgie HE III, et al. Custom total shoulder arthroplasty in inflammatory arthritis. Preliminary results. J Arthroplasty 1992;7:1.
39. Flatow EL, Bigliani LU. Locating and protecting the axillary nerve in shoulder surgery: the tug test. Orthop Rev 1992;21:503.
40. Flatow EL, Connor PD, Levine WN, et al. Coracoacromial arch reconstruction for anterosuperior subluxation after failed rotator cuff surgery: a preliminary report. J Shoulder Elbow Surg 1997; 6:228.
41. Flatow EL, Pollock RG, Bigliani LU. Coracoacromial ligament preservation in rotator cuff surgery. Tech Orthop 1994;9:97.
42. Flatow EL, Soslowsky LJ, Ticker JB, et al. Exclusion of the rotator cuff under the acromion: patterns of subacromial contact. Am J Sports Med 1994;22:779.
43. Flatow EL, Wang VM, Kelkar R, et al. The coracoacromial ligament passively restrains anterosuperior humeral subluxation in the rotator cuff deficient shoulder. Orthop Trans 1996;21:229.
44. Flatow EL, Weinstein DM, Duralde XA, et al. Coracoacromial ligament preservation in rotator cuff surgery. J Shoulder Elbow Surg 1994;3:S73.
45. Franklin JL, Barrett WP, Jackins SE, et al. Glenoid loosening in total shoulder arthroplasty. Association with rotator cuff deficiency. J Arthroplasty 1988;3(1):39.
46. Frich LH, Sojbjerg JO, Sneppen O. Shoulder arthroplasty in complex acute and chronic proximal humeral fractures. Orthopaedics 1991;14:949.
47. Friedman RJ, Hawthorne KB, Genez BM. The use of computerized tomography in the measurement of glenoid version. J Bone Joint Surg Am 1992;74:1032.
48. Garvin KL, Hanssen AD. Infection after total hip arthroplasty. J Bone Joint Surg 1995;77A:1576.
49. Gerber C. Latissimus dorsi transfer for the treatment of irreparable tears of the rotator cuff. Clin Orthop 1992;275:152.
50. Gerber A, Ghalambor N, Warner JJ. Instability of shoulder arthroplasty: balancing mobility and stability. Orthop Clin North Am 2001;32:661.
51. Gerber C, Vinh TS, Hertel R, et al. Latissimus dorsi transfer for the treatment of massive tears of the rotator cuff. Preliminary report. Clin Orthop 1988;232:31.
52. Goss TP. Shoulder infections. In: Bigliani LU, ed. Complications of shoulder surgery. Baltimore, MD, Williams and Wilkins, 1993:202.
53. Green A, Norris TR. Imaging techniques for glenohumeral arthritis and glenohumeral arthroplasty. Clin Orthop 1994;307:7.
54. Gristina AG, Romano RL, Kammire GC, et al. Total shoulder replacement. Orthop Clin North Am 1987;18:445.
55. Hanssen AD, Rand JA, Osmon DR. Treatment of the infected total knee arthroplasty with insertion of another prosthesis: the effect of antibiotic-impregnated bone cement. Clin Orthop 1994;309:44.
56. Harris WH, Schiller AL, Scholler JM, et al. Extensive localized bone resorption in the femur following total hip replacement. J Bone Joint Surg 1976;58A:612.
57. Harryman DT. Shoulders: frozen and stiff. Instr Course Lect 1993;42:247.
58. Hasan SS, Leith JM, Kapil, et al. Characteristics of 141 unsatisfactory shoulder arthroplasties. Proceedings of the 68th Annual Meeting of the American Academy of Orthopaedic Surgeons 2001;2:647.
59. Hawkins JR, Bell RH, Jallay B. Total shoulder arthroplasty. Clin Orthop 1989;242:188.
60. Hawkins RJ, Greis PE, Bonutti PM. Treatment of symptomatic glenoid loosening following unconstrained shoulder arthroplasty. Orthopedics 1999;22:229.
61. Hennigan SP, Iannotti JP. Instability after prosthetic arthroplasty of the shoulder. Orthop Clin North Am 2001;32:649.
62. Hill JM, Norris TR. Long-term results of total shoulder arthroplasty following bone-grafting of the glenoid. J Bone Joint Surg Am 2001;83:877.
63. Isaac GH, Wroblewski BM, Atkinson JR, et al. A tribiological study of retrieved hip prostheses. Clin Orthop 1992;276:115.
64. Jahnke AH Jr., Hawkins RJ. Instability after shoulder arthroplasty: causative factors and treatment options. Semin Arthroplasty 1995;6:289.

65. Jasty MJ, Floyd WE III, Schiller AL, et al. Localized osteolysis in stable, non-septic total hip replacement. J Bone Joint Surg 1986;68A:912.

66. Jensen KL, Toro P, Wirth MA, et al. Salvage of failed glenoid components: conversion to hemiarthroplasty. Proceedings of the 66th Annual Meeting of the American Academy of Orthopaedic Surgeons 1999;39.

67. Karduna AR, Williams GR, Williams JL, et al. Kinematics of the glenohumeral joint before and after total shoulder arthroplasty: effects of component conformity. Trans Orthop Res Soc 1996;21:700.

68. Kelleher IM, Cofield RH, Becker DA, et al. Fluoroscopically positioned radiographs of total shoulder arthroplasty. J Shoulder Elbow Surg 1992;1:306.

69. Kelly IG, Foster RS, Fisher WD. Neer total shoulder replacement in rheumatoid arthritis. J Bone Joint Surg 1987;69B:723.

70. Klemkiewicz JJ, Iannotti JP, Rubash HE, et al. Aseptic loosening of the humeral component in total shoulder arthroplasty. J Shoulder Elbow Surg 1998;7:422.

71. Klepps SJ, Goldfarb C, Flatow E, et al. Anatomic evaluation of the subcoracoid pectoralis major transfer in human cadavers. J Shoulder Elbow Surg 2001;10:453.

72. Klepps S, Hazarti Y, Flatow EL. The management of glenoid bone deficiency during shoulder replacement. Tech Shoulder Elbow Surg 2002 (in press).

73. Lettin AWF, Copeland SA, Scales JT. The Stanmore total shoulder replacement. J Bone Joint Surg Br 1982;64:47.

74. Matsen FA, Iannotti JP, Rockwood CA Jr. Humeral fixation by press-fitting of a tapered metaphyseal stem. A prospective study. J Bone Joint Surg 2003;85:304.

75. McCoy SR, Warren RF, Bade HA III, et al. Total shoulder arthroplasty in rheumatoid arthritis. J Arthroplasty 1989;4:105.

76. McElwain JP, English E. The early results of porous-coated total shoulder arthroplasty. Clin Orthop 1987;218:217.

77. Melzer C, Wallny T, Wirth CJ, et al. Frozen shoulder: treatment and results. Arch Orthop Trauma Surg 1995;114:87.

78. Moeckel BH, Altchek DW, Warren RF, et al. Instability of the shoulder after arthroplasty. J Bone Joint Surg Am 1993;75:492.

79. Murnaghan JP. Frozen shoulder. In: Rockwood Ca Jr., Matsen FA III, eds. The shoulder. Philadelphia, PA, WB Saunders, 1990:837.

80. Neer CS II, Kirby RM. Revision of humeral head and total shoulder arthroplasties. Clin Orthop 1982;170:189.

81. Neer CS II, Morrison DS. Glenoid bone grafting in total shoulder arthroplasty. J Bone Joint Surg Am 1988;70:1154.

82. Neer CS II, Watson KC, Stanton FJ. Recent experience in total shoulder replacement. J Bone Joint Surg 1982;64A:319.

83. Nolan JF, Bucknill TM. Aggressive granulomatosis from polyethylene failure in an uncemented knee replacement. J Bone Joint Surg 1992;74B:23.

84. Norris TR, Lipson SR. Management of the unstable prosthetic shoulder arthroplasty. Instr Course Lect 47 1998:141.

85. Ogilvie-Harris DJ, Biggs DJ, Fitsialos DP, et al. The resistant frozen shoulder: manipulation versus arthroscopic release. Clin Orthop 1995;319:238.

86. Pahle JA, Kvarnes L. Shoulder replacement arthroplasty. Ann Chir Gynaecol 1985;74(198):85.

87. Petersen SA, Hawkins RJ. Revision of failed total shoulder arthroplasty. Orthop Clin North Am 1998;29:519.

88. Petersen SA, Hawkins RJ. Revision shoulder arthroplasty. In: Friedman RJ, ed. Arthroplasty of the shoulder. New York, NY, Thieme Medical Publishers, Inc., 234.

89. Pollock RG, Deliz EB, McIlveen SJ, et al. Prosthetic replacement in rotator cuff deficient shoulders. Presented at the American Shoulder and Elbow Surgeons Annual Meeting, Washington DC, 1992.

90. Pollock RG, Deliz ED, McIlveen SJ, et al. Prosthetic replacement in rotator cuff-deficient shoulders. J Shoulder Elbow Surg 1992;1:173.

91. Post M, Pollock RG. Operative treatment of degenerative and arthritis diseases of the glenohumeral joint. In: Post M, Bigliani LU, Flatow EL, Pollock RG, eds. The shoulder: operative technique. Baltimore, MD, Williams & Wilkins, 1998:73.

92. Ramappa AJ, Gomoll A, Zurakowski D, et al. Failed shoulder hemiarthroplasty: outcome of revision shoulder arthroplasty. Proceedings of the 68th Annual Meeting of the American Academy of Orthopaedic Surgeons 2001;2:648.

93. Ramsey ML, Fenlin JM Jr. Use of an antibiotic impregnated bone cement block in the revision of an infected shoulder arthroplasty. J Shoulder Elbow Surg 1996;5:479.

94. Resch H, Povacz P, Riter E et al. Transfer of the pectoralis major muscle for the treatment of irreparable ruptures of the subscapularis tendon. J Bone Joint Surg Am 2000;82:372.

95. Roper BA, Paterson JMH, Day WH. The Roper-Day total shoulder replacement. J Bone Joint Surg 1990;72B(4):694.

96. Sanchez-Sotelo J, O'Driscoll SW, Torchia ME, et al. Radiographic assessment of cemented humeral components in shoulder arthroplasty. J Shoulder Elbow Surg 2001;10:526.

97. Sanchez-Sotelo J, Wright TW, O'Driscoll, et al. Radiographic assessment of uncemented humeral components in total shoulder arthroplasty. J Arthroplasty 2001;16:180.

98. Schmalzried TP, Jasty M, Harris WH. Periprosthetic bone loss in total hip arthroplasty. Polyethylene wear debris and the concept of the effective joint space. J Bone Joint Surg 1992;74A:849.

99. Seitz WH Jr., Damacen H. Staged exchange arthroplasty for shoulder sepsis. J Arthroplasty 2002;17(Suppl):36.

100. Sochart DH. Relationship of acetabular wear to osteolysis and loosening in total hip arthroplasty. Clin Orthop 1999;363:135.

101. Soghikian GW, Neviaser RJ. Complications of humeral head replacement. In: Bigliani LU, ed. Complications of shoulder surgery. Baltimore, MD, Williams and Wilkins, 1993:81.

102. Sperling JW, Kozak TKW, Hanssen AD, et al. Infection after shoulder arthroplasty. Clin Orthop 2001;382:206.

103. Sperling JW, Potter HG, Craig EV, et al. Magnetic resonance imaging of painful shoulder arthroplasty. J Shoulder Elbow Surg 2002;11:315.

104. Steinmann SP, Cofield RH. Bone grafting for glenoid deficiency in total shoulder replacement. J Shoulder Elbow Surg 2000;9:361.

105. Thomas BJ, Amstutz HC, Cracchiolo A. Shoulder arthroplasty for rheumatoid arthritis. Clin Orthop 1991;265:125.

106. Torchia ME, Cofield RH. Long-term results of Neer total shoulder arthroplasty. Orthop Trans 1994-95;18:977.

107. Torchia ME, Cofield RH, Settergren CR. Total shoulder arthroplasty with the Neer prosthesis: long-term results. J Shoulder Elbow Surg 1997;6:495.

108. Tytherleigh-Strong GM, Levy O, Sforza G, et al. The role of arthroscopy for the problem shoulder arthroplasty. J Shoulder Elbow Surg 2002;11:230.

109. Wang AA, Strauch RJ, Flatow EL, et al. The teres major muscle: an anatomic study of its use as a tendon transfer. J Shoulder Elbow Surg 1999;8:334.

110. Warner JJP, Parsons IM. Latissimus dorsi tendon transfer: a comparative analysis of primary and salvage reconstruction of massive, irreparable rotator cuff tears. J Shoulder Elbow Surg 2001;10:514.

111. Warner JJP, Alien AA, Marks PH, et al. Arthroscopic release of postoperative capsular contracture of the shoulder. J Bone Joint Surg Am 1997;79A:1151.

112. Warren RF, Coleman SH, Dines JS. Instability after arthroplasty: the shoulder. J Arthroplasty 2002;17(4):28.

113. Wiater JM, Levine WN. Revision shoulder arthroplasty. In: Crosby LA, ed. Total shoulder arthroplasty. Rosemont, IL, American Academy of Orthopaedic Surgeons, 2000:47.

114. Wirth MA, Rockwood CA Jr. Complications of shoulder arthroplasty. Clin Orthop 1994;307:47.

115. Wirth MA, Rockwood CA Jr. Current concepts review-complications of total shoulder-replacement arthroplasty. J Bone Joint Surg 1996;78:603.

116. Wirth MA, Rockwood CA. Operative treatment of irreparable ruptures of the subscapularis. J Bone Joint Surg Am 1997;79:722.

117. Wirth MA, Agrawal CM, Mabrey JD, et al. Isolation and characterization of polyethylene wear debris associated with osteolysis following total shoulder arthroplasty. J Bone Joint Surg 1999;81:29.

Arthrodesis and Other Salvage Procedures: When Arthroplasty Is Not Indicated

Robin R. Richards

INTRODUCTION

The advent of total shoulder arthroplasty and the refinement of other reconstructive procedures have narrowed the indications for shoulder arthrodesis.[42] Nevertheless, arthrodesis of the glenohumeral joint continues to provide a valuable method of shoulder reconstruction for specific indications.[14,23,63] During the last decade, I have performed shoulder arthrodesis for the indications listed in Figure 29-1. Although the procedure is infrequently performed, it is a reliable method of providing patients with a stable, strong shoulder. The conventional methods of performing shoulder arthrodesis must be modified for complex and revision problems. These modifications are discussed in this chapter.

Albert[1] first attempted shoulder arthrodesis in 1881. Since then, a voluminous literature has evolved outlining different indications for the procedure and a variety of surgical techniques for performing shoulder arthrodesis. Controversies have developed in the literature regarding the indications for the procedure and the optimum posi-

tion for shoulder arthrodesis,[2,55] and debate has arisen concerning the functional results that can be achieved with the procedure.[10] In this chapter, I discuss the historical perspective of shoulder arthrodesis, the anatomy and biomechanics of the procedure (including the optimum position for placement of the arm), the indications and contraindications for the procedure, the alternative procedures, and my approach to treatment. Complex and revision problems are addressed, and the complications and results of shoulder arthrodesis are discussed.

Arthrodesis is an important method of shoulder reconstruction. The procedure has stood the test of time and continues to deserve a place in the shoulder surgeon's armamentarium. For certain specific indications, it provides the best method of restoring function to the shoulder.

HISTORICAL PERSPECTIVE

Many techniques for shoulder arthrodesis have been reported. Some investigators have used extra-articular arthrodesis, others have reported on methods of intra-articular arthrodesis, and still others have used a combination of the two methods. In reviewing the literature, it is apparent that internal fixation has been used more

R. R. Richards: Surgeon-in-Chief and Professor of Surgery, Sunnybrook and Women's College Health Sciences Center, and the University of Toronto, Toronto, Ontario.

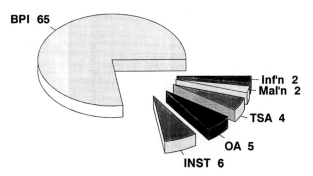

Figure 29-1 Indications for shoulder arthrodesis in 84 cases.

frequently in recent years. Historically, most investigators have recommended external immobilization, although later reports of shoulder arthrodesis without external immobilization have appeared.[29,53] Extra-articular arthrodesis, intra-articular arthrodesis, the use of internal fixation, and the use of external fixators are addressed in the following sections.

Extra-articular Arthrodesis

Extra-articular arthrodesis is primarily a historical procedure that was used before the antibiotic era to treat tuberculous arthritis. This treatment method was used to avoid entering the tuberculous joint and to obliterate motion at the joint without activating and spreading the infection. Watson-Jones[62] described a technique using a Cubbins approach to the shoulder, decorticating the superior and inferior surfaces of the acromion. A bone flap was then cut into the greater tuberosity, and the clavicle and the acromion were osteotomized. The arm was abducted, and the acromion was positioned to lie between the two edges of the bone flap in the proximal humerus. A spica cast was applied for 4 months.

Putti[46] described a technique whereby the spine of the scapula and the acromion were exposed subperiosteally. The spine of the scapula was detached, the acromion was split, and the medial and lateral portions and the upper end of the humerus were exposed. The lateral surface of the humerus was split similar to the method described by Watson-Jones,[62] and the spine of the scapula was driven down into the humerus with the arm abducted. Spica cast immobilization was necessary after this procedure. Neither the Watson-Jones nor the Putti technique was truly extra-articular, because the shoulder joint was usually entered when creating the split in the proximal humerus.

Brittain[7] described a true extra-articular arthrodesis. This arthrodesis used a large tibial graft that was placed between the medial humerus and the axillary border of the scapula. The graft was maintained in position by its arrow shape; the pointed end was inserted into the humerus, and the opposite, notched end was inserted into the axillary border of the scapula. The graft was stabilized by its shape and adduction of the arm, which produced a compressive force along the long axis of the graft. DePalma[13] reports that the failure rate of the arthrodesis was high because of fracture of the long tibial graft.

Intra-articular Arthrodesis

Gill[19] combined intra-articular and extra-articular arthrodesis. Gill used a U-shaped incision centered 2 cm below the acromion combined with a downward limb of the incision. Gill denuded the superior and inferior surface of the acromion and excised the rotator cuff. The glenoid fossa was decorticated, as was the cartilaginous surface of the humeral head. An osseous flap was elevated from the anterolateral surface of the humerus, and a wedge-shaped slice of bone with its base superiorly was removed from the humerus. The arm was then abducted and impacted onto the acromion. The position was maintained by suture of the capsule and rotator cuff to the periosteum on the superior surface of the acromion. This technique is predicated on the assumption that it is desirable to fuse the glenohumeral joint in a large amount of abduction. This can be desirable in children when internal fixation is not used, because with time the amount of abduction decreases. The technique is undesirable in adults because of the likelihood of excessive abduction being retained after arthrodesis.

Makin[34] described a method of shoulder arthrodesis in children that preserved the growth potential of the proximal humeral epiphysis. Makin fused the shoulder in 80 to 90 degrees of abduction, fixing the humerus to the glenoid with Steinmann pins inserted first into the humerus in a proximal to distal direction and then driven in the reverse direction into the glenoid. Makin monitored his pediatric patients until adulthood and noticed that there was only a small loss in humeral length and no change in position of the fused shoulder. He recommended this technique stating that this amount of abduction was necessary to maintain the growth potential of the proximal humeral epiphysis. If this amount of abduction was maintained, the shoulder would be dysfunctional in adulthood.

Moseley[38] reported division of the rotator cuff insertion and excision of the intra-articular portion of the biceps tendon. Moseley advocated suture of the biceps tendon into the bicipital groove after division of its origin. This is an important step in patients who have functioning biceps to avoid the unsightly cosmetic deformity identical to that seen in rupture of the long head of the biceps tendon and to avoid the small loss of elbow flexor power and greater loss of supinator strength that is associated with this pathologic condition. I perform a biceps tenodesis during shoulder arthrodesis in all patients who have a functional biceps. Mosely denuded the inferior surface of the acromion and the articular cartilage of the humeral head and glenoid fossa. This is an important step in performing shoulder arthrodesis, because the humeral head presents such a small area to the glenoid across which fusion can occur.

Beltran and colleagues[5] performed shoulder arthrodesis through an anterior approach. They osteotomized the coracoid and created a tunnel that crossed the humerus and entered the glenoid cavity. They used a screw for internal fixation and a Cloward reamer to position a fibular graft from the proximal humerus into the infraglenoid area. Other techniques for shoulder arthrodesis have been described by May[35] and by Davis and Cottrell.[12]

Internal Fixation

A variety of methods of internal fixation have been advocated for shoulder arthrodesis. It is generally agreed that internal fixation is desirable because it maintains the position of the arthrodesis and can decrease the length of time that plaster immobilization is necessary to obtain an arthrodesis. Makin advocates the use of Steinmann pins in children who are undergoing shoulder arthrodesis at an early age. Carroll[8] described the use of a wire loop to maintain the position of shoulder arthrodesis. Carroll advocated the use of 22-gauge wire passed through the head of the humerus and the anterosuperior lip of the glenoid. He used this method of arthrodesis in 15 patients, and all patients achieved solid bony union between the third and fourth month after surgery. Carroll observed that it was possible to manipulate the shoulder after surgery and change the position of the arthrodesis. As time has gone by, most investigators have advocated more rigid forms of internal fixation. Few surgeons now use a wire loop as a method of internal fixation when performing shoulder arthrodesis. Mohammed[36] reported on the use of a Rush rod combined with a tension band wire to obtain arthrodesis in 4 patients with paralysis caused by brachial plexus injury and in 14 patients with paralysis caused by poliomyelitis.

Other researchers have reported the use of screws to obtain fixation during glenohumeral arthrodesis (Fig. 29-2). May[35] used a single stabilizing wood screw crossing the humerus and entering the glenoid fossa. Davis and Cottrell[12] used a similar technique and added a muscle pedicle bone graft that was fixed in place with wood screws. Cofield and Briggs[11] and Leffert[31] also reported the use of compression screw fixation without the use of a plate. Beltran et al.[5] developed a special fixation device using a screw bolt and washer to obtain shoulder arthrodesis. Beltran and colleagues also used an acromiohumeral screw and a fibular graft as methods of internal fixation.

The Orthopedic Surgical Instruments and Implants (Association for the Study of Internal Fixation [ASIF]) group first advocated the use of plate fixation in 1970. They described this method of arthrodesis as not requiring supplementary plaster immobilization. The AO/ASIF group

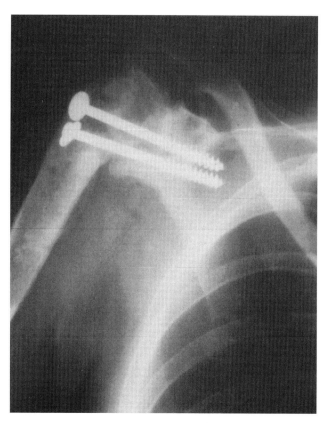

Figure 29-2 Glenohumeral arthrodesis obtained with two compression screws and washers. Although this technique does not provide for fixation to the acromion or the shaft of the humerus, good fixation can be obtained with two screws inserted in this fashion.

advocated the use of two plates for internal fixation.[39] The first plate was applied along the spine of the scapula and then bent down over the humerus, maintaining a position of 70 degrees of abduction between the vertebral border of the scapula and the humerus. The object of this position was to obtain a clinical position of 50 degrees of abduction, 40 degrees of internal rotation, and 25 degrees of flexion. They anchored this plate to the scapula with a long screw placed down through the plate, through the acromion, and into the neck of the glenoid. They observed that fixation could be improved by the insertion of two long screws inserted through the plate, the humeral head, and into the glenoid. If necessary, a second plate applied posteriorly was advocated to improve the internal fixation. I have rarely found it necessary to use two plates when performing shoulder arthrodesis.

Kostiuk and Schatzker[29] described the use of the ASIF technique. They did not use external immobilization postoperatively and reported good results for their patients. Riggins[53] described shoulder fusion without external immobilization in 1976. The AO group and Riggins supplemented their arthrodeses with bone grafts. Riggins treated four patients with the use of a plate for internal fixation.

Two of the patients had above-elbow amputations. The arthrodesis was successful in each case.

My colleagues and I have reported the results of a modified method of shoulder arthrodesis using internal fixation in 14 adult patients with brachial plexus palsy.[48] We first used a single AO/ASIF dynamic compression plate for 4.5-mm screws applied over the spine of the scapula onto the shaft of the humerus. We advocate placement of two cancellous compression screws passing through the plate and proximal humerus into the glenoid to achieve compression at the glenohumeral arthrodesis site. The plate is anchored to the scapula with a long screw passing through the spine of the scapula into the area of the coracoid base. Anchorage of the plate by this method, unlike that of the AO method, which inserts the screw into the glenoid neck, provides good fixation yet leaves room for the large compression screws in the glenoid, which are thought to be more important in obtaining arthrodesis. Initially, we advocated the use of a postoperative spica cast, because adult patients with brachial plexus injuries generally have signif-

icant osteoporosis, poor muscular control, and decreased proprioception resulting from their neurologic injury. Bone grafts were not used in this series, and nonunions did not occur. More recently we have begun to use thermoplastic thoracobrachial orthoses when performing shoulder arthrodesis and no longer use a spica cast.

My colleagues and I reported a modification of the technique described in 1985.[49] The current technique uses a malleable plate for internal fixation. In the modified procedure, a single 10-hole, AO pelvic reconstruction plate for 4.5-mm screws is used for internal fixation. This plate, although weaker than the dynamic compression plate for 4.5-mm screws, is much easier to contour in the operating room and much less prominent as it passes over the acromion onto the shaft of the humerus (Fig. 29-3). None of the 11 patients whose shoulders were fused by this method complained of plate prominence. Fusion was obtained in each instance without the internal fixation device failing. External cast immobilization was used for 6 weeks postoperatively. Plate prominence can also be

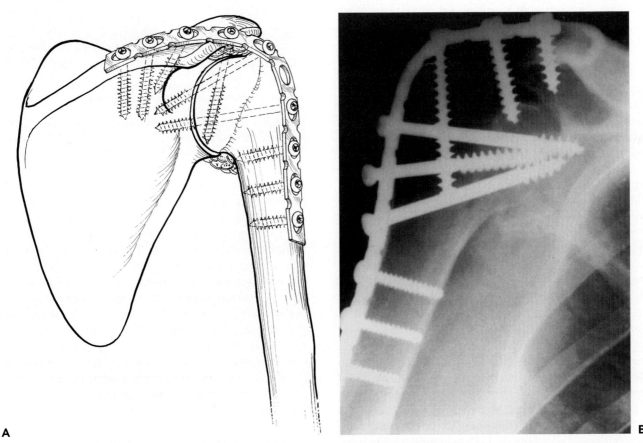

A   B

Figure 29-3 (*A*) Ten-hole AO/Association for the Study of Internal Fixation (ASIF) reconstruction plate applied to stabilize the arthrodesis. The humeral head contacts the acromion and glenoid, and there is cancellous bone graft packed into the interval between the inferior humeral neck and the glenoid. (*B*) Conventional technique for shoulder arthrodesis using a pelvic reconstruction plate. Three compression screws have been inserted from the lateral aspect of the plate into the glenoid to provide compression. One of the screws has backed out slightly as arthrodesis has occurred. The malleable reconstruction plate is easier to contour in the operating room and decreases the frequency with which removal of the internal fixation is required.

decreased postoperatively by notching the acromion laterally where the plate crosses this structure.

External Fixation

Charnley and Houston[9] reported a method of compression arthrodesis of the shoulder using two Steinmann pins. The first Steinmann pin was inserted posterosuperiorly into the base of the acromion and then into the main mass of the scapula just proximal to the glenoid. The second pin is inserted posterolaterally in relation to the shaft of the humerus and perpendicular in relation to the axis of the humerus to transfix the region of the surgical neck. A compression apparatus is then applied to the two pins. After application of the compression apparatus, a plaster spica cast was applied and worn for an average of 4.8 weeks. After removal of the pins and compression clamps, a second plaster cast was applied for an average of 5.3 weeks. Other methods of external fixation have been reported.[24,28,40,59]

The indications for shoulder arthrodesis using external fixation are limited. I have used this method occasionally in

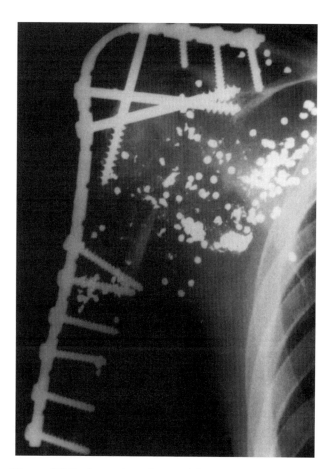

Figure 29-5 Conversion of external fixator to plate fixation to obtain arthrodesis in the same patient as in Figure 29-4.

patients with active septic arthritis of the shoulder and in patients with massive trauma resulting in bone and soft tissue loss (Fig. 29-4). I have used pins placed through the clavicle and acromion and a second set of pins inserted in a separate plane into the spine of the scapula and neck of the glenoid. Two half frames are then constructed to stabilize the shoulder. The two half frames can be cross-connected for increased stability. This technique is desirable if there is an open infected wound draining from the shoulder joint. This method allows dressing changes and care of the soft tissues without the increased dissection and soft tissue disruption necessary to place an internal fixation device. If the soft tissue envelope improves, internal fixation can be used in a delayed fashion (Fig. 29-5).

ANATOMY AND BIOMECHANICS OF SHOULDER ARTHRODESIS

Many positions for glenohumeral arthrodesis have been advocated in the literature. Perusal of the literature reveals that no two surgeons agree on the optimum position for

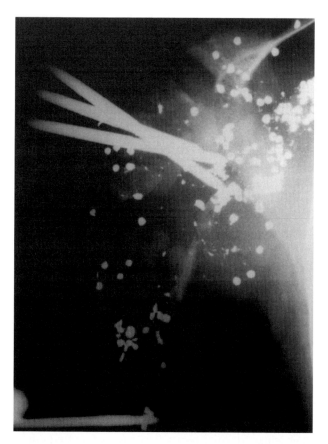

Figure 29-4 Use of external fixator after a shotgun blast to the shoulder. This method of fixation can provide stability while dressing changes are performed. It is usually not chosen as the definitive method of treatment, except in cases of septic arthritis.

shoulder arthrodesis. There was sufficient controversy in the literature that the American Orthopaedic Association established a committee to determine, among other things, the optimum position for shoulder arthrodesis. In 1942, this committee[2] concluded that the optimum position for shoulder arthrodesis was 45 to 50 degrees abduction (measured from the vertebral border of the scapula), 15 to 25 degrees of forward flexion from the plane of the scapula, and 25 to 30 degrees of internal rotation. This report caused a great deal of controversy in the literature after its publication. Part of the controversy revolved around the method of measurement of abduction. Some surgeons recommended using the angle formed by the vertebral border of scapula and the axis of the humerus to determine abduction, and others argued that the angle between the arm and the side of the body was more appropriately measured (i.e., clinical abduction).

In 1974, Rowe[55] noticed that the amount of abduction that had been recommended was excessive for adults. This position had been recommended primarily for patients who had their shoulders fused as children and in whom internal fixation was not used. In this situation, the amount of abduction at the time of surgery was commonly lost during the period required for arthrodesis to become secure and during continued growth. If the same position was used in adults, excessive scapular winging would occur, and the scapula would not comfortably rest at the side. Rowe observed that the measurement of clinical abduction was more practical and recommended this method rather than measuring abduction from the vertebral border of the scapula. Rowe recommended that the arm be placed nearer the center of gravity of the body with enough abduction to clear the axilla and sufficient flexion and internal rotation to bring the hand to the midline of the body.

Other surgeons have recommended a variety of positions for shoulder arthrodesis. All investigators agree that abduction and forward flexion are desirable. Most have recommended internal rotation. I think the optimum position for shoulder arthrodesis is one that brings the hand to the midline anteriorly so that with elbow flexion the mouth can be reached. The amount of abduction should not be excessive so that the arm can rest comfortably at the side. I recommend a position of 30 degrees of abduction (measured clinically), 30 degrees of forward flexion, and 30 degrees of internal rotation. This so-called 30-30-30 position is easily obtained in the operating room and provides patients with the ability to reach the mouth, a front pocket, and a back pocket in most instances (Fig. 29-6). The position cannot always be measured exactly at the time of surgery. I found in a series of shoulder arthrodeses that it is usually possible for the shoulder to undergo arthrodesis within 10 degrees of the described position.

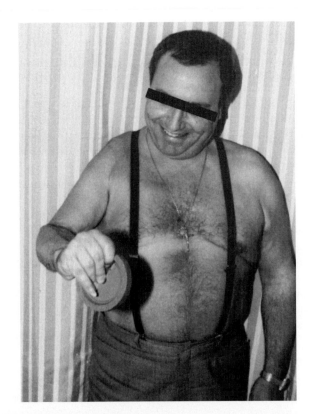

Figure 29-6   Arthrodesis of the shoulder in the 30-30-30 position. The hand can be positioned in space, and the patient can usually reach his or her mouth and front pocket.

INDICATIONS FOR SHOULDER ARTHRODESIS

Shoulder arthrodesis can effectively restore shoulder function to patients with certain disorders. Patient selection is important in determining whether the procedure will be beneficial. The procedure results in the effective sacrifice of all rotation through the glenohumeral joint. However, shoulder arthrodesis does provide strength and stability. When possible, shoulder arthroplasty is preferable to shoulder arthrodesis if there is a choice for the patient between the two procedures. Shoulders can be fused if an arthroplasty fails, although fusion in this situation is a technical challenge. The indications used for surgery in my series are illustrated in Figure 29-1.

Paralysis

All investigators agree that a flail shoulder is an indication for shoulder arthrodesis. Patients with anterior poliomyelitis, patients with severe proximal root and irreparable upper trunk brachial plexus lesions, and some patients with isolated axillary nerve paralysis are candidates for shoulder arthrodesis.[53] These patients have good function in their elbows and hands but are unable to optimize their upper extremity function because of their inability to place their hand in space (Fig. 29-7). If such a patient has good function in the periscapular musculature, particularly the trapezius, levator scapula, and serratus anterior, glenohumeral arthrodesis stabilizes the extremity and allows effective hand function.[50] The patients can then fully use their upper extremity potential and can work effectively at bench level. Many patients with flail shoulders develop inferior subluxation of the glenohumeral joint caused by periarticular paralysis. This condition is uncomfortable and, in some patients, frankly painful. Such patients often find that they must keep their affected arms in slings to avoid injury. Painful inferior subluxation of the shoulder provides another indication for stabilization of the glenohumeral joint.

Patients who have the combination of a flail shoulder and flail elbow need shoulder and elbow reconstruction. In this situation, glenohumeral arthrodesis combined with elbow flexorplasty improves the result of the elbow flexorplasty. Without shoulder stabilization, elbow flexion tends to drive the humerus posteriorly, resulting in shoulder extension rather than elbow flexion. Arthrodesis of the shoulder in some flexion and abduction helps to reduce the effect of gravity and optimize the result that can be achieved with the elbow flexorplasty. Patients with flail shoulders often have a tendency to internally rotate the upper extremity to the chest when some function remains in the powerful internal rotators of the shoulder (e.g., pectoralis major, latissimus dorsi) and no function remains in the external rotators. Shoulder stabilization in the form of arthrodesis or a L'Episcopo tendon transfer reduces this undesirable tendency.

There is great variability in the disability caused by axillary nerve paralysis, and I have seen many patients who have virtually full motion after paralysis of the axillary nerve, providing the rotator cuff musculature is undisturbed (endurance is never normal). Patients with isolated paralysis of the axillary nerve can be treated by muscle or tendon transfer or glenohumeral arthrodesis. Numerous reports exist in the literature on the value of muscle and muscle tendon transfer to restore shoulder function after paralysis of the axillary nerve.[8,20] It is generally agreed that multiple transfers are necessary to restore deltoid function and that significant problems can occur with gliding of transfers over the acromion. It is often necessary to harvest autogenous tissue such as fascia lata to prolong the transfers, and the process of rehabilitation is challenging after such procedures. In my experience, such transfers are indicated primarily for pediatric patients and adult patients who have only partial paralysis of the axillary nerve.[20] However, pediatric patients do well with shoulder arthrodesis, and some investigators believe they are better able to adapt to the procedure.[33] If total paralysis of the axillary nerve exists and significant limitation of shoulder function ensues, I recommend glenohumeral arthrodesis, recognizing that the alternative of muscle transfers may be available in carefully selected patients. Ruhmann et al.[57] reported on the differential function in patients with brachial plexus palsy after reconstruction with either tendon transfer or arthrodesis. I have found glenohumeral arthrodesis to be useful in such patients, provided their symptoms justify the procedure.

Reconstruction After Tumor Resection

En bloc resection of periarticular malignant tumors often requires sacrifice of the rotator cuff or deltoid (Fig. 29-8). When the resection requires sacrifice of these tissues, reconstruction of the shoulder with an arthroplasty is inadvisable because of the high risk of instability if an unconstrained prosthesis is used and the certainty of loosening if a constrained prosthesis is used (Fig. 29-9). Shoulder arthrodesis is the procedure of choice to reconstruct the shoulder after wide resection of periarticular malignancies. Specific techniques have been recommended for shoulder arthrodesis after tumor resection.[32] These include the use of specialized fixation devices and bone grafting techniques. Vascularized bone grafts and massive

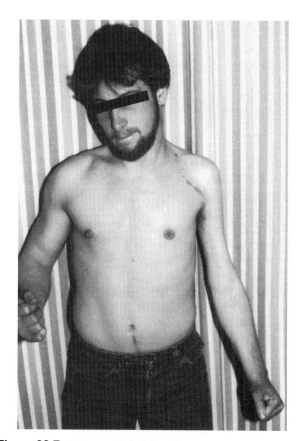

Figure 29-7   Patient with flail shoulder because of an irreparable brachial plexus injury. He has undergone a brachial plexus exploration and nerve grafting and has not recovered function in his shoulder. He does have good hand and wrist function. The restoration of elbow flexion requires reconstruction by flexorplasty.

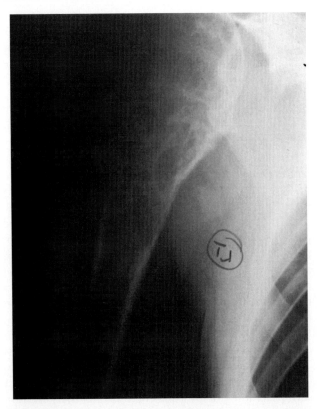

Figure 29-8 Giant cell tumor of the right proximal humerus with a pathologic fracture.

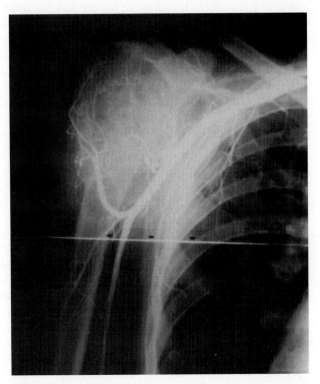

Figure 29-9 Angiogram of the patient shown in Figure 29-8, demonstrating extension of the tumor to the surrounding soft tissues. En bloc resection of the tumor with the surrounding soft tissues is required to prevent recurrence.

allografts are sometimes necessary because of the large defects created by tumor resection.[30] O'Connor et al.[44] reported on the functional results of limb salvage for neoplasms of the shoulder girdle.

Shoulder Joint Destruction Caused by Infection

Destruction of the shoulder joint by septic arthritis remains an indication for shoulder arthrodesis. In the past, tuberculous arthritis was a common indication for shoulder arthrodesis. Worldwide, this condition remains prevalent, although in the Western world it has become extremely uncommon. Septic arthritis continues to occur, and when it does, the shoulder joint can be destroyed, with resultant pain and limitation of function. Most surgeons agree that, in a young patient with shoulder dysfunction for this reason, arthrodesis of the shoulder, instead of total shoulder arthroplasty, is indicated. Although total shoulder arthroplasty can be performed in patients with a remote history of sepsis, with a recent history of sepsis, or who are young, arthrodesis provides a more satisfactory alternative.

Failed Total Shoulder Arthroplasty

I have seen several patients who have had multiple unsuccessful shoulder arthroplasties. Although the results of shoulder arthroplasty are generally good, there are some patients in whom loosening, sepsis, and implant breakage occur. These patients often have severe loss of humeral and glenoid bone stock (Fig. 29-10). In this situation, the surgeon must choose between attempting a repeat revision of the shoulder arthroplasty and obliteration of the shoulder joint by arthrodesis. The results of revision total shoulder arthroplasty are suboptimal when compared with the results of primary arthroplasty for other reasons. The decision between these two alternatives must be made on the basis of the patient's age, the presence or absence of sepsis, the bone stock that remains in the proximal humerus and glenoid, the symptoms the patient is experiencing, the quality and function of the rotator cuff and the deltoid, and the technical experience and expertise of the surgeon. In several patients who were significantly disabled, I performed glenohumeral arthrodesis after multiple failed total shoulder arthroplasties and found it to be a successful procedure. Shoulder arthrodesis must be considered when the reconstructive surgeon is confronted with a patient with a history of multiple failed total shoulder arthroplasties.

Shoulder Instability

Most patients with shoulder instability can be treated by soft tissue or bony reconstructive procedures to stabilize the glenohumeral joint. Rarely, a patient presents with chronic shoulder instability after multiple attempts at sur-

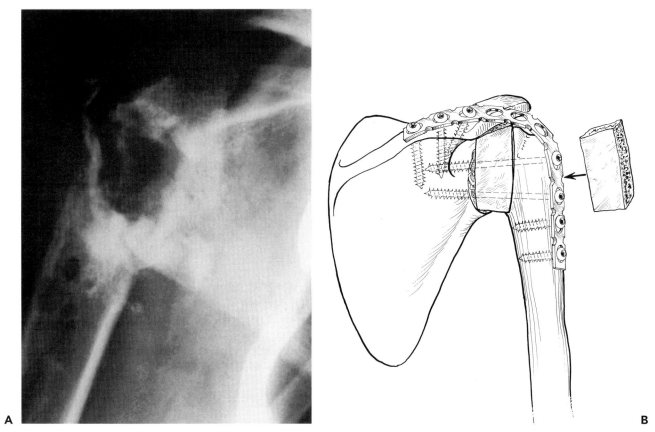

A   B

Figure 29-10   (*A*) Painful glenohumeral joint after resection arthroplasty. There is a significant loss of bone stock in patients with multiple failed glenohumeral arthroplasties. This presents a reconstructive challenge when performing glenohumeral arthrodesis. (*B*) A corticocancellous block of autogenous iliac crest graft can be used to promote a fusion in the setting of proximal humeral deficiency, as may occur after a failed arthroplasty procedure.

gical stabilization. If every surgical therapeutic alternative has been exhausted, the patient's shoulder remains symptomatically unstable, and the patient does not want to wear a thoracobrachial support, arthrodesis can be indicated to restore shoulder stability. In this situation, careful assessment of the patient's psychologic makeup must be carried out, and the physician must be certain the patient has a full understanding of the implications of the procedure. Much has been written about the difficulties in managing such patients, and further elaboration here is unnecessary.[51,56]

Rotator Cuff Tear

Severe shoulder dysfunction can result from massive rotator cuff tears.[16] Most rotator cuff tears can be managed by coracoacromial decompression and repair of the cuff. For patients who have massive rotator cuff tears that cannot be repaired, some surgeons have reported good results with debridement of the cuff tear and coracoacromial decompression.[54] Long-standing rotator cuff tears can lead to cuff tear arthropathy, as reported by Neer et al.[43] Neer et al. report that this difficult pathologic entity can be treated by

prosthetic arthroplasty with cuff reconstruction. This is predicated on the surgeon's ability to repair the cuff by cuff transfer or the use of exogenous materials. Neer et al. report that such patients must have "limited goals," because this is a difficult form of reconstruction. Shoulder arthrodesis should be kept in mind as a possible alternative form of reconstruction in such patients when the technical skill of the surgeon or the available tissues do not permit cuff reconstruction and the patient is sufficiently symptomatic to exchange the loss of glenohumeral motion for the relief of pain. This situation rarely develops.

Malunion

Glenohumeral arthrodesis is rarely indicated for posttraumatic deformity. Most patients with posttraumatic deformities such as osteonecrosis of the humeral head, chronic fracture dislocations, tuberosity impingement, or malunion of the proximal humerus are best treated by shoulder reconstruction using osteotomy, arthroplasty, or a combination of both. If these procedures are not possible, glenohumeral arthrodesis can be considered.

Osteoarthritis

Glenohumeral osteoarthritis in an otherwise normal shoulder is an indication for total shoulder arthroplasty. Naranja and Inanity[41] have reported on the surgical options in the treatment of arthritis of the shoulder. Most patients with glenohumeral osteoarthritis are of sufficient age that they are excellent candidates for total shoulder arthroplasty. If the patient develops osteoarthritis at a relatively young age, glenohumeral arthrodesis should be considered,[3] particularly if the patient is a laborer and modified work is not available to him or her. The results of total shoulder arthroplasty are so much superior that in our experience the operation is rarely indicated for patients with this diagnosis.

Rheumatoid Arthritis

Patients with rheumatoid arthritis affecting the glenohumeral joint commonly have multiple problems in their upper extremity. Shoulder arthrodesis is recognized as a procedure that can decrease pain arising from the glenohumeral joint.[25,47,58] Obliteration of glenohumeral motion has a negative influence on upper extremity function. Frequently, both upper extremities are involved. Patients with rheumatoid arthritis are much more effectively treated by total shoulder arthroplasty.[18] Favorable reports of the combination of shoulder and elbow arthroplasty have appeared in the literature, and I advocate this method of reconstruction for such patients.

CONTRAINDICATIONS TO SHOULDER ARTHRODESIS

Shoulder arthrodesis should not be performed if an alternative method of shoulder reconstruction is available. Many patients are amenable to arthroplastic reconstruction, which preserves glenohumeral motion and has greater potential to restore function. Shoulder arthrodesis places a significant functional demand on the patient and requires a major effort on the part of the patient to rehabilitate the shoulder after surgery and to strengthen the thoracoscapular musculature. The procedure is contraindicated for a patient who cannot cooperate with the program of rehabilitation. I have not performed shoulder arthrodesis on elderly patients for this reason. Similarly, the procedure is contraindicated for any patient with a progressive neurologic disorder who may experience paralysis of the trapezius, levator scapula, or serratus anterior after the procedure. Glenohumeral arthrodesis relies on these muscles to motor the extremity, and significant weakness grossly impairs shoulder function after the procedure.

ALTERNATIVES TO ARTHRODESIS

There are few alternatives to arthrodesis in the subset of patients in whom it is indicated, even in the advent of arthroplasty.[21] Patients with chronic sepsis after shoulder arthroplasty can be treated with exchange arthroplasty using antibiotic-impregnated cement (Fig. 29-11). Some arthroplasties can be salvaged in this manner. If the sepsis is severe, a cement spacer can be constructed with antibiotic-impregnated cement in an effort to control local sepsis. Excision arthroplasty is an alternative to arthrodesis. The results of excision arthroplasty of the glenohumeral joint are somewhat unpredictable. The procedure can be considered for patients who have poor bone stock or whose general medical condition would make them poor candidates for arthrodesis (Fig. 29-12). In some patients, a relatively stable shoulder without significant problems with pain can be achieved, although as a general rule, the results are more consistent after arthrodesis in terms of pain relief and stability. Patients with malignant tumors of the shoulder girdle can be treated with either amputation or limb-salvage procedures. Kneisl[27] has reported on function after amputation, arthrodesis, or arthroplasty for tumors about the shoulder.

TREATMENT

Preferred Approach

The operative technique and postoperative protocol are similar to that previously described. The patient is placed in the semi-sitting position (Fig. 29-13).[4] The arm is free draped. An incision extends from the spine of the scapula to the anterior acromion and down the anterior aspect of the shaft of the humerus. Uematsu[61] recommended a posterior approach when performing shoulder arthrodesis. Other investigators have described arthroscopically assisted shoulder arthrodesis.[37] The deltoid muscle is detached from the anterior acromion, and its fibers are split distally. Because deltoid function is not present in patients with brachial plexus palsy undergoing shoulder arthrodesis, denervation of the muscle is not usually a concern. If deltoid function exists, the incision should be curved over to the deltopectoral interval and the shoulder approached in this fashion. With this approach, deltoid bulk is maintained, and the patient experiences a more satisfactory cosmetic result. Sparing the deltoid may prevent the development of pain from neuromas arising from the axillary nerve postoperatively. The rotator cuff is resected. The glenoid fossa, undersurface of the acromion, and humeral head are decorticated. An attempt is made to obtain arthrodesis of the glenohumeral *and* acromiohumeral articulations because the glenoid fossa offers such a small

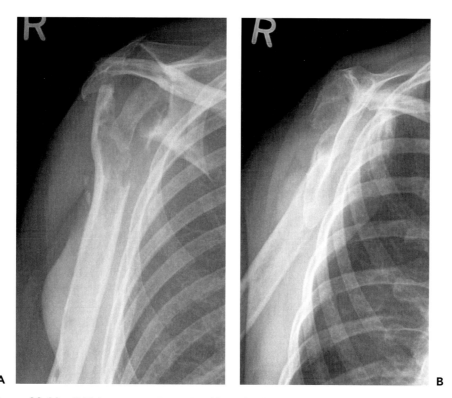

Figure 29-11 *(A,B)* Anteroposterior (AP) and lateral radiographs of the shoulder of a 79-year-old patient after excision of an infected total shoulder arthroplasty and implantation of an antibiotic-impregnated spacer with a Rush rod stem. Such spacers produce high concentrations of antibiotics locally and can be used in an attempt to salvage an infected shoulder arthroplasty by staged reconstruction.

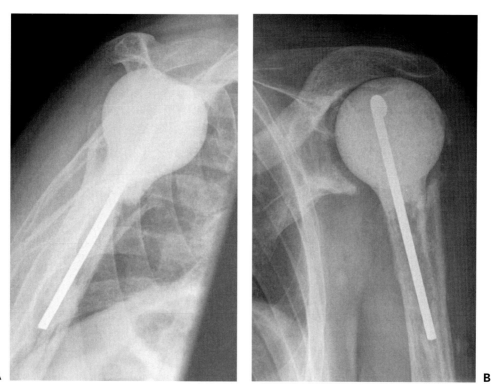

Figure 29-12 *(A,B)* Anteroposterior (AP) and lateral radiograph of the shoulder of a 54-year-old patient with rheumatoid arthritis who had an infected total arthroplasty that became infected. It was not possible to control the sepsis with antibiotics or implantation of an antibiotic-impregnated cement spacer as described previously. Her excision arthroplasty was relatively stable and not unduly painful. After excision arthroplasty there was no further drainage from her shoulder.

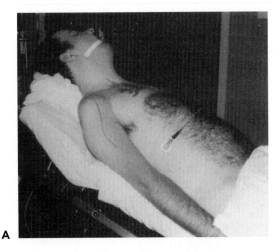

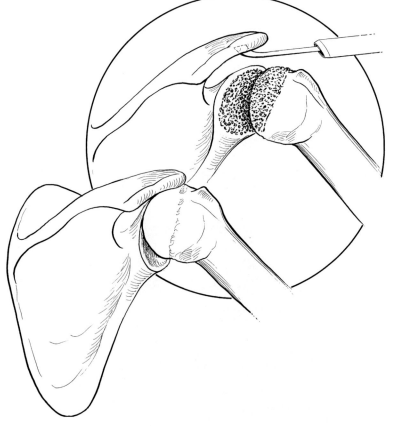

Figure 29-13 (*A*) Placement of the patient in the semi-sitting position preparatory to performing shoulder arthrodesis. The incision site has been marked from the spine of the scapula over the anterior aspect of the acromion and continuing along the lateral aspect of the humerus. (*B*) The glenoid, humeral head, and undersurface of the acromion are decorticated and shaped so that the humeral head has the greatest surface area contact. This technique increases the likelihood of a solid fusion.

B

area for fusion with the humeral head. Decortication of the undersurface of the acromion increases the potential fusion area. A 10-hole, pelvic reconstruction plate for 4.5-mm screws (Synthes, Mississauga, Ontario, Canada, and Wayne, PA) is used for internal fixation during the procedure.

After resection of the rotator cuff and decortication of the joint surfaces, the shoulder is supported in 30 degrees of flexion, 30 degrees of abduction, and 30 degrees of internal rotation. Abduction is measured from the side of the body. This method of measurement does not accommodate for individual variations in muscle mass or body fat. However, clinical experience has shown it to be accurate within 10 degrees in any plane. The humeral head is brought proximally to appose the decorticated undersurface of the acromion. When the humerus is abducted and flexed 30 degrees, the humeral head apposes the undersurface of the acromion and glenoid fossa. The position is maintained by supporting the arm with sterile folded sheets. An assistant is assigned to maintain the position while the plate is contoured. Thirty degrees of internal rotation brings the hand to the midline. I have not found it necessary to measure abduction radiographically.

Handheld bending irons are used to contour the plate along the spine of the scapula, over the acromion, and down onto the shaft of the humerus. The malleable nature

of the plate allows precise intraoperative contouring of the implant to the specific local anatomy in any given patient (Fig. 29-14). The plate must be gently bent 60 degrees over the acromion and twisted 20 to 25 degrees just distal to the bend to appose the shaft of the humerus. The reconstruction plate has holes that allow angulation of the screws as they are passed through the plate.

The screws passing through the plate and the humeral head into the glenoid fossa are inserted first. Two (usually) or three screws can be inserted in this fashion. If the glenoid is dysplastic, only one screw can be used. These screws compress the arthrodesis site. A screw should be directed next from the spine of the scapula into the base of the coracoid process. Because of the cortical bone in this region, care must be taken not to break the drill bit when drilling into the scapula. Another cancellous screw is placed across the acromiohumeral fusion site, and the remaining holes of the plate are secured with cortical screws. The acromion is *not* osteotomized, because it is used to augment fixation of the scapula to the humerus. Creating a notch in the lateral acromion may reduce plate prominence in this area.

Autogenous bone graft is not used routinely. If there is a deficiency of the glenoid or humerus, a bone graft should be used. This is often the situation when the procedure is performed for failed total shoulder arthroplasty.

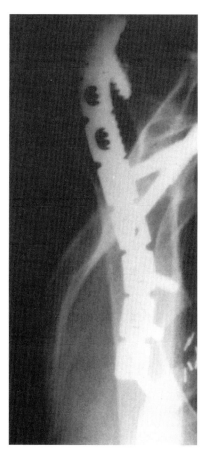

Figure 29-14 Transcapsular radiograph demonstrating contouring of the pelvic reconstruction plate in the sagittal plane.

The arm of the patient is supported postoperatively with a pillow and swathe. A thermoplastic thoracobrachial orthosis is applied 24 hours postoperatively (Fig. 29-15). If possible, the orthosis can be fabricated preoperatively and then adjusted in the postoperative period as necessary. The orthosis is worn for 6 weeks postoperatively. During this time, the orthosis can be removed for short times while the patient showers, provided the arm is supported. Six weeks postoperatively, the patient is examined radiographically, and the stability of the fusion is tested manually in a gentle fashion.

If there is no radiographic sign of loosening of the internal fixation 6 weeks postoperatively, the arm of the patient is placed in a sling. Gentle range-of-motion exercises are allowed until radiographic union is achieved. It is difficult to be certain when fusion occurs radiographically, because the fixation is sufficiently rigid that very little callus forms around the arthrodesis site. Muscle strengthening is encouraged after removal of the thermoplastic thoracobrachial orthosis, but return to strenuous activity is delayed for at least 16 weeks postoperatively. Thoracoscapular strengthening and mobilization exercises can be started 3 months after surgery.

Complex Problems

Complex and revision problems about the shoulder related to shoulder arthrodesis usually consist of various proportions of bone or soft tissue loss. These problems are discussed in turn, although in some cases they must be addressed at the same time.

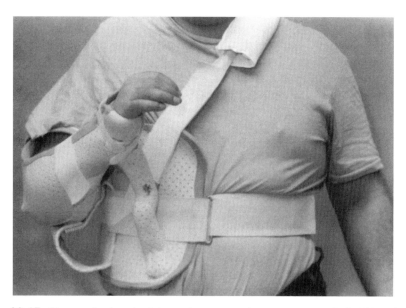

Figure 29-15 Thermoplastic orthosis is used to support the arm postoperatively. This orthosis can be fabricated preoperatively and adjusted in the immediate postoperative period. The orthosis can be removed when the patient bathes. The orthosis is generally worn for 6 weeks postoperatively.

Bone Loss and Bone Grafting

Bone loss can be a significant problem when performing shoulder arthrodesis. The usual causative factors are trauma, previous glenohumeral joint arthroplasty, and tumor resection. The extent of bone loss should be assessed preoperatively by conventional radiographs in every case. It is usually possible and practicable to assess the extent of humeral bone loss on conventional radiographs. It is harder to assess the extent of glenoid bone loss on plain films, and a computed tomographic scan may therefore be required. If the patient has had a previous glenoid replacement or has a scapular tumor, additional imaging is required. If bone loss has occurred, bone grafting must be performed in conjunction with shoulder arthrodesis. The type of bone grafting selected depends on the extent of bone loss determined preoperatively.

Routine bone grafting is advocated by some surgeons during shoulder arthrodesis. The AO/ASIF group recommends prophylactic bone grafting at the termination of a plate if a plate is used for internal fixation. A total of 11 of 71 patients had autogenous bone grafts at the time of their initial procedures in a study performed by Cofield and Briggs.[11] Richards and colleagues[50] obtained successful arthrodesis without primary bone grafts in patients with significant osteoporosis. I do not routinely use bone grafts in adults when performing shoulder arthrodesis. Bone grafting is indicated to fill large defects in patients who are undergoing glenohumeral arthrodesis for complex and revision problems. Bone grafting is also indicated after tumor resection. If large defects have been created after tumor resection, free vascularized bone grafts may be indicated. Nonunion of shoulder arthrodeses should be treated by revision of the arthrodesis combined with bone grafting. An attempt must be made to obtain rigid internal fixation during the arthrodesis. This method of treatment has been successful when used.

Nonstructural Autogenous Bone Grafting

Autogenous bone grafting can be used to provide osteoinductive and osteoconductive material at or in the arthrodesis site to increase the likelihood of successful fusion. Some investigators routinely use cancellous bone harvested from the humeral head when performing shoulder arthrodesis. In complex and revision cases, the humeral head usually is not present, and it is necessary to look elsewhere for autogenous bone. I prefer to harvest bone from the inner aspect of the iliac crest when a nonstructural autogenous graft is required. This is conveniently performed with the patient in the semi-sitting position, unless the patient is obese, in which case the bone graft must be harvested with the table extended and the position changed after closure of the iliac crest wound. I resect the superior and inner cortex of the iliac crest with a sagittal saw. A Capener gauge is then used to excavate strips of cancellous bone. If large amounts of bone are required, it may be necessary to use both iliac crests. If the patient has undergone previous surgery in these areas, a bone graft can be harvested from the posterior aspect of the iliac crest, although the position of the patient must be changed intraoperatively. Alternatively, nonstructural autogenous bone can be obtained from the greater trochanter or provided by morselized rib grafts.

Structural Autogenous Bone Grafting

Structural autogenous bone grafting uses an anatomically intact bone graft such as a full-thickness iliac crest or fibular strut graft. After unsuccessful glenohumeral joint arthroplasty, there is a significant defect related to the often extensive resection of the humeral head and excavation of the proximal humerus. A full-thickness (tricortical) iliac crest graft can be harvested and incorporated into the fusion mass. I have placed such grafts underneath the plate with screws passing through the plate and tricortical iliac crest bone graft into the glenoid. Such a graft maintains the contour of the shoulder and provides autogenous osteoconductive tissue across which fusion can occur. The disadvantage of an anatomically intact graft is the prolonged time required for incorporation. Accordingly, when such a graft is used, it should be supplemented with small chips of cancellous bone. It is usually necessary to harvest the cancellous bone from the other iliac crest. I have not used fibular grafts when performing shoulder arthrodesis, except in conjunction with a vascularized fibular graft. Nonvascularized fibular grafts consist of dense cortical bone, have a limited biologic (but initially a good structural) potential, and probably should not be used in isolation.

Vascularized Autogenous Bone Grafting

Vascularized autogenous bone grafting has the advantage of providing tissue with great biologic potential. The conventional wisdom is that when the surgeon is faced with an intercalary defect of greater than 6 cm, a vascularized bone graft should be considered. After tumor resection, intercalary defects of this magnitude are common, and I have used vascularized fibular bone grafts in this situation. The bone grafting is performed in conjunction with plate fixation. I prefer to use a very long, heavy plate spanning the entire intercalary defect. The vascularized fibular bone graft should be fixed in position with a minimum amount of internal fixation at each bony juncture (Figs. 29-16 and 29-17). Vascularized fibular bone grafts of up to 25 cm can be used to span very large defects. The vascular anastomosis is performed between the peroneal and its vena comitantes and a branch of the axillary or the brachial artery. Vascularized fibular bone grafts should be supplemented with chips

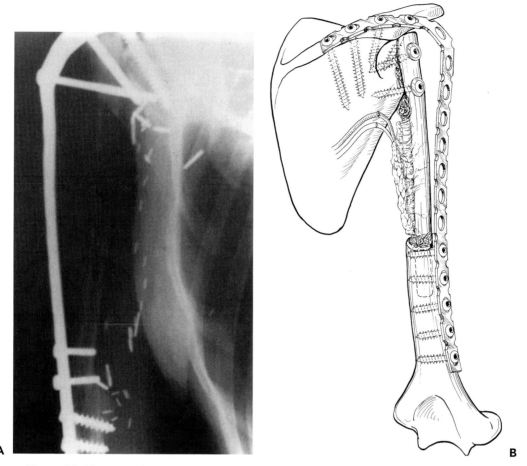

Figure 29-16 (*A*) Vascularized fibular bone graft is used to reconstruct the proximal two thirds of humerus after tumor resection. The plate obtains fixation proximally and distally. Minimal fixation is used in the fibular graft itself. The fibular graft is supplemented with cancellous bone at the proximal and distal bone junctures. (*B*) The technique of a vascularized fibular graft used to span a deficiency of the proximal humerus. Cancellous bone graft has been placed at both ends of the fibular graft.

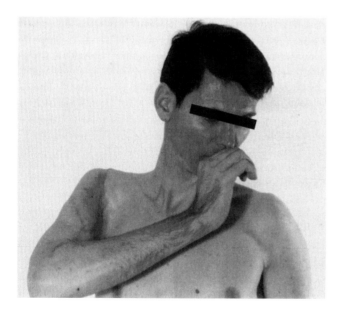

Figure 29-17 Result after reconstruction of the proximal humerus with vascularized fibular bone graft. The patient has a stable upper extremity with good hand function.

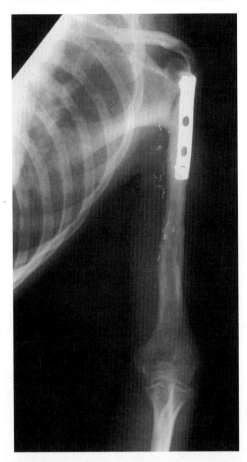

Figure 29-18 Hypertrophy of vascularized fibular graft. Vascular grafts have excellent biologic potential and can hypertrophy over time in response to the stresses placed on them. Such hypertrophy is rarely observed in allografts. Vascularized autogenous grafts are used in preference to allografts when performing glenohumeral arthrodesis.

of autogenous bone at each juncture to maximize the likelihood of fusion occurring (Fig. 29-18).

Vascularized full-thickness iliac crest bone grafts can be used to provide bone and soft tissue. The use of such a bone graft creates a significant donor deficit but can be considered if a bone and soft tissue defect coexists. The shape of the iliac crest limits its usefulness somewhat for long intercalary defects, although the graft can be osteotomized to straighten it. Alternatively, vascularized iliac crest bone grafts can be used in conjunction with a nonvascularized fibular graft or an allograft.

Allograft Reconstruction

Allograft reconstruction can be considered in conjunction with bone grafting when performing shoulder arthrodesis for complex and revision cases.[10] I prefer not to use allograft bone if autogenous bone is available. For instance, if bone grafting is required to supplement a vascularized fibular graft, I would consider using the contralateral fibula or iliac crest graft to supplement the vascularized fibular graft in preference to an allograft. At times, allograft must be used because of the nonavailability of autogenous bone. Both structural and nonstructural allograft bone can be used. More commonly, allograft is used in conjunction with a large implant to perform an arthroplastic reconstruction after tumor resection.

Soft Tissue Loss

Soft tissue loss can be caused by trauma or the necessity to resect soft tissue to obtain clear margins after tumor resection. The most common soft tissue deficiency about the shoulder is related to rotator cuff abnormalities. Isolated rotator cuff deficiency does not require special consideration, and my conventional method of shoulder arthrodesis involves resection of the rotator cuff in its entirety.

Local Flap Techniques

If deltoid resection is required for tumor ablation or if the deltoid has been lost as a result of trauma, consideration should be given to augmentation of the soft tissue envelope. It is important to have well-vascularized muscle surrounding the arthrodesis site. Good muscle coverage is associated with enhanced bone formation and enhanced revascularization of autogenous avascular bone, as seen after bone grafting.[52]

Fortunately, local and free-flap techniques are available to provide a stable soft tissue envelope about the shoulder. The latissimus muscle provides a local source of autogenous tissue that can be rotated to cover the shoulder. The entire latissimus muscle can be elevated on its vascular pedicle and rotated easily to cover the shoulder. The latissimus has an excellent blood supply, and most surgeons are familiar with its dissection. The flap can be rotated as a pure muscle flap or myocutaneous flap, depending on the patient's requirements. If the nerve supply to the latissimus is kept intact, it can also be used for flexorplasty, as described by Zancolli and Mitre.[64] The requirement to use a latissimus flap in this regard may be seen after trauma to the shoulder and proximal humerus resulting in the loss of biceps function. Other local flaps about the shoulder are less reliable. The latissimus flap should be considered the mainstay of treatment when soft tissue is required locally.

Free Tissue Transfer

If a latissimus flap cannot be used, a free tissue transfer can be considered. Such a transfer is required relatively infrequently about the shoulder. The trapezius should not be used to cover a soft tissue defect after shoulder arthrodesis. Good function of the trapezius is required to motor the shoulder girdle after arthrodesis, and its anatomy should not be disturbed.

Hybrid Methods of Reconstruction

Complex and revision problems about the shoulder require special techniques when performing shoulder arthrodesis. In some cases, a combination of techniques is required, and such hybrid methods of treatment are in the patient's best interest when faced with complex bone and soft tissue deficits. For instance, after tumor resection, it may be necessary to perform a vascularized fibular bone graft, a pedicled latissimus muscle flap, an autogenous iliac crest bone graft, and a pectoralis major to scapular transfer (because of long thoracic nerve palsy) to stabilize the shoulder girdle and provide enough tissue so that arthrodesis can occur. The timing and staging of such complex procedures must be assessed on an individual basis (Fig. 29-19).

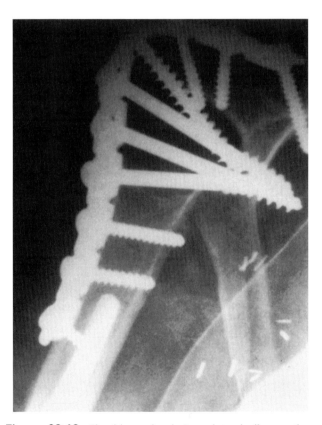

Figure 29-19 Shoulder arthrodesis and total elbow arthroplasty using Mayo-modified Coonrad prosthesis. This patient was involved in a motor vehicle accident and had a flail shoulder and an ankylosed elbow with an associated upper trunk lesion. The upper trunk lesion was reconstructed with nerve grafting to the musculocutaneous nerve. The shoulder was stabilized by arthrodesis. The elbow, which ankylosed because of heterotopic ossification after an intra-articular fracture, was treated by total elbow arthroplasty. Excellent function was restored to this patient's upper extremity.

COMPLICATIONS OF GLENOHUMERAL ARTHRODESIS

Nonunion

Nonunion after shoulder arthrodesis is surprisingly infrequent in view of the magnitude of the procedure, the high stresses across the arthrodesis site, and the difficulty of postoperative immobilization. In Cofield and Briggs's[11] 1979 series of 71 shoulder arthrodeses, only 3 patients went on to have nonunions. All 3 patients' shoulders were successfully fused after second operative procedures. If nonunion occurs after shoulder arthrodesis, a repeat operation with revision of the internal fixation device is indicated. Bone grafting should be used to augment the arthrodesis site if a nonunion has occurred. I have seen a small number of patients who have obtained an acromiohumeral fusion that was not fused solidly at the glenohumeral joint. In one patient, the internal fixation device failed, and bone grafting was necessary.

Infection

Infection is relatively uncommon after shoulder arthrodesis because of the excellent vascularity of the periarticular tissues. Infection after shoulder arthrodesis should be treated with surgical drainage and the appropriate parental antibiotics. The internal fixation should not be removed if it is providing stability at the arthrodesis site. An attempt should be made to obtain solid arthrodesis before removal of any fixation device.

Malposition

Excessive abduction of the extremity during shoulder arthrodesis can place a significant strain on the thoracoscapular musculature. Adult patients have great difficulty adapting to positions of greater than 45 degrees of abduction. Hyperabduction at the arthrodesis site causes significant winging of the scapula to allow the arm to drop to the patient's side. In some patients, the arm does not approximate the trunk if the shoulder has undergone arthrodesis in too much abduction. Women in particular are unhappy with the cosmetic appearance of a shoulder that has been fused in too much abduction because of the significant prominence of the scapula that is created when the arm is adducted.

Fusion of the shoulder in too much internal rotation can occur (Fig. 29-20). If this occurs, the patient cannot easily bring his or her hand to the mouth and cannot reach a front or back pocket. Rotational osteotomy of the humerus may be necessary for patients whose extremities have been positioned in too much internal rotation. I have performed three such osteotomies for this indication. Groh et al.[22] described a reconstructive osteotomy to correct symptomatic

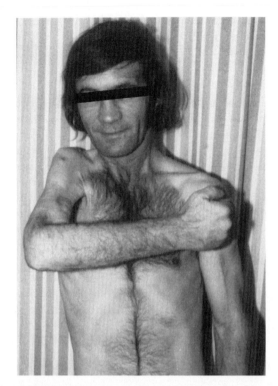

Figure 29-20 Arthrodesis of the shoulder in excessive internal rotation. If the shoulder is malpositioned, a corrective osteotomy below the arthrodesis site may be required.

malposition after arthrodesis of the shoulder. Suprascapular nerve entrapment has been reported after shoulder arthrodesis.[60]

Prominence of the Internal Fixation Device

Many patients who have had internal fixation devices applied over the spine of the scapula have significant skin tenderness in the area of the appliance. This can be particularly troublesome when the patient must wear a prosthetic harness and skin irritation and ulceration have been reported.[48] Cofield and Briggs[11] reported a significant incidence of tenderness over the internal fixation device, which required its removal in 17 of their patients. I have observed a similar experience, although use of a malleable reconstruction plate decreased skin tenderness and reduced the need for removal of internal fixation.[49] The development of appliances specifically designed for shoulder arthrodesis is likely to decrease the incidence of skin tenderness of the skin overlying internal fixation devices even further.

Fracture of the Humerus

Fracture of the humerus at the distal end of the internal fixation device is sufficiently common that the AO group recommended prophylactically bone grafting this area.[39] Cofield and Briggs[11] reported fractures in the fused extrem-

ity occurring in 10 of 71 patients. This complication has occurred in my series in association with significant trauma to the arthrodesed shoulder. If an unstable fracture has occurred at the end of the internal fixation device, I advocate removal of the device together with internal fixation of the fracture if the arthrodesis has solidly healed. If the fracture is relatively undisplaced, it can be treated by closed means, but in my experience, this is uncommon.

FUNCTIONAL OUTCOME AFTER SHOULDER ARTHRODESIS

I have performed 84 shoulder arthrodeses in patients between the ages of 19 and 64 years. Forty-six patients underwent operation for irreparable lesions of the brachial plexus, five patients for recalcitrant shoulder instability, two patients for osteoarthritis, two patients for failed total shoulder arthroplasties, and two patients for sepsis. The technique used was that of combined glenohumeral and acromiohumeral arthrodesis, as described previously. In my home community, tumor surgery is almost exclusively performed by colleagues at the Mount Sinai Hospital in Toronto. I have less experience with shoulder arthrodesis for this indication.

Solid arthrodesis has been obtained in most cases with the primary procedure. Two patients developed only an acromiohumeral fusion, and one of these patients developed a broken screw. This patient had a secondary bone grafting procedure. Infection occurred in only one case. Clinical examination showed all shoulders to be fused within 10 degrees of the desired position. We have not used special techniques to assess the position of the arthrodesis.[26] Eighteen patients required surgery for plate removal, and two patients sustained fractures of the humerus distal to the plate.

Clinical Experience

For a series of 33 patients, my colleagues and I assessed functional outcome in detail.[51] The patients' ability to perform specific activities of daily living after shoulder arthrodesis were ranked as follows:

Working at waist level	29
Getting dressed	29
Sleeping	27
Lifting bags	25
Using knife	25
Washing face	25
Reaching front pocket	23
Working at shoulder level	21
Doing up buttons	21
Reaching opposite axilla	20
Eating	17
Managing toileting	13

Reaching back pocket	11
Bathing	7
Washing back	6
Doing hair	5

The ability to perform activities of daily living depended on the adequacy of hand function in patients with brachial plexus injuries (Fig. 29-21). Regression analysis revealed the underlying indication (preoperative diagnosis) for shoulder arthrodesis to be the single best predictor of the ability of patients to perform the activities of daily living after shoulder arthrodesis. The patient's compensation board status was also a predictor of outcome. Patient satisfaction was highest in those patients undergoing the procedure for a brachial plexus injury, osteoarthritis, and failed total shoulder arthroplasty.

Five patients who had neurogenic pain preoperatively continued to complain of significant neurogenic pain postoperatively. Several other patients who had compensable injuries continued to complain of postoperative pain despite solid arthrodeses. Most patients can reach their front and back pockets after surgery, and many have returned to occupations with fairly heavy labor. These occupations have included tool and dye manufacture, gardening, heavy equipment operation, and brick laying. Patients who had shoulder arthrodesis for compensable injuries did not return to their previous occupations. I have not experienced acromioclavicular joint problems after shoulder arthrodesis. Some surgeons recommend excision arthroplasty of the acromioclavicular joint after arthrodesis in an effort to maximize shoulder motion.[45] I have not found it necessary to perform this adjunctive procedure in this series of patients.

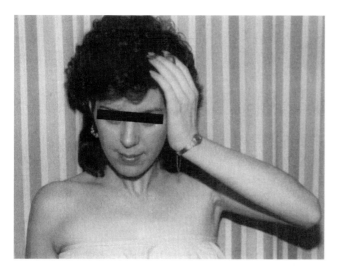

Figure 29-21 After successful shoulder arthrodesis, a patient is usually able to reach his or her mouth, ipsilateral ear, and front pocket. The arm usually comfortably drops down to the side. Patients are able to perform many, but not all, activities of daily living.

Fusion

Fusion rates after shoulder arthrodesis are high. Most older series do not report any nonunions, but later series using internal fixation devices report high union rates. It is often difficult to judge radiographic union in patients who have had internal fixation. The internal fixation device commonly obscures the arthrodesis site, and rigid internal fixation prevents the formation of periarticular new bone. Because I routinely use rigid internal rotation, I tend to arbitrarily discontinue external immobilization by 6 or 8 weeks. I examine the shoulder and, assuming that the patient is comfortable, place the patient's arm in a sling at this time. I avoid any attempt to actively mobilize the thoracoscapular musculature until at least 3 months after arthrodesis. Using this method of postoperative rehabilitation, I have found delayed union or nonunion to be uncommon.

Functional Improvement

The amount of improvement in shoulder function after arthrodesis depends on the degree of function preoperatively. Patients who have flail shoulders experience a significant improvement in glenohumeral function after arthrodesis because they can actively position their extremities in space. Shoulder subluxation is relieved, and function is significantly improved. Most patients can use the extremity to lift, dress, tend to personal hygiene, eat, and comb their hair. In Cofield and Briggs's[11] series, hair combing was the most difficult task to perform after arthrodesis of the glenohumeral joint. El-Gammal et al.[17] reported on the use of shoulder arthrodesis combined with free-functioning gracilis transplantation in patients with elbow and shoulder paralysis caused by poliomyelitis. Doi et al.[15] reported on the restoration of prehension with the double free muscle technique after complete avulsion of the brachial plexus.

Pain Relief

Pain relief is not universal after shoulder arthrodesis. Some pain is commonly experienced by patients who have successfully undergone shoulder arthrodesis. The presence of moderate to severe pain after successful shoulder arthrodesis is difficult to explain but occurs frequently. It is thought that such pain is related to problems with the contiguous soft tissues. Shoulder arthrodesis places a significant strain on the periscapular musculature and requires the patient to make a profound functional adjustment. Pain surrounding successful fusions has also been reported after hip and knee arthrodesis. Most patients experience less pain with longer follow-up periods, and this suggests that with time the periscapular musculature adjusts to the changes imposed on it by glenohumeral arthrodesis.

Patients with neurogenic pain caused by brachial plexus injury do not experience pain relief after glenohumeral arthrodesis. Shoulder function is improved in these patients, but they should understand fully that the procedure is being performed to improve function and not to relieve pain. If function is improved, such neurogenic pain is generally better tolerated by the patient. I concentrate on the restoration of limb function rather than on relief of pain by neurosurgical means.

Acromioclavicular Joint Pain

Acromioclavicular joint pain has been reported after shoulder arthrodesis. Some methods of shoulder arthrodesis require osteotomy of the acromion. Such osteotomies disturb the normal acromioclavicular relation. When pain arises from the acromioclavicular joint postoperatively, excision arthroplasty is indicated if local injections confirm that the pain is arising from the acromioclavicular joint. Some investigators have reported anecdotally that excision arthroplasty of the acromioclavicular joint improves motion after shoulder arthrodesis. In my experience, acromioclavicular joint pain is rare after glenohumeral arthrodesis when the acromion is left in the anatomic position. For this reason, I do not recommend acromial osteotomy to approximate the acromion to the superior surface of the humeral head. I do advocate moving the humerus proximally to appose the acromiohumeral and glenohumeral arthrodesis sites. The glenoid presents a small surface to the humeral head across which arthrodesis can occur. It is for this reason that decortication of the undersurface of the acromion and the glenoid and humeral head is advocated. The presence of a broader surface across which arthrodesis can occur is desirable, and it is believed that this increases the arthrodesis rate.

SUMMARY

Shoulder arthrodesis remains an important procedure that should be part of every shoulder surgeon's armamentarium. The procedure is indicated for patients with paralytic disorders, who require en bloc resection of their glenohumeral joint together with the rotator cuff or deltoid for tumor, and whose shoulder joints have been destroyed by septic arthritis. I have found the procedure useful in a small number of patients with failed total shoulder arthroplasties and shoulder instability. The procedure is rarely indicated for patients with rotator cuff tears, periarticular malunions, osteoarthritis, or rheumatoid arthritis.

Although a variety of different positions for glenohumeral arthrodesis have been advocated in the literature, I recommend a position of 30 degrees of abduction (measured clinically), 30 degrees of flexion, and 30 degrees of internal rotation. This position brings the hand to the midline anteriorly so that with elbow flexion the patient can reach his or her mouth. With the shoulder fused in this position, the arm drops comfortably to the side. I recommend fusion of the acromiohumeral and glenohumeral articulations and the use of internal fixation when performing shoulder arthrodesis. Complications after shoulder arthrodesis are relatively infrequent, and most can be dealt with successfully.

The improvement in shoulder function after shoulder arthrodesis depends on the patient's preoperative shoulder function. Patients with flail shoulders experience a significant improvement in function. Patients with significant mechanical pain in the glenohumeral joint experience relief after the procedure. Shoulder arthrodesis does not relieve neurogenic pain and requires a significant functional adjustment on the part of patients who have undergone the procedure. Shoulder arthrodesis is primarily indicated to restore function. Bone grafting is routinely used for complex and revision procedures. The procedure is contraindicated in any patient with a progressive neurologic disorder affecting the periscapular musculature.

ACKNOWLEDGMENTS

I appreciate the assistance of Mrs. Kim Mason in preparing the references. Several figures were kindly provided by Drs. R.S. Bell and M.D. McKee. Dr. Allan Hudson referred most of the patients with irreparable brachial plexus injuries that were ultimately treated with shoulder arthrodesis. The other patients were referred by my colleagues in the Canadian and Ontario Orthopaedic Associations.

REFERENCES

1. Albert EM. Einige Fälle von kunstlicher Ankylosenbildung an paralytischen Gliedmassen. Wiener medizinische Presse, 1882;23:725. (English translation in: Bick EM, ed. Classics of Orthopaedics. Philadelphia:Lippincott, 1976;52.)
2. Barr J, Freiberg JA, Colonna PC, et al. A survey of end results on stabilization of the paralyzed shoulder: report of the Research Committee of the American Orthopaedic Association. J Bone Joint Surg 1942;24:699.
3. Barton NJ. Arthrodesis of the shoulder for degenerative conditions. J Bone Joint Surg 1972;54A:1759.
4. Bateman JE. The shoulder and neck, 2nd ed. Philadelphia, PA, WB Saunders, 1978;273.
5. Beltran JE, Trilla JC, Barjan R. A simplified compression arthrodesis of the shoulder. J Bone Joint Surg 1975;57A:538.
6. Berger A, Brenner P. Secondary surgery following brachial plexus injuries. Microsurgery 1995;16(1):43.
7. Brittain HA. Architectural principles in arthrodesis, 3rd ed. Edinburgh, E & L Livingstone, 1952.
8. Carroll RE. Wire loop in arthrodesis of the shoulder. Clin Orthop 1957;9:185.
9. Charnley J, Houston JK. Compression arthrodesis of the shoulder. J Bone Joint Surg 1964;46B:614.
10. Cheng EY, Gebhardt MC. Allograft reconstructions of the shoulder after bone tumor resections. Orthop Clin 1991;22:37.
11. Cofield RH, Briggs BT. Glenohumeral arthrodesis. J Bone Joint Surg 1979;61A:668.

12. Davis JB, Cottrell GW. A technique for shoulder arthrodesis. J Bone Joint Surg 1962;44A:657.
13. De Palma AF. Surgery of the shoulder, 3rd ed. Philadelphia, PA, JB Lippincott, 1983;132.
14. De Velasco PG, Cardoso MA. Arthrodesis of the shoulder. Clin Orthop 1973;90:178.
15. Doi K, Muramatsu K, Hattori Y, et al. Restoration of prehension with the double free muscle technique following complete avulsion of the brachial plexus. Indications and long-term results. J Bone Joint Surg Am 2000;82(5):652.
16. Earns CT, Matsen F, Jacking S. Surgical management of complex irreparable rotator cuff deficiency. J Arthroplasty 1991;6:363.
17. El-Gammal TA, El-Sayed A, Kotb MM. Shoulder fusion and free-functioning gracilis transplantation in patients with elbow and shoulder paralysis caused by poliomyelitis. Microsurgery 2002;22(5):199.
18. Freidman RJ, Ewald FC. Arthroplasty of the ipsilateral shoulder and elbow in patients who have rheumatoid arthritis. J Bone Joint Surg 1987;69A:661.
19. Gill AB. A new operation for arthrodesis of the shoulder. J Bone Joint Surg 1931;13:287.
20. Goldner JL. Muscle-tendon transfers for partial paralysis of the shoulder girdle. In: Evarts CMCC, ed. Surgery of the musculoskeletal system. New York, Churchill Livingstone, 1983:167.
21. Gonzalez-Diaz R, Rodriguez-Merchan EC, Gilbert MS. The role of shoulder fusion in the era of arthroplasty. Int Orthop 1997;21(3):204.
22. Groh GI, Williams GR, Jarman RN, et al. Treatment of complications of shoulder arthrodesis. J Bone Joint Surg Am 1997; 79(6):881.
23. Hawkins RJ, Neer CS. A functional analysis of shoulder fusions. Clin Orthop 1987;223:65.
24. Johnson CA, Healy WL, Brooker AF Jr., et al. External fixation shoulder arthrodesis. Clin Orthop 1986;211:219.
25. Jonsson E, Brattstrom M, Lidgren L. Evaluation of the rheumatoid shoulder function after hemiarthroplasty and arthrodesis. Scand J Rheumatol 1988;17:17.
26. Jonsson E, Lidgren L, Rydholm U. Position of shoulder arthrodesis measured with Moire photography. Clin Orthop 1989; 238:117.
27. Kneisl JS. Function after amputation, arthrodesis, or arthroplasty for tumors about the shoulder. J South Orthop Assoc 1995; 4(3):228.
28. Kocialkowski A, Wallace WA. Shoulder arthrodesis using an external fixation. J Bone Joint Surg 1991;73B:180.
29. Kostiuk JP, Schatzker J. Shoulder arthrodesis—AO technique. In: Bateman JE, Welsh RP, eds. Surgery of the shoulder. Philadelphia, PA, CV Mosby, 1984:207.
30. Kumar VP, Satku SK, Mitra AK, et al. Function following limb salvage for primary tumors of the shoulder girdle. Ten patients followed 4 (1–11) years. Acta Orthop Scand 1994;65:55.
31. Leffert RD. Brachial plexus injuries. New York, Churchill Livingstone, 1985;193.
32. Macdonald W, Thrum CB, Hamilton SGL. Designing an implant by CT scanning and solid modelling: arthrodesis of the shoulder after excision of the upper humerus. J Bone Joint Surg 1986;68B:208.
33. Mah JY, Hall JE. Arthrodesis of the shoulder in children. J Bone Joint Surg 1990;72:582.
34. Makin M. Early arthrodesis for a flail shoulder in young children. J Bone Joint Surg 1977;59A:317.
35. May VR. Shoulder fusion: a review of fourteen cases. J Bone Joint Surg 1962;44A:65.
36. Mohammed NS. A simple method of shoulder arthrodesis. J Bone Joint Surg Br 1998;80(4):620.
37. Morgan CD, Casscells CD. Arthroscopic-assisted glenohumeral arthrodesis. Arthroscopy 1992;8:262.
38. Moseley HF. Arthrodesis of the shoulder in the adult. Clin Orthop 1961;20:156.
39. Muller ME, Allgower AM, Willenegger H. Manual of internal fixation, 2nd ed. Berlin, Springer-Verlag, 1979.
40. Nagano A, Okinaga S, Ochiai N, et al. Shoulder arthrodesis by external fixation. Clin Orthop 1989;247:97.
41. Naranja RJ Jr., Inanity JP. Surgical options in the treatment of arthritis of the shoulder: alternatives to prosthetic arthroplasty. Semin Arthroplasty 1995;6(4):204.
42. Neer CS II, Craig EV, Fukada H. Cuff tear arthropathy. J Bone Joint Surg 1983;65A:416.
43. Neer CS II, Watson KC, Stanton FJ. Recent experience in total shoulder replacement. J Bone Joint Surg 1982;64A:319.
44. O'Connor MI, Sim FH, Chao EY. Limb salvage for neoplasms of the shoulder girdle. Intermediate reconstructive and functional results. J Bone Joint Surg 1996;78(12):1872.
45. Pipkin G. Claviculectomy as an adjunct to shoulder arthrodesis. Clin Orthop 1967;54:145.
46. Putti V. Arthrodesis for tuberculosis of the knee and shoulder. Chir Organi Mov 1933;13:217.
47. Raunio P. Arthrodesis of the shoulder joint in rheumatoid arthritis. Reconstr Surg Traumatol 1981;18:48.
48. Richards RR. Operative treatment for irreparable lesions of the brachial plexus. In: Gelberman RH, ed. Operative nerve repair and reconstruction. Philadelphia, PA, JB Lippincott, 1991:1303.
49. Richards RR, Schemitsch EH. The effect of muscle flap coverage on bone blood flow following devascularization of segment of tibia: an experimental investigation in the dog. J Orthop Res 1989; 32:366.
50. Richards RR, Beaton DE, Hudson AR. Shoulder arthrodesis with plate fixation: a functional outcome analysis. J Shoulder Elbow Surg 1993;2:225.
51. Richards RR, Sherman RMP, Hudson AR, et al. Shoulder arthrodesis using a modified pelvic reconstruction plate: a review of eleven cases. J Bone Joint Surg 1988;70A:416.
52. Richards RR, Waddell JP, Hudson AR. Shoulder arthrodesis for the treatment of brachial plexus palsy. Clin Orthop 1985;198:250.
53. Riggins RS. Shoulder fusion without external fixation. J Bone Joint Surg 1976;58A:1007.
54. Rockwood CA, Burkhead WZ. The management of patients with massive rotator cuff defects by acromioplasty and radical cuff debridement. Presented to the Orthopaedic Associations of the English Speaking World, Washington, DC, May 1987.
55. Rowe CR. Re-evaluation of the position of the arm in arthrodesis of the shoulder in the adult. J Bone Joint Surg 1974;56A:913.
56. Rowe CR, Pierce DS, Clark JG. Voluntary dislocation of the shoulder. a preliminary report on a clinical, electromyographic and psychiatric study of twenty-six patients. J Bone Joint Surg 1973;55A:445.
57. Ruhmann O, Gosse F, Wirth CJ, et al. Reconstructive operations of the paralyzed shoulder in brachial plexus palsy: concept of treatment. Injury 1999;30(9):609.
58. Rybka V, Raunio P, Vainio K. Arthrodesis of the shoulder in rheumatoid arthritis: a review of forty-one cases. J Bone Joint Surg 1979;61B:155.
59. Schrader HA, Frandsen PA. External compression arthrodesis of the shoulder joint. Acta Orthop Scand 1983;54:592.
60. Sjostrom L, Mjoberg B. Suprascapular nerve entrapment in an arthrodesed shoulder. J Bone Joint Surg 1992;74B:470.
61. Uematsu A. Arthrodesis of the shoulder: posterior approach. Clin Orthop 1979;139:169.
62. Watson-Jones R. Extra-articular arthrodesis of the shoulder. J Bone Joint Surg 1933;15:862.
63. Wilde AH, Brems JJ, Boumphrey FR. Arthrodesis of the shoulder: current indications and operative technique. Orthop Clin North Am 1987;18:463.
64. Zancolli E, Mitre H. Latissimus dorsi transfer to restore elbow flexion: an appraisal of eight cases. J Bone Joint Surg 1973; 55A:1265.

Miscellaneous Conditions: Nerve Injuries and Soft-Tissue Problems

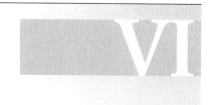

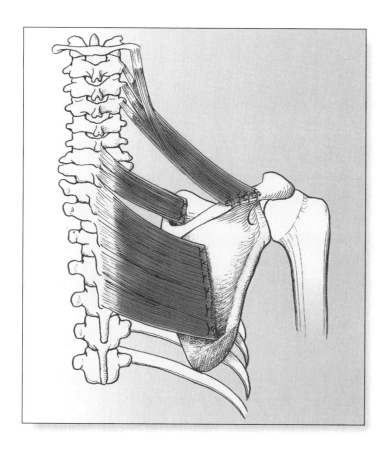

The Painful, Snapping Scapula

30

Peter J. Millett   Philippe Clavert   Jon J. P. Warner

INTRODUCTION

Periscapular pain is not uncommon and is often related to disease of the glenohumeral joint, subacromial bursa, and cervical or dorsal spine. The chest wall is convex, and normally the concave scapula and interposed muscles glide smoothly along this wall. The inferior and superior angles of the scapula are not well cushioned. Even if bony anomalies of this region are rare,[5,6,28,30,33] they may be responsible for inflammation of the surrounding bursa. Although conservative management usually alleviates symptoms, surgical treatment can be performed in the case of refractor pain. Usually this includes an open or arthroscopic resection of the superomedial scapular angle, with a scapulothoracic bursectomy.

HISTORICAL PERSPECTIVE

Symptomatic scapulothoracic bursitis and crepitus are difficult and often poorly understood disorders of the scapulothoracic articulation. Little has been written about arthroscopic or open solutions for refractory pain from this region. The first step[20] is to realize the subtle differences between these two related entities. Historically, several terms have been used to describe various elements of the clinical spectrum, including the snapping scapula,[4,27] scapulothoracic syndrome,[29] washboard syndrome,[9] and rolling scapula.[10] Boinet[4] is generally credited with the first de-

scription of scapulothoracic crepitus in 1867, and Mauclaire[22] later described three subclasses: froissement, frottement, and craquement in 1904. *Froissement* is a gentle physiologic friction sound, *frottement* is a louder grating sound and is usually pathologic, and *craquement* is a consistently pathologic loud snapping sound. Milch[27] added to the understanding in 1961 by differentiating scapulothoracic crepitus into a loud, usually painful grating sound caused by a bony lesion and a less intense sound caused by a soft-tissue lesion such as bursitis. Kuhn et al.[20] extrapolated from Milch, proposing that frottement may represent a soft-tissue lesion or bursitis, whereas craquement represents an osseous lesion as the source of the painful scapulothoracic crepitus. Precise distinction may be difficult even radiographically or surgically. Furthermore, it is crucial to understand that clinically symptomatic bursitis may exist without an audible sound or palpable crepitus. Moreover, isolated crepitus in the absence of pain may be physiologic.

The timing and choice of intervention are influenced by the severity and cause of the symptoms, and an understanding of these two entities will assist the clinician in appropriate diagnosis and treatment.

ANATOMY AND BIOMECHANICS

The anatomy and biomechanics of the scapulothoracic articulation are important to understand when treating these problems. Two major and four minor, or adventitial, bursae have been described in the scapulothoracic articulation (Fig. 30-1).[9,17,18,20,35,36,41] The first major bursa, the infraserratus bursa, is located between the serratus anterior muscle and the chest wall. The second, the supraserratus

P. J. Millett, P. Clavert, and J. J. P. Warner: The Harvard Shoulder Service, Department of Orthopaedic Surgery, Massachusetts General and Brigham and Women's Hospitals, Boston, Massachusetts.

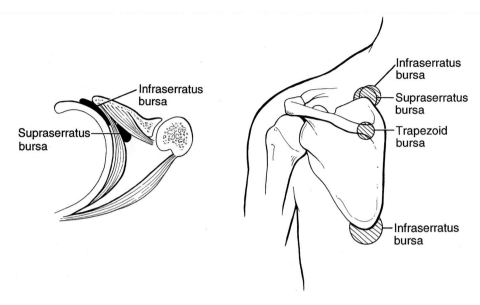

Figure 30-1 Localization of the adventitial bursae of the scapulothoracic articulation. (From: Kuhn JE, Richard JH. Evaluation and treatment of scapular disorder. In: Warner JJP, Iannotti JP, Gerber C, eds. Complex and revision problems in shoulder surgery. 1st edition. Philadelphia, PA, Lippincott-Raven, 1997.)

bursa, is found between the subscapularis and the serratus anterior muscles (Fig. 30-1). The anatomic consistency of these bursae is well documented.[9,17,18,35,36,41] In addition, four minor bursae have been identified.[20,35,41] These, however, have not been consistently found in cadaveric or clinical studies. These bursae have been postulated to be adventitial in nature, arising in response to abnormal biomechanics of the scapulothoracic articulation.[20,35,41] Two have been described at the superomedial angle of the scapula, and historical accounts identify the location to be either infraserratus or supraserratus. A third site of pathology is at the inferior angle of the scapula, thought to be an infraserratus bursa. The fourth location, the trapezoid bursa,[11] is at the medial base of the spine of the scapula, underlying the trapezius muscle. It is usually the bursa in the region of the superior angle of the scapula that is symptomatic[20,35] (Fig. 30-1).

The chest wall is convex and cushioned by several muscles, but especially by the serratus anterior. The concave scapula and interposed muscles glide smoothly along this wall. It is inferred that this condition results from incongruence of the scapulothoracic articulation, which may or may not be associated with bony anomalies of this region.[5,6,28,30,33] Because bony abnormalities are rare, a dynamic compression or maltracking[14,40] is postulated to be responsible for the pathologic contact between the superior angle of the scapula and the ribs that compresses and irritates the bursa between these two structures.[20,41,42] Clinical studies and histologic findings of bursitis, muscle intrafascicular fibrosis, shoulder girdle muscle atrophy, and edema support this hypothesis.[20,33] Rarely, bony abnormalities such as osteochondromas or Luschka's tubercles may be the cause of the crepitus.

The scapular noises encountered in crepitus arise from anatomic changes of the soft tissues in the articulation or from bony incongruity because of the anatomic anomalies of the bones themselves.

DIAGNOSIS

Clinical Evaluation

Clinical evaluation of scapulothoracic bursitis and crepitus begins with a thorough history and physical examination. The history of the problem is similar in both disorders. Patients with bursitis report pain with overhead activity,[36] often with a history of trauma or repetitive overuse in work or recreation.[1,5,20,23,24,36] This constant motion irritates the soft tissues, leading to inflammation and a cycle of chronic bursitis and scarring. This tough, fibrotic bursal tissue can then lead to mechanical impingement and pain with motion, and thus further inflammation. Audible or palpable crepitus may accompany the bursitis. Patients with scapulothoracic crepitus may additionally report a family history, and it is occasionally bilateral.[10]

The physical findings of bursitis include a localized tenderness over the inflamed area. The superomedial border of the scapula is the most common location, but the inferior pole is also a site of pathology. A mild fullness can be palpated, and audible or palpable crepitus may be present. Physical findings in patients with crepitus include point tenderness as well, whereas visual inspection may also reveal a fullness or a compensatory pseudo-winging of the scapula as the individual attempts to avoid the painful bursitis. A mass may be palpable. The scapula will grate as the shoulder is put through a range of motion. In those with winging, it is crucial to perform a careful neuromuscular examination to differentiate compensatory pseudo-winging from true winging. Although some patients may exhibit winging, this may be secondary to pain from the scapulothoracic articulation, and motor examination of the serratus anterior and trapezius will demonstrate normal function of these muscles. If the issue remains unclear, an electromyogram and nerve conduction study may be helpful. Again, crepitus alone in the absence of pain can be physiologic and rarely warrants treatment.

Positive Diagnosis

Selective injections with a corticosteroid and local anesthetic may be very helpful to confirm the diagnosis (Fig. 30-2). The injection can be diagnostic and therapeutic,[5,10,23,33] because immediate symptomatic relief after injection of the local anesthetic helps to confirm the cause of pain and the anatomic location of the bursa in question. If this injection is accurately placed into the scapulothoracic bursa and the patient notes significant pain relief, it confirms the diagnosis.[23,33] The steroid may also afford an anti-inflammatory effect that facilitates a physical therapy program as noted next. The injection should be placed with some caution to avoid a pneumothorax.[5]

Imaging Studies

Radiographs should include tangential scapular views to identify bony anomalies. The role of computed tomography, with or without three-dimensional reconstruction, is still debated[30] (Fig. 30-3), but in patients with suspected osseous lesions and normal x-rays, this additional imaging is often helpful.[30] Magnetic resonance imaging can identify

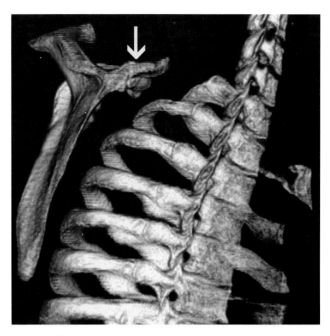

Figure 30-3   Three-dimensional view of a scapula of a patient presenting with a painful snapping scapula. Note Luschka's tubercle.

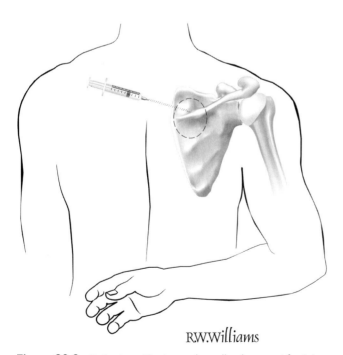

RW.Williams

Figure 30-2   Patient positioning and needle placement for injection of the scapulothoracic articulation.

the size and location of bursal inflammation, but its usefulness is also debated.

Differential Diagnosis

The differential diagnosis of scapulothoracic bursitis includes soft tissue lesions such as atrophied muscle,[27,42] fibrotic muscle,[26,27] anomalous muscle insertions,[13,42] and elastofibroma, a rare but benign soft tissue tumor that is commonly seen in this location and that elevates the scapula.[20]

The differential diagnosis of scapulothoracic crepitus is expansive and includes several anatomic anomalies located between the scapula and the chest wall. Osteochondromas[12,31] can arise from the undersurface of the scapula or the posterior aspect of the ribs. Luschka's tubercle[27] is a prominence of bone at the superomedial aspect of the scapula, and that same region can have an excessively hooked surface that alters scapulothoracic dynamics[27,34] (Fig. 30-3). Malunited fractures of the scapula or the ribs can lead to crepitus.[37] Reactive bone spurs can form from repetitive microtrauma of the periscapular musculature.[2,12,38] Infectious causes such as tuberculosis or syphilis can lead to pathologic changes in the soft tissues.[27] In addition, incongruity of the articulation can exist secondary to scoliosis or thoracic kyphosis, leading to altered biomechanics and crepitus.[10,26] Last, the differential diagnosis of all forms of scapulothoracic pathology must include unrelated disorders, such as cervical spondylosis and radiculopathy, glenohumeral pathology, and periscapular muscle strain.

SCAPULOTHORACIC BURSITIS TREATMENT

Conservative Treatment

Once the diagnosis of scapulothoracic bursitis or crepitus has been made, the initial treatment is nonoperative management. Rest, systemic nonsteroidal anti-inflammatory medications, and activity modification are necessary. Then physical therapy may be initiated. The aim of physical therapy is to restore normal kinematics and prevent sloping of the shoulder.[9,25] Therefore, therapy should emphasize periscapular muscle strengthening, particularly the subscapularis and serratus anterior, which when hypertrophied will elevate the scapula further off the chest wall.[9,25,33] Postural training, figure-of-eight harnesses, taping, or scapulothoracic bracing can serve to minimize thoracic kyphosis, which may be an aggravating factor. Subtle weakness of the serratus anterior muscle may allow the scapula to tilt forward so that its upper border will "washboard" over the ribs and irritate the bursa. Therefore, strengthening of this muscle is very important because it may resolve pain by restoring normal scapular mechanics. As noted previously, injection of a corticosteroid and local anesthetic can assist in treatment and diagnosis.[5,10,23,33] When considering how long to pursue conservative management, the underlying diagnosis is of importance. Scapulothoracic bursal inflammation secondary to overuse and repetitive strain may be treated for quite some time before surgical intervention is needed. In contrast, when there is a structural anatomic lesion such as an osteochondroma, conservative measures alone are unlikely to provide benefit,[12] and the threshold to progress to operative management should be significantly lower.

Surgical Treatment

The majority of patients will improve with conservative measures; for those who do not, a variety of surgical procedures have been described. For those with scapulothoracic bursitis, open bursectomy of the involved region, either the superomedial angle or inferior pole, is a reasonable option that has a proven record of success.[7,16,23,24,26,32,34,36]

Although variations in the techniques are numerous and beyond the scope of this review, the essential steps involve a fairly large exposure and subperiosteal elevation of the medial periscapular musculature (Fig. 30-4), with identification of the pathologic tissue and excision of inflamed bursa, irregular or pathologic bone, or both (Fig. 30-5). The elevated muscle layers are sutured back to bone through drill holes, and the skin is often closed over a drain (Fig. 30-6). Rehabilitation follows a course of early passive motion, active motion by 4 weeks, and strengthening by 8 to 12 weeks.[23,24] Outcomes have generally been good.

Arthroscopic treatment of these disorders have been advocated as an alternative to open surgery in an attempt to

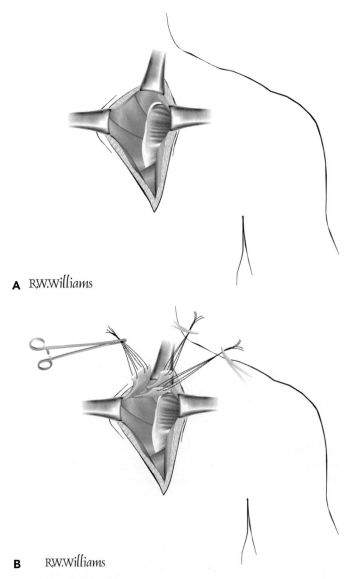

A R.W.Williams

B R.W.Williams

Figure 30-4 Incision and subperiosteal elevation of the medial periscapular muscles.

minimize the morbidity of the exposure with its muscle takedown and to facilitate early rehabilitation and return to preoperative function.[3,9,16,18,21,32] A relative contraindication to the all arthroscopic approach is the patient who has symptomatic crepitus of the trapezoid bursa. This bursa is superficial to the scapulothoracic (infraserratus) bursa, and a bursectomy in this region will fail to remove the pathologic tissue.

Arthroscopic Bursectomy Technique

The surgeon must be skilled in arthroscopy, knowledgeable of the regional anatomy, and proficient in triangulation to perform scapulothoracic bursoscopy in a safe and efficient manner. We perform arthroscopic scapulothoracic bursectomy with the patient in a prone position, with the arm placed behind the back in a position of extension and

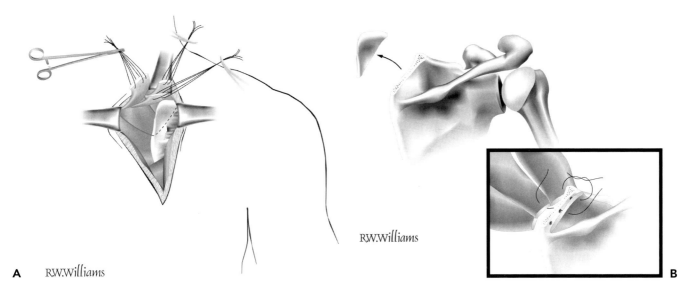

Figure 30-5 Resection of the superior angle of the scapula.

internal rotation (the so-called chicken-wing position). This position results in scapular protraction and winging off the posterior thorax (Fig. 30-7). This facilitates entry of the arthroscopic instruments into the bursal space.

The standard arthroscopic portals are used as shown in Figure 30-8. The initial "safe" portal is placed 2 cm medial to the medial scapular edge at the level of the scapular spine, between the serratus anterior and the posterior thoracic wall. This avoids the dorsal scapular nerve and artery, which course along the medial border of the scapula. The space is localized with a spinal needle and distended with approximately 30 cc of saline, and the portal is created. A blunt obturator is inserted into the subserratus space. Care must be taken to avoid overpenetration through the chest wall or more commonly through the serratus anterior into the sub-

scapular (axillary) space. The 30-degree arthroscope is inserted, and fluid is infiltrated to distend the subserratus space. We prefer to use an arthroscopy pump but keep the pressure low (30 mm Hg) to minimize fluid extravasation or dissection of fluid into the axilla. The second "working" portal can then be localized under direct visualization using a spinal needle. This is placed approximately 4 cm inferior to the first portal. A 6-mm cannula is inserted through this lower portal, and a motorized shaver and bipolar radiofrequency device are used to resect the bursal tissue (Fig. 30-9). The radiofrequency device is particularly useful to minimize bleeding in the vascular, inflamed tissue (Fig. 30-10). Because there are minimal anatomic landmarks for resection, a methodologic approach is essential, ablating from medial to lateral and then from inferior to superior. To facilitate visualization, the surgeon should be prepared to switch viewing portals as needed and to have a 70-degree arthroscope readily available. Spinal needles can be used to help outline

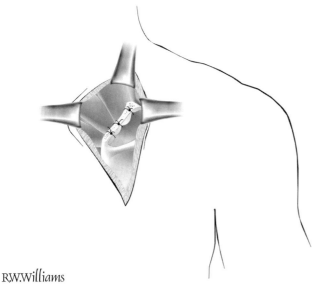

Figure 30-6 Reinsertion of the elevated muscles.

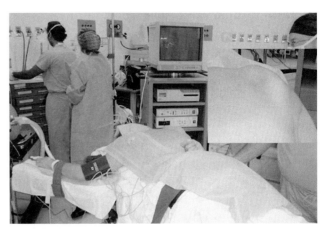

Figure 30-7 Patient in the "chicken-wing position."

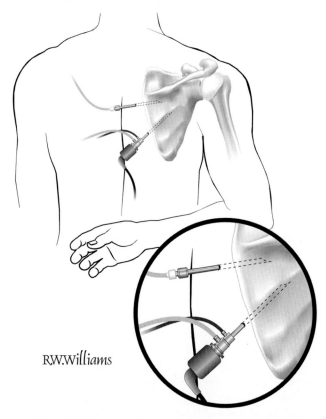

Figure 30-8   Standard arthroscopic portal placement.

the medial border of the scapula, and a probe can be used to palpate the ribs and intercostal muscles inferiorly and the scapula and serratus anterior superiorly. An additional portal may be placed superiorly as needed, although portals superior to the spine of the scapula may place the dorsal scapular neurovascular structures, accessory spinal nerve, and transverse cervical artery at risk.

The superomedial angle of the scapula is then identified by palpation through the skin. The radiofrequency device is

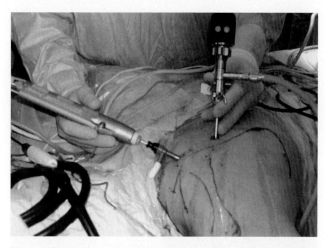

Figure 30-9   Surgeon positioning with an optimal triangulation to perform the scapulothoracic bursectomy.

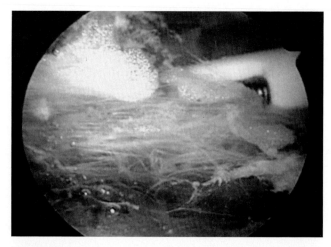

Figure 30-10   Arthroscopic view of an inflamed scapulothoracic bursae.

used to detach the conjoined insertion of the rhomboids, levator scapulae, and supraspinatus from the bone subperiosteally. A partial scapulectomy is then performed using a motorized shaver and a burr. The periosteal sleeve is not repaired and is allowed to heal through scarring. It may sometimes be difficult to fully define the superior scapular angle because of swelling from arthroscopic fluid, and in such cases a small incision allows exposure of the superior scapular angle and its resection. The trapezius muscle is split, and the rhomboids and serratus muscles are removed. The superior angle is resected, and then the rhomboids and serratus are repaired through drill holes to the superior scapula (Fig. 30-5).

Postoperatively the patient is placed in a sling for comfort only, as opposed to a period of 4 weeks for an open approach. Gentle passive motion is initiated immediately to avoid stiffness. At 4 weeks, active and active-assisted range of motion are begun together with isometric exercises, and after 8 weeks strengthening of the periscapular muscles begins (Fig. 30-11).

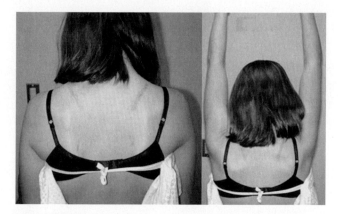

Figure 30-11   Clinical result of a bilateral arthroscopic scapulothoracic bursectomy associated with a bilateral open resection of the superomedial angle of the scapula.

RESULTS

Ciullo and Jones[9] introduced the concept of arthroscopic debridement of the scapulothoracic articulation in 1992, and Harper et al.[16] reported on the first series of arthroscopic bony debridements of the superomedial angle of the scapula in 1999. The arthroscopic anatomy was thoroughly described by Ruland et al.,[35] and two recent alternative arthroscopic portals were introduced by Chan et al. in 2002[8] and Pavlik et al. in 2003.[32] Early results of arthroscopic treatment seem promising, with minimal morbidity and early return to function.[8,16,32] Nevertheless, no large series has been published, and it must be emphasized that this technique is primarily used by the experienced arthroscopists.

Complications of arthroscopic treatment of scapular disorders, although rare, need to be considered. First, failure to resect all pathologic tissues leads to recurrence of the symptoms. For these patients, a new arthroscopic bursectomy or a muscle transfer may be necessary.[24] Then, a pneumothorax may occur because of the localization of the bursa. Neurologic or vascular injury must be taken into account. Because of the relationships of the accessory nerve with the levator scapulae and the medial border of the scapula,[35] it may be at risk during an arthroscopic bursectomy. With correct placement of the portals, the mean distance to the accessory nerve beneath the trapezius is approximately 35 mm.[8] As well, the suprascapular nerve[39] may be at risk when the superior angle of the scapula is resected.

To our knowledge, there are no published reports of these complications, but the experience is still in its infancy.

SCAPULOTHORACIC CREPITUS

Diagnosis

Scapulothoracic crepitus is also inflammation, with or without secondary bursitis, of the scapulothoracic space. Most of the time, patients with scapulothoracic crepitus are able to locate the crepitus. Usually they report overhead activities at work or during their sporting activities.[10,33] A trauma of the shoulder girdle or the upper limb must be noted.[1] Patients may notice that this trauma has precipitated the symptoms. A familial component also may be reported.[10]

The inciting lesion is usually a bony or firm mass, but the differential diagnosis is extensive. Physical findings in crepitus include a fullness or prominence of the involved area, occasionally with a palpable mass. The scapula will grate palpably and/or audibly.

In case of scapulothoracic crepitus, a computed tomography scan with three-dimensional reconstruction may be helpful, especially in case of a palpable or suspected mass.

Treatment

Thirty-five percent of asymptomatic healthy persons have scapulothoracic crepitus.[11,15] This condition is not necessarily a pathologic condition.

Except for patients with clearly defined bony pathology (e.g., an osteochondroma) who will benefit from a resection of that mass, conservative treatment remains the mainstay of the treatment. As for the scapulothoracic bursitis, this conservative treatment will associate a physical therapy program as described for the scapulothoracic bursitis with rest and systemic nonsteroidal anti-inflammatory medications. A local injection of steroid also may be helpful. Surgical treatment is reserved for patients in whom conservative treatment failed; patients with significant psychiatric conditions should be carefully evaluated before any surgery is performed.

Different surgical procedures have been described, such as muscle plasty by Mauclaire[22] or Butters,[5] or partial scapulectomy including resection of the medial border of the scapula[6] or the superomedial angle.[1,10,19,27,34,38,42]

The surgical technique of resection of the superomedial border of the scapula is performed as described previously. Postoperatively, the patient is placed in a regular sling to protect the muscle sutures. Passive assisted range of motion is started immediately. Active assisted range of motion is started at 4 weeks, and strengthening is started at 12 weeks.

RESULTS

In patients undergoing resection of a mass, the results are usually good in terms of pain relief and noise reduction. Patients are able to go back to their activities of daily living and sporting activities.[5,28,31]

Crepitus has been successfully treated with open excision of the superomedial border of the scapula itself.[5,10,19,27,34] The largest series was published by Arntz and Matsen in 1990,[1] who treated approximately 14 shoulders; 86% of the patients obtained complete relief of their pain and crepitus. The bone, postoperatively inspected, appeared to be normal in all cases. This is why some suggest a superomedial scapular angle resection and an open or arthroscopic bursectomy should be performed.[24,36] Our experience also has shown that approximately 85% of patients report marked relief after surgical treatment.

REFERENCES

1. Arntz CT, Matsen FA III. Partial scapulectomy for disabling scapulo-thoracic snapping. Orthop Trans 1990;14:252.
2. Bateman JE. The shoulder and the neck. 2nd edition. Philadelphia, PA, WB Saunders, 1978.
3. Bizousky DT, Gillogly SD. Evaluation of the scapulothoracic articulation with arthroscopy. Orthop Trans 1992–1993;16:822.
4. Boinet J. Snapping scapula. Societe Imperiale de Chirurgie (2nd series). 1987;8:458.

5. Butters KP. The snapping scapula. In: Rockwood CJ, ed. The shoulder. Philadelphia, PA, WB Saunders, 1990:335.

6. Cameron HU. Snapping scapulae: a report of three cases. Eur J Rheumatol Inflamm 1984;7:66.

7. Carlson HL, Haig AJ, Stewart DC. Snapping scapula syndrome: three case reports and an analysis of the literature. Arch Phys Med Rehabil 1997;78:506.

8. Chan BK, Chakrabarti AJ, Bell SN. An alternative portal for scapulothoracic arthroscopy. J Shoulder Elbow Surg 2002;11:235.

9. Ciullo JV, Jones E. Subscapular bursitis: conservative treatment of "snapping scapula" or "wash-board syndrome". Orthop Trans 1992–1993;16:740.

10. Cobey MC. The rolling scapula. Clin Orthop 1969;60:193.

11. Codman EA. The anatomy of the human shoulder. In: Codman E, ed. The shoulder. Malabar, FL, Krieger Publishing, 1984:1.

12. Cuomo F, Blank K, Zuckerman JD, et al. Scapular osteochondroma presenting with exostosis bursata. Bull Hosp Jt Dis 1993;52:55.

13. Edelson JG. Variations in the anatomy of the scapula with references to the snapping scapula. Clin Orthop 1982;322:111.

14. Glousman R, Jobe F, Tibone J, et al. Dynamic electromyographic analysis of the throwing shoulder with glenohumeral instability. J Bone Joint Surg 1988;70(A):220.

15. Grunfeld G. Beitrag zur genese des skapularkrachens und der skapulargerausche. Arch Orthop Unfallchir 1927;24:610.

16. Harper GD, McIlroy S, Bayley JI, et al. Arthroscopic partial resection of the scapula for snapping scapula: a new technique. J Shoulder Elbow Surg 1999;8:53.

17. Hollinshead WH. The back and limbs. In: Hollinshead W, ed. Anatomy for the surgeons. Ed 3. Philadelphia, PA, Harper and Row, 1982:300.

18. Kolodychuk LB, Reagan WD. Visualization of the scapulothoracique articulation using an arthroscope: a proposed technique. Orthop Trans 1993–1994;17:1142.

19. Kouvalchouk JF. Subscapular crepitus. Orthop Trans 1985;9:587.

20. Kuhn JE, Plancher KD, Hawkins RJ. Symptomatic scapulothoracique crepitus and bursitis. J Am Acad Orthop Surg 1998;6:267.

21. Matthews LS, Poehling GC, Hunter DM. Scapulothoracique endoscopy: anatomical and clinical considerations. In: McGinty J, Caspari R, Jackson R, et al. eds. Operative arthroscopy, 2nd edition. Philadelphia, PA, Lippincott-Raven, 1996:813.

22. Mauclaire T. Craquement sous-scapulaire pathologiques traits par l'interposition musculaire interscapulothoracique. Mem Soc Chir Paris 1904;30:164.

23. McCluskey GM III, Bigliani LU. Surgical management of refractory scapulothoracic bursitis. Orthop Trans 1991;15:801.

24. McCluskey GM III, Bigliani LU. Scapulothoracic disorders. In: Andrews J, Wilk K, eds. The athlete's shoulder. New York, Churchill Livingstone, 1994:305.

25. Michele A, Davies JJ, Krueger FJ, et al. Scapulocostal syndrome (fatigue-postural paradox). N Y J Med 1950;50:1353.

26. Milch H. Partial scapulectomy for snapping scapula. J Bone Joint Surg 1950;32(A):561.

27. Milch H. The snapping scapula. Clin Orthop 1961;20:139.

28. Morse BJ, Ebraheim NA, Jackson WT. Partial scapulectomy for snapping scapula syndrome. Orthop Rev 1993;22:1141.

29. Moseley HF. Shoulder lesions 2nd ed. New York, Hocher Publishing, 1953.

30. Mozes G, Bickels J, Ovadia D, et al. The use of three-dimensional computed tomography in evaluating snapping scapula syndrome. Orthopedics 1999;22:1029.

31. Parson TA. The snapping scapula and subscapular exostoses. J Bone Joint Surg 1973;55(B):345.

32. Pavlik A, Ang K, Coghlan J, et al. Arthroscopic treatment of painful snapping of the scapula by using a new superior portal. Arthroscopy 2003;19:608.

33. Percy EL, Birbrager D, Pitt MJ. Snapping scapula: a review of the literature and presentation of 14 patients. Can J Surg 1988;31:248.

34. Richards RR, McKee MD. Treatment of painful scapulothoracic crepitus by resection of the superomedial angle of the scapula: a report of three cases. Clin Orthop 1989;247:111.

35. Ruland LJ III, Ruland CM, Matthews LS. Scapulothoracic anatomy for the arthroscopist. Arthroscopy 1995;11:52.

36. Sisto DJ, Jobe FW. The operative treatment of scapulothoracic bursitis in professional pitchers. Am J Sports Med 1986;14:192.

37. Steindler A. The traumatic deformities and disabilities of the upper extremity. Springfield, MO, Charles C. Thomas, 1946.

38. Strizak AM, Cowen MH. The snapping scapula syndrome: a case report. J Bone Joint Surg 1982;64(A):941.

39. Warner JP, Krushell RJ, Masquelet A, et al. Anatomy and relationships of the suprascapular nerve: anatomical constraints to mobilization of the supraspinatus and infraspinatus muscles in the management of massive rotator-cuff tears. J Bone Joint Surg [Am] 1992;74:36.

40. Warner JJ, Micheli LJ, Arslanian LE, et al. Scapulothoracic motion in normal shoulders and shoulders with glenohumeral instability and impingement syndrome. A study using Moire topographic analysis. Clin Orthop 1992;(285):191.

41. Williams GR, Shakil M, Klimkiewicz J, et al. Anatomy of the scapulothoracique articulation. Clin Orthop 1999;359:237.

42. Wood VE, Verska JM. The snapping scapula in association with the thoracic outlet syndrome. Arch Surg 1989;124:1335.

Scapular Winging Caused by Serratus Anterior Dysfunction: Recognition and Treatment

Philippe Clavert   *Jon J. P. Warner*

INTRODUCTION

Scapular winging may be associated with several neurologic conditions including spinal accessory nerve palsy and fascioscapulohumeral muscular dystrophy; however, it is most commonly associated with isolated paralysis of the long thoracic nerve. Whether of idiopathic or traumatic cause, scapular winging may vary from complete paralysis to paresis, and most cases resolve within 18 months.[56] For this reason, all patients must be treated conservatively when the diagnosis is made, and consideration for surgery is only in the most chronic cases. Diagnosis and surgical management of refractory scapular winging caused by serratus anterior dysfunction will be presented in this chapter.

P. Clavert and J. J. P. Warner: The Harvard Shoulder Service, Department of Orthopaedic Surgery, Massachusetts General Hospital, Boston, Massachusetts.

HISTORICAL PERSPECTIVE

Winslow first reported the clinical presentation of scapular winging in 1777.[66] Velpeau[60] in 1837 was the first to isolate the pathoanatomy of the winging and described a case of an isolated serratus anterior palsy. Subsequently, other authors have reported their experiences in the literature.[10,11,19,22,44,48,50,52,58,63,65,68]

The first surgical treatment was described by Tubby in 1904.[57] He transferred the sternal portion of the pectoralis major to the different digitations of the serratus anterior. But as the serratus was denervated, the graft progressively stretched out and a recurrence of the scapular winging occurred. Others suggested a fascial sling suspension operation as surgical treatment.[4,31,64] As with the prior techniques, the recurrence of scapular winging was high because the graft stretched out[64]; thus, scapulothoracic fusion was proposed and developed.[13,20] Scapulothoracic fusion, however, resulted in more motion loss, so some surgeons developed a method of dynamic scapular stabilization by transferring muscles. Numerous tendon transfers were thus developed, including the pectoralis minor,[10,50,58] pectoralis major or split pectoralis major,[11,44,48,52,63,65] teres major,[19,68] and rhomboideus muscle.[22] Currently, the two techniques routinely used to treat winging caused by long thoracic nerve palsy are the split pectoralis major tendon transfer and scapulothoracic fusion.

Marmor and Bechtol in 1963[38] first described transfer of the sternal head of the pectoralis tendon. Their original technique was with a fascia lata graft extension. This technique requires a large incision over the shoulder and hemithorax as well as a large incision on the lateral thigh. Post[48] and others[11,40,44,48] subsequently refined this technique and reported good success with it. Unfortunately, some patients experienced pain at the donor site of fascia lata graft harvested from the thigh. This morbidity was caused by muscle herniation and development of seromas.

Subsequently, others have described smaller incisions on the shoulder and thorax as well as the use of semitendinosus and gracilis tendons, which may be harvested through a smaller incision with less morbidity.[41,54,63]

SCAPULAR WINGING AND SERRATUS ANTERIOR DYSFUNCTION

Anatomy

The serratus anterior muscle is a large muscle that expands over the lateral aspect of the thorax. Digitations arise from the upper first nine ribs, pass between the scapula and the ribs, and attach to the medial border of the scapula (Fig. 31-1). The long thoracic nerve is the sole innervator of the serratus anterior and is purely a motor nerve. It origi-

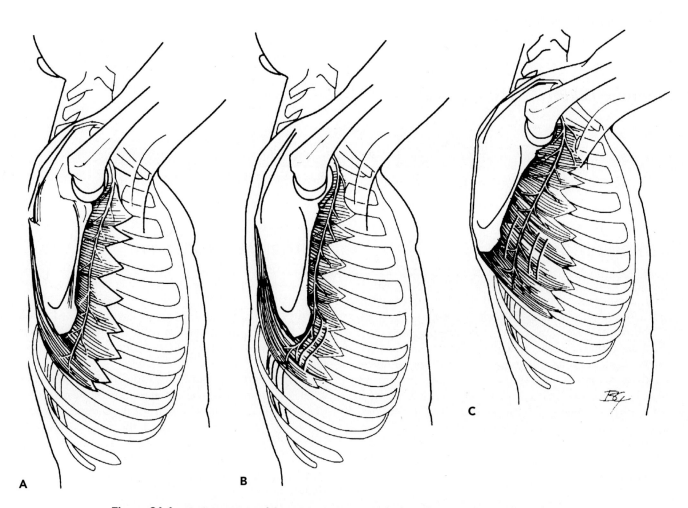

Figure 31-1 *(A–C)* Insertions of the serratus anterior on the lateral aspect of the chest wall and of the long thoracic nerve course. Mechanism of injury of the long thoracic nerve stretched while the arm is protracted. (Reprinted with permission from: Kuhn JE, Hawkins RJ. Evaluation and treatment of scapular disorders. In: Warner JJP, Iannotti JP, Gerber C, eds. Complex and revision problems in shoulder surgery. 1st edition. Philadelphia, PA, Lippincott-Raven, 1997.)

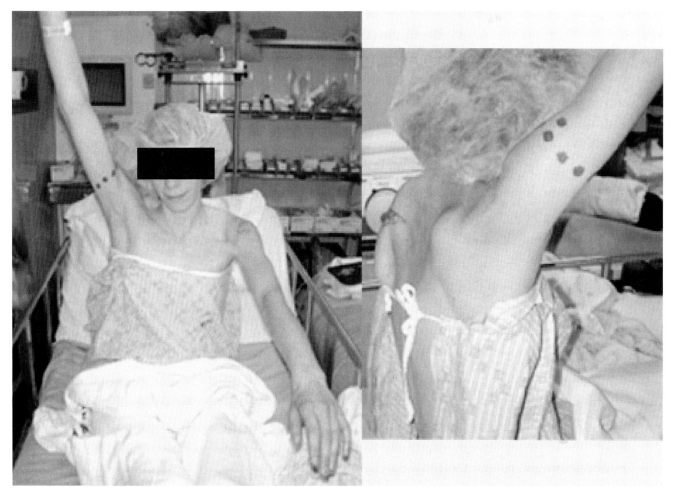

Figure 31-2 *(A,B)* Clinical presentation of a patient presenting a scapular winging.

nates from the ventral rami of the C5 and C6 cervical roots. Some fibers coming from C7 may also participate in the innervation of the serratus anterior. The C5 and C6 roots pass through the scalenus medius muscle and merge before they receive a branch from the seventh cervical root. The long thoracic nerve then courses beneath the clavicle, over the first rib, and beneath the brachial plexus. Once on the chest wall, the long thoracic nerve courses to the serratus anterior muscle slips and ends at the inferior angle of the scapula (Fig. 31-1). This superficial and winding course and its length make this nerve at risk for low-energy compression injuries and stretch injuries.[1,23,25]

Biomechanics

The serratus anterior muscle protracts and rotates the scapula around the thorax. Thus, the scapula is pulled forward during elevation of the arm. This motion is essential to permit full overhead elevation as it tilts the glenoid forward and upward allowing the humeral head to rotate

on a fixed joint platform. An injury to the long thoracic nerve results in paradoxic movement of the scapula away from the chest so that the inferior angle of the scapula rotates toward the midline and the medial border of the scapula becomes prominent. This is observed as winging (Fig. 31-2). The biomechanical consequences of such paradoxic motion are to reduce the arc of motion available to the glenohumeral joint so the humerus cannot move upward because of loss of mechanical advantage of the deltoid and rotator cuff. Furthermore, the humerus will contact the coracoacromial arch, which can cause non-outlet impingement. This may be why a rotator cuff problem is misdiagnosed in some of these patients (Fig. 31-3).

Cause

In most cases, injury to the long thoracic nerve is neurapraxic because of stretching or compression (Fig. 31-1). This explains why most cases improve with conservative treatment. Both traumatic and nontraumatic events may

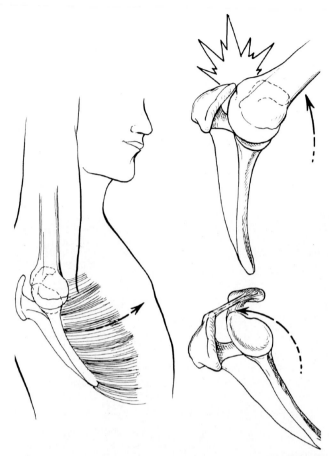

Figure 31-3 Serratus anterior dysfunction and its role in sub-acromial impingement and rotator cuff disease. (Reprinted with permission from: Kuhn JE, Hawkins RJ. Evaluation and treatment of scapular disorders. In: Warner JJP, Iannotti JP, Gerber C, eds. Complex and revision problems in shoulder surgery. 1st edition. Philadelphia, PA, Lippincott-Raven, 1997.)

cause this problem. Described causes include the rare condition of nerve entrapment into the scalenus muscle or by the first rib,[17,18,30] nontraumatic injuries to the long thoracic nerve from compression of the nerve while the arm is abducted,[59] viral illnesses,[15,49] immunization,[5] Parsonage-Turner syndrome,[42] and isolated long thoracic neuritis.[47,49] Iatrogenic lesions of the long thoracic nerve have also been reported, mainly after radical mastectomy, first rib resection for outlet syndrome, and transaxillary sympathectomy.[16,30,59]

Traumatic injuries to the long thoracic nerve occur mainly after sudden traction to the upper limb during a fall or collision, at work, or during sports or daily living activities.[17,37,59,63] The nerve is stretched from its points where it is tethered: first rib, inferior border of the scapula, and first two or last branches of the nerve.[2,17,23,29,67] Finally, in some patients, no cause for serratus anterior palsy can be identified.[44,61,63] No matter what the cause, chronic winging may cause significant shoulder pain and disability.[30]

APPROACH TO DIAGNOSIS

Patient Presentation

Patients may often simply present with pain and/or weakness as the chief complaint, but they may not notice winging. This is why delay in diagnosis is not particularly rare. Indeed, many patients present whose treatments for a variety of other diagnoses have failed, including impingement, instability, and acromioclavicular disease.[45,47,63]

Pain is typically described as posterior around the scapula, and this seems to be caused by compensation of the remaining axioscapular muscles (rhomboids, trapezius). As noted previously, there may be impingement-type symptoms that occur because of a non-outlet impingement mechanism (Fig. 31-3).

Sometimes the patient or a family member may notice the winging when trying to elevate the arm, and in most cases there is difficulty with activities of daily living. More severe pain may indicate an acute plexus neuritis.[49]

Clinical Findings

All patients should be examined with their shirts off and the shoulders viewed from anterior and posterior during elevation of the arms. Muscle atrophy is usually not noticed in these patients, although subtle malpositioning of the scapula may be apparent. Some patients may have a scapula that actually sits in a slightly winged position. If the scapula is ptotic and sits lower than the contralateral side, and if the patient is unable to symmetrically shrug both shoulders, trapezius palsy should be suspected (Fig. 31-4).[63]

While the back of the patient is being viewed, he or she is asked to flex both shoulders, and scapular rhythm and stabilization are observed. Winging may be obvious, although in husky individuals it may still appear to be subtle. Total flexion will be limited in most patients (Fig. 31-2). It may be helpful for the examiner to keep the inferior angle of the scapula between his or her first two fingers to assess the scapulothoracic rhythm and winging. Several maneuvers will enhance winging by placing the serratus anterior at a mechanical disadvantage. The first maneuver is to have the patient place his or her hands on the wall and perform a push-up away from the wall.[55] Winging may be apparent with this motion. The second maneuver is to have the patient resist flexion with the shoulders at 90 degrees, because this will overpower the stronger lower portion of the serratus anterior muscle.[63]

A test that not only confirms winging caused by weakness of the serratus anterior but also predicts success of tendon transfer reconstruction (if needed) is the "scapular stabilizing test."[63] The examiner stabilizes the scapula against the chest wall with his or her hands, with counterpressure on the anterior chest. The patient should have relief of pain and the increased ability to flex his or her arm (Fig. 31-5).

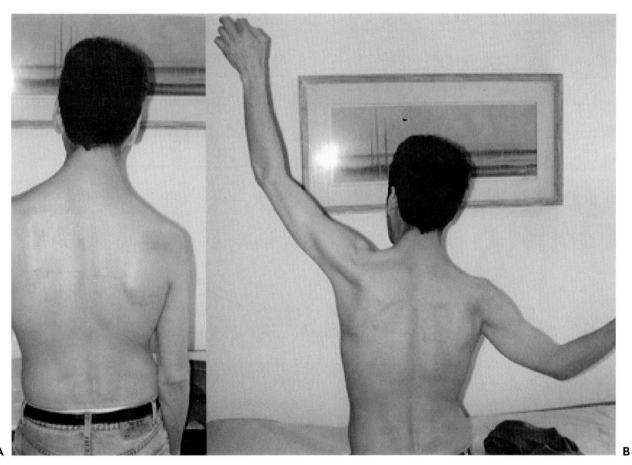

Figure 31-4   *(A,B)* Patient with a trapezius palsy. Note the shoulder ptosis.

Electromyographic Findings

Electrical diagnosis of nerve dysfunction is important; however, not all patients with demonstrable winging caused by serratus anterior dysfunction have clear electromyograph findings. This may be because of the study technique or the direct muscle stretch injury. Nevertheless, electromyograph studies should establish the diagnosis if possible and then be repeated after 6 months to see whether recovery is proceeding.[28,46,63]

Clinical experience has shown that a 1-year trial of conservative management is the minimum to see whether the nerve will recover unless it is clearly established that it has been traumatized by severe compression or actual transection.[30,59]

Differential Diagnosis

As previously stated, trapezius palsy may also cause a type of scapular winging; however, this condition is more rare than long thoracic nerve paralysis, and the pattern of winging differs significantly. This condition is discussed further in Chapter 32. In this condition, the shoulder is depressed and the scapula is translated laterally with the inferior angle rotated laterally (Fig. 31-6). In these cases the patient is unable to shrug his or her shoulders.[6,63]

Others causes of primary winging must be excluded, such as scapulothoracic bursitis,[43] bony abnormalities,[8,12,14,36] rupture or disorder in periscapular muscle, and severe neurologic conditions such as fascioscapulohumeral muscular dystrophy.[3,7,9,13,21,24,26,34,35,39] In the last case, all the scapular stabilizing muscles are weak and dysfunctional so that no useful motion of the scapula is possible (Fig. 31-7).

Scapular winging may also be a secondary phenomenon as the shoulder girdle complex attempts to substitute for glenohumeral or subacromial pathology.[32,55,62] For example, adhesive capsulitis or arthritis results in loss of glenohumeral motion, and the patient compensates by scapulothoracic motion. Patients present in such cases with the appearance of scapular winging and pain in this region because of overload of the axioscapular muscles.

Occasionally, patients may present with winging that is a voluntary ability to contract the axioscapular muscles in an unbalanced fashion. This is similar to voluntary

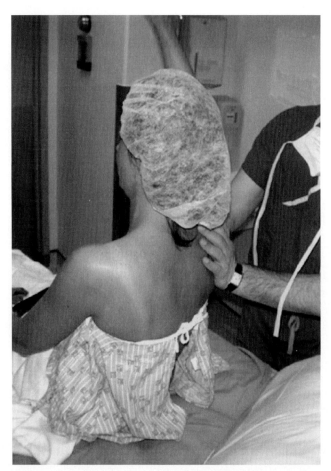

Figure 31-5 Compression test; relief of the pain and ability of the patient to flex his or her arm above 150 degrees.

glenohumeral instability, and it may also be associated with this abnormal motion pattern. This condition is conservatively treated with physical therapy to teach patients not to contract their periscapular muscles during flexion.[51]

TREATMENT

Nonoperative Treatment

Because in most of the cases the patient has a paresis rather than a paralysis, the expectation is for the condition to subside within 1 year and fully recover in 18 months.[56] Thus, all patients should be treated conservatively first. Rest and avoidance of heavy lifting or activities above the level of the scapula are necessary. In fact, we believe that lifting activities or physical therapy attempting to strengthen the serratus anterior muscle may actually stretch the long thoracic nerve more and thus delay recovery. This concept may not always be understood by a worker's insurance carrier, but it is a therapeutic imperative.

The use of an orthosis may help to relieve the pain by controlling the stability of the scapula. This can be accomplished by plastic shell molded and padded to fit against the scapula with a counterpressure strap across the chest. Unfortunately, this brace is often poorly tolerated because it may need to be worn for an extended period.[63]

Surgical Treatment

Tendon Transfer

Most shoulder surgeons would agree that when conservative treatment has failed, and the patient remains symptomatic because of painful loss of motion and winging, a dynamic tendon transfer procedure is indicated. The most commonly used technique is the transfer of the sternal head of the pectoralis major tendon, which is lengthened by autogenous fascia lata graft.[11,48] The author's preference has been to modify this approach to allow for smaller incisions and less donor site morbidity.[48] This

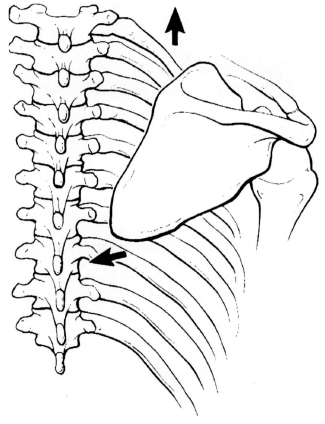

Serratus anterior palsy

Figure 31-6 (A,B) Both types of scapular winging: long thoracic nerve and spinal accessory nerves injury. (Reprinted with permission from: Kuhn JE, Hawkins RJ. Evaluation and treatment of scapular disorders. In: Warner JJP, Iannotti JP, Gerber C, eds. Complex and revision problems in shoulder surgery. 1st edition. Philadelphia, PA, Lippincott-Raven, 1997.)

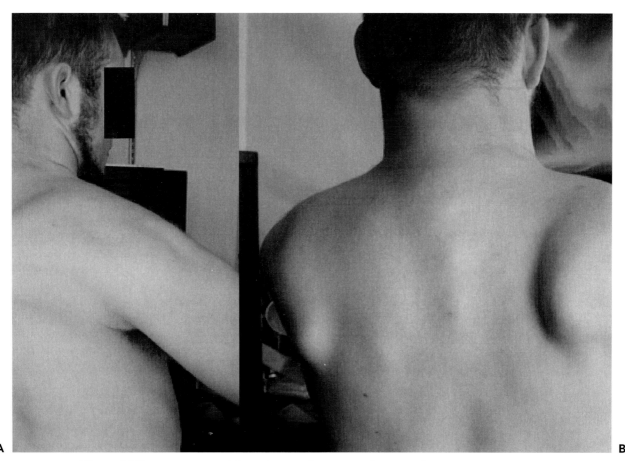

A   **B**

Figure 31-7   *(A,B)* Patient with limited range of motion in relation to a fascioscapulohumeral dystrophy.

is accomplished by harvesting the patient's own hamstrings (semitendinosus and gracilis) through a small incision on the medial aspect of the knee and then mobilizing the pectoralis muscle and transferring it along the chest to a smaller incision over the inferior angle of the scapula.[63]

Scapulothoracic Fusion

This procedure is reserved for failed tendon transfer procedures or for severe axioscapular muscle dysfunction such as occurs with fascioscapulohumeral muscular dystrophy.[9,13,26,34]

Split Pectoralis Major Tendon Transfer: Operative Technique (Author's Method)

The patient is placed on the operating table on the long beanbag in a supine position. After anesthesia, the patient is rolled into a partial lateral decubitus position so that the bean bag can be contoured over the back to allow the scapula free mobility and good exposure for the tendon transfer (Fig. 31-8). The ipsilateral leg is also kept free and

sterilely draped in the operative field. We prefer to use an articulated arm holder (Tenet Spyder, Tenet Medical Engineering, Calgary, Canada) to permit static positioning of the arm into positions needed for dissection and tendon preparation and for tendon transfer (Fig. 31-9).

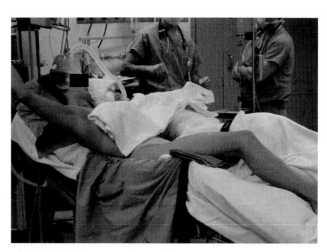

Figure 31-8   Patient positioning on a long bean-bag.

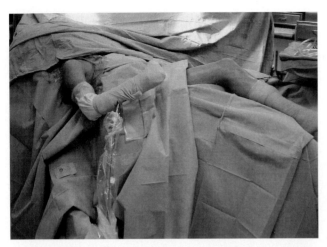

Figure 31-9   Patient draped; uses of a mechanical arm holder.

Tendon Harvest

A sterile pneumatic tourniquet is placed about the upper thigh, and after it is exsanguinated with an Esmarch bandage, it is inflated to 350 mm Hg. Tourniquet time required for this portion of the procedure is usually less than 20 minutes. The technique of harvesting the hamstrings has been described in many prior articles.[41,63] A 4-cm incision is made over the palpable hamstrings medial to the tibial tubercle, and the first layer of the leg is defined. This is divided along the course of the tendons, and the gracilis and semitendinosus are then harvested by means of a tendon stripper (Fig. 31-10). Tendons are then prepared by sewing them side to side and tapering the ends so they can pass into the pectoralis muscle as noted next (Fig. 31-10).

Pectoralis Major Tendon Dissection

An anterior incision is made over the shoulder slightly medial to an incision for a usual deltopectoral approach and also 4 to 5 cm longer (Fig. 31-11). Superficial dissection and undermining of the skin is then performed, and the deltopectoral interval is identified, as is the inferior border of the pectoralis major. The deltopectoral interval is then developed keeping the cephalic vein with the deltoid, and the inferior border of the pectoralis muscle is also dissected free from the surrounding fascia and fat. The insertion of the tendon is defined, and it should be kept in mind that the sternal portion of the tendon courses underneath the clavicular portion to attach to the humeral insertion in a twisting fashion. The interval between the sternal and clavicular head is usually easiest to develop approximately −5 cm medial to the muscle-tendon junction, and a curved clamp is placed in this interval to isolate the sternal head of the muscle. We usually place a Penrose drain around the muscle. Dissection then

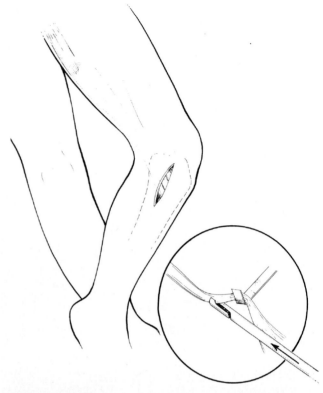

Figure 31-10 Hamstrings tendon harvesting technique. (Reprinted with permission from Warner JJ, Navarro RA. Serratus anterior dysfunction. Recognition and treatment. Clin Orthop 1998;(349):139.)

proceeds laterally toward its insertion, carefully defining the fiber course into the tendon of the sternal head as it attaches to the humerus. The tendon is then sharply detached from the humerus, taking care to protect the long head of the biceps tendon (Fig. 31-12). Several No. 2 braided, non-

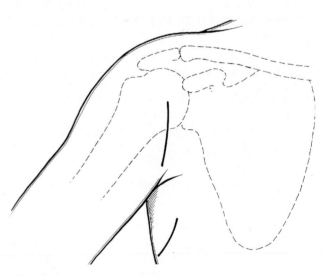

Figure 31-11 Typical incision. (Reprinted with permission from Warner JJ, Navarro RA. Serratus anterior dysfunction. Recognition and treatment. Clin Orthop 1998;(349):139.)

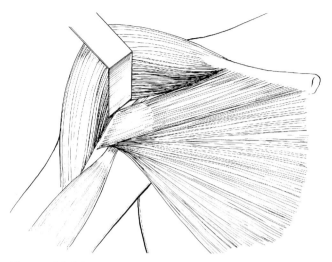

Figure 31-12 Pectoralis major tendon harvesting from the proximal humerus. (Reprinted with permission from Warner JJ, Navarro RA. Serratus anterior dysfunction. Recognition and treatment. Clin Orthop 1998;(349):139.)

absorbable sutures are placed into either edge of the tendon to control it when the hamstrings are brought through it to lengthen it.

The hamstring tendons are then woven through the pectoralis muscle and tendon in a Pulvertaft fashion, and the pectoralis is carefully tubulated around the hamstring graft so that it can easily slide along the chest wall once transferred. We take care to position the hamstring graft so that the pectoralis tendon is lengthened at least 6 cm. This makes it easier to pull the graft through the scapular hole as described next (Fig. 31-13).

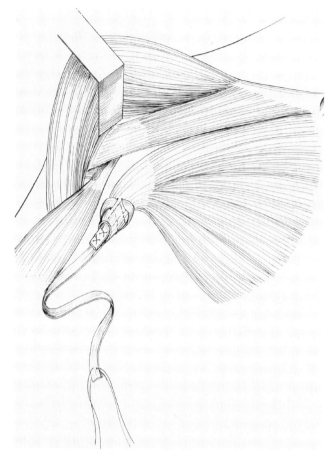

Figure 31-13 Hamstring tendon graft is sewed in a Pulvertaft fashion to the pectoralis major tendon. (Reprinted with permission from Warner JJ, Navarro RA. Serratus anterior dysfunction. Recognition and treatment. Clin Orthop 1998;(349):139.)

Exposure of the Inferior Portion of the Scapula

The arm is placed in forward flexion and adduction to access the inferior scapula. In this position the scapula is pulled forward on the chest wall. We use the mechanical arm holder to maintain the arm in this position because this allows for consistent positioning and avoids the need for an extra assistant. A 4-cm incision is then made over the palpable inferior angle of the scapula and dissection proceeds down to the latissimus muscle. The muscle is then split in line with its fibers both bluntly and with electrocautery until the lateral and inferior angle of the scapula is exposed. It is important to split the muscle sufficiently so that there is good visibility of the inferior scapular angle (Fig. 31-14). Electrocautery then elevates the periosteal sleeve off of the lateral edge of the scapula so that an elevator can strip the teres major off of its fossa as well as the subscapularis. Blunt retractors then expose the inferior angle of the scapula. It is important to note that the lateral and inferior edge of the scapula is thickened and that medially the body of the scapula is very thin. The

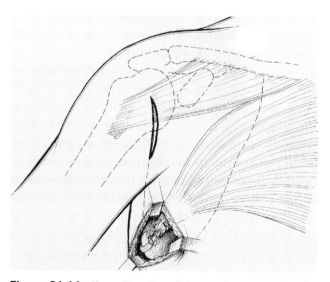

Figure 31-14 Sharp dissection of the muscles surrounding the inferior angle of the scapula. (Reprinted with permission from Warner JJ, Navarro RA. Serratus anterior dysfunction. Recognition and treatment. Clin Orthop 1998;(349):139.)

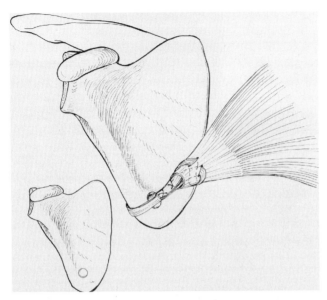

Figure 31-15 Hamstrings tendons are sewn along their course around the inferior angle of the scapula. (Reprinted with permission from Warner JJ, Navarro RA. Serratus anterior dysfunction. Recognition and treatment. Clin Orthop 1998;(349):139.)

hole that will be made will be through this thin area just medial to the thicker cortical bone of the lateral edge of the scapula.

A round burr then makes a hole of sufficient dimension to allow for passage of the hamstring portion of the graft. Typically this is 7 to 8 mm, and this can be checked using a right-angle clamp to palpate the dimensions of the hole.

Tendon Transfer

An interval along the chest wall is created bluntly by developing the soft-tissue tunnel from inferior along the palpable ribs, deep to all the neurovascular elements. This dissection proceeds bluntly from the superior incision along the chest wall as well, and the soft-tissue opening is bluntly dilated with the surgeon's fingers or a curved clamp. A long curved clamp is then used to pull the sutures from the hamstring extension of the pectoralis major down through this soft tissue tunnel and out of the inferior incision. The graft is then pulled along the chest, and care should be taken to ensure that it easily passes without catching in this soft-tissue passage. The hamstring tendons are pulled through the hole created in the inferior scapula, bringing them from the deep surface to the superficial surface. As this maneuver is performed, the scapula is pushed forward along the chest wall so that it slides over the graft until the tip of the pectoralis touches the deep surface of the scapula. The hamstrings are then looped over the lateral angle of the scapula and sewn along their course using No. 2 braided, nonabsorbable sutures (Fig. 31-15). The periosteal sleeve is then closed around the tendons, and a few sutures are placed to reapproximate the muscle fibers of the latissimus dorsi.

Both incisions are then closed in layers finishing with subcuticular absorbable sutures. After sterile dressings are applied, the shoulder is placed into an immobilizer and a cold compression device is applied.

POSTOPERATIVE MANAGEMENT

The patient is usually discharged from the hospital on the first postoperative day and instructed to wear the sling at all times but to begin pendulum exercises. Passive range of motion is instituted during the first week so that the patient's shoulder is moved by a therapist. This ensures that the graft does not become scarred in the soft tissue along the chest wall. After 4 weeks, the shoulder immobilizer is removed and self-assisted exercises and water therapy are instituted to ensure maintenance of motion. The patient is instructed to use his or her arm for daily living routines.

The aim of the physical therapy program is to train the tendon transfer to stabilize the scapula during shoulder flexion. At the 1-month postoperative mark, the patient is supervised by a therapist with an attempt to achieve this substitution pattern of muscle function. A simple biofeedback program is begun after 2 months, and we use a device that the patient may buy or rent (Myotrak, Thought Technology Ltd., Montreal, Quebec, Canada). The patient applies a cutaneous electrode that will give feedback about pectoralis muscle activity by means of an audible signal and a visible change in color (Fig. 31-16). The patient then attempts to maintain pectoralis muscle contraction during elevation of the arm. We have found that this is necessary in some patients and can be very helpful, whereas others activate their pectoralis transfer with little training.[63] Strengthening is begun after 4 months, and return to overhead sports can occur between 4 and 6 months, depending on the appearance of good scapular stabilization.

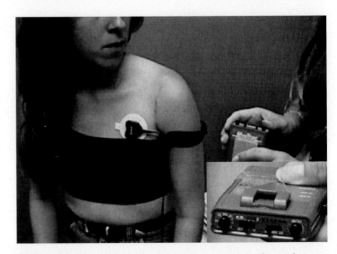

Figure 31-16 Biofeedback training. Cutaneous electrode is applied to the muscle belly.

RESULTS OF SPLIT PECTORALIS MAJOR TRANSFER

Several reports have documented the success of this procedure using techniques similar to the one described in this chapter.[11,44,48,52,63,65] In general, the clinical outcome is very gratifying if the condition is identified and treated before incorrect surgery is performed. In the author's initial experience, most patients referred for treatment had already undergone a surgery for a different diagnosis and winging had been missed. Their ultimate outcome depended more on morbidity of their prior incorrect treatment than on resolution from winging with the definitive procedure.[63]

In most cases the patient regains near normal flexion and good strength (Fig. 31-17). To date, the senior author (J.J.P.Warner) has performed 51 tendon transfer cases. Complications have included only one infection. Two patients continued to have residual pain in their shoulder, although one had complete resolution of winging. One patient had return of her winging, although it was unclear whether this had been the result of a trauma she sustained in an automobile accident 1 year after her surgery.

COMPLICATIONS AND PITFALLS

Few complications after tendon transfer have been reported. An infection occurred in the author's experience, as noted in this chapter.[63] For this patient, a scapulothoracic fusion eliminated pain and improved her function. Post[48] noted that a hematoma spontaneously subsided and that there was one seroma over the thigh where the fascia had been harvested. Connor et al.[11] reported one failure after an initial aggressive physical therapy (use of a rowing machine 2 months after the surgery). Perlmutter and Leffert[44] have had two failures in 16 patients after a new traumatic event; the authors think that the fascial graft was stretched by the injury because of the configuration and preparation of the graft.

SCAPULOTHORACIC FUSION

Scapulothoracic fusion is a procedure with which most orthopedic surgeons have little experience; however, it is a very successful method to treat chronic uncontrollable scapular winging. As indicated in this chapter, scapulotho-

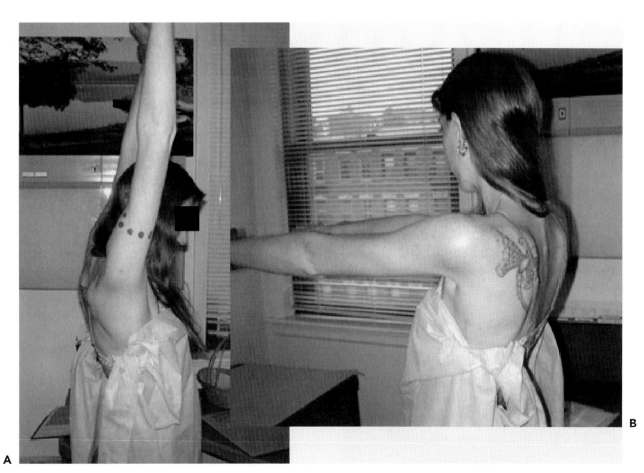

Figure 31-17   (A,B) Postoperative result after a pectoralis tendon transfer for scapular winging.

racic fusion is usually indicated in the case of chronic scapular winging that fails tendon transfer treatment or in patients in whom muscle dysfunction is so severe that tendon transfer is not an option, as in fascioscapulohumeral muscular dystrophy.[3,7,9,13,21,24,26,34,35,39]

Scapulothoracic Fusion Technique

The patient is placed in a prone position, and we prefer to use a Jackson Spine Table (OSI Subsidiary of the Mizuho Group, Union City, CA) (Fig. 31-18). This table is relatively narrow and allows consistent placement of the arms forward and lower than the chest to position the scapula properly for fusion. Care is taken to drape the entire arm and hemithorax free when sterilely preparing and draping the patient, because it will be necessary to bring the arm behind the back of the patient to make the scapula wing away from the chest during the procedure. As with all procedures, intravenous broad-spectrum antibiotics are administered as prophylaxis against infection.

An incision is then made along the medial border of the scapula, and the rhomboids and trapezius are defined. The trapezius is elevated and retracted, and the rhomboids are released from their insertion on the scapula and dissected medially to the spinous process of the thoracic vertebrae. We keep these muscles for repair at the end of the procedure because they will provide a cushion over the wires and plate used. The levator scapulae are also detached. The infraspinatus and supraspinatus are then elevated out of their fossae and retracted laterally. The patient's shoulder is then placed into internal rotation with his or her hand on the lower back, which will cause the scapula to wing away from the chest. The subscapularis is then carefully elevated with electrocautery out of its fossa from medial to lateral. Most of this muscle is resected using electrocautery, being careful to identify large vessels as the muscle is removed. Removal of the

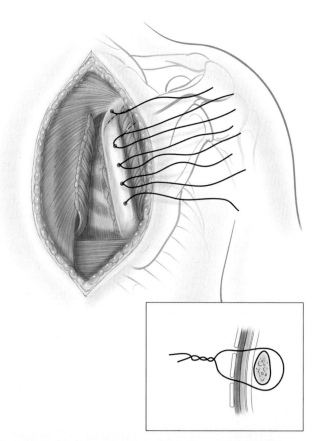

Figure 31-19 Dissection and muscle removal for a scapulothoracic fusion. (Reprinted with permission from: Kuhn JE, Hawkins RJ. Evaluation and treatment of scapular disorders. In: Warner JJP, Iannotti JP, Gerber C, eds. Complex and revision problems in shoulder surgery. 1st edition. Philadelphia, PA, Lippincott-Raven, 1997.)

muscle is necessary to ensure good bony contact of the scapula against the ribs (Fig. 31-19). The soft tissue is then cleared off of the ribs using an electrocautery device, and it may be necessary to remove a portion of the intercostal muscles adjacent to the ribs so that no soft tissue comes between the bony surfaces. Ribs 3, 4, and 5 are then identified, and a subperiosteal dissection is performed around these to allow for passage of 18-gauge wires. We make a wire loop and contour it so it can be carefully passed underneath the rib. Care should be taken not to damage the intercostal vessels and not to penetrate the parietal pleura of the lung. Once all wires are passed, sterile saline is placed over the ribs and the anesthesiologist is asked to administer a positive pressure ventilation to make sure a pneumothorax has not occurred. Such an occurrence has not happened in our patients so far.

A motorized burr is then used to decorticate ribs 3, 4, 5, and 6 as well as the undersurface of the scapula (Fig. 31-20). An AO Dynamic Compression plate (AO-Synthes, Paoli, Pennsylvania) is then taken, cut to three holes, and gently contoured to fit over the scapula just below the

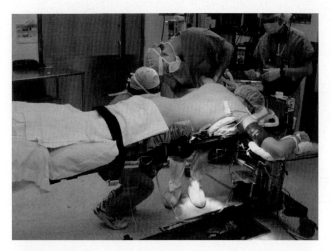

Figure 31-18 Patient installation on a Jackson spine table.

spine. Holes are made through the scapula to correspond to holes in the plate, and a single hole is made in line with these just above the scapular spine in the supraspinatus fossa. The wires around the ribs are then passed through these holes and through the plate, as well as around the spine of the scapula in the case of the upper wire. These are then tightened securely fixing the scapula to the ribs (Fig. 31-21). The muscles are then closed over the plate and scapula, and the incision is closed in layers. The patient is then awakened and rolled into a supine position onto a stretcher bed, and a shoulder immobilizer is applied. A postoperative chest radiograph is always taken in the recovery room.

Aftercare

The shoulder immobilizer is worn for 4 weeks; however, most patients are permitted some use of the arm for elbow flexion. Active motion is begun at 4 weeks, and radiographs are taken to confirm no displacement of fixation. Union is difficult to confirm on plain radiographs, although a computed tomography scan can be ordered if necessary. Most patients are able to use their shoulders after approximately 1 month.

Scapulothoracic fusion has been generally reserved for salvage operation in patients with fascioscapulohumeral muscular dystrophy. Most of the time a fusion is also necessary on the opposite side.[7,31,33] Functional gains are limited (approximately 25 degrees in abduction and

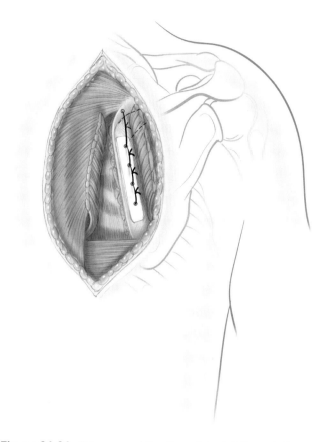

Figure 31-21 Wires around the ribs and the AO Dynamic Compression plate (AO-Synthes, Paoli, Pennsylvania). (Reprinted with permission from: Kuhn JE, Hawkins RJ. Evaluation and treatment of scapular disorders. In: Warner JJP, Iannotti JP, Gerber C, eds. Complex and revision problems in shoulder surgery. 1st edition. Philadelphia, PA, Lippincott-Raven, 1997.)

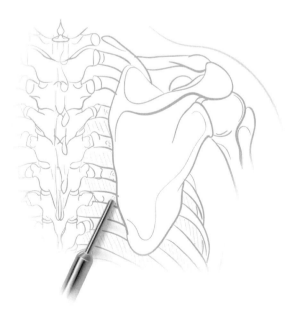

Figure 31-20 Uses of the burr to decorticate the third, fourth, fifth, and sixth ribs. (Reprinted with permission from: Kuhn JE, Hawkins RJ. Evaluation and treatment of scapular disorders. In: Warner JJP, Iannotti JP, Gerber C, eds. Complex and revision problems in shoulder surgery. 1st edition. Philadelphia, PA, Lippincott-Raven, 1997.)

flexion).[7,13,27,31] These reports emphasize that results do not decline over time. Pain relief is the most reasonable expectation of that procedure (Fig. 31-22).[7,13,20,31]

Another possible indication of a scapulothoracic fusion for scapular winging is the laborer who places heavy demand on his or her shoulder.[53]

CONCLUSIONS

Paralysis of the serratus anterior muscle is a rare condition primarily caused by a traumatic injury to the long thoracic nerve. Transfer of the pectoralis major muscle with small incisions is a safe technique and cosmetically acceptable for the patients.

The results are good for pain relief and shoulder function. After 1 year of evolution and repeated electromyography, this surgical procedure is suggested for all patients. In case of failure, a scapulothoracic fusion is proposed.

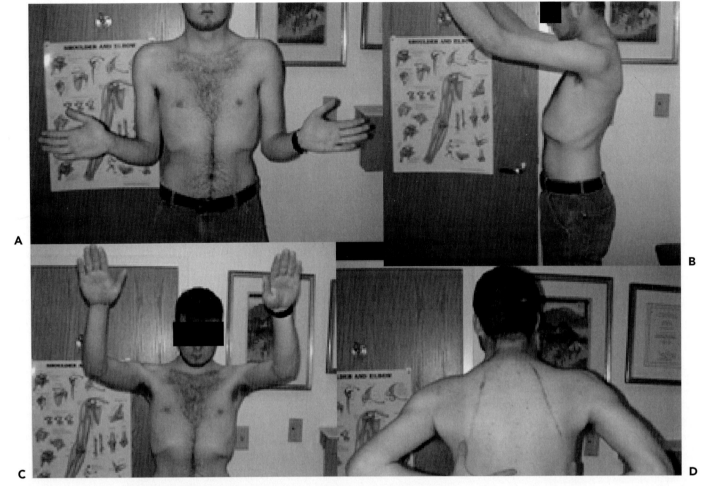

Figure 31-22 *(A–D)* Postoperative motion after a bilateral scapulothoracic fusion for fascioscapulohumeral muscular dystrophy.

REFERENCES

1. Alexandre JH, Kendall HO. Isolated paralysis of the serratus anterior muscle. J Bone Joint Surg 1955;37(A):567.
2. Alexandre JH, Hamonet C, Lacert P, et al. Le nerf du grand dentele. Arch Anat Pathol 1968;16:185.
3. Andrews CT, Taylor TC, Patterson VH. Scapulothoracic arthrodesis for patient with fascioscapulohumeral muscular dystrophy. Neuromuscul Disord 1998;8:580.
4. Atasoy E, Majd M. Scapulothoracic stabilization for winging of the scapula using strips of autologous fascia lata. J Bone Joint Surg 2000;82(B):813.
5. Ball CR. Paralysis following injection of antitetanic serum. Case report with serratus magnus involved. US Naval Med Bull 1939;37:305.
6. Baron OA, Levine WN, Bigliani LU. Surgical management of chronic trapezius dysfunction. In: Warner J, Iannotti J, Gerber C, eds. Complex and revision problems in shoulder surgery. Philadelphia, PA, Lippincott-Raven, 1997:337.
7. Berne D, Laude F, Laporte C, et al. Scapulothoracic arthrodesis in fascioscapulohumeral muscular dystrophy. Clin Orthop 2003; 409:106.
8. Bloch AM, Nevo Y, Ben-Sira L, et al. Winging of the scapula in a child with hereditary multiple exostoses. Pediatr Neurol 2002; 26:74.
9. Bunch WH, Siegel IM. Scapulothoracic arthrodesis in fascioscapulohumeral muscular dystrophy. J Bone Joint Surg 1993;75(A):372.
10. Chavez JP. Pectoralis minor transplant for paralysis of the serratus anterior. J Bone Joint Surg 1951;33(B):228.
11. Connor PM, Yamaguchi K, Manifold SG, et al. Split pectoralis major transfer for serratus anterior palsy. Clin Orthop 1997;12:134.
12. Cooley LH, Torg JS. "Pseudowinging" of the scapula secondary to subscapular osteochondroma. Clin Orthop 1982;162:119.
13. Copeland SA, Howard RC. Thoracoscapular fusion for fascioscapulohumeral dystrophy. J Bone Joint Surg 1978;60(B):547.
14. Danielsson LG, El-Haddad I. Winged scapula due to osteochondroma. Acta Orthop Scand 1989;60:728.
15. Eschner AA. Three cases of paralysis of the serratus magnus (anterior) muscle. N Engl J Med 1930;203:818
16. Fiddian NJ, King RJ. The winging scapula. Clin Orthop 1984; 185:244.
17. Gozna ER, Harris WR. Traumatic winging of the scapula. J Bone Joint Surg 1979;61(A):1230.
18. Gregg JR, Labosky D, Harty M, et al. Serratus anterior paralysis in the young athlete. J Bone Joint Surg 1979;61(A):825.
19. Hass J. Muskelplastik bei serratuslahmung (ersatz des gelahmten musculus serratus anterior durch den musculus teres major). Zetschr Orthop Chir 1931;55:617.
20. Hawkins RJ, Willis RB, Litchfield RB. Scapulothoracic arthrodesis for scapular winging. In: Post M, Morrey B, Hawkins R, eds. Surgery of the shoulder. St. Louis, MO, Mosby-Year Book, 1990:356.

21. Hayes JM, Zehr DJ. Traumatic muscle avulsion causing winging of the scapula. J Bone Joint Surg 1981;63(A):495.
22. Herzmark MH. Traumatic paralysis of the serratus anterior relieved by transplantation of the rhomboidei. J Bone Joint Surg 1951;33(A):235.
23. Hester P, Caborn DN, Nyland J. Cause of long thoracic nerve palsy: a possible dynamic fascial sling cause. J Shoulder Elbow Surg 2000;9:31.
24. Horan FT, Bonefede RP. Bilateral absence of trapezius and sternal head of pectoralis major muscles. J Bone Joint Surg 1977; 59(A):133.
25. Horwitz MT, Tocantin LM. An anatomical study of the role of the long thoracic nerve and the related scapular bursae in the pathogenesis of local paralysis of the serratus anterior muscle. Anat Rec 1938;71:375.
26. Iceton J, Harris WR. Treatment of winged scapula by pectoralis major tendon transfer. J Bone Joint Surg 1987;69(B):108.
27. Jakab E, Gledhill RB. Simplified technique for scapulocostal fusion in fascioscapulohumeral dystrophy. J Pediatr Orthop 1993;13:749.
28. Kaplan PE. Electrodiagnostic confirmation of long thoracic nerve palsy. J Neurol 1980;43:50.
29. Kauppila LI. The long thoracic nerve: possible mechanisms of injury based on autopsy study. J Shoulder Elbow Surg 1993;2:244.
30. Kauppila LI, Vastamaki M. Iatrogenic serratus anterior paralysis: long term outcome in 26 patients. Chest 1996;109:31.
31. Ketenjian AY. Scapulocostal stabilization for scapular winging in fascioscapulohumeral muscular dystrophy. J Bone Joint Surg 1978;60(A):476.
32. Kibler WB, Uhl TL, Maddux JW, et al. Qualitative clinical evaluation of scapular dysfunction: a reliability study. J Shoulder Elbow Surg 2002;11:550.
33. Kocialkowski A, Frostick SP, Wallace WA. One-stage bilateral thoracoscapular fusion using allografts. Clin Orthop 1991; 273:264.
34. Letournel E, Fardeau M, Lytle JO, et al. Scapulothoracic arthrodesis for patients who have fascioscapulo humeral muscular dystrophy. J Bone Joint Surg 1990;72(A):78.
35. Levin SE, Trummer MJ. Agenesis of the serratus anterior muscle: a cause of winged scapula. JAMA 1973;225:748.
36. Lynch AF, Fogarty EE, Dowling FE, et al. Pseudowinging of the scapula due to osteochondroma. J Pediatr Orthop 1985;5:722.
37. Mah JY, Otusko NY. Scapular winging in the young athlete. J Pediatr Orthop 1992;12:245.
38. Marmor L, Bechtol CO. Paralysis of the serratus anterior due to electric shock relieved by transplantation of the pectoralis major muscle: a case report. J Bone Joint Surg 1963;45(A):156.
39. Meythaler JM, Reddy NM, Mitz M. Serratus anterior disruption: a complication of rheumatoid arthritis. Arch Phys Med Rehabil 1986;67:770.
40. Noerdlinger MA, Cole BJ, Stewart M, et al. Results of pectoralis major transfer with fascia lata autograft augmentation for scapular winging. J Shoulder Elbow Surg 2002;11:345.
41. Pagnani MJ, Warner JJP, O'Brien SJ, et al. Anatomic considerations in harvesting the semitendinosus and gracilis tendons and a technique of harvest. Am J Sports Med 1993;12:565.
42. Parsonage M, Turner JW. Neuralgic amyotrophy: the shoulder-girdle syndrome. Lancet 1948;1:973.
43. Percy EL, Birbrager D, Pitt MJ. Snapping scapula: a review of the literature and presentation of 14 patients. Can J Surg 1988;31:248.
44. Perlmutter GS, Leffert RD. Results of transfer of the pectoralis major tendon to treat paralysis of the serratus anterior muscle. J Bone Joint Surg 1999;81(A):377.
45. Perry J. Anatomy and biomechanics of the shoulder in throwing, swimming, gymnastics and tennis. Clin Sports Med 1983;2:247.
46. Petrera JE, Trajaborg W. Conduction studies of the long thoracic nerve in serratus anterior palsy of different etiology. Neurology 1984;34:1033.
47. Post M. Pectoralis major transfer for winging of the scapula. J Shoulder Elbow Surg 1995;4:1.
48. Post M. Orthopaedic management of neuromuscular disorders. In: Post M, Bigliani L, Flatow E, Pollock R, eds. The shoulder: operative technique. Baltimore, MD, Williams and Wilkins, 1998:201.
49. Radin EL. Peripheral neuritis as a complication of infectious mononucleosis: report of a case. J Bone Joint Surg 1967; 49(A):535.
50. Rapp IH. Serratus anterior paralysis treated by transplantation of the pectoralis minor. J Bone Joint Surg 1954;36(A):852.
51. Rowe CR. Unusual shoulder condition. In: Row C, ed. The shoulder. New York, Churchill Livingston, 1988:639.
52. Samter O. Sur le traitement operatoire de la paralysis du grand dentele. J Chir (Paris) 1930;35:299.
53. Segonds JM, Alnot JY, Asfazadourian H. Paralysie isolee du muscle serratus anterieur d'origine traumatique. Rev Chir Orthop 2002;88:751.
54. Solman CG, Pagnani MJ. Hamstring tendon harvesting. Reviewing anatomic relationship and avoiding pitfalls. Orthop Clin North Am 2003;34:1.
55. Tamai K, Ogawa K. Intratendinous tear of the supraspinatus tendon exhibiting winging of the scapula. Clin Orthop 1985; 194:159.
56. Tsairis P, Dyck PJ, Mulder DW. Natural history of brachial plexus neuropathy. Report on 99 patients. Arch Neurol 1972; 27:109.
57. Tubby AH. A case illustrating the operative treatment of paralysis of the serratus magnus by muscle grafting. Br Med J 1904;2:1159.
58. Vastamaki M. Pectoralis minor transfer in serratus anterior paralysis. Acta Orthop Scand 1984;55:293.
59. Vastamaki M, Kauppila LI. Etiologic factors in isolated paralysis of the serratus anterior muscle: a report of 197 cases. J Shoulder Elbow Surg 1993;2:240.
60. Velpeau A. Luxation de l'epaule. Arch Gen Med 1837;14:269.
61. Vukov B, Ukropina D, Bumbasirevic M, et al. Isolated serratus anterior paralysis: a simple surgical procedure to reestablish scapulohumeral dynamics. J Orthop Trauma 1996;10:341.
62. Warner JJP, Micheli LI, Arslanian LE, et al. Scapulothoracic motion in normal shoulders and shoulders with glenohumeral instability and impingement syndrome. A study using Moire topographic analysis. Clin Orthop 1992;285:191.
63. Warner JJP, Navarro RA. Serratus anterior dysfunction. Recognition and treatment. Clin Orthop 1998;349:139.
64. Whitman A. Congenital elevation of the scapula and paralysis of serratus magnus muscle: operation. JAMA 1932;99:1332.
65. Wiater JM, Flatow EL. Long thoracic nerve injury. Clin Orthop 1999;368:17.
66. Winslow M. Sur quelques mouvements extraordinaires des omoplates et des bras, et sur une nouvelle espece de muscles. Mem Acad Royal Sciences. Paris, Chez Panckouke 1777; 1723:98.
67. Wood VE, Frykman GK. Winging of the scapula as a complication of first rib resection: a report of six cases. Clin Orthop 1980; 149:160.
68. Zeier FG. The treatment of winged scapula. Clin Orthop 1973; 91:128.

Scapular Winging: Trapezius Dysfunction

Julie Y. Bishop   Evan L. Flatow

INTRODUCTION

The trapezius is the major suspensory muscle of the shoulder girdle contributing to scapulothoracic rhythm by elevating, rotating, and retracting the scapula. Injury to the spinal accessory (eleventh cranial) nerve can cause significant dysfunction of this muscle.[19,38] Paralysis of the trapezius results in drooping of the entire shoulder girdle, winging and lateral displacement of the scapula, and weakness in forward elevation and abduction.[4,9,22] This constellation of symptoms can lead to considerable pain, deformity, and loss of function.

CAUSE

The spinal accessory nerve is located in the subcutaneous tissue on the floor of the posterior cervical triangle. This superficial location makes it very vulnerable to iatrogenic injury, which is the leading cause of trapezius paralysis.[24,45] In the 1930s, removal of tuberculous lymph nodes in the neck was a common procedure, in which up to 10% of cases were complicated by injury to the spinal accessory nerve.[16,30,47,48] As the incidence of trapezius nerve palsies peaked in the 1950s, concern mounted as it became clear that the morbidity associated with surgery in the posterior cervical triangle was very significant and problematic. Newer techniques and modified procedures have been pro-

J. Y. Bishop: Clinical Shoulder Fellow, Department of Orthopaedic Surgery, Mount Sinai Medical Center, New York, New York.

E. L. Flatow: Lasker Professor of Orthopaedic Surgery, Chief of Shoulder Surgery, Department of Orthopaedic Surgery, Mount Sinai Medical Center, New York, New York.

posed to protect the nerve during head and neck surgery.[2,6] Nevertheless, sacrificing the nerve is sometimes necessary in radical neck dissections for cancer. The spinal accessory nerve may also be injured in anterior neck surgery, such as carotid endarterectomies.[39,40] It has also been used as a graft for facial nerve paralysis and brachial plexus lesions; however, other graft sources are currently preferentially used.[1,32]

Trapezius palsy and dysfunction can also occur after blunt trauma and traction injuries to the spinal accessory nerve. Direct trauma can occur during contact sports, resulting, for example, from a blow from a hockey or lacrosse stick. Traction injuries can occur from motor vehicle accidents, falls from a height, sternoclavicular or acromioclavicular dislocations, or even extended use of an arm sling. Although rare, spontaneous onset of spinal accessory nerve paralysis has been reported.[13,25]

ANATOMY AND BIOMECHANICS

Periscapular Musculature

The scapula floats on the chest wall on a bed of muscles. The trapezius, levator scapulae, rhomboids, and serratus anterior muscles make up the scapular rotator group whose functions include passive support of the shoulder, active elevation of the shoulder, and rotation of the scapula (Fig. 32-1A). Codman[6] was the first to elaborate on the importance of the fine balance among the muscles of the shoulder girdle that support the scapula; he described the concept of scapulohumeral rhythm. Inman et al.[22] later showed the contribution of the trapezius to the

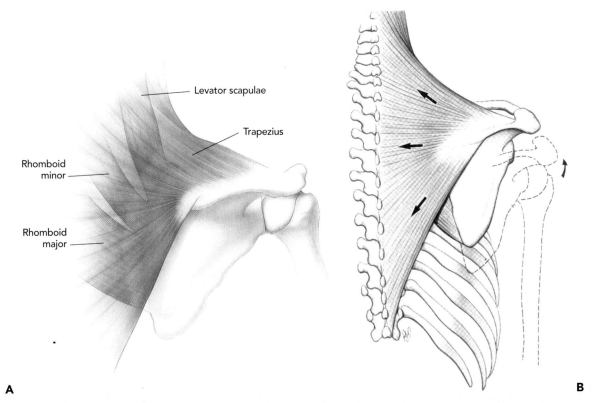

Figure 32-1 (A) Posterior view of the scapula with the trapezius, rhomboids, and levator scapulae muscles. (B) Normal function of the trapezius: the upper portion rotates and elevates the scapula, the middle portion stabilizes and adducts it, and the lower portion rotates the scapula downward and depresses it.

balance of the scapular rotary-force couples. Scapular and humeral motion occur simultaneously during upper extremity movement, and the trapezius is one of the primary movers of the scapula.[22] The trapezius is the largest and most superficial of the scapulothoracic muscles. Its primary origin is the spinous processes of C7 down to T12. Above C7, the upper portion originates from the ligamentum nuchae up to the external occipital protuberance.[23] It is divided into three distinct anatomic components: upper, middle, and lower (Fig. 32-1B). The upper portion inserts on the posterior border of the lateral third of the clavicle and rotates and elevates the scapula. The intermediate portion inserts on the medial acromion and along the superior lip of the spine of the scapula and is responsible for stability and adduction of the scapula. The inferior portion inserts on the base of the spine of the scapula and rotates the scapula downward and depresses it. All three portions of the trapezius work synchronously, and, overall, they work together to elevate, retract, and rotate the scapula. The trapezius is the only muscle to insert on the lateral tip of the scapula; thus, one of its most important functions is to elevate the lateral tip of the scapula and, by extension, the rest of the upper extremity. Therefore, trapezius paralysis will lead to drooping of the entire extremity, because the inferior border of the scapula

rotates laterally.[2,27] The levator scapulae, rhomboids, and serratus anterior are able to compensate to a certain extent, allowing some elevation above the horizontal plane. However, the inferior and laterally positioned scapula places the rhomboids and, to a lesser extent, the levator scapulae at a distinct biomechanical disadvantage, and maximal force generation is compromised.[2,15]

Spinal Accessory Nerve

The spinal accessory nerve, cranial nerve XI, is the sole motor innervation to the trapezius muscle. It also supplies the sternocleidomastoid. It may be joined by proprioceptive branches from the second, third, or fourth cervical nerves.[8,19] After supplying the sternocleidomastoid muscle, the spinal accessory nerve descends obliquely in the posterior triangle of the neck, between the superficial and deep layers of the cervical fascia. The borders of the posterior triangle are the sternocleidomastoid anteriorly, the trapezius posteriorly, and the clavicle inferiorly. It is here in the subcutaneous tissue that the nerve is in contact with the cervical lymph node chain. It then gives off several branches to the upper part of the trapezius muscle before passing under its anterior edge.[8] In the trapezius muscle substance, the nerve continues obliquely as it innervates the lower part of the muscle. It then descends parallel and medial to the vertebral border of the scapula,[24] terminating in the trapezius musculature.

DIAGNOSIS

Trapezius paralysis is frequently misdiagnosed at the initial presentation.[3,4,37] Secondary effects of trapezius dysfunction, such as subacromial impingement, adhesive capsulitis, thoracic outlet syndrome, spasm of the other periscapular muscles, and paresthesias from traction on the brachial plexus, may cloud the diagnosis. Other diagnoses, such as stroke, shoulder dislocations, scoliosis, herniated disks, and progressive neuromuscular disorders, may present with symptoms similar to those of trapezius paralysis and should be ruled out.[3,27,37] However, a detailed patient history and a thorough and careful examination will typically lead to the correct diagnosis.

History

The evaluation at the initial patient presentation begins with a complete medical history. Any recent illnesses, medical problems, history of trauma to the shoulder or neck, or any recent surgical procedures in this area should be elicited, especially in relation to the onset of the current dysfunction. Any deficit caused by traumatic injury to the spinal accessory nerve does not typically become obvious until several days after the initial swelling and pain have subsided. It is then that it becomes apparent that function is abnormal. If the nerve has been injured because of a minor surgical procedure in the area of the posterior cervical triangle, periscapular pain usually develops within several days.[4] The gradual onset of atraumatic weakness and lateral scapular winging should be an alert to investigate possible neurologic or myopathic diseases.[31]

Most patients experience pain with prolonged use of the shoulder, as the other muscles strain and fatigue from overcompensation. This strain often causes significant muscle spasm that adds to the disabling pain some experience.[4] Many also complain of a constant dull ache and heavy feeling about the shoulder. As the condition becomes chronic, the pain may radiate to the hand and forearm, to the face and head, and even to the contralateral extremity.[6,34] As the shoulder droops inferiorly because of the fatigued compensatory muscles, the brachial plexus is placed under tension.[3] This can lead to recurring episodes of radiating pain and paresthesias because of the traction effect, especially when the involved extremity has been unsupported in the early part of treatment.[37] Abnormal scapular rotation, resulting from failure to rotate the scapula out of the way, may cause significant signs of impingement as the greater tuberosity abuts the acromion. This may also be the underlying cause of other associated symptoms such as glenohumeral instability, acromioclavicular joint incongruity, and adhesive capsulitis.[33] Patients experience pain and difficulty with most all

overhead activities, lifting heavy objects, prolonged writing, or driving a car.[3] Unfortunately the pain is so disabling for some that chronic use of narcotic analgesics is necessary.[3,4]

Physical Findings

The physical examination begins with a thorough inspection, which requires males to remove their gown and females to fasten the gown just above the breasts. The examiner can then evaluate the general appearance, posture, and positioning of the extremity. It is important to look for scars, especially in the posterior cervical triangle. It is not infrequent for patients to have forgotten to mention seemingly insignificant past operations, such as lymph node biopsy. The neckline is asymmetric because the trapezius is atrophic on the affected side, which also slopes dramatically (Fig. 32-2). The shoulder droops as the scapula is translated laterally and rotated downward. The patient should be asked to actively elevate both arms in the forward plane, as the rela-

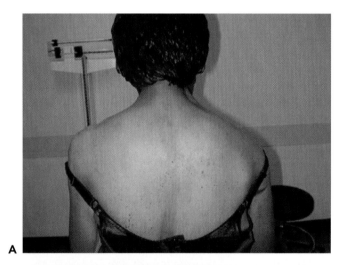

A

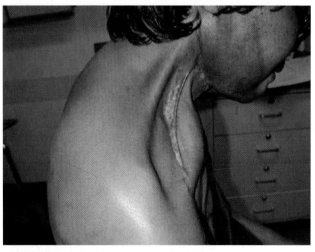

B

Figure 32-2 Woman with long-standing right trapezius paralysis. *(A)* Asymmetric neckline with dramatic downsloping because of atrophic trapezius. *(B)* Significant atrophy of the trapezius musculature.

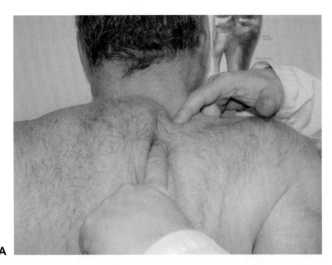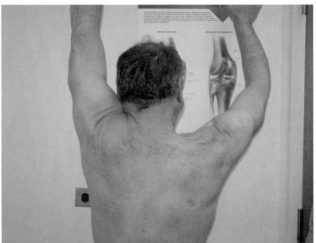

Figure 32-3 Male with trapezius paralysis subsequent to a right radical neck dissection. (A) Atrophic trapezius muscle. (B) Significant difficulty with elevation in the forward plane.

tionship between the scapula and chest wall is observed; 80% of patients have no more than 90 degrees of active abduction, which is generally weak against resistance (Fig. 32-3). Patients will usually be unable to shrug the shoulder, although the levator scapulae can sometimes elevate the scapula enough to mask the shrug deficit.[14] Lateral scapular winging is especially apparent against trapezius muscle resistance (Fig. 32-4). The weight duration test of Neer assesses the onset of fatigue and pain as the patient holds a heavy object at arm's length.[33]

Active and passive range of motion should be assessed to rule out a coexisting adhesive capsulitis, which would be a contraindication to reconstructive surgery. Evidence of any other confounding problem should be sought, such as impingement syndrome. A thorough neurologic examination should be performed of both upper extremities, looking for any cervical spine, brachial plexus, or peripheral nerve injuries. The head and neck should be evaluated to rule out any other disease. A sensory examination of the skin overlying the trapezius should be performed, as a Tinel's sign

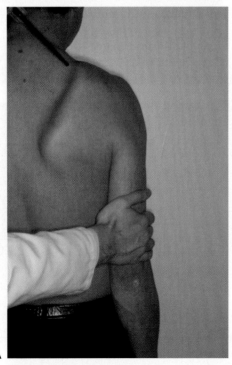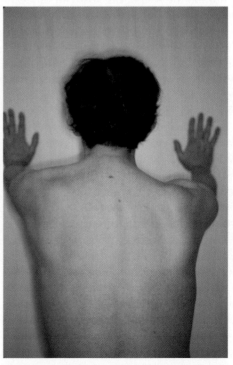

Figure 32-4 Male with trapezius paralysis after blunt injury. Scapular winging deformity is enhanced with resisted abduction (A), not with resisted forward elevation as one would see with serratus anterior paralysis (B).

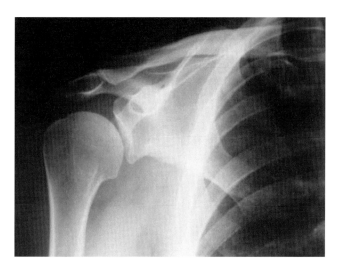

Figure 32-5 Anteroposterior radiograph of the scapula demonstrating a downward and laterally rotated position that is characteristic in trapezius paralysis.

may be elicited. Any associated injuries to the greater auricular or lesser occipital nerves should be sought, because this may also occur during a posterior triangle dissection.[30]

Diagnostic Studies

Although rarely diagnostic, plain radiographs of the shoulder, chest, and cervical spine are obtained. Bony trauma, a lower cervical rib, or any other bony abnormalities can be ruled out. In the case of true paralysis of the trapezius, the scapula will be in a downward and laterally rotated position on the chest radiograph (Fig. 32-5). Magnetic resonance imaging or computed tomography scans are rarely indicated unless another diagnosis such as a herniated cervical disc is being excluded.

The most important tests to confirm the diagnosis of trapezius paralysis caused by spinal accessory nerve palsy are electromyography and nerve conduction studies. The trapezius and sternocleidomastoid are evaluated, and the condition of the surrounding muscles, in particular the rhomboids, serratus anterior, and levator scapulae, is assessed. This allows evaluation of all potentially transferable muscles, as well as assurance that the serratus anterior is intact. Long thoracic nerve palsy, which leads to serratus anterior paralysis, compromises the results of surgical reconstruction for trapezius paralysis.[3]

TREATMENT

Nonoperative Management

Treatment for trapezius palsy is dependent on several factors, including the cause of the initial injury, the duration and severity of symptoms, and the health, age, and activity level of the patient. In patients in whom nerve injury is the result of blunt trauma or traction-induced neuropraxia, ini-

tial treatment should be conservative. Recovery of function is possible in these patients. A baseline electromyograph should be obtained at 3 months, which is the earliest that denervation potentials are seen, and then it should be performed at 6-week intervals to follow any returning function of the nerve. A physical therapy regimen should be instituted in these patients to help maintain glenohumeral motion and prevent adhesive capsulitis. If, at 1 year, trapezius function has not adequately returned and the patient continues to have debilitating symptoms, then it is unlikely that conservative treatment will offer any benefit. At this point, surgery should be considered in the motivated patient.

In nerve injuries that are postsurgical or caused by penetrating trauma, it is unlikely that any spontaneous recovery of the nerve will occur. In these cases, early exploration with possible nerve repair, neurolysis, and/or nerve grafting can be considered. If neurolysis is to be performed, studies have shown a better success rate when performed within the first 6 months of the injury.[4]

Older, more sedentary patients may often benefit from nonsurgical treatment. Often these patients have minimal symptoms, and they are more willing to modify their activity level, especially if the nondominant extremity is involved. However, conservative treatment with rehabilitation in the young, active patient or in those with long-standing paralysis and dysfunction will usually fail.[3,4,36,41] Strengthening the adjacent muscles is mostly inadequate because the muscles are unable to compensate for the loss of function of the trapezius. Few studies exist that detail the results of nonoperative treatment.[4,9,35,36,42] Overall, the results have been poor: seven of eight patients treated nonoperatively in the 1985 study by Bigliani et al.[4] had an unsatisfactory result. Although there are few studies on the use of an orthosis, bracing or use of a sling can provide some benefit to the patient in the short term.[43] Primarily, an orthosis can support the arm and minimize drooping of the shoulder, thus reducing the pull against the levator scapulae and rhomboids and subsequent traction on the brachial plexus. This in turn can help alleviate some of the associated pain caused by traction and muscle fatigue. However, there is little evidence that bracing can improve strength or lead to more overhead use of the arm.

Surgical Treatment

Nerve injuries caused by iatrogenic injury or penetrating trauma may benefit from direct repair, neurolysis, and/or nerve grafting.[1,10,11,46] Overall, the results of these procedures have been variable. However, the success rate seems to be improved if the procedure is performed within 6 to 12 months after the injury.[2,5,9,16,36,38,47]

Historically, several reconstructive procedures have been described for the treatment of spinal accessory nerve paralysis. These can be divided into static and dynamic procedures. Static stabilization includes scapulothoracic fusion, scapulothoracic fasciodesis, and any operation that tethers the scapula to the spine, such as stabilization with fascia lata to the dorsal spine of the thoracic vertebra.[9,17,18,26] The dynamic procedures all involve some form of muscle transfer.[4,20,30] Transfer of the levator scapulae alone has been described,[4,10,44] or more commonly, the Eden-Lange procedure, which involves transfer of the levator scapulae, rhomboid major, and rhomboid minor.[4,12,29] A combination of static and dynamic procedures has also been described that involves transfer of the levator scapulae and stabilization of the scapula to the thoracic spine with fascia lata.[9] Coessens and Wood[7] showed good or excellent results in four of five patients in whom this procedure was performed, although the minimum follow-up was only 14 months. Overall, most procedures that depend on a fascial-sling suspension tend to fail as the fascial attachment stretches over time.[3,4] Transfers that depend solely on the levator scapulae also tend to fail because this muscle is too small to become the sole dynamic substitution for the trapezius. One recent case report involved successful restoration of the trapezius muscle function using a pedicle latissimus dorsi flap.[21] Although this was performed after resection of the trapezius and all surrounding muscles because of a sarcoma, the authors believed that the technique may be extended as a salvage for a failed conventional reconstruction after trapezius paralysis. Overall, dynamic muscle transfers, in particular the Eden-Lange procedure and its modification, have become the most commonly performed technique for trapezius paralysis.[2–4,12,29,45]

Bigliani (Modified Eden-Lange) Procedure

The Eden-Lange procedure involves the lateral transfer of the levator scapulae, rhomboid major, and rhomboid minor to substitute for each part of the trapezius. This lateral transfer of the muscular insertions improves their mechanical advantage to reproduce the functions of the trapezius and support the scapula. The levator scapulae substitutes for the upper part of the trapezius, the rhomboid minor for the middle, and the rhomboid major for the lower part. The original Eden-Lange procedure involved the transfer of the insertion of the rhomboid minor into the infraspinatus fossa.[4] However, this procedure was modified by Bigliani et al.[3] to transfer the insertion of the rhomboid minor cephalad to the scapular spine into the supraspinatus fossa (Fig. 32-6). It was believed that this positional change more closely approximated the function of the middle part of the trapezius and better stabilized the superior angle of the scapula. This is the technique used by the senior author.

Technique

After the induction of general anesthesia, the patient is placed in the lateral decubitus position with a slight forward tilt and then carefully secured. The entire shoulder girdle and upper extremity is draped free to allow manipulation of and complete access to the shoulder. A vertical incision is made midway between the vertebral spinous processes and the medial border of the scapula, extending

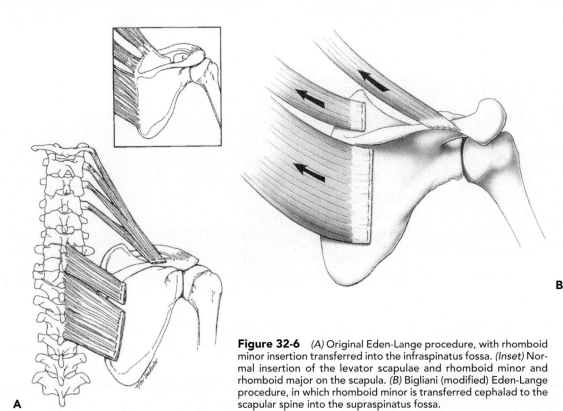

Figure 32-6   *(A)* Original Eden-Lange procedure, with rhomboid minor insertion transferred into the infraspinatus fossa. *(Inset)* Normal insertion of the levator scapulae and rhomboid minor and rhomboid major on the scapula. *(B)* Bigliani (modified) Eden-Lange procedure, in which rhomboid minor is transferred cephalad to the scapular spine into the supraspinatus fossa.

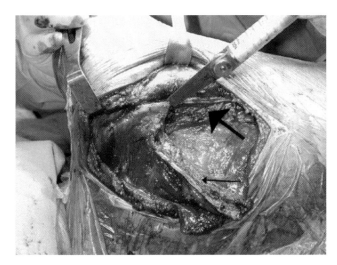
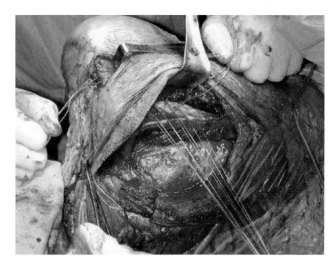

Figure 32-7 Release of levator scapulae and rhomboid minor and major from their insertion on the medial scapula along with a thin portion of bone.

Figure 32-8 After elevation of the supraspinatus and infraspinatus from their respective fossa, drill holes are placed above and below the scapular spine, and heavy, nonabsorbable sutures are passed through.

from just above the superior angle of the scapula down to the inferior scapular angle. The atrophied trapezius is identified and then transected laterally from its insertion on the scapular spine. A more medial transection poses a risk to the rhomboids and is not recommended. The levator scapulae and the rhomboid major and minor are then identified and separated. The muscles are then all sequentially released at their insertion point on the medial scapula along with a thin portion of bone (Fig. 32-7). A thin, narrow osteotome can be used. The muscles are next separated and dissected out 4 to 5 cm medial and proximal toward their origin on the spinous processes.

Next, the supraspinatus and infraspinatus muscle bellies are elevated from their respective fossa approximately 5 to 6 cm or at least half the width of the scapula. The rhomboids are transferred first, with the rhomboid minor cephalad to the scapular spine into the supraspinatus fossa and the rhomboid major into the infraspinatus fossa. Two drill holes are made in the supraspinatus fossa, and four drill holes are made in the infraspinatus fossa (Fig. 32-8). The drill holes are placed 1.5 to 2 cm apart and 4 to 5 cm lateral to the medial scapular border. The transferred muscles will be secured tightly to these drill holes using heavy, nonabsorbable, number 2 sutures passed through the drill holes with a large, curved needle (Fig. 32-9). These sutures are tagged for tying later.

The spine of the scapula is palpated next, and a 4-cm horizontal incision is made, starting 3 cm medial to the posterolateral corner of the acromion and continuing medially. The atrophied trapezius, deltoid, and supraspinatus are dissected and elevated off the scapular spine, taking care to avoid injury to the suprascapular nerve. The medial and lateral wounds are then connected with a tunnel through the atrophied trapezius, in line with its superior fibers. The levator scapulae is then passed through this

tunnel into the lateral wound. Heavy No. 2 nonabsorbable sutures are passed from the levator through three drill holes through the scapular spine approximately 5 to 7 cm medial to the posterolateral corner of the acromion (Fig. 32-10). Transfer more lateral than this can lead to a web neck deformity. If necessary, additional sutures can be used to attach the levator tendon to the deltoid and surrounding soft tissues.

The scapula is held in the reduced position, the upper extremity is held in 90 degrees of abduction, and the sutures holding the three transferred muscles are tied tightly. The supraspinatus and infraspinatus are allowed to fall back over the transferred muscles and are repaired to adjacent fascia. The incisions are then closed in layers over large drains.

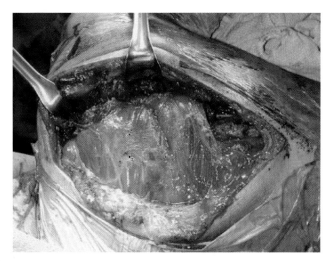

Figure 32-9 Transfer of the rhomboids. The sutures are tied with the scapula held in a reduced position, and the arm is abducted 90 degrees.

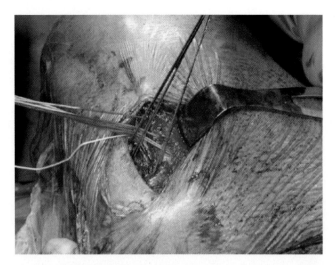

Figure 32-10 Transfer of the levator scapulae, which is tagged with heavy nonabsorbable sutures through three drill holes through the scapular spine.

Postoperative Treatment

Patients are routinely protected in a wedge-type abduction brace for 4 to 6 weeks to maintain the arm in 60 to 70 degrees of abduction.[4] Passive range-of-motion exercises above the level of the brace are started on the first postoperative day to avoid glenohumeral stiffness. The arm is passively elevated approximately 130 degrees in the scapular plane, and passive external rotation is kept at 30 to 40 degrees. The patient is not sent to formal physical therapy at this point; a family member is trained and supervised to perform this early passive motion.

The brace is removed at 4 to 6 weeks and passive range-of-motion exercises are increased. At 3 months, a progressive strengthening program is instituted that is aimed at achieving dynamic scapular stability by strengthening the transferred levator scapulae and rhomboid muscles. Shoulder shrugs are performed with the patient holding a gradually increased amount of weight. Bigliani et al.[3,4] described a special progressive strengthening program that involves the use of rubber tubing, free weights, medicine-ball throws, and overhead throws of 6 kg. All were designed to improve scapulothoracic stability and rhythm.

The transferred muscles are not as large as the trapezius, and thus intensive and consistent strengthening exercises are needed to achieve optimum function. Patients are able to return to athletic activity; however, it has been recommended that patients continuously perform strengthening exercises to maintain this level of function (Fig. 32-11).[45]

Results

The Eden-Lange dynamic muscle transfer has become the procedure of choice for the active and healthy patient with pain and disability from chronic trapezius dysfunction in whom 1 year of conservative treatment has failed. Several early reports documented the success of this procedure.[28,30] In 1973, Langneskiold and Ryoppy[30] reported on three patients who had undergone the Eden-Lange procedure, all with good results, decreased pain, and improved stability. In 1985, Bigliani et al.[4] reported excellent results for five of seven patients followed for more than 2 years after their modification of the Eden-Lange procedure.[4] One patient had a satisfactory result, and one patient had an unsatisfactory result. All patients had improved function and correction of deformity, and six patients had good pain relief. In 1996, as a continuation of the original study, results were reported on 22 patients who underwent the Bigliani transfers, with an average follow-up of 7.5 years.[3] Overall, 13 patients had an excellent result, 6 had a satisfactory result, and 3 had unsatisfactory results. All patients had improved function and correction of the deformity, and 19 patients had good pain relief. Three patients had an additional long thoracic nerve palsy caused by traction after an iatrogenic injury to the spinal accessory nerve. All three patients required transfer of the sternal head of the pectoralis major as well.

Role of Scapulothoracic Fusion

Scapulothoracic fusion or fasciodesis is rarely indicated for patients with isolated trapezius paralysis caused by injury to the spinal accessory nerve. These types of salvage operations are more useful and appropriate for the patient with a neuromuscular disorder, such as fascioscapulohumeral dystrophy, in which there are no transferable muscles. Static stabilization procedures that use a fascial sling eventually fail because the fascial sling stretches out with time.[3,4,37] Scapulothoracic fusion can lead to a significant limitation of motion. In the patient with the isolated trapezius paralysis, in light of the good results with the modified Eden-Lange procedure, this does not seem to be the best choice.

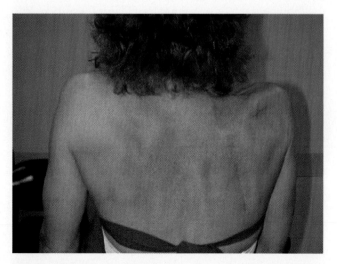

Figure 32-11 Three months after Bigliani Eden-Lange transfer, with satisfactory cosmesis of both scars.

REFERENCES

1. Anderson R, Flowers RS. Free grafts of the spinal accessory nerve during radical neck dissection. Am J Surg 1969;118:796.
2. Barron AO, Levine WN, Bigliani LU. Surgical management of chronic trapezius dysfunction. In: Warner JJP, Iannotti JP, Gerber C, eds. Complex and revision problems in shoulder surgery. Philadelphia, PA, Lippincott-Raven, 1997;377.
3. Bigliani LU, Compito CA, Duralde XA, et al. Transfer of the levator scapulae, rhomboid major, and rhomboid minor for paralysis of the trapezius. J Bone Joint Surg 1996;78A:534.
4. Bigliani LU, Perez-Sanz JR, Wolfe IN. Treatment of trapezius paralysis. J Bone Joint Surg 1985;67A:871.
5. Brandenburg JH, Lee CY. The eleventh nerve in radical neck surgery. Laryngoscope 1981;91:1851.
6. Codman EA. The shoulder. Rupture of the supraspinatus tendon and other lesions in or about the subacromial bursa. Boston, MA, Thomas Todd, 1934.
7. Coessens BC, Wood MB. Levator scapulae transfer and fascia lata fasciodesis for chronic spinal accessory nerve palsy. J Reconstr Microsurg 1995;11:277.
8. Dailiana ZH, Mehdian H, Gilbert A. Surgical anatomy of spinal accessory nerve: is trapezius functional deficit inevitable after division of the nerve? J Hand Surg 2001;26B(2):137.
9. Dewar FP, Harris RI. Restoration of function of the shoulder following paralysis of the trapezius by fascial sling fixation and transplantation of the levator scapulae. Ann Surg 1950;132:1111.
10. Dickson FD. Fascial transplants in paralytic and other conditions. J Bone Joint Surg Am 1937;19:405.
11. Dunn AW. Trapezius paralysis after minor surgical procedures in the posterior cervical triangle. South Med J 1974;67: 312.
12. Eden R. Zur behandlung der trapeziuslähmung mittelst muskelplastik. Dtsch Z Chir 1924;184:387.
13. Eisen A, Bertrand G. Isolated accessory nerve palsy of spontaneous origin. A clinical and electromyographic study. Arch Neurol 1972;27:496.
14. Gabel B, Nunley JA. Spinal accessory nerve. In: Gelberman RH, ed. Operative nerve repair and reconstruction. Philadelphia, PA, JB Lippincott, 1991;445.
15. Garrett WE, Best TM. Anatomy, physiology, and mechanics of skeletal muscle. In: Simon SR, ed. Orthopaedic basic science. Rosemont, IL, American Academy of Orthopaedic Surgeons 1994;89.
16. Hanford JM. Surgical excision of tuberculous lymph nodes of the neck. Report on 131 patients with follow-up results. Surg Clin North Am 1933;13:301.
17. Hawkins RJ, Willis RB, Litchfield RB. Scapulothoracic arthrodesis for scapular winging. In: Post M, Morrey BF, Hawkins RJ, eds. Surgery of the shoulder. St. Louis, MO, Mosby Year Book, 1990;356.
18. Henry AK. An operation for slinging a drooped shoulder. Br J Surg 1927;15:95.
19. Hollinshead WH. Pectoral region, axilla, shoulder and arm. In: Textbook of anatomy. Hagerstown, MD, Harper & Row, 1974:193.
20. Honey PR, Leffert RD. Operative treatment of isolated trapezius paralysis. Orthop Trans 1992–1993;16:761.
21. Ihara K, Katsube K, Misumi H, et al. Successful restoration of the trapezius muscle using pedicle latissimus dorsi. A case report. Clin Orthop 2000;371:125.
22. Inman VT, Saunders JB, Abbott LC. Observations of the function of the shoulder joint. J Bone Joint Surg 1944;26:1.
23. Jobe CM. Gross anatomy of the shoulder. In: Rockwood CA Jr., Matsen FA III, eds. The shoulder. Ed 2. Philadelphia, PA, WB Saunders Company, 1998;34.
24. Jobe CM, Kropp WE, Wood VE. The spinal accessory nerve in a trapezius splitting approach. J Shoulder Elbow Surg 1996;5:206.
25. Kayamori T, Orii K. Schmidt syndrome due to idiopathic accessory nerve paralysis. Electromyogr Clin Neurophysiol 1991;31:199.
26. Ketenjian AY. Scapulocostal stabilization for scapular winging in fascioscapulohumeral muscular dystrophy. J Bone Joint Surg 1978;60A:476.
27. Kuhn JE, Plancher KD, Hawkins RJ. Scapular winging. J Am Acad Orthop Surg 1995;3:319.
28. Lange M. Die behandlung der irreparablem trapeziusmahlung. Langenbecks Arch Klin Chir 1951;270:437.
29. Lange M. The operative treatment of irreparable trapezius paralysis [in German]. Tip Fakult Mecmausi (Istanbul) 1959;22:137.
30. Langneskiold A, Ryoppy S. Treatment of paralysis of the trapezius muscle by the Eden-Lange operation. Acta Orthop Scand 1973;44:383.
31. Leffert RD. Neurologic problems. In: Rockwood CA Jr., Matsen FA III, eds. The shoulder. 2nd ed. Philadelphia, WB Saunders, 1998:965.
32. McKenzie KG, Alexander E. Restoration of facial function by nerve anastomosis. Ann Surg 1950;132:411.
33. Neer CS II. Anatomy of shoulder reconstruction. In: Shoulder reconstruction. Philadelphia, WB Saunders, 1990:1, 421.
34. Norden A. Peripheral injuries to the spinal accessory nerve. Acta Chir Scand 1946;94:515.
35. Ogino T, Sugawara M, Minami A, et al. Accessory nerve injury: conservative or surgical treatment? J Hand Surg (Br) 1991;16(5):531.
36. Olarte M, Adams D. Accessory nerve palsy. J Neurol Neurosurg Psychiatry 1977;40:1113.
37. Post M. Orthopaedic management of neuromuscular disorders. In: Post M, Bigliani LU, Flatow EL, Pollock RG, eds. The shoulder: operative technique. Baltimore, MD, Williams and Wilkins, 1998;201.
38. Roy PH, Beahrs OH. Spinal accessory nerve in radical neck dissections. Am J Surg 1969;118:800.
39. Swann KW, Heros RC. Accessory nerve palsy following carotid endarterectomy. J Neurosurg 1985;63:630.
40. Tucker JA, Gee W, Nicholas GG, et al. Accessory nerve injury during carotid endarterectomy. J Vasc Surg 1987;5:440.
41. Valtonen EJ, Lilius HG. Late sequelae of iatrogenic spinal accessory nerve injury. Acta Chir Scand 1974;140:453.
42. Vastamaki M, Solonen KA. Accessory nerve injury. Acta Orthop Scand 1984;55:296.
43. Villanueva R. Orthosis to correct shoulder pain and deformity after trapezius palsy. Arch Phys Med Rehabil 1977;58(1):30.
44. Whitman A. Congenital elevation of the scapula and paralysis of the serratus magnus muscle. JAMA 1932;9:1332.
45. Wiater JM, Bigliani LU. Spinal accessory nerve injury. Clin Orthop 1999;368:5.
46. Woodhall B. Trapezius paralysis following minor surgical procedures in the posterior cervical triangle: results following cranial nerve suture. Ann Surg 1952;136:375.
47. Wright TA. Accessory spinal nerve injury. Clin Orthop 1975;108:15.
48. Wulff HB. Treatment of tuberculous cervical lymphoma: late results in 230 cases treated partly surgically, partly radiologically. Acta Chir Scand 1941;84:343.

Nerve Lesions: Suprascapular, Axillary, Thoracic Outlet, and Brachial Plexus

Scott H. Kozin

INTRODUCTION

Nerve injuries about the shoulder encompass a gamut of problems with varied treatment algorithms. Accurate diagnosis requires an understanding of the complex anatomy, a careful history of the events necessitating evaluation, and an astute physical examination. Imaging studies can be helpful in certain instances and provide valuable information regarding muscle quality. Electrodiagnostic testing can confirm the diagnosis, expel other causes, provide information regarding the extent of nerve damage, and gauge the status of recovery.

Nerve injuries vary with regard to severity. Classification systems have been developed to grade the extent of nerve injury and reflect the prognosis. Seddon's classification is most commonly used and provides a basis for treatment (Table 33-1).[97] The gradation of nerve injury begins with neuropraxia, extends to axonotmesis, and culminates in neurotmesis. A neuropraxia is a segmental demyelination with maintenance of intact nerve fibers and axonal sheath.

Demyelination causes a temporary conduction block without axonal damage and wallerian degeneration; electrodiagnostic studies demonstrate a decrease in nerve conduction without electromyographic changes of denervation within the muscle.[15] Complete recovery occurs over the ensuing days to weeks as remyelinization is completed. An axonotmesis is a disruption of nerve fiber integrity with preservation of the axonal sheath and framework. Wallerian degeneration and nerve fiber regeneration are necessary for recovery. Wallerian degeneration is characterized by the proliferation of Schwann cells that phagocytose myelin and axon debris. The axons distal to the injury degrade from lack of nutrition and loss of blood supply. Electrodiagnostic studies exhibit a decrease in nerve conduction and electromyographic changes of muscle denervation (insertional activity, fibrillations, positive sharp waves, and reduction in amplitude of motor-evoked potentials).[15] These electromyographic changes are apparent 3 weeks after injury. The regeneration rate is approximately 1 mm per day or 1 inch per month. This slow regeneration process delays return of function and often results in incomplete recovery. This slow recovery also means that distal nerve injuries have a better prognosis because the extent of wallerian degeneration is decreased and the proximity to the motor end plates is increased. In addition, prolonged

S. H. Kozin: Associate Professor, Department of Orthopaedic Surgery, Temple University and Hand Surgeon, Shriners Hospitals for Children, Philadelphia, Pennsylvania.

TABLE 33-1
SEDDON'S CLASSIFICATION OF NERVE INJURY

Type	Definition	Outcome
Neuropraxia	Interruption of nerve conduction; some segmental demyelination; axon continuity intact	Reversible
Axonotmesis	Axon continuity disrupted; neural tube intact	Wallerian degeneration; incomplete recovery
Neurotmesis	Complete disruption of nerve continuity; loss of axons and neural tubes	No spontaneous recovery; surgery required

muscle denervation lasting more than 18 to 24 months results in irreversible motor end-plate degradation and muscle fibrosis. This irreversible motor end-plate demise prevents continued muscle reinnervation. In contrast, the encapsulated sensory receptors retain their capacity for reinnervation for many years. A neurotmesis is a disruption of both nerve fiber and axonal sheath integrity. Transection is the classic example, but severe traction or contusion can produce a similar injury with severe intraneural scarring. Electrodiagnostic studies exhibit a loss of nerve conduction and subsequent electromyographic changes of denervation 3 weeks after injury. The prognosis is bleak without surgical resection of the intervening scar and nerve coaptation by direct repair or graft interposition.

This chapter discusses specific nerve injuries about the shoulder with regard to diagnosis, treatment, and outcome. Surgical indications, operative details, and reported outcomes are enumerated for the treating physician.

SUPRASCAPULAR NERVE INJURY

Anatomy

The suprascapular nerve originates from the upper trunk of the brachial plexus, which is formed by the union of C5 and C6 roots.[50,88] The nerve travels in a lateral direction across the posterior cervical triangle and deep to the trapezius muscle. The nerve passes through the suprascapular notch beneath the superior transverse scapular ligament (Fig. 33-1). In contrast, the suprascapular artery and vein course superficial to the ligament. The suprascapular nerve supplies one or two main branches to the supraspinatus muscle and travels into the infraspinatus fossa by descending around the lateral margin of the scapular spine (spinoglenoid notch). The suprascapular nerve supplies the infraspinatus muscle through two or more motor branches.[9] The suprascapular nerve is predominantly a motor nerve, although sensory fibers from the adjacent glenohumeral and acromioclavicular joints and a cutaneous branch to the lateral shoulder may be present.

The configuration of the suprascapular notch is variable. A narrow or encased notch may predispose the suprascapular nerve to injury.[85] Six types of scapular notch morphology have been classified (Fig. 33-2). Partial or complete osseous bridging has been detected in 12% to 23% of the population.

The proximity of the suprascapular nerve to the glenohumeral joint is approximately 3.0 cm from the supra-

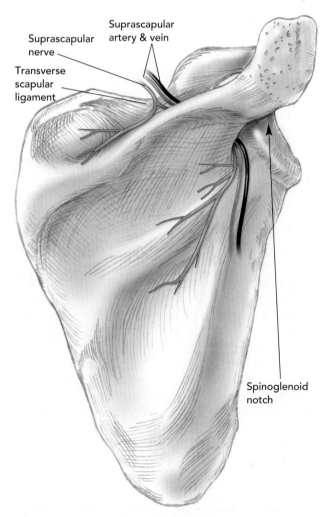

Figure 33-1 Suprascapular nerve passes below the transverse scapular ligament and around lateral margin of the scapular spine (spinoglenoid notch).

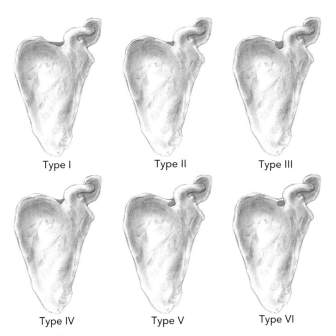

Type I Type II Type III

Type IV Type V Type VI

Figure 33-2 Classification of suprascapular notch morphology. In type I, the entire superior border of the scapula shows a depression (8% of specimens). In type II, there is a wide, blunted, V-shaped notch (31%). In type III, the notch is symmetrical and U-shaped (48%). In type IV, there is a very small V-shaped notch (3%). Type V is similar to type III but with partial ossification of the medial portion of the transverse scapular ligament (6%). In tye VI, the transverse scapular ligament is completely ossified, resulting in a foramen of variable size (4%). (Adapted from Rengachary SS, Burr D, Lucas S, et al. Suprascapular entrapment neuropathy: a clinical, anatomical, and comprehensive study. Part 2: anatomical study. Neurosurgery 1979;5:447.)

glenoid tubercle at the suprascapular notch and 1.8 cm from the glenoid rim at the base of the scapular spine.[9] The inferior transverse scapular ligament (aka spinoglenoid ligament) spans the spinoglenoid notch and has been reported with variable prevalence. The variation depends on the interpretation of a spinoglenoid ligament. Cummins and colleagues[25] studied the anatomy and histology of the spinoglenoid ligament in 112 shoulder cadavers. Two different types of ligaments were identified. A type I ligament was a thin fibrous band, and a type II ligament was a distinct well-formed structure. According to this characterization, 60% of specimens had a type I ligament and 20% had a type II ligament. The remaining 20% had no definable spinoglenoid ligament. The presence of a spinoglenoid ligament forms a fibro-osseous canal at the level of the spinoglenoid notch that may narrow during combined cross-body adduction and internal rotation. In individuals who perform rigorous overhead activities, this motion can compress the underlying suprascapular nerve.

Cause

Suprascapular neuropathy is an uncommon cause of shoulder pain. The differential diagnosis includes rotator cuff

TABLE 33-2
CAUSE OF SUPRASCAPULAR NEUROPATHY

Repetitive microtrauma	Overhead activities (e.g., volleyball, tennis, weight lifting)
Direct trauma	Glenohumeral dislocation, scapular fracture, proximal humerus fracture, iatrogenic injury (e.g., posterior shoulder surgery, distal clavicle resection, transglenoid arthroscopic shoulder stabilization, and rotator cuff surgery)
External compression	Patient positioning during spine surgery
	Glenohumeral ganglion or cyst
Infection	Brachial neuritis (Parsonage-Turner syndrome)

disease, impingement syndrome, shoulder instability, acromioclavicular joint arthritis, and cervical disk disease. Isolated suprascapular neuropathy can be secondary to traction (repetitive microtrauma), direct trauma, and/or external compression (Table 33-2).[27,31,87,99,100,117] In addition, suprascapular neuropathy can be part of a generalized brachial plexus disorder after trauma or infection.[65]

Traction or repetitive microtrauma usually damages the suprascapular nerve at the suprascapular notch. Extreme repetitive movements of the shoulder can cause traction across the nerve. This susceptibility is related to the limited excursion of the nerve as it passes through the suprascapular notch.[88,107] In contrast, external compression secondary to a glenohumeral cyst can injure the nerve along its course from the suprascapular notch through the spinoglenoid notch (Fig. 33-3).[107] The most common location is adjacent to a posterior-superior capsular-labrum junction.[108] At this location, the suprascapular nerve is compressed before innervation of the infraspinatus muscle.[107] On rare occasions, cyst compression may occur at the suprascapular notch and interfere with innervation to both the supraspinatus and infraspinatus muscles.

Iatrogenic injury after rotator cuff surgery is the result of extensive lateral mobilization of a large and retracted cuff tear.[117] The suprascapular nerve is stretched over the lateral margin of the suprascapular notch or injured directly by surgical dissection too far medial to the glenoid rim.

Diagnosis

Patient Presentation

Signs and symptoms of suprascapular neuropathy are more prominent with involvement at the suprascapular notch compared with the spinoglenoid notch. Patients with

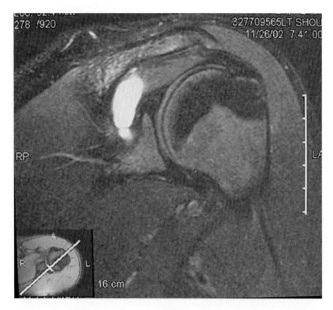

Figure 33-3 Magnetic resonance imaging (MRI) of glenohumeral cyst emanating from the posterior-superior capsular-labrum junction and compressing the suprascapular nerve before innervation of the infraspinatus muscle.

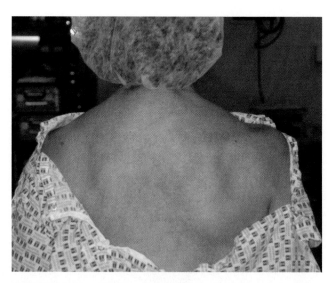

Figure 33-4 A 30-year-old woman with right suprascapular notch neuropathy and diffuse atrophy of both the supraspinatus and infraspinatus muscles.

suprascapular notch neuropathy experience a dull aching pain over the posterior and/or lateral aspect of the shoulder.[88] The pain is poorly localized and may radiate up the neck, down the arm, or across the chest wall mimicking cervical disc disease. Patients with spinoglenoid notch neuropathy may experience similar pain or present with painless wasting of the infraspinatus muscle.[34]

Physical Examination

Clinical diagnosis is difficult without muscle atrophy. Patients with suprascapular notch neuropathy may have tenderness about the notch. Chronic neuropathy results in diffuse atrophy of both the supraspinatus and infraspinatus muscles with weakness in shoulder abduction and external rotation, respectively (Fig. 33-4).

Patients with spinoglenoid notch neuropathy may have pain to palpation about the spinoglenoid notch. Provocative maneuvers, such as cross-body adduction, may increase the pain.[88] Chronic neuropathy results in atrophy of the infraspinatus muscle and weakness in external rotation. Gradual loss of the infraspinatus muscle, however, allows secondary hypertrophy of the posterior deltoid and teres minor muscles, which diminishes the expected weakness in external rotation.[34]

Electrodiagnostic Studies

Electrodiagnostic testing is useful in the diagnosis of suprascapular neuropathy.[5,80] The examination should confirm the diagnosis and exclude other causes of neuro-

genic shoulder pain, such as cervical disc disease. In suprascapular neuropathy, nerve conduction studies reveal prolonged motor latencies across the suprascapular nerve. Chronic suprascapular neuropathy yields electromyographic changes within the supraspinatus and/or infraspinatus muscles. Findings consistent with muscle denervation include insertional activity, fibrillation potentials, and positive sharp waves.

Imaging

Imaging studies may be useful in validating the diagnosis. Plain x-rays and an anteroposterior x-ray angled 15 to 30 degrees in the caudal direction can detect scapular fractures that involve the suprascapular notch.[81] Computed tomography (CT) provides higher bony resolution and better depicts the suprascapular notch.

Magnetic resonance imaging (MRI) is the modality of choice for identifying soft tissue lesions that can compress the nerve. MRI can readily identify ganglion cysts with characteristic high signal intensity on T2-weighted images (Fig. 33-3).[5,88,107] The size and extent of the cyst can also be appreciated. MRI can also evaluate the rotator cuff and provide information regarding muscle atrophy of the supraspinatus and/or infraspinatus.[5,119] Abnormal MRI signal changes within denervated muscles may be evident before clinical or electrodiagnostic findings.[119]

Treatment

Suprascapular Notch Neuropathy

The treatment of suprascapular notch neuropathy varies with the duration of symptoms, the cause of neuropathy,

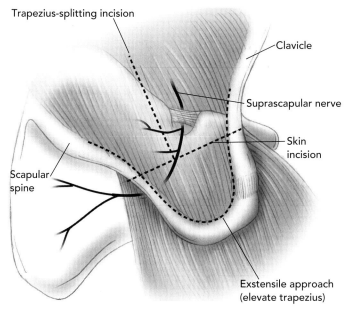

Figure 33-5 Superior trapezius-splitting approach for decompression of suprascapular notch neuropathy.

and the extent of nerve/muscle involvement.[64,80,87,88] Nonoperative treatment is indicated for nerve irritation or traction-type symptoms without substantial nerve or muscle damage.[64] Treatment consists of avoiding extreme overhead activity that may precipitate suprascapular neuropathy while maintaining full shoulder motion. Exercises are prescribed to correct any postural abnormalities, including scapular retraction exercises and strengthening of the parascapular muscles. Prolonged recovery is common and may require more than 1 year of dedicated treatment.

Operative treatment is indicated for symptoms refractory to nonoperative techniques (usually after 6 months), neuropathy attributed to a ganglion cyst, and marked muscle atrophy.[5,81,88] The operative treatment of suprascapular notch neuropathy requires decompression of the nerve. Multiple techniques have been proposed with a trend toward a superior trapezius-splitting approach (Fig. 33-5).[5,88] The patient is placed in a beach-chair position, and a saber incision is performed over the top of the shoulder 2 cm medial to the acromioclavicular joint. The skin flaps are elevated, and the underlying trapezius muscle is identified. The trapezius muscle is split in line with its fibers for a distance of 5 cm. The supraspinatus muscle is retracted in a posterior direction to visualize the superior aspect of the scapula. The notch and suprascapular neurovascular structures are isolated. The suprascapular artery and vein are mobilized away from the notch. A right-angle clamp is placed beneath the superior transverse ligament to protect the nerve. The superior transverse ligament is resected, and the notch is examined for persistent compression or tethering. Persistent notch encroachment requires removal of its osseous edges using a small rongeur.

Spinoglenoid Neuropathy

The treatment of spinoglenoid neuropathy also varies with the duration of symptoms, the cause of neuropathy, the extent of nerve/muscle involvement, and the degree of disability.[34,88] Nonoperative treatment is indicated for nerve irritation or minimal impairment. Treatment consists of avoiding extreme overhead activity, strengthening the external rotators, and preserving shoulder motion. Hypertrophy of the teres minor and posterior deltoid muscle can compensate for weakness of the infraspinatus muscle.[34] Operative treatment is indicated in patients with refractory symptoms, a compressive lesion, or considerable muscle atrophy that interferes with activities.

The operative treatment of neuropathy attributed to a ganglion requires cyst excision with or without glenohumeral joint arthroscopy for suspected labral tears.[5,88] Arthroscopy is usually performed because a high incidence of labral tears has been reported with spinoglenoid cysts.[5,88,108] Cyst decompression without glenohumeral joint exploration, however, has been associated with excellent results.[71] Cyst excision requires a posterior approach to the shoulder.[88] This exposure allows direct visualization of the suprascapular nerve around the spinoglenoid notch. A deltoid-splitting approach is performed through a 5-cm incision beginning from the posterolateral aspect of the acromion (Fig. 33-6). The superior edge of the infraspinatus is identified and retracted in an inferior direction. The presence of a ganglion cyst requires circumferential isolation of the mass and complete removal. The suprascapular neurovascular structures must be isolated and protected. Any overlying spinoglenoid ligament requires excision during nerve decompression. The suprascapular nerve is freed until it divides into motor branches that innervate the infraspinatus muscle.

Another, more sophisticated approach involves arthroscopic decompression of the cyst.[5,47] This technique allows treatment of the intra-articular abnormalities (e.g., labral

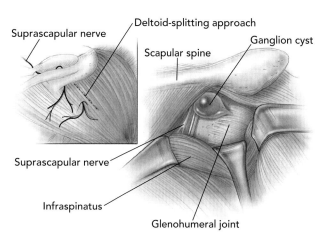

Figure 33-6 Posterior approach to the shoulder for isolation of the suprascapular nerve and excision of glenohumeral cyst.

tears) and cyst decompression with diminished morbidity associated with open surgery. The cyst is decompressed through a surgical defect created in the capsule adjacent to the glenoid site of cyst origin. This procedure is technically challenging and requires proficient technique for safe cyst decompression.

Clinical Results

Nonoperative Treatment

Martin et al.[64] published the results of nonoperative treatment of suprascapular neuropathy in 15 patients without a distinct compressive lesion. A program of physical therapy was used to improve the range of motion and strengthen muscles; 33% of patients had excellent results, and 47% had good results. Three patients who did not respond to nonoperative treatment required surgery. Of this group, one patient had an excellent result, one patient had a good result, and one patient had a poor result. The authors concluded that in the absence of a lesion producing mechanical compression of the suprascapular nerve, patients should be treated without surgery. Recalcitrant symptoms, however, require decompression before substantial atrophy.

Ferretti et al.[34] reported on 38 cases of isolated atrophy of the infraspinatus muscle in volleyball players; 35 of these athletes had no pain and were treated with exercises to strengthen the external rotators. The remaining three patients underwent surgery because of pain at the posterior aspect of the shoulder. Only 16 of the 35 players who were treated nonoperatively were reviewed. Thirteen were still involved in volleyball, three had retired without symptoms, and all had persistent atrophy of the infraspinatus muscle. All three patients who underwent surgery were able to play volleyball at their pre-injury levels. The authors concluded that suprascapular nerve at the spinoglenoid notch is usually a painless syndrome and that surgical treatment is indicated in cases of persistent pain after nonoperative management.

Operative Treatment

Numerous authors have reported consistent results after suprascapular nerve decompression.[5,14,47,71,80,81,87,113] Callahan et al.[14] reported long-term relief of pain and resolution of weakness in 20 of 23 patients (87%), although 3 required repeat decompression 2 to 4 years after the index procedure. Vastamäki and Göransson[113] reported the outcome in 54 patients. Pain relief was reported in 39 patients (72%), and resolution of supraspinatus atrophy occurred in 15 of 16 patients. Atrophy of the infraspinatus resolved in 15 of 26 muscles.

Post[80] reported on a cohort of 39 patients after surgery. Twenty-seven patients had excellent results and returned to work in an average of 3.3 months. Eleven patients had

good results, and one patient had a fair result. Earlier surgical treatment resulted in resolution of both shoulder pain and muscle atrophy. Delayed surgical treatment resulted in subsidence of pain but persistent muscle atrophy.

Successful arthroscopic treatment has also been reported.[5,33,47] Fehrman et al.[33] reported complete pain relief in the short-term outcome of six patients treated with combined arthroscopic management of intra-articular lesions and open resection of the ganglia. Iannotti and Ramsey[47] described the technique of arthroscopic decompression of a ganglion cyst and successful surgery in three patients.

Antoniou et al.[5] reported a comparison series of functional outcome after operative and nonoperative treatments. Fifty-three patients were followed for a minimum of 1 year after treatment. Thirty-six were treated with surgery, and 17 were managed with conservative measures. Decompression was performed for suprascapular notch neuropathy (7 patients) and spinoglenoid neuropathy without a ganglion cyst (7 patients). Cyst excision was performed by open excision (7 patients) or arthroscopic decompression (10 patients). Comparison of all causes of suprascapular nerve injury revealed a significant improvement in the operative and nonoperative groups with a greater degree of improvement in the operative group. Spinoglenoid cysts responded significantly better to operative treatment than to nonoperative treatment. Open and arthroscopic treatments were equally effective, and no recurrence was seen in either group.

AXILLARY

Anatomy

The axillary nerve is the terminal branch of the posterior cord and is composed of fibers from C5 and C6 roots.[12,50,102] The nerve travels across the inferolateral portion of the subscapularis muscle to enter the quadrilateral space along with the posterior humeral circumflex artery (Fig. 33-7).[102] The subscapularis muscle forms the anterior border of the quadrilateral space. The inferior boundary is the teres major and latissimus muscles, and the lateral margin is the long head of the triceps. The superior margin is the teres minor muscle. Within the quadrilateral space, the axillary nerve is in close proximity to the inferior glenohumeral joint capsule.

After the axillary nerve exits the quadrilateral space, the anterior trunk travels beneath the deltoid and innervates the anterior and middle sections of the deltoid muscle. The posterior trunk traverses in a posterior direction to innervate the posterior portion of the deltoid muscle and teres minor muscle (Fig. 33-7).[12,75] A superior lateral cutaneous emerges from the posterior trunk to supply sensation to the lateral portion of the upper arm. The axillary nerve is susceptible to injury at several sites including the origin of the nerve from the posterior cord, the anteroinferior juncture

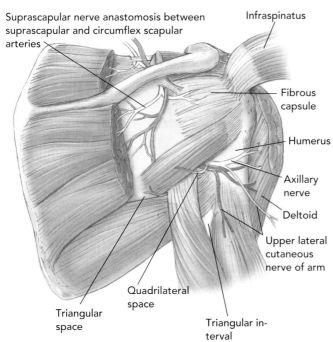

Suprascapular nerve anastomosis between suprascapular and circumflex scapular arteries

Infraspinatus

Fibrous capsule

Humerus

Axillary nerve

Deltoid

Upper lateral cutaneous nerve of arm

Quadrilateral space

Triangular interval

Triangular space

Figure 33-7 Posterior view of quadrilateral space with axillary nerve and posterior humeral circumflex artery.

TABLE 33-3
CAUSE OF AXILLARY NEUROPATHY

Repetitive Microtrauma	Quadrilateral Space Syndrome
Direct trauma	Glenohumeral fracture and/or dislocation
	Iatrogenic injury (e.g., shoulder instability surgery, rotator cuff surgery, arthroscopy, and capsular shrinkage)
	Penetrating trauma
	Gunshot injury
Infection	Brachial neuritis (Parsonage-Turner syndrome)
External compression	Tumor or aneurysm

of the subscapularis muscle and shoulder capsule, the quadrilateral space, and beneath the deltoid muscle. The axillary nerve is tethered between the posterior cord and the deltoid muscle, which limits its mobility and increases its susceptibility to injury.

Cause

Axillary nerve injury is usually secondary to trauma (Table 33-3).[75,102] Fracture and/or dislocation about the shoulder joint is the most common cause of isolated axillary neuropathy. Direct trauma to the shoulder can also injure the axillary nerve beneath the deltoid muscle.[75] Penetrating trauma, such as a stab or gunshot wound, can cause injury to the axillary nerve as part of a brachial plexopathy. Iatrogenic damage to the axillary nerve has been reported after surgical insult or anesthesia-related injury.[17,39,75] A less common cause of axillary neuropathy is repetitive microtrauma and compression within the quadrilateral space.[35,102] Lastly, axillary neuropathy can be secondary to brachial neuritis, the exact cause of which remains unknown.[29,111]

Diagnosis

Patient Presentation

Clinical history is an essential part of the evaluation in a patient with axillary neuropathy. A history of trauma usually dates the onset of nerve injury. In many patients, nerve in-

jury may be initially overlooked because the joint and/or bony injury dominates the clinical picture. Treatment for injury and development of muscle weakness and/or atrophy is vital information. Prolonged atrophy indicates considerable nerve damage and motor end-plate degeneration. In contrast, return of function indicates mild nerve injury and preservation of the motor end plates.

Patients with quadrilateral space syndrome present with diffuse, dull, aching pain about the shoulder.[13,35,75] The pain may awaken them at night and interfere with activities. Frank weakness and atrophy are uncommon, and electromyography is usually normal.

Acute brachial neuritis or Parsonage-Turner syndrome presents quite differently from other causes of axillary neuropathy.[29,111] Typically, severe radiating pain around the shoulder girdle precedes the onset of weakness. The intense pain may persist for a few hours up to 3 weeks. Subsequently, the pain abates and loss of function is noted. The degree of weakness is related to the number of nerves involved. The axillary nerve is most commonly involved (up to 70% of patients), followed by the suprascapular, long thoracic, and musculocutaneous nerves.[111] Multiple nerve involvement is more disabling than single nerve affliction (Fig. 33-8).

Physical Examination

Initial physical examination includes observation for muscle loss. Subtle asymmetry is more apparent during comparison to the unaffected side (Fig. 33-9). Active and passive motions about the shoulder are measured and recorded. Strength in abduction, adduction, external rotation, and internal rotation is graded according to the medical research scale (Table 33-4).[2] The degree of motion loss and effect on function after isolated axillary nerve injury are variable. The deltoid muscle provides approximately 50%

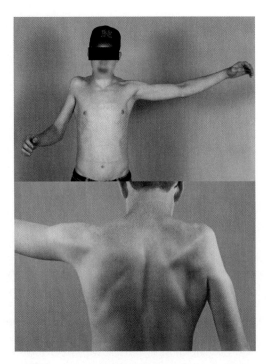

Figure 33-8 An 8-year-old boy with Parsonage-Turner syndrome involving the suprascapular and axillary nerves with marked atrophy of the supraspinatus, infraspinatus, and deltoid muscles, resulting in limited abduction.

TABLE 33-4
MUSCLE GRADING CHART

Muscle Grade	Description
5: Normal	Full range of motion against gravity with full resistance
4: Good	Full range of motion against gravity with some resistance
3: Fair	Full range of motion against gravity
2: Poor	Full range of motion with gravity eliminated
1: Trace	Slight contraction without joint motion
0: Zero	No evidence of contraction

of the abduction torque as determined by selective nerve blocks.[23,46] The limitation of abduction motion, however, is related to the degree of nerve damage, status of the rotator cuff, and time from injury. In fact, children may be able to compensate for complete deltoid paralysis and perform all activities of daily living (Fig. 33-10).[75] Sports that require extreme overhead motion, such as swimming and throwing, may be limited by fatigue.

The other nerves about the shoulder, including the spinal accessory, suprascapular, long thoracic, and axillary nerves, are routinely examined. A generalized brachial plexus injury requires a more detailed examination. The

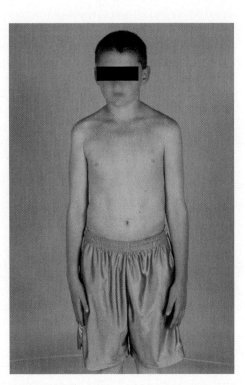

Figure 33-9 A 9-year-old boy with blunt trauma to the right shoulder and axillary neuropathy. Loss of shoulder contour is noted.

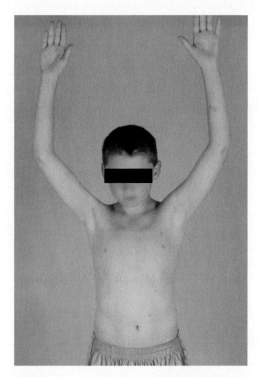

Figure 33-10 Full range of motion despite profound axillary neuropathy.

sensibility along the lateral aspect of the shoulder and upper arm is assessed, although patients with complete axillary nerve injuries may have no deficit.[102]

Electrodiagnostic Studies

Electrodiagnostic testing is useful in the diagnosis of axillary neuropathy.[75,102] The examination can determine the extent of nerve and muscle involvement. Testing can also differentiate an isolated axillary neuropathy from a more generalized nerve injury, such as a brachial plexus palsy.

In axillary neuropathy, nerve conduction studies reveal prolonged motor latencies across the axillary nerve. Severe axillary neuropathy (i.e., axonotmesis or neurotmesis) causes electromyographic changes within the deltoid and/or teres minor muscles. Findings consistent with muscle denervation include insertional activity, fibrillation potentials, and positive sharp waves.[15,75]

Imaging

Plain x-rays are used to identify fractures and/or dislocations about the shoulder. Anteroposterior and axillary views provide biplanar evaluation and assessment of joint reduction. CT images provide higher bony resolution and better delineation of fracture pattern. MRI is used for soft tissue evaluation including the status of the rotator cuff and deltoid musculature. Muscle atrophy and altered signal within the deltoid are indicative of muscle damage.[81,112] Abnormal MRI signal changes within denervated muscles may be detectable before clinical or electrodiagnostic findings.[81]

Arteriogram

Arteriography may be useful to diagnose quadrilateral space syndrome. Occlusion of the posterior humeral circumflex artery with the arm positioned in less than 60 degrees of abduction is considered positive.[13,102]

Treatment

The treatment of axillary neuropathy depends on the cause and extent of nerve damage. The natural history is variable and dependent on a variety of factors.

Traumatic Axillary Neuropathy

Open trauma to the axillary nerve is treated according to the mechanism of injury and physical examination. Most gunshot wounds do not disrupt nerve continuity and partially recover over time. The blast effect may cause a neuropraxia or axonotmesis, which does not require surgical management. Nonoperative treatment is the general course of management. Surgery is an option when there is no clinical or electrodiagnostic evidence of recovery 3 months after injury.

Penetrating sharp trauma requires a different treatment algorithm, because nerve laceration is likely. Early exploration is warranted to assess nerve continuity and the potential for nerve repair. Nerve conduction studies can be helpful because absent conduction immediately after injury (within the first week) implies laceration.[102] Direct nerve repair is difficult because of the zone of nerve injury, the confines of the brachial plexus, and the difficulties in exposure. Therefore, even after sharp laceration, primary nerve grafting is usually required.

Closed trauma to the axillary nerve requires a combination of nonoperative and operative treatment depending on the extent of recovery. Axillary nerve injury after a fracture or dislocation often recovers over time. Prompt reduction of the shoulder dislocation may enhance the chances of spontaneous nerve recovery.[76] The reported incidence of isolated axillary nerve injury after dislocation varies greatly from 5% to 54%. This wide variation is due to numerous factors, including the inclusion criteria and the possibility of subclinical injury to the axillary nerve.[41,110] Neurologic complications after shoulder dislocation occur more frequently in patients older than 50 years of age.[41,110]

The initial treatment is directed at maintaining shoulder motion until nerve regeneration. Passive- and active-assisted range-of-motion exercises are instituted to prevent joint contracture. The timing of mobilization varies with concomitant injuries. There is controversy regarding the appropriate time for surgical exploration after isolated axillary nerve injury. Operative treatment is usually recommended when there is no clinical or electrodiagnostic evidence of recovery after 3 months. This timing is based on the rate of axillary nerve recovery and the distance from the nerve injury to the deltoid muscle. Considering these factors, one should expect signs of renervation within 3 to 4 months after an axonotmesis nerve injury. This treatment algorithm allows sufficient duration for signs of spontaneous recovery and ample time for nerve regeneration after surgery before endplate demise.

Surgical Techniques

Surgical techniques for axillary neuropathy include neurolysis, neurorrhaphy, nerve grafting, and nerve transfer. Neurolysis and direct neurorrhaphy are seldom used after traumatic axillary nerve injury. Retraction, scarring, and inherent anatomy preclude primary nerve repair, unless the injury is acute and viable cut ends can be readily approximated. Disruption of nerve continuity by traction (aka neurotmesis) prevents neurolysis and requires nerve grafting, which is the preferred method of surgical treatment for isolated axillary nerve disruption.[4,6,22,77,110] The interposition source for nerve grafting is usually the sural nerve. Nerve transfer is an alternative technique that requires coaptation of an adjacent motor nerve directly into the distal end of the severed axillary nerve.[20,26] This technique is most commonly used for multiple nerve lesions, such a brachial plexus injury. Nerve transfer encourages nerve regeneration using a different source of axons; potential donor nerves include the thoracodorsal, phrenic, radial spinal accessory, and intercostal nerves. The choice of donor often depends on the concomitant nerve injuries.

Nerve Grafting Technique

Exploration of the axillary nerve through the quadrilateral space usually requires an anterior and a posterior exposure to the shoulder.[4,6,22,75,77,102,110] The patient is placed in a lateral decubitus position. The ipsilateral lower extremity is prepped for harvesting the sural nerve. A deltopectoral incision is performed, and the conjoined tendon is isolated from the coracoid. The pectoralis minor is tagged and released from the coracoid. The underlying brachial plexus and axillary vessels are isolated. Careful dissection is performed to isolate the axillary, radial, musculocutaneous, and ulnar nerves. Intraoperative nerve stimulation of viable nerves can facilitate proper identification. The axillary nerve is recognized by its course over the subscapularis and into the quadrilateral space. Proximal dissection to the posterior cord can assist in isolation of the axillary and radial nerves. The axillary nerve must be dissected in a proximal direction until normal nerve is encountered. Distal dissection toward the quadrilateral space will reveal dense scar formation about the nerve, indicative of injury and loss of viable fascicles. Discriminating injured from viable fascicles is exceedingly difficult even with intraoperative nerve stimulation and magnification. In rare cases, intact nerve can be separated from disrupted nerve, and a partial nerve graft can be placed across the disrupted segment. Usually, complete nerve disorganization is present that is consistent with a neurotmesis, which requires neuroma resection and grafting. The neuroma is resected in a proximal direction until viable fascicles are encountered.

A posterior shoulder incision is necessary to identify the axillary nerve exiting from the quadrilateral space. An incision is performed from the acromion to the posterior axillary crease. The quadrilateral space is exposed inferior to the teres minor muscle. The axillary nerve and posterior humeral circumflex vessels are isolated. Viable axillary nerve distal to the quadrilateral space is identified. The defect between the axillary nerve in the anterior and posterior incisions is measured for graft distance. This distance is calculated with the arm in abduction and external rotation to grafting without tension.

Sural nerve graft is harvested from the leg under tourniquet control. Usually two or three grafts between 4 and 8 cm in length are required. The nerve grafts are connected across the defect within the axillary nerve. Fibrin glue is used to facilitate this process. The nerve grafts are cut to the appropriate length, and the ends are glued together on the back table. The excess glue is cut from each end, and the grafts are placed through the quadrilateral space. The conjoined nerve graft ends are coaptated to the proximal and distal ends of the axillary nerve using a combination of suture and fibrin glue.

Standard closure is performed, and the limb is immobilized in a sling with an abduction pillow. Active and gentle passive motion are instituted 1 week after surgery. Full abduction and external rotation are avoided for the first month.

Acute Brachial Neuritis or Parsonage-Turner Syndrome

Brachial neuritis is usually a benign disease that is self-limited (Fig. 33-8). Treatment is nonoperative with analgesics to control the initial pain and physical therapy to maintain motion until nerve regeneration. Therapy and exercises are used to prevent joint contracture, with passive and active-assisted range of motion the mainstays of management. Corticosteroids have been used as part of the treatment regimen, but their efficacy is unknown.[111] Electromyography may be useful to define the extent of involvement and to assess for signs of recovery. Gradual improvement is often the case, although incomplete recovery and persistent impairment can occur. Rates of complete recovery have been estimated to be 36% within 1 year, 75% within 2 years, and 89% within 3 years.[111]

Quadrilateral Space Syndrome

Treatment of quadrilateral space syndrome is usually nonoperative, and most patients improve over time. Avoidance of aggravating factors and analgesics are the principles of management. Persistent symptoms and evidence of muscle loss are indications for surgical decompression, which involves decompression of the axillary nerve with the quadrilateral space.[13,35] Release of the compressive fascia and fibrous bands around the axillary nerve and posterior humeral circumflex vessel is the standard treatment.

Late Treatment

Nerve surgery is not an option after irreversible motor endplate degeneration (usually 24 months). Patients with satisfactory motion and slight activity limitations do not require surgery. Restricted motion that interferes with function is an indication for surgery; however, the options are limited. Abduction is a difficult motion to reestablish, especially with rotator cuff dysfunction. Tendon transfer is the primary alternative with a variety of donor muscles suggested, including the trapezius and latissimus dorsi.[8,32,48,53]

Severe shoulder impairment without available donors for transfers precludes reconstruction. Persistent pain, instability, or arthritis can only be remedied by shoulder

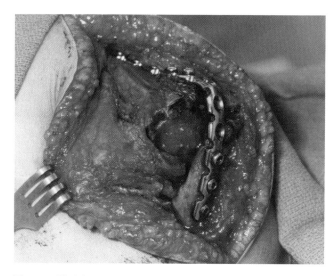

Figure 33-11 An 11-year-old patient with axillary and suprascapular nerve injury creating a flail shoulder. Patient was treated with shoulder arthrodesis using plate fixation along scapular spine and humerus.

arthrodesis (Fig. 33-11).[86] Functioning scapular muscles, however, are a prerequisite to prevent progressive scapulothoracic winging after shoulder arthrodesis.

Clinical Results

Nonoperative Treatment

Axillary nerve injury attributed to trauma, especially fracture and/or dislocation, has a good to excellent chance of recovery. Blom and Dahlbäck[10] studied 73 patients with fracture or dislocation of the proximal humerus. Twenty-four patients had electrodiagnostic evidence of partial or complete axillary neuropathy (9 complete and 15 partial). All patients recovered over the ensuing 1 to 2 years without objective loss of function. Gumina and Postacchini[41] reported on 108 elderly patients after shoulder dislocation. Ten patients had axillary nerve injury, and all cases resolved within 1 year.

Toolanen et al.[110] reported a high incidence of axillary nerve injury after shoulder dislocation in patients more than 40 years of age. Electrodiagnostic studies revealed moderate to severe denervation in 28 of 55 patients. After 3 years, no patient had persistent deficits. In contrast, Leffert and Seddon[59] reported a small series of six patients with dislocation, and only one achieved good functional recovery of the deltoid muscle.

Quadrilateral Space Decompression

Reports after surgical decompression for quadrilateral are scant, although the results are generally good. Cahill and Palmer[13] reported decompression of the quadrilateral space in 18 patients. Eight patients achieved substantial relief of symptoms, and eight patients noted partial diminution of pain. Two patients were not improved. Francel et al.[35] reported a small series of five patients, and all noted improvement with respect to sensory deficits, pain, and active motion.

Nerve Reconstruction

Because the axillary nerve is primarily composed of motor fibers and is relatively close to its motor end plates, the prognosis for recovery after surgical repair and grafting is good. The results of nerve reconstruction, however, vary with the timing of surgery and the procedure performed. Coene and Narakas[22] reported on 66 patients with axillary neuropathy isolated or combined with other nerve lesions. Nerve grafting within 6 months was performed on 27 patients. Eighteen of these patients regained strength graded as M4 or M5. Delayed grafting was performed in six patients, and only one achieved M4 strength. Petrucci and colleagues[77] reported on 15 patients who underwent sural nerve grafting at an average of 5.8 months after injury. Fourteen of the patients regained M4 or M5 muscle strength. Alnot et al.[4] reported on 28 patients with isolated axillary nerve injuries; 23 underwent nerve grafting, 4 had neurolysis, and 1 had primary nerve repair. Good to excellent results were reported in 57%.

Nerve Transfers

Reports after nerve transfer to the axillary nerve often include other aspects of brachial plexus reconstruction. Chuang et al.[20] reviewed their results for restoration of shoulder abduction by nerve transfers using a variety of donor nerves. The spinal accessory or phrenic nerve was most commonly used, and the results were similar. The average improvement in abduction was 45 degrees. Dai et al.[26] described nerve transfer of the thoracodorsal nerve to the axillary nerve and reported good results in two patients.

Tendon Transfers

The results after tendon transfers about the shoulder for abduction are less predictable and have a variable success rate.[8,32,48,53] The status of the rotator cuff and degree of preoperative abduction are important factors. Surgery to improve abduction is more predictable than surgery to obtain abduction. Aziz et al.[8] treated 27 shoulders with trapezius transfers after brachial plexus injuries and noted an average abduction gain of 45 degrees. Kotwal et al.[53] reported an average increase of 60 degrees in eight patients after trapezius transfer. Itoh et al.[48] described the technique of bipolar latissimus transfer and noted a marked improvement in forward flexion (average = 102 degrees), although average abduction was less impressive (38 degrees).

THORACIC OUTLET SYNDROME

Anatomy

The thoracic outlet begins just distal to the spinal intervertebral foramina and extends to the coracoid process.[7,58,73,82,125] The outlet is bordered by anatomic constraints that encompass the brachial plexus and associated vessels (subclavian and axillary). These structures include muscles (anterior and middle scalene muscles), bones (first rib, cervical ribs, clavicle, and coracoid), and fascial bands. The most common sites of compression in thoracic outlet syndrome are at the superior thoracic outlet, scalene interval or triangle, costoclavicular space, or subcoracoid area (Fig. 33-12).[58,73,82] This compression can be static and constant or dynamic and dependent on posture, limb position, and activity level.[58]

The superior thoracic outlet is defined by sternum (anterior), first rib (lateral), and thoracic vertebrae (posterior).[101] The inferior trunk must ascend from its intervertebral foramina to maneuver over the first rib. This route can result in compression or stretching of the inferior trunk over the first rib. The scalene triangle is formed by the anterior and middle scalene insertions on the first rib. The triangle has a narrow base (~1–2 cm) and elongated sides.[82] The upper roots (C5–C7) descend, whereas the inferior roots (C8 and T1) and subclavian artery must ascend to advance through the scalene triangle. The presence of a cervical rib or a fibrous band extending from an incomplete cervical rib to the first rib elevates the base of the scalene triangle and narrows its confines. This compels the inferior roots and subclavian artery to further ascend to enter the scalene triangle. In addition, the anterior or middle scalene can attach to these anomalous ribs and further narrow the scalene interval.[58] The incidence of cervical ribs is between 0.5% to 1% of individuals, and bilateral cervical ribs are present 50% to 80% of the time (Fig. 33-13).[79,101] The presence of an anomalous rib, however, does not establish or exclude the diagnosis of thoracic outlet syndrome. The width of the scalene triangle can also be narrowed by anterior or middle scalene muscle hypertrophy or anomaly, which can cause thoracic outlet compression.[106]

The costoclavicular interval is located between the clavicle and first rib. Depression of the clavicle reduces this space and compresses the brachial plexus or adjacent subclavian or axillary vessels. Hypertrophy of the subclavius muscle or abundant callus about a clavicle fracture can narrow the costoclavicular space. The subcoracoid area can compress the brachial plexus and vascular structure behind the coracoid, which provides a fulcrum for the neurovascular structures when the arm is positioned in abduction and

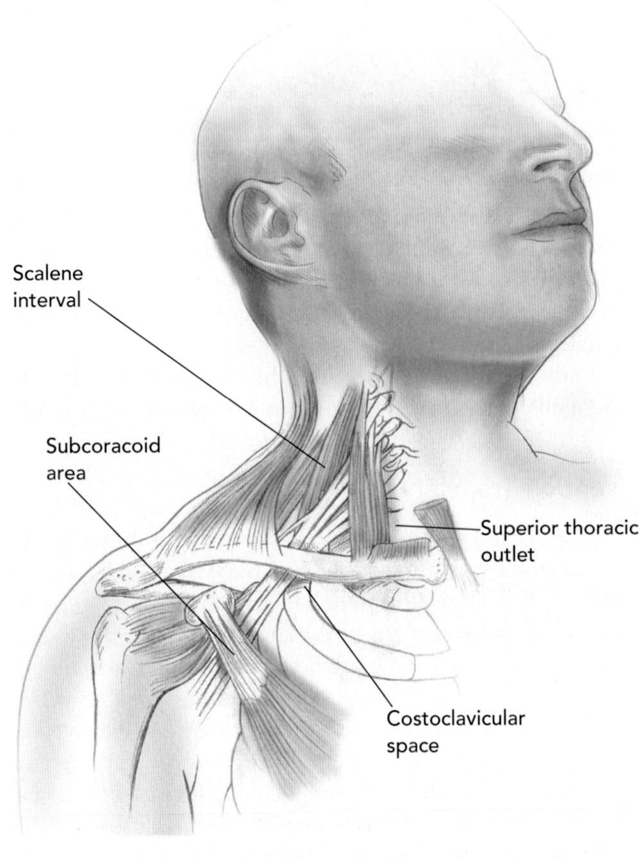

Scalene
interval

Subcoracoid
area

Superior thoracic
outlet

Costoclavicular
space

Figure 33-12 Common sites of compression within the thoracic outlet include the superior thoracic outlet, scalene interval, costoclavicular space, and subcoracoid area.

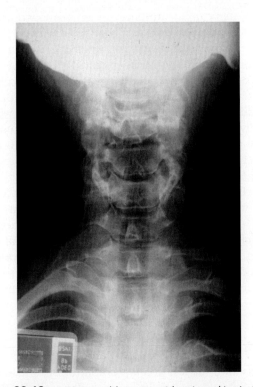

Figure 33-13 A 50-year-old woman with pain and intrinsic atrophy in left hand; x-ray shows bilateral cervical ribs.

external rotation.[103] Excessive arm elevation, therefore, can cause a traction or compressive neuropathy across the coracoid process. The pectoralis minor muscle and conjoined tendon can further contribute to compression behind the coracoid process.

Cause

The cause of thoracic outlet syndrome is often multifactorial. The majority of patients present with neurologic symptoms (~94% to 97% cases), with preferential involvement of the lower plexus. Venous and arterial thoracic outlet syndromes are much less common, appearing in 2% to 3% and 1% to 2%, respectively.[7,73] The potential sites of compression have been described in the preceding anatomy section. Anomalous anatomy, poor posture, and/or injury to the supporting musculature often can incite these potential sites of compression. For example, poor posture or injury to the trapezius muscle can result in descent of the scapula and irritation of the nerves within the thoracic outlet.[58,66,73] In addition, shoulder muscle atrophy can depress the entire limb and cause the inferior trunk to be compressed within the superior thoracic outlet against the first rib. Further narrowing of the costoclavicular space can occur from downward pressure on the shoulder girdle from heavy backpacks or pendulous breasts.[49,58] In predisposed persons, repetitive motion may play a factor, although this remains speculative.[63,93]

Arterial signs and symptoms can be induced by compression along the thoracic outlet. Pressure can be from the tip of a cervical rib, a fibrous band, or costoclavicular narrowing. Subclavian or axillary artery stenosis may occur, which can rarely advance to mural thrombus formation, emboli, and distal ischemia.[7]

Diagnosis

Patient Presentation

The history and physical examination are the cornerstones of diagnosis. A spectrum of signs and symptoms exist, dependent on the elements involved and the degree of compression. Typically, the symptoms of thoracic outlet syndrome are vague, and the signs are subtle unless severe compression is present.[58,72,73] Females are more commonly affected (4:1).[58] Virtually all patients with thoracic outlet compression present with neurologic symptoms affecting the lower plexus (C8 and T1). Therefore, the distribution of pain or paresthesias is the medial side of the arm and ulnar digits (ring and small). Difficulty with overhead use and carrying objects is a common complaint. Loss of dexterity during fine manipulation can occur secondary to intrinsic muscle weakness. Vascular thoracic outlet syndrome is much less common (<5%) and can affect venous outflow or arterial inflow.[73] Venous thoracic outlet syn-

drome is more common than arterial involvement, which yields bluish discoloration or edema. Arterial compression may produce pain, cold intolerance (similar to Raynaud's phenomenon), and claudication.[93]

Physical Examination

A thorough examination with provocative maneuvers is required for accurate diagnosis. The physical examination begins with an assessment of the posture of the patient, especially the scapula and shoulder girdle. A malpositioned scapula and poor posture can narrow the thoracic outlet and provoke symptoms. A standard cervical spine and peripheral nerve evaluation is routine to exclude additional sites of compression that can lead to a double crush neuropathy (e.g., carpal or cubital tunnel syndrome).[121] The area of reported diminished sensibility should be delineated and defined by two-point discrimination or Semmes-Weinstein monofilament testing. A careful manual muscle test is performed for objective signs of motor weakness that can occur in long-standing thoracic outlet syndrome.[2] Special attention is devoted to the trapezius, parascapular muscles, and ulnar innervated muscles. Edema, venous distension, or cyanosis may indicate a venous thoracic outlet syndrome, whereas pallor, splinter hemorrhages, or ischemic changes suggest arterial involvement from vessel constriction and/or embolization.[7,95]

The supraclavicular region is palpated for areas of tenderness. Percussion is performed in an attempt to evoke a Tinel's sign, which indicates underlying nerve irritation. Provocative maneuvers are instrumental for the diagnosis of thoracic outlet syndrome, but they must be interpreted with caution. To be noteworthy, a positive test result must elicit the expected outcome and reproduce the patient's symptoms. These provocative maneuvers narrow the anatomic constraints of the thoracic outlet and attempt to compress the neural and/or vascular elements. The Adson test is performed with the patient seated, placing the arm at the side, and palpating the radial pulse.[1] The patient extends the head and rotates the neck toward the affected side while taking a deep breath. This movement narrows the scalene triangle. A positive test result is diminution or obliteration of the radial pulse with a corresponding reproduction of the patient's symptoms. The Wright hyperabduction test consists of placing the arm in 90 degrees of abduction and external rotation.[123] As in the Adson test, the loss of a radial pulse and the reproduction of symptoms are considered positive results. The overhead exercise stress test and 3-minute stress test are similar and performed by instructing the patient to abduct and externally rotate the shoulder to place the arms above shoulder level. Active opening and closing of the hands is then executed, and a positive response will reproduce symptoms such as paresthesias or fatigue.[58,89]

The uncertainty with provocative maneuvers for thoracic outlet syndrome is based on the significant rate of false-positive results that occur in both asymptomatic volunteers and in other common entrapment neuropathies.[73,84] For example, shoulder abduction and external rotation applies traction across the lower plexus at the level of the first rib, narrows the costoclavicular space, drags the plexus around the coracoid process, and increases the pressure within the cubital tunnel.

Electrodiagnostic Studies

The role of electrodiagnostic studies in the diagnosis of thoracic outlet syndrome is controversial. Certainly, severe compression will produce denervation of the affected muscles, usually the intrinsic muscles of the hand.[15] Most patients, however, do not present with atrophy and electromyographic findings. Slowing of the nerve conduction across the affected segment would seem to be a reliable indicator of thoracic outlet syndrome. Unfortunately, standard orthodromic nerve conduction tests and somatosensory-evoked potentials have been relatively difficult to perform, interpret, and reproduce.[15,58,62] Dynamic or positional recording of nerve conduction across the brachial plexus during provocative maneuvers is logical but is also difficult to perform in a reproducible manner.[92]

Other Imaging Studies

Numerous imaging studies have been recommended to assist in the diagnosis of thoracic outlet syndrome. Plain x-ray films of the cervical spine are used to identify cervical ribs or elongated transverse processes, although cervical ribs may be present in asymptomatic individuals.[79,101] Angiography, venography, or noninvasive studies may be used in patients suspected with vascular thoracic outlet, although false-negative and false-positive results have been reported.[7,58,114]

Treatment

Nonoperative (Natural History)

The principal treatment for thoracic outlet syndrome is conservative management. Correction of abnormal shoulder girdle alignment and alleviation of aggravating factors are the mainstays of treatment.[72] Poor posture and weakness of the parascapular muscles often result in descent of the scapula and narrowing of the thoracic outlet. Postural reeducation exercises and patient education are instituted to correct this altered position and improve overall body mechanics. Ergonomic modification, aimed at the decrease of overhead activity and elimination of any downward force on the shoulder girdle, is part of the treatment regimen. An exercise program, directed at selective muscle strengthening of the shoulder girdle with maneuvers designed to stretch the scalene muscles and relax the first rib,

is included. Supervision is required to selectively exercise and strengthen the parascapular muscles (trapezius, levator scapulae, and rhomboids) without further compression of the thoracic outlet.[58,72] A variety of additional therapeutic modalities (ultrasound, biofeedback, and electrical stimulation) have been proposed with ambivalent success.[7]

Factors that may contribute to thoracic outlet syndrome are also addressed. Obese patients are encouraged to lose weight. Women with macromastia are instructed to wear better breast support and may benefit from reduction mammoplasty.[49,58] Conservative treatment is effective for improving symptoms in most patients, although patients will not experience relief within the first 2 months.[58] Only 10% to 30% of patients fail nonoperative treatment and are potential candidates for surgical intervention.[73,95]

Surgical Treatment

Indications for surgical treatment are failure of a supervised nonoperative program, intractable pain, a considerable neurologic deficit, or vascular compromise.[58] The surgery for thoracic outlet syndrome has considerable risks, and mild discomfort from limited compression is better treated without surgery. The operative procedure is directed at decompression of the thoracic outlet and release of any anatomic constrictions. There is no consensus as to the most efficacious approach or procedure to alleviate thoracic outlet syndrome.[58] The fundamental components of the described procedures include cervical rib resection, first rib resection, scalenotomy, scalenectomy, excision of anomalous fascial bands, claviculectomy, pectoralis minor release, or a combination of these. Resection of the first rib, with or without anterior scalenectomy, has become the preferred procedure for thoracic outlet syndrome by most surgeons.[1,38,58,73,90]

The procedure can be accomplished by a variety of approaches, including a supraclavicular, transclavicular, subclavicular, axillary, posterior, or combined approach. The supraclavicular approach favors scalenectomy and upper plexus exploration, but sacrifices posterior first rib exposure. The axillary route is more cosmetic and affords the best access to the first rib.[58,90] Cervical ribs can usually be removed through the axillary approach, and the pectoralis minor tendon can be divided for suspected subcoracoid compression. The axillary exposure also allows scalenotomy but precludes formal exploration of the upper plexus. The posterior approach offers extensile exposure of the posterior portion of the first rib but requires sectioning of the muscles supporting the scapula including the trapezius muscle.[1,58] The transclavicular approach is best used in patients with fracture or nonunion of the clavicle. A combined supraclavicular and transaxillary method is reserved for complicated or recurrent cases.[83] Persistent long-standing venous or arterial thrombosis may require thrombectomy or bypass grafting and an extensile exposure.

Clinical Results

The results of thoracic outlet surgery are difficult to accumulate and compare. The reported outcome is divergent, with success rates dependent on the procedure used, the surgeon, and the interpretation of success. Isolated anterior scalenotomy has a 50% failure rate, with a significant recurrence rate.[38,58] The results of first-rib resection are successful (improvement of symptoms) in 37% to 92% of individuals, with lower recurrence rates than scalenotomy.[11,60,89] Scalenectomy alone or combined with first-rib resection has a reported success rate between 68% and 86%.[7,83,94,95,122] Improvement after thoracic outlet surgery may require 2 years or longer, and continued rehabilitation is necessary to maintain postural alignment and proper shoulder mechanics.[7,58]

Surgery for thoracic outlet syndrome is fraught with potential complications. Vascular injury can occur during the dissection and result in considerable blood loss. Pulmonary injury is frequent during rib resection, and chest tube placement is necessary. Phrenic nerve injury during anterior scalenectomy can cause hemidiaphragm paralysis and dyspnea. Long thoracic nerve injury during middle scalenectomy will produce further alterations in scapular motion.[122] Cervicothoracic ganglion injury during lower trunk mobilization can result in Horner's syndrome.

BRACHIAL PLEXUS INJURIES

Anatomy

The brachial plexus originates from the fifth to eighth cervical (C5–C8) and the first thoracic (T1) spinal nerves.[50] Small contributions may emanate from the fourth cervical (C4) and second thoracic (T2) nerves. The dorsal and ventral rootlets (six to eight rootlets per level) exit the spinal cord and merge to form the spinal nerves, which leave the intervertebral foramina and divide into dorsal and ventral rami (Fig. 33-14). The small dorsal rami travel posterior to innervate the skin and muscles of the neck and are not considered part of the brachial plexus. The ventral rami emerge between the anterior and middle scalene muscles and are designated as the nerve roots of the brachial plexus. The motor cell bodies of the nerve roots are located within the ventral horn of the spinal cord gray matter. In contrast, the sensory cell bodies are situated outside the spinal cord within the dorsal root ganglia (Fig. 33-14). The dorsal root ganglia transfer afferent fibers to the spinal cord through the dorsal rootlets. This difference in anatomic location of cell bodies between motor and sensory fibers is meaningful for the accurate diagnosis and treatment of brachial plexus injuries.

The ventral rami of C5 and C6 combine to form the superior trunk, the C7 ramus continues alone as the middle trunk, and C8 and T1 unite to form the lower trunk

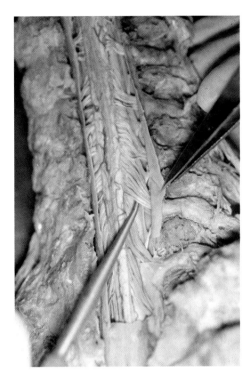

Figure 33-14 Dorsal rootlets exiting the spinal cord beneath the probe. Forceps holding dura matter. Dorsal root ganglion is lateral to the forceps and situated outside the spinal cord.

(Fig. 33-15). Each trunk divides into anterior and posterior divisions and proceeds behind the clavicle. The divisions then merge into three cords named in relation to the axillary artery. The anterior divisions of the upper and middle trunks combine to form the lateral cord. The three posterior

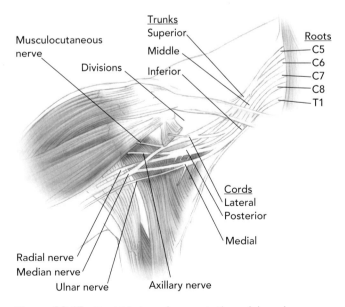

Figure 33-15 Brachial plexus from roots through branches.

divisions converge to form the posterior cord, and the anterior division of the inferior trunk continues as the medial cord. The cords proceed behind the pectoralis minor muscle into the axilla, and each divide into two terminal branches. The lateral cord terminates as the musculocutaneous nerve and a branch to the median nerve. The posterior cord divides into the axillary and radial nerves. The medial cord continues as the ulnar nerve and supplies a branch to the median nerve.

Several branches arise from the roots, trunks, and cords of the brachial plexus. The condition of these intermediate nerves provides important information with reference to the location of nerve injury.

There are variability and asymmetry in the neural and vascular anatomy of the brachial plexus.[50] The plexus is termed *prefixed* when there is a relatively large contribution from C4 and a small allotment from T1. Similarly, a *postfixed* plexus has substantial contribution from T2 with little from C5. There are also variations in cord separation and peripheral branchings of nerves that may or may not affect segmental innervation.

Cause

Brachial plexus injuries affect a wide range of individuals from newborns to the elderly. Brachial plexus birth palsies can occur during passage through the birth canal, whereas adolescent and adult injury may be secondary to domestic violence, vehicular trauma, athletic endeavors, or systemic disease.[54,118] The causes can be divided into trauma (penetrating and nonpenetrating), entrapment, and infection. This section will discuss traumatic plexus injuries in the adult population.

Nonpenetrating Trauma

Nonpenetrating trauma is the principal cause of injury to the brachial plexus. Traction produces tension across the brachial plexus.[103] The traction mechanism is variable and may be from pulling the extremity, forcible head rotation away from the shoulder, or direct depression of the shoulder girdle.[103] A traction injury yields a stretch along the nerve beyond its physiologic limits. There is a direct reduction of intraneural blood flow with increasing strain. A 15% elongation will reduce blood flow approximately 80% to 100%.[21,54,61,124] Continued elongation causes profound ischemia and cessation of nerve metabolism. Persisted traction will ultimately tear nerve fibers and disrupt nerve continuity. Therefore, traction can cause a spectrum of nerve injury, ranging from a transient disruption in nerve fiber conduction (neuropraxia) to functional discontinuity of the nerve sheath and/or fibers (axonotmesis or neurotmesis).

Various factors influence the portion of the plexus injured and the extent of damage incurred. These determinants include the magnitude and duration of the force applied and the position of the extremity and head at time of accident.[103] The upper and middle trunks descend beneath the clavicle, whereas the lower trunk ascends over the first rib to form the lower trunk. The upper plexus is taut with the arm hanging at the side, which predisposes this part of the plexus to traction injury. In contrast, the lower plexus is strained with the arm abducted and elevated.

Adult Traction Injuries

The majority of adult brachial plexus traction injuries occur after motor vehicle accidents, especially motorcycle mishaps.[70,91] Brachial plexus injury is more prevalent in regions that rely on motorcycles as the principal mode of transportation. The incidence of brachial plexus injury after a motorcycle accident has been approximated to be 2%, with predominance in young males.[69,70] Associated head trauma and fractures/dislocations of the cervical spine, shoulder, forearm, and hand are common.

Less common causes of brachial plexus injuries are bicycle, sporting, and pedestrian accidents. Minor stretch injuries (aka burners or stingers) of the plexus are common in contact sports, especially football or rugby, because tackling forces the shoulder downward and the neck toward the contralateral side.[44] Immediate burning pain and paresthesias that radiate into the arm are characteristic symptoms. Transient weakness and sensory abnormalities can be present, although these symptoms should resolve over a few minutes. Persistent complaints, physical findings, neck pain, or restricted neck mobility warrant further evaluation to exclude a cervical spine fracture/dislocation, substantial brachial plexus injury, or spinal cord injury.

Penetrating Trauma

Penetrating trauma to the brachial plexus occurs after a gunshot wound or stabbing. Gunshot wounds occur at a time of war and during domestic violence.[44,74] A bullet rarely transects a nerve, but rather causes nerve damage through a blast effect.[44] The projectile's path creates a shock wave or temporary cavity that resonates and causes a variable degree of nerve injury. The extent of blast effect is related to the deformation, fragmentation, orientation, and velocity of the bullet. In contrast, stab wounds directly transect a part or portions of the plexus with or without an associated vascular injury.[30] Stab wounds tend to injure the upper and middle portion of the plexus as the clavicle protects the lower elements.

Classification

Brachial plexus injuries are classified according to the anatomic location and extent of nerve involvement. The location of nerve injury can be at the root level, which disrupts the rootlet connection with the spinal cord and is called an *avulsion* injury.[54,69] This separates the motor cell body in the spinal cord from its axons, whereas the sensory cell body located in the dorsal root ganglion remains connected to its axons (Fig. 33-14). Subsequently, the motor portion of the nerve undergoes wallerian degeneration, with degradation of the axons and myelin sheaths. In contrast, the sensory fibers are spared from wallerian degeneration but have been irreversibly detached from the spinal cord. The injury will cause a clinical motor and sensory loss, whereas electrodiagnostic studies will reveal absent motor conduction with intact sensory conduction. An injury distal to the root can affect the trunks, divisions, cords, and/or branches. Complete disruption along these segments is termed a *rupture*, which separates both motor and sensory cell bodies from their axons and results in wallerian degeneration and interrupts both motor and sensory nerve conduction. The differentiation between avulsion and rupture is an important element in the treatment algorithm of brachial plexus traction injuries. Avulsion injuries are irreparable, although experimental work is being performed in root reimplantation.[16] Ruptures along the brachial plexus can be treated by a variety of surgical techniques to reestablish nerve continuity.

Supraclavicular lesions account for most brachial plexus injuries (~75%) and are also subdivided into groups according to the pattern of involvement (Table 33-5).[3,54] The Erb-Duchenne palsy involves C5 and C6 roots or the upper trunk. Motor loss is characterized by weakness of shoulder abduction and external rotation, loss of elbow flexion, and deficient forearm supination. Sensory deficit is apparent in the corresponding dermatome (radial side of forearm and thumb). A C7 injury can accompany an Erb's palsy (extended upper brachial plexus lesion) and adds paralysis of elbow extension, wrist extension, and finger extension. The Dejerine-Klumpke palsy involves C8 and T1, or lower trunk, and is characterized by absent intrinsic hand musculature and finger flexors with intact shoulder, elbow, and wrist function. Sensory deficit is situated over the ulnar side of the forearm and hand. This isolated lower plexus palsy is uncommon in both adults and children. A global or total palsy affects the entire plexus (C5, C6, C7, C8, and T1) and causes a flail and anesthetic arm.

Diagnosis

Patient Presentation

Adult brachial plexus injuries are usually not evaluated in the acute setting, but rather referred after treatment of any life-threatening injuries. A history of the mechanism of injury and degree of trauma are important details. The force incurred (direction, magnitude, and duration), position of extremity, and concomitant injuries (fractures, dislocations, visceral damage, head trauma, and vascular disruptions) relate to the degree of nerve damage. Many patients, however, cannot recall the particulars of the accident, which are obscured by loss of consciousness, associated injuries, or amnesia.[69]

Physical Examination

The physical examination should include the head, neck, thorax, injured extremity, and neurovascular systems. Accurate knowledge of brachial plexus anatomy and concomitant muscle innervation is required for an accurate diagnosis. A thorough physical examination is the foundation that will dictate the treatment algorithm. The goal of this evaluation is to precisely define the location and extent of nerve injury. A severe brachial plexus injury often involves a combination of neuropraxia, axonotmesis, and neurotmesis, which complicates accurate diagnosis and predictions for recovery.

Observation of the limb posture provides information regarding the segment of brachial plexus involved. Complete brachial plexus palsy has a flail limb and postures in a limp position. In contrast, partial palsy will position according to the functioning muscles that overcome weak or absent antagonists. A detailed motor and sensory examination requires an inventory of the muscles innervated by the brachial plexus. Physical findings should be recorded on a data sheet, including the gradation of muscle strength and status of sensation (Table 33-6).[2] This documentation ensures detail and allows serial examinations to be performed by different individuals.

Examination of the muscles innervated by the proximal branches of the brachial plexus will help define the proximity of the plexus lesion to the spinal cord (Table 33-7). Disruption of the dorsal rami (paraspinal muscles), dorsal scapular (rhomboids and levator scapulae), long thoracic (serratus anterior), and phrenic nerves are suggestive of an avulsion injury. The presence of Horner's syndrome (drooped eyelid, constricted pupil, sunken globe, and deceased sweating) implies an avulsion injury at C8 and T1. Horner's syndrome, however, has both a false-positive rate (10%) and false-negative occurrence (28%).[43]

TABLE 33-5
PATTERNS OF BRACHIAL PLEXUS INJURIES

Pattern	Roots Involved
Upper brachial plexus (Erb-Duchenne)	C5 and C6
Extended upper brachial plexus	C5, C6, and C7
Lower brachial plexus (Dejerine-Klumpke)	C8 and T1
Total brachial plexus lesion	C5, C6, C7, C8, and T1

TABLE 33-6
BRACHIAL PLEXUS EXAMINATION SHEET

Muscle Tested	Date		Date		Date	
	R	L	R	L	R	L
Trapezius (C3, C4, XI)						
Levator scapulae (<u>C3</u>, <u>C4</u>, C5)						
Rhomboids (C4, <u>C5</u>)						
Supraspinatus (<u>C5</u>, C6)						
Infraspinatus (<u>C5</u>, C6)						
Serratus anterior (<u>C5</u>, <u>C6</u>, <u>C7</u>)						
Teres major (C5, C6)						
Subscapularis (C5, C6)						
Pectoralis major clavicle (C5, <u>C6</u>, C7)						
Pectoralis major sternocostal (C6, <u>C7</u>,<u>C8</u>, T1)						
Latissimus dorsi (C6,<u>C7</u>, C8)						
Biceps and brachialis (<u>C5</u>, C6)						
Deltoid (<u>C5</u>, C6)						
Teres minor (<u>C5</u>, C6)						
Pronator quadratus (C7,<u>C8</u>,T1)						
Pronator teres (<u>C6</u>, <u>C7</u>)						
Flexor carpi radialis (<u>C6</u>, <u>C7</u>)						
Flexor digitorum profundus II, III (C7, <u>C8</u>, T1)						
Flexor digitorum superficialis (C7, <u>C8</u>, T1)						
Flexor pollicis longus (C7, <u>C8</u>, T1)						
Abductor pollicis brevis (C6, C7, <u>C8</u>,<u>T1</u>)						
Opponens pollicis (<u>C8</u>, <u>T1</u>)						
Lumbricals (<u>C8</u>, <u>T1</u>)						
Triceps (C6, <u>C7</u>, C8)						
Supinator (<u>C5</u>, C6)						
Brachioradialis (<u>C5</u>, C6)						
Extensor carpi radialis longus (<u>C6</u>, <u>C7</u>)						
Extensor carpi radialis brevis (<u>C6</u>, <u>C7</u>,C8)						
Extensor carpi ulnaris (<u>C7</u>, C8)						
Extensor digitorum communis (<u>C7</u>, C8)						
Extensor digiti minimi (<u>C7</u>, C8)						
Extensor indicis (<u>C7</u>, C8)						
Extensor pollicis longus (<u>C7</u>, C8)						
Extensor pollicis brevis (C6, <u>C7</u>)						
Abductor pollicis longus (C6, <u>C7</u>)						
Flexor carpi ulnaris (C7, <u>C8</u>, T1)						
Flexor digitorum profundus IV, V (C7, <u>C8</u>, T1)						
Abductor digiti minimi (C8, <u>T1</u>)						
Abductor pollicis (C8, <u>T1</u>)						
Opponens digiti (C8, <u>T1</u>)						
Interossei (<u>C8</u>, <u>T1</u>)						

Examination of the muscles innervated by the intermediate and terminal branches of the brachial plexus will help localize postganglionic lesions. The status of the suprascapular (suprascapular and infrascapular muscles), thoracodorsal (latissimus dorsi muscle), subscapular (subscapularis and teres major muscles), and pectoral (pectoralis major and minor muscles) nerves should further localize the injury. A peripheral vascular examination is a standard part of the evaluation because damage to the axillary or subclavian vessels can occur. Decreased or absent peripheral pulses warrant arteriography.[30,54,104]

Electrodiagnostic Studies

Electrodiagnostic testing is helpful in the diagnosis and formulation of a treatment plan, although the precise role is controversial.[15,28] Electrodiagnostic methods to evaluate the brachial plexus injuries include nerve conduction ve-

TABLE 33-7

INDICATORS OF AVULSION INJURIES

Finding	Inference
Denervation paraspinal muscles	Dorsal rami injury
Denervation rhomboid muscles	Dorsal scapular (C5) injury
Scapular winging	Long thoracic (C5, C6, C7) injury
Horner's syndrome	Cervicothoracic sympathetic injury
Hemidiaphragm paralysis	Phrenic nerve injury
Pseudomeningocele	Dura and arachnoid avulsion injury
Anesthesia and intact conduction velocity	Dorsal ganglion intact (avulsion from cord)

locity, electromyography, somatosensory-evoked potentials (SEPs), and nerve action potentials (NAPs).

The integrity of the peripheral nerve is determined by the measurement of the conduction velocity. The motor or sensory latency can be measured depending on the recording of the compound motor action potential (CMAP) or the sensory nerve action potential (SNAP). The status of the SNAP and corresponding sensory nerve conduction velocity is helpful in differentiating a preganglionic avulsion injury from a postganglionic lesion. The presence of an intact sensory conduction velocity in an anesthetic part of the arm indicates a preganglionic injury, because the sensory nerve is not separated from its cell body (i.e., dorsal root ganglion). The CMAP or motor nerve conduction velocity is absent in both preganglionic and postganglionic injuries and is not a distinguishing factor.

A normal muscle is silent at rest and active during contraction with progressive recruitment of motor units. A denervated muscle will exhibit spontaneous electrical discharge (insertional activity, fibrillations, and positive sharp wave) when the needle is inserted.[15,28] These spontaneous discharges are not present until 2 to 4 weeks after denervation. A reinnervated muscle will show polyphasic low-amplitude recordings before the clinical detection of muscle activity. Therefore, electromyography of the muscles innervated by the brachial plexus can provide valuable information about the degree of injury and early recovery. Unfortunately, electromyography cannot predict the extent of muscle recovery, which creates confusion regarding timing of surgery.

Somatosensory-evoked potentials and NAPs are primarily used intraoperatively to assess lesions in continuity. Somatosensory-evoked potential recordings from the roots or trunks to the brain and spinal cord indicate lesions without nerve root avulsion. The absence of SEPs on nerve root stimulation indicates a root avulsion and is a contraindica-

tion for nerve grafting.[56,67] Intraoperative stimulating and recording of a nerve proximal and distal to a neuroma can identify the presence or absence of axonal continuity.[51] The presence of NAPs indicates some viable nerve fibers and may assist in the decision between neurolysis or excision and interposition grafting. This method has drawbacks that include the inability to provide quantitative data and the incapacity to distinguish motor from sensory axons.

Treatment

Natural History

The natural history after a brachial plexus injury varies greatly with the location of injury (avulsion versus rupture), degree of nerve involvement (neuropraxia, axonotmesis, and neurotmesis), and extent of plexus injured (Erb's, extended Erb's, and global). A neuropraxia or minor stretch injury, such as burners or stingers, has a favorable prognosis for complete recovery because the axons are uninjured. An axonotmesis of the upper plexus has a guarded prognosis because reinnervation is usually incomplete and permanent deficits are likely. A neurotmesis, root avulsion, and global plexus injury all indicate poor prognosis for spontaneous recovery and usually require surgery to restore some nerve continuity.

Role of Surgical Exploration

Immediate surgical intervention for brachial plexus injuries is uncommon and primarily performed for vascular injuries to the axillary or subclavian vessels. Concurrent inspection of the plexus can be performed with identification of the injured segments. The treatment of the nerve injuries will vary with the mechanism of injury. Sharp transections can be managed by immediate repair or graft interposition. A clean transection can be repaired by primary neurorrhaphy if the cut ends can be approximated without excessive tension.[30,96]

Delayed management is preferred after a traction or blast injury to allow a better assessment of the zone of injury. Similar to other closed nerve injuries, the decision to intercede with surgical intervention is not always straightforward. Surgery is indicated for nerve injuries that have a poor chance of spontaneous recovery. A neurotmesis, root avulsion, and global plexus are standard indications for surgery. Serial examinations, supplemented by ancillary studies, are used to determine the extent of injury. Insufficient recovery after 1 month warrants further study to better define the location of the lesion. Methodology to differentiate an avulsion from a rupture includes CT myelogram, MRI, and electrodiagnostic testing. Unfortunately, no single study reproducibly defines the location and extent of the lesion, and surgery remains the gold standard. Contrast enhancement has improved the diagnostic accuracy of CT scanning, although the number of avulsed roots tends to be overestimated.[42,68] In contrast, MRI tends to underestimate the number of individual nerve root avulsions.

In general, loss of nerve continuity (avulsion, rupture, and laceration) will not exhibit considerable evidence of improvement at 3 months. In these lesions, surgery is recommended between 3 and 6 months after injury. This time frame ensures the viability of motor end plates to sprouting axons after nerve reconstruction. A further delay in surgery may jeopardize the integrity of the motor end plates and prevent functional recovery, despite satisfactory nerve repair, grafting, or transfer. Surgical exploration affords the opportunity to graft nerve ruptures and perform nerve transfers to circumvent nerve root avulsions.

Role of Nerve Grafting

Nerve grafting is the preferred technique for most lesions (i.e., ruptures) with loss of continuity. Root avulsion prohibits use of the involved segment for grafting.[16,54] The interposition of nerve segments links the proximal and distal axons and serves as a conduit for axons to bridge the defect created by the injury. The donor nerves are usually one or both sural nerves, harvested at the time of brachial plexus exploration. Other potential donors are the ipsilateral medial antebrachial cutaneous and superficial radial nerves. The donor nerve graft is divided into sections that span the defect until a comparable cross-sectional area is obtained for interpositional grafting. The nerve grafts are secured between the proximal and distal stumps by epineural sutures and/or biologic adhesives, such as fibrin glue (Fig. 33-16).[30,36,69,96]

Nerve grafts are preferably directed toward shoulder and elbow muscles for reinnervation because the distance to the muscle is short and axonal regrowth can occur before irreversible muscle damage.[54,69] In addition, the plexus fascicular anatomy shifts rapidly over relatively short distances, which encourages inaccurate growth of axons. Therefore, nerve-grafting strategy should attempt to direct the axons to achieve a defined function. For example, grafts that connect to the musculocutaneous, axillary, and suprascapular nerves have less inclination for axonal dropout and misdirection compared with grafts placed into the divisions.

Role of Nerve Transfer

Nerve transfer is indicated for avulsion injuries and large or extensive defects of the brachial plexus. The indications for nerve transfer increases as the number of avulsed roots multiplies. In addition, long nerve grafts (>10 cm) are limited by available donor nerves and have less chance for recovery.[19] Nerve transfers use a variety of axonal sources depending on the level of injury. Options include the spinal accessory nerve, intercostal nerves, a portion of the ulnar nerve, medial pectoral nerve, phrenic nerve, and contralateral C7 nerve root.[18-20,54,55] The donor nerves are transferred to the recipient nerve while maintaining their proximal connection. Transfer of the spinal accessory to the suprascapular nerve, transfer of the intercostal nerves to the musculocutaneous nerve, and transfer of a portion of the ulnar nerve to the musculocutaneous nerve are popular techniques for avulsion injuries involving C5, C6, and C7 (Fig. 33-17).[18-20,57] The spinal accessory nerve is divided distal to the sternocleidomastoid and upper trapezius innervation to preserve some function in the trapezius. When the intercostal nerves are transferred, two to four nerves are used to provide increased motor fibers to the musculocutaneous nerve.[55] Transfer of an ulnar nerve fascicle to the musculocutaneous nerve is an effective treatment for upper

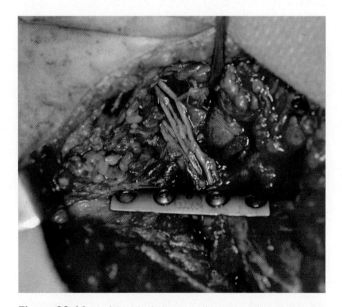

Figure 33-16 Left brachial plexus exploration and sural nerve interposition grafting from C5 and C6 to anterior and posterior divisions of upper trunk. Plate across osteotomy of the clavicle.

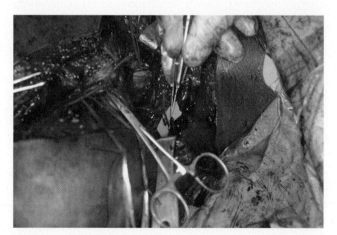

Figure 33-17 Spinal accessory nerve held with forceps before transfer to the suprascapular nerve.

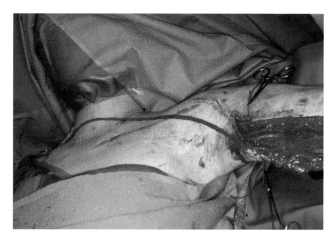

Figure 33-18 An 18-year-old patient treated with complete avulsion of the brachial plexus after scapulothoracic dissociation. Contralateral C7 nerve transfer to the median nerve using an ipsilateral and vascularized ulnar nerve graft.

root avulsions (C5 and C6). Clinical recovery of elbow flexion tends to occur relatively early (2–5 months) secondary to proximity of transfer to the motor end plates. Transient ulnar nerve paresthesias can occur, but no permanent loss of sensibility is apparent.[57]

Contralateral C7 nerve transfer has been used in total root avulsions because of the considerable deficiency in viable axons (Fig. 33-18).[18,115] C7 nerve transfer does not result in permanent donor deficit and possesses a large number of nerve fibers for reinnervation. C7 is usually transferred to the median nerve and is often combined with other nerve transfers to enhance the likelihood of muscle recovery (e.g., spinal accessory nerve to musculocutaneous nerve). The clinical results of C7 root transfer to the median nerve have been encouraging with reference to return of sensibility but disappointing with regard to forearm and hand motor recovery.[115] This outcome is related to the distance and time required for axonal regeneration, which results in irreversible changes in the neuromuscular junction and motor end plates.

Prioritization in Severe Brachial Plexus Injuries

A priority list must be established in severe brachial plexus injuries. Nerve grafts are preferred for nerve reconstruction with viable proximal and distal stumps. Inadequate proximal inflow (i.e., avulsion injuries) requires nerve transfer. The roster of importance is based on function and prognosis after nerve reconstruction. Nerve reconstruction directed toward the proximal musculature achieves better results. Elbow flexion against gravity is the highest priority in brachial plexus injuries to allow limb positioning hand-to-mouth use. Shoulder balance and stability is the next priority for reconstruction, because an unstable, dislocated, or contracted shoulder will impede use of the entire ex-

tremity. Elbow extension is next on the priority list, because nerve grafting or nerve transfer can reliably regain triceps function by coaptation to the radial nerve, which also addresses the wrist and finger extensors. Parascapular stabilization by serratus anterior (long thoracic nerve) and pectoralis muscles (lateral and medial pectoral nerves) reinnervation is then attempted followed by the forearm flexors and digital sensibility (median nerve). The ulnar-innervated structures are the last priority because of the poor prognosis for recovery in adults.[69,70]

Role of Shoulder Fusion and Tendon Transfers

Shoulder function is impaired in upper brachial plexus lesions with paralysis of the deltoid and rotator cuff muscles. The flail shoulder can lead to inferior subluxation and pain. A flail shoulder without any inherent stability despite nerve reconstruction often requires arthrodesis (Fig. 33-11). The lack of proximal stability impairs limb use and can cause pain.[86] Absent scapular control is a contraindication for shoulder fusion. The optimum position for fusion should allow hand-to-mouth function with active elbow flexion (Fig. 33-19). This position is usually 30 degrees of abduction, internal rotation, and forward flexion.[86] Numerous operative techniques have been described for shoulder fusion. Currently, rigid internal fixation is preferred to limit the postoperative immobilization and achieve consistent union.

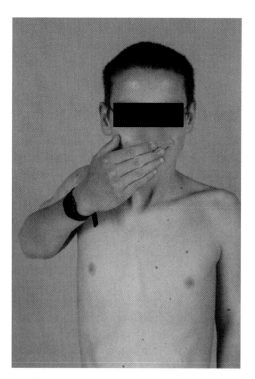

Figure 33-19 A 16-year-old patient after right shoulder fusion, positioned to allow hand-to-mouth function.

The shoulder can also be unbalanced secondary to asymmetric muscle forces. In general, internal rotation dominates over external rotation through activity of the subscapularis, pectoralis major, latissimus dorsi muscle, or teres major muscle(s). Paralysis or weakness of the infraspinatus and teres minor muscles fails to provide adequate external rotation. Over time, a fixed internal rotation contracture will develop, limiting workable space and limb use.[36,37] A severe internal rotation contracture greater than 45 degrees, combined with active abduction less than 80 degrees, makes hand-to-mouth function impossible.[120]

Tendon transfer can treat a stable shoulder that lacks external rotation as long as passive motion is present. The most common tendon transfer used is relocation of the latissimus dorsi and teres major tendons to the infraspinatus insertion to restore external rotation.[45,78] The surgery often involves release or lengthening of the pectoralis major and subscapularis muscles.

The stable shoulder can also lack sufficient abduction. In this case, tendon transfer is less predictable than transfer for external rotation because the complex interaction between the rotator cuff and deltoid muscle is difficult to reproduce. The primary donor muscles for abduction are the trapezius transferred with a portion of the acromion and the latissimus dorsi transferred on its neurovascular pedicle by using a bipolar technique.[8,32,48,53]

Clinical Results

Primary Neurorrhaphy

Primary neurorrhaphy is usually not performed in brachial plexus injury. However, when primary repair of the upper trunk is performed, most patients regain strength to overcome gravity in the shoulder and elbow muscles.[30,52]

Nerve Grafting

Nerve grafting results are better with upper plexus lesions, shorter graft length, and surgery within 6 to 9 months after injury.[18,19,24,43,98] Sufficient antigravity proximal muscle strength returns in approximately 50% to 80% of cases.[3,24,98,109] Nerve grafting for lower plexus lesions in adults is uniformly unsuccessful but may provide some mild return of extrinsic muscle function and protective sensation.

Nerve Transfer

Nerve transfer results are variable, with good results for reinnervation of proximal muscles. Better results are achieved when the nerve transfer is performed early, placed into a peripheral nerve, and without an intervening graft. Return of elbow flexion against gravity is achieved in 60% to 88% of cases.[18,19,40,55,57,67,116] The results for return of shoulder function are more variable when using a nerve transfer to the suprascapular nerve or axillary nerve to achieve stability and abduction. The results of transfer for suprascapular and axillary function are currently approximately 80% and 40% successful, respectively.[18,20,70,105] Simultaneous nerve transfer to the suprascapular and axillary nerves obtains more reliable shoulder abduction.[20] The inferior results for restoration of shoulder function compared with elbow flexion are, in part, secondary to mass innervation.[69] Shoulder function is a coupled movement of scapulothoracic and glenohumeral motion to achieve abduction. Simultaneous contraction of the reinnervated shoulder muscles prevents synchronous motion and diminishes effective abduction. Nerve transfer for forearm and hand function is less successful, with some return of extrinsic function, but not intrinsic activity.[115]

Tendon Transfer

Tendon transfers to restore shoulder external rotation have good to excellent success in the majority of cases, with the ability to achieve hand-to-mouth function in most patients.[45,78] Restoration of external rotation by transfer also balances the shoulder and may prevent progressive deformity and posterior shoulder subluxation.

Tendon transfers to restore shoulder abduction have limited success.[8,32,48,53] The complex movements of the shoulder prohibit restoration of synchronous movement.

The amount of abduction obtained varies between 40 and 60 degrees.[8,48,53]

Shoulder Fusion

Shoulder arthrodesis can correct painful subluxation and provide stability to the extremity, which allows better use of the extremity.[86] Shoulder arthrodesis is often combined with other tendon transfers to improve distal function.

REFERENCES

1. Adson AW, Coffey JR. Cervical rib. A method of anterior approach for relief of symptoms by division of the scalenus anticus. Ann Surg 1927;85:839.
2. Aids to the investigation of peripheral nerve injuries, ed 2. (Medical Research Council War Memorandum, vol. 7.) London, His Majesty's Stationery Office, 1943:48.
3. Alnot JY. Traumatic brachial plexus lesions in the adult. Indications and results. Hand Clin 1995;11:623.
4. Alnot JY, Liverneaux P, Silberman O. Lesions to the axillary nerve. Rev Chir Orthop Reparatrice Appar Mot 1996;82:579.
5. Antoniou J, Suk-Kee T, Williams GR, et al. Suprascapular neuropathy. Variability on the diagnosis, treatment, and outcome. Clin Orthop 2001;386:131.
6. Artico M, Salvati M, D'Andrea V, et al. Isolated lesion of the axillary nerves: surgical treatment and outcome in twelve cases. Neurosurgery 1991;29:697.
7. Atasoy E. Thoracic outlet syndrome. Orthop Clin North Am 1996;27:265.

8. Aziz W, Singer RM, Wolff TW. Transfer of the trapezius for flail shoulder after brachial plexus injuries. J Bone Joint Surg 1990;72B:701.

9. Bigliani L, Dalsey RM, McCann PD, et al. An anatomical study of the suprascapular nerve. Arthroscopy 1990;6:301.

10. Blom S, Dahlbäck LO. Nerve injuries in dislocations of the shoulder joint and fractures of the neck of the humerus: a clinical and electromyographical study. Acta Chir Scand 1970;136:461.

11. Brown SCW, Charlesworth D. Results of excision of a cervical rib in patients with the thoracic outlet syndrome. Br J Surg 1988;75:431.

12. Burkhead WZ Jr., Scheinberg RR, Box G. Surgical anatomy of the axillary nerve. J Shoulder Elbow Surg 1992;1:31.

13. Cahill BR, Palmer RE. Quadrilateral space syndrome. J Hand Surg 1983;8:65.

14. Callahan JD, Scully, Shapiro SA, et al. Suprascapular nerve entrapment. A series of 27 cases. J Neurosurg 1991;74:893.

15. Campion D. Electrodiagnostic testing in hand surgery. J Hand Surg 1996;21A:947.

16. Carlsted T, Grane P, Hallin RG, et al. Return of function after spinal cord implantation of avulsed spinal nerve roots. Lancet 1995;346:1323.

17. Cheney FW, Domino KB, Caplan RA, et al. Nerve injury associated with anesthesia: a closed chain analysis. Anesthesiology 1999;90:1062.

18. Chuang DC. Neurotization procedures for brachial plexus injuries. Hand Clin 1995;11:633.

19. Chuang DC, Epstein MD, Yeh MC, et al. Functional restoration of elbow flexion in brachial plexus injuries: results in 167 patients (excluding obstetric brachial plexus injury). J Hand Surg 1993;18A:285.

20. Chuang DC, Lee GW, Hashem F, et al. Restoration of shoulder abduction by nerve transfer in avulsed brachial plexus injury: evaluation of 99 patients with various nerve transfers. Plast Reconstr Surg 1995;96:122.

21. Clark WL, Trumble TE, Swiontkowski MF, et al. Nerve tension and blood flow in a rat model of immediate and delayed repairs. J Hand Surg 1992;17A:677.

22. Coene LNJEM, Narakas AO. Operative management of lesions of the axillary nerve, isolated or combined with other lesions. Clin Neurol Neurosurg 1992;94(Suppl):S64.

23. Colachis SC Jr., Strohm BR, Brechner VL. Effects of axillary nerve block on muscle force in upper extremity. Arch Phys Med Rehabil 1969;50:647.

24. Comtet JJ, Sedel L, Fredenucci JF, et al. Duchenne-Erb palsy. Experience with direct surgery. Clin Orthop 1988;237:17.

25. Cummins CA, Anderson K, Bowen M, et al. Anatomy and histological characteristics of the spinoglenoid ligament. J Bone Joint Surg 1998;80A:1622.

26. Dai SY, Lin DX, Han Z, et al. Transference of thoracodorsal nerve to the musculocutaneous or axillary nerve in old traumatic injury. J Hand Surg 1990;15A:36.

27. De Laat EA, Visser CP, Coene LN, et al. Nerve injuries in primary shoulder dislocations and humeral neck fractures: a prospective clinical and EMG study. J Bone Joint Surg 1994;76B: 381.

28. Deletis V, Morota N, Abbott IR. Electrodiagnosis in the management of brachial plexus surgery. Hand Clin 1995;11:555.

29. Dillin L, Hoaglund FT, Scheck M. Brachial neuritis. J Bone Joint Surg 1985;67A:878.

30. Dunkerton MC, Boome RS. Stab wounds involving the brachial plexus. J Bone Joint Surg 1988;70B:566.

31. Edeland HG, Zachrisson BE. Fracture of the scapular notch associated with lesion of the suprascapular nerve. Acta Orthop Scand 1975;46:758.

32. Egloff DV, Raffoul W, Bonnard C, et al. Palliative surgical procedures to restore shoulder function in obstetrical brachial palsy. A critical analysis of Narakas' series. Hand Clin 1995;11:597.

33. Fehrman DA, Orwin JF, Jennings RM. Suprascapular nerve entrapment by ganglion cysts: a report of six cases with arthroscopic findings and review of the literature. Arthroscopy 1995;11:727.

34. Ferretti A, De Carli A, Fontana M. Injury of the suprascapular nerve at the spinoglenoid notch. The natural history of infraspinatus atrophy in volleyball players. Am J Sports Med 1998;26:759.

35. Francel TJ, Dellon AL, Campbell JN. Quadrilateral space syndrome: diagnosis and operative decompression technique. Plast Reconstr Surg 1991;87:911.

36. Gilbert A. Long-term evaluation of brachial plexus surgery in obstetrical palsy. Hand Clin 1995;11:583.

37. Gilbert A, Romana C, Ayatta R. Tendon transfers for shoulder paralysis in children. Hand Clin 1988;4:633.

38. Gockel M, Vastamaki M, Alaranta H. Long-term results of primary scalenotomy in the treatment of thoracic outlet syndrome. J Hand Surg 1994;19B:229.

39. Greis PE, Burks RT, Schickendantz MS, et al. Axillary nerve injury after thermal capsular shrinkage of the shoulder. J Shoulder Elbow Surg 2001;10:231.

40. Gu YD, Ma MK. Use of the phrenic nerve for brachial plexus reconstruction. Clin Orthop 1996;323:119.

41. Gumina S, Postacchini F. Anterior dislocation of the shoulder in elderly patients. J Bone Joint Surg 1997;79B:540.

42. Hems TEJ, Birch R, Carlstedt T. The role of magnetic resonance imaging in the management of traction injuries to the adult brachial plexus. J Hand Surg 1999;24B:550.

43. Hentz VR, Narakas A. The results of microneurosurgical reconstruction in complete plexus palsy. Assessing outcome and predicting results. Orthop Clin North Am 1988;19:107.

44. Hershman E. Brachial plexus injuries. Clin Sports Med 1990;9:311.

45. Hoffer MM, Wickendon R, Roper B. Brachial plexus palsies. Results of tendon transfers to the rotator cuff. J Bone Joint Surg 1978;69:691.

46. Howell SM, Imobersteg AM, Seger DH, et al. Clarification of the role of the supraspinatus muscle in shoulder function. J Bone Joint Surg 1986;68A:398.

47. Iannotti JP, Ramsey ML. Arthroscopic decompression of a ganglion cyst causing suprascapular nerve compression. Arthroscopy 1996;12:739.

48. Itoh Y, Sasaki T, Ishiguro T, et al. Transfer of latissimus dorsi to replace a paralysed anterior deltoid. A new technique using an inverted pedicled graft. J Bone Joint Surg 1987;69B:647.

49. Kaye BL. Neurologic changes with excessively large breasts. South Med J 1972;65:177.

50. Kerr AT. The brachial plexus of nerves in man, the variations in its formation and branches. Am J Anat 1918;22:285.

51. Kline DG. Civilian gunshot wounds to the brachial plexus. J Neurosurg 1989;70:166.

52. Kline DG, Judice DJ. Operative management of selected brachial plexus lesions. J Neurosurg 1983;58:631.

53. Kotwal PP, Mittal R, Malhotra R. Trapezius transfer for deltoid paralysis. J Bone Joint Surg 1998;80B:114.

54. Kozin SH. Injuries of the brachial plexus. In: Iannotti JP, Williams GR, eds. Disorders of the shoulder: diagnosis and management. Philadelphia, PA, Lippincott Williams & Wilkins, 1999;847.

55. Krakauer JD, Wood MB. Intercostal nerve transfer for brachial plexopathy. J Hand Surg 1994;19A:829.

56. Landi A, Copeland SA, Wynn Parry CB, et al. The role of somatosensory evoked potentials and nerve conduction studies in the surgical management of brachial plexus injuries. J Bone Joint Surg 1980;62B:492.

57. Leechavengvongs S, Witoonchart K, Uerpairojkit C, et al. Nerve transfer to biceps muscle using a part of the ulnar nerve in brachial plexus injury (upper arm type): a report of 32 cases. J Hand Surg 1998;23A:711.

58. Leffert RD. Thoracic outlet syndrome. J Am Acad Orthop Surg 1994;2:317.

59. Leffert RD, Seddon H. Infraclavicular brachial plexus injuries. J Bone Joint Surg 1965;7B:9.

60. Lepantalo M, Lindgren K-A, Leino E. Long-term outcome after resection of the first rib for thoracic outlet syndrome. Br J Surg 1989;76:1255.

61. Lundborg G, Rydevik B. Effects of stretching the tibial nerve of the rabbit. A preliminary study of the intraneural circulation and the barrier function of the perineurium. J Bone Joint Surg 1973;55B:390.

62. Machleder HI, Moll F, Nuwer M, et al. Somatosensory evoked potentials in the assessment of thoracic outlet syndrome. J Vasc Surg 1987;6:177.

63. Mandel S. Neurologic syndromes from repetitive trauma at work. Postgrad Med 1987;82:87.

64. Martin DM, Warren RF, Martin TL, et al. Suprascapular neuropathy. J Bone Joint Surg 1997;79A:1159.

65. McCarty EC, Tsairis P, Warren RF. Brachial neuritis. Clin Orthop 1999;368:37.

66. Mulder DS, Greenwood FAH, Brooks CE. Posttraumatic thoracic outlet syndrome. J Trauma 1973;13:706.

67. Nagano A, Ochiai S. Restoration of elbow flexion in root lesions of brachial plexus injuries. J Hand Surg 1992;17A:815.

68. Nakamura T, Yabe Y, Horiuchi Y, et al. Magnetic resonance myelography in brachial plexus injury. J Bone Joint Surg 1997;79B:764.

69. Narakas A. Surgical treatment of traction injuries of the brachial plexus. Clin Orthop 1978;133:71.

70. Narakas AO. The treatment of brachial plexus injuries. Int Orthop 1985;9:29.

71. Nevasier TJ, Ain BR, Nevaiser RJ. Suprascapular nerve denervation secondary to attenuation by a ganglionic cyst. J Bone Joint Surg 1986;68A:627.

72. Novak CB, Mackinnon SE, Patterson GA. Evaluation of patients with thoracic outlet syndrome. J Hand Surg 1993;18A:292.

73. Oates SD, Daley RA. Thoracic outlet syndrome. Hand Clin 1996;12:705.

74. Omer GE. Injuries to nerves of the upper extremity. J Bone Joint Surg 1974;56A:1615.

75. Perlmutter GS. Axillary nerve injury. Clin Orthop 1999;368:28.

76. Perlmutter GS, Apruzzese W. Axillary nerve injury in contact sports: recommendations for treatment and rehabilitation. Sports Med 1998;26:351.

77. Petrucci FS, Morelli A, Raimondi PL. Axillary nerve injuries: 21 cases treated by nerve graft and neurolysis. J Hand Surg 1982;7:271.

78. Phipps GJ, Hoffer MM. Latissimus dorsi and teres major transfer to rotator cuff for Erb's palsy. J Shoulder Elbow Surg 1995;4:124.

79. Pollack EW. Surgical anatomy of the thoracic outlet syndrome. Surg Gynecol Obstet 1980;150:97.

80. Post M. Diagnosis and treatment of suprascapular neuropathy. Clin Orthop 1999;368:92.

81. Post M, Mayer J. Suprascapular nerve entrapment: diagnosis and treatment. Clin Orthop 1987;23:126.

82. Pratt NE. Neurovascular entrapment in the regions of the shoulder and posterior triangle of the neck. Phys Ther 1986;66:1894.

83. Qvarfordt PG, Ehrenfeld WK, Stony RJ. Supraclavicular radical scalenectomy and transaxillary first rib resection for the thoracic outlet syndrome. Am J Surg 1984;70:111.

84. Rayan GM, Jensen C. Thoracic outlet syndrome: provocative examination maneuvers in a typical population. J Shoulder Elbow Surg 1995;4:113.

85. Rengachary SS, Burr D, Lucas S, et al. Suprascapular entrapment neuropathy: a clinical, anatomical, and comprehensive study. Part 2: anatomical study. Neurosurgery 1979;5:447.

86. Richards RR, Waddel JP, Hudson AR. Shoulder arthrodesis for the treatment of brachial plexus palsy. Clin Orthop 1985;250:250.

87. Ringel SP, Treihaft M, Carry M, et al. Suprascapular neuropathy in pitchers. Am J Sports Med 1990;18:80.

88. Romeo AA, Rotenberg D, Bach BR Jr. Suprascapular neuropathy. J Am Acad Orthop Surg 1999;7:358.

89. Roos DB. Congenital anomalies associated with thoracic outlet syndrome: anatomy, symptoms, diagnosis, and treatment. Am J Surg 1976;132:771.

90. Roos DB. The place for scalenectomy and first rib resection in thoracic outlet syndrome. Surgery 1982;92:1077.

91. Rosson JW. Closed traction lesions of the brachial plexus: an epidemic among young motorcyclists. Injury 1988;19:4.

92. Sadler TR, Rainer WG, Twobley G. Thoracic outlet compression. Application of positional arteriographic and nerve conduction studies. Am J Surg 1975;130:704.

93. Sallstrom J, Schmidt H. Cervicobrachial disorders in certain occupations with special reference to compression in the thoracic outlet. Am J Ind Med 1984;6:45.

94. Sanders RJ, Monsour JW, Gerber WF, et al. Scalenectomy versus first rib resection for treatment of the thoracic outlet syndrome. Surgery 1979;85:109.

95. Sanders RJ, Pearce WH. The treatment of thoracic outlet syndrome: a comparison of different operations. J Vasc Surg 1989;10:626.

96. Seddon HJ. Nerve grafting. J Bone Joint Surg 1963;45B:447.

97. Seddon HJ. Surgical disorders of peripheral nerve injuries. 2nd ed. Edinburgh, Churchill-Livingstone, 1972.

98. Sedel L. The results of surgical repair of brachial plexus injury. J Bone Joint Surg 982;64B:54.

99. Shaffer BS, Conway J, Jobe FW, et al. Infraspinatus splitting incision in posterior shoulder surgery: an anatomic and electromyographic study. Am J Sports Med 1994;22:113.

100. Shishido H Kikuchi S. Injury of the suprascapular nerve in shoulder surgery: an anatomic study. J Shoulder Elbow Surg 2001;10:372.

101. Singh HK. Incidence of congenital rib anomalies. Indian J Chest Dis 1973;15:157.

102. Steinman SP, Moran EA. Axillary nerve injury: diagnosis and treatment. J Am Acad Orthop Surg 2001;9:328.

103. Stevens JH. The classic. Brachial plexus paralysis. Clin Orthop 1988;237:4.

104. Sturm J, Cicero J. The clinical diagnosis of ruptured subclavian artery following blunt thoracic trauma. Ann Emerg Med 1983;12:17.

105. Sungpet A, Suphachatwong C, Kawinwonggowith V. Restoration of shoulder abduction in brachial plexus injury with phrenic nerve transfer. Aust N Z J Surg 2000;70:783.

106. Thomas GI, Jones TW, Stavney LS, et al. The middle scalene muscle and its contribution to the thoracic outlet syndrome. Am J Surg 1983;145:589.

107. Ticker JB, Djurasovic M, Strauch RJ, et al. The incidence of ganglion cysts and other variations in anatomy along the course of the suprascapular nerve. J Shoulder Elbow Surg 1998;7:472.

108. Tirman PFJ, Feller JF, Janzen DL, et al. Association of glenoid labral cysts with labral tears and glenohumeral instability: radiologic findings and clinical significance. Radiology 1994;190:653.

109. Tonkin MA, Eckersley JR, Gscwind CR. The surgical treatment of brachial plexus injuries. Aust N Z J Surg 1996;66:29.

110. Toolanen G, Hildingsson C, Hedlund T, et al. Early complications after anterior dislocation of the shoulder in patients over 40 years. Acta Orthop Scand 1993;64:549.

111. Tsairis P, Dyck PJ, Mulder DW. Natural history of brachial plexus neuropathy. Report on 99 patients. Arch Neurol 1972:27:109.

112. Tuckman GA, Devlin TC. Axillary nerve injury after anterior glenohumeral dislocation: MR findings in three patients. Am J Roentgenol 1996;167:695.

113. Vastamäki M, Göransson H. Suprascapular nerve entrapment. Clin Orthop 1993;297:135.

114. Vin F, Koskas F, Levy D, et al. Thoracic outlet syndrome. Value of non-invasive arterial studies. Presse Med 1986;15:1709.

115. Waikakul S, Orapin S, Vanadurongwan V. Clinical results of contralateral C7 root neurization to the median nerve in brachial plexus injuries with total root avulsions. J Hand Surg 1999;24B:556.

116. Waikakul S, Wongtragul S, Vanadurongwan V. Restoration of elbow flexion in brachial plexus avulsion injury: comparing spinal accessory nerve transfer with intercostal nerve transfer. J Hand Surg 1999;24A:571.

117. Warner JJP, Krushell RJ, Masquelet A, et al. Anatomy and relationships of the suprascapular nerve: anatomical constraints to mobilization of the supraspinatus and infraspinatus muscles in the management of massive rotator-cuff tears. J Bone Joint Surg 1992;74A:36.

118. Waters PM. Obstetric brachial plexus injuries: evaluation and management. J Am Acad Orthop Surg 1997;5:205.

119. West GA, Haynor DR, Goodkin R, et al. Magnetic resonance imaging signal changes in denervated muscles after peripheral nerve injury. Neurosurgery 1994;35:1077.

120. Wickstrom J. Birth palsies of the brachial plexus. Treatment of defects in the shoulder. Clin Orthop 1962;23:187.

121. Wood VE, Biondi J. Double-crush compression in thoracic-outlet syndrome. J Bone Joint Surg 1990;72A:85.

122. Wood VE, Frykman GK. Winging of the scapula as a complication of first rib resection: a report of six cases. Clin Orthop 1980;149:160.

123. Wright IS. The neurovascular syndrome produced by hyperabduction of the arms. Am Heart J 1945;29:1.

124. Wright TW, Glowczewskie F, Wheeler D, et al. Excursion and strain of the median nerve. J Bone Joint Surg 1996;78A:1897.

125. Young HA, Hardy DG. Thoracic outlet syndrome. Br J Hosp Med 1983;29:459.

Deltoid Injuries

34

Jerry S. Sher   Joseph P. Iannotti

INTRODUCTION

Injuries to the deltoid muscle occur relatively infrequently compared with other, more common shoulder disorders such as those involving the rotator cuff. Regardless of the cause, these injuries can often result in significant shoulder dysfunction. An understanding of the functional anatomy of the deltoid and the mechanisms of injury can help to minimize iatrogenic causes and enable the formulation of optimal treatment strategies.

ANATOMY AND FUNCTION

The importance of the deltoid in providing active elevation of the arm is readily appreciated when considering the compromised function associated with pathologic conditions affecting this muscle. Approximately 60% of the strength in abduction and elevation in both the coronal and scapular planes, respectively, is attributed to the deltoid, as determined after anesthetic block of the axillary nerve. Progressive loss of muscle force with increased abduction and early fatigue further compromises shoulder function in such individuals.[16]

Some reports cite sporadic cases of functional elevation of the arm in patients with isolated and complete paralysis of the deltoid.[3,19,36,58] Preservation of active elevation was attributed to the compensatory action of the rotator cuff, pectoralis major, trapezius, and serratus anterior muscles.[3] Despite the ability to raise the unweighted arm, consider-

able deficits in abduction strength occurred in addition to abnormal scapulohumeral mechanics, impairment of humeral extension, and early fatigability.[3,19,58]

Anatomically, the deltoid comprises three distinct heads: the anterior, the middle, and the posterior portions, which vary in both structure and function. Its extensive origin forms a horseshoe-type configuration arising from the distal one-third of the clavicle, the acromion, and the lateral one-third of the spine of the scapula. Distally, the muscle converges to insert on the deltoid tuberosity of the mid-diaphysis of the humerus. Its broad origin, which is derived from the mobile scapula and clavicle, affords the deltoid a mechanical advantage by allowing the muscle to maintain its resting length at various arm positions. The bipennate structure of the large middle head contributes to abduction strength through contraction of its fibers at an angle to the line of pull, which also serves to maintain muscle fiber resting length and improve efficiency. In contrast, muscles with a parallel fiber arrangement such as the anterior and posterior deltoid, by virtue of their structural configuration, result in considerably decreased strength during contraction.[21]

Differences in activity of the deltoid's three portions, relative to arm position, have also been observed through electromyographic analysis.[57] The anterior and middle heads remain active at all angles of abduction and in multiple planes (coronal, scapular, and parasagittal), whereas the posterior deltoid, also an important shoulder extensor, contributes to elevation when the arm is above 110 degrees.[57] Abduction in the coronal rather than scapular plane effects a relative increase in posterior deltoid function and a decrease in anterior deltoid activity.[31] When the arm is in abduction, the posterior deltoid functions as a secondary external rotator, and its clinical importance is increased in patients with massive rotator cuff tears involving the infraspinatus tendon. Its function as a secondary external rotator is greatest with the arm posterior to the plane of the scapula and at 90 degrees of abduction.

J. S. Sher: Clinical Assistant Professor, Department of Orthopaedics and Rehabilitation, University of Miami School of Medicine, Miami Beach, Florida.
J. P. Iannotti: Professor and Chairman, Department of Orthopaedic Surgery, The Cleveland Clinic Foundation, Cleveland Clinic Lerner Foundation, Cleveland Clinic Lerner College of Medicine, Cleveland, Ohio.

Neural innervation is afforded by the axillary nerve, which takes a circuitous path before entering the deltoid muscle. It arises from the posterior cord of the brachial plexus and courses across the inferolateral border of the subscapularis approximately 3 to 5 mm medial to the musculotendinous junction.[37] It passes inferior to the glenohumeral axillary recess and exits the quadrangular space where it divides into two trunks. The posterior trunk splits and innervates the teres minor and posterior deltoid before terminating as the superior lateral cutaneous nerve. The anterior trunk winds around the humerus and innervates the remaining deltoid muscle. It becomes subfascial and intramuscular at a point between the anterior and middle heads.[13] It is generally located one-third the distance from the lateral acromion to the deltoid tuberosity, which in most patients is 4.4 cm from the lateral acromion.

Cause

Although a host of disorders can affect the function of the deltoid, this chapter focuses on lesions isolated to the axillary nerve and those affecting the musculotendinous integrity of the deltoid. For the purpose of completeness, Table 34-1 has been included and represents a comprehensive list of causative factors that can contribute to deltoid muscle dysfunction.

DETACHMENT OF THE DELTOID ORIGIN

Cause

Surgical techniques that use open methods of rotator cuff repair and acromioplasty often require detachment of a portion of the deltoid origin to facilitate exposure.

TABLE 34-1
CAUSES OF DELTOID INJURIES

Cause	Nerve
Muscle	Iatrogenic
Iatrogenic	Incomplete injury
Detachment of origin	Complete injury (transection, traction,
Soft tissue	compression)
Lateral acromionectomy	Trauma
Complete acromionectomy	Glenohumeral dislocation
Infection	Fracture
Necrosis/fibrosis	Blunt trauma
Posttraumatic injury	Penetrating trauma
Fracture/dislocation	Entrapment
Blunt	Quadrilateral space syndrome
Penetrating	Cervical radiculopathy
Contracture	Brachial plexopathy
Inflammatory	Infection
Polymyositis	Upper motor neuron disease
Dermatomyositis	Lower motor neuron disease
Infection	Myoneural junction (myasthenia gravis)
Candida	
Mycoplasma	
Trichinosis	
Toxoplasmosis	
Viral	
Other	
Metabolic/endocrine	
Hypothyroidism	
Acromegaly	
Other	
Steroid myopathy	
Alcoholic myopathy	
Electrolyte imbalance (hypokalemia)	
Muscular dystrophy	
Amyloidosis	
Spontaneous detachment of the deltoid origin (chronic massive rotator cuff tear)	

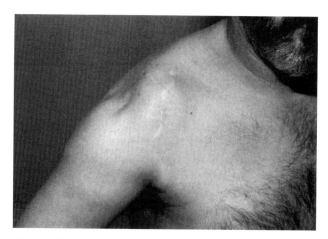

Figure 34-1 Shoulder with middle deltoid detachment 2 years after anterior acromioplasty and rotator cuff repair.

Although many patients demonstrate an uneventful postoperative course, a few develop complications related to dehiscence of the deltoid repair, which can manifest as a residual defect at the muscle's origin (Fig. 34-1). Similar but less frequent occurrences have been reported after deltopectoral, deltoid splitting, and axillary surgical approaches for instability, degenerative, and traumatic conditions of the shoulder.[25] Factors thought to contribute to this postoperative complication include inadequate surgical repair of the deltoid origin, osteoporotic bone unable to withstand the tension afforded by transosseous sutures, poor tissue quality, overzealous retraction, and patient noncompliance. This outcome is avoidable in most cases, but when it does occur, it is typically associated with considerable morbidity and disability.[6,20,25,32,45,46,55,56,64]

Recent reports have implicated arthroscopic acromioplasty as a potential cause of detachment of the deltoid origin (Fig. 34-2).[10,34,59] In an anatomic study, Torpey and colleagues[59] noted that the anterior and anterolateral

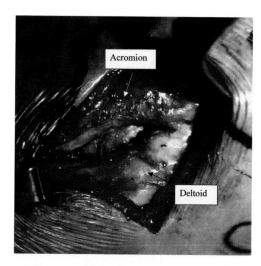

Figure 34-2 Chronic defect in the anterior deltoid origin, seen at the time of revision open repair, secondary to an excessive detachment of the deltoid origin during an arthroscopic acromioplasty.

acromion have a direct tendinous attachment of the deltoid muscle, whereas the muscle attaches to the dorsal side of the acromion through a periosteal attachment. Mathematical models indicate that an anterior inferior acromioplasty of 4 and 6 mm would release 41% and 69% of the tendinous origin, respectively.[16,59] Another report[10] confirms detachment of the deltoid origin during an arthroscopic subacromial decompression and highlights this complication, which is likely underreported. Although most patients do satisfactorily after arthroscopic acromioplasty, caution is warranted in performing aggressive bone resection. Moreover, although the anterior deltoid origin may be weakened after this procedure, superior fibers remain in continuity preserving deltoid function.

Atraumatic or Spontaneous Deltoid Origin Detachment

Sporadic cases of spontaneous rupture of the deltoid origin have been described in the literature.[7,43,48] The senior author has described a deltoid origin rupture in the absence of any iatrogenic event in four shoulders of three patients.[7] All cases were associated with chronic massive tears of the rotator cuff and cephalad migration of the humeral head (Fig. 34-3). Poor shoulder function was evident throughout, and a maximum of 30 degrees of arm elevation was evident in one patient. Notably, weakness rather than pain was the predominant symptom. Another report cites two cases of spontaneous deltoid rupture involving the middle head of the muscle.[43] Both cases also had concomitant massive rotator cuff tears.

Some common findings included advanced age more than 60 years in all cases and involvement of the middle head of the deltoid in most cases. Repeated cortisone injections are also believed to play a causative role in some instances. One proposed explanation for spontaneous rupture includes increased friction or mechanical impingement of the greater tuberosity against the proximal deltoid. Absence of a functional rotator cuff can cause cephalad migration of the humeral head with resultant abnormal or excessive contact between the deltoid and greater tuberosity (Fig. 34-4). Chronic mechanical deltoid impingement, decreased muscle mass, and repeated corticosteroid injections may all contribute to this uncommon occurrence. These cases highlight that a new onset of shoulder weakness in the presence of an existing massive rotator cuff tear may be secondary to deltoid rupture rather than extension of the rotator cuff tear.

Diagnosis

Assessment of an affected patient should include consideration of the individual's overall complaints, precipitating factors, functional status, and associated pathologic conditions. Evaluation may reveal symptomatic arthritis of the glenohumeral or acromioclavicular joints, failure of rotator cuff repair, inadequate acromioplasty, excessive acromion

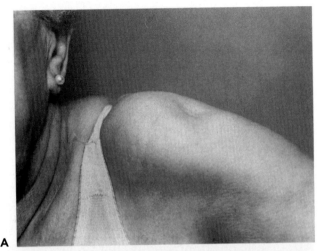

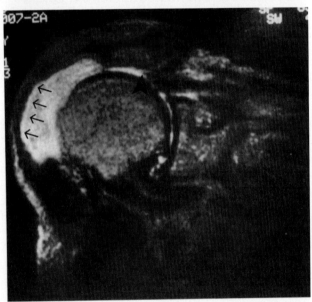

Figure 34-3 *(A)* Spontaneous middle deltoid origin detachment in a patient with a massive chronic rotator cuff tear. *(B)* Magnetic resonance scan demonstrates the deltoid origin disruption *(arrows)* and rotator cuff tear *(arrowhead).*

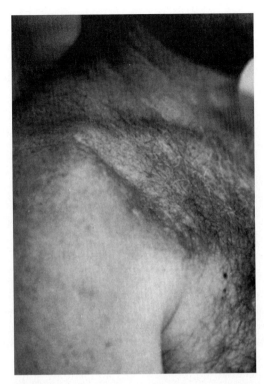

Figure 34-5   Postoperative anterior deltoid detachment.

resection (acromionectomy), or neurologic impairment in association with deltoid detachment. Pain at the anterolateral aspect of the shoulder, for example, could be related to a refractory rotator cuff disorder, disruption of the deltoid origin, or both. This may also hold true for a patient's inability to elevate the arm. Evaluation may reveal functional deficits secondary to rotator cuff dysfunction, deltoid dysfunction, or both.

Patients with disruption and retraction of the deltoid origin frequently display a defect and a loss of normal muscle contour at the sight of detachment with enlargement (bulge) of the deltoid distal to the site (Fig. 34-5). This deformity is best seen with the arm in abduction against gravity or resistance. The deformity may be difficult to see in obese patients. Smaller deficiencies may not be readily apparent with

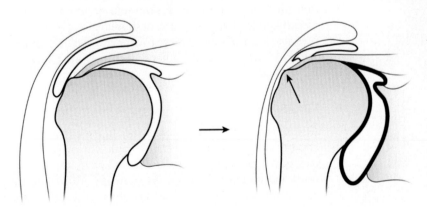

Figure 34-4   Mechanism of wear on the undersurface of the deltoid muscle in a shoulder without *(left)* and with *(right)* a rotator cuff tear. A deficient rotator cuff allows for cephalad migration of the humeral head with chronic abrasion of the greater tuberosity against the deltoid muscle. (Reproduced with permission from Morisawa K, Yamashita K, Asami A, et al. Spontaneous rupture of the deltoid associated with massive tearing of the rotator cuff. J Shoulder Elbow Surg 1997;6:556.)

the arm at the side, but they can often be appreciated when the humerus is actively abducted. Palpation along the acromion border can facilitate assessment of the size of the defect and the degree of retraction. Frequently, focal tenderness can be elicited at the detachment site. Atrophy of the deltoid or rotator cuff may also be evident and can represent disuse, muscle or tendon injury, or neurologic impairment.

Although a thorough history and examination can reliably generate a diagnosis, additional studies are often helpful in excluding alternate sources of shoulder pain. Plain radiographs can facilitate the assessment of acromion morphology, the adequacy of decompression, and the presence of a prior acromionectomy (Fig. 34-6). Diagnoses of glenohumeral and acromioclavicular joint arthritis or cervical spondylosis may be realized. Cephalad migration of the humeral head can confirm any chronic tearing or dysfunction of the rotator cuff. Electrodiagnostic studies can provide objective confirmation of neurologic dysfunction and are generally indicated to rule out deltoid denervation. Arthrograms and magnetic resonance images can aid in the evaluation of rotator cuff integrity. Magnetic resonance imaging can also demonstrate deltoid detachment. It helps define the degree of muscle atrophy and retraction that can correlate with the ability to achieve a successful primary repair (Fig. 34-7).

Functional Outcome

Many investigators have confirmed the overall poor results of rotator cuff repair when the abnormality was associated with detachment of the deltoid ori-

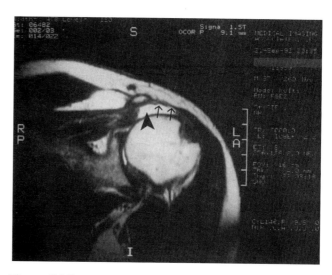

Figure 34-7 Postoperative magnetic resonance image demonstrates a detachment of the middle deltoid (arrows) and full-thickness tear of the supraspinatus tendon (arrowhead).

gin.[6,20,25,45,46,55,56,64] In some cases, function is satisfactory although not normal (Fig. 34-8). In these patients, the deltoid detachment is often small, and there is evidence of intact rotator cuff with minimal pain. Bigliani and colleagues[6] reported a series of 31 patients who underwent reoperation for failed rotator cuff repairs. At follow-up, 15 individuals had unsatisfactory results, and 9 of these demonstrated associated deformities of the deltoid origin. Overall, 13 of the 31 individuals had deltoid detachments.[6] Neviaser and Neviaser[46] published the results of 50 patients who underwent repeated surgery for failed repairs of the rotator cuff. Six of 17 patients who had less than 90 degrees of active elevation before reoperation still had poor active motion (<90 degrees) postoperatively. All 6 of the patients had deltoid deficiencies. Closer analysis of this group revealed that 4 had irreparable detachments of the deltoid origin, 1 had deltoid fibrosis as a result of a previous postoperative infection, and 1 had a permanent axillary nerve palsy.[46]

Groh and colleagues[25] further confirmed the expected poor results in a series of 36 patients with iatrogenic deltoid injuries. Functional impairment was observed in all individuals, regardless of the presence or absence of associated shoulder disorders. Coexisting shoulder problems that were thought to be symptomatic were found in 42% of patients. Overall, there were 86% unsatisfactory, 14% good, and no excellent results when patients were rated on their ability to perform activities of daily living.[25]

In these studies, the poor outcome associated with deltoid detachment in the setting of a rotator cuff defect is clearly demonstrated. Both the rotator cuff defect and the deltoid detachment play important roles in the poor functional outcome. A small deltoid detachment in the setting of an intact rotator cuff may have minimal functional deficit.

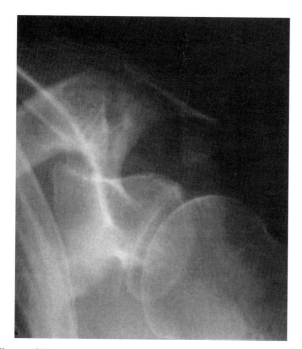

Figure 34-6 Lateral acromionectomy in a patient with a middle deltoid detachment.

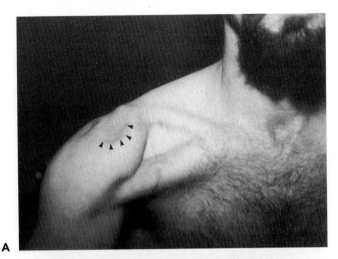

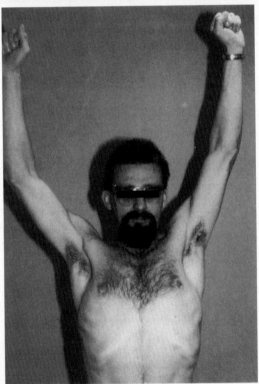

Figure 34-8 *(A)* Postoperative detachment of the middle deltoid origin *(arrowheads)* in a patient and *(B)* good overhead function of the shoulder.

On the basis of limited reports[6,20,25,45,46,55,64] and the authors' experience, it is apparent that individuals who demonstrate an iatrogenic deltoid injury and failure of rotator cuff repair present a complex problem for which attempt at salvage is difficult and success is limited. Bigliani and associates[6] observed the poorest results in six of seven patients who had lateral acromionectomies before attempted salvage operations. Of six patients who had detached deltoids but intact acromions, three demonstrated satisfactory results after mobilization and repair of the scarred and retracted muscle's origin. Neer and Marberry[45]

pointed out that acromionectomy weakens the deltoid by removing the muscle's mechanical fulcrum and by contributing to contracture of the tendinous origin. The retracted deltoid commonly adheres to the underlying rotator cuff and humerus, resulting in stiffness and pain.[45] Although earlier investigations[2,28,63] have reported favorable results after complete acromionectomy for the surgical treatment of rotator cuff conditions, there is no role currently for this overly aggressive form of management in light of abetter understanding of impingement syndrome, as introduced by Neer.[44]

Treatment

Prevention of postoperative deltoid complications remains a critical factor related to the success of operations that use mobilization of this muscle. McShane et al.[42] compared three techniques of open acromioplasty and observed that the most favorable results were associated with methods that used the least disruption of the deltoid. Further confirmation was achieved by Bigliani and coworkers,[5] who observed that deltoid complications that occurred early in their experience were avoided after a modification in surgical technique consisting of the reflection of a small portion of anterior deltoid. They emphasized preservation of the bulk of the deltoid's attachment to bone by splitting the origin in line with its fibers at a point overlying the bony margin of the anterior acromion.[5] Attention to surgical technique with secure transosseous repair of the deltoid to the acromion, with No. 2 nonabsorbable braided suture, minimizes the chance for dehiscence and allows for early mobilization.

Factors related to the success of deltoid repair after a dehiscence has occurred include the size of the defect, the duration of detachment, the osseous integrity of the acromion, the quality of the soft tissues, and the degree of soft tissue deficiency. It is not uncommon to find an iatrogenic deltoid injury associated with other shoulder abnormalities.[25] Typically, the deltoid suffers the role of the "innocent bystander" after previous operative attempts of other shoulder disorders. A thorough evaluation for other potential sources of pain and dysfunction cannot be overemphasized and is paramount to the initiation of appropriate treatment.

In selected cases, repair of the long-standing deltoid deformity may be indicated (Fig. 34-9). However, patient education regarding the likely events of prolonged postoperative immobilization and rehabilitation and about the unpredictability of outcome should be emphasized. The surgical method requires accurate identification of the detached muscular segment, adequate mobilization, and secure transosseous repair. The viable muscle borders of the detached segment are not always readily identified because the tissues may be bound in abundant scar. Caution is warranted in handling the overlying skin, because it is typically

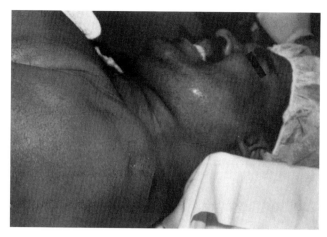

Figure 34-9   Postoperative deltoid detachment involving the anterior and middle deltoid.

thin, attenuated, and prone to postoperative wound complications, especially if an excessive acromion resection had been previously performed.[45] Full-thickness skin flaps should be developed without undue undermining of tissue. Electrocautery set at a low conductive level can facilitate demarcation of the detached segment's viable muscular border by stimulating contraction without untoward thermal effects. Division of scar and tendon approximately 1 cm proximal to the muscular margin provides a sufficient cuff of tissue for repair to the remaining acromion. Blunt and sharp dissection is often necessary above and deep to the muscle in an attempt to mobilize the muscle adequately for repair with minimal tension. Anterior and posterior relaxing incisions may be required to mobilize a retracted and scarred muscle. In cases with a small area of detachment (<4 cm) and minimal retraction (<4 cm), a side-to-side closure of the deltoid may be considered or a direct repair to the acromion may be accomplished using

heavy nonabsorbable suture (Fig. 34-10). Other methods of reconstruction include direct repair and rotational deltoidplasty in which the middle deltoid is typically mobilized anteriorly to allow for closure of the defect (Figs. 34-11 and 34-12). The acromion is often soft, osteoporotic, and foreshortened because of disuse and prior surgery; therefore, it may be of less than ideal quality for sustaining transosseous sutures. Most important, appreciation of the course of the axillary nerve is vital to avoid any further morbidity to an already violated muscle.

For large chronic tears with middle deltoid involvement, shoulder immobilization is recommended with the use of an abduction pillow or abduction brace at 30 degrees for 6 weeks. After brace immobilization, transition to the arm by the side in the brace over the next 2 weeks. The period of immobilization depends in part on the quality of tissue, the size and tension of the repaired defect, and any concomitant repair of the rotator cuff. Active exercises are not initiated until at least 6 weeks, and passive range of motion within a safe arc may be initiated before this time, depending on the circumstances of the reconstruction.

Clinical Outcome

Few data are available regarding the results of surgical treatment for deltoid origin detachment. Surgical repair can be difficult and frequently meets with failure. In a multicenter series of 24 patients surgically treated for this problem,[56] satisfactory results were achieved in only 33% at a mean follow-up of 39 months. All patients had undergone a direct repair or a rotation deltoidplasty, depending on the size and chronicity of the defect. All patients who had evidence of a prior lateral acromionectomy uniformly demonstrated poor results. The size of the preoperative deltoid defect did not correlate with outcome unless the middle deltoid was also involved. Factors associated with satisfac-

A 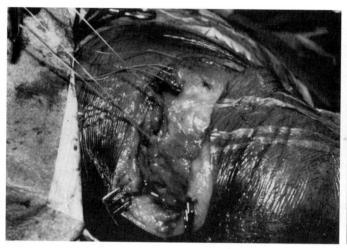 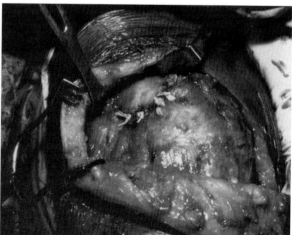 B

Figure 34-10   (A) Mobilization of the detached deltoid muscle. (B) A 1-cm cuff of tendon and scar tissue proximal to the viable muscle border is preserved for subsequent transosseous repair to the acromion.

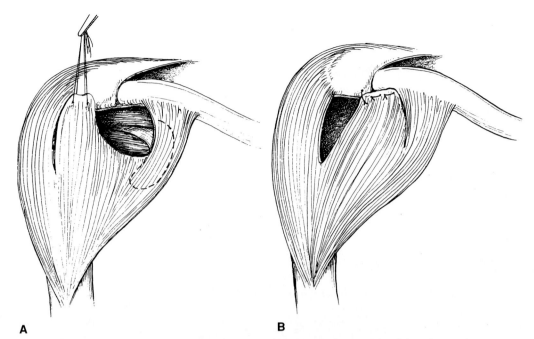

A   B

Figure 34-11 Rotational deltoidplasty for treatment of an anterior deltoid detachment that cannot be repaired primarily. (A) A portion of the deltoid origin posterior to the defect is mobilized, (B) rotated anteriorly, and reattached to fill the defect. The newly created defect is closed side to side.

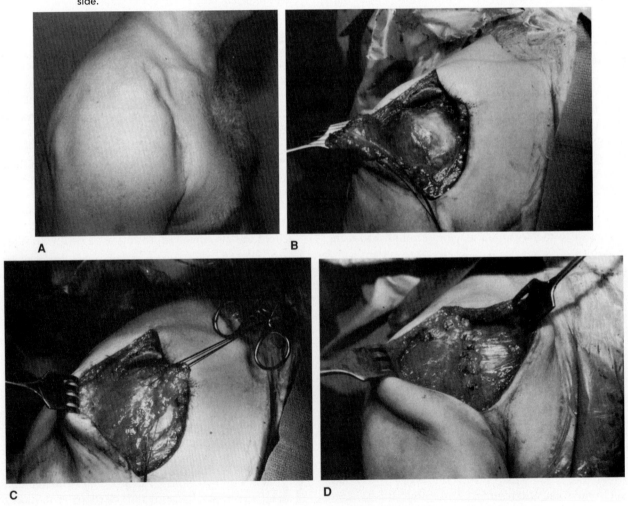

A   B

C   D

Figure 34-12 Postoperative deltoid detachment of the anterior deltoid treated by rotational deltoidplasty. (A) The preoperative photograph demonstrates the defect. Intraoperative photographs demonstrate the (B) anterior defect, (C) lateral deltoid flap, and (D) repaired flap into the deltoid defect. (continued)

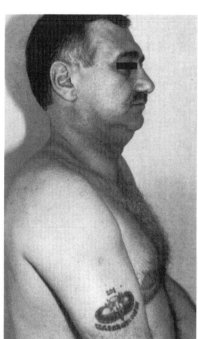
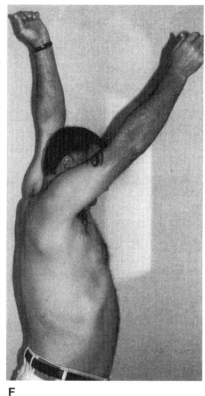

E   F

Figure 34-12 *(continued) (E,F)* Postoperative photographs demonstrate restoration of the anterior deltoid of the shoulder and good postoperative deltoid function.

tory outcomes included isolated disruptions of the anterior deltoid, an intact acromion, preservation of rotator cuff function, and evidence of a healed deltoid reconstruction. Conversely, poor results were associated with prior lateral acromionectomy, involvement of the middle deltoid, concomitant and poorly compensated massive rotator cuff tear, and duration of symptoms longer than 12 months.[56] Success of deltoidplasty is more predictably achieved when the dehiscence is in the acute phase. Early recognition and prompt repair avoid the associated scarring and fixed retraction seen in chronic situations.[38]

AXILLARY NERVE INJURY

Anatomy and Incidence

The proximity of the axillary nerve to the glenohumeral capsule predisposes this neural structure to injury through iatrogenic and traumatic mechanisms. Open shoulder operations that require anterior capsulotomy can inadvertently injure the nerve if care is not taken to identify its location and protect it during dissection. Lateral deltoid-splitting approaches, commonly used for the management of rotator cuff disorders, can also result in nerve injury if the dissection is brought below a critical margin relative to the acromion. Abbott and colleagues[1] demonstrated that the nerve traverses the deltoid muscle at approximately 5 cm below the

lateral tip of the acromion. However, Burkhead and associates,[13] in a cadaveric investigation, observed that the nerve can occupy a position as close as 3.1 cm from the tip of the acromion and that in 20% of specimens it was less than the generally accepted 5-cm distance. Posterior approaches to the shoulder, which are used infrequently, may also result in nerve injury if dissection is mistakenly carried out in the interval between the teres minor and major.

Traumatic injuries, such as dislocations of the glenohumeral joint, can result in axillary nerve lesions in 2% to 25% of cases.[12,21,40,41,53,61] The nerve may be subjected to excessive compression and traction with luxation of the humeral head.[39] Patient age, duration of dislocation, and degree of trauma at the time of injury influence the incidence and prognosis of nerve injury.[8,49] Proximal humerus fractures, blunt trauma, and gunshot injuries have all been associated with axillary nerve palsy.

The possibility of a more proximal nerve lesion should be entertained, and if present, it can often be detected by careful examination. Excessive traction on the extremity during surgery, especially in patients with cervical spondylosis, may result in cervical root or brachial plexus lesions producing demonstrable deltoid dysfunction, in addition to other findings. Individuals undergoing manipulation, under anesthesia, for restriction of shoulder motion may also be at an increased risk for neural stretch injuries, especially if overzealous techniques are used. These patients may demonstrate complete or partial deltoid paralysis, muscle weakness, or paresthesias of the skin overlying the lateral aspect of the proximal humerus. Poor function, prolonged rehabilitation, and patient dissatisfaction can be expected if significant nerve injury has occurred.

Idiopathic brachial plexus neuropathies (Parsonage-Turner syndrome, viral brachial plexopathy) results in weakness or paralysis of multiple muscles around the shoulder but often affects the deltoid most severely. The most commonly affected nerves in this disorder are the axillary, long thoracic, spinal accessory, and suprascapular nerves. The problem typically begins as a spontaneous atraumatic onset of pain that is at first severe. The severe pain decreases over the next several days to a mild to moderate pain with mild to severe weakness and atrophy. Recovery occurs over the next 6 to 12 months and can be incomplete. Rarely is the paralysis permanent.

Segmental denervation of the anterior deltoid can occur during lateral deltoid-splitting approaches for treatment of rotator cuff disorders. Either a neuropraxia or division of the nerve can result from overzealous muscle retraction or excessive inferior dissection, respectively. Exposure of the rotator cuff can be difficult, especially in muscular individuals, and requires adequate anesthetic muscle relaxation, proper use of retractors, and a complete understanding of the local anatomy to minimize the potential for nerve injury.

More recently, axillary nerve palsy after thermal capsular shrinkage of the shoulder has been reported. Injury to the nerve believed to be mediated by heat penetration through the inferior capsule during thermal capsulorrhaphy. Motor and sensory deficits were evident in two of four cases, and only sensory findings were found in the remainder of the patients.[24] Thermocouples placed along the axillary nerve in cadaveric specimens further confirmed that heating of the nerve can occur beyond desired proportions when thermal capsulorrhaphy is performed using radiofrequency probes.[26] Reducing power settings when probing the axillary recess, maintaining motion of the probe, and "painting" a grid pattern rather than probing the entire surface of the inferior capsule are a few measures that can minimize iatrogenic injury.

Management

Prevention efforts remain the best form of management. Similar to iatrogenic disruption of the deltoid origin, careful attention to surgical technique and appreciation of normal shoulder anatomy can minimize the potential for iatrogenic injury to the axillary nerve.

Neuropraxic injuries can be initially managed expectantly. Although specific data do not exist for axillary nerve recovery after iatrogenic mechanisms, neural regeneration usually can be anticipated over 4 to 6 months after contusions to the axillary nerve.[60] Return of deltoid function after axillary palsy associated with glenohumeral dislocation has occurred within 6 months in 67% of 15 patients, between 6 and 12 months in 20%, and not at all in the

remainder.[62,63] Electrodiagnostic tests obtained at approximately 3 weeks after the injury may aid in confirming deltoid denervation and providing a baseline study with which to monitor potential recovery if return of function remains equivocal.

Surgical management is indicated for those in whom nerve transection has occurred or when clinical or electrodiagnostic signs of recovery are not evident after 3 to 6 months. In keeping with peripheral nerve lesions elsewhere in the body, surgical exploration before 6 months from the onset of injury seems preferable.[50] A more recent study has supported this recommendation and demonstrated 85% satisfactory results after grafting of isolated axillary nerve lesions in 121 patients. Results were significantly better when nerve grafting was performed within 5.3 months from the time of injury.[9] Early decompression may halt progressive deterioration of function and minimize the potential for irreversible changes of the nerve and muscle.

Literature describing the management of iatrogenic axillary nerve lesions is scarce. This may be explained, in part, by the relative infrequency of occurrence or the reluctance to report the devastating complication. More commonly, nerve palsy occurs secondary to trauma, which can include displaced proximal humeral fractures, dislocations, and blunt and penetrating injuries. Management of isolated posttraumatic axillary nerve lesions has been described, but the data are limited, and valid conclusions regarding the optimal indications and timing of surgery cannot be drawn.[23,50] Petrucci and colleagues[50] published their results after neurolysis with and without nerve grafting in 21 patients who had incurred isolated axillary nerve palsies. Although only 12 patients were evaluated 1 year postoperatively, the surgeons reported encouraging results and suggested that neurolysis and grafting remain a viable alternative in selected patients. Factors thought to be related to their success included the youth of the patient population, the relatively short course of the axillary nerve, and the fascicular composition of predominantly motor fibers.[50] Friedman and coworkers[23] also reported encouraging results after axillary neurolysis and sural nerve grafting in three patients who experienced a traumatic infraclavicular brachial plexus lesion and who were left with a residual axillary nerve palsy. The physicians observed that the nerve was typically stretched over several centimeters just anterior to the quadrilateral space, and that both anterior and posterior approaches were required for adequate exposure and repair. From 7 to 13 months postoperatively, all three patients demonstrated signs of deltoid reinnervation and functional improvement.[23]

Alternative treatment options to nerve exploration and repair remain limited. Individuals with chronic deltoid paralysis may be suitable candidates for muscle transfers or glenohumeral arthrodesis. Although fusion may offer gains in shoulder strength and function, this typically occurs at the expense of waist-level motion and function.[27] Clinical experience has demonstrated that few patients are receptive to the possibility of a shoulder arthrodesis as an initial procedure, regardless of the circumstances. Muscle transfers may improve active motion but are generally associated with decreased shoulder strength compared with the normal, uninvolved side. Numerous muscle transpositions have been described in the literature and include deltoid substitution with the trapezius, latissimus dorsi, teres major, coracobrachialis, biceps, triceps, pectoralis major, and posterior deltoid for anterior deltoid paralysis.[4,15,17,18,27,29,30,33,35,36,47,52]

Itoh and associates[30] reported their experience with a rotational transfer of the latissimus dorsi about its neurovascular pedicle and over the paralyzed deltoid in 10 patients. Active flexion beyond 90 degrees was achieved in six of them. Although the operation was complex and technically demanding, transfer of the latissimus dorsi was thought to restore a long mechanical lever arm, approximating that of the normal deltoid, and the lost soft tissue contour at the proximal portion of the arm.[30] One of the authors (J.P.I.) has performed a bipolar latissimus transfer in four patients with isolated paralysis of the deltoid muscle. Three of these patients demonstrated marked improvement in function with active flexion above 160 degrees (Fig. 34-13), and one patient demonstrated improvement at 120 degrees. Proper patient selection was thought to be the single most important factor responsible for the satisfactory results. An intact rotator cuff and a mobile glenohumeral joint without capsular contracture and normal scapulothoracic function in a physiologically young patient provides the best results.

The prolonged rehabilitation and the magnitude of the operation can place significant demands on the patient, but these are necessary for optimal results. At least partial func-

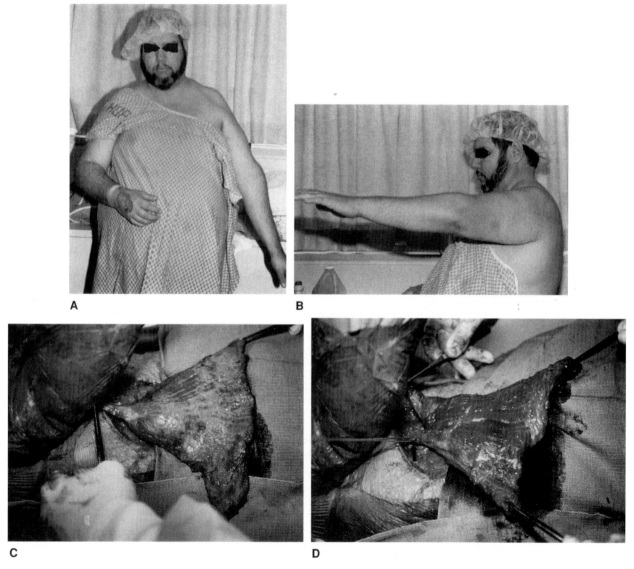

Figure 34-13 *(A)* Preoperative maximum elevation in a patient with an axillary nerve palsy 2 years after an anterior shoulder dislocation without any return of function. *(B)* The condition was treated with a bipolar latissimus transfer. *(C)* Latissimus insertion and origin. *(D)* The mobilized latissimus is flipped 180 degrees such that the neurovascular bundle is superficial *(arrow)*. *(continued)*

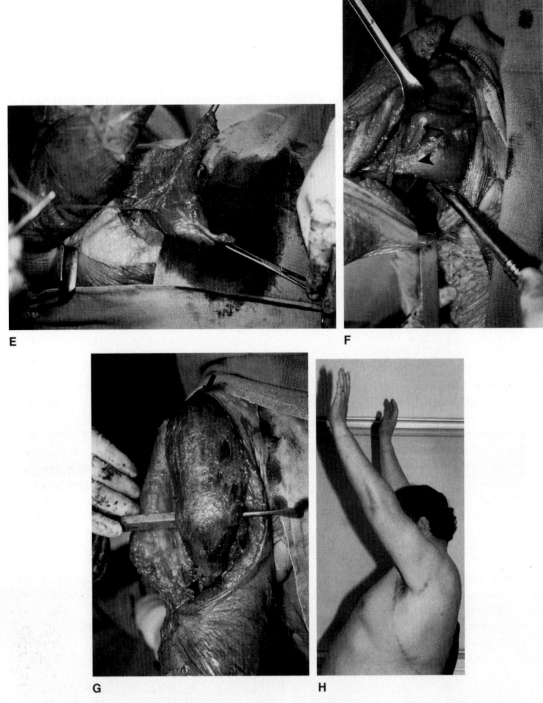

Figure 34-13 *(continued)* *(E)* Latissimus is then rotated 180 degrees such that the origin is proximal and the original tendinous insertion site is distal *(arrow)*. *(F)* Anterior aspect of the shoulder wound, axillary sheath *(arrow)*, and pectoralis major *(arrowhead)* are dissected. *(G)* Latissimus is then transferred to the anterior wound and passed under the pectoralis major. Its origin is sutured to the acromion *(arrow)*, and its insertion is sutured to the deltoid tuberosity *(arrowhead)*. *(H)* Postoperative maximum elevation 4 years after the bipolar latissimus transfer.

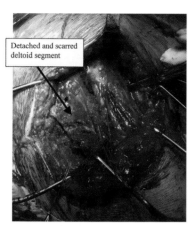
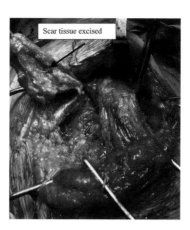
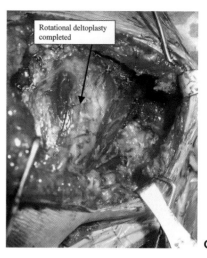

A,B   **C**

Figure 34-14 *(A,B)* Scar tissue is identified and excised from a chronic detachment of the anterior deltoid origin with 6 cm retraction. *(C)* The middle and posterior deltoid origin is detached and transposed to create a new anterior and middle deltoid.

tion of the rotator cuff is required if a successful outcome is to be achieved.[30] Biofeedback and external electrical stimulation of the transferred muscle have been useful in maintaining muscle mass and improving synchronous contraction of the transferred muscle with active forward elevation.

Other transfers that include use of the trapezius,[4,27,33] the pectoralis major,[15,35] and the biceps and triceps[47] have been reported to yield satisfactory results, but the patient populations are typically small and heterogenous, making it difficult to draw reliable conclusions.

Patients with isolated paralysis of the anterior portion of the deltoid may benefit from transfer of the remaining viable middle and posterior functioning muscle's origin to the anterior acromion (Fig. 34-14).[25,30] A rotational deltoplasty can potentially improve functional arm elevation by restoring the important anterior deltoid if electromyographic studies confirm activity in the anterior muscle head at all angles of abduction in various planes.[48] The authors' experience is limited to three cases, with all three cases demonstrating improved function. In all cases the rotator cuff was intact or the tear was small and limited to the supraspinatus insertion site.

Axillary nerve injury after rotator cuff repair through a deltoid split should be approached in much the same way (Fig. 34-15). Often, muscle paralysis anterior to the incision will occur. Neuropraxic injuries can be managed conservatively and confirmed through electrodiagnostic studies. If a neurotmesis has occurred within the muscle substance, then exploration and attempt at repair should not be considered. However, the nerve does begin to arborize at approximately the anterior and middle third muscular junction, making identification and repair of the transected nerve endings impossible. Rotational deltoidplasty

can be considered in those cases with residual isolated anterior deltoid dysfunction. Some patients may demonstrate a small longitudinal cleft-like defect deep to the mini-open skin incision. This is usually a result of focal myonecrosis and secondary to prolonged or excessive retraction of the interval rather than denervation or detachment. Failure to adequately close the deltoid fascia or epimysium may also contribute to this finding. Mild symptoms occur in most patients, but fortunately, most of the types of deltoid injury do not result in significant pain or weakness.

Although muscle transfers for deltoid paralysis may have a role in some patients, further investigation is warranted to better define the indications and assess the

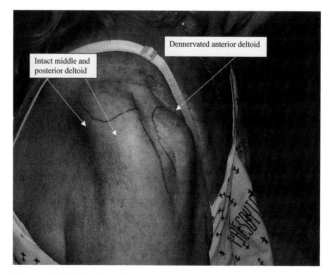

Figure 34-15 Clinical example of an intraoperative deltoid denervation of the anterior deltoid secondary to a distal split of the middle deltoid fibers at the time of rotator cuff repair.

long-term outcomes. Adversaries of such procedures have considered the transposed muscles to act as a tenodesis that can stretch with time and demonstrate insufficient contractility.[11] The limited functional capacity of the shoulder requires consideration, because transfer of a viable remaining motor, if unsuccessful, may further compromise an already disabled patient.

QUADRILATERAL SPACE SYNDROME

Although quadrilateral space syndrome represents an entrapment neuropathy rather than an iatrogenic injury of the axillary nerve, it is briefly discussed here because its clinical presentation shares a few features with operative injuries to the nerve. Initially described by Cahill and Palmer,[14] this disorder represents an uncommon entity for which the diagnosis is often difficult and frequently overlooked. Symptoms that characterize the disorder include poorly localized shoulder pain, paresthesias not necessarily of a dermatomal distribution, and focal tenderness overlying the quadrilateral space (Fig. 34-16).[14,22] Symptoms may be exacerbated with forward flexion or abduction and external rotation of the arm.[14] These patients often present with focal tenderness to deep palpation over the quadrilateral space. Deltoid weakness or atrophy is not always present because pain may precede any objective decrease in deltoid strength or mass. Such findings can demonstrate considerable variability among individuals and are probably related to the degree and duration of nerve compression.

Individuals between 22 and 35 years of age are typically affected, and their symptoms may be mistaken for thoracic outlet syndrome or other shoulder disorders.[14] Quadrilateral space syndrome secondary to an enlarging paralabral cyst has been reported.[54] This disorder has also been observed in throwing athletes with shoulder pain and paresthesias.[51] Diagnostic studies may include electrodiagnostic tests, arteriograms, and magnetic resonance imaging. The role of arteriograms is not clearly established in the literature but may be of value in selected cases (Fig 34-17). Cahill and Palmer[14] demonstrated radiographic evidence of occlusion of the posterior humeral circumflex artery when the affected shoulder was in an abducted and externally rotated position. This finding was thought to be diagnostic and was not present in the uninvolved contralateral extremity when studied for comparison.[14] Francel and colleagues[22] were able to confirm the diagnosis in the absence of arteriograms and suggested that this study may be of limited value, because it provides only indirect evidence of neuropathy.

The authors' experience includes six patients who presented with persistent nonfocal shoulder pain with mild evidence of deltoid weakness or atrophy on physical examination. Clinical evaluation of these patients included magnetic resonance imaging that revealed fatty streaking of the deltoid and a decrease in deltoid cross-sectional area consistent with muscle degeneration and atrophy (Fig. 34-18). Further confirmation of deltoid dysfunction was attained through electrodiagnostic studies, and arteriograms were not obtained. Surgical exploration of the quadrilateral space in three patients demonstrated compression of the axillary nerve by fibrous bands of connective tissue in two (Fig. 34-19) and by an arteriovenous malformation with multiple vascular branches and few fibrous bands in one. In some cases, release of the upper portion of the teres major insertion may improve exposure and decompress the quadrangular space. A careful and meticulous neurolysis was performed in all cases, with excellent results achieved in the former two patients and an unsatisfactory result at-

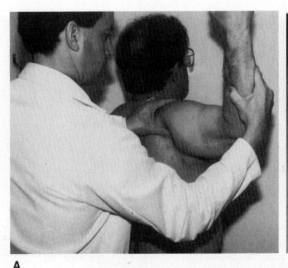
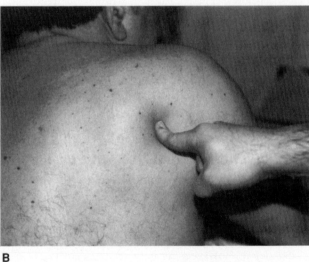

A   **B**

Figure 34-16 (A) The patient described pain in the posterior aspect of the shoulder that was often localized to the quadrangular space. (B) Abduction, external rotation, and compression of the quadrangular space reproduces the patient's symptoms.

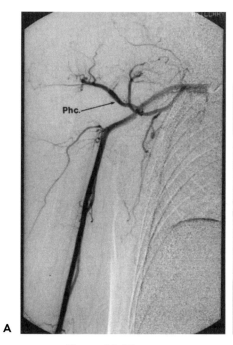

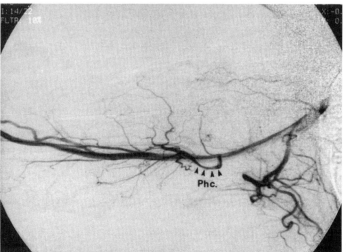

Figure 34-17 Arteriograms demonstrate *(A)* blood flow *(arrow)* through the posterior humeral circumflex (Phc.) artery when the arm is in neutral position and *(B)* occlusion *(arrowheads)* of the artery when the arm is positioned in abduction and external rotation.

tained in the latter patient. In such instances, an arteriogram may be of diagnostic, prognostic, and therapeutic benefit; however, because of the rarity of quadrilateral space syndrome, the limited experience among experts, and the invasiveness and added expense of this test, further study is warranted to define its role in the evaluation of patients with this disorder.

Electrodiagnostic studies are helpful in confirming the presence of axillary nerve compression when results are positive; however, a negative electromyographic study result does not preclude the diagnosis. Few patients were found to have quadrilateral space syndrome despite normal electromyographic findings.[14,22,51] Magnetic resonance imaging can provide useful information, especially when the diagnosis is equivocal. It can help to exclude alternate sources of shoulder pain and can aid in revealing early deltoid atrophy that is not otherwise discernible on clinical examination.

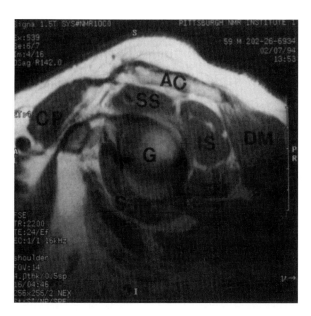

Figure 34-18 Magnetic resonance scan of the deltoid and teres minor muscles demonstrates marbling of the muscles that is consistent with fatty infiltration. AC, acromion; G, glenoid.

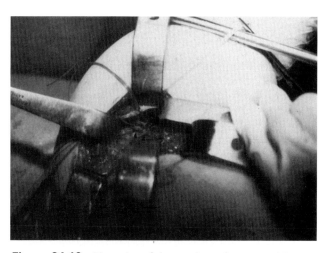

Figure 34-19 Dissection of the quadrangular space with exposure of the axillary nerve and posterior circumflex artery *(arrows)*.

Because of the infrequency of the diagnosis and the fact that many patients do not demonstrate sufficient symptoms to warrant neurolysis, few individuals may ultimately require surgical intervention. However, many symptomatic patients may have significant delays in diagnosis. Patients with clinical evidence of this syndrome who do not have findings of deltoid denervation or dysfunction sufficient to warrant surgical intervention may benefit from activity modification and stretching exercises alone (e.g., throwing athletes). Those with symptoms refractory to conservative measures or manifestations of deltoid denervation and positive electromyographic or arteriographic results should be considered as candidates for nerve decompression. Optimal timing of surgical decompression becomes difficult to outline in light of the variable stages of presentation and the indeterminate natural history of this disorder. However, nerve exploration within 6 months from the time of injury is generally preferred, because it may minimize the potential for irreversible changes within the deltoid muscle and axillary nerve.[50]

Surgical decompression of the axillary nerve can be adequately achieved through a posterior approach without detachment of the deltoid origin from the scapular spine.[22] With the arm in abduction, the posterior border of the deltoid can be easily identified and gently retracted cephalad to expose the underlying quadrilateral space. Care should be taken to avoid injury to the posterior humeral circumflex artery on exploration. Initial reports by Cahill and Palmer[14] demonstrated satisfactory results in 16 of 18 patients after nerve decompression using a more extensible surgical approach.

Postoperative complications to the deltoid are associated with denervation and detachment of the deltoid origin. The functional deficits associated with these problems often result in chronic pain. Prevention of these injuries can usually be accomplished by careful surgical techniques and postoperative rehabilitation. Unpreventable accidents may occur in the early postoperative period because of poor-quality tissue. When the deltoid detachment occurs in the postoperative period, early recognition and repair are recommended to improve the functional outcome.

Quadrilateral space syndrome is a rare cause of shoulder pain and weakness. It should be considered if the clinical symptoms suggest this diagnosis. Electromyography, arteriography, and magnetic resonance imaging are helpful in defining the pathologic anatomy associated with this problem.

REFERENCES

1. Abbott LC, Saunders JBM, Hagey H, et al. Surgical approaches to the shoulder joint. J Bone Joint Surg 1949;31-A:235.
2. Armstrong JR. Excision of the acromion in the treatment of the supraspinatus syndrome. Report of ninety-five excisions. J Bone Joint Surg 1949;31-B:436.
3. Babcock JL, Wray JB. Analysis of abduction in a shoulder with deltoid paralysis due to axillary nerve injury. Clin Orthop 1970;68:116.
4. Bateman JE. Transplant of the trapezius for abductor paralysis of the shoulder. J Bone Joint Surg 1948;30-B:221.
5. Bigliani LU, Cordasco FA, McIlveen SJ, et al. Operative repair of massive rotator cuff tears: long-term results. J Shoulder Elbow Surg 1992;1:120.
6. Bigliani LU, Cordasco FA, McIlveen SJ, et al. Operative treatment of failed repairs of the rotator cuff. J Bone Joint Surg 1992;74-A:1505.7.
7. Blazar PE, Williams GR, Iannotti JP. Spontaneous detachment of the deltoid muscle. J Shoulder Elbow Surg 1998;7:389.
8. Blom S, Dahlback LO. Nerve injuries in dislocations of the shoulder joint and fractures of the neck of the humerus. Acta Chir Scand 1970;136:461.
9. Bonnard C, Anastakis DJ, Van Melle G, et al. Isolated and combined lesions of the axillary nerve. A review of 146 cases. J Bone Joint Surg 1999;81:212.
10. Bonsell S. Detached deltoid during arthroscopic subacromial decompression. Arthroscopy 2000;16:745.
11. Brems JJ, Wilde AM. Shoulder arthroplasty: principles. In: Watson MS, ed. Surgical disorders of the shoulder. New York, Churchill Livingstone, 1991.
12. Brown JT. Nerve injuries complicating dislocation of the shoulder. J Bone Joint Surg 1952;34B:526.
13. Burkhead WZ, Scheinberg RR, Box G. Surgical anatomy of the axillary nerve. J Shoulder Elbow Surg 1992;1:31.
14. Cahill BR, Palmer RE. Quadrilateral space syndrome. J Hand Surg 1983;8-A:65.
15. Chun-lin H, Yong-hua T. Transfer of upper pectoralis major flap for functional reconstruction of deltoid muscle. Chinese Med J 1991;104:753.
16. Colachis SC, Strohm BR, Brechner VL. Effects of axillary nerve block on muscle force in the upper extremity. Arch Phys Med Rehabil 1969;50:647.
17. Davidson WD. Traumatic deltoid paralysis treated by muscle transplantation. J Am Med Assoc 1936;106:2237.
18. Dawson CW. Use of the Ober transplant for deltoid muscle paralysis. Clin Orthop 1955;5:207.
19. Dehne E, Hall RM. Active shoulder motion in complete deltoid paralysis. J Bone Joint Surg 1959;41-A:745.
20. DeOrio JK, Cofield RH. Results of a second attempt at surgical repair of a failed initial rotator-cuff repair. J Bone Joint Surg 1984;66-A:563.
21. DePalma AF. Biomechanics of the shoulder. In: DePalma, ed. Surgery of the shoulder. Third ed. Philadelphia, PA, T.P. Lippincott Co., 1983.
22. Francel TJ, Dellon AL, Campbell JN. Quadrilateral space syndrome: diagnosis and operative decompression technique. Plast Reconstr Surg 1991;87:911.
23. Friedman AH, Nunley JA, Urbaniak JR, et al. Repair of isolated axillary nerve lesions after infraclavicular brachial plexus injuries: case reports. Neurosurgery 1990;27:403.
24. Greis PE, Burks RT, Schickendantz MS, et al. Axillary nerve injury after capsular shrinkage of the shoulder. J Shoulder Elbow Surg 2001;10:231.
25. Groh GI, Simoni M, Rolla P, et al. Loss of the deltoid after shoulder operations: an operative disaster. J Shoulder Elbow Surg 1994;3:243.
26. Gryler EC, Greis PE, Burks RT, et al. Axillary nerve temperatures during radiofrequency capsulorrhaphy of the shoulder. Arthroscopy 2001;17:567.
27. Haas SL. The treatment of permanent paralysis of the deltoid muscle. J Am Med Assoc 1935;104:99.
28. Hammond G. Complete acromionectomy in the treatment of chronic tendinitis of the shoulder. J Bone Joint Surg 1971;53-A:173.
29. Harmon PH. Anterior transplantation of the posterior deltoid for shoulder palsy and dislocation in poliomyelitis. Surg Gynecol Obstet 1947;84:117.
30. Itoh Y, Sasaki T, Ishiguro T, et al. Transfer of latissimus dorsi to replace a paralyzed anterior deltoid. J Bone Joint Surg 1987;69-B:647.
31. Jobe CM. Gross anatomy of the shoulder. In: Rockwood CA, Matsen FA, eds. The shoulder. Philadelphia, PA, WB Saunders, 1990.

32. Karas EH, Iannotti JP. Failed repair of the rotator cuff. Evaluation and treatment of complications. J Bone Joint Surg 1997;79-A:784.
33. Karev A. Trapezius transfer for paralysis of the deltoid. J Bone Joint Surg 1986;11-B:81.
34. Kumar VP, Satku K, Liu J, et al. The anatomy of the anterior origin of the deltoid. J Bone Joint Surg 1997;79:680.
35. La Chapelle EH. Pectoralis major transfer for deltoid paralysis. J Bone Joint Surg 1961;43-B:192.
36. Leffert RD. Neurological problems. In: Rockwood CA, Matsen FA, eds. The shoulder. Philadelphia, PA, WB Saunders, 1990.
37. Levy HJ, Uribe JW, Delaney LG. Arthroscopic assisted rotator cuff repair: preliminary results. Arthroscopy 1990;6:55.
38. Matsen FA, Arntz CT. Rotator cuff tendon failure. In: Rockwood CA, Matsen FA, eds. The shoulder. Philadelphia, PA, WB Saunders, 1990:644.
39. Matsen FA, Thomas SC, Rockwood CA. Anterior glenohumeral instability. In: Rockwood CA, Matsen FA, eds. The shoulder. Philadelphia, PA, WB Saunders, 1990: 526.
40. McLaughlin HL, Cavallaro WU. Primary anterior dislocation of the shoulder. Am J Surg 1950;80:615.
41. McLaughlin HL, MacLellan DI. Recurrent anterior dislocation of the shoulder: II. A comparative study. J Trauma 1967;7:191.
42. McShane RB, Leinberry CF, Fenlin JM. Conservative open anterior acromioplasty. Clin. Orthop 1987;223:137.
43. Morisawa K, Yamashita K, Asami A, et al. Spontaneous rupture of the deltoid associated with massive tearing of the rotator cuff. J Shoulder Elbow Surg 1997;6:556.
44. Neer CS. Anterior acromioplasty for the chronic impingement syndrome. A preliminary report. J Bone Joint Surg 1972;54-A:41.
45. Neer CS, Marberry TA. On the disadvantages of radical acromionectomy. J Bone Joint Surg 1981;63-A:416.
46. Neviaser RJ, Neviaser TJ. Reoperation for failed rotator cuff repair: analysis of fifty cases. J Shoulder Elbow Surg 1992;1:283.
47. Ober FR. An operation to relieve paralysis of the deltoid muscle. J Am Med Assoc 1932;99:2182.
48. Panting AL, Hunter MH. Spontaneous rupture of the deltoid. J Bone Joint Surg 1983;65B:518.
49. Pasila M, Jaroma H, Kiviluoto O, et al. Early complications of primary shoulder dislocations. Acta Orthop Scand 1978;49:260.
50. Petrucci FS, Morelli A, Raimondi PL. Axillary nerve injuries—21 cases treated by nerve graft and neurolysis. J Hand Surg 1982; 7-B:271.
51. Redler MR, Ruland LJ, McCue FC. Quadrilateral space syndrome in a throwing athlete. Am J Sports Med 1986;14:511.
52. Roper B, Brooks D. Restoration of function following paralysis of the deltoid and spinati. J Bone Joint Surg 1972;54-B:172.
53. Rowe CR. Prognosis in dislocations of the shoulder. J Bone Joint Surg 1956;38-A:957.
54. Sanders TG, Tirman PF. Paralabral cyst: an unusual cause of quadrilateral space syndrome. Arthroscopy 1999;15:632.
55. Satterlee CC, Neer CS. Reoperation for failed rotator cuff repairs. J Shoulder Elbow Surg 1993;2:S10.
56. Sher JS, Warner JJP, Groff Y, et al. Surgical treatment of postoperative deltoid origin disruption. Clin Orthop 1997;343:93.
57. Shevlin MG, Lucci JA. Electromyographic study of the function of some muscles crossing the glenohumeral joint. Arch Phys Med Rehabil 1969;50:264.
58. Staples OS, Watkins AL. Full active abduction in traumatic paralysis of the deltoid. J Bone Joint Surg 1943;25:85.
59. Torpey BM, Ikeda K, Wang M, et al. The deltoid muscle origin. Histological characteristics and effects of subacromial decompression. Am J Sports Med 1998;26:379.
60. Turek SL. Orthopaedic neurology. In: Turek SL, ed. Orthopaedics. Principles and their application. Third ed. Philadelphia, PA, JB Lippincott Co., 1977.
61. Watson-Jones R. Dislocation of the shoulder joint. Proc R Soc Med 1936;29:1060.
62. Watson-Jones R. Fracture in the region of the shoulder joint. Proc R Soc Med 1930;29:1058.
63. Wilson JN, ed. Watson-Jones fractures and joint injuries. Edinburgh, Churchill Livingstone, 1976.
64. Wolfgang GL. Surgical repairs of tears of the rotator cuff of the shoulder. Factors influencing the result. J Bone Joint Surg 1974; 56-A:14.

Index